Add : no, colle . Vol 2 .

Handbuch der experimentellen Pharmakologie

Handbook of Experimental Pharmacology

Heffter-Heubner New Series

Herausgegeben von/Edited by

O. Eichler (Heidelberg) · A. Farah (Rensselaer, NY) · H. Herken (Berlin) · A. D. Welch (New Brunswick, NJ)

Volume XXVIII/2

Concepts in Biochemical Pharmacology

Part 2

Contributors

H. S. Ackerman, M. W. Anders, J. Axelrod, P. Bommer, T. R. Bosin, E. Boyland, B. B. Brodie, A. K. Cho, A. H. Conney, R. H. Cox, Jr., P. A. Dahm, J. W. Daly, G. J. Dutton, E. G. Erdös, R. W. Estabrook, H. M. Fales, J. R. Fouts, H. V. Gelboin, J. R. Gillette, T. E. Gram, A. M. Guarino, R. Kuntzman, B. N. La Du, J. L. Leong, R. P. Maickel, H. G. Mandel, G. J. Mannering, R. E. McMahon, V. T. Oliverio, A. B. Roy, E. A. Smuckler, H. Snady, W. R. Snodgrass, S. Spector, Hj. Staudinger, E. O. Titus, S. Udenfriend, V. Ullrich, F. M. Vane, M. Vogt, L. W. Wattenberg, W. W. Weber, E. K. Weisburger, J. H. Weisburger, R. T. Williams, E. A. Zeller

Editors

B. B. Brodie and J. R. Gillette

Assistant Editor

Helen S. Ackerman

With 137 Figures

Springer-Verlag Berlin · Heidelberg · New York 1971

Dr. Bernard B. Brodie — Dr. James R. Gillette
Department of Health, Education and Welfare,
National Institutes of Health, Bethesda, MD 20014/USA

ISBN 3-540-05389-1 Springer-Verlag Berlin Heidelberg New York
ISBN 0-387-05389-1 Springer-Verlag New York Heidelberg Berlin

Druck: Joh. Roth sel. Ww., München

Preface

This volume of the Handbook of Experimental Pharmacology (Concepts in Biochemical Pharmacology) will show that pharmacology has finally arrived as a true discipline in its own right, and is no longer the handmaiden of organic chemistry and physiology. Instead it is an amalgam of all the biological sciences including biochemistry, biophysical chemistry, physiology, pathology and clinical medicine. In the volumes that make up Concepts in Biochemical Pharmacology we hope to convince Medical Schools what should now be obvious, that pharmacology is no longer that dull topic bridging the basic sciences with medicine, but is probably the most important subject in the medical curriculum.

We are grateful for the advice of Dr. Byron Clark, Director of the Pharmacology-Toxicology Program at the National Institutes of Health whose support made possible much of the work described in this volume.

Contents

Section Four: Methods of Studying the Metabolism of Drugs
Subsection A. Assay of Drugs and Their Metabolites

Contents of Part 1

List of Contributors

ACKERMAN, HELEN S., Laboratory of Chemical Pharmacology, National Heart and Lung Institute, National Institutes of Health, Bethesda, MD 20014/USA
ANDERS, M.W., Department of Pharmacology, University of Minnesota, Minneapolis, MN 55455/USA
AXELROD, J., Laboratory of Clinical Science, National Institute of Mental Health, Bethesda, MD 20014/USA
BOMMER, P., Hoffmann-La Roche Inc., Basel/Switzerland
BOSIN, T.R., Department of Pharmacology, Medical Sciences Program, Indiana University, Bloomington, IN 47401/USA
BOYLAND, E., Chester Beatty Research Institute, Institute of Cancer Research, Royal Cancer Hospital, Fulham Road, London, S.W. 3/England
BRODIE, B.B., Laboratory of Chemical Pharmacology, National Heart and Lung Institute, National Institutes of Health, Bethesda, MD 20014/USA
CHO, ARTHUR K., Department of Pharmacology, UCLA Center for the Health Sciences, Los Angeles, CA 90024/USA
CONNEY, A.H., The Wellcome Research Laboratories, Burroughs Wellcome & Co., (US) Inc., Tuckahoe, NY 10707 and Department of Biochemistry, Hoffmann-La Roche Inc., Nutley, NJ 07110/USA
COX, RAYMOND H., JR., Laboratory of Psychopharmacology, Departments of Pharmacology and Psychology, Indiana University, Bloomington, IN 47401/USA
DAHM, PAUL A., Department of Zoology and Entomology, Iowa State University, Ames, IA 50010/USA
DALY, JOHN W., Laboratory of Chemistry, National Institute of Arthritis and Metabolic Diseases, Bethesda, MD 20014/USA
DUTTON, G.J., Biochemistry Department, The University, Dundee/Scotland
ERDÖS, E.G., Department of Pharmacology, University of Oklahoma Medical Center, Oklahoma City, OK 73104/USA
ESTABROOK, R.W., Department of Biochemistry, The University of Texas (Southwestern) Medical School, Dalles, TX 75235 / USA
FALES, H.M., Laboratory of Chemistry, National Heart and Lung Institute, National Institutes of Health, Bethesda, MD 20014/USA
FOUTS, J.R., Pharmacology and Toxicology Branch, National Institute of Environmental Health Sciences Research Triangle Park, NC 27709/USA
GELBOIN, HARRY V., Chemistry Branch, National Cancer Institute, National Institutes of Health, Bethesda, MD 20014/USA
GILLETTE, J. R., Laboratory of Chemical Pharmacology, National Heart and Lung Institute, National Institutes of Health, Bethesda, MD 20014/USA
GRAM, THEODORE E., Pharmacology and Toxicology Branch, National Institute of Environmental Health Sciences Research Triangle Park, NC 27709/USA
GUARINO, A.M., Laboratory of Chemical Pharmacology, National Cancer Institute, Bethesda, MD 20014/USA
KUNTZMAN, RONALD, Biochemistry Department, Hoffmann-La Roche Inc., Nutley, NJ 07110/USA

La Du, B.N., Stella and Charles Guttman Laboratories for Human Pharmacology and Pharmacogenetics, Department of Pharmacology, University Medical School, New York, NY 10016/USA
Leong, J. Lionel, Department of Pathology, University of Minnesota, Medical School, Minneapolis, MN 55455/USA
Maickel, Roger P., Laboratory of Psychopharmacology, Departments of Pharmacology and Psychology, Indiana University, Bloomington, IN 47401/USA
Mandel, H. George, Department of Pharmacology, The George Washington University, School of Medicine, Washington, DC 20005/USA
Mannering, G.J., Department of Pharmacology, University of Minnesota, Minneapolis, MN 55455/USA
McMahon, Robert E., The Lilly Research Laboratories, Indianapolis, IN 46206/USA
Oliverio, Vincent T., Laboratory of Chemical Pharmacology, National Cancer Institute, National Institutes of Health, Bethesda, MD 20014/USA
Roy, Alexander B., Department of Physical Biochemistry, The John Curtin School of Medical Research, P.O. Box 334, Canberra City, A.C.T. 2601/Australia
Smuckler, E.A., Department of Pathology, School of Medicine, University of Washington, Seattle, WA 98105/USA
Snady, H., Stella and Charles Guttman Laboratories for Human Pharmacology and Pharmacogenetics, Department of Pharmacology, University Medical School, New York, NY 10016/USA
Snodgrass, Wayne R., Laboratory of Psychopharmacology, Departments of Pharmacology and Psychology, Indiana University, Bloomington, IN 47401/USA
Spector, Sydney, Department of Physiological Chemistry, Roche Institute of Molecular Biology, Nutley, NJ 07110/USA
Staudinger, Hj., Institut für Biochemie der Universität Gießen, 63 Gießen
Titus, E.O., Laboratory of Chemical Pharmacology, National Heart and Lung Institute, National Institutes of Health, Bethesda, MD 20014/USA
Udenfriend, Sidney, Roche Institute of Molecular Biology, Nutley, NJ 07110/USA
Ullrich, V., Institut für Biochemie der Universität Gießen, 63 Gießen
Vane, F.M., Hoffmann-La Roche Inc., Nutley, NJ 07110/USA
Vogt, Marthe, Agricultural Research Council, Institute of Animal Physiology, Babraham, Cambridge/England
Wattenberg, Lee W., Department of Pathology, University of Minnesota Medical School, Minneapolis, MN 55455/USA
Weber, Wendell, W., Stella and Charles Guttman Laboratories for Human Pharmacology and Pharmacogenetics, Department of Pharmacology, New York University Medical School, New York, NY 10016/USA
Weisburger, Elizabeth K., Experimental Pathology Branch, National Cancer Institute, National Institutes of Health, Bethesda, MD 20014/USA
Weisburger, J.H., Experimental Pathology Branch, National Cancer Institute, National Institutes of Health, Bethesda, MD 20014/USA
Williams, R.T., Department of Biochemistry, St. Mary's Hospital Medical School, London W 2/Great Britain
Zeller, E.A., Department of Biochemistry, The Medical School, Northwestern University, Chicago, IL 60611/USA

Section Four: Methods of Studying the Metabolism of Drugs

Subsection A. Assay of Drugs and Their Metabolites

Chapter 22

Basic Principles in Development of Methods for Drug Assay

BERNARD B. BRODIE

With 2 Figures

A. Introduction

The availability of simple methods for the assay of drugs and their active metabolites in biological materials have greatly facilitated the study of their physiological disposition upon which sound therapy must be based. Such methods have led to an understanding of the principle pathways of drug metabolism and the quantitative importance of each metabolite. They have also been essential in elucidating mechanisms of drug action, since the interpretation of studies with a therapeutic agent *in vitro* is open to question unless the concentration of the agent is also known in the living animal.

I was first faced with the problem of devising a simple scheme for the development of analytical procedures for the estimation of a diversity of organic compounds in connection with an antimalarial screening program (BRODIE et al., 1947a). The principles involved in this scheme are still applicable today, although the availability of other assay procedures have been greatly expanded by the development of more sensitive analytical tools.

In this scheme basic drugs are separated from their metabolic derivatives and from normally occurring substances by extraction from alkalinized plasma or tissue homogenates into an organic solvent and then concentrated in a small aqueous phase by shaking the solvent phase with acid. The drug is then assayed either directly or after conversion to a derivative by nonspecific procedures which take advantage of physiochemical properties, such as fluorescence and absorption of light. A general technique of appraising specificity was developed based on comparison of the solubility characteristics of the material extracted from the biological material with those of the pure compound. Data obtained from this comparison may be used to modify the extraction procedure so that interfering drug metabolites may be separated from the unchanged drug.

B. Principles of Developing a Method

The application of this systematic approach includes a number of discrete steps described below.

I. Selection of Method of Assay

The simplicity, speed and sensitivity of fluorometry recommend it as the method of choice when possible. At one time, the successful application of this technique was limited by instruments which confined the wavelength of the activating radiation to the 365, 405 and 436 mμ lines of the mercury arc lamp (BRODIE et al., 1947b). The possibilities of fluorescence have been vastly expanded by the development of spectrophotofluorometers which permit the assay of compounds activated at wavelengths ranging from 200—600 mμ and by the discovery that fluorescence efficiency may often be vastly increased by activation in solvents having low dielectric constants (UDENFRIEND, 1969). Some compounds can be converted to fluorophores by suitable treatment, such as oxidation, hydrolysis, ultraviolet irradiation or reaction with suitable fluorescent reagents (BRODIE et al., 1947c).

If fluorescence techniques cannot be applied, a coupling reaction to form a dye may next be tried. Aromatic amines can often be diazotized and coupled with N-(1-naphthyl) ethylenediamine, particularly if the position para to the amino group is free (BRODIE et al., 1947d). Certain primary amines, such as 2,6-diaminopyridine, which do not easily form diazonium salts may be coupled with diazonium salts of other amines. The above reactions are not subject to interference by organic extractable substances normally present in biological material, hence a high degree of sensitivity may be achieved by extraction of the azo dye into a microvolume before photometric assay.

Most organic bases form methyl orange salts, which are highly soluble in certain organic solvents, but relatively insoluble in water. Bases may, therefore, be assayed indirectly by extraction of the methyl orange drug complexes into an organic solvent and measurement of the methyl orange in the organic phase photometrically (BRODIE et al., 1947e). The sensitivity of this reaction is limited by the interference of small amounts of naturally occurring substances in plasma.

Although spectrophotometry in the UV region lacks the sensitivity of the assay methods previously described, it is useful as a final means of assay in certain instances and as will be described later, as an aid in developing procedures which eventually involve other principles of assay (JOSEPHSON et al., 1947). The absorption spectrum of a base in 0.1 N H_2SO_4 is investigated to determine the wavelength of maximum absorption ($>$ 240 mμ).

In recent years a number of additional techniques of assay have been developed, especially gas-liquid chromatography, but even with this method preliminary separation by solvents as described above greatly facilitates the ease of assay and interpretation of results.

II. Choice of Solvent for Extraction of Drug

In choosing a solvent, advantage is taken of the fact that drugs are almost invariably converted by the body to derivatives that are less lipid soluble and therefore have lower distribution coefficients between organic solvents and water. The solvents are usually heptane, benzene, ethylene dichloride or isobutanol in order of increasing polarity. For example, heptane extracts only the most lipid-soluble nonpolar substances; in contrast, isobutanol extracts many polar substances that would not be removed by heptane. In other words, compounds that are extractable from an aqueous phase into a nonpolar solvent are also extractable into more polar ones. For this reason the solvent of choice is the least polar one which completely extracts the compound to be analyzed but leaves a large fraction of the relatively polar metabolites behind in the initial extraction. This decreases the chance of extracting not only interfering metabolites but also normally occurring substances that might interfere with the assay.

To select the solvent and to define the pH for the extraction, the fraction of the compound extracted from water is measured at various pH values (1—14) with

Table 1. *Distribution of quinine and one of its metabolic derivatives between water and solvents at various pH values.* The fraction of the compound extracted at various pH values is expressed as the ratio of the amount of compound in the organic phase to total compound after shaking the buffered solution with an equal volume of solvent (BRODIE et al., 1947a)

pH	Petroleum ether-water system		Benzene-water system		Ethylene dichloride-water system	
	Quinine	Quinine metabolic product	Quinine	Quinine metabolic product	Quinine	Quinine metabolic product
6	0.02	0	0.12	0	0.31	0
7	0.04	0	0.36	0	0.80	0
8	0.05	0	1.00	0.06	0.98	0
9	0.13	0	1.00	0.10	1.00	0.27
10	0.26	0	1.00	0.14	1.00	0.31
11	0.31	0	1.00	0.13	1.00	0.37
14 (1 N NaOH)	0.28	0	1.00	0.14	1.03	0.29

each solvent. A simple way of doing this is to extract relatively large amounts of the drug (about 10 μg/ml) with equal volumes of solvent and buffer and then to measure the unextracted drug by UV spectrophotometry.

Table 1 shows the importance of the choice of the proper solvent. Quinine is metabolized in man to a product containing an additional oxygen in the quinuclidine ring. The fractions of quinine and its metabolite extracted from aqueous solution by various solvents at various pH values are compared in Table 1. The data indicate that the least polar solvent which achieves complete extraction of quinine is benzene at pH 8 or higher. Moreover, the extraction of the metabolite is relatively slight with benzene, though appreciable with ethylene dichloride. Thus, benzene is the solvent of choice, since it extracts quinine quantitatively, but very little of the metabolite. The fraction of the metabolite which does pass into the benzene may be removed by aqueous alkaline washes.

III. Adsorption of Drugs by Glass Surfaces

The adsorption of compounds from organic solvents onto glass surfaces constitutes a major source of error because of the micro amounts involved. The extent of this adsorption depends on the properties of the compound, and the polarity of the solvent, the adsorption being greatest from the least polar solvents. This loss

Table 2. *Adsorption of chloroquine onto glass from various organic solvents.* Duplicate 10 γ samples of chloroquine were extracted from alkaline aqueous solution into 100 ml of solvent. After separation of the phases, 1.5 ml of isoamyl alcohol were added to the organic phase of one sample, the other being used as a control. The aqueous phase was discarded, and 15 ml aliquots of solvent were removed at intervals and analyzed for chloroquine. The recovery of chloroquine at zero time is arbitrarily designated as 100 per cent (BRODIE et al., 1947a)

Time	Per cent recovery of chloroquine					
	From ethylene dichloride		From benzene		From heptane	
Minutes	Without isoamyl alcohol	With isoamyl alcohol	Without isoamyl alcohol	With isoamyl alcohol	Without isoamyl alcohol	With isoamyl alcohol
0	100	100	100	100	100	100
5	98	101	96	100	94	97
15	99	100	100	104	81	104
30	97	98	100	106	76	103
60	100	99	106	100	75	97

is minimized by the addition of 1.5% isoamyl alcohol to the solvent before or subsequent to the initial extraction. The extent of adsorption of chloroquine from various solvents with and without the presence of the alcohol is shown in Table 2. The data indicate that more of the drug is adsorbed onto glass from heptane, the least polar solvent, and that isoamyl alcohol minimizes this adsorption. Organic bases are usually adsorbed onto glass from neutral or alkaline aqueous solutions. For this reason, standards are routinely made up in acid solution.

IV. Recoveries of Known Amounts of Compound from Biological Material

Known amounts of compound are extracted from biological materials with the selected solvent and assayed by the method found to be most suitable. The amount of compound to be carried through the procedure will depend on the sensitivity of the final measurement and the concentration of drug expected in the biological tissues after administration to animals or man.

Plasma or Urine. The extraction procedure varies somewhat with the solvent used. As a rule, with ethylene dichloride, 1—10 ml of plasma is alkalized with 1 ml of 2.5 N NaOH and shaken for 10 min in a glass-stoppered bottle containing 20—30 ml of solvent. The phases are separated by transferring the contents of the bottle to a test tube, centrifuging at 3000 rpm, and removing the aqueous phase by aspiration. With larger volumes of plasma, extraction with ethylene dichloride sometimes results in the formation of a gel in the organic phase. The formation of these gels is minimized by adding the ethylene dichloride to the bottle first and carefully layering the plasma over the solvent without preliminary mixing, and by shaking the mixture gently. This prevents the formation of air bubbles at the interface of the two liquids.

With benzene as the solvent, the procedure is the same as with ethylene dichloride, except that it is not necessary to transfer to a tube for centrifugation, as the two phases usually separate easily when bottle and contents are centrifuged directly at low speed.

When heptane is used, the plasma is diluted with an equal volume of 0.1 N NaOH and the mixture is shaken for 30 min. Dilution of plasma is necessary, since otherwise it becomes quite viscous. This may result in incomplete extraction of the base because of the inefficient mixing of the two phases. With heptane, as with benzene, the two phases separate easily on centrifugation of the bottle and contents at low speed.

Certain drugs may be determined directly in plasma filtrates after protein precipitation. This type of procedure, which has been described for the fluorometric determination of quinine, has the advantages of speed and simplicity. But it lacks specificity, since interfering metabolic derivatives of the compound are not removed. In addition, a drug may be dragged down by the protein precipitate. This method may sometimes be used routinely as a semi-quantitative procedure, provided the magnitude of error involved has been assayed by comparison with an extraction procedure of known specificity.

Tissues. Up to 2 g of tissue are added to 5 ml of 0.1 N HCl and ground to a fine suspension in an electrically driven homogenizer. Since homogenates are more homogeneous at neutral pH, 5 ml of buffer may be used with drugs which are not rapidly metabolized. An aliquot of the suspension, diluted if necessary with water, is then extracted as described above.

Occasionally, recoveries from plasma are incomplete, even though recoveries from water are quantitative. This is due to binding on plasma constituents.

The following should be tried. (a) Since binding of organic bases onto plasma protein is minimized at lower pH values, the plasma is adjusted to the lowest pH which will permit complete extraction of the compound from water. For instance, a large series of dialkylaminomethyl derivatives of phenanthrene methanol, *e.g.*, SN 1796 (α-(diamylaminomethyl)-9-(1,2,3,4-tetrahydrophenanthrenemethanol)) can be extracted quantitatively from alkaline aqueous solutions, but not from alkaline plasma. However, the salts of these bases are soluble in organic solvents, and, since the plasma binding is reversed in an acid medium, complete extraction is achieved from acidified plasma. (b) Longer shaking up to 1 h may result in complete extraction. (c) Extraction is carried out with a more polar solvent. The resulting loss of specificity may be corrected, if necessary, by returning the compound from the solvent to acid, from which the compound may be extracted, after alkalization, into a less polar solvent.

V. Assessment of Sensitivity

After adequate recoveries of the compound from biological material are achieved, the next step is to determine whether the method is sensitive enough to assay tissue levels after a prescribed dose. The drug is administered in the required dosage and the tissue concentrations determined. If the amounts in a particular tissue are too small for estimation, the procedure must be revised by changing the assay method, the size of the sample or the volume of the final aqueous extract.

VI. Assessment of Specificity

The specificity of a method may be examined by the pH partition technique (Brodie and Udenfriend, 1945). In this technique the sample of apparent substance is distributed between the organic solvent and a series of buffers of various pH values. The proportions of the apparent substance extracted from the organic phase are then compared with the proportions of a sample of authentic substance extracted in a similar series of distributions between the solvent and buffers. Differences in the distribution of the authentic and apparent substances indicate the presence of an interfering metabolite. When this occurs the method must be modified, usually by washing the extract with buffer at a suitable pH. If no differences in the distribution of the authentic and apparent substances are found, the method is probably specific. Various chromatographic procedures are then usually used to further verify the specificity. For example, a volume of plasma from a patient receiving chloroquine, containing about 5—10 μg of apparent chloroquine, was diluted with one volume of 0.1 N NaOH and shaken for 1 h with 6 volumes of heptane containing 1.5% isoamyl alcohol. As much of the solvent as possible was separated and the drug returned to 10 ml of 0.1 N HCl. Aliquots of the acid solution were set aside for direct analysis; other aliquots were neutralized by the addition of 1 ml of 0.1 N NaOH; 15 ml of the appropriate buffer and 15 ml of heptane were added and the mixture shaken for 15 min. The heptane phase was assayed for chloroquine as described in the method for 4-aminoquinolines (Brodie et al., 1947c) and the fraction of apparent drug extracted at each pH calculated.

Table 3 compares the partition coefficients of pure chloroquine with those of the apparent chloroquine extracted from plasma. Since the distribution of the authentic and apparent chloroquine differ, the heptane extract of plasma must contain material that is more water soluble than authentic chloroquine. These data suggest that an alkaline wash of the heptane extract of the plasma will confer additional specificity to the analytical procedure.

Table 3. *Distribution of chloroquine and apparent chloroquine between water and heptane at various pH values.* The apparent chloroquine was obtained by extraction, with heptane, of the plasma of a patient receiving the drug. The compound was then returned to dilute acid. Aliquots of this solution and of a chloroquine solution were adjusted to various pH values and shaken with equal volumes of heptane. The fraction of the compound extracted at the various pH values is expressed as the ratio of the amount of compound in the organic phase to total compound (BRODIE et al., 1947a)

pH	Chloroquine, aqueous control (a)	Apparent chloroquine from plasma extract: Without alkali wash of solvent phase (b)	Apparent chloroquine from plasma extract: With alkali wash of solvent phase (c)
6	0	0	0
7	0	0.02	0
8	0.11	0.09	0.12
8.5	0.43	0.28	0.44
9	0.71	0.56	0.70
9.5	0.83	0.62	0.85
10	0.94	0.75	0.95
11	0.96	0.77	0.98
13 (0.1 N NaOH)	0.96	0.80	0.98
14 (1 N NaOH)	0.97	0.78	0.99

Column (a) authentic chloroquine; column (b) apparent chloroquine from plasma extracted into heptane and returned to dilute acid; column (c) apparent chloroquine from plasma extracted into heptane and returned to dilute acid after removal of drug metabolites by washing the heptane phase with 0.1 N NaOH.

The effect of the introduction of an alkaline wash was shown as follows: Plasma was extracted with heptane (containing 2.5% isoamyl alcohol) as described above and the heptane phase separated from the aqueous phase. Two volumes of 0.1 N NaOH were added to the heptane and the mixture shaken 10 min. The heptane phase was separated and the wash was repeated two more times. Chloroquine in the washed heptane phase was then returned to 0.1 N H_2SO_4. Aliquots of the solution were set aside for direct analysis, and other aliquots were shaken with a series of buffer solutions as described above. As expected the results in Table 3 indicate that the treatment with an alkali wash removes chloroquine metabolites from the heptane phase, leaving behind a substance with solubility characteristics similar to those of chloroquine.

The pH partition technique is more readily applied when the metabolic products are available as shown by DINGELL et al. (1964) in the fluorometric assay of imipramine and its main metabolite, desipramine. The brain tissue of rats receiving imipramine was homogenized with four volumes of water, the homogenate was adjusted to pH 12 and the imipramine and DMI extracted with heptane. Figure 1 shows the partition ratios of imipramine and DMI between heptane (1.5% isoamyl alcohol) and water at various pH values. From the data it is evident that virtually no hydroxyimipramine is extracted into heptane at pH 12 and that DMI may be returned from the heptane phase to an aqueous phase at pH 6.0. This procedure removes about 80—90% of the DMI but leaves most of the imipramine in the heptane phase. The imipramine is then extracted from the heptane phase into 0.1 N HCl. The aqueous phases are then made alkaline and measured fluorometrically. It is noteworthy that the separation of the three compounds would not have been possible if the more polar solvent ethylene dichloride had been used. At pH 12, almost all the hydroxyimipramine would have been extracted into this organic solvent (Fig. 2) and thus there would have been no simple way to separate hydroxyimipramine from DMI.

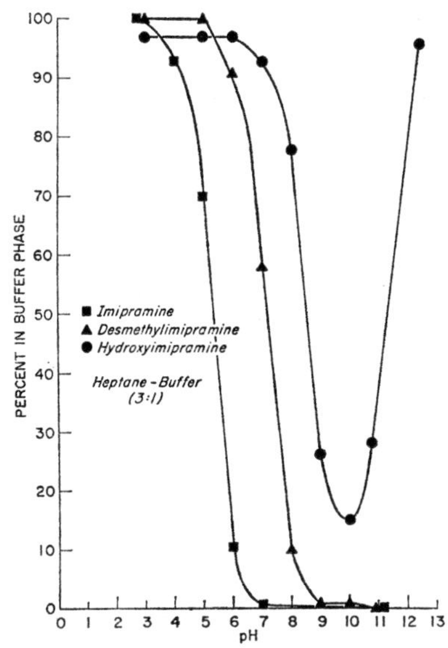

Fig. 1. Distribution of imipramine and its metabolites between heptane and water buffers of various pH

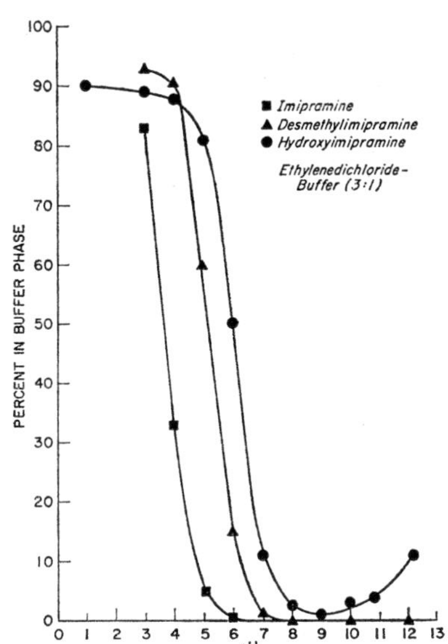

Fig. 2. Distribution of imipramine and its metabolites between ethylene dichloride and buffers of various pH

Similar considerations have been applied to the assay of chlorpromazine and its metabolites by CURRY (1968). In this procedure, chlorpromazine and its relatively nonpolar metabolites, the monomethylated derivative and chlorpromazine sulfoxide were extracted from alkalinized plasma into n-heptane. From the partition ratios between heptane and water at various pH values, it was evident that the sulfoxide could be removed from the heptane phase by extraction with buffer adjusted to pH 8 and the monomethyl analogue of chlorpromazine by extraction with buffer at pH 5.6. The chlorpromazine then remains behind in the heptane phase. In Curry's procedure the various samples were assayed by gas-liquid chromatography.

It must be emphasized that an indication of specificity in the case of plasma does not necessarily indicate a similar specificity for urine and tissues. Many methods which have been found to be specific for plasma require an additional step to remove interfering drug metabolites and endogenous substances present in urine and organ tissues. Furthermore, a particular method may be specific for one species of animal but not for another.

References

BRODIE, B. B., UDENFRIEND, S.: The estimation of basic organic compounds and a technique for the appraisal of specificity. J. biol. Chem. **158**, 705—714 (1945).

— — BAER, J. E.: The estimation of basic organic compounds in biological material. I. General principles. J. biol. Chem. **168**, 299—309 (1947a).

— — DILL, W.: The estimation of basic organic compounds in biological material. V. Estimation by salt formation with methyl orange. J. biol. Chem. **168**, 335—339 (1947e).

— — — CHENKIN, T.: The estimation of basic organic compounds in biological material. III. Estimation by conversion to fluorescent compounds. J. biol. Chem. **168**, 319—325 (1947c).

— — — DOWNING, G.: The estimation of basic organic compounds in biological material. II. Estimation of fluorescent compounds. J. biol. Chem. **168**, 311—318 (1947b).

— — TAGGERT, J. V.: The estimation of basic organic compounds in biological material. IV. Estimation by coupling with diazonium salts. J. biol. Chem. **168**, 327—334 (1947d).

CURRY, S. H.: Determination of nanogram quantities of chlorpromazine and some of its metabolites in plasma used gas-liquid chromatography with an electron capture detector. Anal. Chem. **40**, 1251—1255 (1968).

DINGELL, J. V., SULSER, F., GILLETTE, J. R.: Species differences in the metabolism of imipramine and desmethylimipramine (DMI). J. Pharmacol. exp. Ther. **143**, 14—22 (1964).

JOSEPHSON, E. S., UDENFRIEND, S., BRODIE, B. B.: The estimation of basic organic compounds in biological material. VII. Estimation by ultraviolet spectrophotometry. J. biol. Chem. **168**, 341—344 (1947).

UDENFRIEND, S.: Fluorescence assay in biology and medicine, Vol. II. New York: Academic Press 1969.

Chapter 23

Absorption Spectrophotometry[1]

R. P. MAICKEL and T. R. BOSIN

Absorption spectrophotometry is based on the ability of a substance to absorb radiation, particularly in the wavelength region between 0.2 and 30 microns (μ). Measurement of the degree of absorption at various discrete wavelengths yields a pattern of absorbance relative to wavelength — an absorption spectrum — characteristic of the light-absorbing substance. Such absorption spectra may be used to identify or characterize unknown compounds. In addition, the amount of absorbance of monochromatic light is often proportional to the amount of absorbing substance, thus yielding a method for quantitative estimation of the substance.

In practical laboratory applications, three regions of the spectrum lend themselves to ready use: the ultraviolet region (UV), the visible region (VIS), and the infrared region (IR). In Table 1, we have briefly summarized some of the important

Table 1. *Characteristics of absorption spectrometry techniques*

Characteristics	Ultraviolet (UV)	Visible (VIS)	Infrared (IR)
Wavelength	200—400 mμ	400—750 mμ	750 mμ to 20 μ
Sensitivity			
usual	1—10 μg/ml	1—10 μg/ml	50—200 μg/ml
maximal	0.1—1 μg/ml	0.1—1 μg/ml	10—50 μg/ml
Application possibilities			
characterization	good	poor	excellent
quantitation	excellent	excellent	fair
Problems and difficulties	solvent absorption fluorescence light-scattering	few molecules absorb	water interferes poor sensitivity

characteristics of each of these areas of spectrophotometry; we will now examine each area in turn with regard to actual and potential applications to pharmacological research.

A. Ultraviolet Absorption Spectrophotometry

The basic wavelength limits for UV absorption are set by the transmission limit of air — 190 mμ (LADENBURG et al., 1932) — and by the arbitrarily designated beginning of the "visible" region — 400 mμ. The historical development of the relationship of light absorption to atomic and molecular structure has been extensively reviewed by HOFFMAN (1947). While quantum mechanics as a field of science has grown by leaps and bounds, the structural complexity of most drugs is such that quantum calculations relating structure to absorption phenomena are virtually

1 Supported in part by USPHS grants MH-14658 and HD-03037 and by Research Development Award KO2-MH-41083 (to R. P. MAICKEL).

impossible. Thus, most relationships between structural characteristics and UV absorption properties of compounds have been obtained by empirical means.

I. Chromophores

Basically, the UV absorption of a compound is made up of contributions from certain specific groups of atoms (chromophores) and from the molecule as a whole. In the case of chromophoric groups, the electronic configurations responsible for the absorption of light are spatially restricted to the locus of the atoms comprising the structural groups. By contrast, electrons in unsaturated bonds may be influenced by changes in other parts of the molecule. A list of common chromophoric groups and their usual absorption maxima is seen in Table 2; this list is meant to be exemplary rather than all-inclusive, and the absorption bands given are approximate.

There are a number of ways in which chromophoric groups may interact with each other or with another portion of a molecule resulting in considerable deviations from the values described in Table 2. Since these are common occurrences, it is worthwhile considering each of these interactions briefly.

1. Chromophore Coupling with Electron Fusing

When two or more chromophores are joined so that their electrons may intimately interact with each other, the combination may be considered to be a new chromophore. For example, benzene has a number of small absorption peaks in the region 245—275 mμ. However, the absorption spectrum of naphthalene is not simply a doubling of that of benzene — rather, a new spectrum is produced, with maxima in the region of 250—290 mμ and with more than 5 times the absorbance of benzene.

2. Chromophore Coupling by a Saturated Link

In contrast to the electron fusing situation described above, when two chromophores are joined by a saturated link (such as a methylene group), the linkage prevents interaction of the electrons and acts as a buffer. Thus, toluene has absorption peaks in the region 250—275 mμ; diphenylethylene has a similar absorption spectrum with approximate doubling of absorbance at the peaks.

Table 2. *Absorption bands of some representative chromophores*

Structure	Absorption (λ) mμ
R—COOH	205—215
C—(C=C—)$_2$C—	210—225
R—COO—R′	220—235
—SH	220—230
R—COS—R′	220—270
R—CSO—R′	230—240
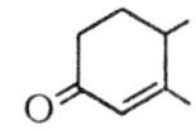	230—240
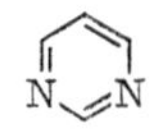	245—265
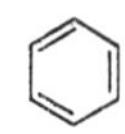	245—260
C-(C=C-)$_3$-C-	250—265
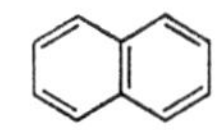	250—290
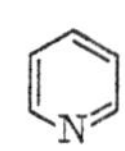	255—265
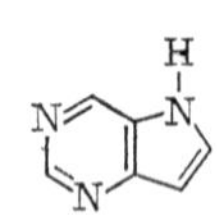	255—275
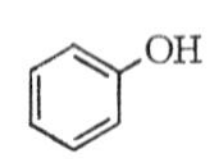	265—290
—O—NO$_2$	270—300
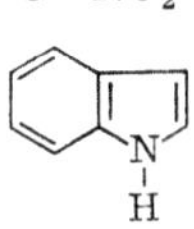	270—295
>C=O	275—285
C-(C=C-)$_4$C-	280—300
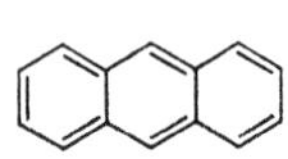	305—380
>C=S	320—340
-NO$_2$	355—375

3. Chromophore Coupling by Conjugated Systems

If two chromophores are joined by a conjugated system (—C=C—) the individual absorbances are altered considerably. Generally, the changes are so great that it is difficult to see any of the original absorption characteristics in the final structure. LEWIS and CALVIN (1939) have studied this phenomena in some detail, considering molecules as linear oscillators. In this regard, it is also of interest that ROE and BEALE (1953) found that the *cis*- and *trans*-isomers of stilbene have significantly different absorptions. The *cis*-isomer has absorption maxima (λ_{max}) at 225 mμ and 280 mμ, with the absorbance at 225 mμ about 2.3 times greater than that at 280 mμ. In contrast, the *trans*-isomer has a dual peak at 290—310 mμ and a single peak at 230 mμ, with the longer wavelength peak about twice as intense.

4. Effect of Tautomerism

One of the useful applications of UV spectrophotometry is in the identification of structural components. However, tautomeric shifts may cause changes in absorption bands; contributions expected from chromophores may not appear or unexpected contributions may be present. This effect is particularly noticeable in compounds where keto-enol shifts occur, such as acetylacetone (HENRI, 1932) and thio esters (LYNEN, 1953).

II. Environmental Influences

In addition to perturbations caused by interactions of atoms or bonds within the molecule, there are many environmental factors that also influence the absorption characteristics of molecules. A consideration of these environmental influences is extremely pertinent to this review.

1. Effects of Solvent

Since the absorption properties of molecules may be altered by interaction with other molecules, it is obvious that spectrophotometric measurements will be greatly influenced by the choice of solvent. An excellent review of this phenomena has been written by KLOTZ (1947). In applying the principles expressed in that review to actual experimental procedures, two very basic points should be emphasized.

First, when UV spectra are being determined, the zero absorbance (100% transmission) point of the instrument should be set with a cuvette containing the same solvent used to dissolve the solute to be studied. This is necessary to assure that contributions from trace contaminants in the solvent will be eliminated as much as possible. In addition, care must be taken to insure that the contributions from the solvent are kept as constant as possible by using similar batches or aliquots from the same pool.

Second, the solvent sample to be used as a "blank" should be treated in precisely the same manner as the sample solution. For example, when quantitative assay procedures require multiple extractions, *e.g.*, acidified aqueous phase to organic solvent to alkalinized aqueous phase, a quantity of the solvent should be run through the entire procedure with only the drug or biological sample not included. When spectra are determined by a double-beam, ratio recording instrument, such a reagent "blank" should be used as the comparison sample.

2. Effects of Ionic Strength

The possible errors in UV spectrophotometric measurements due to differences in ionic strength of sample solutions are the subject of some controversy (SCOTT,

1955). Generally, it may be assumed that most drug molecules are small enough to be largely unaffected by differences in ionic strength. It is only when one reaches the dimensions of macromolecules, such as proteins or nucleic acids, that ionic strength becomes important. Again, consistency in composition of the solvent phase used for spectrophotometric measurements should eliminate problems due to variability in ionic strength.

III. Applications of Ultraviolet Spectrophotometry to Drug Assay

The applications of UV absorption spectrophotometry to studies of drugs in biological materials are many and varied. Two classic papers describing general aspects of methodology in this area are those of BRODIE et al. (1947a) and JOSEPHSON et al. (1947). It would not be within the realm of this review to attempt to list all possible applications of UV spectrophotometry; numerous reviews and books are available in this area (SCOTT, 1964; JAFFE and ORCHIN, 1962). There are, however, several specialized aspects that will be mentioned briefly.

1. Assays Based on a Change in pH

From the discussion of the role of tautomerism above, it should be readily apparent that chromophores may be influenced by changes in ionization. A constant pH must be maintained in different samples to assume comparability; for many compounds, even slight changes in pH (0.1—0.2 units) may cause drastic changes in absorbance.

This change in absorbance with pH may be used to determine the pK of compounds with great accuracy, often requiring a smaller quantity of the compound than would be needed for a titrimetric procedure. The technique requires the determination of λ_{min}, λ_{max}, or the intensity of absorption at a specific wavelength at various values of pH. A suitable plot of the data obtained *vs* pH then yields a multiphasic curve, with the pK determined from the midpoint of the sloping portion, just as in a titrimetric procedure (SCOTT, 1955).

Another application of pH effects on absorption is a technique involving the use of difference spectra. This method has been given great impetus by recent work with barbiturates (BUSH, 1961; BUSH et al., 1961). The general procedure involves measuring the UV absorbancy differences between two samples, differing only in pH. For example, when barbital is examined in this manner, using pH 6.25 as the reference and pH 10 as the sample, a $\lambda_{max} = 300$ mμ is seen; the height of this absorption peak is directly proportional to the concentration of barbital. Thiobarbital, under similar conditions, shows a differential absorption peak at $\lambda_{max} = 236$ mμ. The use of this pH-varying technique confers added sensitivity and specificity on UV assay.

2. Assays Based on a Change of Redox State

Here again, it seems obvious that changes in the oxidation-reduction state of a molecule may readily influence the contributions of various chromophores to the overall absorption characteristics of the molecular system. One of the earliest demonstrations of this effect was the work of WARBURG and CHRISTIAN (1936) with diphosphopyridine nucleotide (DPN). In the oxidized state, DPN (NAD) has a single UV absorption peak, occurring at 260 mμ. However, on reduction to DPNH (NADH), the absorption at 260 mμ decreases slightly and a new peak appears at 345 mμ. This 345 mμ absorbance peak of DPNH is directly proportional to the concentration of the nucleotide; this was first reported for the lactic dehydrogenase system (KOBOWITZ and OTT, 1943) and has since formed the basis for numerous enzymatic assays. Some drugs containing a hydroxyl group sensitive to alcohol dehydrogenase (ethanol, steroids) can be determined indirectly by the DPNH produced in this reaction (THEORELL and BONNICHSEN, 1951; THEORELL and CHANCE, 1951).

3. Assays Based on Production of UV Absorption by Chemical Reaction

A rather unique application of UV spectrophotometric technique may be seen in the method developed by BRODIE et al. (1949) for the determination of antipyrine in biological material. While antipyrine itself has a poor UV absorption, 4-nitrosoantipyrine has a good absorption peak at 350 mμ. After isolation of antipyrine from biological material, the compound in dilute acid (0.07 N H_2SO_4) solution is placed in the spectrophotometer cuvette and absorbance is measured at 350 mμ. A small amount of $NaNO_2$ solution is added to each cuvette yielding HONO which nitrosates the antipyrine to produce 4-nitrosoantipyrine; the absorbance at 350 mμ is determined after a few minutes. The Δ absorbance of each cuvette is proportional to the concentration of antipyrine present.

4. Blank Correction by Differential Wavelength Readings

In many cases, endogenous constituents of biological materials have UV absorbance characteristics that would interfere with the measurement of a desired drug. For example, barbiturates such as hexobarbital show a UV absorbance peak at 245 mμ, with a λ_{min} at 260 mμ. The blank material extracted from biological samples has a broad, flat absorbance, identical in quantity at both 245 mμ and 260 mμ. COOPER and BRODIE (1955) developed an assay procedure for hexobarbital based on this difference. After appropriate extractions, the absorbance of each sample is determined in pH 11.8 buffer at 245 mμ and 260 mμ. The Δ absorbance (λ_{245} to λ_{260}) is proportional to the concentration of hexobarbital. A similar procedure has been reported for thiopental (BRODIE et al., 1950).

5. Estimation of Drug and Metabolite at Differential Wavelengths

Because of the basic principles regarding interaction of chromophoric groups, it is sometimes possible to develop methodology for determining a drug in the presence of a metabolite. This is best illustrated with chlorpromazine and its sulfoxide metabolite. As reported by SALZMAN and BRODIE (1956), the UV absorption spectra of chlorpromazine and chlorpromazine sulfoxide are considerably different. When studied in 0.1 N HCl, chlorpromazine has a major absorption peak at $\lambda_{max} =$ 260 mμ, with λ_{min} at about 280 mμ and a weak absorption "hump" at 290—330 mμ. In contrast, chlorpromazine sulfoxide has four absorption peaks — a major one at $\lambda_{max} = 240$ mμ, and minor peaks at 275, 300 and 340 mμ. In addition, the sulfoxide has λ_{min} at 260 mμ, 285 mμ and 310—320 mμ. Thus, it is possible to determine chlorpromazine and chlorpromazine sulfoxide in the same sample by using UV absorption readings at several wavelengths and an appropriate set of simultaneous equations.

In summary, UV absorption spectrophotometry is a very useful technique for the quantitative estimation of many drugs. In addition, changes in the UV absorption spectrum of a compound may be a useful indicator of metabolically-induced changes in the drug molecule. However, this latter application is limited considerably by the difficulties inherent in interpreting changes in electronic spectra (SCOTT, 1955).

B. Visible Absorption Spectrophotometry

I. General

The wavelength range from 400—750 mμ (0.4—0.75 μ) is generally referred to as the visible (VIS) absorption range, since the human eye is sensitive to these wavelengths. Indeed, the earliest quantitative applications of colorimetry employed visual techniques in which the investigator estimated the concentration of a solute by comparing the depth of color in an unknown with that of a series of known concentrations of the absorbing substance. The early development of VIS absorption technology is reviewed by Gibb (1942). Within the last 25 years, visible absorption spectrophotometry has increased in sensitivity, accuracy and reproducibility; consequently, many simple VIS absorption techniques are still used, although generally classified as colorimetry.

As with UV absorption, a number of factors influence the spectral characteristics of compounds containing VIS chromophoric groups. In general, only those compounds appearing as colored to the naked eye will possess significant absorbance in the VIS absorption region. Thus, most drugs will not be directly determinable, as the majority of therapeutic agents are colorless substances. But as discussed below, there are a number of ways to introduce a chromophoric group into a molecule. In this section we will briefly consider several aspects of the use of visible absorption for drug assay.

II. Application of Visible Spectrophotometry to Drug Assay

1. Assays Based on Changes in pH

Since many compounds contain ionizable groups, it seems obvious that the pH of the solution being studied may influence the absorption characteristics of the solute. Indeed, the color change seen in litmus test paper is an example of this property; the natural coloring matter from lichens such as *Variolaria* is red at pH < 4.5 and blue at pH > 8.3 (Beecken et al., 1961). This change in color, due to a change in the λ_{max} and λ_{min} of the VIS absorption spectrum, is the basis for acid-base titrimetry (Kolthoff and Rosenblum, 1937).

The importance of these pH phenomena in the application of VIS absorption spectrophotometry to the determination of drugs may be seen, for example, in the determination of aniline as described by Mayer et al. (1959). In this case, the dyestuff, absorbing at 570 mμ, which is formed by coupling aniline with N-1-naphthylethylenediamine (Brodie and Axelrod, 1948), can be concentrated by extraction from alkaline solutions into a small volume of benzene containing 1.5% isoamyl alcohol. However, in basic or neutral solutions, the dyestuff exists as a faint yellow (leuco) form, with a weak λ_{max} at 380 mμ. On addition of a small amount of trichloroacetic acid to the benzene extract, the 570 λ_{max} reappears, with excellent sensitivity. It is obvious from this and other similar situations that the pH of samples to be compared must be the same.

2. Assays Based on Changes of Redox State

Many organic compounds show different VIS absorption characteristics when in different states of oxidation, a principle which is also important in oxidation-reduction titrimetry (Clark, 1925). One of the most common examples of a compound which undergoes a shift in VIS absorption peaks with redox state is methylene blue. This dye has a reduced (leuco) form which is colorless; on oxidation, two strong VIS absorption bands are formed with λ_{max} at 609 mμ and 668 mμ.

3. Production of Visible Absorption by Chemical Reaction

We have previously mentioned that few drugs contain VIS chromophoric groups, i.e., few are naturally colored. It is therefore obvious that in order to apply visible absorption methods to drugs, chromophoric groups absorbing in the VIS region must be introduced into the drug molecules. Various reactions may be used for this purpose, depending on the nature of the reactive groups in the particular drug. The methods described in the following sections are typical examples of general procedures. All of these procedures are meant to be applied after preliminary physical separation of the drugs from biological material (Brodie et al., 1947a).

a) Aromatic Amines. Diazotization and Coupling. Many aromatic amines can be converted to reactive diazonium salts in solution, then coupled immediately with suitable reagents to form dyes (Brodie et al., 1947a). This procedure was first applied to drugs by Bratton and Marshall (1939), who used N-1-naphthylethylenediamine to react with diazotized aniline structures in the determination of sulfonamides in biological samples. This reaction has subsequently been applied to numerous compounds with good sensitivity and precision. In some cases, a preliminary hydrolytic reaction may be needed to free the aromatic amine, as in the case of acetanilide-aniline system described by Brodie and Axelrod (1948). In a similar fashion, the compound 4-amino-antipyrine may be converted to a diazonium salt and coupled with α-naphthol to yield a dye with λ_{max} about 540 mμ; the details of this assay have been reported by Brodie and Axelrod (1950).

The basic principles of these diazotization and coupling procedures are similar. The amine-containing compound is separated from biological material by appropriate procedures. A solution of the compound in dilute acid ($\sim$ 0.5 N) is chilled to 0—4° C and treated with an excess of $NaNO_2$, producing HNO_2 *in situ* and converting the aromatic amine to a diazonium salt. Excess, unreacted HNO_2 is destroyed by addition of ammonium sulfamate, after which the coupling agent is added and the pH adjusted to promote dye formation.

b) Phenols and Aromatic Amines. Coupling with Diazonium Salts. When the drug to be studied cannot easily be converted to a diazonium salt (such as 2,6-diaminopyridine), it is often possible to react it with a stable diazonium salt. A general procedure of this type has been described by Brodie et al. (1947c) for the estimation of pamaquine. In this case, the diazonium salt used is that of sulfanilic acid, one that can be readily prepared as described in the preceding section. The preliminary requirements for the application of this kind of procedure are the presence of a reactive position on the drug molecule (often the para position of the amine or phenol) and the availability of a suitable chromophore-generating diazonium salt.

c) Aromatic Aminophenols. Conversion to Indophenols. Brodie and Axelrod (1948) reported the use of a simple process for conversion of *p*-aminophenol into an indophenol with VIS absorption at $\lambda_{max} = 620$ mμ. After the *p*-aminophenol is separated from biological material and extracted into dilute acid, it is converted by the addition of phenol and aqueous NaOBr into an indophenol dye, which has a λ_{max} at 620—625 mμ. This method is also useful for other compounds capable of undergoing the indophenol reaction.

d) Aromatic Amines. Salt Formation with Methyl Orange. The indicator dye methyl orange (the sodium salt of *p*-dimethylaminoazobenzenesulfonic acid) has the property of forming salts with many organic bases. These salts are poorly soluble in water but quite soluble in many organic solvents (Brodie and Udenfriend, 1945). Thus, it is possible to extract an amine-containing drug from aqueous solution into an organic solvent phase as the methyl orange salt. When the organic solvent is subsequently extracted with an acidic aqueous phase, the methyl orange is quantiatively transferred; the amount of methyl orange (as determined by VIS absorption spectrophotometry) is stoichiometrically related to the amount of drug originally present. This procedure has been used for the determination of cinchonine (BRODIE et al., 1947b), amphetamine (AXELROD, 1954) and other compounds.

e) Complex Formation and Chelation. The formation of complexes or chelates between organic compounds and metallic ions often leads to the production of specific chromophores that may be useful in VIS absorption spectrophotometry. Generally, the overall procedure is similar to others described in this chapter, i.e., isolation of the drug from interfering biological material followed by reaction to form the chromophore. An excellent example is found in the method reported by BRODIE et al. (1944) for the determination of salicylic acid. In this procedure, the drug is extracted into chloroform from acidified biological material; the chloroform phase is then shaken with an acidified aqueous solution of $Fe(NO_3)_3$. The absorbance of the violet-colored ($\lambda_{max} = 570$ mμ) salicylate-Fe^{+++} complex in the aqueous phase is proportional to the concentration of salicylate, since Fe^{+++} in acid medium has a yellow color with a λ_{max} about 430 mμ.

An interesting variation on this technique may be seen in an assay for ascorbic acid reported by MAICKEL (1960). In this procedure, excess Fe^{+++} is added to a solution containing an unknown quantity of ascorbic acid in H_3PO_4. The ascorbate reduces the Fe^{+++} to Fe^{++}; subsequent addition of excess *a,a'*-dipyridyl forms a chelate with the Fe^{++} with λ_{max} at 525 mμ. The absorbance of the chelate is proportional to the quantity of Fe^{++} which has been reduced on a mole-for-mole basis by the ascorbic acid.

From this discussion of various methods for introducing chromophoric groups into drugs, it should be readily apparent that VIS absorption techniques can be adapted to the quantitative estimation of drugs in biological samples. However, the lack of endogenous absorption in the 400—750 mμ region, as well as the obvious nonspecificity of the color producing reagents, precludes the application of such techniques to the identification of drugs, with the exception of a very few highly specific substances.

4. Other Factors Affecting Visible Absorption

Colloidal substances have been shown to influence visible absorption in some instances. SORENSON (1909) was the first to report that solutions of various indicators showed marked color changes when proteins were added, despite rigorous control of pH. More recently, HISKEY and DOWNEY (1954) were able to demonstrate an interaction between micellar formation and VIS absorption characteristics of methyl orange. This compound usually exhibits a λ_{max} at 500—520 mμ in aqueous solution at pH 1.1, with a shift of λ_{max} to about 460 mμ at pH 12. However, when 0.015 M octadecyltrimethylammonium chloride was added to the solution, the λ_{max} at both pH 1.1 and 12 was about 425 mμ. Similarly, CARROLL and THOMAS (1949) demonstrated marked changes in the VIS absorption spectrum of methyl orange in the presence of colloidal aluminium hydroxide. These effects on the methyl orange spectrum must be considered important in view of the applications of this dyestuff in drug methods (BRODIE et al., 1947b).

In addition, it is important to remember that a number of substances normally present in biological material also contain chromophoric groups absorbing in the VIS region of the spectrum. Thus, if extraction procedures fail to remove these interferences, the principles described above in the section on blank correction may also be applied to VIS absorption procedures.

C. Infrared Absorption Spectrophotometry

In the previous two sections of this chapter, we have been concerned with methods which are used primarily for the quantitative estimation of compounds by measurement of the interaction of radiation with chromophoric structures within a molecule. It is often said that UV and VIS absorption spectra are "electronic" spectra since they result from the interaction of light with the electronic configurations of molecules or portions of molecules. By contrast, infrared (IR) absorption spectra characterize a molecule by describing, in terms of absorption bands, its vibrational and rotational energy states. Most IR spectra contain numerous sharp absorption bands — so numerous that they may be considered as "fingerprints" of the molecule. Although brief reference will be made to the use of IR absorption as a quantitative technique, it should be strongly emphasized that the primary value of IR absorption studies lies in identification and structure characterization of compounds.

A basic difficulty in the use of IR techniques arises from the fact that special materials must be used to transmit radiation of wavelength 0.75—20 μ. Since glass and quartz do not effectively transmit wavelengths longer than 2—3 μ, sample containers must be made from crystals of NaCl, CaF_2, KBr, AgCl, or other such inorganic materials. Water in any form is generally avoided, because it causes deterioration of cells and prisms and has significant absorption in the IR region. Thus, Nujol mulls and KBr pellets have usually been preferred as media for the sample compound.

The first report on the use of aqueous solutions in IR absorption spectrophotometry was that of Gore et al. (1949). These authors studied the absorption of aqueous solutions of organic acids and found H_2O to be relatively transparent in some regions, especially if used in a thin layer cell. Interestingly, they also found that D_2O was transparent where H_2O absorbed and *vice versa*; thus, they were able to cover the region from 2.5—14.3 μ (4000 cm^{-1} to 700 cm^{-1}) by using some samples in H_2O and others in D_2O. Subsequent work by Blout (1957) suggests that aqueous solutions may be useful in IR studies of proteins and perhaps in studies of enzymatic reactions.

The selection of a suitable "transparent" solvent is an important problem in obtaining IR spectra of drugs. Several solvents, notably CCl_4 and CS_2, are virtually transparent in the wavelength range 2—15 μ when used in thickness of 1.0 mm or less, and thus these may be used to dissolve many compounds (Carol, 1957). Similarly, the advent of the KBr disc technique has also improved the potential for studies of drugs by reducing the amount of compound needed to 1 mg or less (Stimson and O'Donnell, 1952; Schiedt and Reinwein, 1952).

The unique characteristic of an IR absorption spectrum is that it may be used for a functional group analysis of an unknown compound. By referring to absorption bands known to be associated with specific functional groups, it is possible to deduce the chemical structure of an unknown group. One of the earliest compilations of specifically assigned IR absorption bands was made by Colthup (1950); since then, many similar tables have been published in general references for IR work (Bellamy, 1959; Kendall, 1966; Conley, 1966). A good example of the use of IR spectra for identification of pharmaceuticals may be seen in the report of Pleat et al. (1951). Janot et al. (1951) used characteristic wave number assignments to elucidate the structure of holstiine, while Thompson et al. (1949) were able to learn a great deal about the structure of penicillin from IR spectra. In addition to the tables of IR absorption bands mentioned above, several other sources

Table 3. *Sources of infrared absorption data*

Pre-1944 data:	Infrared Spectroscopy, Industrial Applications and Bibliography. Ed. by R. B. BARNES, R. C. GORE, U. LIDDEL and V. Z. WILLIAMS. New York, N.Y.: Reinhold Publishing Company.
Looseleaf collections of spectra:	Catalog of Infrared Spectrograms, American Petroleum Institute, API Research Project 44. Pittsburgh, Pennsylvania: Carnegie Institute of Technology. The Sadtler Standard Spectra, Sadtler Research Laboratories, Philadelphia, Pennsylvania.
Punched card collection of spectra:	American Association for Testing Materials, Philadelphia, Pa. Commission on Infrared Absorption Spectroscopy, National Research Council, National Bureau of Standards, Washington, D.C.

of IR absorption data are listed in Table 3. CLARK and CHIANTA (1957) have discussed some of the problems involved in searching the literature for IR spectral information.

In a few instances, IR absorption has been used for quantitative drug assays. For example, CAROL (1954) used the IR absorption band of atropine at 9.66 μ (1035 cm^{-1}) to determine then content of the drug in tablets. WASHBURN and KRUEGER (1949) have measured the absorbance of standard solutions of aspirin, phenacetin and caffeine in chloroform solutions at 5.70 μ (1750 cm^{-1}), 6.05 μ (1650 cm^{-1}) and 6.63 μ (1510 cm^{-1}). By using suitable determinants, they were able to measure these three compounds in mixed samples. More recently, ERLEY et al. (1960) have used IR absorption to measure the level of various organic compounds in blood, after a suitable solvent extraction procedure. Similar applications are reviewed by various authors (CONLEY, 1966; KENDALL, 1966; NAKANISHI, 1962). In conclusion, however, it must be emphasized that the use of IR absorption as a quantitative tool is still extremely limited.

References

AXELROD, J.: Studies on sympathomimetic amines. II. The biotransformation and physiological disposition of D-amphetamine, D-p-hydroxyamphetamine and D-methamphetamine J. Pharmacol. exp. Ther. **110**, 315—326 (1954).

BEECKEN, H., GOTTSCHALK, E. M., GIZYCKI, U. V., KRAEMER, H., MAASSEN, D., MATTHICS, H. G., MUSSO, H., RATHJEN, C., ZAHORSZKY, U. I.: Orcein and Litmus. Angew. Chem. **73**, 665—673 (1961).

BELLAMY, L.: The Infrared Spectra of Complex Molecules. New York: John Wiley and Sons 1959.

BLOUT, E. R.: Aqueous solution infrared spectroscopy of biochemical polymers. Ann. N.Y. Acad. Sci. **69**, 84—93 (1957).

BRATTON, A. C., MARSHALL, E. K., JR.: A new coupling component for sulfanilamide determination. J. biol. Chem. **128**, 537—550 (1939).

BRODIE, B. B., AXELROD, J.: The estimation of acetanilide and its metabolic products, aniline, N-acetyl-p-aminophenol and p-aminophenol (free and total conjugated) in biological fluids and tissues. J. Pharmacol. exp. Ther. **94**, 22—28 (1948).

— — The fate of aminopyrine in man and methods for the estimation of aminopyrine and its metabolites in biological material. J. Pharmacol. exp. Ther. **99**, 171—184 (1950).

— — SOBERMAN, R., LEVY, B. B.: The estimation of antipyrine in biological materials. J. biol. Chem. **179**, 25—29 (1949).

— MARK, L. C., PAPPER, E. M., LIEF, P. A., BERNSTEIN, E., ROVENSTINE, E. A.: The fate of thiopental in man and a method for its estimation in biological material. J. Pharmacol. exp. Ther. **98**, 85—96 (1950).

— UDENFRIEND, S.: The estimation of basic organic compounds and a technique for the appraisal of specificity. Application to the cinchona alkaloids. J. biol. Chem. **158**, 705—714 (1945).

Brodie, B.B., Udenfriend, S., Baer, J.E.: The estimation of basic organic compounds in biological material. I. General principles. J. biol. Chem. **168**, 299—309 (1947a).

— — Coburn, A.F.: Determination of salicylic acid in plasma. J. Pharmacol. exp. Ther. **80**, 114—117 (1944).

— — Dill, W.: The estimation of basic organic compounds in biological material. V. Estimation by salt formation with methyl orange. J. biol. Chem. **168**, 335—339 (1947b).

— — Taggart, J.V.: The estimation of basic organic compounds in biological material. IV. Estimation by coupling with diazonium salts. J. biol. Chem. **168**, 327—334 (1947c).

Bush, M.T.: Extraction and identification of barbiturates. Microchem. J. **5**, 73—90 (1961).

— Mazel, P., Chambers, J.: The metabolic fate of thiobarbiturates. Thiobarbital in man. J. Pharmacol. exp. Ther. **134**, 110—116 (1961).

Carol, J.: The application of infrared methods to parmaceutical analysis. Ann. N.Y. Acad. Sci. **69**, 190—193 (1957).

— Report on analysis of drugs by infrared spectrophotometry. J. Ass. off. agric. Chem. **37**, 692—697 (1954).

Carroll, B., Thomas, A.W.: Spectral changes of dyes in colloidal solutions of hydrous oxides. J. Chem. Phys. **17**, 1336 (1949).

Clark, C., Chianta, M.: A bibliography of infrared spectra of biochemicals. Ann. N.Y. Acad. Sci. **69**, 205—253 (1957).

Clark, M.: Recent studies on reversible oxidation-reduction in organic systems. Chem. Rev. **2**, 127—178 (1925).

Colthup, N.B.: Spectra-structure correlations in the infrared region. J. Opt. Soc. Amer. **40**, 397—400 (1950).

Conley, R.T.: Infrared Spectroscopy. Boston: Allyn and Bacon 1966.

Cooper, J.R., Brodie, B.B.: Enzymatic metabolism of hexobarbital (Evipal). J. Pharmacol. exp. Ther. **114**, 409—417 (1955).

Erley, D.S., Blake, B.H., Potts, W.J.: Small volume long path infrared cell for liquids. Appl. Spectros. **14**, 108—109 (1960).

Gibb, T.R.P., Jr.: Optical Methods of Chemical Analysis. New York: McGraw-Hill 1942.

Gore, R.C., Barnes, R.B., Petersen, E.: Infrared absorption of aqueous solutions of organic acids and their salts. Anal. Chem. **21**, 382—386 (1949).

Henri, V.: Tables Annuelles de Constantes et Donnees Numerique. New York: McGraw-Hill 1932.

Hiskey, C.F., Downey, T.: The colloid error of indicators. J. Phys. Chem. **58**, 835—340 (1954).

Hoffman, B.: The Strange Story of the Quantum. New York: Harper 1947.

Jaffe, H.H., Orchin, M.: Theory and Applications of UV Spectroscopy. New York: John Wiley and Sons 1962.

Janot, M.M., Goutarel, R., Bosly, J.: Holstiine, an alkaloid from Strychnos holstii. Compt. Rend. **323**, 853—855 (1951).

Josephson, E.S., Udenfriend, S., Brodie, B.B.: The estimation of basic organic compounds in biological material. VI. Estimation by ultraviolet spectrophotometry. J. biol. Chem. **168**, 341—344 (1947).

Kendall, D.N. (ed.): Applied Infrared Spectroscopy. New York: Reinhold 1966.

Klotz, I.M.: The effects of salts and proteins on the spectra of some dyes and indicators. Chem. Rev. **41**, 373—399 (1947).

Kobowitz, F., Ott, P.: Isolierung und Kristallisation eines Gärungsfermentes aus Tumoren. Biochem. Z. **314**, 94—117 (1943).

Kolthoff, I.M., Rosenblum, C.: Acid-Base Indicators. New York: Macmillan 1937.

Ladenburg, R., Voorhis, C.C. van, Boyce, J.C.: Absorption of oxygen in the region of short wavelengths. Physiol. Rev. **40**, 1018—1020 (1932).

Lewis, G.N., Calvin, M.: The color of organic substances. Chem. Rev. **24—25**, 273—328 (1939).

Lynen, F.: Functional group of coenzyme A and its metabolic relations, especially in the fatty acid cycle. Fed. Proc. **12**, 683—691 (1953).

Maickel, R.P.: A rapid procedure for the determination of adrenal ascorbic acid. Application of the Sullivan and Clarke method to tissues. Anal. Biochem. **1**, 498—501 (1960).

Mayer, S., Maickel, R.P., Brodie, B.B.: Kinetics of penetration of drugs and other foreign compounds into cerebrospinal fluid and brain. J. Pharmacol. exp. Ther. **127**, 205—211 (1959).

Nakanishi, K.: Infrared Absorption Spectroscopy — Practical. San Francisco: Holden-Day, Inc. 1962.

Pleat, G.B., Harley, J.H., Wiberley, S.E.: Use of infrared spectra in the quantitative determination of alkaloids. J. Amer. pharm. Ass., sci. Ed. **40**, 107—110 (1951).

Roe, E.M.F., Beale, R.N.: Ultraviolet absorption spectra of trans- and cis- stilbenes and their derivatives. I. Trans- and cis- stilbenes. J. Chem. Soc. 2755—2763 (1953).

SALZMAN, N. P., BRODIE, B. B.: Physiological disposition and fate of chlorpromazine and a method for its determination in biological material. J. Pharmacol. exp. Ther. **118**, 46—54 (1956).
SCHIEDT, U., REINWEIN, H.: The infrared spectroscopy of amino acids. I. A new preparation technique for the infrared spectroscopy of amino acids and other polar compounds. Z. Naturforsch. **76**, 270—277 (1952).
SCOTT, A. I.: Interpretation of the Ultraviolet Spectra of Natural Products. New York: Macmillan 1964.
SCOTT, J. E.: Ultraviolet absorption spectrophotometry. In: Physical Techniques in Biological Research, Vol. I, pp. 131—205 (G. OSTER and A. W. POLLISTER, eds.). New York: Academic Press 1955.
SORENSON, S. P. L.: Enzymstudien. II. Mitteilung. Über die Messung und die Bedeutung der Wasserstoffionen-Konzentration bei enzymatischen Prozessen. Biochem. Z. **21**, 131—200 (1909).
STIMSON, M. M., O'DONNELL, M. J.: The infrared and ultraviolet absorption spectra of cytosine and isocytosine in solid state. J. Amer. chem. Soc. **74**, 1805—1808 (1952).
THEORELL, H., BONNICHSEN, R.: Studies on liver alcohol dehydrogenase. I. Equilibria and initial reaction velocities. Acta chem. scand. **5**, 1105—1126 (1951).
— CHANCE, B.: Studies on liver alcohol dehydrogenase. II. The kinetics of the compound of hose liver alcohol dehydrogenase and reduced diphosphopyridine nucleotide. Acta chem. scand. **5**, 1127—1144 (1951).
THOMPSON, H. W., BRATTAIN, R. R., RANDALL, H. M., RASMUSSEN, R. S.: Infrared spectroscopic studies on the structure of penicillin. In: The Chemistry of Penicillin, pp. 382—414 (H. T. CLARKE, J. R. JOHNSON and R. ROBINSON, eds.). Princeton: University Press 1949.
WARBURG, O., CHRISTIAN, W.: Pyridine, the hydrogen-transferring component of the fermentation enzymes (Pyridine nucleotide). Biochem. Z. **287**, 291—328 (1936).
WASHBURN, W. H., KRUEGER, E. O.: Infrared determination of aspirin, phenacetin and caffeine. J. Amer. pharm. Ass., sci. Ed. **38**, 623—625 (1949).

Chapter 24

Fluorometry

HELEN S. ACKERMAN and SIDNEY UDENFRIEND

With 1 Figure

A. Introduction

Fluorescence assay originated as an adjunct to colorimetry with the realization that various colorless drugs such as quinine could be determined from their characteristic emission during irradiation with UV light. It has since become clear, however, that fluorometry is a highly sophisticated tool, far more sensitive and versatile than colorimetry, more descriptive of molecular structure than absorptiometry, more convenient and, in some cases, more sensitive than radioassay.

An appreciation of the specificity of fluorometry awaited the development of a spectrofluorometer (BOWMAN et al., 1955), able to monitor and record both excitation and emission spectra over a wide spectral range (230—600 mμ). The sensitivity of the technique has steadily improved with increases in light source intensity and detector sensitivity, so that determination of substances in concentrations as low as nanograms (10^{-9} g) per ml is now common.

Luminescence techniques have achieved even greater sophistication with the development of methods for the measurement of fluorescence polarization, direct determination of fluorescence lifetimes, measurement of absolute quantum yield, excited state ionization, and many types of energy transfer, as well as the development of phosphorescence assay. These advances are extensively reviewed by UDENFRIEND (1969) and will be mentioned here only as they relate to drug assay.

The mechanism of fluorescence and the various processes that influence its character underlie the rational development of fluorescence assay procedures. A detailed treatment and many additional references are given by UDENFRIEND (1962, 1969). A brief outline of these principles follows.

B. Principles

Early observations of atomic spectra revealed that the energy of an atom can vary only in discrete intervals which are characteristic of the structure of the particular atom. For complex molecules, one may imagine that the interactions of many nuclei and electrons can be summed, resulting in a series of specific energy states in which a given molecule may exist. Figure 1 is a schematic representation of the three lowest energy states of a hypothetical organic molecule, the ground state (S_0), the first excited state (S^*) and the first triplet state (T). In the ground state, most stable organic molecules have an even number of electrons distributed in pairs, with spins opposed, in the lowest available molecular orbitals. Since the multiplicity[1] of an energy state in which all electrons are paired is one, the ground state is a singlet, designated in the figure as S_0.

---

[1] Multiplicity is a term denoting the orbital angular momentum of a given state and is equal to $(2S + 1)$, where S is electron spin and has the values $\pm\ ^1/_2$. When all electrons are paired, $S = (+^1/_2 - ^1/_2) = 0$; when two electrons are unpaired, $S = (+^1/_2 + ^1/_2) = 1$.

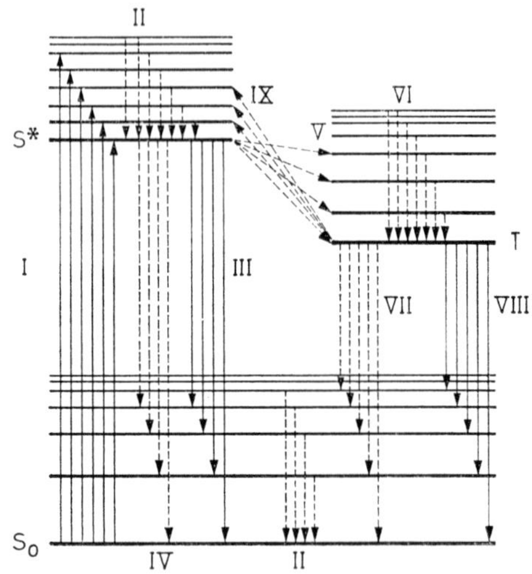

Fig. 1. Energy level diagram of typical organic molecule including only ground singlet (S_0), first excited singlet (S*) and its corresponding triplet state (T). Solid lines indicate radiational transitions and dashed lines indicate nonradiational transitions. See text for definition of Roman numerals. After Winefordner et al. (1969). Reprinted by permission of Academic Press

Many aromatic molecules absorb ultraviolet or visible light (see chapter 23, this volume); the energy of light in this spectral region is about 100 Kcal/mole and corresponds to the energy required for an electronic transition within the molecule in which the most loosely bound electron, usually in a π or n orbital, is promoted to an orbital of higher energy, usually π^*. The promoted electron may remain spin-paired with its former partner, in which case the excited electronic state will be a singlet, S*; if the spin of the promoted electron is reversed, the molecule will contain two unpaired electrons. Since the multiplicity[1] will now be 3, the new state will be a triplet, T. In most aromatic molecules, the triplet state is lower in energy than the corresponding singlet state, so the energy of T is less than that of S*. Each electronic state has associated with it many closely spaced states corresponding to the various vibrational modes of the molecule. Low energy photons (infrared) or moderate heat (.5 Kcal/mole) are sufficient to raise the molecule to a higher vibrational level of a given electronic state.

The various processes involved in absorption and luminescence are shown in Fig. 1 and include:

Process I. *Absorption*, an electronic transition from the ground state, S_0, to some vibrational level of S*.

Process II. A radiationless "*vibrational cascade*" to the lowest vibrational level of S*, brought about by collisions with solvent molecules which drain off excess vibrational energy as heat.

Process III. *Fluorescence*, a radiational return from the lowest vibrational level of S* to some vibrational level of the ground state by the emission of energy as a photon of light.

Process IV. *Quenching*, a radiationless return to the ground state. The probabilities of Process IV versus III depend on the disposition of the energy levels of a particular molecule. Both fluorescence and quenching are followed by a vibrational cascade to the lowest vibrational level of the ground state, in which the great majority of a population of molecules exists at biological temperatures.

Process V. *Intersystem crossing*, a radiationless transition from the excited singlet to the triplet state, involving a change in multiplicity, i. e., an electron spin reversal. This process is "forbidden" according to quantum mechanical selection rules, but in complex molecules it is often observed because of magnetic interaction of the spin and orbital angular momenta of the electron (spin-orbit coupling).

Process VI. *Vibrational cascade*, following Process V, to the lowest vibrational level of T.

Process VII. *Quenching*, a radiationless transition from T to S_0.

Process VIII. *Phosphorescence*, a radiational transition from the triplet state to the ground state by the emission of a photon. Both VII and VIII require intersystem crossing.

Process IX. A radiationless transition from the triplet state back to the excited singlet state, involving another intersystem crossing. Since S* is a higher energy state than T, this transition requires thermal energy; after loss of excess vibrational energy (II), it can be followed by any process III—VIII. If the molecule drops back to the ground state by emitting radiation (III), this emission is termed "*E-type delayed fluorescence*"[2].

The exact energy which a molecule can absorb and emit is determined by its own energy level spacing. In a fluorescence spectrometer, a fluorphor is normally irradiated at the wavelength of maximum absorption and the intensity of emission is determined at different wavelengths to obtain a *fluorescence spectrum*. Since fluorescence is directly dependent on absorption, an *excitation spectrum* is obtained when the intensity of emission at the fluorescence maximum is plotted while the wavelength of the exciting light is varied. The excitation spectrum is theoretically identical to the absorption spectrum for a particular molecule, and observed shifts are due to instrumental factors. Figure 1 shows that because vibrational energy is lost (Process II) before and after the fluorescence transition (Process III), the photons emitted as fluorescence are lower in energy and therefore have a longer wavelength than those absorbed. Thus, a given fluorophor has *two* characteristic spectra, excitation and emission, and both can contribute to the specificity of fluorescence assay. Although a compound may exhibit more than one absorption or excitation band, corresponding to transitions to several higher singlet states, radiationless deactivation between higher states (internal conversion) is so probable in liquids and solids that fluorescence almost invariably takes place from the first excited singlet state; thus fluorescence can be excited at any absorption band of a fluorophor and fluorescence spectra normally have only one maximum. Quinine, which seems to be an exception, will be discussed below. It can also be seen from Fig. 1 that the wavelength of phosphorescence will be longer than that of fluorescence, since it originates from a lower energy state. Delayed fluorescence, on the other hand, will be at the same wavelength as fluorescence.

Absorption and the vibrational cascade in S* are very rapid (10^{-15} sec), but the probabilities of the fluorescence and phosphorescence transitions are sufficiently low that the molecule will spend a measurable length of time in the excited state. The lifetime of the excited state, τ, is the length of time necessary for luminescence intensity to decay to $1/e$ of its initial value after removal of the exciting light[3], and is inversely proportional to the probability of the lumines-

2 Other types of delayed fluorescence, resulting from interaction of the excited molecule with other molecules, are described by UDENFRIEND (1969).

3 Since e, the base of Napierian logarithms, is 2.718..., $1/e = 0.368$, and τ is therefore the time required for the luminescence intensity to drop to 36.8% of its initial value.

cence transition in question. Since these probabilities are functions of the energy spacing of the molecule, τ is a true molecular property and is potentially useful for quantitative assay. Fluorescence lifetimes range from 10^{-6} to 10^{-9} sec, while phosphorescence and delayed fluorescence, which involve forbidden transitions (low probability), have lifetimes of 10^{-4} to 100 sec.

Both phosphorescence and delayed fluorescence can be distinguished from fluorescence by means of a phosphoroscope, which momentarily blocks out the exciting light and allows observation of the long-lived emission; fluorescence decays so rapidly that it is not detected in the absence of the exciting light. When fluorescence and phosphorescence take place in the same system, both should be seen in emission spectra. In practice, however, phosphorescence is usually observed only at low temperatures in rigid media, since the extended lifetime of the triplet state makes it extremely sensitive to deactivation by collision quenching. The phosphorescope can also be used to measure the lifetime of phosphorescence (WINEFORDNER, 1969, p. 93). Fluorescence lifetimes are much more difficult to measure directly, but the recent development of nanosecond flash and phase fluorometers (UDENFRIEND, 1969, p. 160) have made these measurements feasible.

An additional molecular property can be determined by measuring *fluorescence polarization*. The part of a molecule responsible for a given electronic transition can be thought of as an electric oscillator with a definite axis of oscillation. When a fluorophor in solution is irradiated by polarized light[4], those molecules whose absorption oscillators are parallel to the plane of the light will be preferentially excited. If the molecules are in a viscous medium or attached to a macromolecule, their free rotation in the solution may be restricted sufficiently that they will remain oriented during the lifetime of the excited state; under these conditions the fluorescence emitted will be polarized. The plane of polarized emission will be at some angle to the plane of the exciting light depending on the spacial relationship within the molecule between the particular absorption and emission oscillators. When polarization, a function of this angle, is plotted against the wavelength of exciting or emitted light, the resulting polarization spectra will show regions of constant polarization, characteristic of one absorption or emission band, and regions of rapidly changing polarization that reflect the overlap of two neighboring bands. These spectra can therefore distinguish electronic transitions which may be hidden beneath broad bands in excitation or emission spectra. For example, it has recently been shown (CHEN, 1967a) that the fluorescence efficiency of quinine changes with the wavelength of the exciting light. By measuring polarization spectra, CHEN explained this observation by demonstrating that quinine emits from *two* excited singlet states. This is important because quinine is often used as a standard in quantum efficiency determinations.

The *quantum efficiency*, Φ, of a luminescence process is the ratio of quanta emitted to quanta absorbed per unit time[5]. Although a few compounds are highly fluorescent with quantum efficiencies close to one (Φ of fluorescein in 0.1 N NaOH = 0.92, WEBER and TEALE, 1957), most compounds that absorb UV or visible light have low yields of fluorescence or do not fluoresce at all because of competing processes of energy deactivation. These quenching processes may be i) intramolecular or ii) intermolecular.

4 Strangely enough, because of geometric considerations, polarized fluorescence can also be excited by nonpolarized light. See UDENFRIEND, 1969, p. 33.

5 Methods for measuring Φ in solution are discussed by UDENFRIEND (1962, 1969). These methods are frequently comparative and many discrepancies appear in the literature when absolute quantum efficiencies of standards are in doubt.

i) *Intramolecular quenching:* Radiationless loss of excitation energy occurs by internal conversion (Process IV, Fig. 1) when the particular energy level spacing of a molecule provides a route for the loss of energy in small vibrational steps, that is, as heat. Intersystem crossing (Processes V, VII, VIII, IX) also diminishes fluorescence yield and is enhanced by any factor facilitating spin-orbit coupling, such as the presence of bromo, iodo, nitro, or azo groups. Thus, uranine (sodium fluorescein) has a fluorescence Φ of 0.70, while that of the iodinated derivative, tetraiodouranine, is only 0.02 (BOWEN and WOKES, 1953).

Some molecules absorb light of an energy that exceeds the energy of their weakest chemical bond. In this case, the bond may be broken in a predissociative transition, dissipating the excitation energy in the process. For example, butadiene, which contains a C=C bond (125 Kcal/mole), absorbs light at 210 mμ (140—160 Kcal/mole) and does not fluoresce; in contrast, decapentaene, containing the same kind of bond, absorbs light at 300 mμ (95 Kcal/mole) and does fluoresce (UDENFRIEND, 1962, p. 23).

It should be emphasized that any environmental factor that influences the energy level spacing of a molecule, such as solvent-solute hydrogen binding or solvent polarity, can change fluorescence efficiency by increasing or decreasing internal conversion, intersystem crossing, or predissociative transitions. MATAGA et al. (1956) pointed out that the lowest excited singlet state of quinoline is π, π^* in polar solvents and n, π^* in nonpolar solvents. Accordingly, VAN DUUREN (1963) demonstrated that the fluorescence yield of quinoline is almost 1000 times greater in water than in benzene. Chemical interaction with the solvent can also increase fluorescence yield. For example, although aromatic aldehydes are non-fluorescent, acetal formation in methanolic HCl results in considerable fluorescence (CROWELL and VARSEL, 1963).

The pH of solutions can also profoundly influence the fluorescence of many compounds, indeed fluorescence indicators are used in acid-base titrations (UDENFRIEND, 1962). This effect occurs because the excited state energy levels of the ionized and nonionized forms of a molecule differ; one form may fluoresce and the other not. Thus, phenol, catechol, resorcinol and quinol fluoresce when undissociated but not when ionized. Anisole, the methyl ether of phenol, cannot be ionized and therefore fluoresces even in strongly alkaline solutions. On the other hand, heterocyclic and polycyclic phenols, such as α-naphthol and *p*-hydroxydiphenyl, fluoresce only in the ionized form, although these structures can rearrange to quinoid resonance forms, which may be the actual fluorophors (WILLIAMS, 1959).

Any marked change in fluorescence efficiency caused by ionization would be expected to occur at a pH that coincides with the pKa of the compound in question. This should be accompanied by a slight shift in excitation and emission maxima, reflecting a different energy level spacing for the ionized compared to the unionized species. This is usually the case, but occasionally a change in fluorescence intensity and a shift in the fluorescence spectrum, but not in the absorption spectrum, will be detected at pH values that do not coincide with the pKa because of *excited state ionization.* In some phenolic and arylammonium compounds, the acidic proton is apparently bound more loosely in the excited molecule than in the ground state and thus the excited species will be a stronger acid. For example, fluorescence of the ionic form of β-naphthol (pKa 9.46) can be seen at pH 5 (HERCULES, 1966). Conversely, carboxylate groups may become stronger bases in the excited state.

ii) *Intermolecular quenching:* Fluorescence efficiency can also be diminished by interaction of the excited molecule with other molecules to form nonfluorescent dimers, by transfer of excitation energy to other molecules, or by collisional deactivation of the fluorophor by other solutes. All these processes are diffusion controlled and thus depend on the temperature and viscosity of the solutions and on the concentrations of the solutes involved. Some types of collisional quenching depend on the structure of the fluorophor and the quencher and are therefore very specific.

From the above discussion of the factors which affect fluorescence yield, it is apparent that fluorophors possess certain properties. Fluorescent compounds must absorb light in the ultraviolet or visible regions; those with the highest molecular extinction are potentially the most fluorescent. Absorption and fluorescence are enhanced in compounds containing conjugated unsaturated systems capable of a high degree of resonance. Thus aromatic rings substituted with electron donating groups, such as phenols and arylamines, would be expected to fluoresce. When ionization leads to an increase in resonance energy, as in the quinoid resonance forms of α-naphthol cited above, the ionized species should be more highly fluorescent than the undissociated form. Fluorescence is diminished by the introduction of electron accepting groups into the ring, e.g., iodination of tyrosine or acetylation of phenols and arylamines. In addition, many polycyclic compounds, both homocyclic and heterocyclic, are fluorescent; the latter group includes numerous drugs, such as quinine, pamaquine, chlorpromazine, lysergic acid diethylamine and reserpine. Furthermore, substances that are nonfluorescent or weakly fluorescent can usually be converted to highly fluorescent derivatives by suitable chemical procedures.

C. Practical Considerations

I. Concentration

Fluorescence intensity is proportional to the concentration of the fluorescence species only in rather dilute solutions because collision quenching with other solute molecules becomes significant at high concentrations. Furthermore, fluorescence may also be diminished in a concentrated solution by an "inner filter" effect in which a high percentage of the activating photons are absorbed as they enter the solution. For these reasons dilute solutions which absorb less than 5% of the exciting light are usually necessary to maintain linearity (Bowen and Wokes, 1953). Phosphorescence is routinely measured in rigid media to avoid collisional deactivation, but it is nevertheless subject to inner filter effects at high sample concentrations.

II. Background Fluorescence

Since fluorescence assay is frequently employed near the limits of sensitivity, it is often very important to reduce background interference from traces of fluorescent materials in solvents and reagents. Spectral grade solvents are commercially available, although even these may sometimes require further purification by appropriate procedures. Other possible sources of background fluorescence are detergents used to wash glassware, traces of stopcock grease, rubber or cork stoppers, filter paper, and chromatographic materials. All these possibilities should be checked if the blank is high. The interested reader should consult Udenfriend (1962) for a detailed discussion.

III. Surface Adsorption of Fluorophors

Fluorophors, especially when dissolved in organic solvents, occasionally adsorb to glass surfaces, decreasing their concentration (see chapter 22, this volume). This loss, which can be significant in highly dilute solutions, can often be reduced by the addition of a small amount of a polar solvent such as isoamyl alcohol to organic phases during extraction procedures (BRODIE et al., 1947a). The fluorescent solute may also adsorb to protein surfaces during protein precipitation steps. When this problem occurs in a given procedure, various precipitating agents should be tested until the most suitable one is found (UDENFRIEND, 1962, p. 103) or the fluorescent compound should be extracted directly into an organic solvent without prior precipitation of the protein.

IV. Scattered Light

Light scatter can be a major problem in fluorescence spectrometry. Several types of scatter are frequently encountered in fluorescence spectra and can be distinguished by their spectral properties. *Tyndall* scatter occurs at the wavelength of excitation and results from the reflection of light from colloidal particles in solutions; it is particularly troublesome when tissues or intact cells are studied. *Raleigh* scatter involves an interaction of the exciting photons with solvent or other molecules in the light path. Since this interaction is described as perfectly elastic, no transfer of energy takes place and the photon leaves the encounter with its energy unchanged. Thus, Raleigh scatter, like Tyndall scatter, is observed in fluorescence emission spectra at the wavelength of excitation.

Raman scatter is also the result of the interaction of light with solvent molecules, but in this case the encounter is not perfectly elastic; energy, corresponding to that between two vibrational modes of the molecule, may be added or subtracted from the photon and hence Raman scatter appears in the fluorescence emission spectrum separated from the wavelength of excitation by an energy difference which is determined by the vibrational spacing of the solvent molecule. Since molecules at room temperature and below are almost always found at their lowest possible vibrational level, energy is usually transferred from the photon to the molecule; the Raman scatter peak therefore appears at a longer wavelength than the excitation band.

All types of scatter can be diminished by narrowing the slits that define the excitation and emission beams, or by appropriate filters, but these methods reduce sensitivity as well. Since scattered light tends to be highly polarized, it can also be reduced by the use of polarizers. However, a polarizer in the emitted beam may distort the fluorescence spectrum, while polarizers in both the exciting and emitted beams will seriously reduce sensitivity (CHEN, 1966). CHEN has demonstrated (1966) that because of the right angle optics of most spectrofluorometers, scatter can be satisfactorily controlled by the use of a single horizonal polarizer in the *excitation* beam.

Other problems encountered in fluorescence assay, such as oxidation and photodecomposition of samples, are usually described in detail in particular methods.

D. Luminescence Analysis

Studies of the disposition of drugs in the body require the most exacting of analytical methods. Fluorescence procedures are often an extremely attractive answer to this challange since, when properly designed, they can be highly sensitive and specific, simple, rapid, and free of the hazards which attend radioassay and the complications of sample preparation necessary for gas chromatography. Modern commercial spectrofluorometers are standard equipment in most research laboratories; they are easy to operate, calibrate, and maintain. Fluores-

Table 1

Fluorescence Assay	Reference
Antimalarials	
Quinine	BRODIE and UDENFRIEND (1943a)
	BRODIE et al. (1947b)
Quinacrine (atabrine)	BRODIE et al. (1947b)
Pamaquine	IRVIN and IRVIN (1948)
	UDENFRIEND (1969 p. 505)
Chloroquine	BRODIE et al. (1947c)
	RUBIN et al. (1965)
Hydroxychloroquine	RUBIN et al. (1965)
Antibiotics	
Penicillin	SCUDI and JELINEK (1946)
Chlortetracycline	SALTZMAN (1950)
Tetracyclines (except oxytetracycline)	KOHN (1961)
Tetracycline, chlortetracycline, N-pyrrolidinomethyltetracycline, demethylchlortetracycline, oxytetracycline	HAYES and DU BUY (1964)
Oxytetracycline	IBSEN and URIST (1962)
Streptomycin and dihydrostreptomycin	FAURE and BLANQUET (1964)
Antimycin A	SEHGAL et al. (1965)
Griseofulvin	BEDFORD et al. (1959)
Antitubercular Drugs	
5-*n*-Heptyl-2-thiohydantoin	AUERBACH and ANGELL (1958)
Isoniazid	PETERS (1960)
	MOMOSE et al. (1960)
	HEDRICK et al. (1962)
Iproniazid	HEDRICK et al. (1962)
Antiparasitic Drugs	
Emetine	DAVIS et al. (1962)
Amprolium	KANORA and SZALKOWSKI (1964)
Carcinostatic Agents	
Aminopterin and Methotrexate	ZAKRZEWSKI and NICHOL (1953)
Methotrexate	FREEMAN (1958)
8-Azaquanine	MARKHAM and SMITH (1952)
Podophyllotoxin (extraction)	UDENFRIEND et al. (1957)
Sarcolysine	CHIRIGOS and MEAD (1964)
1,3-Diamino-5-methylphenazinium chloride	ANSTALL et al. (1964)
NSC-35847 (2-Nitro-4′,4″-di-2-imidazolin-2-yl-terephthalanilide, 2 HCl)	CHIRIGOS et al. (1963)
Analgesics	
Dromoran	UDENFRIEND et al. (1957)
Presidon	DERITTER et al. (1949)
Morphine	NADEAU and SOBOLEWSKI (1958)
	KUPFERBERG et al. (1964)
Codeine and codethyline	BALATRE et al. (1961)
Salicylate	CHIRIGOS and UDENFRIEND (1959)
	POTTER and GUY (1964)
Salicyluric acid	TRUITT et al. (1955)
Sedatives and Tranquilizers	
Pentobarbital	HOLLISTER et al. (1963)
Amobarbital	SWAGZDIS and FLANAGAN (1964)
Mephenesin	BRADSHAW and DOUGLAS (1962)

Table 1 (continued)

Fluorescence Assay	Reference
Chlorpromazine and other phenothiazines	MELLINGER and KEELER (1963, 1964)
	RAGLAND and KINROSS-WRIGHT (1964)
	RAGLAND et al. (1965)
Chlorprothixene	MELLINGER et al. (1964)
Reserpine	GORDON and CAMPBELL (1957)
	JAKOVLJEVIC et al. (1962)
	HESS et al. (1954)
Antidepressants	
Imipramine and desmethylimipramine	GILLETTE et al. (1960)
	DINGELL et al. (1964)
Iproniazid metabolites, benzylhydrazine and isopropylhydrazine	ROTH and RIEDER (1962)
Hallucinogenic Agents	
Lysergic acid diethylamide (LSD)	AXELROD et al. (1957)
	GENEST and FARMILIO (1964)
	DAL CORTIVO et al. (1966)
	AGHAJANIAN and BING (1964)
N-Diethyltryptamine	SZARA (1963)
Parasympathetic Agents	
Atropine	YAMAZAKI (1963)
	OGAWA et al. (1965)
d-Tubocurarine	COHEN (1963)
Antihistamines	
Diphenhydramine	GLAZKO et al. (1962)
Cardiovascular Agents	
Quinidine	EDGAR and SOKOLOW (1950)
	GELFMAN and SELIGSON (1961)
	CRAMER and ISAKSSON (1963)
Yohimbine	UDENFRIEND (1962 p. 431)
Metaraminol	SHORE and ALPERS (1964)
	COULSON et al. (1965)
L-Methyldopa and Metabolites	SCHÜMANN et al. (1965)
Dipyridamole	LABADIE (1964)
Cardiac glycosides	JENSEN (1952, 1953, 1956)
	WELLS et al. (1961)
	SILBERMAN and THORP (1954)
	PESEZ (1950)
	FRÈREJACQUE and DE GRAEVE (1963)
Digoxin	JELLINEK and WILLMAN (1963)
Digitoxin and Digoxin	JAKOVLJEVIC (1963)
Naphthionine	EISENBRAND and MEYER (1960)
Hydrastine	BROCHMANN-HANSSEN and EVERS (1951)
Miscellaneous Drugs	
Alloxan	ARCHIBALD (1945)
	LOUBATIÈRES and BOUYARD (1954)
Stilbamidine	SALTZMAN (1947)
Diethylstilbestrol	GOODYEAR and JENKINS (1960, 1961)

cence assay is also amenable to automation and instrumentation is available for this purpose. Sophisticated instruments can be obtained which automatically provide corrected spectral data, but this is not usually necessary for quantitative analysis. Detailed descriptions of available instrumentation and instructions for calibration of typical spectrofluorometers are given by UDENFRIEND (1962, 1969).

Fluorescence procedures have been developed for many drugs in common use and methods are continually being introduced or refined. Table 1 provides only a sample of this vast literature; for specific procedures the reader should consult the references mentioned in the table or those listed by Udenfriend in *Fluorescence Assay in Biology and Medicine*, Vol. I, chapter 13 and Vol. II, chapter 17.

Every fluorescence procedure is founded on the principles outlined above in Section B; the remainder of this chapter is devoted to specific examples of various types of luminescence assay based on these principles. A brief discussion of phosphorescence analysis is also included.

I. Types of Fluorescence Assay Procedures

1. *Native fluorescence — simple extraction procedures:* Among the earliest applications of fluorescence to drug assay were methods developed for quinine and related anti-malarials by Brodie and Udenfriend (1943a, b; Brodie et al., 1947b, c). Quinine, long known to be highly fluorescent, is an alkaloid which can be separated from its polar metabolites by extraction into organic solvents as the free base; it fluoresces maximally, however, in its ionized form and is thus returned to acid aqueous media as the salt for fluorescence determination. The following procedure for estimating quinine in biological samples is based on these properties (Brodie et al., 1947b).

A sample of plasma, urine or tissue homogenate, containing up to 1 μg of quinine, is shaken with 0.1 *N* NaOH and benzene and centrifuged. To minimize adsorption onto glass surfaces, a small amount of isoamyl alcohol is dissolved in the benzene before the extraction step. An aliquot of the organic layer is then extracted with 0.1 *N* H_2SO_4. After centrifugation, the fluorescence of the acid layer is measured at 450 mμ and compared with reagent and tissue blanks, as well as with quinine standards, carried through the entire procedure. Quinine is usually excited at 350 mμ, one of its three absorption peaks. The native fluorescence of this drug is so intense that as little as 0.001 μg/ml can be determined. It should be noted that quinine is maximally fluorescent in 0.1 *N* H_2SO_4, but its fluorescence is almost totally quenched by chloride ion in 0.1 *N* HCl.

2. *Fluorescence produced by chemical conversion:* The carcinostatic folic acid antagonist, methotrexate, is naturally fluorescent, but can be converted to the much more intense fluorophor, pteroyl-6-carboxylic acid, by oxidation. This fact was utilized by Freeman (1958) in the following procedure for the determination of methotrexate in tissues.

A plasma sample containing 0.06—1 μg methotrexate is diluted with water, and plasma proteins are precipitated by the addition of 15% trichloracetic acid. After centrifugation, an aliquot of the supernatant layer is mixed with 3.24% NaOH and 5 M acetate buffer, pH 5, and the fluorescence is measured (A). Potassium permanganate solution is then added to the cuvette and allowed to react for 5 min. Excess permanganate is then destroyed by the addition of 3% H_2O_2. Three minutes later fluorescence is again measured at the same wavelength settings (B). The increase in fluorescence due to oxidation (B—A), is directly proportional to the amount of methotrexate originally present in the sample. The oxidation step makes this procedure so sensitive and specific that as little as 0.005 μg/ml of the drug in the final solution can be determined. Freeman has applied this method to the absorption, distribution, and excretion of methotrexate in man.

Although morphine is naturally fluorescent in its unionized form in acid solution (excitation maxima, 245, 285 mμ; fluorescence maximum, 350 mμ), this fluorescence is apparently neither specific nor intense enough to be used for assay in tissues. However, the condensation of two molecules of morphine to yield the highly fluorescent pseudomorphine is accomplished in basic solution in the presence of potassium ferricyanide. Pseudomorphine has entirely different fluorescent characteristics than morphine; it is maximally fluorescent between pH 7 and 12 at 440 mμ with excitation maxima at 250, 280 and 320 mμ. The following procedure utilizing the conversion of morphine to pseudomorphine was published by Kupferberg et al. (1964).

A plasma sample containing morphine is mixed with sodium bicarbonate and then shaken with a solution of *n*-butanol in chloroform. After centrifugation, the morphine is extracted from the organic phase into 0.01 *N* HCl. An aliquot of this acid phase is treated with potassium ferriferrocyanide reagent in pyrophosphate buffer at pH 8.5. After 10 min fluorescence is measured (excitation, 250 mμ; fluorescence, 440 mμ). This procedure is specific for morphine in the presence of related drugs; the sensitivity is as high as 0.003 μg/ml in the final extract.

3. *Fluorescence dye procedures:* Many drugs are organic bases and can be reacted with water soluble acidic dyes to form complexes which are soluble in organic solvents. Thus the extraction of a dye-drug complex into an organic phase and comparison of the resulting color with that of known standards is the basis of many colorimetric assays (see chapter 2, this volume). Use of fluorescent dyes in such procedures can greatly increase the sensitivity and specificity of these assays. Glazko et al. (1962) have found that the fluorescent acid dyes, Xylene Red B[6] and Tinopal GS[7], can be used for the determination of a variety of basic drugs. They developed the following procedure for the antihistamine, diphenhydramine, which they report is sensitive enough to determine between 0.08 and 0.5 μg/ml of the drug in plasma.

Diphenhydramine is extracted into heptane from alkalinized plasma samples containing 0.2—2 μg of the drug. A small amount of ethanol is added to the heptane layer to prevent adsorption of the drug onto glass surfaces. The drug is then extracted back into aqueous solution as the acid salt by shaking an aliquot of the heptane layer with 0.1 *N* HCl. After centrifugation, the drug in the acid layer is extracted into a mixture of 0.5 *N* NaOH in half-saturated sodium carbonate and 1,2-dichloroethane. The dichloroethane phase is then carefully transferred to another tube, a small amount of 10% Tinopal GS in 0.1 M citric acid is added, and the tube is shaken and centrifuged. The dye combines stochiometrically with the drug in the organic solvent and thus the fluorescence of the organic phase (excitation, 365 mμ; fluorescence, 450 mμ) is directly proportional to the amount of drug present, after correction by subtraction of blanks which are carried through the entire procedure. Absolute concentrations are determined by comparison with standards, also carried through the procedure.

The reaction of dimethylaminonaphthalene sulfonyl chloride (dansyl chloride) with the terminal amino groups in protein hydrolyzates to yield highly fluorescent dansyl derivatives has been used for a number of years in protein structure studies (Gray and Hartley, 1963). Since this reagent also reacts with drugs containing primary and secondary amino groups, an attempt has recently been made to develop a simple dansyl chloride assay procedure which could be applied to the analysis of many basic drugs in biological fluids (Krishna and Moskowitz, 1969). Amphetamine, used as a model drug, was added to human plasma.

6 Sandoz Inc., Basle, Switzerland.
7 Geigy, A.G., Industrial Chemicals Division, Basle, Switzerland.

The sample was made alkaline with NaOH (pH 10) and the drug was quantitatively extracted as the free base into 10 volumes of benzene and then back into aqueous solution (0.01 *N* HCl) as the acid salt. The acid solution was neutralized with 1 *N* NaOH, and 0.1 M $NaHCO_3$ buffer and dansyl chloride in acetone (0.5 mg/ml) were added. After 6 h incubation at room temperature, the dansyl drug derivative was extracted into chloroform and the fluorescence measured. Chloroform was used for the final extraction because it greatly enhances the fluorescence of the dansyl derivative over its fluorescence in more polar solvents. This is in accord with CHEN's finding (1967b) that the fluorescence of dansyl derivatives decreases as the polarity of the solvent increases, probably because excited state energy is lost in dipole-dipole interaction between the excited molecule and solvent molecules. Unfortunately, the sensitivity of the method for amphetamine is limited to 100 ng/ml by a high blank in the dansyl reagent and the $NaHCO_3$ buffer, but if this blank can be reduced 10-fold this simple method is potentially useful for a variety of basic drugs.

4. *Fluorescence of drug-metal ion complexes:* The antibiotic, oxytetracycline, fluoresces in alkaline solutions at 520 mμ upon excitation at 390 mμ. When magnesium ions are added the excitation maximum shifts to 405 mμ and the fluorescence intensity increases. These properties were utilized by IBSEN et al. (1963) to determine oxytetracycline in tissues. The drug in acidified, deproteinized tissue samples is extracted first into amyl alcohol and then into 7 *N* ammonium hydroxide. An aliquot of the ammonium hydroxide phase is transferred to a cuvette containing $MgCl_2$ and fluorescence is measured at 520 mμ with excitation at 405 mμ. Ethylenediaminetetraacetate is then added to the cuvette to degrade the drug-Mg complex and fluorescence is again measured at the same settings. The resulting decrease in fluorescence intensity is proportional to the amount of drug present. It was noted that photodecomposition of oxytetracycline occurs in alkaline solution and thus excessive exposure to light must be avoided after the drug is extracted into ammonium hydroxide.

5. *Fluorescence produced by photochemical means:* GOODYEAR and JENKINS (1960, 1961) have developed an assay which can distinguish the synthetic estrogen, diethylstilbestrol, from other tissue phenols by photochemical conversion of the drug to an unidentified fluorescent derivative. The drug is extracted from a tissue homogenate into an organic solvent, the solvent is evaporated, and the residue is dissolved in ethanol. An aliquot of this solution is then irradiated with ultraviolet light for a controlled length of time, and the fluorescence of the resulting photoproduct is measured and compared with a non-irradiated sample. The increment in fluorescence caused by irradiation is proportional to the concentration of diethylstilbestrol in the sample. To make the assay even more specific, NaOH is added to both the irradiated and nonirradiated samples and fluorescence is remeasured. The photoproduct of the drug displays a characteristic shift in its fluorescence maximum upon the addition of alkali.

II. Phosphorescence Analysis

Phosphorimetry has not yet been extensively used for drug analysis, but several methods recently reported by WINEFORDNER and his colleagues are presented here to suggest the possibilities of this type of luminescence assay.

Since phosphorescence and fluorescence are alternate routes for excited state deactivation (see Fig. 1), compounds which do not fluoresce may phosphoresce strongly. For example, aspirin is only weakly fluorescent and must be hydrolyzed before fluorescence assay, but it is intensely phosphorescent and can be determined directly in plasma or serum by the following procedure, which the authors state can be completed in 10 min (WINEFORDNER and LATZ, 1963).

Aspirin is extracted from acidified plasma into chloroform. An aliquot of the chloroform phase is evaporated to dryness and the residue dissolved in EPA[8]. The solution is placed in a quartz cuvette and cooled in a special Dewar flask to 77°K by liquid nitrogen; the phosphorescence is measured and compared with blanks and standards. The authors found that the optimum concentration range for this method was 5—50 mg of aspirin per 100 ml of blood serum or plasma.

MOYE and WINEFORDNER (1965) have developed a phosphorescence method for the analysis of urinary *p*-nitrophenol, the major metabolic product of the insecticide, parathion. They report that this procedure is rapid, accurate, and 1000 times more sensitive than any previously reported. A sample of urine is hydrolyzed with concentrated HCl and extracted with ether. This extract is concentrated by evaporation and subjected to thin layer chromatography with ether as the developing solvent. The spot corresponding to *p*-nitrophenol is scraped into a vial and extracted with 0.1 M HCl and then re-extracted several times into ether. The ether extracts are combined, cooled to 77°K, and the phosphorescence is measured at 525 mμ (excitation, 265 mμ) and compared with standards and blanks carried through the procedure. The blank phosphorescence in this procedure was equivalent to only 1.3 μg of *p*-nitrophenol per 100 ml of urine.

A method based on the native phosphorescence of several sulfonamides (sulfadiazine, sulfamerizine, sulfamethazine and sulfacetamide) was reported by HOLLIFIELD and WINEFORDNER (1966) to be simple, selective, and sensitive enough to measure serum concentrations of the drugs as low as 0.1 μg/ml. The drugs were added *in vitro* to serum to determine the feasibility of the method. Serum samples were deproteinized by the addition of absolute alcohol, followed by centrifugation. The ethanol solution, diluted further with absolute alcohol, forms a transparent amorphous solid when cooled to liquid nitrogen temperatures and is thus suitable for direct measurement of phosphorescence.

Several authors have evaluated the potentialities and limitations of phosphorimetry as an analytical technique. A particularly complete discussion by WINEFORDNER et al. (1969) has recently appeared. Earlier, FREED and SALMRE (1958) and FREED and VISE (1963) concluded that solvent purity is the major limitation in phosphorescence assay. PARKER and HATCHARD (1962) emphasized that phosphorescence efficiency is so diminished in liquid solutions at room temperature that analytical procedures will probably always require the measurement of phosphorescence in rigid solutions at very low temperatures. This complication can be troublesome, since glasses formed by solvents at low temperatures are prone to crack. Yet phosphorimetry is highly selective and free from the problems of scattered light, which is removed by the phosphoroscope. These authors concluded that phosphorimetry could be useful when fluorometry was insensitive or nonspecific. HOLLIFIELD and WINEFORDNER (1967) also pointed out that the high selectivity of phosphorimetry could sometimes overshadow the simpler methodology of fluorometry.

KEIRS et al. (1957) also reviewed the possibilities of phosphorescence analysis. They showed that mixtures of phosphors can be analyzed without physical separation by varying the speed of the phosphoroscope to resolve compounds

8 EPA, a mixture of ethanol, isopentane and diethyl ether (2:5:5), forms a transparent amorphous solid (a "glass") on cooling to liquid nitrogen temperatures and is widely used as a solvent in phosphorimetry.

with differing phosphorescence decay times, by varying the excitation wavelength to preferentially excite one phosphor, or by varying the wavelength at which phosphorescence is observed. Simultaneous equations can be used if the resolution is incomplete. (Of course, excitation and emission resolution can be applied to fluorometric analysis as well.) St. John and Winefordner (1967) have also described a method for the resolution of two phosphors with different phosphorescence decay times in which the concentration of each component is determined from a plot of the log of the decay time of the mixture versus time after termination of excitation.

III. Application of Fluorescence Analysis to Drug Metabolism Studies

Studies of drug metabolism necessitate assay techniques which are sensitive and specific enough to distinguish very low concentrations of drug metabolites, often in the presence of the parent compound. Several examples will be presented in this section to illustrate the application of fluorescence techniques to this problem.

1. *Assay of the hydroxylated metabolites of 3,4-benzpyrene:* The hydroxylation of 3,4-benzpyrene by liver microsomes is monitored by a fluorescence technique and provides by far the most sensitive measurement presently available of the activity of hepatic microsomal enzymes. Kuntzman et al. (1966) used the following procedure modified from the method of Wattenberg et al. (1962).

Whole liver homogenate samples are incubated for 15 min at 37°C with an acetone solution of 3,4-benzpyrene and a NADPH cofactor generating system. The resulting metabolites, as well as the remaining parent drug, are extracted into a solution of acetone and hexane. The hydroxylated metabolites are then separated from the parent hydrocarbon by extraction into 1.0 *N* NaOH. The fluorescence of the metabolites in the alkaline phase is measured (excitation, 382 mμ; fluorescence, 510 mμ) exactly 10 min after the NaOH is added to the organic solvent. Timing is critical here since the fluorescence of the metabolites in alkaline solution decreases with time. The authors note that these metabolites are also subject to photodecomposition, hence the entire procedure must be carried out in dim light.

2. *Assay of some phenothiazines and their sulfoxide metabolites:* Udenfriend (1962, p. 437) noted that although the native fluorescence of chlorpromazine (excitation, 350 mμ; fluorescence, 480 mμ) is probably too weak to be useful for analysis in biological materials, the fluorescence of its sulfoxide metabolite is intense and easily distinguished from that of the parent drug by its spectral characteristics (excitation 335 mμ, fluorescence 400 mμ). These properties were utilized by Ragland et al. (1965) to develop an assay for several phenothiazines and their sulfoxide metabolites in tissues. In their procedure the parent drug and its sulfoxide metabolite are extracted from alkaline tissue homogenates into a solution of heptane and isoamyl alcohol. The sulfoxide metabolite is then separated from an aliquot of the organic layer by extraction into buffer, pH 5.0. Another aliquot of the organic layer is shaken with 50% acetic acid to extract the parent phenothiazine. The parent drug in this extract (sample 1) is oxidized to the more intensely fluorescent sulfoxide by the addition of 3% H_2O_2. The pH 5.0 buffer solution (sample 2) containing the sulfoxide is also treated with 3% H_2O_2 after acidification with glacial acetic acid. Both samples are heated for 10 min in a boiling water bath, cooled immediately to room temperature, and measured for fluorescence. Their fluorescence is compared with that of blanks and standards

carried through the procedure. This assay was sufficiently sensitive to measure chlorpromazine levels in tissues of 1 μg/ml and thioridazine levels of 0.05 μg/ml.

3. *Assay of imipramine and desmethylimipramine:* The tricyclic antidepressant imipramine is demethylated in the body to the even more active agent, desmethylimipramine (DMI). Both compounds fluoresce maximally in strongly basic solution at 415 mμ upon excitation at 295 mμ. DINGELL et al. (1964) developed the following procedure for the measurement of both compounds in tissue extracts.

The parent drug and metabolite are extracted into heptane containing 1.5% isoamyl alcohol from alkaline tissue samples. The organic extract is shaken with 0.2 M phosphate buffer, pH 5.9, which extracts about 80% of the DMI but only about 10% of the imipramine. The organic phase is shaken again with phosphate buffer to remove the last traces of DMI and then with 0.1 *N* HCl, which extracts the imipramine. An aliquot of this acidic phase is treated with 3 *N* NaOH and the imipramine fluorescence measured. The pH 5.9 buffer phase containing DMI is washed with the heptane-isoamyl alcohol solvent to remove any remaining imipramine, made basic with 3.0 *N* NaOH, and measured for DMI fluorescence. Total levels of imipramine and its metabolites were determined by combining the final extracts, measuring the combined fluorescence of imipramine and DMI, and comparing it with blanks and alkalinized imipramine standards carried through the procedure. Using this method, GILLETTE et al. (1960) were able to measure plasma levels of 0.1—0.6 μg/ml of imipramine in rats receiving 150—300 mg of the drug.

An interesting note in the DINGELL et al. report described the visualization of imipramine and its metabolites on paper chromatograms by their phosphorescence, seen when the chromatograms were cooled with liquid nitrogen and irradiated by an ultraviolet lamp.

4. *Assay of α-methylnorepinephrine in the presence of norepinephrine:* When two compounds with similar fluorescence characteristics cannot be easily separated, it is sometimes possible to analyze each one in the presence of the other by using a combination of methods and simultaneous equations. For example, α-methylnorepinephrine, the active metabolite of α-methyldopa, can be separated chromatographically from the parent drug and its other major metabolite, α-methyldopamine (SCHÜMANN et al., 1965). The α-methylnorepinephrine fraction, however, also contains norepinephrine. This fraction is therefore subjected to two fluorescence procedures. Norepinephrine is first estimated in one aliquot of the mixture by the trihydroxyindole method for norepinephrine in which the catecholamine is oxidized to the aminochrome and subsequently converted by the addition of alkaline ascorbic acid to the highly fluorescent trihydroxyindole (UDENFRIEND, 1962, p. 141). In this procedure α-methylnorepinephrine gives only 10% the fluorescence of norepinephrine. A second aliquot of the mixture is treated with 4.5 *N* NaOH and 1% *o*-phthaldialdehyde in methanol and finally with 3 *N* HCl to form the highly fluorescent aldehyde condensation product. In this procedure norepinephrine produces only 33% the fluorescence of α-methylnorepinephrine. The concentration of both can thus be estimated from these measurements and the appropriate simultaneous equations.

Many other examples of the use of differential fluorometry could be given. In the trihydroxyindole method for catecholamines, for example, epinephrine and norepinephrine can be estimated in a mixture by taking advantage of the fact that although both amines are oxidized to the aminochrome at pH 6.5, only epinephrine undergoes significant oxidation at pH 3.5. Thus by carrying out the procedure under both pH conditions and using simultaneous equations, one can determine both compounds.

Another interesting example of the fluorometric resolution of a mixture is the determination of 2- and 4-hydroxybiphenyl, the products of the metabolism of biphenyl by liver microsomes (CREAVEN et al., 1965). Both hydroxylated metabolites are unionized in acid solution, but at pH values as low as two, 2-hydroxybiphenyl exhibits the fluorescence characteristic of its ionic form (415 mμ) because of excited state ionization, while 4-hydroxybiphenyl exhibits the fluorescence of the unionized form (340 mμ). Hence, the two metabolites can be estimated in a mixture without separation.

IV. The Application of Fluorescence Spectroscopy to Drug Binding Studies

The transport of drugs by plasma proteins, their localization in tissues, their transformation by metabolic enzymes, as well as the actual mechanisms of drug action at receptor sites, are all related in one way or another to the binding of drug molecules to macromolecules. Since these interactions may change the fluorescence characteristics of the drug, the macromolecule, or a fluorescent probe attached to the macromolecule, fluorescence techniques have proved to be powerful tools for studying drug-macromolecule interactions (CHIGNELL, 1970a; see also chapter 9, this volume). This subject has been recently reviewed by CHIGNELL (1970a) and CHEN and CHIGNELL (1971) and only a few examples will be cited here to suggest the scope of this application of fluorescence technology.

The fluorescence characteristics of a fluorophor are highly sensitive to changes in the immediate surroundings. As discussed in Section B, changes in the polarity of the solvent may change the nature of the emitting state and thus influence both the intensity and wavelength of the emission. Shifts of fluorescence maxima to longer wavelengths (red shifts) are often observed as the polarity of the solvent increases, presumably because the energy of the excited state is lowered by dipole-dipole interactions or hydrogen binding between the excited molecule and the solvent. In an analogous manner, shifts in fluorescence maxima of small molecules upon binding to proteins or nucleic acids may provide information on the polarity of the binding sites. For example, the fluorescence peaks of the dyes ANS (1-anilinonaphthalene-8-sulfonic acid) and TNS (2-*p*-toluidinylnaphthalene-6-sulfonic acid) exhibit a blue shift, as well as a marked increase in intensity, when these compounds bind to serum albumin, suggesting that the dye binding sites are nonpolar (EDELMAN and MCCLURE, 1968).

The fluorescence of the macromolecule may also be affected by the binding of a drug. If the fluorescence maxima of one species (A) coincides with an absorption band of another species (B), the excitation energy of A can be transferred to B, quenching the fluorescence of A (FÖRSTER, 1951). This type of energy transfer from the single tryptophan residue of human serum albumin to the phenylbutazone analog, 4-butyl-1-(*p*-nitrophenyl)-2-phenyl-3,5-pyrazolidinedione, with the consequent quenching of the tryptophan fluorescence has been used by CHIGNELL (1970a) to study the binding of the drug to the protein.

LE PECQ and PAOLETTI (1967) have shown that the fluorescence of the trypanocidal dye ethidium bromide is greatly enhanced when the drug complexes to DNA or RNA. Since the drug seems to interact specifically with the base-paired regions of the helical nucleic acids, the authors suggested that the drug molecules were intercalated between the base pairs. Later work by BURNS (1969) showed that excitation energy can be transferred from the nucleic acids to the bound dye and, furthermore, that only the intercalated dye molecules can act as acceptors in this energy transfer.

Since the binding of a fluorescent drug to a macromolecule is usually accompanied by a marked increase in the polarization of the fluorescence emitted by the drug, fluorescence polarization studies can be used to monitor drug-macromolecule interactions, if the drug is fluorescent both before and after binding. TELLER et al. (1968) have used this technique to study the binding of chlorpromazine to human serum albumin.

A fluorescent probe attached to a macromolecule may be used to study the binding of nonfluorescent drugs. Thus CHIGNELL (1969a, b, 1970b) has studied the binding of phenylbutazone, flufenamic acid and dicoumarol to human serum albumin by observing the decrease in the fluorescence of dansylglycine as it was competitively displaced from the protein by the drugs.

Fluorescence studies have already yielded much data concerning the extent of drug binding and the nature of binding sites and forces. These applications of fluorescence spectroscopy will undoubtedly gain in importance as pharmacologists probe more deeply into the intimate mechanisms of drug metabolism and action.

References

AGHAJANIAN, G.K., BING, O.H.L.: Persistence of lysergic acid diethylamide in the plasma of human subjects. Clin. Pharmacol. Ther. **5**, 611—614 (1964).

ANSTALL, H.B., PETERSON, D.M., TRUJILLO, J.M., SAMUELS, M.L.: Spectofluorimetric measurement of 1,3-diamino-5-methylphenzinium chloride (NSC-33419) in urine. Cancer Chemother. Abstr. **43**, 43—45 (1964).

ARCHIBALD, R.M.: Methods for the determination of alloxan, together with observations of certain properties of alloxan. J. biol. Chem. **158**, 347—373 (1945).

AUERBACH, M.E., ANGELL, E.: A fluorimetric assay for minute amounts of some thiohydantoins. J. Pharm. Pharmacol. **10**, 776—779 (1958).

AXELROD, J., BRADY, R.O., WITKOP, B., EVARTS, E.V.: The distribution and metabolism of lysergic acid diethylamide. Ann. N.Y. Acad. Sci. **66**, 435—444 (1957).

BALATRE, P.H., TRAISNEL, M., DELCAMBRE, J.P.: Micro-dosage halofluorique de la codeine et de la codethyline. Ann. pharm. franç. **19**, 171—174 (1961).

BEDFORD, C., CHILD, K.J., TOMICH, E.G.: Spectrophotofluorometric assay of griseofulvin. Nature (Lond.) **184**, 364—365 (1959).

BOWEN, E.J., WOKES, F.: Fluorescence of Solutions. London: Longmans-Green 1953.

BOWMAN, R.L., CAULFIELD, P.A., UDENFRIEND, S.: Spectrophotofluorometric assay in the visible and ultraviolet. Science **122**, 32—33 (1955).

BRADSHAW, W.H., DOUGLAS, J.F.: Fluorometric determination of 3-o-tolyloxy-1,2-propanediol (mephenesin) using the 580 mμ fluorescent peak. Anal. Chem. **34**, 1172 (1962).

BROCHMANN-HANSSEN, E., EVERS, J.A.: A fluorometric method for the determination of hydrastine in hydrastis. J. Amer. pharm. Ass., Sci. Ed. **40**, 620—622 (1951).

BRODIE, B.B., UDENFRIEND, S.: The estimation of atabrine in biological fluids and tissues. J. biol. Chem. **151**, 299—317 (1943a).

— — The estimation of quinine in human plasma with a note on the estimation of quinidine. J. Pharmacol. exp. Ther. **78**, 154—158 (1943b).

— — BAER, J.E.: The estimation of basic organic compounds in biological material. I. General principles. J. biol. Chem. **168**, 299—309 (1947a).

— — DILL, W., CHENKIN, T.: The estimation of basic organic compounds in biological material. III. Estimation by conversion to fluorescent compounds. J. biol. Chem. **168**, 319—325 (1947c).

— — — DOWNING, G.: The estimation of basic organic compounds in biological material. II. Estimation of fluorescent compounds. J. biol. Chem. **168**, 311—318 (1947b).

BURNS, V.W.F.: Fluorescence delay time characteristics of the complex between ethidium bromide and nucleic acids. Arch. Biochem. **133**, 420—424 (1969).

CHEN, R.F.: Reduction of light scatter in fluorometry by the use of horizontally polarized excitation. Analyt. Biochem. **14**, 497—499 (1966).

— Some characteristics of the fluorescence of quinine. Analyt. Biochem. **19**, 374—387 (1967a).

— Fluorencence of dansyl amino acids in organic solvents and protein solutions. Arch. Biochem. **120**, 609—620 (1967b).

— CHIGNELL, C.F.: Fluorescence techniques. In: Methods in Pharmacology, Vol. II, Physical Methods. C.F. CHIGNELL, ed. New York: Appleton-Century-Crofts 1971.

CHIGNELL, C.F.: Studies of drug protein complexes. II. The interaction of phenylbutazone and its analogs with human serum albumin. Molec. Pharmacol. **5**, 244—252 (1969a).
— Studies of drug protein complexes. III. The interaction of flufenamic acid and other N-arylanthranilates with serum albumin. Molec. Pharmacol. **5**, 455—462 (1969b).
— Fluorescence studies of drug interactions with biological systems — a review. Fluorescence News **5**, No. 2. Silver Spring, Maryland, USA: American Instrument Co. 1970a.
— Optical studies of drug protein complexes. IV. The interaction of warfarin and dicoumarol with human serum albumin. Molec. Pharmacol. **6**, 1—12 (1970b).
CHIRIGOS, M.A., MEAD, J.A.R.: Experiments on determination of melphalan by fluorescence interaction with protein and various solutions. Analyt. Biochem. **7**, 259—268 (1964).
— UDENFRIEND, S.: A simple fluorometric procedure for determining salicyclic acid in biologic tissues. J. Lab. clin. Med. **54**, 769—772 (1959).
— VENDITTI, J.M., FANNING, G.R.: Extraction and fluorometric determination of a terephthalanilide in biological tissues. Cancer Chemother. Abstr. **32**, 1—5 (1963).
COHEN, E.N.: Fluorescent analysis of d-tubocurarine hydrochloride. J. Lab. clin. Med. **61**, 338—345 (1963).
COULSON, W.F., SMITH, A.D., JEPSON, J.B.: Fluorometric determination of m-hydroxylphenylethylamine (m-tyramine) and its analogs. Analyt. Biochem. **10**, 101—107 (1965).
CRAMER, G., ISAKSSON, B.: Quantitative determination of quinidine in plasma. Scand. J. clin. Lab. Invest. **15**, 553—556 (1963).
CREAVEN, P.J., PARKE, D.V., WILLIAMS, R.T.: A fluorimetric study of the hydroxylation of biphenyl *in vitro* by liver preparations of various species. Biochem. J. **96**, 879—885 (1965).
CROWELL, E.P., VARSEL, C.S.: Spectrophotofluorometric studies of some aromatic aldehydes and their acetals. Anal. Chem. **35**, 189—192 (1963).
DAL CORTIVO, L.A., BROICH, J.R., DIHRBERG, A., NEWMAN, B.: Identification and estimation of lysergic acid diethylamide by thin layer chromatography and fluorometry. Anal. Chem. **38**, 1959—1960 (1966).
DAVIS, B., DODDS, M.G., TOMICH, E.G.: Spectrophotofluorometric determination of emetine in animal tissues. J. Pharm. Pharmacol. **14**, 249—252 (1962).
DERITTER, E., JAHNS, F.W., RUBIN, S.H.: Fluorometric determination of ketotetrahydropyridines. An improved method for urine. J. Amer. pharm. Ass. Sci. Ed. **38**, 319—321 (1949).
DINGELL, J.V., SULSER, F., GILLETTE, J.R.: Species differences in the metabolism of imipramine and desmethylimipramine (DMI). J. Pharmacol. exp. Ther. **143**, 14—22 (1964).
EDELMAN, G.M., MCCLURE, W.O.: Fluorescent probes and the conformation of proteins. Accounts Chem. Res. **1**, 65—70 (1968).
EDGAR, A.L., SOKOLOW, M.: Experiences with the photofluorometric determination of quinidine in blood. J. Lab. clin. Med. **36**, 478—484 (1950).
EISENBRAND, J., MEYER, H.: Fluorimetry. III. Fluorimetric determination of naphthionic acid by using short-wave ultraviolet light. Z. Anal. Chem. **174**, 414—418 (1960).
FAURE, F., BLANQUET, P.: Microdosage fluorometrique de la streptomycine et de la dihydrostreptomycine par la reaction au β-naphtoquinone-4-sulfonate de sodium en milieu alcalin. Clin. chim. Acta **9**, 292—300 (1964).
FÖRSTER, T.: In: Fluoreszenz Organische Verbindungen, p. 83. Göttingen: Vanderhoeke und Rupprecht 1951.
FREED, S., SALMRE, W.: Phosphorescence spectra and analyses of some indole derivatives. Science **128**, 1341—1342 (1958).
— VISE, M.H.: On phosphorimetry as quantitative microanalysis with application to some substances of biochemical interest. Analyt. Biochem. **5**, 338—344 (1963).
FREEMAN, M.V.: The fluorometric measurement of the absorption, distribution and excretion of single doses of 3-amino-10-methyl pteroylglutamic acid (amethopterin) in man. J. Pharmacol. exp. Ther. **122**, 154—162 (1958).
FRÈREJACQUE, M., DE GRAEVE, P.: Reactions colorees et reactions de fluorescence des digitaliques. Ann. pharm. franç. **21**, 509—528 (1963).
GELFMAN, N., SELIGSON, D.: Quinidine. Amer. J. clin. Path. **36**, 390—392 (1961).
GENEST, K., FARMILIO, C.G.: The identification and determination of lysergic acid diethylamide in narcotic seizures. J. Pharm. Pharmacol. **16**, 250—257 (1964).
GILLETTE, J.R., DINGELL, J.V., QUINN, G.P.: Physiological distribution and metabolism of imipramine (tofranil). Fed. Proc. **19**, 137 (1960).
GLAZKO, A.J., DILL, W.A., FRANSWAY, R.L.: Determination of diphenhydramine blood levels using a new fluorescent dye-salt procedure generally applicable to basic organic compounds. Fed. Proc. **21**, 269 (1962).
GOODYEAR, J.M., JENKINS, N.R.: New method for the detection of fractional P.P.M. quantities of diethylstilbestrol. Anal. Chem. **32**, 1203—1204 (1960).
— — Irradiation fluorometric method for estimation of diethylstilbestrol in beef liver tissue. Anal. Chem. **33**, 853—856 (1961).

GORDON, J.A., CAMPBELL, D.J.: Fluorometric determination of 11-desmethoxyreserpine. Anal. Chem. **29**, 488—491 (1957).

GRAY, W.R., HARTLEY, B.S.: The structure of chymotryptic peptide from Pseudomonas cytochrome C-551. Biochem. J. **89**, 379—380 (1963).

HAYES, J.E., JR., DU BUY, H.G.: A simple method for quantitative estimation of tetracycline antibiotics. Analyt. Biochem. **7**, 322—327 (1964).

HEDRICK, M.T., RIPPON, J.W., DECKER, L.E., BERNSOHN, J.: Fluorometric determination of isonicotinic acid hydrazide in serum. Analyt. Biochem. **4**, 85—98 (1962).

HERCULES, D.M. (ed.): Fluorescence and Phosphorescence Analysis, chapter I. New York: Wiley Interscience 1966.

HESS, S., SHORE, P.A., BRODIE, B.B.: Persistence of reserpine action after the disappearance of drug from brain: effect on serotonin. J. Pharmacol. exp. Ther. **118**, 84—89 (1956).

HOLLIFIELD, H.C., WINEFORDNER, J.D.: A phosphorimetric investigation of several sulfonamide drugs: A rapid direct procedure for the determination of drug levels in pooled human serum with specific application to sulfadiazine, sulfamethazine, sulfamerazine and sulfacetamide. Anal. chim. Acta **36**, 352—359 (1966).

— — Fluorescence and phosphorescence characteristics of anticoagulants — a new approach to direct measurements of drugs in whole blood. Talanta **14**, 103—107 (1967).

HOLLISTER, L.E., KANTER, S.L., CLYDE, D.J.: Studies of prolongedaction medication. III. Pentobarbital sodium in prolongedaction form compared with conventional capsules: Serum levels of drug and clinical effects following acute doses. Clin. Pharmacol. Ther. **4**, 612—618 (1963).

IBSEN, K.H., SAUNDERS, R.L., URIST, M.R.: Fluorometric determination of oxytetracycline in biological material. Analyt. Biochem. **5**, 505—514 (1963).

— URIST, M.R.: Complexes of calcium and magnesium with oxytetracycline. Proc. Soc. exp. Biol. (N.Y.) **109**, 797—801 (1962).

IRVIN, J.L., IRVIN, E.M.: A fluorometric method for the determination of pamaquine, SN-13276, and SN-3294. J. biol. Chem. **174**, 589—596 (1948).

JAKOVLJEVIC, I.M.: New fluorometric micromethod for the simultaneous determination of digitoxin and digoxin. Anal. Chem. **35**, 1513—1516 (1963).

— FOSE, J.M., KUZEL, N.R.: New fluorometric micromethod for the determination of reserpine. Anal. Chem. **34**, 410—413 (1962).

JELLINEK, M., WILLMAN, V.L.: Fractionation and fluorometric quantitation of digoxin and its metabolites from human urine. Fed. Proc. **22**, 186 (1963).

JENSEN, K.B.: Fluorimetric determination of gitoxigenin. Acta pharmacol. (Kbh.) **8**, 101—109 (1952).

— Fluorimetric determination of digitoxigenin. Acta pharmacol. (Kbh.) **9**, 66—74 (1953).

— A paper-chromatographic and fluorimetric method for determining the cardiac glycosides and aglycones of digitalis purpurea. Acta pharmacol. (Kbh.) **12**, 27—46 (1956).

KANORA, J., SZALKOWSKI, C.R.: Fluorometric method for the determination of amprolium in feeds. J. Ass. Offic. Agr. Chemists **47**, 209—213 (1964).

KEIRS, R.J., BRITT, R.D., JR., WENTWORTH, W.E.: Phosphorimetry. A new method of analysis. Anal. Chem. **29**, 202—209 (1957).

KOHN, K.W.: Determination of tetracyclines by extraction of fluorescent complexes — Application to biological materials. Anal. Chem. **33**, 862—866 (1961).

KRISHNA, G., MOSKOWITZ, J.: Development of simple, sensitive methods for assay of drugs in body fluids. Annual Report, 1969, Heart and Lung Institute, National Institutes of Health, Bethesda, Maryland.

KUNTZMAN, R., MARK, L.C., BRAND, L., JACOBSON, M., LEVIN, W., CONNEY, A.H.: Metabolism of drugs and carcinogens by human liver enzymes. J. Pharmacol. exp. Ther. **152**, 151—156 (1966).

KUPFERBERG, H., BURKHALTER, A., WAY, E.L.: A sensitive fluorimetric assay for morphine in plasma and brain. J. Pharmacol. exp. Ther. **145**, 247—152 (1964).

LABADIE, P.: Dosage fluorimetrique de la 2,6-bis (diethanolamino)-4,8 dipiperidino-pyrimido (5,4-d) pyrimidine libre dans la plasma et dans les globules. Path. Biol. Paris Semaine Hop. **12**, 24—31 (1964).

LE PECQ, J.B., PAOLETTI, C.: A fluorescent complex between ethidium bromide and nucleic acids. Physical-chemical characterizations. J. molec. Biol. **27**, 87—106 (1967).

LOUBATIÈRES, A., BOUYARD, P.: L'etude des spectres d'absorption et de fluorescence des produits d'extraction du sang et de l'intestinole diabetique apporte-t-elle des arguments en faveur du role biologique l'animal normal ou physiopathologique de l'alloxane. J. Physiol. (Paris) **46**, 437—441 (1954).

MARKHAM, R., SMITH, J.D.: The structure of ribonucleic acids. Biochem. J. **52**, 552—557 (1952).

MATAGA, N., KAIFU, Y., KOIZUMI, M.: On the base strength of some nitrogen heterocycles in the excited state. Bull. Chem. Soc. Japan **29**, 373—378 (1956).

Mellinger, T.J., Keeler, C.E.: Spectrofluorometric identification of phenothiazine drugs. Anal. Chem. **35**, 554—558 (1963).

— — Factors influencing spectrofluorometry of phenothiazine drugs. Anal. Chem. **36**, 1840—1847 (1964).

— Mellinger, E.M., Smith, W.T.: Urine tests for chlorprothixene. Amer. J. Psychiat. **120**, 1111—1114 (1964).

Momose, T., Uedo, Y., Mukai, Y., Watanabe, K.: Organic analysis XIX. Microfluorometric estimation of isonicotinic acid hydrazide. J. pharm. Soc. Japan (Yakugaku Zasshi) **80**, 225—228 (1960).

Moye, H.A., Winefordner, J.D.: Determination of urinary *p*-nitrophenol by thin-layer chromatography and phosphorimetry. J. Agr. Food Chem. **13**, 533—536 (1965).

Nadeau, G., Sobolewski, G.: Une nouvelle methode de dosage de tres petites quantities de morphine. Canad. J. Biochem. **36**, 625—631 (1958).

Ogawa, S., Morita, M., Nishiura, K., Fujisawa, K.: Studies on the fluorometry of drugs. I. Fluorometric determination of atropine with eosine Y (tetrabromofluoresceine). J. pharm. Soc. Japan (Yakugaku Zasshi) **85**, 650—653 (1965).

Parker, C.A., Hatchard, C.G.: The possibilities of phosphorescence measurement in chemical analysis: Tests with a new instrument. Analyst **87**, 664—676 (1962).

Pesez, M.: Dosage fluorometrique du gitoxoside. Ann. pharm. franç. **8**, 746—750 (1950).

Peters, J.H.: Studies on the metabolism of isoniazid I. Development and application of a fluorometric procedure for measuring isoniazid in blood plasma. Amer. Rev. resp. Dis. **81**, 485—497 (1960).

Potter, G.D., Guy, J.L.: A micro method for analysis of plasma salicylate. Proc. Soc. exp. Biol. (N.Y.) **116**, 658—660 (1964).

Ragland, J.B., Kinross-Wright, V.J.: Spectrofluorometric measurement of phenothiazines. Anal. Chem. **36**, 1356—1359 (1964).

— — Ragland, R.S.: Determination of phenothiazines in biological samples. Analyt. Biochem. **12**, 60—69 (1965).

Roth, M., Rieder, J.: Spektrofluorometrische Bestimmung von Hydrazinen und deren Anwendung zur quantitativen Bestimmung von Benzylhydrazin in biologischen Proben. Anal. chim. Acta **27**, 20—26 (1962).

Rubin, M., Zvaifler, N., Bernstein, H.N., Sister Agnes Mansour: In: Drugs and Enzymes, Proc. 2nd Inter. Pharmac. Meeting, p. 467. Oxford: Pergamon Press 1965.

Saltzman, A.: Fluorophotometric estimation of stilbamidine in urine and blood. J. biol. Chem. **168**, 699—703 (1947).

— Fluorophotometric estimation of aureomycin in blood and urine. J. Lab. clin. Med. **35**, 123—128 (1950).

Schümann, H.J., Grobecker, H., Schmidt, K.: Über die Wirkung von Alpha-methyl-dopa auf den Brenzcatechinamingehalt von Meerschweinchenorganen. Naunyn-Schmiedeberg's Arch. exp. Path. Pharmak. **251**, 48—61 (1965).

Scudi, J.V., Jelinek, V.C.: A rapid micromethod for the fluorometric determination of penicillin. J. biol. Chem. **164**, 195—201 (1946).

Sehgal, A.N., Singh, K., Vezina, C.: Spectrophotofluorometric assay of antimycin A. Analyt. Biochem. **12**, 191—195 (1965).

Shore, P.A., Alpers, H.S.: Fluorometric estimation of metaraminol and related compounds. Life Sci. **3**, 551—554 (1964).

Silberman, H., Thorp, R.H.: The estimation of the component cardiac glycosides in digitalis plant samples. Part II. The estimation of the desgluco-glycosides and some observations on the production of ultra-violet fluorescence with trichloracetic acid. J. Pharm. Pharmacol. **6**, 546—551 (1954).

St. John, P.A., Winefordner, J.D.: Time-resolved phosphorimetry as a method of simultaneous analysis of two-component mixtures. Anal. Chem. **39**, 500—503 (1967).

Swagzdis, J.E., Flanagan, T.L.: Spectrophotofluorometric determination of low concentrations of amobarbital in plasma. Analyt. Biochem. **7**, 147—151 (1964).

Szara, S.: Enzymatic formation of a phenolic metabolite from lysergic acid diethylamide by rat liver microsomes. Life Sci. **9**, 662—670 (1963).

Teller, D.N., Levine, R.J.C., Denber, H.C.B.: Binding of chlorpromazine and thioproperazine *in vitro*. II. Fluorometric measurement of stoichiometry and alteration of protein structure. Agressologie **IX**, 167—188 (1968).

Truitt, E.B., Jr., Morgan, A.M., Little, J.M.: Determination of salicylic acid and two metabolites in plasma and urine using fluorimetry for directly measuring salicyluric acid. J. Amer. pharm. Ass. **44**, 142—148 (1955).

Udenfriend, S.: Fluorescence Assay in Biology and Medicine, Vol. I. New York-London: Academic Press 1962.

UDENFRIEND, S.: Fluorescence Assay in Biology and Medicine, Vol. II. New York-London: Academic Press 1969.

— DUGGAN, D.E., VASTA, B.M., BRODIE, B.B.: A spectrophotofluorometric study of organic compounds of pharmacological interest. J. Pharmacol. exp. Ther. **120**, 26—32 (1957).

VAN DUUREN, B.L.: Effects of the environment on the fluorescence of aromatic compounds in solution. Chem. Rev. **63**, 325—354 (1963).

WATTENBERG, L.W., LEONG, J.L., STRAND, P.J.: Benzpyrene hydroxylase activity in the gastrointestinal tract. Cancer Res. **22**, 1120—1126 (1962).

WEBER, G., TEALE, F.W.J.: Determination of the absolute quantum yield of fluorescent solutions. Trans. Faraday Soc. (Brit. J.) **53**, 646—655 (1957).

WELLS, D., KATZUNG, B., MEYERS, F.H.: Spectrofluorometric analysis of cardiotonic steroids. J. Pharm. Pharmacol. **13**, 389—395 (1961).

WILLIAMS, R.T.: Fluorescence of some aromatic compounds in aqueous solution. J. roy. Inst. Chem. **83**, 611—626 (1959).

WINEFORDNER, J.D., LATZ, H.W.: Phosphorimetry as a means of chemical analysis — The analysis of aspirin in blood serum and plasma. Anal. Chem. **35**, 1517—1522 (1963).

— ST. JOHN, P.A., MCCARTHY, W.J.: Phosphorimetry as a means of chemical analysis. In: Fluorescence Assay in Biology and Medicine, Vol. II. by S. UDENFRIEND. New York-London: Academic Press 1969.

YAMAZAKI, T.: Fluorescence analysis of alkaloids. I. A new fluorometry of atropine. J. Pharm. Soc. Japan (Yakugaku Zasshi) **83**, 402—405 (1963).

ZAKRZEWSKI, S.F., NICHOL, C.A.: The separation and determination of pteroylglutamic acid and related compounds. J. biol. Chem. **205**, 361—368 (1953).

Chapter 25

Radioactive Techniques: The Use of Labeled Drugs[1]

R. P. MAICKEL, W. R. SNODGRASS and R. KUNTZMAN

With 2 Figures

A. Introduction

HEVESY (1923) opened broad new vistas of research when he reported the first use of radioactive substances in biological research — a study of the absorption and translocation of lead in plants. Ten years later, GETTLER and NORRIS (1933) reported a death by radium poisoning, corroborating their findings with autoradiographic studies of human bone. Meanwhile, UREY et al. (1932) described the characteristics of a newly discovered isotope of hydrogen (^2H) and named it deuterium. Within a few years, SCHOENHEIMER and RITTENBERG (1935) demonstrated the use of this stable isotope in tracing pathways of intermediary metabolism. The next major step forward in biomedical applications of isotopes awaited the isolation of small quantities of ^{13}C by HUTCHISON et al. (1940). RITTENBERG and BLOCH (1944) then used ^2H and ^{13}C to demonstrate the successive condensations of two-carbon units during the normal biosynthesis of long chain fatty acids.

A new era of biomedical research began with the preparation of the radioactive isotope ^{11}C in the cyclotron. RUBEN et al. (1939) prepared this radioisotope, then used it to demonstrate the assimilation of CO_2 by barley. In the next two years, CO_2 fixation in animal metabolism was demonstrated by isolation of ^{11}C-labeled α-ketoglutarate from a pigeon liver system exposed to $^{11}CO_2$ (EVANS and SLOTIN, 1940, 1941). While these reports were able to provide actual data to replace speculation, the short half life (20.5 min) of ^{11}C made these studies extremely difficult.

Previously, KURIE (1934a,b) had suggested the existence of ^{14}C, a longer-lived radioisotope. RUBEN and KAMEN (1940) isolated this longer-lived (5.77×10^3 years) radiocarbon and subsequently BARKER and KAMEN (1945) reported the biosynthesis of ^{14}C-labeled acetic acid, proceeding from cyclotron-produced ^{14}C. As ^{14}C became available from the USAEC atomic pile in Oak Ridge, Tennessee, it was rapidly put to use. MURRAY et al. (1947) used this new item to prepare quantities of ^{14}C-carboxyl nicotinic acid and nicotinamide by chemical means, while GEILING et al. (1948) using a biosynthetic approach, grew plants in an atmosphere of $^{14}CO_2$, then isolated the desired compounds from the plants.

In 1934, the bombardment of deuterium (^2H) targets with accelerated deuterium nuclei led to the production of a still heavier isotopic form of hydrogen, namely ^3H or tritium (OLIPHANT et al., 1934). This hydrogen isotope is of even greater use in labeling studies than ^2H because it is unstable, emitting a weak β-radiation. Many of the general experimental designs useful for studies of compounds containing ^2H can easily be revised to permit use of ^3H with a consequent increase in sensitivity.

1 Supported in part by USPHS grants MH-14658, HD-03037 and by Research Development Award KO2-MH-41083 to R. P. MAICKEL.

For example, GLASCOCK and DUNCOMBE (1952), and EIDINOFF et al. (1953) showed that the incorporation of ^{2}H and ^{3}H from drinking water into rat liver fatty acids was similar. VERLY et al. (1952) studied the incorporation of methyl groups from $^{14}CH_3OH$, C^2H_3OH and C^3H_3OH into choline and creatinine in rats *in vivo* and found essentially the same results as those previously reported (DU VIGNEAUD et al., 1951) for methanol labeled with ^{14}C or ^{2}H. At about this same time, a number of tritiated compounds were prepared, using a diversity of chemical procedures, including gaseous exchange (WILZBACH, 1957), reduction with ^{3}H gas (FUKUSHIMA et al., 1950) or NaB^3H_4 (SMITH et al., 1955), exchange with $^{3}H_2O$ (CONDON, 1951), metal catalyzed exchange with $^{3}H_2O$ or CH_3COO^3H (VAN HEYNINGEN et al., 1938; EIDINOFF and KNOLL, 1953) or hydrolysis using $^{3}H_2O$ (WAGNER and STEVENSON, 1950; BOYER et al., 1951).

In addition to ^{14}C and ^{3}H, there are several other radioisotopes useful in the preparation of labeled drugs, including ^{32}P, ^{35}S, ^{36}Cl, ^{125}I and ^{131}I. A discussion of synthetic methods using these compounds may be found in ROTHCHILD (1965). A comparison of the characteristics of the various isotopes is seen in Table 1. From

Table 1. *Radioisotopes useful for labeling pharmacological compounds*

Isotope	Half-Life	Principal Radiation Type	MEV	Raw Material	Specific Activity Common mc/mmol	High mc/mmol
^{3}H	12.5 years	β^-	.018	H_2	25—500	>1,000
^{14}C	5,570 years	β^-	.115	$BaCO_3$	1—5	20—45
^{32}P	14.3 days	β^-	1.70	H_3PO_4	5—25	>100
^{35}S	89 days	β^-	.167	H_2SO_4	5—25	>100
^{36}Cl	308,000 years	β^-	.714	HCl	.01	0.2
^{125}I	57.4 days	β^- X-ray	.035 .027	NaI	25—100	>1,000
^{131}I	8.0 days	β^- γ	.608 .364	NaI	25—100	>1,000

these figures, several advantages and disavantages are readily apparent. For example, with respect to half lives, those of ^{131}I and ^{32}P are so short as to make experimental use more complex than desired. With regard to the radiation produced, only the iodine isotopes yield other than β-radiation, but the energy of the β-radiation produced by ^{36}Cl and ^{32}P is sufficiently "hard" to require special safety precautions. Finally, the low specific activities achievable with ^{36}Cl also make this isotope less desirable. Since it is reasonable to conclude from these considerations that ^{3}H and ^{14}C are the most useful radioisotopes available for the majority of pharmacological studies with labeled compounds, the present review will strongly emphasize these two isotopes.

B. Synthesis of Labeled Compounds

There are two general types of synthetic procedures that may be used to produce labeled compounds such as drugs: (1) chemical synthesis and (2) biosynthesis. Each of these has a number of advantages and disadvantages; the actual selection of a method of choice rests upon many factors depending upon the specific situation.

I. Chemical Synthesis Procedures

1. Procedures for ^3H

a) *Reduction of Appropriate Precursors.* An easy and efficient means of introducing ^3H into a molecule is catalytic reduction of a carbon-carbon double bond, using ^3H gas (ROTHCHILD, 1965). The use of hydroxylic solvents should be avoided as considerable loss of ^3H may occur through solvent exchange. Thus, steroids such as pregn-11-ene-3,20-dione can be reduced by ^3H enriched hydrogen gas in hexane solution to pregnane-3,20-dione-11α,12α-^3H (GUT and HAYANO, 1962). Many compounds not amenable to catalytic reduction with ^3H gas can be readily reduced by use of NaB^3H_4, or $LiAl^3H_4$, often with highly specific insertion of ^3H into the molecule (SMITH et al., 1955).

b) *Acid Catalyzed Exchange Reactions.* Many compounds, of diverse structures, will exchange their ^1H atoms for ^3H when exposed to the proper conditions. The use of a $^3H_3PO_4$-BF_3 catalyst system has been strongly recommended for this purpose (YAVORSKY and GORIN, 1962). More recently, ROTHCHILD (1965) and others have suggested the use of CF_3COO^3H for this type of exchange process. In general, the structural requirements for successful acid-catalyzed exchange demand the presence of an aromatic system to permit exchange of compound hydrogens for protonic ^3H.

c) *Metal Catalyzed Exchange in Hydroxylic Solvents.* When the compound of interest is sufficiently temperature insensitive, random labeling with ^3H can be achieved by exposure to solvents such as ^3H_2O, CH_3COO^3H or $CH_3CH_2O^3H$ in the presence of metallic catalysts like platinum, palladium, ruthenium or nickel (GARNETT, 1962; GARNETT and SOLLICH, 1965). The mechanism of this exchange is probably via a π-complex adsorption process (CALF et al., 1968).

d) *Wilzbach Tritium Gas Exposure.* This extremely simple technique was first described by WILZBACH (1957). It involves placing the compound to be labeled and a supply of $^3H_2$ gas in a sealed tube for some period of time. The efficiency of incorporation varies widely; the fraction of ^3H incorporated per day has been reported to range from 10^{-6} to 10^{-2} (ROSENBLUM, 1959). Various methods have been employed to accelerate the exchange, including exposure to ultraviolet light, X-irradiation or electrical discharges (MAICKEL and WEISSBACH, 1962). The Wilzbach process has been used to produce numerous ^3H-labeled compounds, including meprobamate (ROTH et al., 1959), digitoxin (SPRATT et al., 1957) and normorphine (MISRA et al., 1961a, b). While the Wilzbach procedure is simple, it suffers from two drawbacks. The formation of high specific activity impurities or breakdown products may make it difficult to obtain a high purity labeled compound (WILZBACH, 1957). In addition, some carbon-carbon double bonds will be reduced during the course of the $^3H_2$ gas exposure (ROSENBLUM and MERIWETHER, 1963).

e) *Synthesis of ^3H-Labeled Compounds from ^3H-Labeled Intermediates.* In general, this type of process requires similar precautions and poses difficulties similar to syntheses of compounds containing ^{14}C. Added care must be taken however, since oxidative conditions or extreme pH values may lead to loss of ^3H from the molecule (ROTHCHILD, 1965).

2. Procedures for ^{14}C

In general, the procedures used for ^{14}C-labeling are those of synthetic organic chemistry. The label is usually introduced into the overall synthetic process as late as possible in order to minimize losses and increase yield of useful label. The problems of running reactions and isolating products on a semimicro scale have been reviewed by CATCH (1961). A collection of synthetic procedures has been compiled by MURRAY and WILLIAMS (1958). If the molecule to be labeled is complex, it is generally more feasible to label on a side chain portion of the structure, rather than to attempt to include the ^{14}C atom somewhere in the middle of a polycyclic structure.

II. Biosynthesis Procedures

1. *In Vivo* Procedures

a) *Use of Microorganisms.* If an appropriate microorganism is available, many labeled compounds can be produced merely by including $^{3}H_2O$, $^{14}CO_2$ or ^{14}C-acetate in the atmosphere or culture medium. For example, the primary source of commercial ^{14}C-labeled amino acids is the protein of *Chlorella*, grown in a $^{14}CO_2$ environment. ^{3}H-Puromycin has been prepared by fermentation of *S. rimosus* in a medium containing $^{3}H_2O$ (OBER et al., 1962).

b) *Use of Plants.* Early work by GEILING and coworkers demonstrated the feasibility of producing ^{14}C-labeled compounds by isolation from the appropriate plants grown in an atmosphere of $^{14}CO_2$ (GEILING et al., 1948; OKITA et al., 1954). A standardized unit for this type of work has been described by LARSON and HARLOW (1958); the application of this system has recently been discussed by STEPKA and LARSON (1965). The use of this procedure has yielded compounds such as ^{14}C-nicotine (sp. act. 120 μc/mmol) from tobacco plants and ^{14}C-digitoxin (sp. act. 492 μc/mmol) from digitalis plants.

2. *In Vitro* Procedures

a) *Use of Crude Tissue Preparations.* A number of uses of crude tissue prepara tions to convert labeled precursors into ^{3}H- or ^{14}C-labeled compounds have been reported. For example, BAUER et al. (1965), have prepared and isolated ^{3}H- or ^{14}C-labeled insulin after incubation of pancreatic islets with ^{14}C-glucose or ^{3}H-leucine. Similarly, VAN DEN BOSCH and VAN DEENEN (1966) have prepared single or multiple-labeled lecithins by incubation of rat liver slices with appropriate substrates.

b) *Use of Purified Enzymes.* A highly specific synthesis of glucose-3-^{3}H and glucose-4-^{3}H has recently been reported, using a series of glycolytic enzymes (ROGNSTAD et al., 1965). More recently, MCMAHON and MARSHALL (1968) have suggested that methyl transferases may be useful to transfer a labeled methyl group from S-adenosylmethionine to various compounds.

C. Stability of Labeled Compounds

One great problem in the use of labeled compounds is the fact that chemical instability is often enhanced by or may even be produced by the presence of radiation. Thus, the energy produced by ionizing radiation can easily be absorbed by molecules, converted internally into rotational or vibrational energy, transferred to other molecules directly, or radiated as photons. Excited molecules can decompose into fragments, or can polymerize with each other. If they fragment, the portions produced may combine with each other, may react with other unexcited molecules, or may further fragment (BURTON, 1959). Radiation-induced damage may be particularly severe if the conditions are such that free radicals can be formed, since these will readily propagate. In order to facilitate stability of labeled compounds during the time between synthesis and experimental use, several general rules may be formulated. For example, the compounds should be stored at low temperatures; radiation-induced decomposition proceeds more slowly at 0° C than at 30° C and more slowly at —30° C than at 0° C. Similarly, the storage form of the compound should be as stable a derivative as possible. Salts such as iodides, benzoates and acetates have been suggested as likely to improve stability (TOLBERT, 1963). The solvent used to dissolve the labeled compound should also be carefully chosen. Aromatic compounds such as benzene are particularly useful, while water should be avoided if at all possible. Finally, the presence of oxygen should be avoided due to the possibilities of free radicals being generated by the radiation. If radioactive decomposition is suspected, repurification should be performed immediately prior to the use of the radioisotope (BAYLY and EVANS, 1966, 1967).

D. Measurement of Labeled Drugs

There are two basic types of procedures by which the quantity of radioactivity can be determined in a biological sample: (1) autoradiography, and (2) counting procedures. In line with the previous portions of this chapter, we shall continue to emphasize ^{3}H and ^{14}C labeled compounds in this discussion.

a) *Autoradiography*. Many different types of autoradiographic procedures have been devised and reported. For example, ULLBERG (1954, 1962) has described the use of whole-body autoradiography, in which whole frozen mice (killed by immersion in hexane at dry ice temperature) are mounted in carboxy-methyl-cellulose ice. Sagittal sections (20 μ thick) are cut at —10° C and placed in apposition to an appropriate photographic film sheet. Many techniques have been described for higher resolution autoradiography such as that required for organ sections; these have been mentioned by STUMPF and ROTH (1965) (see also chapter 16 in this volume). It is obvious from the criticisms of these and other authors that the techniques are far from perfect. In addition, a major problem with the use of autoradiographic techniques is the inability to distinguish between parent drug and metabolites. The photographic emulsion is sensitive to any and all radiation; it is incapable of discriminating between two or more compounds containing the same radioisotope. If, however, the compound of interest is not metabolized, or if metabolic products are known to be present in only trace quantities, autoradiography may be especially useful for subcellular localization studies. This is particularly true if the radioisotope being used is ^{3}H. The soft β-radiation of ^{3}H penetrates $< 2\,\mu$ into photographic emulsions, thus limiting the activation of the emulsion to an area about 1 μ distant from the labeled locus (FITZGERALD et al., 1951).

b) *Counting Procedures*. A large number of counting procedures have been and are being used for the determination of radioisotopes. However, for the majority of labeled drugs (usually labeled with ^{3}H, ^{14}C or ^{35}S) the primary method is liquid scintillation spectrometry (MAICKEL and WEISSBACH, 1962). Basically, this technique requires that the labeled compound be dissolved (or suspended) in a "cocktail" consisting of a solvent, a primary solute, and a secondary solute or "wavelength shifter". By a process of energy transfer:

$$\beta\text{-radiation} \rightarrow \text{solvent} \rightarrow 1^\circ \text{ solute} \rightarrow 2^\circ \text{ solute}$$

the energy of a β-emission is converted into a photon of light ($\lambda = 3700$—4200 Å) capable of being "seen" by an appropriate photomultiplier tube. As with autoradiography, the system is incapable of determining what compound contained the radioisotope — it can only measure the amount of radiation being emitted.

E. Specific Procedures for the Analysis of Labeled Compounds

A number of papers in the literature have described the application of specific analytical procedures to the determination of labeled compounds in animals. In general, almost any method having suitable specificity may be used. A recent paper by MAICKEL et al. (1969) describes the procedures used for two compounds: d-amphetamine-^{3}H and pentobarbital-2-^{14}C. A description of these procedures exemplify some of the problems that must be solved to permit successful application of a method; therefore, a brief discussion of each procedure seems appropriate at this time.

d-Amphetamine-^{3}H is a generally labeled compound with ^{3}H at various points throughout the molecule. The compound is chemically and isotopically stable when stored in dilute aqueous acid solutions (0.1 N HCl) at temperatures below

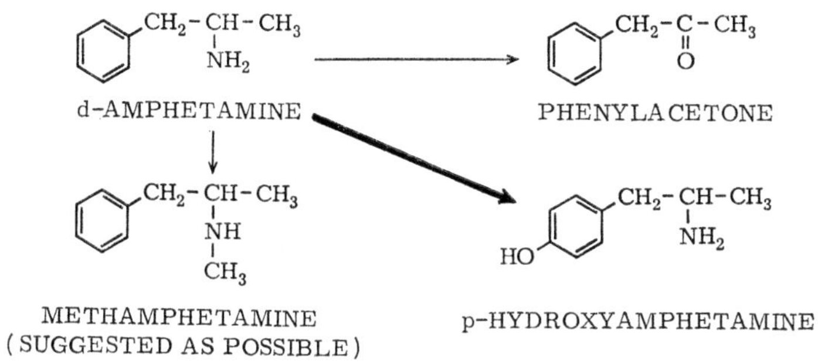

Fig. 1

+10° C. Figure 1 shows the metabolites which are formed from amphetamine in mammals. Since the molecule is generally labeled, all of the metabolites would contain ^{3}H. Thus a suitable analytical procedure must separate the unchanged drug from the metabolic products.

The methyl orange method used by AXELROD (1954) to measure unlabeled d-amphetamine by a colorimetric procedure can be readily adapted for use with ^{3}H-d-amphetamine. Tissue (homogenized in dilute acid) or plasma samples are made strongly alkaline (pH > 12) with aqueous NaOH. Extraction with benzene removes all of the unchanged d-amphetamine, some of the phenylacetone and any N-methylamphetamine, leaving the p-hydroxyamphetamine and its conjugates behind. A wash of the benzene with dilute aqueous alkali removes most of the phenylacetone and further cleans the benzene. After washing, the benzene is extracted with dilute aqueous acid (1 N HCl), selectively removing d-amphetamine and any N-methylamphetamine which might be present. The purity of this final aqueous phase is confirmed by thin layer chromatography; no evidence for N-methyl-amphetamine was found (MAICKEL et al., 1969). Thus, the acid aqueous phase contains only d-amphetamine-^{3}H and may be counted by liquid scintillation techniques. A similar procedure has been described by KUNTZMAN (1969) for studies of triprolidine-^{14}C.

Pentobarbital-2-^{14}C is a specifically labeled compound with the ^{14}C-atom in a metabolically inert site. When stored as a dry powder at temperatures below + 10° C, chemical and radiochemical stability is quite satisfactory. The major metabolic routes in mammals are shown in Fig. 2.

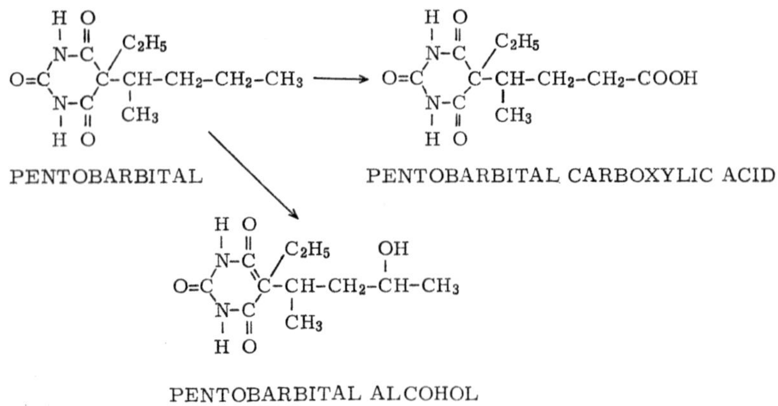

Fig. 2

BRODIE et al. (1953) reported a method for the measurement of pentobarbital in biological materials by liquid-liquid extraction and ultraviolet absorption spectrophotometry. This method lends itself readily to the measurement of pentobarbital-2-^{14}C as follows (MAICKEL et al., 1969). Tissues (homogenized in dilute acid) or plasma samples are added to pH 5.5 phosphate buffer. The solutions are saturated with solid NaCl, and the pentobarbital and small amounts of pentobarbital alcohol are extracted into n-heptane (containing 1.5% isoamyl alcohol) by shaking. After washing with a fresh portion of salt-saturated pH 5.5 buffer to remove more alcohol metabolites, the unchanged pentobarbital-2-^{14}C may be extracted from the heptane phase by shaking with pH 11.0 phosphate buffer. Aliquots of the alkaline buffer may then be added to liquid scintillation cocktail for assay of the ^{14}C content. As with the d-amphetamine-^{3}H, TLC studies of the final aqueous phase reveal only a single component — pentobarbital-2-^{14}C (MAICKEL et al., 1969).

Numerous other methods have been applied to the determination of labeled compounds; a partial listing of references is given in Table 2. In these studies, the labeled drug present in biological material was first separated from its metabolites

Table 2. *Some studies of drug distribution using labeled compounds*

Drug	Type	Reference
hydroxyurea-^{14}C	leukemia chemotherapy	ADAMSON et al. (1965)
etorphine-^{3}H and dihydromorphine-^{3}H	analgesic	BLANE and DOBBS (1967)
pentaerythritol- and pentaerythritol tetranitrate	smooth muscle relaxants	DICARLO et al. (1965)
thiazesim-^{14}C	antidepressant	DREYFUSS et al. (1968a)
mineral oil-^{3}H	inert drug solvent	EBERT et al. (1966)
d-propoxyphene-^{14}C	analgesic	EMMERSON et al. (1967)
guanethidine-^{14}C, ^{3}H	antihypertensive	FURST (1968)
dimethylsulfoxide-^{35}S	analgesic	HUCKER et al. (1966a)
indomethacin-^{14}C	analgesic	HUCKER et al. (1966b)
d,l-acetylmethadol-^{14}C	narcotic	MCMAHON et al. (1965a)
cyclazocine-^{3}H	analgesic	MULÉ and GORODETZKY (1966)
thalidomide-^{14}C	hypnotic	NICHOLLS (1966)
epsilon amino caproic acid-^{3}H	coagulant	OBIANWU (1967)
neostigmine-^{14}C	anticholinesterase	ROBERTS et al. (1965b)
dihydromorphine-^{3}H	analgesic	SANNER and WOODS (1965)
salicylic acid-^{14}C	analgesic	STURMAN et al. (1968)

before quantitation. This separation was obtained for each individual drug by solvent extraction alone or in conjunction with chromatography.

Since specificity is obtained by the separation step(s), they are, therefore, of utmost importance. For example, TITUS and WEISS (1955) showed that, after administration of pentobarbital-2-^{14}C to a dog, paper chromatography of the urine followed by radioautographic localization of the ^{14}C-containing spots on the paper chromatogram demonstrated the presence of unaltered pentobarbital and *nine* metabolites. Thus, mere measurement of radioactivity in plasma or tissues, no matter how sophisticated the measuring technique, cannot be used as an indicator of the level of any one compound.

F. Use of Labeled Compounds to Study Drug Metabolism

Anyone who has worked in the field of drug metabolism *in vivo* is familiar with the book "*Detoxication Mechanisms*" (WILLIAMS, 1959). Many of the metabolic pathways described in this book were worked out, often laboriously, prior to the availability of labeled compounds. Some idea of the importance of labeled compounds in elucidating metabolic pathways can be seen from a statement by Dr. D. V. PARKE of Williams' laboratory, "Isotopic labeling has been responsible, probably more than any other single new technique, for transforming the study of the metabolism of foreign compounds from a semi-quantitative estimate to a fully quantitative discipline" (PARKE, 1965). An excellent example of the validity of this statement can be seen in studies of the metabolism of benzene and phenol. Early work with unlabeled benzene had shown that, after administration to rabbits, 20—30% of the dose was excreted in the urine as phenol, catechol, quinone and hydroxyquinone (PORTEOUS and WILLIAMS, 1949) and the minor metabolites, L-phenyl-mercapturic acid (PARKE and WILLIAMS, 1951) and trans-trans-muconic acid (PARKE and WILLIAMS, 1952). An additional 40% of the benzene dose was excreted unchanged in the expired air (PARKE and WILLIAMS, 1950). Thus, only 60—70% of the administered dose could be accounted for. However, the availability of ^{14}C-benzene permitted PARKE and WILLIAMS (1953a) to restudy this problem and account for 90—100% of the administered dose. In addition, these later studies confirmed the presence of trans-trans-muconic acid as a metabolic product of benzene (PARKE and WILLIAMS, 1953a) but not of phenol (PARKE and WILLIAMS, 1953b).

Another interesting application of labeled compounds to the determination of metabolic pathways can be seen in work on aniline. SMITH and WILLIAMS (1949) showed that 40—45% of a dose of unlabeled aniline administered to rabbits was excreted as conjugates of o- and p-aminophenol; an additional 50% was excreted as a labile compound, thought to be aniline-N-glucuronide. However, subsequent studies of the fate of aniline-^{14}C by PARKE (1960) clearly demonstrated that while 75—85% of the dose was excreted in the urine, only about 6% was excreted as aniline-N-glucuronide.

Other compounds studied in this manner include: nitrobenzene-^{14}C (PARKE, 1956), m-dinitrobenzene-^{14}C (PARKE, 1961), phenylhydrazine-^{14}C (McISAAC et al., 1958), cyclohexane-^{14}C (ELLIOT et al., 1959), tetralin-1-^{14}C (Elliot et al., 1964), ethylene glycol-2-^{14}C (GESSNER et al., 1961), indole-2-^{14}C (KING et al., 1963), dehydroacetic acid-^{14}C (BARMAN et al., 1963) and coumarin-3-^{14}C (KAIGHEN and WILLIAMS, 1961).

Of particular interest are some studies with labeled insecticides. In the case of aldrin and dieldrin, the isotope used to label the compounds was ^{36}Cl. While no

Table 3. *Some studies of drug metabolism using labeled compounds*

Drug	Major Metabolites	Reference
hydroxyurea-^{14}C	urea	ADAMSON et al. (1965)
4-acetamido-2-morpholino-1,3,5-triazine-^{14}C	6-hydroxy derivative	ANGELUCCI et al. (1965)
pyridostigmine-^{14}C	3-hydroxy-N-methylpridinium	BIRTLEY et al. (1966)
α-3,4-dimethoxyphenylethylamine-^{14}C	3,4-dimethoxyphenyl acetic acid	CHARALAMPOUS and TANSEY (1967)
2-(o-phenoxyphenyl)-amino-4-amino-1,3,5-triazine-^{14}C	2-(o-phenoxyphenyl)-amino-4-amino-6-hydroxy-1,3,5-triazine	CRESSERI et al. (1966)
protocatechuic acid-^{14}C	vanillic acid	DACRE and WILLIAMS (1968)
homoprotocatechuic acid-^{14}C	homovanillic acid	DACRE et al. (1968)
5,5′-methylene-disalicylic acid-^{14}C	no metabolites	DAVISON and WILLIAMS (1968)
prazepam-^{14}C	oxazepam glucuronide	DICARLO et al. (1969)
thiazesim-^{14}C	o-hydroxy-thiazesim	DREYFUSS et al. (1968a, b)
d-amphetamine-^{14}C	p-hydroxy-d-amphetamine glucuronide and hippuric acid	ELLISON et al. (1966)
thalidomide-^{14}C	2-(o-carboxybenzamido)-glutarimide and 2-(o-carboxybenzamido)-glutaric acid	HAGUE et al. (1967)
dihydromorphine-^{3}H	dihydromorphine glucuronide	HUG and MELLETT (1965)
dimethylsulfoxide-^{3}H	dimethylsulfone	HUCKER et al. (1966a)
3-hydroxyphenyltrimethylammonium (PTMA)-^{14}C and neostigmine-^{14}C	PTMA glucuronide and PTMA	HUSAIN et al. (1969)
dextromethorphan-^{3}H	d-3-hydroxy-N-methylmorphinan glucuronide and d-3-hydroxy-N-methyl morphinan	KAMM et al. (1967)
chlordiazepoxide-^{14}C	7-chloro-1,3-dihydro-5-phenyl-2H-1,4-benzodiazepin-2-one-4-oxide and (N-2-amino-5-chloro-β-phenylbenzylidine) glycine-N-oxide	KOECHLIN et al. (1965)
d,l-acetylmethadol-^{14}C	1-noracetylmethadol	MCMAHON et al. (1965a)
acetohexamide-^{14}C	trans-3-hydroxyhexamide	MCMAHON et al. (1965b)
cyclazocine-^{3}H	cyclazocine glucuronide	MULÉ et al. (1968)
β-phenethylbiguanide-^{14}C	p-hydroxy-β-phenethylbiguanide and p-hydroxy-β-phenethylbiguanide glucuronide	MURPHY and WICK (1968)
neostigmine-^{14}C	m-hydroxyphenyltrimethylammonium	ROBERTS et al. (1965a)
diethylpropion-^{14}C	hippuric acid	SCHREIBER et al. (1968)
diazepam-^{3}H	7-chloro-1,3-dihydro-3-hydroxy-5-phenyl-2H-1,4-benzodiazepin-2-one	SCHWARTZ et al. (1965)
3,5-dimethylpyrazole-^{14}C	conjugated 4-hydroxy-3,5-dimethylpyrazole	SMITH et al. (1965)
5-methylpyrazole-3-carboxylic acid-^{14}C	conjugated 5-methylpyrazole-3-carboxylic acid	SMITH et al. (1967)
pentobarbital-^{14}C	pentobarbital alcohol	TITUS and WEISS (1955)
thiabendazole-^{14}C,^{3}H,^{35}S	5-hydroxythiabendazole	TOCCO et al. (1965)
thiabendazole-^{14}C	5-hydroxythiabendazole glucuronide and sulfate esters	TOCCO et al. (1966)

metabolites of dieldrin-^{36}Cl were detected, the study confirmed that aldrin is metabolized into dieldrin *in vivo* and also demonstrated a considerable localization of both compounds in the mammalian body (HUNTER et al., 1960). The veterinary anthelmintic hexachloroethane has also been studied after being labeled in both carbon atoms with ^{14}C. High localization of this compound was demonstrated by the fact that by 3 days after administration to rabbits, less than 30% of the dose had been excreted, 5% in the urine as metabolites and about 24% in the expired air as unchanged hexachloroethane-^{14}C (JONDORF et al., 1957).

Finally, a similar approach has been used to study the metabolism of two interesting drugs, thiambutosine and thalidomide. The antileprotic drug, thiambutosine-^{35}S, was found to be metabolized with only a small amount ($<$ 10% of the dose) of desulfuration (SMITH and WILLIAMS, 1961). This is incontrast to the metabolic pathways of other diaryl- and monoarylthioureas, some of which lead to toxic products because of metabolism via desulfuration (WILLIAMS, 1961; SCHELINE et al., 1960). With regard to thalidomide, it has been shown that, merely on standing in aqueous solution, thalidomide-^{14}C breaks down to twelve hydrolysis products (WILLIAMS, 1963). Without the use of labeled material, this study would have been impossible. Some additional significant studies of drug metabolic pathways using labeled drugs are given in Table 3.

G. Discussion of Basic Principles

From the presentations made in this chapter, it is obvious that the availability of radioisotopes, especially ^{3}H and ^{14}C, has facilitated the study of drug metabolism in animals. Anyone who has attempted to investigate the metabolism of a drug *in vivo* or *in vitro* can easily grasp the significance of being able to measure submicrogram quantities with accuracy. While the future of biochemical pharmacology has been considerably brightened by this recent development in technology, many facets of the use of labeled compounds must be kept in mind. It is especially pertinent to remember that the actual measurement process is non-specific. The radioactivity detector measures only ^{3}H or ^{14}C — it does not differentiate between different compounds containing the same isotope. One may group the factors important for successful use of isotopically labeled compounds into several categories:

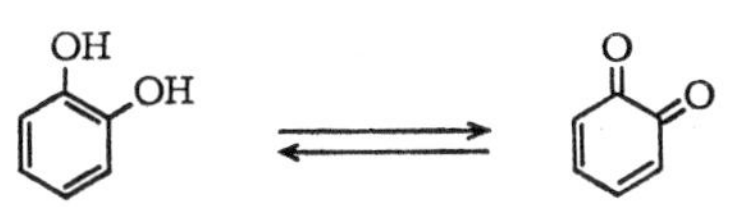

a) *Chemical Stability of the Labeled Atom.* A primary factor in preparation of a labeled compound or in purchase of a suitable compound from a commercial supplier is the position of the labeled atom. This position should be selected with regard to both chemical and biological stability. From the point of view of chemical stability, it is undesirable to have ^{3}H atoms on an aromatic ring containing hydroxyl groups which are capable of quinone-type resonance forms:
as the resonance would facilitate hydrogen exchange with hydrophilic substances. Similarly, it should be obvious that ^{3}H in labile or ionizable hydroxyl groups should be avoided; mere solution in solvents such as water would cause loss of radioactivity. If ^{14}C is the preferable atom, care should be taken to avoid putting it in thermosensitive positions such as those carboxyl groups that readily decarboxylate under appropriate conditions of pH or temperature. Finally, one must remember that all radioisotopes give off radiation; self-absorption of such energy may cause breakdown of the compounds on storage.

b) *Biological Stability of the Labeled Atom.* If a labeled compound is to be used in a metabolic study, it is essential that the label be in a metabolically stable position. For example, ^{3}H-tyrosine, labeled in the 3- or 5-positions of the benzene ring, would be a poor choice to study the synthesis of epinephrine from tyrosine. In converting the tyrosine to 3,4-dihydroxyphenylalanine, the enzymatic placement of a hydroxyl group would remove the ^{3}H, thus leaving a mixture of unlabeled and labeled compounds. Similarly, the N-methyl positions of imipramine would be lost in enzymatic N-dealkylation:

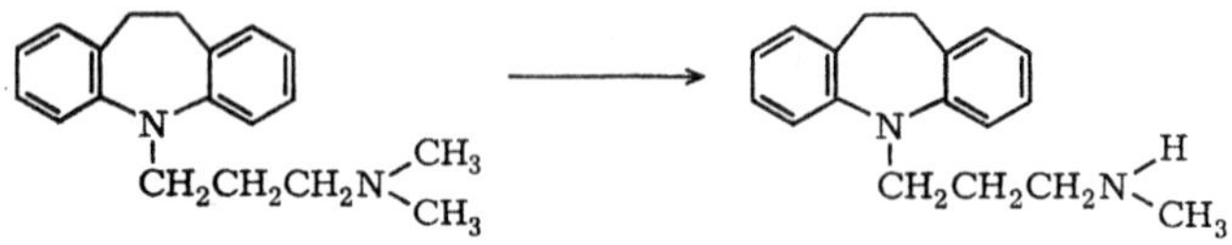

reducing the specific activity by 50% at the very least.

c) *Methodological Specificity.* Methods used to measure radioactivity do not specify the compound containing the labeled atom. Thus, prior to measurement of radioactivity, suitable techniques of separation (paper or thin layer chromatography, vapor-phase chromatography, or liquid-liquid extraction) must be applied to isolate the specific compound one desires to measure. The problem of specificity is the major difficulty in interpreting autoradiographic studies. Unless one has a non-metabolized compound, the autoradiogram will measure both unchanged drug and metabolic products, without discrimination.

From the above considerations, it should be obvious that radioisotopes, improperly employed, can lead to extremely misleading results. However, one must remember that when employed properly, radioisotopes can be the almost ideal solution for many knotty problems in drug metabolism. Perhaps the most significant point that should be emphasized is the sensitivity of measurement obtainable. Many ^{14}C-compounds are available with specific activities of 20 mc/mmol; at this level, the minimal quantity of a compound (molecular weight = 200) that can be measured with good accuracy and precision is $< 10^{-9}$ g. Many ^{3}H-labeled compounds are obtainable at specific activities of more than 1 c/mmol; at this level the minimum measurable amount of a compound of molecular weight = 200 is $< 10^{-10}$ g. It is obvious that such sensitivities make possible applications that were formerly almost impossible. The ultimate limitations in present and future applications of the technology reviewed in this chapter are in the physical techniques required to separate the specific compound one desires to measure. Future developments in these areas may carry to even further lengths the usefulness of labeled compounds in pharmacological research.

References

Adamson, R.H., Ague, S.L., Hess, S.M., Davidson, J.D.: The distribution, excretion and metabolism of hydroxyurea-^{14}C. J. Pharmacol. exp. Ther. **150**, 322—327 (1965).

Angelucci, R., Artini, D., Cresseri, A., Giraldi, P.N., Logemann, W., Nannini, G., Valzelli, G.: Some aspects of the metabolism of triazine derivatives active in experimentally induced virus infections. Brit. J. Pharmacol. **24**, 274—281 (1965).

Axelrod, J.: Studies on symptomimetic amines. II. The biotransformation and physiological disposition of D-amphetamine, D-p-hydroxyamphetamine and D-methamphetamine. J. Pharmacol. exp. Ther. **110**, 315—326 (1954).

Barker, H.A., Kamen, M.D.: Carbon dioxide utilization in the synthesis of acetic acid by clostridium thermoaceticum. Proc. nat. Acad. Sci. (Wash.) **31**, 219—225 (1945).

Barman, T.E., Parke, D.V., Williams, R.T.: The metabolism of dehydroacetic acid (DHA). Toxicol. appl. Pharmacol. **5**, 545—568 (1963).

BAUER, G.E., LINDALL, A.W., LAZAROW, A.: The biosynthesis of [^{14}C-] and [^{3}H-] labeled insulin. In: Advances in Tracer Methodology, Vol. 2, pp. 73—81. Ed. by S. ROTHCHILD. New York: Plenum Press 1965.

BAYLY, R.J., EVANS, E.A.: Stability and storage of compounds labeled with radioisotopes. J. labld Compds **2**, 1—34 (1966).

— — Storage and stability of compounds labeled with radioisotopes. Part II. J. labld Compds **3**, 349—374 (1967).

BIRTLEY R.D.N., ROBERTS, J.B., THOMAS, B.H., WILSON, A.: Excretion and metabolism of ^{14}C-pyridostigmine in the rat. Brit. J. Pharmacol. **26**, 393—402 (1966).

BLANE, G.F., DOBBS, H.E.: Distribution of tritium-labeled etorphine (M99) and dihydromorphine in pregnant rats at term. Brit. J. Pharmacol. **30**, 166—172 (1967).

VAN DEN BOSCH, H., VAN DEENEN, L.L.M.: Synthesis of ^{32}P-, ^{14}C-, and ^{3}H-labeled lecithins and their use in studies on lipid metabolism. In: Advances in Tracer Methodology, vol. 3, pp. 61—67. Ed. by S. ROTHCHILD. New York: Plenum Press 1966.

BOYER, W.M., BERNSTEIN, R.B., BROWN, T.L., DIBELER, V.H.: Investigation of the deuterohaloform synthesis. A new preparation of chloroform-d. J. Amer. chem. Soc. **73**, 770—772 (1951).

BRODIE, B.B., BURNS, J.J., MARK, L.C., LIEF, P.A., BERNSTEIN, E., PAPPER, E.M.: The fate of pentobarbital in man and dog and a method for its estimation in biological material. J. Pharmacol. exp. Ther. **109**, 26—34 (1953).

BURTON, M.: Development of current concepts of elementary processes in radiation chemistry. J. chem. Educ. **36**, 273—278 (1959).

CALF, G.E., GARNETT, J.L., SOLLICH, W.A.: Recent developments in labeling by catalytic exchange — the application of π-complex theory to the prediction of isotopic hydrogen orientation in molecules labeled by heterogeneous techniques. In: Advances in Tracer Methodology, Vol. 4, pp. 11—27. Ed. by S. ROTHCHILD. New York: Plenum Press 1968.

CATCH, J.R.: Carbon-14 compounds. London: Butterworth 1961.

CHARALAMPOUS, K.D., TANSEY, L.W.: Metabolic fate of β-(3,4,dimethoxyphenyl)-ethylamine in man. J. Pharmacol. exp. Ther. **155**, 318—329 (1967).

CONDON, F.E.: Synthesis and mass spectra of some hexa-, hepta- and octadeuterated derivatives of propane. J. Amer. chem. Soc. **73**, 4675—4678 (1951).

CRESSERI, A., GIRALDI, P.N., LOGEMANN, W., TOSOLINI, G., VALZELLI, G.: Some aspects of the metabolism of triazine derivatives active in experimentally induced virus infections. Brit. J. Pharmacol. **27**, 486—490 (1966).

DACRE, J.C., SCHELINE, R.R., WILLIAMS, R.T.: The role of the tissues and gut flora in the metabolism of [^{14}C] homoprotocatechuic acid in the rat and rabbit. J. Pharm. Pharmacol. **20**, 619—625 (1968).

— WILLIAMS, R.T.: The role of the tissues and gut micro-organisms in the metabolism of [^{14}C] protocatechuic acid in the rat. Aromatic dehydroxylation. J. Pharm. Pharmacol. **20**, 610—618 (1968).

DAVISON, C., WILLIAMS, R.T.: The metabolism of 5,5-methylene-disalicylic acid in various species. J. Pharm. Pharmacol. **20**, 12—18 (1968).

DICARLO, F.J., CREW, M.C., MELGAR, M.D., HAYNES, L.J.: Prazepam metabolism by dogs. J. pharm. Sci. **58**, 960—962 (1969).

— HARTIGAN, J.M., COUTINHO, C.B., PHILLIPS, G.E.: Absorption, distribution and excretion of pentaerythritol and pentaerythritol tetranitrate by mice. Proc. Soc. exp. Biol. (N.Y.) **118**, 311—315 (1965).

DREYFUSS, J., COHEN, A.I., HESS, S.M.: Metabolism of thiazesim, 5-(2-dimethylaminoethyl)-2,3-dihydro-2-phenyl-1,5-benzothiazepin-4-(5H)-one, in the rat *in vivo* and *in vitro*. J. pharm. Sci. **57**, 1505—1511 (1968b).

— SWOAP, J.R., CHINN, C., HESS, S.M.: Excretion and distribution of thiazesim-^{14}C with its biotransformation *in vivo* and *in vitro*. J. pharm. Sci. **57**, 1497—1505 (1968a).

DU VIGNEAUD, V., VERLY, W.G.L., WILSON, J.E., RACHELE, J.R., RESSLER, C., KINNEY, J.M.: One-carbon compounds in the biosynthesis of the "biologically labile" methyl group. J. Amer. chem. Soc. **73**, 2782—2785 (1951).

EBERT, A.G., SCHLEIFER, C.R., HESS, S.M.: Absorption, disposition and excretion of ^{3}H-mineral oil in rats. J. pharm. Sci. **55**, 923—929 (1966).

EIDINOFF, M.L., KNOLL, J.E.: The introduction of isotopic hydrogen into purine ring systems by catalytic exchange. J. Amer. chem. Soc. **75**, 1992—1993 (1953).

— PERRI, G.C., KNOLL, J.E., MARANO, B.J., ARNHEIM, J.: The fractionation of hydrogen isotopes in biological systems. J. Amer. chem. Soc. **75**, 248—249 (1953).

ELLIOTT, T.H., HANAM, J., PARKE, D.V., WILLIAMS, R.T.: The metabolism of [^{14}C]tetralin. Biochem. J. **92**, 52P—53P (1964).

— PARKE, D.V., WILLIAMS, R.T.: The metabolism of cyclo [^{14}C]hexane and its derivatives. Biochem. J. **72**, 193—200 (1959).

ELLISON, T., GUTZAIT, L., VAN LOON, E.J.: The comparative metabolism of d-amphetamine-^{14}C in the rat, dog and monkey. J. Pharmacol. exp. Ther. **152**, 383—387 (1966).
EMMERSON, J.L., WELLES, J.S., ANDERSON, R.C.: Studies on the tissue distribution of d-propoxyphene. Toxicol. appl. Pharmacol. **11**, 482—488 (1967).
EVANS, E.A., SLOTIN, L.: The utilization of carbon dioxide in the synthesis of α-ketoglutaric acid. J. biol. Chem. **136**, 301—302 (1940).
— — Carbon dioxide utilization by pigeon liver. J. biol. Chem. **141**, 439—450 (1941).
FITZGERALD, P.J., EIDINOFF, M.L., KNOLL, J.E., SIMMEL, E.B.: Tritium in radioautography. Science **114**, 494—498 (1951).
FUKUSHIMA, D.K., LIEBERMAN, S., PRAETZ, B.: Preparation of deuterated steroids. J. Amer. chem. Soc. **72**, 5205—5211 (1950).
FURST, C.J.: Studies on the distribution and excretion of a metabolite of guanethidine in the rat. Brit. J. Pharmacol. **32**, 57—64 (1968).
GARNETT, J.L.: Catalytic tritium labeling attractive for organics. Nucleonics **20**, 86—91 (1962).
— SOLLICH, W.A.: Catalytic deuterium exchange reactions with organics. XII. Characteristic reactions of the Group VIII transition metals. Aust. J. Chem. **18**, 1003—1008 (1965).
GEILING, E.M.K., KELSEY, F.E., MCINTOSH, B.J., GANZ, A.: Biosynthesis of radioactive drugs using carbon 14. Science **108**, 558—559 (1948).
GESSNER, P.K., PARKE, D.V., WILLIAMS, R.T.: The metabolism of ^{14}C-labeled ethylene glycol. Biochem. J. **79**, 482—489 (1961).
GETTLER, A.O., NORRIS, C.: Poisoning from drinking radium water. J. Amer. med. Ass. **100**, 400—402 (1933).
GLASCOCK, R.F., DUNCOMBE, W.G.: Biological fractionation of hydrogen isotopes in mammary gland and other tissues. Biochem. J. **51**, xl (1952).
GUT, M., HAYANO, M.: Some aspects of stereoselectivity in the introduction of tritium into steroids. In: Advances in Tracer Methodology, Vol. 1, pp. 60—63. Ed. by S. ROTHCHILD. New York: Plenum Press 1962.
HAGUE, D.E., FABRO, S., SMITH, R.L.: The fate of [^{14}C]thalidomide in the pregnant hamster. J. Pharm. Pharmacol. **19**, 603—607 (1967).
VAN HEYNINGEN, W.E., RITTENBERG, D. SCHOENHEIMER, R.: The preparation of fatty acids containing deuterium. J. biol. Chem. **125**, 495—500 (1938).
HEVESY, G.: The absorption and translocation of lead by plants. A contribution to the application of the method of radioactive indicators in the investigation of the change of substance in plants. Biochem. J. **17**, 439—445 (1923).
HUCKER, H.B., AHMAD, P.M., MILLER, E.A.: Absorption, distribution and metabolism of dimethylsulfoxide in the rat, rabbit and guinea pig. J. Pharmacol. exp. Ther. **154**, 176—184 (1966a).
— ZACCHEI, A.G., COX, S.V., BRODIE, D.A., CANTWELL, N.H.R.: Studies on the absorption, distribution and excretion of indomethacin in various species. J. Pharmacol. exp. Ther. **153**, 237—249 (1966b).
HUG, C.C., JR., MELLETT, L.B.: Tritium-labeled dihydromorphine: Its metabolic fate and excretion in the rat. J. Pharmacol. exp. Ther. **149**, 446—453 (1965).
HUNTER, C.G., ROSEN, A., WILLIAMS, R.T., REYNOLDS, J.G., WORDEN, A.N.: Proc. 12th Int. Conf. World Crop Protection, pp. 1296 —1303 (1960).
HUSAIN, M.A., ROBERTS, J.B., THOMAS, B.H., WILSON, A.: Metabolism and excretion of 3-hydroxyphenyltrimethylammonium and neostigmine. Brit. J. Pharmacol. **35**, 344—350 (1969).
HUTCHISON, C.A., STEWART, D.W., UREY, H.C.: The concentration of ^{13}C. J. chem. Phys. **8**, 532—537 (1940).
JONDORF, W.R., PARKE, D.V., WILLIAMS, R.T.: The metabolism of [^{14}C]hexachloroethane. Biochem. J. **65**, 14P—15P (1957).
KAIGHEN, M., WILLIAMS, R.T.: The metabolism of [3-^{14}C]coumarin. J. med. pharm. Chem. **3**, 25—43 (1961).
KAMM, J.J., TADDEO, A.B., VAN LOON, E.J.: Metabolism and excretion of tritiated dextromethorphan by the rat. J. Pharmacol. exp. Ther. **158**, 437—444 (1967).
KING, L.J., PARKE, D.V., WILLIAMS, R.T.: The metabolism of [2-^{14}C] indole. Biochem. J. **88**, 66P (1963).
KOECHLIN, B.A., SCHWARTZ, M.A., KROL, G., OBERHANSLI, W.: The metabolic fate of ^{14}C-labeled chlordiazepoxide in man, in the dog, and in the rat. J. Pharmacol. exp. Ther. **148**, 399—411 (1965).
KUNTZMAN, R.: Application of tracer techniques in drug metabolism. In: Fundamentals of Drug Metabolism and Disposition. Ed. by B. LA DU. Baltimore: Williams and Wilkins 1969 [in press].

KURIE, F.N.D.: A new mode of disintegration induced by neutrons. Phys. Rev. **45**, 904—905 (1934a).
— Disintegration with the emission of protons induced by neutrons. Phys. Rev. **45**, 330 (1934b).
LARSON, P.S., HARLOW, E.S.: Some current applications of carbon-^{14} to animal and human physiological research. Studies with tobacco and its constituents. In: Radioisotopes in Scientific Research, vol. III, pp. 62—78. Ed. by R.C. EXTERMANN. London: Pergamon Press 1958.
MAICKEL, R.P., COX, R.H., MILLER, F.P., SEGAL, D.S., RUSSELL, R.W.: Correlation of brain levels of drugs with behavioral effects. J. Pharmacol. exp. Ther. **165**, 216—224 (1969).
— WEISSBACH, H.: Recent developments in chemical and biochemical assay techniques applicable in pharmacology. Ann. Rev. Pharmacol. **2**, 399—414 (1962).
McISAAC, W.M., PARKE, D.V., WILLIAMS, R.T.: The metabolism of phenylhydrazine and some phenylhydrazones. Biochem. J. **70**, 688—697 (1958).
McMAHON, R.E., CULP, H.W., MARSHALL, F.J.: The metabolism of α-dl-acetylmethadol in the rat. The identification of the probable active metabolite. J. Pharmacol. exp. Ther. **149**, 436—445 (1965a).
— MARSHALL, F.J.: The preparation of N-methyl ^{14}C-labeled drugs. In: Advances in Tracer Methodology (S. ROTHCHILD, ed.). Vol. 4, pp. 29—39. New York: Plenum Press 1968.
— — CULP, H.W.: The nature of the metabolites of acetohexamide in the rat and in the human. J. Pharmacol. exp. Ther. **149**, 272—279 (1965b).
MISRA, A.L., JACOBY, H.I., WOODS, L.A.: The preparation of tritium-labeled normorphine and its physiological disposition in dog and monkey. J. Pharmacol. exp. Ther. **132**, 311—316 (1961a).
— MULÉ, S.J., WOODS, L.A.: The preparation of tritium nuclear-labeled morphine and evidence for its *in vivo* biotransformation to normorphine in the rat. J. Pharmacol. exp. Ther. **132**, 317—322 (1961b).
MULÉ, S.J., CLEMENTS, T.H., GORODETZKY, C.W.: The metabolic fate of ^{3}H-cyclazocine in dogs. J. Pharmacol. exp. Ther. **160**, 387—396 (1968).
— GORODETZKY, C.W.: Physiologic disposition of ^{3}H-cyclazocine in nontolerant, tolerant and abstinent dogs. J. Pharmacol. exp. Ther. **154**, 632—645 (1966).
MURPHY, P.J., WICK, A.N.: Metabolism of β-phenethylbiguanide. J. pharm. Sci. **57**, 1125—1127 (1968).
MURRAY, A., FOREMAN, W.W., LANGHAM, W.: The halogen-metal interconversion reaction and its application to the synthesis of nicotinic acid labeled with isotopic carbon. Science **106**, 277 (1947).
— WILLIAMS, D.L.: Organic synthesis with isotopes. New York: Interscience 1958.
NICHOLLS, P.J.: A note on the absorption and excretion of ^{14}C-labelled thalidomide in pregnant mice. J. Pharm. Pharmacol. **18**, 46—48 (1966).
OBER, R.E., FUSARI, S.A., COFFEY, G.L., GWYNN, G.W., GLAZKO, A.J.: Preparation of tritium-labelled paromomycin ("Humatin") by fermentation in a medium containing tritiated water. Nature (Lond.) **193**, 1289—1290 (1962).
OBIANWU, H.O.: Disposition of epsilon-amino caproic-^{3}H acid and its investigation with adrenergic neurones. Brit. J. Pharmacol. **31**, 244—252 (1967).
OKITA, G.T., KELSEY, F.E., WALASZEK, E.J., GEILING, E.M.K.: Biosynthesis and isolation of carbon-14 labelled digitoxin. J. Pharmacol. exp. Ther. **110**, 244—250 (1954).
OLIPHANT, M.L.E., HARTECK, P., RUTHERFORD, L.: Transmutation effects observed with heavy hydrogen. Proc. roy. Soc. B **144**A, 692—703 (1934).
PARKE, D.V.: The metabolism of [^{14}C] nitrobenzene in the rabbit and guinea pig. Biochem. J. **62**, 339—346 (1956).
— The metabolism of [^{14}C]aniline in the rabbit and other animals. Biochem. J. **77**, 493—503 (1960).
— The metabolism of m-dinitro[^{14}C]benzene in the rabbit. Biochem. J. **78**, 262—271 (1961).
— Radioisotopes in the study of the metabolism of foreign compounds. In: Isotopes in Experimental Pharmacology (L.J. ROTH, ed.), pp. 315—342. Chicago: University of Chicago Press 1965.
— WILLIAMS, R.T.: The metabolism of benzene. (a) The determination of benzene. (b) The elimination of unchanged benzene by rabbits. Biochem. J. **46**, 236—243 (1950).
— — The metabolism of benzene. (a) The determination of phenylmercapturic acid in urine. (b) Mercapturic acid excretion by rabbits receiving benzene. Biochem. J. **48**, 624—629 (1951).
— — The metabolism of benzene. The muconic acid excreted by rabbits receiving benzene. Determination of the isomeric muconic acids. Biochem. J. **51**, 339—348 (1952).
— — The metabolism of benzene containing [^{14}C]benzene. Biochem. J. **54**, 231—238 (1953a).
— — The metabolism of benzene. (a) The formation of phenylglucuronide and phenylsulphuric acid from [^{14}C]benzene. (b) The metabolism of [^{14}C]phenol. Biochem. J. **55**, 337—340 (1953b).

PORTEOUS J.W., WILLIAMS, R.T.: The metabolism of benzene. I (a) The determination of phenol in urine with 2:6-dichloroquinonechloroimide. (b) The excretion of phenol, glucuronic acid and ethereal sulphate by rabbits receiving benzene and phenol. (c) Observations on the determination of catechol, quinol, and muconic acid in urine. Biochem. J. **44**, 46—55 (1949).
RITTENBERG, D., BLOCH, K.: The utilization of acetic acid for fatty acid synthesis. J. biol. Chem. **154**, 311—312 (1944).
ROBERTS, J.B., THOMAS, B.H., WILSON, A.: Metabolism of neostigmine-^{14}C in the rat. Brit. J. Pharmacol. **25**, 763—770 (1965a).
— — — Distribution and excretion of neostigmine-^{14}C in the rat and hen. Brit. J. Pharmacol. **25**, 234—242 (1965b).
ROGNSTAD, R., KEMP, R.G., KATZ, J.: Enzymatic synthesis of glucose-4-tritium and glucose-3-tritium. Arch. Biochem. **109**, 372—375 (1965).
ROSENBLUM, C.: The chemistry and application of tritium labelling. Nucleonics **17**, 80—83 (1959).
— MERIWETHER, H.T.: Experiences with tritiated compounds produced by exposure to tritium gas. In: Advances in Tracer Methodology (S. ROTHCHILD, ed.). Vol. 1, pp. 12—17. New York: Plenum Press 1963.
ROTH, L.J., WILZBACH, K.E., HELLER, A., KAPLAN, L.: Tritium-labelled meprobamate. J. Amer. pharm. Ass. **48**, 415—416 (1959).
ROTHCHILD, S.: Chemical synthesis of isotopically labelled drugs. In: Isotopes in Experimental Pharmacology (L.J. ROTH, ed.), pp. 12—22. Chicago: University of Chicago Press 1965.
RUBEN, S., HASSID, W.Z., KAMEN, M.D.: Radioactive carbon in the study of photosynthesis. J. Amer. chem. Soc. **61**, 661—663 (1939).
— KAMEN, M.D.: Radioactive carbon of long half-life. Phys. Rev. **57**, 549 (1940).
SANNER, J.H., WOODS, L.A.: Comparative distribution of tritium-labeled dihydromorphine between maternal and fetal rats. J. Pharmacol. exp. Ther. **148**, 176—184 (1965).
SCHELINE, R.R., WILLIAMS, R.T., WIT, J.G.: Biological dehydroxylation. Nature (Lond.) **188**, 849—850 (1960).
SCHOENHEIMER, R., RITTENBERG, D.: Deuterium as an indicator in the study of intermediary metabolism. Science **82**, 156—517 (1935).
SCHREIBER, E.C., MIN, B.H., ZEIGER, A.V., LANG, J.F.: Metabolism of diethylpropion-1-^{14}C hydrochloride by the human. J. Pharmacol. exp. Ther. **159**, 372—378 (1968).
SCHWARTZ, M.A., KOECHLIN, B.A., POSTMA, E., PALMER, S., KROL, G.: Metabolism of diazepam in rat, dog, and man. J. Pharmacol. exp. Ther. **149**, 423—435 (1965).
SMITH, D.L., FORIST, A.A., GERRITSEN, G.C.: Metabolism of 3,5-dimethylpyrazole-^{14}C in the rat. J. Pharmacol. exp. Ther. **150**, 316—321 (1965).
— WAGNER, J.G., GERRITSEN, G.C.: Absorption, metabolism, and excretion of 5-methylpyrazole-3-carboxylic acid in the rat, dog, and human. J. pharm. Sci. **56**, 1150—1157 (1967).
SMITH, J.N., WILLIAMS, R.T.: The fate of aniline in the rabbit. Biochem. J. **44**, 242—250 (1949).
SMITH, N.H., WILZBACH, K.E., BROWN, W.G.: The synthesis of tritium-labelled methyl iodide and acriflavine. J. Amer. chem. Soc. **77**, 1033—1035 (1955).
SMITH, R.L., WILLIAMS, R.T.: The metabolism of arylthioureas. V. The metabolism of 1-(p-butoxyphenyl)-3-(p-dimethylaminophenyl)-2-thiourea (Ciba-1906, thiambutosine). J. med. pharm. Chem. **4**, 163—176 (1961).
SPRATT, J.L., OKITA, G.T., GEILING, E.M.: In vivo radiotracer stability of a tritium "self-radiation"-labelled compound. Int. J. appl. Radiat. **2**, 167—168 (1957).
STEPKA, W., LARSON, P.S.: Biosynthesis of ^{14}C-labelled compounds with higher plants. In: Isotopes in Experimental Pharmacology (L.J. ROTH, ed.), pp. 7—13. Chicago: University of Chicago Press 1965.
STUMPF, W.E., ROTH, L.J.: Dry-mounting high-resolution autoradiography. In: Isotopes in Experimental Pharmacology (L.J. ROTH, ed.), pp. 133—143. Chicago: University of Chicago Press 1965.
STURMAN, J.A., DAWKINS, P.D., MCARTHUR, N., SMITH, M.J.H.: The distribution of salicylate in mouse tissues after intraperitoneal injection. J. Pharm. Pharmacol. **20**, 58—63 (1968).
TITUS, E., WEISS, H.: The use of biologically prepared radioactive indicators in metabolic studies: metabolism of pentobarbital. J. biol. Chem. **214**, 807—820 (1955).
TOCCO, D.J., EGERTON, J.R., BOWERS, W., CHRISTENSEN, V.W., ROSENBLUM, C.: Absorption, metabolism and elimination of thiabendazole in farm animals and a method for its estimation in biological materials. J. Pharmacol. exp. Ther. **149**, 263—271 (1965).
— ROSENBLUM, C., MARTIN, C.M., ROBINSON, H.J.: Absorption, metabolism and excretion, of thiabendazole in man and laboratory animals. Toxicol. appl. Pharmacol. **9**, 31—39 (1966).

TOLBERT, B. M.: Radiation self-decomposition of labelled compounds. In: Advances in Tracer Methodology (S. ROTHCHILD, ed.). Vol. 1, pp. 64—68. New York: Plenum Press 1963.
ULLBERG, S.: Studies on distribution and fate of ^{35}S-labelled benzylpenicillin in body. Acta radiol. (Stockh.), Suppl. **118**, 1—110 (1954).
— Autoradiographic localization in the tissues of drugs and metabolites. Biochem. Pharmacol. **9**, 29—36 (1962).
UREY, H. C., BRICKWEDDE, F. G., MURPHY, G. M.: A hydrogen isotope of mass 2. Phys. Rev. **39**, 164—165 (1932).
VERLY, W. G., RACHELE, J. R., DU VIGNEAUD, V., EIDINOFF, M. L., KNOLL, J. E.: A test of tritium as a labelling device in a biological study. J. Amer. chem. Soc. **74**, 5941—5943 (1952).
WAGNER, C. D., STEVENSON, D. P.: The preparation and purification of methane-d, ethane-d, propane-1-d, propane-2-d, n-butane-1-d, n-butane-2-d, isobutane-1-d′ and isobutane-2-d′. J. Amer. chem. Soc. **72**, 5785 (1950).
WILLIAMS, R. T.: Detoxication mechanisms. The mechanism and detoxication of drugs, toxic substances and other organic compounds. 2nd edition. New York: John Wiley and Sons, Inc., 1959.
— The metabolism and toxicity of arylthioureas. Biochem. J. **80**, 1P—2P (1961).
— Teratogenic effects of thalidomide and related substances. Lancet **1963 1**, 723—724.
WILZBACH, K. E.: Tritium-labelling by exposure of organic compounds to tritium gas. J. Amer. chem. Soc. **79**, 1013 (1957).
YAVORSKY, P. M., GORIN, E.: New reagent for labelling organic compounds with tritium. J. Amer. chem. Soc. **84**, 1071—1072 (1962).

Chapter 26

Radioactive Techniques: Radioactive Isotope Derivatives of Nonlabeled Drugs[1]

R. Kuntzman, R.H. Cox, Jr., and R.P. Maickel

A required course for most graduate students in chemistry is one which explores the facets of semi-micro qualitative organic analysis. This is not a new area of study; the first book on the subject was published some 48 years ago (Kamm, 1922). The basic principles are simple. After using appropriate physical methods to separate components of a mixture, each compound is treated with a suitable reagent to yield a specific derivative, preferably a crystalline material, which can then be purified and characterized by a specific physical property such as its melting point. With the advent of radioisotopes, these principles become the basis for an entirely new approach to analytical chemistry. If one uses a derivatizing agent labeled with a radioactive atom, the derivative can be used to quantitatively estimate the original substance, often with extremely high sensitivity. The use of appropriate physical and/or chemical separations, before or after the derivatizing reaction, can easily confer the desired degree of specificity upon the overall analytical procedure.

Although this approach seems extremely reasonable, only a relatively few examples are seen to date. The first reported applications of labeled derivatizing agents was that of Keston and coworkers (1949, 1950) who used this technique to measure amino acids. More recently, Kliman and Peterson (1960) described the use of acetic anhydride labeled with ^{3}H or ^{14}C to determine submicrogram amounts of steroids such as aldosterone in biological materials. The use of ^{3}H-acetic anhydride, ^{14}C-methyliodide and ^{63}Ni as radioactive reagents has recently been applied to the quantitation of drugs in biological materials.

I. Estimation of Primary or Secondary Amines

Hammer and Brodie (1967) first applied ^{3}H-acetic anhydride to determine drug amines. Basically, such procedures may be described by a schematic flow sheet, as follows:

a) biological sample containing amine

↓ 1. adjust to alkaline pH
2. extract amine into organic solvent (e.g., hexane)
3. wash organic phase to remove interfering metabolites of the drug

b) organic phase containing amine

↓ add ^{3}H-acetic anhydride + catalyst (pyridine)

c) organic phase containing ^{3}H-acetylated amine + unreacted ^{3}H-acetic anhydride

↓ remove unreacted ^{3}H-acetic anhydride

1 Supported in part by USPHS grants MH-14658 and HD-03037 and by Research Development Award KO2-MH-41083 (to R.P. Maickel).

d) organic phase containing ^{3}H-acetylated amine
↓ further purification (see references below for specific details for each drug)

e) measure radioactivity.

Since the specific activity of the ^{3}H-labeled reagent is known, use of suitable standards permits accurate estimation of the quantity of unlabeled drug present in the original sample. Applications of this technique may be seen in methods reported for desmethylimipramine (HAMMER and BRODIE, 1967), norchlorcyclizine (KUNTZMAN et al., 1967), phenmetrazine (QUINN et al., 1967), and pseudoephedrine (KUNTZMAN et al., 1969). The sensitivity obtained permits accurate measurement of as little 10^{-8} g of drug per ml plasma.

II. Estimation of Tertiary Amines

Tertiary amines cannot be determined by the procedures described in the previous section, as the lack of replaceable hydrogen prevents reaction with ^{3}H-acetic anhydride. KUNTZMAN and TSAI (1967) suggested a two-step procedure in which the tertiary amine is first demethylated *in vitro* by incubation with lyophilized liver microsomes in the presence of a TPNH generating system. Then, the secondary amine formed by this process may be extracted, reacted with ^{3}H-acetic anhydride, and determined as previously described (KUNTZMAN et al., 1967). This two-step procedure has a serious limitation as it can be used only when the conversion of tertiary amine to secondary amine by the liver microsomes is considerably faster than any further metabolism of the secondary amine (KUNTZMAN et al., 1969).

More recently, HARRIS et al. (1968) have reported a method for the determination of tertiary amines by quaternization with ^{14}C-methyl iodide. The quaternary amine derivative, labeled with a ^{14}C-methyl group, can be easily and accurately measured after removal of excess ^{14}C-methyl iodide. By using this technique to measure imipramine, in combination with the ^{3}H-acetic anhydride procedure of HAMMER and BRODIE (1967) for desmethylimipramine, HARRIS et al. (1968) have been able to accurately follow the conversion of imipramine to desmethylimipramine *in vivo* in the dog.

III. Estimation of Drugs by Chelation

A recently reported technique (KUNTZMAN, 1969) may be useful in the development of another area of derivative technology. For many years, it has been known that chelates of Co^{+3}, Al^{+3}, Cr^{+3} or Mn^{+3} form readily with organic compounds such as acetylacetone (URBAIN and DEBIERNE, 1899; ASTBURY, 1926). Such metal-organic chelates are usually soluble in organic solvents, permitting the extraction of the metal from an aqueous solution into an immiscible organic solvent. The complexes of Cu^{+2} and straight chain fatty acids are extremely soluble in organic solvents (PICKERING, 1912); this phenomenon has been utilized by DUNCOMBE (1963) to determine long chain fatty acids in blood plasma by a colorimetric procedure.

Compounds such as B.W. 356C61 (3-ethoxy-2-keto-butyraldehydedithiosemicarbazone) form chelates with Cu^{+2} that are extractable from aqueous solutions into diethyl ether. However, attempts to measure colorimetrically the amount of Cu^{+2} extracting in complex with B.W. 356C61 were unsuccessful as the sensitivity of the colorimetric procedure was insufficient. Further study indicated that B.W. 356C61 formed a chelate with Ni^{+3} that was also ether extractable. A method was thus developed in which $^{63}Ni^{+3}$ was added to plasma containing B,W, 356C61: the ether extractable radioactivity (^{63}Ni, $\beta^{-} = 0.067$ MEV) was directly proportional to the plasma content of B.W. 356C61. Less than 2×10^{-8} g of B.W. 356C61 could be accurately determined in 1.0 ml of plasma by this procedure (KUNTZMAN, 1969).

IV. Estimation of Steroids as Radioactive Derivatives

Many naturally-occurring steroids are also used as therapeutic agents. Since the first description of the use of ^{3}H-acetic anhydride for the double-isotope derivative analysis of aldosterone and other steroids (KLIMAN and PETERSON, 1960) many variations utilizing this principle have been developed. Recently KARMEN et al. (1963) reported a determination of testosterone as the ^{14}C-acetate derivative. A list

Table 1. *Radiolabeled derivative techniques for steroids*

Reference	Derivatizing Agent	Steroids
KLIMAN et al. (1960)	H^3-acetic anhydride	Aldosterone
FISHMAN et al. (1967)	H^3-acetic anhydride	Estrogen metabolites
WIEST (1967)	H^3-acetic anhydride	Progesterone 20-α-Hydroxypregn-4-en-3-one
NOWACZYNSKI et al. (1967)	H^3-acetic anhydride	Aldosterone
STACHENKO et al. (1964)	H^3-acetic anhydride	Aldosterone, corticosterone, cortisol
PETERSON (1962)	H^3-acetic anhydride	Cortisol, 11-desoxycortisol corticosterone, 11-desoxy-corticosterone, aldosterone
BOJESEN et al. (1967)	S^{35}-sulfonylating reagents	Estrone, estradiol, cortisol, cortisone, 11-desoxycortisol, corticosterone, aldosterone

of radiolabeled derivative techniques is given in Table 1; although the original methods were designed for naturally-occurring compounds such as aldosterone or hydrocortisone, the procedures should be easily adaptable for use in determining synthetic steroids.

V. Enzymatic Production of Labeled Derivatives

Recently, the potential of using the isotope derivative technique for the enzymatic production of labeled products has been explored. With this process, one simply measures the appearance of a labeled product following incubation of an unlabeled substrate with a labeled cofactor and the appropriate enzyme.

Using this technique, SAELENS et al. (1967) developed an enzyme assay for norepinephrine in brain tissue. Phenylethanolamine-N-methyltransferase catalyzes the transfer of the methyl-^{14}C group of S-adenosylmethionine-methyl-^{14}C specifically to the primary amine nitrogen of norepinephrine. The rate of formation of epinephrine-N-methyl-^{14}C is linearly related to the concentration of substrate (norepinephrine) over a range of 0.1—5.0 μg norepinephrine/ml. Thus, the specificity of the enzyme and the linearity of the reaction produces a useful assay.

More recently, ENGLEMAN et al. (1968) developed a double-isotope derivative technique making it possible to determine either norepinephrine or epinephrine. In this procedure, the catecholamines are converted to ^{14}C-metanephrines by incubating with S-adenosylmethionine-methyl-^{14}C and catechol-O-methyltransferase in the presence of tracer amounts of 7-^{3}H-norepinephrine. Using this procedure, one can obtain a reading of 6 $\times$ blank with only 1.0 ng of catecholamine.

The current fluorometric procedures for norepinephrine can detect as little as 2—3 ng but the reading is often less than 2 $\times$ blank resulting in poor accuracy.

Thus, applying the isotope derivative technique, one can work with a selective and much more sensitive method.

VI. Potential Applications of Radiolabeled Derivatizing Reagents

The future of the type of methodology described in this chapter appears very bright. One need only leaf through the classical textbooks of semimicro organic analysis (Kamm, 1922; Shriner and Fuson, 1948; McElvain, 1953; Chernois and Entrekin, 1947) to see the myriad of potential reaction procedures available.

Table 2. *Possible applications of radiolabeled derivatizing reagents*

Derivatizing Reagent	Reactive Groups	Products
aniline	—COOH	anilides
p-bromoaniline		p-bromoanilides
p-toluidine		p-toluidides
p-nitrobenzoyl chloride	—OH	p-nitrobenzoates
3,5-dinitrobenzoyl chloride		3,5-dinitrobenzoates
3-nitrophthalic anhydride	—OH	3-nitrophthalates
2,4-dinitrophenyl hydrazine	—CHO, —C=O	2,4-dinitrophenyl hydrazones
p-nitrophenyl hydrazine		p-nitrophenyl hydrazones
acetic anhydride	$—NH_2$, —NHR	amides
methyl iodide	$—NR_2$	quaternary amines
benzenesulfonyl chloride	$—NH_2$	sulfonamides
p-toluenesulfonyl chloride		
fluoro-2,4-dinitrobenzene	$—NH_2$	2,4-dinitrophenylamines
monochloroacetic acid	—OH (phenol)	aryloxyacetates
chloro-2,4-dinitrobenzene	—SH	2,4-dinitrophenylthioethers

A collection of some of the more promising reactions is given in Table 2 — while far from complete, it is evident that numerous functional groups on organic compounds should be amenable to this approach.

Basically, the procedures are extremely simple. The compound or compounds of choice may either be separated from possible interfering substances prior to reaction with the radiolabeled derivatizing agent, or the derivatization step may be carried out first on a crude tissue preparation, followed by suitable extraction procedures. The derivatizing reaction, when carried out under suitable conditions, gives stoichiometric reaction so that the specific activity of the derivative is directly proportional to the specific activity of the radiolabeled reagent. Thus, the quantitative measurement of the radioactivity in the derivative will yield a quantitative estimate of the amount of compound present in the sample, with the sensitivity limit dependent on the specific activity of the radiolabeled reagent and the degree of removal of the excess reagent.

References

Astbury, W.T.: The structure and isotrimorphism of the tervalent metallic acetylacetones. Proc. roy. Soc. **112**A, 448—467 (1926).

Bojesen, E., Svendsen, O.B.R., Thurneberg, L.: Isotope derivative methods for the determination of steroid hormones with ^{35}S-sulfonylating reagents. In: Steroid hormone analysis. Vol. 1, pp. 1—53. New York: Marcel Dekker, Inc., 1967.

Chernois, N.D., Entrekin, J.B.: Semi-micro qualitative organic analysis. New York: N.Y. Crowell Co. 1947.

Duncombe, W.G.: The colorimetric micro-determination of long-chain fatty acids. Biochem. J. **88**, 7—10 (1963).

ENGLEMAN, K., PORTNOY, B., LOVENBERG, W.: A sensitive and specific double-isotope derivative method for the determination of catecholamines in biological specimens. Amer. J. med. Sci. **255** (4), 259—268 (1968).

FISHMAN, J., GURNY, O., ROSENFELD, R.S., GALLAGHER, T.T.: Analysis of estrogen metabolites by isotope derivative and by fluorimetry. Steroids **10**, 317—327 (1967).

HAMMER, W., BRODIE, B.B.: Application of isotope derivative technique to assay of secondary amines. Estimation of desipramine by acetylation with H^3-acetic anhydride. J. Pharmacol. exp. Ther. **157**, 503—508 (1967).

HARRIS, S.R., EFRON, D., GAUDETTE, L.: Radioactive derivative formation for the simultaneous estimation of plasma imipramine and desimipramine. Pharmacologist **10**, 166 (1968).

KAMM, O.: Qualitative organic analysis. New York: John Wiley and Sons 1922.

KARMEN, A., MCCAFFREY, I., KLIMAN, B.: Derivative ratio analysis. A new method for measurement of steroids and other compounds with specific functional groups using radioassay by gas-liquid chromatography. Analyt. Biochem. **6**, 31—38 (1963).

KESTON, A.S., UDENFRIEND, S., CANNON, R.K.: A method for the determination of organic compounds in the form of isotopic derivatives. I. Estimation of amino acids by the carrier technique. J. Amer. chem. Soc. **71**, 249—257 (1949).

— — LEVY, M.: Determination of organic compounds as isotope derivatives. II. Amino acids by paper chromatographic and indicator techniques. J. Amer. chem. Soc. **72**, 748—753 (1950).

KLIMAN, B., PETERSON, R.E.: Double isotope derivative assay of aldosterone in biological fluids. J. biol. Chem. **235**, 1639—1648 (1960).

KUNTZMAN, R.: Application of tracer techniques in drug metabolism studies. In: Fundamentals of Drug Metabolism and Disposition. Baltimore/Md.: Williams and Wilkins Co. 1969 [in press].

— SERNATINGER, E., TSAI, I., KLUTCH, A.: New methodology for studies of drug metabolism. In: Importance of fundamental principles in drug evaluation (D.H. TEDESCHI and R.E. TEDESCHI, eds.), pp. 87—103. New York: Raven Press 1969.

— TSAI, I.: A sensitive radiochemical method for the assay of some tertiary amines. Pharmacologist **9**, 240 (1967).

— — BURNS, J.J.: Importance of tissue and plasma binding in determining the retention of norchlorcyclizine and norcyclizine in man, dog and rat. J. Pharmacol. exp. Ther. **158**, 332—339 (1967).

MCELVAIN, S.M.: The characterization of organic compounds. New York: Macmillan 1953.

NOWACZYNSKI, W., SILAH, J., GENEST, J.: Procedure for determination of aldosterone in human peripheral plasma by double-isotope derivative assay, and its application for measurement of secretory rate and urinary excretion. Canad. J. Biochem. **45** (**12**), 1919—1936 (1967).

PETERSON, R.E.: Use of radioisotopes in steroid methodology. Atomlight **24**, 2—8 (1962).

PICKERING, S.U.: Copper salts and their behaviour with alkalis. J. chem. Soc. **101**, 174—192 (1912).

QUINN, G.P., COHN, M.M., REID, M.B., GREENGARD, P., WEINER, M.: The effect of formulation on phenmetrazine plasma levels in man studied by a sensitive analytic method. Clin. Pharmacol. Ther. **8**, 369—373 (1967).

SAELENS, J.K., SCHOEN, M.S., KOVACSICS, G.B.: An enzyme assay for norepinephrine in brain tissue. Biochem. Pharmacol. **16**, 1043—1049 (1967).

SHRINER, R.L., FUSON, R.C.: The systematic identification of organic compounds. 3rd edition. New York: John Wiley and Sons 1948.

STACHENKO, J., LAPLANTE, C., GIROUD, C.J.P.: Double isotope derivative assay of aldosterone, corticosterone, and cortisol. Canad. J. Biochem. **42** (**9**), 1275—1291 (1964).

URBAIN, G., DEBIERNE, A.: Sur quelques acetylacetonates. C.R. Soc. Biol. (Paris) **129**, 302—305 (1899).

WIEST, W.G.: A double isotope derivative assay for progesterone and 20α-hydroxypregn-4-en-3-one. Steroid **10**(**3**), 257—278 (1967).

Chapter 27

Gas Chromatography

M. W. ANDERS

With 18 Figures

I. Introduction

Gas chromatography is one of the most powerful analytical tools currently available to the biochemical pharmacologist. By this technique it is possible to quantitatively and qualitatively analyze drugs in biological samples at the microgram and submicrogram level. It is of interest to note that the first reports describing gas chromatography dealt with applications to biological problems, specifically the analysis of fatty acids (JAMES and MARTIN, 1952) and amines (JAMES et al., 1952). Indeed, to look for a moment into the earlier history of chromatography we find that the feasibility of gas chromatography was suggested by MARTIN and SYNGE (1941) in their classical description of paper chromatography. Again the application was biologically oriented, specifically to the analysis of amino acids. During the years between about 1952 and 1960 many advances were made in gas chromatography. Instruments were improved to include sensitive detectors and associated electronics, improved techniques for column preparation were described and thermostable liquid phases permitting chromatography of high molecular weight compounds were made available.

The potential applicability of gas chromatography to pharmacological investigations was shown by several publications reporting the chromatography of morphine alkaloids (LLOYD et al., 1960), barbiturates (PARKER and KIRK, 1961) and phenothiazine tranquilizers (ANDERS and MANNERING, 1962b). These reports were followed by others in which gas chromatography was applied to the analysis of drugs in biological tissues. Since that time gas chromatography has been successfully employed in many pharmacological investigations. It has proved to be particularly useful in the study of drug metabolism.

The purpose of this chapter is to acquaint the biochemical pharmacologist with the theory of gas chromatography and its applications to problems in his field. Particular emphasis will be placed on applications involving biological systems since it is here that gas chromatography is often of greatest use. A number of detailed discussions of the theory and applications of gas chromatography are available (ANDERS and MANNERING, 1967; BURCHFIELD and STORRS, 1962; DAL NOGARE and JUVET, 1962; ETTRE and ZLATKIS, 1967; GUDZINOWICZ, 1967a; KEULEMANS, 1959; PECSOK, 1959; PURNELL, 1962).

One final point to be noted is that the following discussion will treat only packed gas chromatographic columns. Capillary columns, which have been widely employed in the analysis of hydrocarbons, have found minimal application to pharmacological problems; the properties of these columns are described in the sources cited above.

II. Theory of Gas Chromatography

Chromatography is a separating technique in which the components of the sample (solutes) are distributed between two phases, one mobile and the other stationary. Gas chromatography, or more specifically gas-liquid chromatography, is a form of chromatography in which the mobile phase is a gas and the stationary phase a liquid. Movement of the mobile phase along with distribution of the solute molecules between the two phases results in migration of solutes along the chromatographic column. The movement of the solute molecules along the column is termed *elution* and involves the continuous passage of the mobile phase through the gas chromatograph. A sample introduced into the chromatographic column will be distributed between the gas and liquid phases according to its *partition coefficient*. Only those solute molecules present in the gas phase will migrate along the column. In many cases, sample components are separated (depending on partition coefficients) and eluted from the column at different times as symmetrical peaks. In some cases, peaks will be distorted due to non-linear absorption isotherms or instrumental or operational reasons.

It is important in a discussion of the theory of gas chromatography to distinguish between efficiency or peak sharpness and the ability of the column to separate two solutes. These considerations are illustrated in Fig. 1. In both chromato-

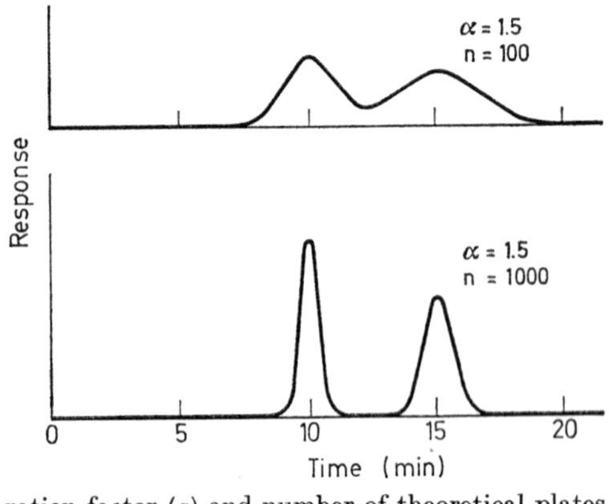

Fig. 1. Effect of separation factor (a) and number of theoretical plates (n) on the separation of two compounds

grams, the separation factor (a) is the same. However, the lower chromatogram is clearly more desirable due to increased peak sharpness or, in other words, to increased efficiency.

Two general theories have evolved which describe the efficiency of the gas chromatographic process. These are the *plate theory* and the *rate theory*.

The *plate theory* describes the chromatographic column as operating in a fashion similar to a distillation column. It assumes that the column is made up of many theoretical plates and that equilibrium occurs on each plate. Thus in passing one theoretical plate, the solute molecules are visualized as having attained equilibrium between the gas and liquid phases on that plate. The sharpness of a chromatographic peak is determined by the number of theoretical plates in a column. The number of theoretical plates, n, present in a column can be computed from the data available on the chromatogram as shown in Fig. 2: $n = 16\,(t_R/\Delta t)^2$. The height equivalent to a theoretical plate, HETP, can be obtained from: HETP = column

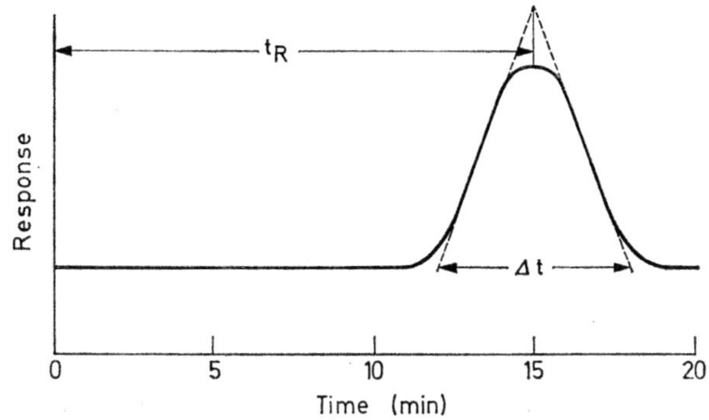

Fig. 2. Parameters required for the computation of theoretical plates. t_R = retention time

length/n. The lower the HETP, the more efficient the column. The plate theory is useful in evaluating column efficiency; unfortunately, it does not detail the factors that constitute efficiency and thus gives no clues as to improvement of efficiency.

The *rate theory*, described by VAN DEEMTER et al. (1956), does consider the many factors that determine column efficiency and, thus, peak sharpness. The complete van Deemter equation is shown in Equation 1.

$$\mathrm{HETP} = 2\lambda dp + \frac{2\gamma D_{gas}}{u} + \frac{8k'}{\pi^2(1+k')^2} \frac{d_f^2}{D_{liq}} u \tag{1}$$

The equation is frequently written in an abbreviated form as shown in Equation 2.

$$\mathrm{HETP} = A + B/u + Cu \tag{2}$$

HETP has previously been defined as the height equivalent to a theoretical plate and u is the carrier gas velocity.

The "A" term ($A = 2\lambda dp$) is called the *eddy diffusion* or *multipath term*. The components of this term include λ, a quantity characteristic of the column packing, and dp, the average particle diameter. The eddy diffusion term is defined by the irregular paths the solute molecules take as they pass through the packed chromatographic column. Because of the non-uniformity of a column packed with small particles, paths of differing lengths and cross sections are present and contribute to peak broadening.

The "B" term ($B = 2\gamma D_{gas}$) is called the *molecular diffusion term* and is inversely related to gas velocity. The contribution of this term is considerable at low gas velocities and is the result of diffusion of solute molecules in the mobile phase. The components of this term include γ, a correction factor for the tortuosity of the interparticle spaces and, D_{gas}, the diffusion coefficient of the solute molecules in the gas phase. In a properly operated gas chromatographic column, the contribution of the "B" term is minimal.

The "C" term ($C = 8k'/\pi^2 [1 + k']^2 \cdot d_f^2/D_{liq}$) is called the *resistance to mass transfer term* and is directly proportional to gas velocity. This term relates to the factors involved in the partitioning of solute molecules between the gas and liquid phases. Its components include k', a value relating to the fraction of the solute in the liquid and gas phases (partition coefficient) and to the relative volumes occupied by gas and liquid in the column, d_f, the thickness of the liquid film and D_{liq}, the diffusion coefficient of solute molecules in the liquid phase.

Both the molecular diffusion and resistance to mass transfer terms are related to gas velocity; the eddy diffusion term is independent of gas velocity. Examination of Eq. 1 and 2 shows that, if other factors are constant, there will be an optimum

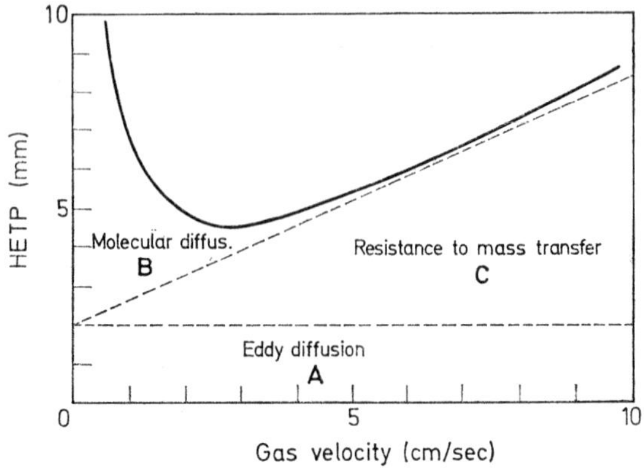

Fig. 3. Relationship between carrier gas velocity and column efficiency (HETP)

gas velocity resulting in a minimal HETP. This is shown graphically in Fig. 3. At low flow rates, molecular diffusion is an important determinant of HETP while at flow rates above the optimum, the resistance to mass transfer term predominates.

The real value of the rate theory of VAN DEEMTER is that it describes the factors contributing to column efficiency and, therefore, permits the chromatographer to operate his instrument most effectively. The predictive value of the van Deemter equation is illustrated in Table 1.

Table 1. *Qualitative predictions from rate theory*[a]

Change	Partial Effects	Effect on HETP
Particle Size		
Increase	Increase dp, decrease λ ?	?
Narrow range	Decrease λ, γ	Decrease
Spherical	Decrease λ, γ	Decrease
Carrier Gas		
Increase density	Decrease D_{gas}	Decrease
Increase pressure	Decrease D_{gas}	Decrease
Increase flow rate		Minimum at optimum flow rate
Temperature		
Increase	Increase D_{gas}, D_{liq}, decrease k'	?
Liquid		
Decrease amount	Decrease k', d_f	Decrease
Decrease viscosity	Increase D_{liq}	Decrease

[a] Reproduced with permission of the publisher from PECSOK (1959).

Finally, it should be noted that the van Deemter equation as presented above has been found to be a somewhat inadequate description of the gas chromatographic process in view of recent studies. These deficiencies are primarily related to non-equilibrium conditions and exert prominent effects on the resistance to mass transfer term; these have been discussed in detail by GUDZINOWICZ (1967a).

While efficiency is an important consideration in the chromatographic process, the separating ability of the column must not be overlooked; clearly, the purpose of employing chromatographic techniques is to separate compounds. The separation of two solutes can be described by their relative retention (a) or relative volatility as shown in Equation 3. By convention, solute 1 has the

$$a = t_{R2}/t_{R1} \tag{3}$$

shorter retention time and a is always greater than unity; t_R is the retention time. It is useful to express, in a quantitative manner, the degree of separation obtained;

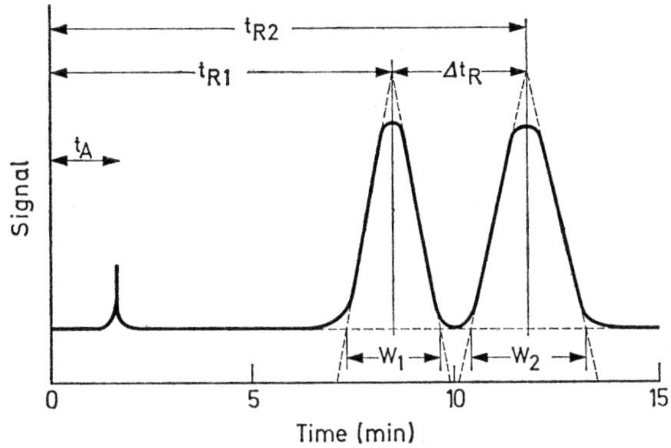

Fig. 4. Parameters required for the computation of resolution (R)

this is *resolution*, R. Resolution is computed by Equation 4 from data obtained from the chromatogram as shown in Fig. 4;

$$R = 2(t_{R2}—t_{R1})/(W_1 + W_2) \tag{4}$$

W is the width at the peak at the base line. Peaks are considered to be completely resolved (99.7% separated) when R = 1.5; for most purposes R = 1 (98% separation) is sufficient. It should be noted that resolution is proportional to the square root of the plate number. Thus, while the space separating two peaks is proportional to column length, the peak width increases in proportion to the square root of the column length. For these reasons, peak separation is greater than peak spreading as the column length is increased.

A number of factors contribute to the relative retention of two solutes. By analogy to distillation, the relative volatility of the two solutes may be a factor. However, solute-liquid phase interactions are often more important and, consequently, the selectivity of the liquid phase is of importance. Therefore, the affinity of the liquid phase for the solutes, which may involve hydrogen bonding, van der Waals forces and so forth, is a major consideration in separations.

III. Columns

The column is the most important component of the gas chromatograph and should receive the most attention. Care in the selection and preparation of the column packing material and column tubing composition is of paramount importance.

The composition of the column tubing material can exert prominent effects on the chromatography of many drugs. Metal columns, in particular, may catalyze the degradation or rearrangement of injected solutes. This may result in the complete loss of the injected solute or in the appearance of degradation peaks on the chromatogram. Studies dealing with the effect of column tubing composition on the chromatography of various compounds have shown that glass or quartz columns give the best results (BECKMAN and BEVENUE, 1963; LEVINS and OTTENSTEIN, 1967). It appears to be particularly important that the sample injector area be constructed of glass. Indeed, a packed glass injector port followed by a stainless steel column has been used successfully in the author's laboratory for the analysis of many compounds.

The column packing material consists of the solid support and the liquid or stationary phase. Ideally, the *solid support* should be completely inert and serve only to retain the liquid phase in the column. This ideal is not realized, however, because of the tendency of support materials to interact with solutes during chromatography. The usual support material for gas-liquid chromatography is a preparation of diatomaceous earth. This siliceous material has a very large specific surface (m^2/g) and good thermal stability; on the other hand, it lacks mechanical strength and is not completely chemically inert. Indeed, it is this lack of inertness that is one of the most troublesome characteristics of solid supports. For this reason, the solid support will tend to adsorb solutes during chromatography producing peak distortions (tailing). Available evidence suggests that the adsorptive properties of solid supports are due to the presence of silanol (Si-OH) groups on the surface. These groups are acidic and polar. Consequently, inactivation of support materials is usually aimed at masking the silanol groups. This is effected by treating the support material with a silanizing agent which serves to convert the silanol groups into inert trimethylsilyl ethers. OTTENSTEIN (1968) studied several methods of support inactivation and concluded that acid-washing followed by treatment with dimethyldichlorosilane produced the most inert support material. The results of this study showed that dimethyldichlorosilane was more effective than hexamethyldisilizane which was more suitable than trimethylchlorosilane.

A number of materials in addition to diatomaceous earths have been employed as support materials. Included are powdered Teflon, glass beads and powdered detergents (Tide) among others. OTTENSTEIN (1963) has discussed in detail the properties of column support materials.

There is a wide variety of *liquid phases* available for use in gas chromatography. Fortunately, the choice of a liquid phase is not as difficult in gas chromatography as in paper or thin-layer chromatography. Indeed, most biochemical pharmacologists employing gas chromatography would probably not require more than six different liquid phases. While the selection of a suitable liquid phase may involve considerable trial and error experimentation, certain predictions can be made. This is possible because of the availability of quantitative estimations of column polarity and interactions. An important contribution was made by ROHRSCHNEIDER (1966) who classified the polarity of liquid phases on the basis of the retention behavior of benzene, ethanol, 2-butanone, nitromethane and pyridine. The magnitude of the Rohrschneider constants is a measure of the interaction of the liquid phase and the solute being chromatographed and, consequently, of the retention time. For example, the Rohrschneider constants of Carbowax 4000 for ethanol and 2-butanone are 5.46 and 3.86, respectively. This indicates that on a Carbowax 4000 column, 2-butanol would have a longer retention time than 2-butanone and this is the result obtained when these compounds are analyzed. On the other hand, the Rohrschneider constants of OV-210 (Table 2) for ethanol and 2-butanone are 2.13 and 3.55, respectively. This column would then be expected to retain the ketone longer than the alcohol. Clearly, this type of information is useful in identifying metabolites since the order of elution can be predicted by selection of appropriate columns.

Table 2. *Liquid phases for gas chromatography*

Liquid Phase	Composition	Polarity	Maximum Temperature °C
SE-30	Methyl silicone	Non-polar	300
DC-200	Methyl silicone	Non-polar	250
OV-1	Methyl silicone	Non-polar	350
OV-7	Methylphenyl silicone (20% phenyl)	Moderately polar	350
OV-17	Methylphenyl silicone (50% phenyl)	Polar	375
OV-210	Trifluoropropyl silicone	Polar	275
OV-225	Cyanopropylphenyl silicone	Polar	275
Carbowax 4000	Polyethylene glycol	Polar	200
Neopentyl glycol succinate	Ester	Polar	225
1,2,3-Tris(2-cyano-ethoxy)propane	Nitrile	Very polar	175

The most widely used liquid phases for biochemical problems are the silicones. Many of these materials are suitable for high-temperature chromatography and are available in differing polarities. Non-polar silicones (SE-30, DC-200, OV-1) provide a separation based primarily on molecular weight and polarity of the solutes. Other polar silicones (OV-17, OV-210, OV-225) interact with functional groups present in the solute and can be very useful in achieving difficult separations. Another useful group of liquid phases are the polyethyleneglycols (Carbowaxes). These are particularly suitable for the chromatography of alcohols, amines and ketones. Some of the commonly employed liquid phases are shown in Table 2.

The preparation of the column packing material is one of the most critical steps in gas chromatographic analysis. There are several techniques employed for coating the solid support with the liquid phase. Included are batch coating, in-place coating and filtration coating. In the *batch technique*, the solid support is suspended in a solution of the liquid phase in a volatile solvent. The solvent is then evaporated in a hood or, alternatively, a rotary evaporator may be employed to hasten solvent removal. This method has the advantages of ease and simplicity and that the liquid/support ratio can be readily and accurately determined. *In-place coating* of the support is accomplished by passing a solution of the liquid phase through the column already packed with uncoated solid support. Purging the column with an inert gas removes the excess solvent. This technique is somewhat laborious and does not permit ready determination of the liquid/support ratio. On the other hand, in-place coating should result in a uniform coating of the solid support and, consequently, a column that would perform well. At any rate, the method appears to be only infrequently employed. The most widely used procedure for biochemical problems is the *filtration technique* (Horning et al., 1959). In this technique, the solid support is suspended in a solution of the liquid phase in a volatile solvent. The suspension is then degassed to insure uniform coating and the solvent filtered off with the aid of vacuum. The coated material is then dried and packed into the column. The liquid/support ratio can be determined by evaporating the excess solvent and weighing the residue or by exhaustively extracting a sample of the coated support material.

In some cases it is desirable to *subcoat* the solid support before applying the liquid phase. This is usually done to enhance the chromatographic properties of highly polar solutes. For example, application of a coating of a non-volatile organic acid (terephthalic acid, trimer acid) improves the performance of the column while chromatographing acidic solutes. Conversely, bases (potassium hydroxide, Alkaterge T) are used to subcoat columns for the analysis of amines. Beckett and Rowland (1964) used a column of 10% polyethylene glycol 6000 and 5% potassium hydroxide for the analysis of amphetamine in urine.

IV. Detectors

One of the major advances in gas chromatographic analysis has been the development of highly sensitive detectors. These are, in most cases, ionization devices that measure the solutes as they are eluted from the chromatographic column. The development of sensitive detectors has necessitated a standardized basis for comparing detector performance. Because of fundamental differences in the mode of operation, quantitative comparisons are not always readily obtainable. Gudzinowicz (1967a, b) has discussed the problem of detector sensitivity in detail. One expression of sensitivity that is commonly seen in manufacturer's literature is the lower limit of detection, L. This depends on the amount of solute entering the detector per unit of time and is based on a recorder deflection of twice the noise level. It is computed from Equation 5 where: L = lower limit of

$$L = 2CFR/I \tag{5}$$

detection, g/sec; C = concentration of solute in carrier gas, g/ml; F = carrier gas flow rate, ml/sec; R = noise level, mV; and I = detector voltage in mV produced by CF (g/sec) of solute. Another parameter of detector performance is the linear range or the range over which detector response is a linear function of the solute content of the carrier gas entering the detector. This is seldom a limiting factor, however, since the linear ranges of most commercially available detectors are at least 50 or greater.

Gudzinowicz (1967a, b) has presented a detailed discussion of the theory and design of gas chromatographic detectors.

The *thermal conductivity detector* (Fig. 5) has been widely employed in gas chromatographic analysis. While this device lacks sensitivity, it is almost a universal detector in that it will detect virtually all materials different from the carrier gas. Because of its lack of sensitivity, the thermal conductivity detector is seldom employed in drug analysis.

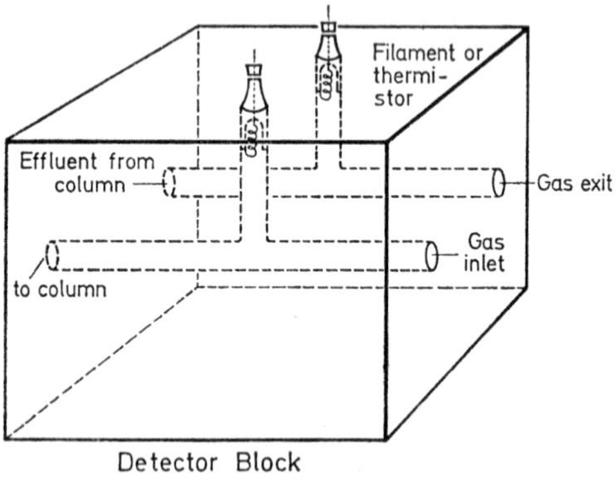

Fig. 5. Thermal conductivity detector

The *argon ionization detector* (Fig. 6) was the first sensitive detector to be made commercially available. With this detector it is possible to measure microgram and

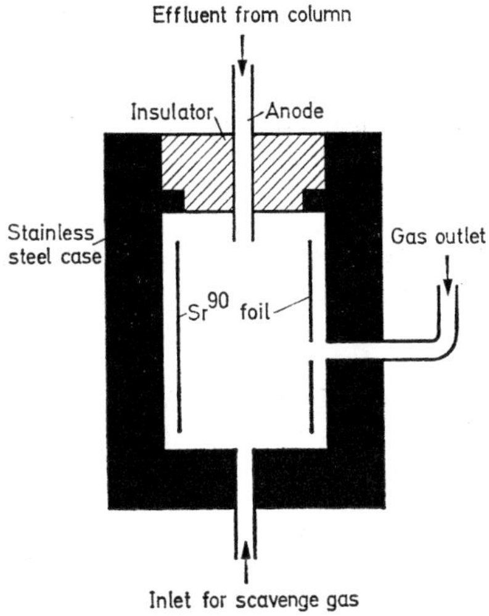

Fig. 6. Argon ionization detector

submicrogram quantities of solutes. In this detector, argon is used as the carrier gas. A β-ray source serves to excite argon to a metastable state. Upon collision of metastable argon with organic molecules, ions are produced and the resulting increase in current is measured by appropriate electronics.

The *flame ionization detector* (Fig. 7) is probably the most widely employed detector today. These detectors are sensitive and stable and require minimum maintenance. The basis for operation of this detector is the observation that a high

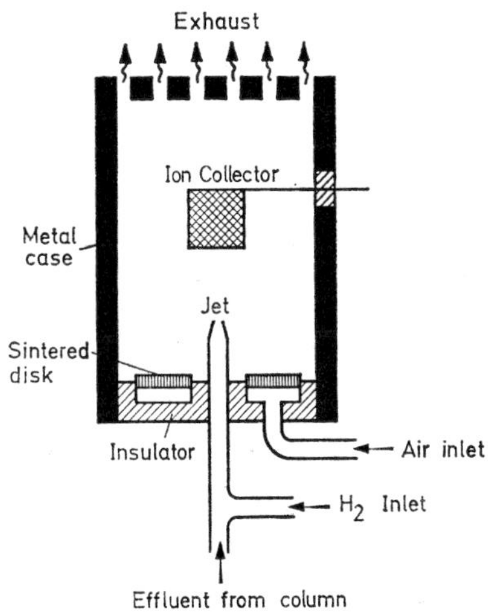

Fig. 7. Flame ionization detector

yield of ions is obtained, compared to a hydrogen-oxygen flame, when organic compounds are combusted in an atmosphere of hydrogen and oxygen or air. The ions formed in the detector are collected at the anode and the resulting change in current is displayed on a recorder after amplification. Flame ionization detectors can be operated at a variety of column flow rates although hydrogen and oxygen flow rates must be standardized. The sensitivity (L) of a typical detector is 9×10^{-13} (hydrocarbon) g/sec and the linear range is 3×10^7; the upper temperature limit is 400° C. In addition the detector is not affected by temperature changes and is insensitive to inorganic gases permitting the use of a variety of carrier gases. In this connection it is important to note that the sensitivity of the flame ionization detector varies with the thermal conductivity of the carrier gas employed (HOFFMANN and EVANS, 1966). Carbon dioxide, with a lower thermal conductivity than helium, gives a ninefold increase in detector sensitivity when substituted for helium as the carrier gas. Because of its availability, it is of practical importance to note that the use of nitrogen will result in a considerable increase in detector sensitivity compared to helium.

The *electron capture* or *electron affinity detector* is based on the property of certain compounds to capture free electrons (LOVELOCK and LIPSKY, 1960). In practice, the detector employs tritium or Ni^{63} as a source of ionizing radiation and nitrogen or methane/argon as the carrier gas. Under these conditions the ions formed by the radiation of the carrier gas can be collected at the anode by applying a small potential across the detector cell. When the effluent entering the cell contains a solute with a high affinity for electrons a decrease in the current flowing across the cell is observed. This change in current is then amplified and displayed on a recorder. The electron capture detector is very sensitive and specific. Nanogram and picogram quantities of certain compounds can be detected by this tool. The sensitivity of a typical electron capture detector employing a Ni^{63} source is 5×10^{-14} (CCl_4) g/sec with a linear range of 50; the temperature limit for Ni^{63} is 400° C. Types of compounds showing a high affinity for electrons include: halogenated hydrocarbons, nitro compounds, conjugated carbonyl groups, 1,2-diketones and quinones.

Many detecting devices in addition to those described above have been employed. These have been discussed by GUDZINOWICZ (1967b). One deserves special mention, however, because of the great potential it offers. This is the use of a mass spectrometer as a detector for a gas chromatograph. By use of this combination it is possible to confirm or establish the identity of peaks appearing on the gas chromatogram inasmuch as organic compounds possess predictable and unique mass spectra. Two critical features of this combination include the scan time of the mass spectrometer and the separator for enhancing the sample-to-carrier gas ratio. Early studies employed the time-of-flight mass spectrometer which is capable of very rapid scans. Conventional magnetic deflection spectrometers generally have comparatively slow scan times but have been adapted to fast scans. The recently introduced quadropole mass spectrometer is also capable of very rapid scans. A number of separators have been described for use in gas chromatography-mass spectrometry (KRUEGER and MCCLOSKEY, 1969; RYHAGE, 1964; WATSON and BIEMANN, 1965). All serve to remove a portion of the carrier gas and permit transfer of the desired solute to the ionization chamber of the mass spectrometer. It would appear that the art of separator design is in its infancy and that substantial improvements will be made in the future.

V. Techniques in Gas Chromatography

The purpose of gas chromatographic analysis is to determine sample composition. Very frequently in pharmacological problems, the task is simplified in that only a limited number of compounds are usually present in any given sample. For example, it may be desirable to quantitatively measure the appearance of one or two metabolites of a drug after incubation with cell fractions or to measure the disappearance of a single compound from the blood of an experimental animal.

A number of approaches are available for the qualitative identification of a compound by gas chromatography. If authentic reference materials are available, the problem is simplified considerably. In this case, retention times of the known compound and that extracted from biological material can be compared. While these values must, of course, be the same, agreement of retention times alone does not conclusively show identity. However, chromatographing the samples on several columns, containing liquid phases of differing polarities, will frequently suggest with considerable certainty that the compounds are the same. In addition, if the compounds contain appropriate functional groups, derivatives can be prepared and their retention behavior examined. Finally, gas chromatography can be used in conjunction with other techniques to show the qualitative identity of the peaks. Trapping the sample in the effluent of the gas chromatograph and subjecting it to further analysis is also feasible. For example, it is possible to trap microgram quantities of compounds and obtain excellent infrared spectra (ANDERS and MANNERING, 1967). Similarly, ultraviolet or visible spectra can be obtained. Furthermore, the collected sample can be examined by other chromatographic techniques such as paper or thin-layer chromatography. Finally, the most conclusive approach for qualitative identification of a peak is the use of the combined gas chromatograph-mass spectrometer. By this technique it is possible to determine the identity of the compound in question with a great deal of certainty.

Gas chromatography can be effectively employed for quantitative analysis. Indeed, in pharmacological studies this is often the most suitable method for the quantitative determination of drugs in biological samples. Two problems must be considered in the quantitative evaluation of a chromatogram. First, the peak in question must be measured in a quantitative manner and second, the concentration of the compound in the sample determined. In the quantitative measurement of peaks two approaches can be employed, namely, the determination of peak area or height. In many cases, peak area measurements are the more desirable; frequently, however, this measurement is difficult to obtain accurately. Methods commonly employed for the estimation of peak areas include the use of automatic integrators, planimeters, cutting out the peaks and weighing the paper, multiplication of peak height by peak width at half-height and triangulation. ETTRE (1967) has discussed these and additional methods in detail. It should be noted that all of these techniques are employed successfully and that the choice of method is largely a matter of personal preference and availability of equipment (integrator or planimeter). Furthermore, measurement of peak height will suffice for many quantitative applications. This technique requires that peaks lack appreciable tailing or other distortions to be used successfully. However, when applicable this is the simplest approach available.

The concentration of compound in the sample can be determined by several means. One approach is to prepare standards containing known amounts of drug and inject appropriate aliquots into the gas chromatograph. Comparison of peak areas or heights of the known and unknown samples permits quantitative evaluation. While this is a straightforward approach, it requires care in that volumes must be accurately measured and that sample changes (for example, due to evaporation of the solvent) must be avoided. A second technique, the *internal standard method*, is widely employed in gas chromatographic analysis. In this technique, the area or height of the unknown peak is related to that of a known compound added to the sample. Advantages of this approach are that exact sample volumes need not be known and that calibration curves are easily prepared and are quite independent of minor instrumental variables. In the internal standard technique, a calibration curve is prepared by chromatographing samples containing a fixed amount of the internal standard and varying amounts of the compound to be analyzed. The ratio (peak area or height) of the unknown/internal standard is plotted against concentration of unknown (Fig. 8). Samples are then analyzed after adding the internal standard and chromatographing. Quantitative evaluation is then made by direct reference to the standard curve. The requirements for a

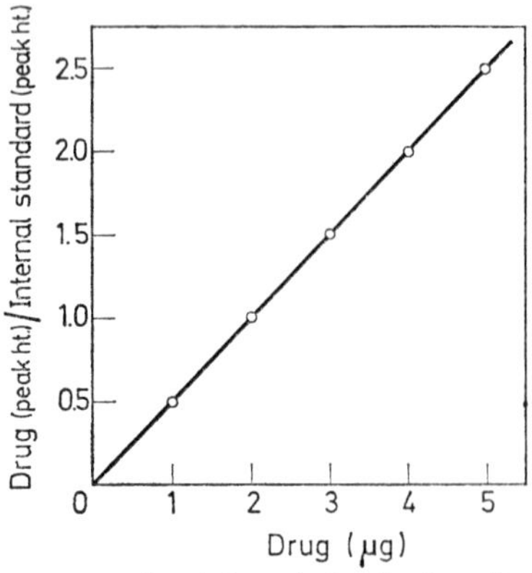

Fig. 8. Calibration curve using internal standard method of quantitation

suitable internal standard are that it be cleanly separated from the unknown compound (and any other peaks on the chromatogram) and that symmetrical peaks be obtained. In most cases of drug analysis, selection of internal standards is straightforward because of the availability of closely related analogues of drugs by different pharmaceutical houses.

Derivative formation has been widely employed in gas chromatographic analysis. The usual purpose of forming derivatives is to improve the chromatographic properties of the solutes or to permit separation of certain compounds. In some cases, derivatives are formed to enhance the sensitivity of the determination. Specifically, electron capturing derivatives may be formed to permit detection at the nanogram level.

Although often overlooked, derivative formation is a useful tool in the identification of compounds. Formation of several derivatives of an unknown and known compound followed by comparison of retention values provides firm evidence for the identity of the two compounds. Indeed, this approach is similar to the classical technique of derivative formation in organic chemistry where melting points and mixed melting points are compared rather than retention data.

Table 3 summarizes derivatives that have been formed with various functional groups. It should be noted that Table 3 is not an exhaustive compilation of derivatives that have been formed but rather presents the types of approaches that have been employed. Discussions of derivative formation have been presented by ANDERS and MANNERING (1967), CAVAGNOL and BETKER (1967) and VANDENHEUVEL and HORNING (1968).

Certain techniques employed in derivative formation require special comment. In most cases, derivatives have been formed outside the gas chromatograph followed by injection of the reaction mixture into the column. ANDERS and MANNERING (1962a) observed that derivatives could be formed "on-column" by injection of the compound and derivatizing agent. This approach was termed the "peak-

Table 3. *Derivatives useful in gas chromatographic analysis*

Functional Group	Derivative Formed	Derivatizing Agent(s)	Reference
Carboxylic acid	Ester, methyl	Diazomethane, BF_3/methanol. methanolic HCl	BURCHFIELD and STORRS (1962)
	Ester, trimethylsilyl	Various silylating agents	PIERCE (1969)
	Ester, halomethyldimethylsilyl[a]	Chloro- or bromomethyldimethylchlorosilane	BACHE et al. (1968)
Ketones	N,N-Dimethylhydrazones	N,N-Dimethylhydrazine	VANDENHEUVEL and HORNING (1963)
	Methoxime	Methoxyamine	FALES and LUUKKAINEN (1965)
	Ethylene-thioketal	Ethanedithiol/p-toluenesulfonic acid	ZMIGROD and LINDNER (1966)
	Iodoform (methyl ketones only)	I_2/KI/NaOH	STEVENS and VAN MIDDELEM (1966)
Amines (excluding tertiary amines)	*Dinitrophenyl*	2,4-Dinitrofluorobenzene	WALLE (1968)
	Schiff base (primary amines only)	Acetone and other ketones	VANDENHEUVEL et al. (1964)
	Amides (*fluorinated amides*)	Anhydrides and perfluorinated anhydrides	VANDENHEUVEL et al. (1964)
	Carbamates	Methyl chloroformate, methyl chlorothioformate	VANDENHEUVEL et al. (1964)
	Methanesulfonamide	Methanesulfonyl chloride	VANDENHEUVEL et al. (1964)
	N-Trimethylsilyl	Various silylating agents	PIERCE (1969)
Hydroxyl	Ester (*fluorinated esters*)	Anhydride and perfluorinated anhydrides	VANDENHEUVEL and HORNING (1961)
	Chloroacetate	Chloroacetic anhydride	ARGAUER (1968)
	Carbonates	Methyl chloroformate, methyl chlorothioformate	VANDENHEUVEL et al. (1965)
	Methanesulfonate	Methanesulfonyl chloride	VANDENHEUVEL et al. (1965)
	Ether, trimethylsilyl	Various silylating agents	PIERCE (1969)
	Ether, halomethyldimethylsilyl	Chloro- or bromomethyldimethylchlorosilane	BACHE et al. (1968)

[a] Italicized derivatives possess electron capturing properties.

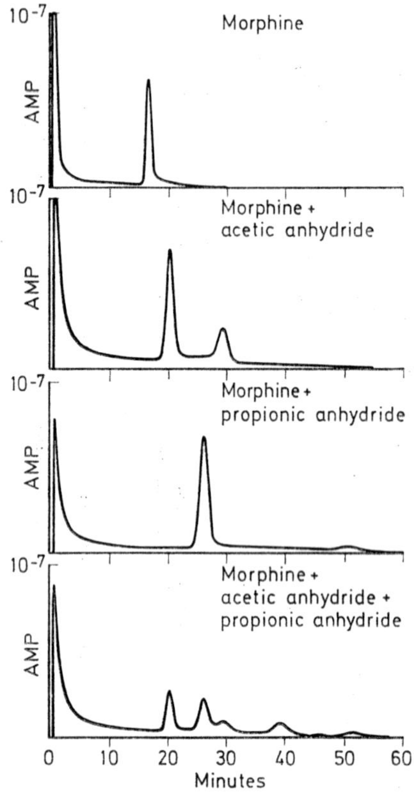

Fig. 9. Peak-shift of morphine after treatment with acetic and propionic anhydride. Top chromatogram: 30 μg of morphine. Second chromatogram: 30 μg of morphine followed by 5 μl of acetic anhydride. Third chromatogram: 30 μg of morphine followed by 5 μl of propionic anhydride. Bottom chromatogram: 30 μg of morphine followed by a mixture of 5 μl of acetic anhydride and 5 μl of propionic anhydride. Reproduced with permission from ANDERS and MANNERING (1962a)

shift technique". In this method, the injection of the parent compound was followed within seconds by an injection of acetic, propionic or trifluoroacetic anhydride. Using this technique, it was found that esters and amides were formed with alcohols and phenols as well as primary and secondary amines, respectively. The results obtained with morphine using this technique are shown in Fig. 9. ELLIOTT et al. (1964) and MULÉ (1964) have applied the peak-shift technique to the analysis of morphine and congeners in biological materials. ANDERS et al. (1966) utilized the peak-shift technique to identify a metabolite of SKF 525-A (2-diethylaminoethyl 2,2-diphenylvalerate HCl). In these experiments, the formation of the deethylated analog of SKF 525-A, SKF 8742-A (2-ethylaminoethyl 2,2-diphenylvalerate HCl), was suggested because of acetaldehyde formation. Comparison of the retention behavior of the acetamide, propionamide and trifluoroacetamide derivatives, formed on the column, of authentic SKF 8742-A and the isolated metabolite indicated that the compounds were identical. This conclusion was supported by thin-layer chromatographic evidence.

A number of derivatives can be formed "on-column". ESPOSITO (1968) reported the formation of trimethylsilyl (TMS) esters and ethers by an on-column technique and STREET (1969) extended this approach to the analysis of drugs. STEVENSON (1966) showed that N-methylated derivatives of barbiturates could be formed on-column by injecting a mixture of the barbiturate and tetramethylammonium hydroxide. This approach was later extended by BROCHMANN-HANSSEN and OKE (1969) who used trimethylanilinium hydroxide as the derivatizing agent. This reagent reacted on-column to form methylated derivatives of barbiturates, phenolic alkaloids and xanthines. The formation of Schiff bases derivatives of primary amines by on-column reaction with acetone has been described by FALES and PISANO (1962).

VI. Analytical Applications of Gas Chromatography in Pharmacology

Gas chromatography has seen wide application in the field of drug analysis. In many cases it has proved to be the analytical method of choice because of sensitivity, specificity and ease of analysis. Many of the problems encountered in the application of gas chromatography to drug analysis in biological tissues and fluids are not unique to this analytical method. The task of quantitatively isolating microgram or submicrogram amounts of drugs from biological samples is present whatever the analytical method finally employed; in many cases this is the limiting factor in drug analysis. Fortunately, the specificity of gas chromatographic analysis often permits analyses to be performed that would be impossible by other techniques. In this regard it is of interest to note that the subtractive function of the column is probably very important in the analysis of drugs in biological samples. By subtractive function of the column is meant the ability of the column (more specifically, the column packing material) to adsorb polar compounds present in the injected sample. These will then be deposited in the injection port and will not be eluted from the column.

In the analytical methods to be summarized below, primary emphasis will be given to those describing the use of gas chromatography in the analysis of drugs in biological materials. References to the chromatographic properties of drugs are cited in many of the analytical papers and will not be repeated here. ANDERS and MANNERING (1967) have presented a detailed discussion of many analytical procedures employing gas chromatography and the monograph by GUDZINOWICZ (1967a) is devoted entirely to drug and pesticide analysis.

Urine contains a large number of compounds derived from both intermediary metabolism and metabolism of ingested foreign compounds. The pattern of excretion of these substances is potentially useful both as a diagnostic tool and in studying the effects of drug treatment on the metabolism of endogenous substances. DALGLIESH et al. (1966) have described a technique in which phenolic, alcoholic and acidic functional groups are derivatized and the sample examined by programmed temperature gas chromatography. With this procedure the excretion pattern of fatty acids, di- and tri-carboxylic acids, hydroxyacids, polyhydroxy compounds, sugar alcohols and aromatic hydroxy and acidic compounds can be measured. In addition, glycine conjugates, mercapturic acids and glucuronides can be detected; the method is not suitable for sulfate conjugates. COWARD and SMITH (1969) have also described methods for preparing urinary extracts suitable for gas chromatographic analysis. These approaches should prove to be useful in many pharmacological studies.

Gas chromatography has been widely employed for the determination of *volatile organic compounds* in biological materials. In particular, blood and urine alcohol determinations, both for research and forensic purposes, are well suited to

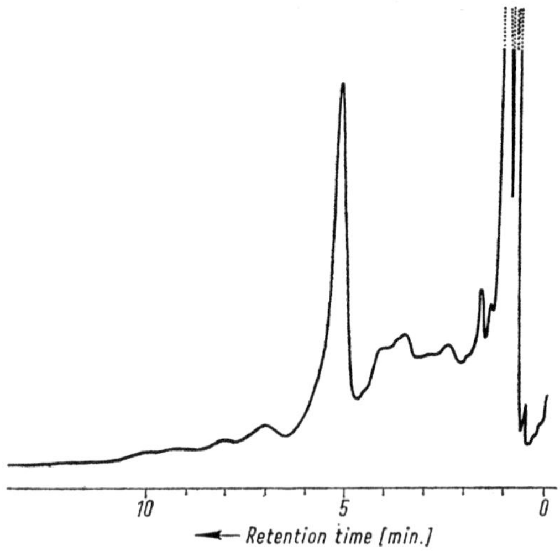

Fig. 10. Typical chromatogram of an assay mixture. Injected volume: 12.5 μl (max. 50 μl) of the deproteinized supernatant. Cyclohexanol appears as a peak with a retention time of 5.2 min. Reproduced with permission from ULLRICH (1969)

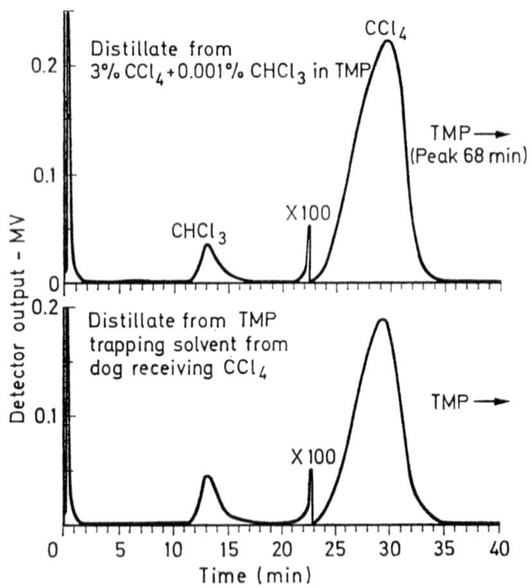

Fig. 11. Gas chromatograms of samples of 2,2,4-trimethylpentane (TMP) containing $CHCl_3$ and CCl_4. In the lower record the sample was a distillate from the solvent through which had passed the expired air of a dog that had received CCl_4. For comparison the upper record shows a chromatogram of a synthetic mixture subjected to all of the manipulations routinely used for preparing trapping solvents for chromatography. At the designated points, as CCl_4 was beginning to leave the column, the sensitivity of recording was reduced to $^1/_{100}$. TMP left the column later, and the peak due to this component is not included on the record. Reproduced with permission from BUTLER (1961)

Table 4. *Gas chromatographic determination of volatile organic compounds*

Compound(s) analyzed	Comment	Ref.
Ethanol and other volatiles	Compounds isolated by distillation	1
Ethanol	Blood ethanol extracted with butanol before analysis	2
Ethanol and other volatiles	Direct injection method, 56 volatiles in blood studied	3
Ethanol and other volatiles	Direct injection method, authors employed interchangeable inlets to prevent column contamination	4
Cyclohexanol	Measured the microsomal oxidation of cyclohexane to cyclohexanol, direct injection method	5
Ethanol	Head-space method	6
Ethanol	Head-space method	7
Methoxyflurane	Anesthetic agent isolated by distillation	8
Ether	Ether extracted with cyclohexane	9
Cyclopropane, halothane, methoxyflurane, ether and nitrous oxide	Direct injection method	10
Halothane	Head-space analysis employed	11
Ether, halothane, methoxyflurane, nitrous oxide and cyclopropane	Head-space analysis employed	12
Carbon tetrachloride and chloroform	Metabolism *in vivo* and *in vitro* studied	13

Reference. 1. Fox (1958); 2. Laessig (1968); 3. Parker et al. (1962); 4. Baker et al. (1969); 5. Ullrich (1969); 6. Machata (1964); 7. Bassette and Glendenning (1968); 8. Gadsden et al. (1962); 9. Northington and Owens (1964); 10. Yokota et al. (1967); 11. Purchase (1963); 12. Yamamura et al. (1966); 13. Butler (1961).

gas chromatographic analysis. Similarly, volatile anesthetics can readily be measured in blood or tissue samples.

Table 4 summarizes methods describing the determination of volatile organic compounds in biological samples. These techniques differ in the method of sample preparation and in the chromatographic conditions employed. Methods of sample preparation include: distillation, extraction, head-space analysis and direct injection techniques. While the direct injection technique is widely employed, its use results in the deposition of precipitated tissue components in the column. This problem is circumvented by the head-space method in which the sample is heated in a closed container to drive the volatile material into the vapor phase; an aliquot of the vapor phase in then injected into the gas chromatograph for analysis. It should be noted that Table 4 does not comprise a complete listing of all methods described for the determination of volatile compounds. A large number of procedures have been described, many representing minor modifications of previously described analytical techniques.

Figure 10 shows gas chromatographic analysis of cyclohexanol produced by the microsomal hydroxylation of cyclohexane (Ullrich, 1969). The analysis of chloroform produced by the *in vivo* reduction of carbon tetrachloride is illustrated in Fig. 11 (Butler, 1961).

Applications describing the use of gas chromatography for the analysis of barbiturates and anticonvulsants are summarized in Table 5. The use of gas chromatography for the analysis of these compounds permits quantitative microdeterminations to be made with a specificity not readily attainable by ultraviolet spectrophotometry or paper and thin-layer chromatography. Indeed, it is possible to quantitatively measure the barbiturate content of as little as 0.1 ml of blood (Jain et al., 1964; Anders, 1966). This permits pharmacokinetic studies to be conducted in individual laboratory rodents, as illustrated in Figs. 12 and 13.

Table 5. *Gas chromatographic analysis of barbiturates and anticonvulsants in biological materials*

Compound(s) analyzed	Comment	Ref.
Barbiturates	Compounds estimated in blood, urine and tissue	1
Barbiturates	Urinary excretion of barbiturates and metabolites studied	2
Thiopental	Metabolism in human subjects reported	3
Barbiturates	Micromethod requiring 0.1 ml blood reported	4
Barbiturates	Identified certain barbiturates by bromination or permanganate oxidation	5
Hydroxyamobarbital	Measured hydroxyamobarbital in urine as TMS derivative	6
Barbiturates	Methylated (dimethyl sulfate) before analysis	7
Barbiturates	A gas chromatographic method was employed to study the effect of diuresis on barbiturate intoxication	8
Barbiturates	Compounds estimated in blood and liver	9
Methohexital	Distribution and excretion studied in man	10
Barbiturates	Rapid micromethod (0.1 ml blood) described	11
Secobarbital	Metabolism in cell fractions studied	12
Barbiturates	Compounds determined in blood (0.5 ml sample required)	13
Barbiturates	Compared methods of extraction and gas, paper and thin-layer chromatographic analytical methods	14
Barbiturates, neutral and acidic drugs	Compared results obtained by gas chromatographic and UV methods	15
Barbiturates	Estimation in biological materials reported	16
Diphenylhydantoin	Diphenylhydantoin methylated with diazomethane prior to analysis	17
Primidone and phenobarbital	Conversion of primidone to phenobarbital in human subjects reported	18
Hexobarbital	Method applied to microsomal metabolism of hexobarbital	19
Amobarbital and hydroxyamobarbital	Compounds determined in serum after TLC clean-up	20
Anticonvulsants	Estimation in plasma, urine and CSF reported	21
Diphenylhydantoin and hydroxydiphenylhydantoin	Blood levels studied, compounds methylated with diazomethane before analysis	22
Diphenylhydantoin	Metabolic diposition in human subjects studied	23
Diphenylhydantoin	Method applied to blood, no derivatives formed	24

References: 1. Parker and Kirk (1961); 2. Svendsen and Brochmann-Hanssen (1962); 3. Furano and Greene (1963); 4. Jain et al. (1964); 5. Reith et al. (1965); 6. Kamm and Van Loon (1966); 7. Martin and Driscoll (1966); 8. Bloomer (1966); 9. McMartin and Street (1966); 10. Sunshine et al. (1966); 11. Anders (1966); 12. Ide et al. (1967); 13. Jain and Kirk (1967c); 14. Sunshine et al. (1968b); 15. Leach and Toseland (1968); 16. Machata and Battista (1968); 17. Sandberg et al. (1968); 18. Bogan and Smith (1968); 19. Den Tonkelaar et al. (1969); 20. Balasubramaniam et al. (1969); 21. Pippenger and Gillen (1969); 22. Grimmer et al. (1969); 23. Glazko et al. (1969); 24. Sabih and Sabih (1969).

Table 6 presents methods in which gas chromatography has been employed for the estimation of narcotic analgesics in biological materials. Again, the specificity and sensitivity of gas chromatography makes its use in this area possible for studying the metabolism and excretion of these compounds.

Gas chromatography can be effectively employed for the measurement of sympathomimetic amines as summarized in Table 7. The analysis of these compounds in biological materials is a challenge to the chemist in that the dose given is very small and, consequently, the tissue levels are very low. The extraction procedure outlined by Beckett and Rowland (1965) is very useful for analyzing urine for the presence of organic bases in general; its use in amine analysis is illustrated in Fig. 14. It has been employed in the author's laboratory for the estimation of strychnine and various bases in urine. Analysis of amphetamine and related compounds in blood has been made possible by derivative formation and electron capture detection.

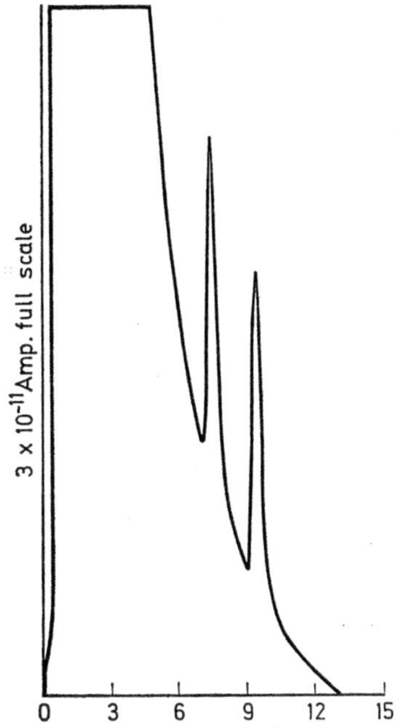

Fig. 12

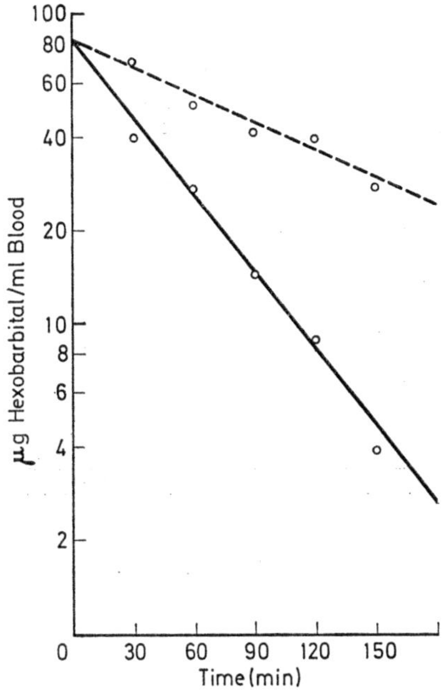

Fig. 13

Fig. 12. Gas chromatogram of hexobarbital extracted from rat blood. Peaks represent duplicate injections of the same sample. Reproduced with permission from Anders (1966)

Fig. 13. Blood hexobarbital levels after administration of hexobarbital or hexobarbital and SKF 525-A to rats. Lower line. Hexobarbital sodium, 82.5 mg/kg (320 µmol/kg) administered intraperitoneally. Hexobarbital half-life estimated from the plot was 35.8 min. Upper line. Hexobarbital sodium, 82.5 mg/kg (320 µmol/kg) given 45 min after an injection of 12.4 mg/kg (32 µmol/kg) SKF 525-A. Both drugs were administered intraperitoneally. Hexobarbital half-life estimated from the plot was 98.0 min. Reproduced with permission from Anders (1966).

Table 6. *Gas chromatographic determination of narcotic analgesics in biological materials*

Compound(s) analyzed	Comment	Ref.
Natural and synthetic analgesics	Compounds estimated in human tissues and fluids	1
Narcotic analgesics	Compounds measured in urine	2
Morphine	Compound measured in urine	3
Codeine and metabolites	Measurement of codeine in plasma and codeine, norcodeine and morphine in urine is described	4
Morphine and nalorphine	Procedures for the analysis of bases in urine, blood and tissues are described	5
Narcotic analgesics and other alkaloids	Compounds determined in blood (0.5 ml sample required)	6
Propoxyphene	Estimation in human plasma reported	7
Morphine	Compound measured in plasma or CSF as TMS[a] derivative	8
Fentanyl	Metabolic fate of fentanyl reported	9
Morphine	Morphine analyzed in urine as TMS[a] derivative	10

References: 1. Mulé (1964); 2. Elliott et al. (1964); 3. Yoshimura et al. (1966); 4. Schmerzler et al. (1966); 5. Street (1967); 6. Jain and Kirk (1967a); 7. Wolen and Gruber (1968); 8. Wilkinson and Way (1969); 9. Maruyama and Hosoya (1969); 10. Ikekawa et al. (1969).

[a] Trimethylsilyl

Table 7. *Gas chromatographic determination of sympathomimetic amines in biological materials*

Compound(s) analyzed	Comment	Ref.
Amphetamine	Compound isolated from urine by distillation	1
Amphetamine	Versatile extraction procedure described for isolation of bases from urine	2
Ephedrine and related amines	Compounds identified by derivative formation with acetone	3
Amphetamine and related drugs	Gas chromatography employed in conjunction with thin-layer chromatography for analysis in urine	4
Amphetamine	Trichloroacetamide derivative and election capture detector employed for blood amphetamine analysis	5
Amphetamine and related amines	Heptafluorobutyramide derivative and electron capture detector employed for blood level analysis	6
Amphetamine	Compound measured in urine after conversion to N-acetyl derivative	7

References: 1. BECKETT and ROWLAND (1964); 2. BECKETT and ROWLAND (1965); 3. BECKETT and WILKINSON (1965); 4. CARTONI and CAVALLI (1968); 5. NOONAN et al. (1969); 6. BRUCE and MAYNARD (1969); 7. TOSELAND and SCOTT (1969).

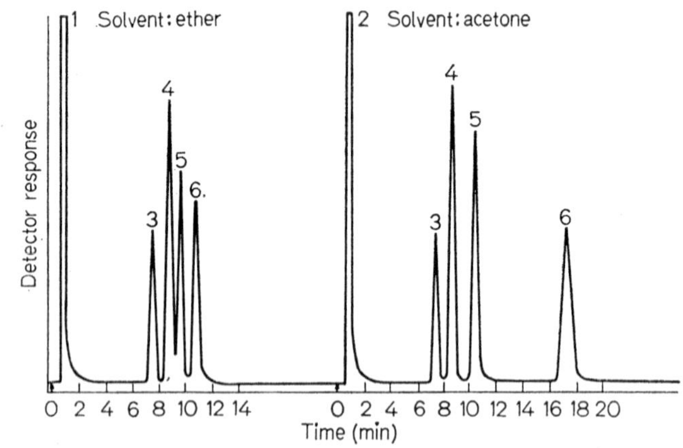

Fig. 14. Chromatograms of amphetamine, methylamphetamine, β-phenylethylamine and N,N-dimethylaniline in the absence and presence of acetone: 1. ether, 2. acetone, 3. N,N-dimethylaniline (t_R 7.5 min), 4. methylamphetamine (t_R 8.7 min), 5. amphetamine (t_R 9.5 min in ether, 10.4 in acetone), 6. β-phenylethylamine (t_R 10.8 min in ether, 17.4 min in acetone). Reproduced with permission from BECKETT and ROWLAND (1965)

Table 8 lists gas chromatographic procedures for the determination of various CNS depressants in biological materials. Included are phenothiazine tranquilizers, propanediol dicarbamates and related compounds and various other non-barbiturate depressants. Considerable attention has been given to the phenothiazine tranquilizers, particularly chlorpromazine, because of their use in the therapy of various mental disorders. HAMMAR et al. (1968) have applied gas chromatography-mass spectrometry to the analysis of chlorpromazine metabolites in blood. A new approach, termed *mass fragmentography*, was employed in these studies. First the fragmentation pattern of the metabolites was determined by mass spectrometry. Then the mass spectrometer was focused on up to three fragments which were unique to these compounds. The output of the mass spectrometer, which is being employed as a detector for the gas chromatograph, then gives superimposable tracings representing the mass numbers being detected. By this technique the

Table 8. *Gas chromatographic determination of miscellaneous central nervous system depressants in biological materials*

Compound(s) analyzed	Comment	Ref.
Chlorpromazine	Chlorpromazine, demethylated metabolites and sulfoxides measured in urine	1
Chlorpromazine	Chlorpromazine and metabolites estimated in urine	2
Phenothiazine tranquillizers and other agents	Method for determination in blood described	3
Chlorpromazine	Chlorpromazine and metabolites determined in blood using mass spectrometry-gas chromatography	4
Chlorpromazine	Chlorpromazine and metabolites identified in blood	5
Chlorpromazine	Parent compound and metabolites estimated in blood using electron capture detector	6
Thioridazine	Method for the routine assay of drug in plasma described	7
Glutethimide	Identification and estimation in blood described	8
Glutethimide	Rapid method for determination in biologic fluids described	9
Glutethimide	Gas and thin-layer chromatographic analysis compared	10
Glutethimide	Estimation in blood and urine described	11
Meprobamate	Estimation in urine and plasma reported	12
Meprobamate	Meprobamate measured in plasma and urine	13
Mebutamate, carisoprodol and tybamate	Compounds measured in plasma and urine	14
Diazepam	Parent compound and demethylated metabolite measured in blood after hydrolysis to 2-methylamino-5-chlorobenzophenone and 2-amino-5-chlorobenzophenone, resp.	15
Ro 5-3350[a]	Compound measured in blood after hydrolysis to 2-amino-5-bromobenzoylpyridine	16
Diazepam	Compound measured in blood and urine after hydrolysis to 2-methylamino-5-chlorobenzophenone	17
Thalidomide	Serum levels estimated	18
Chloral hydrate	Parent compound and trichloroethanol, trichloroacetic acid and trichloroethanol glucuronide measured in urine	19
Ethchlorvynol	Compound measured in blood	20
Methaqualone	Estimation in plasma described	21

References: 1. Driscoll et al. (1964); 2. Johnson et al. (1965); 3. Jain and Kirk (1967d); 4. Hammar et al. (1968); 5. Hammar and Holmstedt (1968); 6. Curry (1968); 7. Curry and Mould (1969); 8. Korzun et al. (1966); 9. Winsten and Brody (1967); 10. Rejent and Klendshoj (1968); 11. Sunshine et al. (1968a); 12. Maddock and Bloomer (1967); 13. Douglas et al. (1967); 14. Douglas et al. (1969); 15. De Silva et al. (1964); 16. De Silva and Kaplan (1966); 17. Cano et al. (1967a, b); 18. Sandberg et al. (1964); 19. Garrett and Lambert (1966); 20. Hedley-Whyte and Laasberg (1969); 21. Berry (1969).

[a] 7-Bromo-1,3-dihydro-5-(2-pyridyl)-2H-1,4-benzodiazepin-2-one

identity of a peak can be determined with great certainty. In addition, the technique is very sensitive since as little as 10^{-12} g of chlorpromazine can be detected.

Gas chromatography has been employed for the determination of many compounds in biological materials in addition to those listed above. Table 9 shows some of these applications. In some cases, compounds have been degraded to yield ketones with electron capturing properties to permit detection of the agents in blood. This approach was employed by Bruce et al. (1968) for the analysis of the antihistamine, brompheniramine, in blood (Fig. 15) and by Vessman and Strömberg (1969) for the detection of the antianginal agent, terodiline, in blood.

The use of gas chromatography for the analysis of drug conjugates has been studied and these results are summarized in Table 10. While these compounds are non-volatile, suitable derivatives can be prepared that permit gas chromatographic measurements to be made. In general, methyl esters and trimethylsilyl (TMS) ethers have been employed for the analysis of glucuronides but other deri-

Table 9. *Gas chromatographic determination of miscellaneous drugs in biological materials*

Compound(s) analyzed	Comment	Ref.
Lidocaine and prilocaine	Agents estimated in blood, plasma, serum, urine or tissue homogenate	1
Lidocaine	Compound measured in blood and urine	2
Mepivacaine	Estimation in blood reported	3
Lidocaine and prilocaine	Compounds determined in whole blood	4
Bupivacaine, lidocaine and mepivacaine	Estimation in blood reported	5
Mepivacaine	Compound measured in blood, as little as 0.2 ml of sample required	6
Nicotine	Compound estimated in urine	7
Nicotine and cotinine	Nicotine and its metabolite, cotinine, measured in urine after smoking	8
Antihistamines	Compounds measured in blood	9
Brompheniramine	Estimation in urine and blood after oxidation to p-bromophenyl 2-pyridyl ketone reported	10
5,5-Dimethyl-2,4-oxazolidinedione (DMO)	Compound measured in plasma, urine and skeletal muscle	11
Caffeine	Estimation in plasma reported	12
Acetylsalicylic acid	Compound chromatographed as methyl ester	13
Acetylsalicylic and salicylic acid	Compounds analyzed in plasma as TMS[a] derivatives	14
Terodiline[b]	Estimation in serum after oxidation to benzophenone using electron capture detector reported	15

References: 1. SVINHUFVUD et al. (1965); 2. BECKETT et al. (1965); 3. PRATT et al. (1967); 4. KEENAGHAN (1968); 5. REYNOLDS and BECKETT (1968); 6. ASLING et al. (1969); 7. MCNIVEN et al. (1965); 8. BECKETT and TRIGGS (1966); 9. JAIN and KIRK (1967b); 10. BRUCE et al. (1968); 11. SARDINI and MARZO (1969), MARZO and SARDINI (1969); 12. GRAB and REINSTEIN (1968); 13. CRIPPEN and FREIMUTH (1964); 14. ROWLAND and RIEGELMAN (1967); 15. VESSMAN and STRÖMBERG (1969).

[a] Trimethylsilyl
[b] N-*tert*-Butyl-1-methyl-3,3-diphenylpropylamine

Table 10. *Gas chromatographic analysis of drug conjugates*

Compound(s) analyzed	Comment	Ref.
Steroidal glucuronides	Analyzed as methyl esters-TMS ethers	1
Ethyl glucuronide	Compound shown to be a metabolite of ethanol in the rat and man	2
Ester, ether, N- and S-glucuronides	Compounds analyzed as methyl esters — acetyl, methyl and TMS derivatives. Method for measurement of glucuronides in urine described	3
Glucuronides	General method for isolation and derivatization described	4
Mercapturic and hippuric	Compounds analyzed as methyl esters	5

References: 1. JAAKONMAKI et al. (1967a); 2. JAAKONMAKI et al. (1967b); 3. IMANARI and TAMURA (1967); 4. KNAAK et al. (1967); 5. JAMES et al. (1967).

vatives have also been investigated. Gas chromatography-mass spectrometry has been applied to these compounds with considerable success; JAAKONMAKI et al. (1967b) employed this technique to identify ethyl glucuronide in the urine of individuals given ethanol. Figure 16 shows the gas chromatographic analysis of glucuronide conjugates.

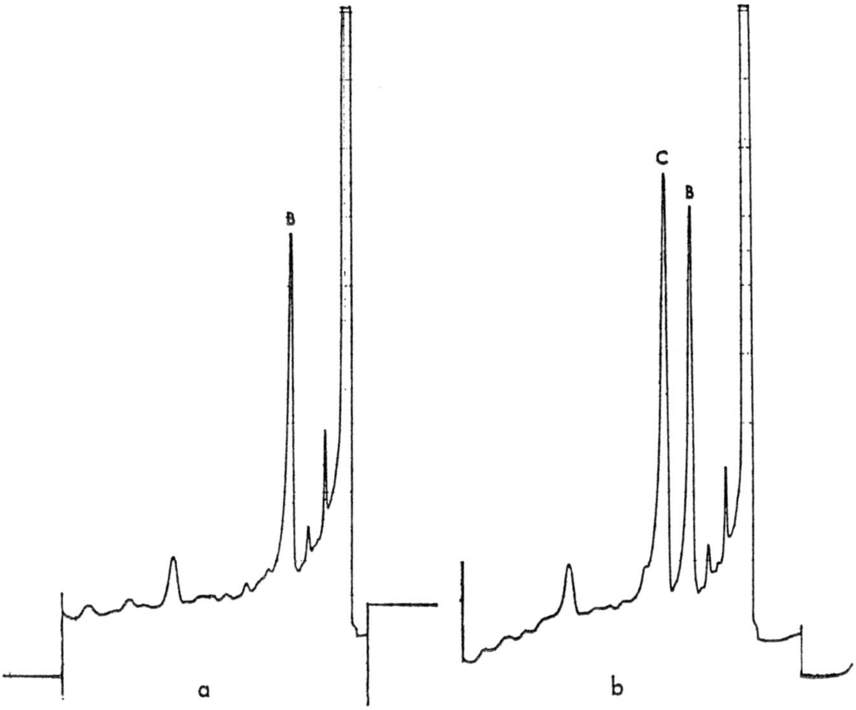

Fig. 15. Gas chromatograms obtained for (a) control blood to which chlorpheniramine (B) had been added and (b) from a subject 6.5 hours after receiving 8 mg of brompheniramine (C). Volume injected, 10 μl in each case. Reproduced with permission from BRUCE et al. (1968)

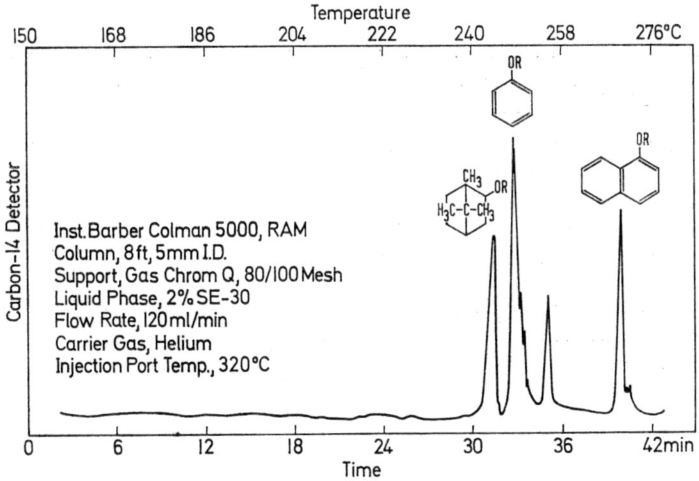

Fig. 16. Composite gas chromatogram of methyl-bornyl-2,3,4-tri-trimethylsilyl-β-D-glucuronate-C^{14}, methyl-phenyl-C^{14}-2,3,4-tri-trimethylsilyl-β-D-glucuronate, and methyl-1-naphthyl-1-C^{14}-2,3,4-tri-trimethylsilyl-β-D-glucuronate. Reproduced with permission from KNAAK et al. (1967)

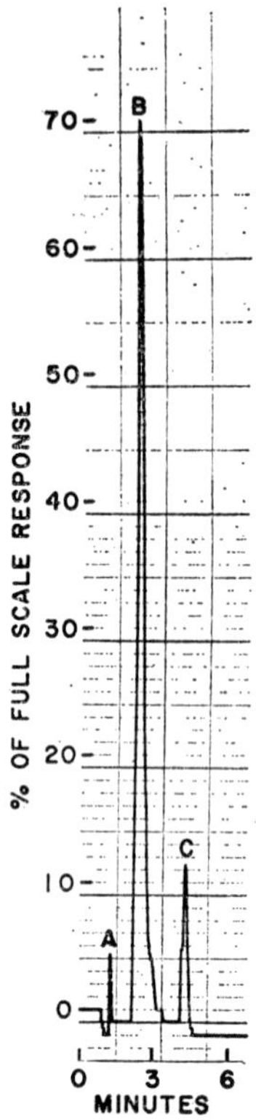

Fig. 17. Chromatogram at X2 attenuation produced by 222 ng ethanol (equivalent to 710 ng acetylcholine) derived from the reaction of borohydride with the acetylcholine present in an extract of rat brain. Brain weight 1.9 g; volume of extract 100 μl, 10 μl injected at 0 time. A, unknown; B, ethanol; C, water. Reproduced with permission from STAVINOHA and RYAN (1965)

The use of gas chromatography for the detection of neurotransmitter substances presents special problems in that the compounds are present in tissue only in small amounts. STAVINOHA et al. (1964) described a method for the measurement of acetylcholine in which the compound is reduced to ethanol by action of potassium borohydride; the ethanol is measured gas chromatographically. This method was employed for estimating the acetylcholine content of rat brain by STAVINOHA and RYAN (1965) as shown in Fig. 17; levels determined by this technique and by bioassay showed good agreement. JENDEN et al. (1968) have described a technique for the microestimation of acetylcholine. In this method acetylcholine is demethylated to yield dimethylaminoethyl acetate by treatment with benzenethiolate ion. The method is sensitive in the submicrogram range and can be applied to other choline esters. Pyrolysis-gas chromatography has been employed for the determination of acetylcholine, choline and choline esters by SZILAGYI et al. (1968). The products of the reaction are demethylated derivatives that can be detected at the nanogram level. The method is applicable to dilute solutions since the material can be concentrated on the pyrolyzing ribbon prior to pyrolysis and chromatography.

Gas chromatographic analysis of catecholamines and their metabolites in biological materials has been reported. KAWAI and TAMURA (1967, 1968a, b) have described methods for the derivatization and gas chromatography of catechol-

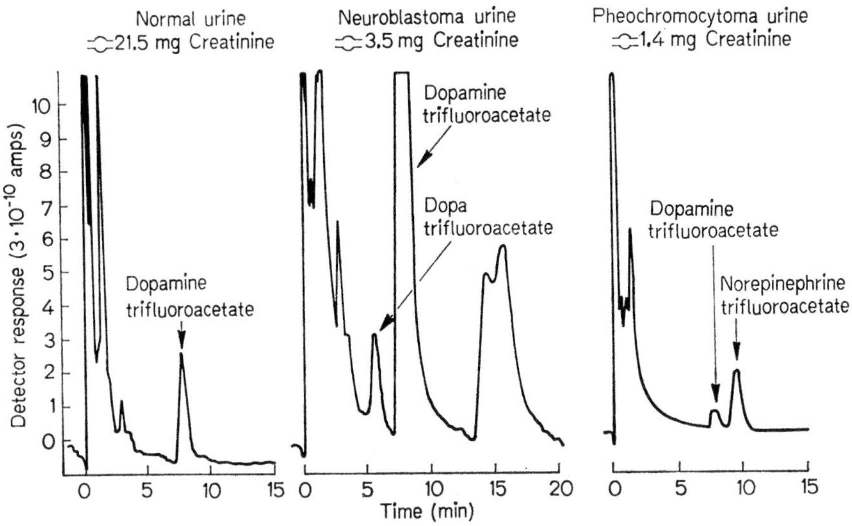

Fig. 18. A comparison of chromatograms from normal urine with those from a patient with neuroblastoma (center) and pheochromocytoma (right). Column: 6% QF-1 coated on Anakrom ABS 60/70 mesh; Column temperature: 160°C; Nitrogen flow rate: 65 ml/min; Current: 3×10^{-10} amps; Voltage: 50 v. The peak labeled norepinephrine trifluoroacetate may also represent epinephrine trifluoroacetate since these compounds are not separated on the column employed. Reproduced with permission from Clarke et al. (1967)

amines and metabolites; these techniques were applied to the determination of catecholamines in urine and tumor tissue (Kawai and Tamura, 1968b). Gas chromatography has been used to study the excretion of catecholamine metabolites in patients with catecholamine producing tumors (pheochromocytoma, neuroblastoma). Wilk et al. (1965) described a quantitative method for the estimation of urinary vanillylmandelic acid and Clarke et al. (1967) measured dopamine in urine at the nanogram level (Fig. 18). The estimation of urinary 3-methoxy-4-hydroxyphenylethylene glycol by gas chromatography was reported by Wilk et al. (1967) and 3-methoxytyramine, normetanephrine and metanephrine levels in urine were measured gas chromatographically after derivatization by Greer et al. (1968). A number of authors have studied the derivatization of catecholamines and catecholamine metabolites (Fales and Pisano, 1962; Sen and McGeer, 1963; Lindstedt, 1964; Brooks and Horning, 1964; Horning et al., 1964; Kawai et al., 1966; Capella and Horning, 1966; Horning et al., 1967; Frere and Verly, 1967; Änggård and Sedvall, 1969).

The gas chromatographic determination of histamine metabolites in urine has been reported by Tham (1966).

References

Anders, M.W.: Rapid micromethod for gas chromatographic determination of blood barbiturates. Analyt. Chem. **38**, 1945—1947 (1966).

— Alvares, A.P., Mannering, G.J.: Inhibition of drug metabolism. II. Metabolism of 2-diethylaminoethyl 2,2-diphenylvalerate HCl (SKF 525-A). Molec. Pharmacol. **2**, 328—334 (1966).

— Mannering, G.J.: New peak shift technique for gas-liquid chromatography. Preparation of derivatives on the column. Analyt. Chem. **34**, 730—733 (1962a).

— — Gas chromatography of some pharmacologically active phenothiazines. J. Chromat. **7**, 258—260 (1962b).

Anders, M.W., Mannering, G.J.: Application of gas chromatography to toxicology. Progr. chem. Toxicol. **3**, 121—218 (1967).
Änggård, E., Sedvall, G.: Gas chromatography of catecholamine metabolites using electron capture detection and mass spectrometry. Analyt. Chem. **41**, 1250—1256 (1969).
Argauer, R.J.: Rapid procedure for the chloroacetylation of microgram quantities of phenols and detection by electron-capture gas chromatography. Analyt. Chem. **40**, 122—124 (1968).
Asling, J.H., Shnider, S.M., Wilkinson, G.R., Way, E.L.: Gas chromatographic determination of mepivacaine in capillary blood. Anesthesiology **31**, 458—461 (1969).
Bache, C.A., St. John, L.E., Jr., Lisk, D.J.: Gas chromatographic analysis of insensitive pesticides as their halomethyldimethylsilyl derivatives. Analyt. Chem. **40**, 1241—1242 (1968).
Baker, R.N., Alenty, A.L., Zack, J.F., Jr.: Simultaneous determination of lower alcohols, acetone and acetaldehyde in blood by gas chromatography. J. chrom. Sci. **7**, 312—314 (1969).
Balasubramaniam, K., Mawer, G.E., Rogers, E.M.: The estimation of amylobarbitone and hydroxyamylobarbitone in serum by gas liquid chromatography. Brit. J. Pharmacol. **37**, 546P—547P (1969).
Bassette, R., Glendenning, B.L.: Analysis of blood alcohol by direct head space gas sampling and gas chromatography. Microchem. J. **13**, 374—380 (1968).
Beckett, A.H., Boyes, R.N., Parker, J.B.R.: Determination of lignocaine in blood and urine in human subjects undergoing local analgesic procedures. Anaesthesia **20**, 294—298 (1965).
— Rowland, M.: A specific method for the determination of amphetamine in urine. J. Pharm. Pharmacol. **16**, Suppl., 27T—31T (1964).
— — Determination and identification of amphetamine in urine. J. Pharm. Pharmacol. **17**, 59—60 (1965).
— Triggs, E.J.: Determination of nicotine and its metabolite, cotinine, in urine by gas chromatography. Nature (Lond.) **211**, 1415—1417 (1966).
— Wilkinson, G.R.: Identification and determination of ephedrine and its congeners in urine by gas chromatography. J. Pharm. Pharmacol. **17**, Suppl., 104S—106S (1965).
Beckman, H., Bevenue, A.: The effect of the column tubing composition on the recovery of chlorinated hydrocarbons by gas chromatography. J. Chromat. **10**, 231—233 (1963).
Berry, D.J.: Gas chromatographic determination of methaqualone, 2-methyl-3-*o*-tolyl-4(3H)-quinazolinone, at therapeutic levels in human plasma. J. Chromat. **42**, 39—44 (1969).
Bloomer, H.A.: A critical evaluation of diuresis in the treatment of barbiturate intoxication. J. Lab. clin. Med. **67**, 898—905 (1966).
Bogan, J., Smith, H.: The relation between primidone and phenobarbitone blood levels. J. Pharm. Pharmacol. **20**, 64—67 (1968).
Brochmann-Hanssen, E., Oke, T.O.: Gas chromatography of barbiturates, phenolic alkaloids and xanthine bases: Flash-heater methylation by means of trimethylanilinium hydroxide. J. pharm. Sci. **58**, 370—371 (1969).
Brooks, C.J.W., Horning, E.C.: Gas chromatographic studies of catecholamines, tryptamines, and other biological amines. Part I. Catecholamines and related compounds. Analyt. Chem. **36**, 1540—1545 (1964).
Bruce, R.B., Maynard, W.R., Jr.: Determination of amphetamine and related amines in blood by gas chromatography. Analyt. Chem. **41**, 977—979 (1969).
— Pitts, J.E., Pinchbeck, F.M.: Determination of brompheniramine in blood and urine by gas-liquid chromatography. Analyt. Chem. **40**, 1246—1250 (1968).
Burchfield, H.P., Storrs, E.E.: Biochemical applications of gas chromatography. New York-London: Academic Press 1962.
Butler, T.C.: Reduction of carbon tetrachloride *in vivo* and reduction of carbon tetrachloride and chloroform *in vitro* by tissues and tissue constituents. J. Pharmacol. exp. Ther. **134**, 311—319 (1961).
Cano, J.P., Vignoli, L., Viala, A.: Détermination du diazépam dans le sang et l'urine par chromatographie en phase gazeuse. I. Matérial et méthode. Ann. pharm. franç. **25**, 697—703 (1967a).
— — — Détermination du diazépam dans le sang et l'urine par chromatographie en phase gazeuse. II. Applications pharmacologiques et toxicologiques. Ann. pharm. franç. **25**, 821—828 (1967b).
Capella, P., Horning, E.C.: Separation and identification of derivatives of biologic amines by gas-liquid chromatography. Analyt. Chem. **38**, 316—321 (1966).
Cartoni, G.P., Cavalli, A.: Detection of doping by thin-layer and gas chromatography. J. Chromat. **37**, 158—161 (1968).
Cavagnol, J.C., Betker, W.R.: Sampling: Preparation of volatile derivatives and sample introduction. In: L.S. Ettre and A. Zlatkis: The practice of gas chromatography. New York: Interscience 1967.

CLARKE, D.D., WILK, S., GITLOW, S.E., FRANKLIN, M.J.: Gas chromatographic determination of dopamine at the nanogram level. J. Gas Chromat. **5**, 307—310 (1967).

COWARD, R.F., SMITH, P.: Some easily prepared urinary extracts suitable for gas chromatography. J. Chromat. **39**, 496—500 (1969).

CRIPPEN, R.C., FREIMUTH, H.C.: Determination of aspirin by gas chromatography. Analyt. Chem. **36**, 273—275 (1964).

CURRY, S.H.: Determination of nanogram quantities of chlorpromazine and some of its metabolites in plasma using gas-liquid chromatography with an electron capture detector. Analyt. Chem. **40**, 1251—1255 (1968).

— MOULD, G.P.: Gas chromatographic identification of thioridazine in plasma and a method for routine assay of the drug. J. Pharm. Pharmacol. **21**, 674—677 (1969).

DALGLIESH, C.E., HORNING, E.C., HORNING, M.G., KNOX, K.L., YARGER, K.: A gas-liquid chromatographic procedure for separating a wide range of metabolites occurring in urine or tissue extracts. Biochem. J. **101**, 792—810 (1966).

DAL NOGARE, S., JUVET, R.S., JR.: Gas-liquid chromatography. New York: Interscience 1962.

VAN DEEMTER, J.J., ZUIDERWEG, F.J., KLINKENBERG, A.: Longitudinal diffusion and resistance to mass transfer as a cause of non-ideality in chromatography. Chem. Eng. Sci. **5**, 271—289 (1956).

DOUGLAS, J.F., KELLY, T.F., SMITH, N.B., STOCKAGE, J.A.: Gas chromatographic determination of meprobamate, 2-methyl-2-propyl-1,3-propanediol dicarbamate, in plasma and urine. Analyt. Chem. **39**, 956—958 (1967).

— SMITH, N.B., STOCKAGE, J.A.: Gas chromatographic determination of mebutamate, carisoprodol and tybamate in plasma and urine. J. pharm. Sci. **58**, 145—146 (1969).

DRISCOLL, J.L., MARTIN, H.F., GUDZINOWICZ, B.J.: A gas chromatographic method for the quantitative analysis of some urinary metabolites of chlorpromazine. J. Gas Chromat. **2**, 109—114 (1964).

ELLIOTT, H.W., NOMOF, N., PARKER, K., DEWEY, M.L., WAY, E.L.: Comparison of the nalorphine test and urinary analysis in the detection of narcotic use. Clin. Pharmacol. Ther. **5**, 405—413 (1964).

ESPOSITO, G.G.: On-column formation and analysis of trimethylsilyl derivatives. Analyt. Chem. **40**, 1902—1904 (1968).

ETTRE, L.S.: The interpretation of analytical results; Qualitative and quantitative analysis. In: L.S. ETTRE and A. ZLATKIS: The practice of gas chromatography. New York: Interscience 1967.

— ZLATKIS, A., eds.: The practice of gas chromatography. New York: Interscience 1967.

FALES, H.M., LUUKKAINEN, T.: O-Methyloximes as carbonyl derivatives in gas chromatography, mass spectrometry and nuclear magnetic resonance. Analyt. Chem. **37**, 955—957 (1965).

— PISANO, J.J.: Gas chromatography of biologically important amines. Analyt. Biochem. **3**, 337—342 (1962).

FOX, J.E.: Gas chromatographic analysis of alcohol and certain other volatiles in biological material for forensic purposes. Proc. Soc. exp. Biol. (N.Y.) **97**, 236—237 (1958).

FRERE, J.M., VERLY, W.G.: On the use of an acetylated derivative of normetanephrine for gas chromatographic analysis. J. Chromat. **30**, 397—404 (1967).

FURANO, E.S., GREENE, N.M.: Metabolic breakdown of thiopental in man determined by gas chromatographic analysis of serum barbiturate levels. Anesthesiology **24**, 796—800 (1963).

GADSDEN, R.H., MCCORD, W.M., WOODS, E.F., BAGWELL, E.E.: Gas chromatographic determination of methoxyflurane in blood. Anesthesiology **23**, 831—836 (1962).

GARRETT, E.R., LAMBERT, H.J.: Gas chromatographic analysis of trichloroethanol, chloral hydrate, trichloroacetic acid, and trichloroethanol glucuronide. J. pharm. Sci. **55**, 812—817 (1966).

GLAZKO, A.J., CHANG, T., BAUKEMA, J., BILL, W.A., GOULET, J.R., BUCHANAN, R.A.: Metabolic disposition of diphenylhydantoin in normal human subjects following intravenous administration. Clin. Pharmacol. Ther. **10**, 498—504 (1969).

GRAB, F.L., REINSTEIN, J.A.: Determination of caffeine in plasma by gas chromatography. J. pharm. Sci. **57**, 1703—1706 (1968).

GREER, M., SPRINKLE, T.J., WILLIAMS, C.M.: Determination of urinary 3-methoxytyramine, normetanephrine and metanephrine in pheochromocytoma and neuroblastoma by gas chromatography. Clin. chim. Acta **21**, 247—253 (1968).

GRIMMER, G., JACOB, J., SCHAFER, H.: Die gaschromatographische Bestimmung von 5,5-diphenylhydantoin und 5-(p-hydroxyphenyl)-5-phenylhydantoin im Blut. Arzneimittel-Forsch. **19**, 1287—1290 (1969).

GUDZINOWICZ, B.J.: Gas chromatographic analysis of drugs and pesticides. New York: Dekker 1967a.

Gudzinowicz, B.J.: Detectors. In: L.S. Ettre and A. Zlatkis: The practice of gas chromatography. New York: Interscience 1967b.
Hammar, C.G., Holmstedt, B.: The identification of chlorpromazine metabolites in human blood by gas liquid chromatography. Experientia (Basel) **24**, 98—100 (1968).
— — Ryhage, R.: Mass fragmentography. Identification of chlorpromazine and its metabolites in human blood by a new method. Analyt. Biochem. **25**, 532—548 (1968).
Hedley-Whyte, J., Laasberg, L.H.: Ethchlorvynol poisoning: Gas-liquid chromatography in management. Anesthesiology **30**, 107—111 (1969).
Hoffmann, R.L., Evans, C.D.: Thermal conductivity effect of carrier gases on flame-ionization detector sensitivity. Science **153**, 172—173 (1966).
Horning, E.C., Horning, M.G., Vandenheuvel, W.J.A., Knox, K.L., Holmstedt, B., Brooks, C.J.W.: Gas chromatographic studies of catecholamines, tryptamines and other biological amines. Part II. Tryptamine-related amines and catecholamines. Analyt. Chem. **36**, 1546—1549 (1964).
— Moscatelli, E.A., Sweeley, C.C.: Polyester liquid phases in gas-liquid chromatography. Chem. Ind. (Lond.) 751—752 (1959).
Horning, M.G., Moss, A.M., Horning, E.C.: A new method for the separation of the catecholamines by gas-liquid chromatography. Biochim. biophys. Acta (Amst.) **148**, 597—600 (1967).
Ide, H., Yoshimura, H., Tsukamoto, H.: Metabolism of drugs. LII. Enzymatic study on secobarbital metabolism. Chem. pharm. Bull. **15**, 411—419 (1967).
Ikekawa, N., Takayama, K., Hosoya, E., Oka, T.: Determination of morphine in urine by gas chromatography. Analyt. Biochem. **28**, 156—163 (1969).
Imanari, T., Tamura, Z.: Gas chromatography of glucuronides. Chem. pharm. Bull. **15**, 1677—1681 (1967).
Jaakonmaki, P.I., Knox, K.L., Horning, E.C., Horning, M.G.: The characterization by gas-liquid chromatography of ethyl β-D-glucosiduronic acid as a metabolite of ethanol in rat and man. Europ. J. Pharmacol. **1**, 63—70 (1967b).
— Yarger, K.A., Horning, E.C.: Gas-liquid chromatographic separation of human urinary steroid glucuronides. Biochim. biophys. Acta (Amst.) **137**, 213—216 (1967a).
Jain, N.C., Fontan, C.R., Kirk, P.L.: Rapid extraction method for barbiturates from blood for gas-liquid chromatographic analysis. Microchem. J. **8**, 28—34 (1964).
— Kirk, P.L.: Systemic applications of gas-liquid in toxicology. I. Extraction procedure and the alkaloids. Microchem. J. **12**, 229—241 (1967a).
— — Systematic application of gas-liquid chromatography in toxicology. II. The antihistamines. Microchem. J. **12**, 242—248 (1967b).
— — Systematic applications of gas-liquid chromatography in toxicology. III. The barbiturates. Microchem. J. **12**, 249—255 (1967c).
— — Systematic applications of gas-liquid chromatography in toxicology. IV. The tranquilizers. Microchem. J. **12**, 256—264 (1967d).
James, A.T., Martin, A.J.P.: Gas-liquid partition chromatography: The separation and micro-estimation of volatile fatty acids from formic acid to dodecanoic acid. Biochem. J. **50**, 679—690 (1952).
— — Smith, G.H.: Gas-liquid partition chromatography: The separation and micro-estimation of ammonia and the methylamines. Biochem. J. **52**, 238—242 (1952).
James, S.P., Waring, R.H., White, D.A.: Separation and mercapturic acids and related compounds by gas chromatography and a method for the determination of hippuric acid. J. Chromat. **26**, 255—258 (1967).
Jenden, D.J., Hanin, I., Lamb, S.I.: Gas chromatographic microestimation of acetylcholine and related compounds. Analyt. Chem. **40**, 125—128 (1968).
Johnson, D.E., Rodriguez, C.F., Burchfield, H.P.: Determination by microcoulometric gas chromatography of chlorpromazine metabolites in human urine. Biochem. Pharmacol. **14**, 1453—1469 (1965).
Kamm, J.J., Van Loon, E.J.: Amobarbital metabolism in man. Clin. Chem. **12**, 789—796 (1966).
Kawai, S., Nagatsu, T., Imanari, T., Tamura, Z.: Gas chromatography of catecholamines and related compounds. Chem. pharm. Bull. **14**, 618—621 (1966).
— Tamura, Z.: Gas chromatography of catecholamines using dimethyl sulfoxide as an effective solvent for trimethylsilylation. Chem. pharm. Bull. **15**, 1493—1497 (1967).
— — Gas chromatography of catecholamines as their trifluoroacetates. Chem. pharm. Bull. **16**, 699—701 (1968a).
— — Gas chromatography of the catecholamines as their trifluoroacetates in urine and tumor. Chem. pharm. Bull. **16**, 1091—1094 (1968b).
Keenaghan, J.B.: The determination of lidocaine and prilocaine in whole blood by gas chromatography. Anesthesiology **29**, 110—112 (1968).

KEULEMANS, A.I.M.: Gas chromatography, 2nd ed. New York: Reinhold 1959.
KNAAK, J.B., ELDRIDGE, J.M., SULLIVAN, L.J.: Systematic approach to preparation and identification of glucuronic acid conjugates. J. Agr. Food Chem. **15**, 605—609 (1967).
KORZUN, B.P., BRODY, S.M., KEEGAN, P.G., LUDERS, R.C., REHM, C.R.: Rapid chromatographic method for the identification and estimation of glutethimide (Doriden) in blood. J. Lab. clin. Med. **68**, 333—339 (1966).
KRUEGER, P.M., MCCLOSKEY, J.A.: Porous stainless steel as a carrier gas separator interface material for gas chromatography-mass spectrometry. Analyt. Chem. **41**, 1930—1935 (1969).
LAESSIG, R.H.: Submicro sampling and solvent extraction system for rapid gas chromatographic determination of blood alcohol. Analyt. Chem. **40**, 2205—2207 (1968).
LEACH, H., TOSELAND, P.A.: The determination of barbiturates and some related drugs by gas chromatography. Clin. chim. Acta **20**, 195—203 (1968).
LEVINS, R.J., OTTENSTEIN, D.M.: The effect of the tubing material in the gas chromatography of polyols and vanillins. J. Gas Chromat. **5**, 539—542 (1967).
LINDSTEDT, S.: Gas chromatography of adrenalin, noradrenalin and related amines as their trimethylsilyl ethers. Clin. chim. Acta **9**, 309—310 (1964).
LLOYD, H.A., FALES, H.M., HIGHET, P.F., VANDENHEUVEL, W.J.A., WILDMAN, W.C.: Separation of alkaloids by gas chromatography. J. Amer. chem. Soc. **82**, 3791 (1960).
LOVELOCK, J.E., LIPSKY, S.R.: Electron affinity spectroscopy — A new method for the identification of functional groups in chemical compounds separated by gas chromatography. J. Amer. chem. Soc. **82**, 431—433 (1960).
MACHATA, G.: Über die gaschromatographische Blutalkoholbestimmung. Analyse der Dampfphase. Mikrochim. Acta 262—271 (1964).
— BATTISTA, H.J.: Gaschromatographische Barbituratbestimmung. Mikrochim. Acta 866—874 (1968).
MADDOCK, R.K., JR., BLOOMER, H.A.: Gas chromatography of meprobamate. Clin. Chem. **13**, 333—338 (1967).
MARTIN, A.J.P., SYNGE, R.L.M.: A new form of chromatogram employing two liquid phases. Biochem. J. **35**, 1358—1368 (1941).
MARTIN, H.F., DRISCOLL, J.L.: Gas chromatographic identification and determination of barbiturates. Analyt. Chem. **38**, 345—346 (1966).
MARZO, A., SARDINI, D.: Quantitative gas chromatographic determination of 5,5-dimethyl-2,4-oxazolidinedione. J. Chromat. **44**, 611—613 (1969).
MARUYAMA, Y., HOSOYA, E.: Studies on the fate of fentanyl. Keio J. Med. **18**, 59—70 (1969).
MCMARTIN, C., STREET, H.V.: Gas-liquid chromatography of submicrogram amounts of drugs. II. Analysis of barbiturates and related drugs in biological media. J. Chromat. **23**, 232—241 (1966).
MCNIVEN, N.L., RAISINGHANI, K.H., PATASHNIK, S., DORFMAN, R.I.: Determination of nicotine in smokers' urine by gas chromatography. Nature (Lond.) **208**, 788—789 (1965).
MULÉ, S.J.: Determination of narcotic analgesics in human biological materials. Analyt. Chem. **36**, 1907—1914 (1964).
NOONAN, J.S., MURDICK, P.W., RAY, R.S.: A method for detecting amphetamine using gas chromatography of a halogenated derivative. J. Pharmacol. exp. Ther. **168**, 205—209 (1969).
NORTHINGTON, M.S., OWENS, G.: Determination of blood ether levels by gas-liquid chromatography. Analyt. Biochem. **9**, 48—53 (1964).
OTTENSTEIN, D.M.: Column support materials for use in gas chromatography. J. Gas Chromat. **1**, 11—23 (1963).
— Comparison of support deactivation in gas chromatography. J. Gas Chromat. **6**, 129—134 (1968).
PARKER, K.D., FONTAN, C.R., YEE, J.L., KIRK, P.L.: Gas chromatographic determination of ethyl alcohol in blood for medicolegal purposes. Analyt. Chem. **34**, 1234—1236 (1962).
— KIRK, P.L.: Separation and identification of barbiturates by gas chromatography. Analyt. Chem. **33**, 1378—1381 (1961).
PECSOK, R.L., ed.: Principles and practice of gas chromatography. New York: Wiley 1959.
PIERCE, A.E.: Silylation of organic compounds. Rockford: Pierce Chemical Co. 1969.
PIPPENGER, C.E., GILLEN, H.W.: Gas chromatographic analysis for anticonvulsant drugs in biologic fluids. Clin. Chem. **15**, 582—590 (1969).
PRATT, E.L., WARRINGTON, H.P., GREGO, J.: The gas chromatographic determination of mepivacaine in blood with a note on other local anesthetics. Anesthesiology **28**, 432—437 (1967).
PURCHASE, I.F.H.: Estimation of halothane tensions in blood by gas chromatography. Nature (Lond.) **198**, 895—896 (1963).
PURNELL, J.H.: Gas chromatography. New York: Wiley 1962.
REITH, J.F., VAN DER HEIDE, R.F., ZWALL, R.F.A.: Herkenning en bepaling van barbitalen in bloed door middel van gaschromatografie. Pharm. Weekbl. Ned. **100**, 219—227 (1965).

REJENT, T.A., KLENDSHOJ, N.C.: Rapid determination of glutethimide in biological fluids. A comparison of the thin-layer-chromatographic method with gas-chromatographic methods. Clin. Toxic. **1**, 143—148 (1968).
REYNOLDS, F., BECKETT, A.H.: The determination of bupivacaine, lignocaine and mepivacaine in human blood. J. Pharm. Pharmacol. **20**, 704—708 (1968).
ROHRSCHNEIDER, L.: Eine Methode zur Charakterisierung von gaschromatographischen Trennflüssigkeiten. J. Chromat. **22**, 6—22 (1966).
ROWLAND, M., RIEGELMAN, S.: Determination of acetylsalicylic acid and salicylic acid in plasma. J. pharm. Sci. **56**, 717—720 (1967).
RYHAGE, R.: Use of a mass spectrometer as a detector and analyzer for effluents emerging from high temperature gas liquid chromatography columns. Analyt. Chem. **36**, 759—764 (1964).
SABIH, K., SABIH, K.: Gas chromatographic method for determination of diphenylhydantoin blood level. Analyt. Chem. **41**, 1452—1454 (1969).
SANDBERG, D.H., BOCK, S.A., TURNER, D.A.: Quantitative measurement of thalidomide by gas-liquid chromatography. Analyt. Biochem. **8**, 129—132 (1964).
— RESNICK, G.L., BACALLAO, C.Z.: Measurement of serum diphenylhydantoin by gas-liquid chromatography. Analyt. Chem. **40**, 736—738 (1968).
SARDINI, D., MARZO, A.: Gas chromatographic evaluation of 5,5-dimethyl-2,4-oxazolidinedione (DMO) for determination of intracellular pH. J. Pharm. Pharmacol. **21**, 477 (1969).
SCHMERZLER, E., YU, W., HEWITT, M.I., GREENBLATT, I.J.: Gas chromatographic determination of codeine in serum and urine. J. pharm. Sci. **55**, 155—157 (1966).
SEN, N.P., MCGEER, P.L.: Gas chromatography of phenolic and catecholic amines as the trimethylsilyl ethers. Biochem. biophys. Res. Commun. **13**, 390—393 (1963).
SILVA, J.A.F. DE, KAPLAN, J.: Determination of 7-bromo-1,3-dihydro-5-(2-pyridyl)-2H-1,4-benzodiazepin-2-one (Ro 5-3350) in blood by gas-liquid chromatography. J. pharm. Sci. **55**, 1278—1283 (1966).
— SCHWARTZ, M.A., STEFANOVIC, V., KAPLAN, J., D'ARCONTE, L.: Determination of diazepam (Valium) in blood by gas liquid chromatography. Analyt. Chem. **36**, 2099—2104 (1964).
STAVINOHA, W.B., RYAN, L.C.: Estimation of the acetylcholine content of rat brain by gas chromatography. J. Pharmacol. exp. Ther. **150**, 231—235 (1965).
— — TREAT, E.L.: Estimation of acetylcholine by gas chromatography. Life Sci. **3**, 689—693 (1964).
STEVENS, R.D., VAN MIDDELEM, C.H.: Analysis of Bidrin as iodoform by electron capture-gas-liquid chromatography. J. Agr. Food Chem. **14**, 149—152 (1966).
STEVENSON, G.W.: On-column methylation of barbituric acids. Analyt. Chem. **38**, 1948—1949 (1966).
STREET, H.V.: Gas-liquid chromatography of submicrogram amounts of drugs. III. Analysis of alkaloids in biological media. J. Chromat. **29**, 68—79 (1967).
— Gas-liquid chromatography of submicrogram amounts of drugs. IV. Identification of barbiturates, hydantoins, amides, imides, carbamates, phenylbutazone, carboxylic acids and hydrazine derivatives by direct derivative formation within the gas chromatograph. J. Chromat. **41**, 358—366 (1969).
SUNSHINE, I., MAES, R., FARACCI, R.: Determination of glutethimide (Doriden) and its metabolites in biologic specimens. Clin. Chem. **14**, 595—609 (1968a).
— — FINKLE, B.: An evaluation of methods for the determination of barbiturates in biological materials. Clin. Toxic. **1**, 281—296 (1968b).
— WHITWAM, J.G., FIKE, W.W., FINKLE, B., LEBEAU, J.: Distribution and excretion of methohexitone in man. Brit. J. Anaesth. **38**, 23—28 (1966).
SVENDSEN, A.B., BROCHMANN-HANSSEN, E.: Gas chromatography of barbiturates. II. Application to the study of their metabolism and excretion in humans. J. pharm. Sci. **51**, 494—495 (1962).
SVINHUFVUD, G., ÖRTENGREN, B., JACOBSSON, S.E.: The estimation of lidocaine and prilocaine in biological material by gas chromatography. Scand. J. clin. Lab. Invest. **17**, 162—164 (1965).
SZILAGYI, P.I.A., SCHMIDT, D.E., GREEN, J.P.: Microanalytical determination of acetylcholine, other choline esters and choline by pyrolysis-gas chromatography. Analyt. Chem. **40**, 2009—2013 (1968).
THAM, R.: Gas chromatographic analysis of histamine metabolites in urine. Quantitative determination of ring methylated imidazole-acetic acids in healthy man. J. Chromat. **23**, 207—216 (1966).
TONKELAAR, E.M. DEN, KLAP-VAN DIJK, A., WIT, S.L.: Determination of rat liver hexobarbital oxidase activity with a gas chromatographic method. Biochem. Pharmacol. **18**, 262—265 (1969).

TOSELAND, P. A., SCOTT, P. H.: Determination of amphetamine as its N-acetyl derivative by gas-liquid chromatography. Clin. chim. Acta **25**, 75—78 (1969).
ULLRICH, V.: On the hydroxylation of cyclohexane in rat liver microsomes. Hoppe-Seyler's Z. physiol. Chem. **350**, 357—365 (1969).
VANDENHEUVEL, W. J. A., GARDINER, W. L., HORNING, E. C.: Characterization and separation of amines by gas chromatography. Analyt. Chem. **36**, 1550—1560 (1964).
— — — Gas chromatographic behavior of long chain alcolhols and their derivatives. J. Chromat. **19**, 263—276 (1965).
— HORNING, E. C.: Gas chromatographic separations of sugars and related compounds as acetyl derivatives. Biochem. biophys. Res. Commun. **4**, 399—403 (1961).
— — Gas-chromatographic characterization of steroid ketones as N,N-dimethylhydrazones. Biochim. biophys. Acta (Amst.) **74**, 560—563 (1963).
— — Gas-liquid chromatographic (GLC) methods for the analysis of steroids and their derivatives. Med. Res. Eng. **7**, 10—22 (1968).
VESSMAN, J., STRÖMBERG, S.: Determination of terodiline (Bicor) in serum by gas chromatography and electron capture detection of benzophenone formed by chromic acid oxidation. Acta pharm. suec. **6**, 505—518 (1969).
WALLE, T.: Quantitative gas chromatography of picogram quantities of amines as 2,4-dinitrophenyl derivatives. Acta. pharm. suec. **5**, 367—384 (1968).
WATSON, J. T., BIEMANN, K.: Direct recording of high resolution mass spectra of gas chromatographic effluents. Analyt. Chem. **37**, 844—851 (1965).
WILK, S., GITLOW, S. E., CLARKE, D. D., PALEY, D. H.: Determination of urinary 3-methoxy-4-hydroxyphenylethylene glycol by gas-liquid chromatography and electron capture detection. Clin. chim. Acta **16**, 403—408 (1967).
— — MENDLOWITZ, M., FRANKLIN, M. J., CARR, H. E., CLARKE, D. D.: A quantitative assay for vanillylmandelic acid (VMA) by gas-liquid chromatography. Analyt. Biochem. **13**, 544—551 (1965).
WILKINSON, G. R., WAY, E. L.: Sub-microgram estimation of morphine in biological fluids by gas-liquid chromatography. Biochem. Pharmacol. **18**, 1435—1439 (1969).
WINSTEN, S., BRODY, D.: Rapid determination of glutethimide (Doriden) by gas-liquid chromatography. Clin. Chem. **13**, 589—594 (1967).
WOLEN, R. L., GRUBER, C. M., JR.: Determination of propoxyphene in human plasma by gas chromatography. Analyt. Chem. **40**, 1243—1246 (1968).
YAMAMURA, H., WAKASUGI, B., SATO, S., TAKEBE, Y.: Gas chromatographic analysis of inhalation, anesthetics in whole blood by an equilibration method. Anesthesiology **27**, 311—317 (1966).
YOKOTA, T., HITOMI, Y., OHTA, K., KOSAKA, F.: Direct injection method for gas chromatographic measurement of inhalation anesthetics in whole blood and tissues. Anesthesiology **28**, 1064—1073 (1967).
YOSHIMURA, H., OGURI, K., TSUKAMOTO: Detection of morphine in urine. Chem. pharm. Bull. **14**, 62—67 (1966).
ZMIGROD, A., LINDNER, H. R.: Gas-chromatographic separation of ketosterioids as ethylenethioketal derivatives. Steroids **8**, 119—132 (1966).

Chapter 28

Enzymatic Assays in Pharmacology

A.K. Cho

With 4 Figures

I. Introduction

Enzymatic methods of analysis can be considered a modification of the bioassay where the concentration of a product formed by an enzyme is measured instead of a biological response such as a muscle contraction or death. Since enzymes usually have very specific substrate or inhibitor requirements, they are excellent reagents for the analysis of biochemicals that are present in complex mixtures (Bergmeyer, 1963).

This chapter describes enzymatic methods that have been used for the analysis of pharmacological agents. In these methods drugs are analyzed as substrates or as inhibitors in a variety of reactions. Drugs have also been assayed by competitive protein binding techniques utilizing a specific interaction between a drug and a protein, similar to that between an enzyme and substrate, but without a subsequent chemical reaction. The methods are discussed with emphasis on specificity, separation procedures, the chemistry of the reaction and the applications of the assay.

Information from the literature is also presented on enzymes or proteins that might be used in future analyses because of their specificity for small molecules.

II. Enzymatic Assays with Pharmacological Agents as Substrates

In the analyses described here pharmacological agents are assayed by their enzymatic conversion to an isotopically labeled derivative. The most frequently used source of isotope has been S-adenosylmethionine-C^{14} (SAM), a cofactor that donates a methyl-C^{14} group to a functional group whose structure depends on the enzyme being used. In the assays the reaction is carried out under conditions where the rate of product formed per unit of time is proportional to the initial substrate or drug concentration. A standard curve is prepared using carefully defined reaction conditions.

The procedures usually involve a purification step where the compound to be analyzed is freed from other potential substrates. After the incubation another purification step is frequently used to remove traces of other products as well as the S-adenosylmethionine-C^{14}. The extent of the purification varies depending on the enzyme specificity and the substrate.

A highly sensitive assay for histamine has been described (Snyder et al., 1966) in which histamine-N-methylase, isolated from guinea pig brain, is used to convert histamine to N-methyl-C^{14} histamine with S-adenosylmethionine-C^{14}. The specificity of this assay is based on the high substrate specificity of the enzyme for histamine and the selective extraction of the N-methylhistamine formed into chloroform. Other possible substrates are not present in tissues or do not yield products extractable into chloroform from alkaline solution. A simple purification of the tissue extract is required primarily to remove tissue S-adenosylmethionine, since the specific activity of the methylating cofactor is the basis of the quantitation. In the assay procedure, a sample of boiled tissue extract is incubated with methylating enzyme and C^{14}-S-adenosylmethionine. After incubation the formed methylhistamine is extracted into chloroform and counted. One problem encountered with this enzyme was a nonlinear standard curve, reflecting different rate constants for the reaction at different substrate levels. This problem was solved with a double isotope technique in which small amounts of H^3-histamine were carried through the assay as an internal standard. Levels of histamine in a variety of rat tissues and various parts of the frog brain were determined by this procedure and were found to compare favorably with those determined by the fluorometric procedure of SHORE et al. (1959). The sensitivity of this enzymatic assay is 2 ng histamine per 25 μl of tissue homogenate.

An enzymatic assay for acetylcholine has been described by FEIGENSON and SAELENS (1969). Their assay involves the hydrolysis of acetylcholine and reacetylation of the choline formed with acetyl-CoA-C^{14} and cholineacetylase followed by isolation of the product. This assay requires the complete removal of choline before the initial hydrolysis of the acetylcholine. By operating on a micro scale, it were possible to use paper electrophoresis to isolate the acetylcholine both before the hydrolysis step and after acetylation of choline with labeled acetyl-CoA. This method has been used for measurement of acetylcholine levels in various areas of mouse brain, since only 20 μl of tissue extract was needed. However, the concentration of acetylcholine in the 20 μl sample must be at least 0.4 μg/ml.

More recently, REID and co-workers (1970) have developed an enzymatic assay for acetylcholine in which the neurohormone is isolated by high voltage paper electrophoresis, hydrolyzed to choline, enzymatically phosphorylated to labeled phosphorylcholine by choline phosphokinase and ATP^{32}, and the P^{32}-phosphorylcholine isolated by column chromatography. The choline phosphokinase, partially purified from a homogenate of Ehrlich's ascites tumor cells, is stable at —5° C. The method is able to measure as little as 0.003 μg of acetylcholine or choline in 70 mg of brain tissue and can be applied to larger numbers of tissue samples.

Several different enzymatic assays for norepinephrine have been reported. The first method (SAELENS et al., 1967) utilizes the enzyme phenylethanolamine-N-methyl transferase (PMT) (Table 1). In this procedure a small volume (15 μl) of tissue extract was incubated with enzyme and S-adenosylmethionine C^{14}. The reaction products were separated by paper chromatography and the resulting C^{14}-epinephrine counted. The small volumes used in this assay permitted the separate analysis of different parts of the mouse brain. The specificity of the method is due in part to the relative values of the Michaelis constants for possible substrates. The K_m for norepinephrine is 9.1×10^{-6}M (SAELENS et al., 1967), and the values for other phenethanol amines are all greater than 10^{-4}. As the tissue concentrations of these other amines are about 10^{-5}M, norepinephrine is the predominant amine methylated under the conditions of the incubation. Paper chromatography was used to separate the epinephrine-C^{14} formed from other radioactive materials such as SAM. With added epinephrine as carrier, the recovery of added norepinephrine was quantitative.

ENGELMAN and co-workers (1968) have reported an enzymatic assay using catechol-O-methyltransferase (COMT) (Fig. 1). This method measures norepinephrine and epinephrine together in plasma and urine by converting the catecholamines to their O-methyl ethers, which are then oxidized to toluene-extractable vanillin derivatives, i.e.,

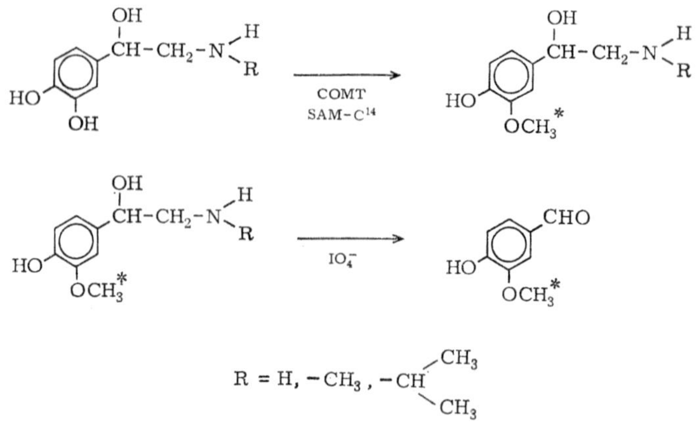

Fig. 1

Table 1. *Substrate requirements for methylating enzymes*

1. Catechol-O-methyl transferase (COMT)
Source--Rat liver,

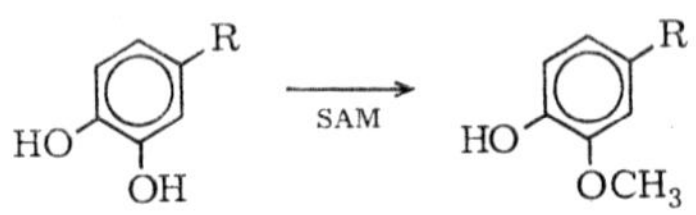

(Axelrod and Tomchick, 1958)

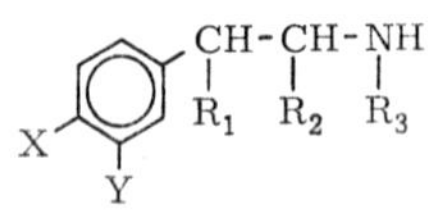

X	Y	R_1	R_2	R_3	Relative efficiency at substrate concentration of 10^{-4} M
OH	OH	OH	H	CH_3	100
OH	OH	OH	H	H	106
OH	OH	H	H	H	110
OH	OH	H	COOH	H	90
OH	OH	H	H	CH_3	105
OH	OH	OH	CH_3	H	100
OH	OH	H	CH_3	H	110
OH	H	OH	H	CH_3	0
H	OH	OH	H	$(CH_3)_2$	0
OH	H	H	CH_3	H	0
OH	H	OH	CH_3	CH_3	0
OH	H	H	COOH	H	0
OH	H	H	H	H	0
Catechol					160

In the determination of the catecholamines in urine, the catecholamines were first adsorbed onto a cationic exchange resin, washed, and eluted. The eluate, containing concentrated amines, was then subjected to the methylation and oxidation.

Table 1 (Continued)

2. Phenol-O-methyltransferase
   Source--Rabbit liver microsomes

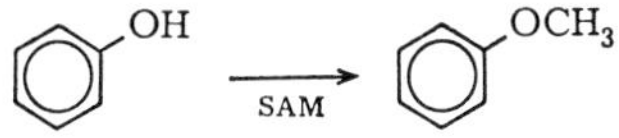

(Axelrod and Daly, 1968)

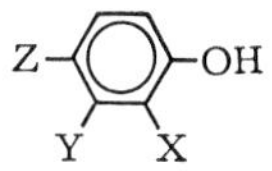

X	Y	Z	Relative efficiency at substrate concentration of 10^{-3} M	Relative levels of enzyme	
H	H	H	100	Guinea Pig	48
H	H	Cl	150	Mouse	27
H	Cl	H	140	Rabbit	15
Cl	H	H	62	Rat	9
H	Br	H	80		
H	NO_2	H	40		
H	H	CH_3	160		
H	CH_3	H	80		
CH_3	H	H	7.5		
H	H	Et	110		
H	H	H			
H	H	N-$COCH_3$	60		
OCH_3	H	H	70		
H	OCH_3	H	100		
H	H	OCH_3	30		
Tyramine			0		
a-Methyltyramine			0		
2,6-Dichlorophenol			0		

The specificity of the assay is based on the substrate requirements of COMT and the *β*-hydroxyl group required for the periodate oxidation. The substrate specificity of the enzyme was examined by AXELROD and TOMCHICK (1958) and, as seen in Table 1, the enzyme methylates all catechols. However, all but *β*-hydroxylated amines are eliminated by the removal of non-basic compounds by ion exchange, followed by reaction with periodate which selectively oxidizes the *β*-hydroxylated amines to neutral compounds which can be extracted with toluene. The major interfering substances observed were *a*-methyl-*l*-norepinephrine and *d,l*,-isoproterenol, both of which appear only after drug administration. Recovery of the catecholamines is monitored by the addition of tracer amounts of H^3-NE to the urine or plasma in the initial step of the assay.

COMT was also utilized by NIKODIJEVIC and co-workers (1969) for the analysis of norepinephrine in heart tissue. In this procedure, an acid extract of tissue was incubated with COMT and S-adenosylmethionine-C^{14} and the methylated catecholamines extracted directly into organic solvents for counting. This method does not distinguish between the catecholamines and is satisfactory for norepinephrine in the heart only because it is the sole catecholamine present in significant levels (UDENFRIEND, 1962, p. 158). The brains of rats and guinea pigs contain high levels of dopamine and the adrenal glands contain high levels of epinephrine, so this assay is not suitable for these tissues. Coupling the assay with a chromatographic separation of products as the authors suggest should provide the desired specificity.

Table 1 (Continued)

3. Polyphenol-O-transmethylase
Source--Streptomyces - timosus
Reaction

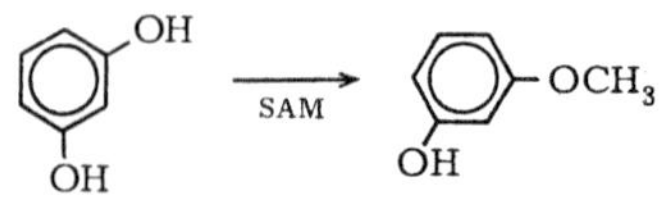

(Gatenbeck and Brunsberg, 1964)

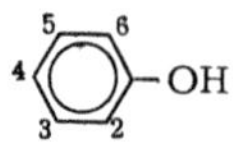

2	3	4	5	6	Relative efficiency at substrate concentration of 5×10^{-4}M
H	OH	H	H	H	100
H	OH	Cl	H	H	120
OH	H	H	H	H	140
OH	CH_3	H	H	H	98
OH	H	CHO	H	H	245
OH	OH	H	H	H	200
OH	OCH_3	H	H	H	140
OCH_3	OH	H	H	H	500
OH	OH	CH_3CO	H	H	190
OH	OH	H	Et	H	130

All of the three methods described are highly sensitive. The PMT assay can analyze levels of NE of 1 ng in a volume of 15 μl or a concentration of 0.07 μg/ml. The COMT assay of ENGELMAN et al. (1968) has a lower limit of 1 ng in 100 λ sample or 10 ng/ml. The method of NIKODIJEVIC is sensitive to 0.3 μg NE. However, the fluorometric analysis of catecholamines has comparable sensitivity and the fluorescence is more specific for each compound. For example, levels of 5 ng of norepinephrine in 1 ml can be assayed with fluorescence techniques (LAVERTY and TAYLOR, 1968). One advantage of the enzymatic methods is in the capability they provide for the analysis of small pieces of tissue (SAELENS et al., 1967).

COMT and S-adenosylmethionine have also been used to analyze urine and plasma for 3,4-dihydroxymandelic acid (SATO and DE QUATTRO, 1969), an oxidative metabolite of norepinephrine and epinephrine. Catechol derivatives are separated from the urine or tissue extract by adsorption onto alumina columns. After elution the catechol acids are selectively extracted into ethyl acetate. After evaporation of ethyl acetate the catechol acid is converted to its O-methyl-C^{14} ether, and subsequently oxidatively degraded to vanillin for extraction and counting (Fig. 2).

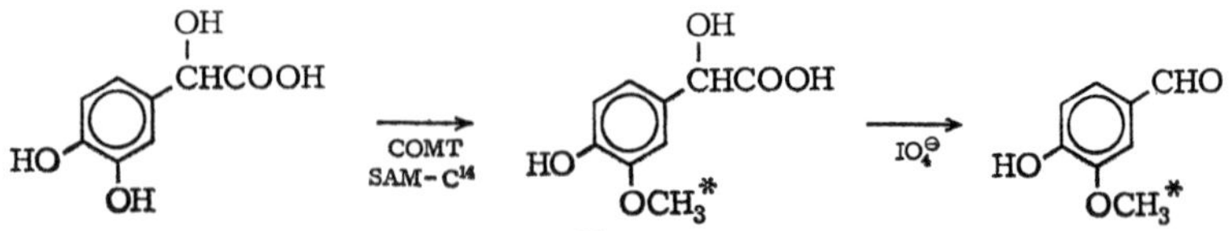

Fig. 2

Because of the lack of specificity of the methylation reaction, the dihydroxymandelic acid was separated from the catechol amines by extraction with ethylacetate before methylation and oxidation. The assay is sensitive to levels of

Table 1 (Continued)

4. Phenylethanolamine-N-methyltransferase (PMT)
Source--Rabbit Adrenal.

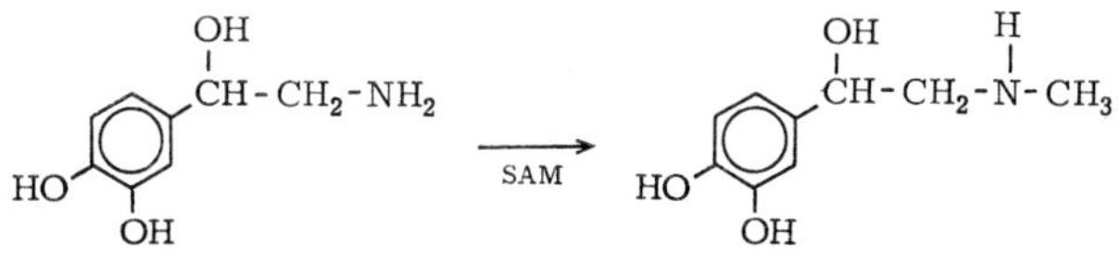

(Axelrod, 1962)

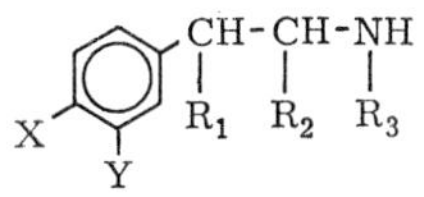

X	Y	R_1	R_2	R_3	Enan-tiomen	Relative efficiency at substrate concen-tration of 10^{-3} M
OH	OCH_3	OH	H	H	—	100
OH	OCH_3	H	H	H	—	0
H	H	OH	H	H	—	72
H	H	H	H	H	—	0
OH	H	OH	H	H	—	18
OH	H	H	H	H	—	0
H	OH	OH	H	H	—	60
OH	OH	OH	H	H	(l)	21
OH	OH	OH	H	H	(d)	15
OH	OH	H	H	H	—	0
OH	OCH_3	OH	H	CH_3	—	4
OH	OH	OH	H	CH_3	(l)	4
H	OH	OH	H	CH_3	—	20
H	H	OH	H	H	(l)	14
H	H	H	CH_3	H	(dl)	0
OH	H	OH	CH_3	H	(dl)	18
OH	OH	OH	H	H	(dl)	18
Tryptamine						0
Serotonin						0

10—20 ng per 50 ml sample, and levels of dihydroxymandelic acid in human urine and plasma as well as animal hearts may be determined by this method.

Phenylethanolamine N-methyltransferase was also used with S-adenosyl-methionine^{14}C to assay octopamine (Molinoff and Axelrod, 1969, Fig. 3). In this

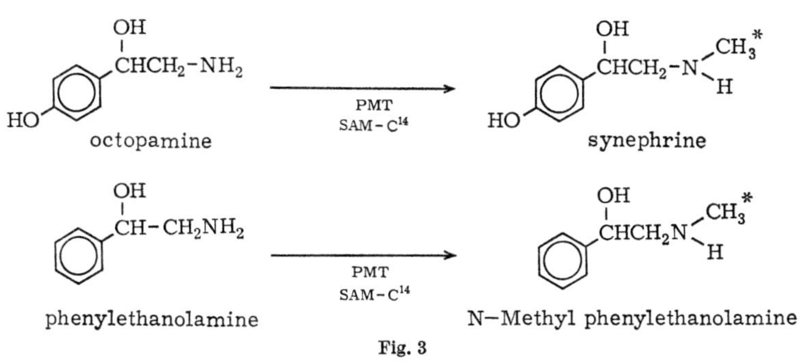

Fig. 3

Table 1 (Continued)

5. Tyramine methylphorase
Source--Barley seedlings

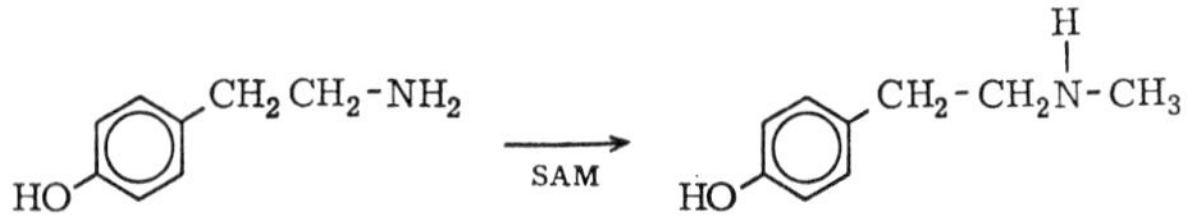

(Mann and Mudd, 1963).

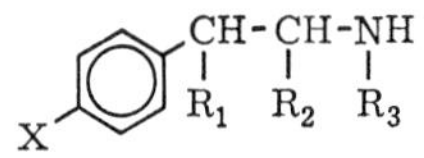

X	R_1	R_2	R_3	Relative efficiency at substrate concentration of 5×10^{-4} M
OH	H	H	H	100
OH	H	CH_3	H	53
OH	OH	H	H	6
OH	H	H	CH_3	2
H	H	H	H	108
H	OH	H	H	23
Cl	H	H	H	28
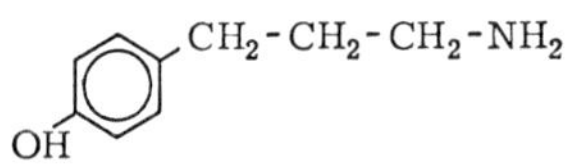				0
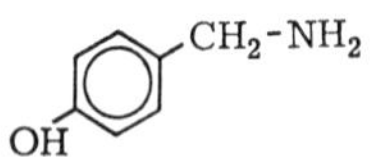				0

method the supernatant from a boiled tissue homogenate was incubated with PMT and S-adenosylmethionine. The reaction mixture was extracted with a toluene-amyl alcohol mixture at pH 10 to remove the synephrine while keeping epinephrine in the aqueous phase. The toluene-amyl alcohol extract was then evaporated and counted. Analysis of the toluene-amyl alcohol extract by thin-layer chromatography revealed that some dimethylation had occurred, but it did not affect the assay. The method was used to determine levels of octopamine in sympathetically innervated tissues before and after monoamine oxidase inhibition. This method can detect 1 ng octopamine in 1 ml of tissue homogenate.

Phenylethanolamine was assayed by a slight modification of the octopamine procedure (Molinoff et al., 1969). Lacking a phenolic hydroxyl group, phenylethanolamine is more volatile but less polar than octopamine so the evaporation step of the assay was eliminated and 3% amyl alcohol in toluene was used for the extraction of the methylated product instead of the 20% amyl alcohol toluene solution used for octopamine. The methylation product of octopamine was not extractable into this less polar toluene solution.

Most of the enzymes used in these assays have general substrate requirements (Table 1) so steps must be taken to assure the specificity of the assay. The fraction of the reaction mixture to be counted must be examined to identify the radioactivity as coming from the substrate being analyzed. Chromatographic procedures are most frequently used for this purpose. The specificity of the assay should be

Table 1 (Continued)

6. Indole (ethyl)amine-N-methyltransferase
Source--Chick brain

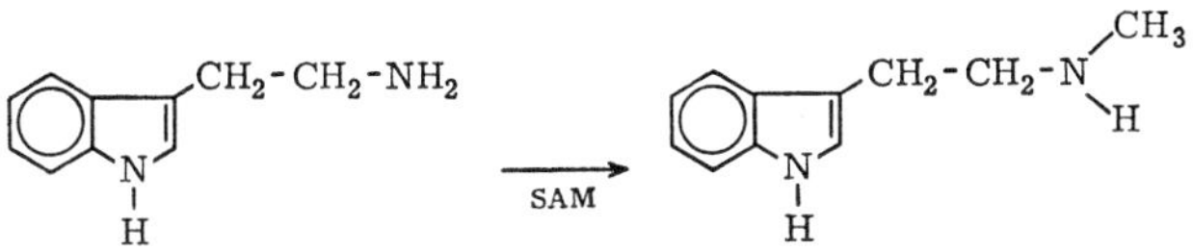

(Morgan and Mandell, 1969)

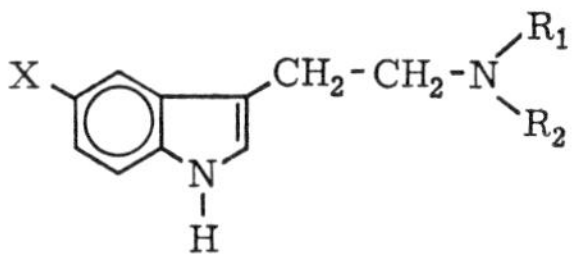

X	R_1	R_2	Relative efficiency at substrate concentration of 10^{-2} M
OH	H	H	100
OCH_3	H	H	88
H	H	H	60
H	H	CH_3	47
OH	CH_3	CH_3	0

7. Indoleamine-N-methylase
Source--Rabbit lung

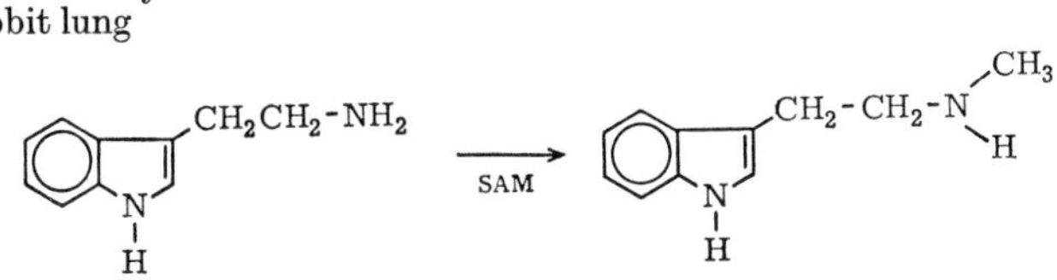

(Axelrod, 1961)

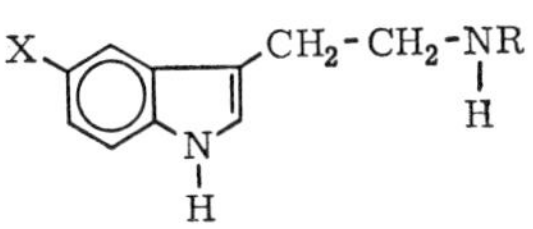

X	R	Relative efficiency at substrate concentration of 10^{-3} M
OH	H	100
OH	CH_3	70
H	H	90
OH	CH_3	25

established for each tissue, since levels of interfering substances can vary with tissue (e.g. COMT assay of NIKODIJEVIC). The effect of drugs on the specificity of the assay should also be considered. For example, amphetamine and p-hydroxyamphetamine form significant levels of α-methyloctopamine (p-hydroxynorephedrine), also a substrate of phenethanolanine methyltransferase. If octopamine were being assayed after administration of either of these compounds, errors could result from the extraction of the N-methylated hydroxynorephedrine.

The enzymes used in these assays are readily available. COMT is purified from the soluble fraction of rat liver by ammonium sulfate precipitation techniques (Axelrod and Tomchick, 1958). Phenethanolamine N-methyl transferase (PMT) has been purified from rabbit adrenal tissue by ammonium sulfate precipitation (Saelens et al., 1967). PMT is now commercially available[1] but is contaminated with a monoamine oxidase and therefore a monoamine oxidase inhibitor is routinely added to the reaction mixture.

Other enzymes that alkylate substrates with S-adenosylmethionine have been reported (Mudd and Cantoni, 1964). The substrate specificity of those enzymes that might act on pharmacological agents are listed in Table 1. In all cases the data reflect relative effectiveness at one substrate concentration, not at the optimum concentration for each compound tested.

III. Enzymatic Assays with Drugs as Inhibitors

Drugs such as the anticholinesterases in very low concentrations have been shown to inhibit enzymes and this feature has been used in their analysis. The anticholinesterase insecticides, which are generally organic esters of phosphoric acid, are analyzed with acetylcholinesterase. These compounds are readily separated from tissue components by extraction into organic solvents; the organic extract is then analyzed for its ability to inhibit the hydolysis of acetylcholine by cholinesterase (Giang, 1963). Since the compounds are non-competitive inhibitors of the enzyme the inhibition is not reversed by excess substrate. The specificity of this assay is based on the solubility of the insecticides in organic solvents. Cholinesterase is inhibited by a variety of compounds ranging from tetramethylammonium ion to organic phosphate esters and care must be taken to insure that the only substance inhibiting the enzymes is the agent being analyzed. The organic solvents do not extract most tissue constituents which could interfere in enzymatic reactions. Giang measured the hydrolysis of acetylcholine manometrically in a Warburg apparatus but constant pH titrations have also been employed to follow the hydrolysis rate and are more convenient (e.g. Cho et al., 1962). The sensitivity of this method permits the assay of 3 ng in a 6 ml reaction volume.

The inhibitory action of DDT on carbonic anhydrase has been used in an assay for DDT (Keller, 1963). This substance is a potent noncompetitive inhibitor of the enzyme at levels of 10 ng/ml. The high liposolubility of DDT is used to make the assay specific, i.e., the insecticide is extracted into an organic solvent, the solvent evaporated and the residue analyzed for inhibitory action. A manometric method was used to follow enzymatic activity but more recently a convenient spectrophotometric method has been described in which the hydrolysis of *p*-nitrophenylacetate by the enzyme is used to monitor inhibition (Armstrong et al., 1966). These workers also point out that acetazolamide (5-acetamido-1,3,4,-thiadiazole-2-sulfonamide) is a noncompetitive inhibitor of carbonic anhydrase with a K_i of 3×10^{-7}M. This inhibitory constant should permit the analysis of very low concentrations of this drug.

The inhibition of enzymes is classified as competitive or non-competitive, depending on the effect of varying the substrate concentration. The sensitivity of an assay for non-competitive inhibitors is independent of the concentration of the substrate. In the examples above, the inhibition is noncompetitive and occurs at

---

1 Gallard-Schlesinger Chemical Manufacturing Corporation, 584 Mineola Avenue, Carle Place, Long Island, New York 11514.

inhibitor concentrations of about 10^{-6}M. The enzyme monoamine oxidase is also noncompetitively inhibited by some of its inhibitors (FULLER, 1968) at concentrations of 10^{-6} to 10^{-8}M, and might be used for analytical purposes. Irreversible monoamine oxidase inhibitors such as iproniazid (isonicotinic acid 2-isopropylhydrazide) and pargyline (methyl propargylbenzylamine) could be assayed with this enzyme since they are effective at concentrations of 10^{-6} to 10^{-8}M.

In contrast, the sensitivity of an assay for competitive inhibitors depends on the substrate concentration used in the assay, since a high substrate concentration will prevent the competitive inhibitor from binding to the enzyme. This type of inhibition is the basis of a recently described isotope dilution assay for adenosine and guanosine-3′,5′-cyclic monophosphate (BROOKER et al., 1968) in which the rate of enzymatic hydrolysis of cyclic phosphate-H^3 of known specific activity is measured after the addition of an unknown quantity of carrier cyclic phosphate. The unlabeled substrate acts as a competitive inhibitor of the hydrolysis of labeled substrate and the reaction is followed by determining the amount of labeled nucleotide formed. The cyclic monophosphate is hydrolyzed in two steps, catalyzed by brain phosphodiesterase (I) and snake venom 5′-nucleotidase (II) (Fig. 4).

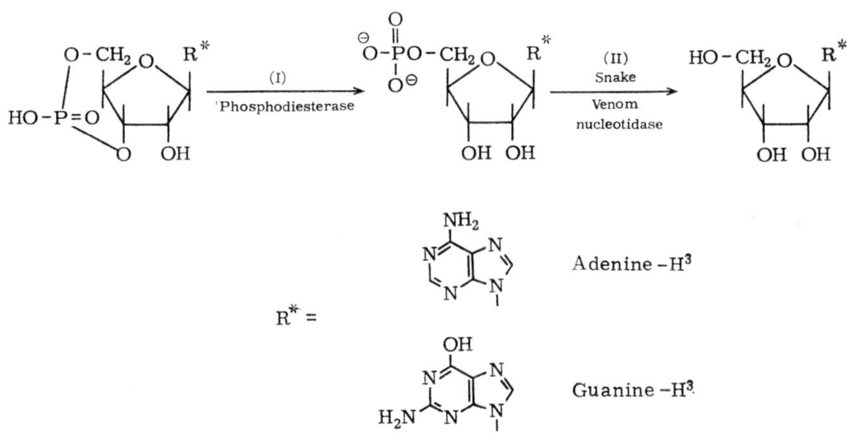

Fig. 4

In the procedure, carrier cyclic phosphate, isolated from tissue, is added to a standard incubation mixture containing labeled cyclic phosphate. The two enzymes remove the phosphate group, converting the strongly acidic nucleotide to the weakly basic nucleoside. The reactions are carried out in a counting vial and stopped by the addition of anionic exchange resin. The unreacted phosphate nucleotide is absorbed by the resin while the formed nucleoside remains in solution where it is counted after addition of scintillation phosphor.

The rat brain phosphodiesterase (I) is the rate limiting enzyme since only 30% of the substrate is hydrolyzed in the incubation. The snake venom nucleotidase (II) converts all of the 5′-monophosphate formed to the corresponding nucleoside which does not adsorb onto the anion exchange resin because of its very weak acidic properties. The phosphodiesterase has two K_m values for 3′,5′-cyclic AMP, 10^{-4} and 10^{-6}M; the lower K_m is used in the assay. There is only one K_m for 3′,5′-cyclic GMP, about 5×10^{-6}M. Phosphodiesterase is purified by an ammonium sulfate precipitation of a 30,000 $\times$ g supernate from rat brain homogenate (BROOKER, et al., 1968). Snake venom, the source of the 5′ nucleotidase, is commercially available. A standard curve relating dpm to the amount of added carrier nucleotide is used and the technique is sensitive to concentrations of 10^{-7}M nucleotide. The method has been used to measure the cyclic AMP content of skeletal muscle, where levels of 40×10^{-12} moles/50 mg tissue were assayed.

This type of analytical method is rapid, highly sensitive and precise but has limitations in its applicability. The enzyme for such an assay must have a low K_m and labeled substrate must be available with high specific activity. Because of the dilution in the assay the lower practical concentration limit of the unknown is about 0.1 the K_m value of the enzyme. As the method is based on an apparent competitive inhibition the K_m values must be known and the assay performed with substrates at concentrations in the vicinity of the K_m or above.

Newsholme and Taylor (1968) have used this same principle to assay serum glycerol with glycerol kinase. This enzyme has a K_m for glycerol of 4.6×10^{-5}M and serum glycerol concentrations as low as 7 μM were assayed by their procedure.

The inhibition of histidine decarboxylase has been used to analyze plasma levels of the inhibitors, brocresine (4-bromo-3-hydroxybenzyloxy amine) and MK 785 (*D*-2-hydrazino-3-4 (5) imidazoleproprionic acid) (Wustrack and Levine, 1969). The mechanism of the inhibition has not been defined but under a selected set of conditions the inhibition was proportional to inhibitor concentration over 0.1—50 μM. In the procedure 0.8 ml of plasma is incubated directly with histidine decarboxylase prepared from whole fetal rats. Since untreated plasma has no inhibitory action it was assumed that the inhibition was due to the administrated drug. No attempt was made to eliminate metabolites with inhibitory activity. Levels of activity corresponding to 0.05 μM (about 10 ng/ml) were detected in plasma.

IV. Competitive Protein Binding Analysis

Recently, the high affinity of certain plasma proteins for nonpeptide hormones has been utilized to analyze for these hormones and structurally related compounds (Murphy, 1964). While no chemical modifications of the bound molecules occur, the specificity and nature of the binding is analogous to the interaction of an enzyme and its substrate. The displacement of labeled hormone by added nonlabeled steroid is the basis for the assay.

There are globulins in plasma which bind thyroxine and cortisol with a high affinity (Desgrez and De Traverse, 1966). These proteins, called thyroxin binding globulin (TBG) and cortisol binding globulin (CBG), are involved in the transport of the hormones and, because of their high affinity for their ligand, maintain very low levels of the free hormones in the plasma. The affinity constant of TBG for thyroxine has been estimated to be about 10^9 and the affinity constant of CBG for cortisol is about 10^7. The protein bound hormone is in readily reversible equilibrium since exchange of labeled hormone for carrier occurs *in vitro* within a minute. This exchange is utilized in the assay.

The procedure consists of separation of the hormone from tissue by extraction into organic solvent, evaporation of the solvent, and the addition of a solution of tritiated steroid-protein complex to the residue. After equilibration is attained, the non-bound steroid is separated from the bound by a variety of different methods and the radioactivity bound to protein is determined. The loss in bound radioactivity is proportional to the amount of added steroid and the quantitation is based on a standard curve.

Different techniques have been used for the separation of free from bound steroid. Initially, an equilibrium dialysis procedure was used, but this was changed in favor of the more rapid gel filtration procedure. Although the cortisol-CBG complex is sufficiently stable to withstand gel filtration, not all steroids have such a high affinity. Peets et al. (1969) have shown that the testosterone-protein complex is decomposed on Sephadex. Other adsorbing materials such as Fullers' earth, Florisil, and charcoal coated with a dextran have been employed for the separation of bound from free steroid.

The sensitivity of the method is in the nanogram range and it utilizes 10—100 μl of solution for the analysis. In a comparison with the double isotope assay for cortisol, BOWMAN and DELŪNA (1968) found the competitive binding analysis to be statistically indistinguishable and the method of choice for cortisol analysis because of its rapidity and simplicity. SNART (1969) used the binding assay to determine the binding capacity and endogenous steroid levels of human plasma.

The protein source for these assays can be unfractionated plasma or the commercially available rabbit α-globulin (BOWMAN and DELŪNA, 1968). The compounds that have been assayed by this technique are shown in Table 2.

Table 2. *Displacement analysis of steroid hormones and thyroxin*

Compound analyzed	Compound displaced	Ref.
Hydrocortisone	Cortisol-^{3}H	(A)
	Corticosterone-^{3}H	(A)
Progesterone	Corticosterone-^{3}H	(A)
17-hydroxyprogesterone	Corticosterone-^{3}H	(A)
Corticosterone	Corticosterone-^{3}H	(A)
Cortisone	Corticosterone-^{3}H	(A)
Thyroxin	Thyroxin-^{131}I	(D, F)
Testosterone	Estradiol-^{3}H	(B, C.)
Testosterone	Testosterone-^{3}H	(C, F.)

(A) (MURPHY, 1967); (B) (PIZARRO and ARRENDONDO, 1969); (C) (ROSENFIELD et al., 1969); (D) (SPARAGANA et al., 1969); (F) (MURPHY and PATTEE, 1964); (F) (HEYNS et al., 1969).

As many drugs displace each other from plasma proteins (BRODIE, 1966), this type of assay might be used to quantitate drugs also. SOLOMON and co-workers (1968) have demonstrated competitive binding on albumin between labeled phenylbutazone and warfarin, tolbutamide, indomethacin, sulfomethoxypyridine, and chlorphenoxyisobutyric acid. The binding was followed by means of equilibrium dialysis since gel filtration separates the bound drug from the protein. Since warfarin can be determined fluorometrically (CORN and BERBERICH, 1967), however, the displacement of warfarin by the other drugs could be used to assay any of these drugs.

V. Conclusion

The use of enzymes as an analytical tool has been restricted primarily to the determination of natural substances and it is likely that the main use of this technique will be in the measurement of these compounds. The rapid quantitation of biogenic substances such as hormones and neurohormonal agents in tissues and body fluids is a vital step in the understanding of the mechanism of action of drugs. Biogenic substances are often highly reactive, polar compounds that are readily oxidized and difficult to extract into organic solvents. Therefore, enzymatic assays that analyze only specific chemicals in partially purified aqueous tissue extracts are of great value.

The isotope dilution in the competitive substrate assay for cyclic nucleotides has been useful in the analysis of small quantities of this biogenic material. The previous methods of analysis for cyclic 3′,5′-AMP were extremely complicated and time consuming. As the analysis becomes more rapid, more information on the dynamics of this important chemical can be obtained.

Enzymatic methods might also be used for the analysis of drug metabolites since these materials occur in small quantities and are difficult to extract into organic solvents because of their polarity. As seen in Table 1, the substrate requirements for many of the enzymes are sufficiently general that many drugs or drug metabolites may be potential substrates (see Shapiro and Schlenk, 1965). The isotope derivative technique is adaptable for work on a microscale and permits the use of small samples of tissues. Microtechniques for extraction and paper partition techniques for the separation of substrates and products can be used to impart the desired specificity to the assay.

References

Armstrong, J. McD., Myers, D.V., Verpoorte, J.A., Edsall, J.T.: Purification and properties of human erythrocyte carbonic anhydrases. J. biol. Chem. **241**, 5137—5149 (1966).

Axelrod, J.: Enzymatic formation of psychotomimetic metabolites from normally occurring compounds. Science **134**, 343 (1961).

— Purification and properties of phenylethanolamine-N-methyl transferase. J. biol. Chem. **237**, 1657—1660 (1962).

— Daly, J.: Phenol-O-methyltransferase. Biochim. biophys. Acta (Amst.) **159**, 472—478 (1968).

— Tomchick, R.: Enzymatic O-methylation of epinephrine and other catechols. J. biol. Chem. **233**, 702—705 (1958).

Bergmeyer, H.V.: Methods of Enzymatic Analysis. New York: Academic Press 1963.

Bowman, R.E., DeLüna, R.F.: Assessment of a protein binding method for cortisol determination. Analyt. Biochem. **26**, 461—469 (1968).

Brodie, B.B.: In: Transport Function of Plasma Proteins (P. Desgrez and P.M. DeTraverse, ed.). Amsterdam/London, N.Y.: Elsevier Publishing Co. 1966.

Brooker, G., Thomas, L.J., jr., Appleman, M.M.: The assay of adenosine 3′,5′-cyclic monophosphate and guanosine 3′,5′-monophosphate in biological materials by enzymatic radioisotope displacement. Biochemistry **7**, 4177—4181 (1968).

Cho, A.K., Haslett, W.L., Jenden, D.J.: The peripheral actions of oxotremorine, a metabolite of tremorine. J. Pharmacol. exp. Ther. **138**, 249—257 (1962).

Corn, M., Berberich, R.: Rapid fluorometric assay for plasma warfarin. Clin. Chem. **13**, 126—131 (1967).

Desgrez, P., DeTraverse, P.M.: Transport Function of Plasma Proteins. Amsterdam/London, N.Y.: Elsevier Publishing Co. 1966.

Engelman, K.B., Portnoy, B., Lovenberg, W.: A sensitive and specific double-isotope derivative method for the determination of catecholamines in biological agreements. Amer. J. med. Sci. **285**, 259—269 (1968).

Feigenson, M.E., Saelens, J.K.: An enzyme assay for acetylcholine. Biochem. Pharmacol. **18**, 1479—1486 (1969).

Fuller, R.W.: Kinetic studies and effects *in vivo* of a new monoamine oxidase inhibitor, N-[2-(O-chlorophenoxy)-ethyl]-cyclopropylamine. Biochem. Pharmacol. **17**, 2097—2106 (1968).

Gatenbeck, S., Brunsberg, U.: A polyphenol-O-transmethylase isolated from *Streptomyces rimosus*. Acta chem. scand. **18**, 2061—2068 (1964).

Giang, P.A.: Organophosphorus Insecticides. In: Methods of Enzymatic Analysis (H.U. Bergmeyer). New York: Academic Press 1963.

Heyns, W., Verhoeven, G., van Baelen, H., De Moor, P.: Measurement of testosterone in plasma by competitive protein binding. Ann. Endocr. (Paris) **30**, 153—158 (1969).

Keller, H.: Di(p-Chlorphenyl)trichloroesthane (DDT). In: Methods of Enzymatic Analysis (H.V. Bergmeyer, ed.), pp. 626—632. New York: Academic Press 1963.

Laverty, R., Taylor, T.M.: The fluorometric assay of catecholamines and related compounds. Improvements and extensions to the hydroxyindole technique. Analyt. Biochem. **22**, 269—279 (1968).

Mann, J.D., Mudd, S.H.: Alkaloids and Plant Metabolism. IV. The tyramine methylphorase of barley roots. J. biol. Chem. **238**, 381—385 (1963).

Molinoff, P., Axelrod, J.: Octopamine. Normal occurrence in sympathetic nerves of rats. Science **164**, 428—429 (1969).

MOLINOFF, P.B., LANDSBERG, L., AXELROD, J.: An enzymatic assay for octopamine and other β-hydroxylated phenylethylamines. J. Pharmacol. exp. Ther. **170**, 253—261 (1969).
MORGAN, M., MANDELL, A.J.: Indol(Ethyl)amine N-methyltransferase in the brain. Science **165**, 492 (1969).
MUDD, S.H., CANTONI, G.L.: Group transfer reactions (7). Biological transmethylation, methyl group neogenisis and other "one carbon" metabolic reactions dependent on tetrahydrofolic acid. Comprehensive Biochemistry. Vol. 15, p. 1. Ed. by H. FLORKIN and E.H. STOTZ. Amsterdam: Elsevier Publishing Co. 1964.
MURPHY, B.E.P.: Application of the property of protein binding to the assay of minute quantities of hormones and other substances. Nature (Lond.) **201**, 679—681 (1964).
— Some studies of the protein binding of steroids and their application to the routine micro and ultramicro measurement of various steroids in body fluids by competitive protein-binding radio assay. J. clin. Endocr. **27**, 973—990 (1967).
— PATTEE, C.J.: Determination of thyroxine utilizing the property of protein binding. J. clin. Endocr. **24**, 187—196 (1964).
NEWSHOLME, E.A., TAYLOR, K.: A new principle for the assay of metabolites involving the combined effects of isotope dilution and enzymatic catalysis. Biochim. biophys. Acta (Amst.) **158**, 11—24 (1968).
NIKODIJEVIC, B.Z., DALY, J., CREVELING, C.R.: Catechol-O-methyltransferase. An enzymatic assay for cardiac norepinephrine. Biochem. Pharmacol. **18**, 1577—1584 (1969).
PEETS, E.A., STAUB, M., SYNCHOWICZ, S.: Plasma binding of beta-methanone-^{3}H, dexamethazone-^{3}H and cortisol-^{14}C. A comparative study. Biochem. Pharmacol. **18**, 1655—1663 (1969).
PIZARRO, M.A., ARRENDONDO, R.: Measurement of plasma testosterone by competitive protein binding. Ann. Endocr. (Paris) **30**, 159—164 (1969).
REID, W.D., HAUBRICH, D.R., KRISHNA, G.: An enzymatic radioassay for acetylcholine and choline in brain. Analyt. Biochem. (1970), in press.
ROSENFIELD, R.L., EBERLEIN, W.R., BONGIOVANNI, A.M.: Measurement of plasma testosterone by means of competitive protein binding analysis. J. clin. Endocr. **29**, 854—859 (1969).
SAELENS, J.K., SCHOEN, M.S., KOVACSICS, G.B.: An enzyme assay for norepinephrine in brain tissue. Biochem. Pharmacol. **16**, 1043—1049 (1967).
SATO, T., DE QUATTRO, V.: Enzymic assay for 3,4-dihydroxymandelic acid (DOMA) in human urine and tissues. J. Lab. clin. Med. **74**, 672—681 (1969).
SHAPIRO, S.K., SCHLENK, F.: Transmethylation and methionine. Biosynthesis. Chicago/Ill.: University of Chicago Press 1965.
SHORE, P.A., BURKHALTER, A., COHN, V.H.: A method for the fluorometric assay of histamine in tissue. J. Pharmacol. exp. Ther. **127**, 182—186 (1959).
SNART, R.S.: Determination of binding capacity and endogenous concentration of steroids. Biochem. J. **111**, 254—255 (1969).
SNYDER, S.H., BALDESSARINI, R.J., AXELROD, J.: A sensitive and specific enzymatic isotropic assay for tissue histamine. J. Pharmacol. exp. Ther. **153**, 544—549 (1966).
SOLOMON, H.M., SCHROGIE, J.J., WILLIAMS, D.: The displacement of phenylbutazone-^{14}C and warfarin-^{14}C from human albumin by various drugs and fatty acids. Biochem. Pharmacol. **17**, 143—151 (1968).
SPARAGANA, M., PHILLIPS, G., KUCERA, L.: Serum thyroxin by competitive protein binding analysis; clinical, statistical and comparative evaluation. J. clin. Endocr. **29**, 191—199 (1969).
UDENFRIEND, S.: Fluorescence assay in biology and medicine, p. 158. New York, N.Y.: Academic Press 1962.
WUSTRACK, K.O., LEVINE, R.J.: Assay of histidine decarboxylase inhibitors in human plasma. Biochem. Pharmacol. **18**, 2465—2471 (1969).

Chapter 29

Bioassay

MARTHE VOGT

With 2 Figures

Bioassays are looked upon by many as unspecific, inaccurate, tedious and exasperating to perform, not amenable to automation, obsolete and altogether superfluous in the age of scintillation counting, N.M.R., and gas-chromatography/mass-spectroscopy. The object of this article is to show which of these attributes are justified and which are mistaken. It will show that with the development of new techniques some substances drop out from the range of compounds for which bioassays are unavoidable, while new ones keep entering the field because no physical or chemical methods are known for the estimation of what are usually substances of great biological interest, occurring in tantalizingly small quantities.

There is no doubt that bioassays are often tedious and exasperating to perform, yet there are several reasons why pharmacologists and physiologists cannot dispense with them: one is that they often surpass in sensitivity the best available physical or chemical methods; another that they are at present the only methods known for the estimation of some compounds such as certain proteins, polypeptides and acids. Finally, they may be necessary for the detection of substances which are rapidly inactivated after release into the circulation. A special form of bioassay, the 'blood-bathed organ technique' was devised by VANE (1958) for this purpose. The technique and its applications have been reviewed (VANE, 1969).

The shift of compounds for which, at different times, bioassays were considered suitable is well illustrated by a toxicological monograph (FÜHNER, 1923) describing detection and estimation, on tissues or whole animals, of some 60 'poisonous' substances; very few of these 'bioassays' have survived, particularly since the development of chromatography; yet the possibility described by FÜHNER of detecting 1 ng of hyoscine on the frog heart, or eserine in a concentration of 10 ng g/ml on the dorsal muscle of the leech, might still be useful nowadays. Whereas FÜHNER used the leech muscle for the detection of eserine, the very same preparation is now used for estimating acetylcholine; this assay makes use of FÜHNER's (1917) observation that eserine greatly sensitizes the leech muscle to acetylcholine.

A. General Considerations

Before surveying the bioassays which, to the sorrow of those using them, have not yet been superseded by equally sensitive chemical methods, a few general remarks are required about their supposed lack of specificity, accuracy and amenability to automation.

I. Specificity

No chemical reaction used to measure a compound is specific; for example, the reduction of tetrazolium is used for the quantitative estimation by colorimetry of innumerable compounds, whose only common property is their ability to act as reducing agents. Furthermore, fluorescence, even within narrow bands of activating and emitted light, is usually not the property of a single substance, but of whole groups of more or less related substances. This, in fact, leads to the well-known phenomenon that the sensitivity of fluorimetric methods is more dependent on achieving low blanks than on the intensity of the fluorescence induced. The way to make any method specific is the same for chemical and biological estimations: purification of the material, be it tissue extract or body fluid, till all contaminants which might give the same final reaction have been removed. The more refined the physical methods are, the greater is the need for preliminary purification, as is well known from such methods as gas-chromatography or infrared spectroscopy. Errors may occur in bioassays if unsuspected compounds are contained in the material to be tested, but this is equally true of chemical estimations. The best check is to compare two methods which have as little as possible in common; and here identical results obtained by chemical and by biological means are particularly convincing because they usually depend on different properties of the molecules in question. Such a comparison has, for example, been used for the identification of adrenaline in brain (JUORIO and VOGT, 1970).

With the discovery of increasing numbers of drug antagonists the specificity of a bioassay is no longer dependent only on prior purification of the material. Drug antagonists are not completely specific in their action, and it is important to remember that the specificity is highest when the dose of the antagonist is smallest. If one uses the lowest concentration which will abolish or diminish the response to a dose of authentic agonist giving a response similar in size to that of

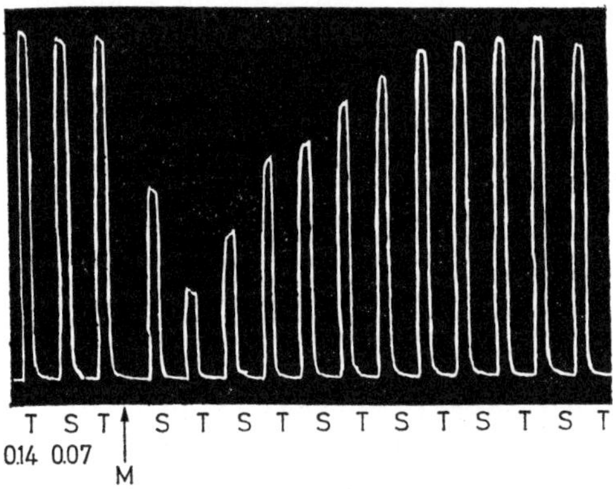

Fig. 1. Alternating doses of the histamine fraction from a urinary extract (T), and of histamine standard (S), which give identical responses on the guinea-pig ileum, are seen to become less effective after a single dose of 2 ng of mepyramine maleate (arrow M) and to recover activity at the same rate. (From ROBERTS and ADAM, 1950; by permission of Brit. J. Pharmacol.)

the unknown, then a *pari passu* reduction and recovery of the effects of the unknown and authentic compound are very strong support for their identity. Thus, in the assay of histamine (carried out in the presence of atropine to exclude the interference of choline esters) the histamine antagonist mepyramine is employed to show whether it reduces the effect of the unknown and of authentic histamine in parallel. The fact that the antagonism is reversible is helpful since its application does not terminate the experiment. Fig. 1 (ROBERTS and ADAM, 1950) illustrates the use of mepyramine in the identification of histamine in an extract of urine.

As pointed out in 1933 by CHANG and GADDUM, the specificity of bioassays is further enhanced if estimations are carried out on two or more different organs and can be shown to agree quantitatively. Thus discrepancies in the results of 'parallel assays' gave CANNON and URIDIL (1921) the idea that sympathin, the transmitter of impulses in what are now called adrenergic nerves, was not identical with adrenaline; and agreement in parallel assays against noradrenaline suggested to GADDUM and GOODWIN (1947) that sympathin might be noradrenaline.

II. Accuracy

The accuracy of bioassays can be calculated by standard statistical methods. It depends on the slope of the dose-response curve, the variability of tissue responses to the same dose of drug, and, to some extent, on the amount of material available for assay. It is often expressed by λ, the index of precision (standard error over slope). BOURA et al. (1954) have calculated the error of a histamine estimation done by the so-called four point-assay illustrated in Fig. 2. This consists of assaying

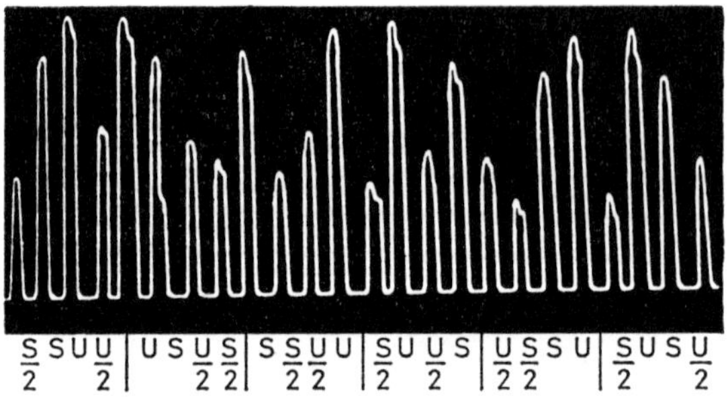

Fig. 2. S is a standard solution of histamine and U the unknown; both cause contractions of the ileum of the same order of magnitude. By giving S, U, 0.5 S and 0.5 U six times each in random order, six values for each dose are obtained and the potency of the unknown and the error of the estimation can be calculated. (From BOURA et al., 1954; by permission of Brit. J. Pharmacol.)

in random order, unknown and standard in two doses differing by a factor of 2. They found errors ranging between 3 and 10%. In contrast to this high accuracy, estimations of, for example, ACTH on quartered adrenals have errors which may occasionally exceed 50% (SAFFRAN and SCHALLY, 1955). Most bioassays have errors between these extremes. For assays with large errors it is useful to give the con fidence limits ($P > 0.05$) with every estimation.

III. Automation

When the assay is carried out either by immersing a piece of tissue in an organ bath or 'superfusing' it with a slow drip of fluid (in order to reduce the amount of material necessary to obtain a response), automatic machines can be used which give the required doses and carry out the washing of the tissue at suitable intervals. Such equipment reduces errors by guaranteeing accurate timing. It usually operates with the help of telephone relays which compress or release pieces of tubing connected to fluid reservoires. The early version described by SCHILD (1946) has been greatly elaborated (BOURA, et al., 1954). Figure 2 is a record obtained with this newer model. An arrangement suited for adrenaline assays on the rat uterus has been described by GADDUM and LEMBECK (1949), and the assay shown to have great accuracy (λ of 0.062); this is only slightly less than the λ of

0.043 for the assay of histamine discussed earlier. Furthermore, the authors show that parallel assays for the purpose of determining the proportion of adrenaline and noradrenaline in a mixture may be subject to great errors, and should be avoided if possible. A more accurate procedure in these circumstances will be discussed later.

When estimation is done on tissue suspended in air and 'superfused', a modified automatic machine may be used such as that described for histamine assays by ADAM et al. (1954). By superfusing the ileum instead of immersing it in a bath they increased the sensitivity of the method by a factor of 100 without loss of accuracy ($\lambda = 0.03$). Unfortunately the sensitivity of tissues towards many other agents is not spectacularly increased by superfusion.

It may be useful to recall three important rules governing the use of bioassay.

1. Assays of mixtures of active substances should be avoided unless the 'contaminant' can be safely inactivated by a potent antagonist which does not interfere with the action of the compound to be determined. Thus histamine can be assayed with impunity in a mixture containing acetylcholine and 5-hydroxytryptamine if atropine and bromolysergic acid diethylamide are present as antagonists. There is, however, no justification in assaying mixtures of related substances such as adrenaline and noradrenaline since the results are inaccurate and easy chromatographic methods exist to separate these substances. The same is true of mixtures of choline esters, or of histamine and its methyl derivatives, or of the different prostaglandins.

2. If enough material and apparently satisfactory chemical methods are available for the determination of a compound, it may still be desirable to check the chemical results by comparing them with a bioassay whenever the composition of the original material is not fully known. Thus certain procedures for the estimation of noradrenaline by fluorescence which give satisfactory results in some types of cerebral tissue, give erroneous results in others. If a check of the values ob tained by fluorimetry against results of a bioassay shows up discrepancies, it is usually possible to improve the purification of the extract before the fluorimetry is carried out, so that agreement between chemical and biological estimations is achieved (see SHARMAN and VOGT, 1965). Because such checks are not always made the literature contains many erroneously high figures for the noradrenaline content of certain parts of the brain which contain only traces of that amine.

3. In order to avoid unpleasant surprises, results of bioassays should, whenever possible, be checked for specificity by using an antagonist known to show good specificity. Figure 2 illustrates the use of a reversible antagonist for this purpose. If there is no readily reversible antagonist, the assay should be performed and then the experiment terminated by watching the effect of a more persistent antagonist, such as d-tubocurarine (for acetylcholine on leech preparation) or phentolamine (for noradrenaline on rat blood pressure) on the response to authentic and presumptive compound side by side. Phentolamine can also be used as an antagonist of the pressor action of adrenaline if the preparation has first been treated with a β-blocker such as pronethalol (see later).

B. Individual Assays

I. Assays Used on Grounds of Sensitivity or Specificity

When small quantities of *acetylcholine*, such as are released by nerve stimulation, have to be estimated, the use of FÜHNER's (1917) preparation, the eserinized dorsal muscle of the leech (*hirudo medicinalis*), is still unavoidable, although there is hope that radioactive techniques may supersede the bioassay. This assay is more sensitive and specific than that on the more rapidly contracting and therefore more convenient frog rectus abdominis. d-Tubocurarine as a selective antagonist of nicotinic responses to acetylcholine can be used to further increase specificity, and GADDUM's microbath to raise sensitivity (GADDUM, 1964; SZERB, 1961). STRAUGHAN (1958) described a more convenient assay utilizing the depressor effect of acetylcholine on the rat blood pressure; special tests of specificity are required and are explained in his article.

Histamine assays have been illustrated in the general section; the only problem of specificity is posed by biologically active derivatives, such as β-N-methyl-histamines. These can be separated from histamine by chromatography (ADAM and HYE, 1966).

The rat stomach preparation (VANE, 1957) detects single doses of as little as 0.05 ng *5-hydroxytryptamine*. At present it is the only method sensitive enough to detect the release of this amine from nervous tissue. Antagonists belonging to the group of lysergic acid derivatives are highly specific.

The most sensitive assay for *adrenaline* which lends itself to automation (GADDUM and LEMBECK, 1949) is on the rat uterus preparation; the tissue is stimulated by carbachol at regular intervals and the response temporarily decreased by the addition of adrenaline. The preparation is at least 75 times less sensitive to noradrenaline, so that it will determine adrenaline in a mixture of the two compounds without previous separation of the amines, provided the adrenaline contributes at least 10% to the total catecholamines. ARMIN and GRANT (1955) have described a more sensitive *in vivo* test for adrenaline on the rabbit's ear, but the experimental conditions are too exacting for routine purposes. A less sensitive, but much more rapid assay for adrenaline utilizes the pressor effect on the pithed rat. A single dose of 0.5—1.0 ng can be detected provided the rat has been injected with a drug which blocks the β-receptors. Thus a dose of pronethalol 2 mg/kg transforms the biphasic blood pressure response to adrenaline which has a very poor dose-response relationship to a pure pressor response with a good dose-response curve (VANOV and VOGT, 1963). Noradrenaline assays may be done on the same preparation; the sensitivity of the pressor response is almost identical for the two compounds. It is therefore obvious that preliminary separation of the two amines is essential; a convenient method of paper chromatography has been described (VOGT, 1952; for a summary of the procedures see also SHARMAN, in the press). Another bioassay of noradrenaline (DE LA LANDE and HARVEY, 1965) utilizes the vasoconstriction produced in a perfused segment of the rabbit ear artery. According to DE LA LANDE and GLOVER (1966) it detects concentrations down to 0.5 ng/ml, one ml being the smallest volume which will give a perceptible rise in perfusion pressure.

II. Assays Used for Confirmation of Biological Activity (Steroids)

Cortical hormones, androgens, oestrogens and progestins were all discovered by bioassay. However, for all steroidal substances of known chemical composition chemical or physical methods are now available which are far more sensitive, accurate and specific than bioassays. Thus bioassays of steroids are now used only to determine whether a new synthetic compound or a metabolite is biologically active. Methods can be found in the endocrinological literature.

III. Assays Used Because Chemical Methods are not yet Available

Like the substances dealt with in the previous sections, all compounds falling in this category were discovered by some form of bioassay. While the search for physical or chemical methods is going on, new active compounds are being discovered all the time.

The *prostaglandins* are unsaturated hydroxyacids which contract a variety of smooth muscles; some of them occur in the brain but their role in this and other tissues is still a matter of conjecture. They can be extracted by organic solvents and separated chromatographically from biologically active compounds belonging to other chemical groups: however, since the different prostaglandins have distinctive biological actions, but not all of them have a characteristic chromatographic behaviour, each member of a mixture must in the end be assayed biologically on one or several smooth muscle preparations. (For details see HORTON and THOMPSON, 1964; HORTON and MAIN, 1967; HORTON and JONES, 1969). It is to be hoped that gas chromatography will eventually replace this complicated procedure.

Certain *polypeptides* are among the most important compounds with strong biological action. Although they can be synthesized once their aminoacid sequence is known, methods of estimation are entirely biological. When these substances are used medicinally, they have to be assayed by methods specified by the diverse pharmacopoeias; these methods, which do not concern us here, are reviewed in DORFMAN (1969). The following examples will only be concerned with methods outside the framework of the pharmacopoeias.

By combining preliminary extraction with sensitive bioassay preparations, it has now become possible to follow accurately the secretion of *oxytocin* and *vasopressin* into the blood stream (BISSET et al., 1967a; BISSET et al., 1967b; BISSET et al., 1970). Oxytocin is detected by retrograde arterial injection into the mammary gland of the lactating rat, and vasopressin by the antidiuresis produced in the ethanol-anaesthetized hydrated rat. A new synthetic antagonist of oxytocin (1-N-carbamylhemicystine-20-methyltyrosine-oxytocin) has added to the specificity of the test. 5 μ units of oxytocin give a clear increase in milk-ejection pressure.

Angiotensin is a physiologically important polypeptide; its pressor effect on the rat blood pressure is adequate for its assay in pure solutions, but more specific and sensitive procedures are needed if its release into, and fate in, the blood stream are to be examined. A radioimmunoassay has been developed (BOYD et al., 1969) which can detect 0.04 ng angiotensin in plasma.

The polypeptides called *kinins* cause wound pain and contract uterine muscle but, in contrast to angiotensin, they dilate blood vessels. They are formed from precursors in plasma or tissue by enzymatic means as well as by simple procedures such as contact of plasma with glass or kaolin. The nonapeptide bradykinin contracts the rat uterus while relaxing the rat duodenum (HORTON, 1959), the smallest concentrations required being 10^{-10}M and 10^{-9}M respectively (KEELE, 1969); this combination of effects is highly specific and can be used to identify the material, particularly if it can also be shown to be depressor. In practice, the identity of a kinin will not be in doubt in experiments in which the factors controlling its formation are under investigation.

The polypeptide chains of *glucagon* and *parathyroid hormone* are larger than those of the peptides hitherto discussed; the aminoacid sequence is fully known only for glucagon. Both have been assayed by their principle physiological actions, e.g. glucagon by its elevation of blood glucose in cats, and parathyroid hormone by its hypercalcaemic action in dogs. None of these methods are sensitive or very specific, but suffice for assay of medicinal preparations. However, plasma concentration of both hormones can now be determined by radio-immunoassay (UNGER et al., 1961; UNGER et al., 1963; BERSON et al., 1963). The thresholds lie at 0.05 ng/ml for glucagon and 0.025—0.1 ng (0.15—0.6 m units) for parathyroid hormone. The method was originally devised for the assay of insulin (see below).

The bioassay of '*substance P*' (v. EULER and GADDUM, 1931) has had a checkered career. The structure of this polypeptide is only partially known, and its function is still obscure. At one time its potent vasodilator activity made it a candidate for the transmitter of impulses at sensory synapses. It was discovered by its depressor effect on rabbit blood pressure and its stimulation of rabbit intestine. Its distribution in tissue, i.e. in brain and gastro-intestinal tract, has usually been estimated by its power to contract the guinea-pig ileum; atropine and mepyramine are added to the bath to exclude the effects of acetylcholine and histamine (DOUGLAS et al., 1951). Usually 5-hydroxytryptamine is removed in the extraction procedure; if necessary the tissue can be desensitized to 5-hydroxytryptamine with the help of tryptamine. However, as shown by GADDUM (1961) and CLEUGH et al. (1964), assays of tissue extracts containing substance P on four different isolated tissues did not give concordant results. There might have been several reasons for this: the presence of other polypeptides in the extracts for which there were no known antagonists, and the fact that 'substance P' itself consists of more than one active compound. The authors concluded that assays on the guinea-pig ileum were more specific than estimations on other tissues, provided the antagonists listed above were present in the bath. GADDUM et al. (1964) also showed that a frequent contaminant of substance P which could be separated from it by chromatography on alumina had some anti-strychnine activity but had little effect on the guinea-pig ileum.

Very recently, convenient bioassays have been developed for small quantities of the polypeptides *gastrin* and *urogastrone*. The first stimulates, and the second inhibits gastric secretion; both effects can be determined with confidence limits of $\pm$ 30% by a method using the rat's stomach *in vivo*. Recirculation of a small volume of buffer through the stomach and recording of the cumulative changes in pH allow the estimation of 10—20 ng of synthetic human gastrin or the amount of urogastrone present in 50—100 ml of human urine (SMITH et al., 1970; LAWRENCE et al., 1970).

IV. Proteins

Traditionally, the term bioassay of protein hormones is usually applied to the determination of insulin and of the hormones of the anterior lobe of the pituitary. There is no logical reason why the determination should not include, for example, the assay of the 'releasing factors', such as corticotrophin-releasing factor etc., but there are good practical grounds for omitting them at present: their chemical identity is still controversial, and the assay procedures have very large errors and are constantly being improved. There is competition between *in vivo* and *in vitro* assays and the question is not settled whether the two determine the same substances.

The clinically acceptable assays for *insulin* are well established; the latest survey (1969) is found in DORFMAN's *Methods in Hormone Research*. The possibility of determining concentrations of circulating insulin by radio-immunoassay is a recent development (YALOW and BERSON, 1960; BERSON et al., 1963). The method utilizes the fact that blood insulin competitively inhibits the binding of ^{131}I-labeled crystalline beef insulin to specific antibody formed in animals against insulin. Like all immunoassays it is strictly speaking not a bioassay, except that it depends on antibody formation in the living animal; from this step it is carried on in the test tube. Less than a microunit of insulin in 10—20 μl plasma can be determined by this method.

The actions of the different hormones derived from the *anterior lobe* of the *pituitary*, in contrast to those of most of the polypeptides or amines discussed earlier, are highly specific, so that the problem of excluding inactive contaminants is far less serious than, for example, in an assay utilizing smooth muscle contraction as its indicator. On the other hand, a complication is introduced by the synergism existing between certain pairs of these hormones, notably the pairs follicle-stimulating and luteinizing hormone, and prolactin and growth hormone. There is also in some instances a lack of suitable standard preparations. Whereas there are international or national standards for corticotrophin, chorionic gonadotrophin, pregnant mare serum, prolactin, thyrotrophin and melanophore-stimulating hormone, no such preparations exist for human follicle-stimulating hormone, luteinizing hormone and growth hormone. These hormones, particularly growth hormone, are highly species specific, so that there is a need for a standard from human pituitaries.

The well-established assay procedures for pituitary hormones are based strictly on the specific properties of the particular hormone: thus growth hormone may be measured on the gain in weight of young hypophysectomized rats, or thyrotrophic hormone on the release of previously ^{131}I-labeled thyroid hormone in mice in which endogenous release has been suppressed by thyroxin. Melanophore-stimulating activity may be assayed on isolated pieces of frog skin with good precision ($\lambda = 0.08$, Rigler and Holzbauer, 1956). An excellent up-to-date summary by Astwood of useful methods is found in Goodman and Gilman (1965). Radioimmuno assays are available for growth hormone and chorionic gonadotrophin and may soon be devised for all anterior pituitary hormones so that tissue and blood concentration can be measured.

An unusual tissue for bioassay is used to estimate a group of proteins called nerve growth factors; sensory ganglia are extirpated from chick embryos and the outgrowth of nerve fibres measured as an index of activity (Cohen et al., 1954). This is but one example in which substances which determine embryological or post-natal development have to be traced by their activity *in vivo* long before their composition becomes known.

C. Conclusion

There is no doubt that, in the future, bioassays will continue to lead to the discovery of new physiologically important compounds and help in elucidating the role of substances of known identity but unknown function. For the less affluent parts of the world, bioassays have the advantage of rarely requiring expensive equipment. For the future it is hoped that in routine determinations of biologically active compounds one will be able to dispense with bioassays except in those circumstances where the compounds are available only in trace amounts.

References

Adam, H.M., Hardwick, C.D., Spencer, K.E.V.: Assay of histamine on the isolated guinea-pig intestine by the method of superfusion. Brit. J. Pharmacol. **9**, 360—366 (1954).

— Hye, H.K.A.: Concentration of histamine in different parts of the brain and hypophysis of cat and its modification by drugs. Brit. J. Pharmacol. **28**, 137—152 (1966).

Armin, J., Grant, R.T.: Vasoconstrictor activity in the rabbit's blood and plasma. J. Physiol. (Lond.) **128**, 511—540 (1955).

BERSON, S.A., YALOW, R.S., AURBACH, G.D., POTTS, J.T.: Immunoassay of bovine and human parathyroid hormone. Proc. nat. Acad. Sci. (Wash.) **49**, 613—617 (1963).
BISSET, G.W., CLARK, B.J., HALDAR, J.: Blood levels of oxytocin and vasopressin during suckling in the rabbit and the problem of their independent release. J. Physiol. (Lond.) **206**, 711—722 (1970).
— — — HARRIS, M.C., LEWIS, G.P., ROCHA E SILVA, M., JR.: The assay of milk-ejecting activity in the lactating rat. Brit. J. Pharmacol. **31**, 537—549 (1967a).
— HILTON, S.M., POISNER, A.M.: Hypothalamic pathways for independent release of vasopressin and oxytocin. Proc. roy. Soc. B **166**, 422—442 (1967b).
BOURA, A., MONGAR, J.L., SCHILD, H.O.: Improved automatic apparatus for pharmacological assays on isolated preparations. Brit. J. Pharmacol. **9**, 24—30 (1954).
BOYD, G.W., LANDON, J., PEART, W.S.: The radio-immuno-assay of angiotensin. II. Proc. roy. Soc. B **173**, 327—338 (1969).
CANNON, W.B., URIDIL, J.E.: Studies on the conditions of activity in endocrine glands. VIII. Amer. J. Physiol. **58**, 353—364 (1921).
CHANG, H.C., GADDUM, J.H.: Choline esters in tissue extracts. J. Physiol. (Lond.) **79**, 255—285 (1933).
CLEUGH, J., GADDUM, J.H., MITCHELL, A.A., SMITH, M.W., WHITTAKER, V.P.: Substance P in brain extracts. J. Physiol. (Lond.) **170**, 69—85 (1964).
COHEN, S., LEVI-MONTALCINI, R., HAMBURGER, V.: A nerve growth-stimulating factor isolated from sarcomas 37 and 180. Proc. nat. Acad. Sci. (Wash.) **40**, 1014—1018 (1954).
DORFMAN, R.I. (Editor): Methods in Hormone Research, 2nd Ed., Vol. IIA, Bioassay. New York and London: Academic Press 1969.
DOUGLAS, W.W., FELDBERG, W., PATON, W.D.M., SCHACHTER, M.: Distribution of histamine and substance P in the wall of the dog's digestive tract. J. Physiol. (Lond.) **115**, 163—176 (1951).
EULER, U.S. v., GADDUM, J.H.: An unidentified depressor substance in certain tissue extracts. J. Physiol. (Lond.) **72**, 74—87 (1931).
FÜHNER, H.: Untersuchungen über den Synergismus von Giften. IV. Arch. exp. Pathol. Pharmakol. **82**, 51—80 (1917).
— Nachweis und Bestimmung von Giften auf pharmakologischem Wege. In: Handbuch der biologischen Arbeitsmethoden. Hrsg. von ABDERHALDEN. Abt. IV, Teil 7, p. 421—612. Berlin: Urban und Schwarzenberg 1923.
GADDUM, J.H.: The technique of superfusion. Brit. J. Pharmacol. **8**, 321—326 (1953).
— Symposium on substance P (ed. P. STERN). Proc. Sci. Soc. Bosnia Herzegovinia **1**, 7—14 (1961).
— An improved microbath. Brit. J. Pharmacol. **23**, 613—619 (1964).
— GOODWIN, L.G.: Experiments on liver sympathin. J. Physiol. (Lond.) **105**, 357—369 (1947).
— LEMBECK, F.: The assay of substances from the adrenal medulla. Brit. J. Pharmacol. **4**, 401—408 (1949).
— RANDIĆ, M., SMITH, M.W.: An antistrychnine extract from horse intestine. J. Physiol. (Lond.) **172**, 207—215 (1964).
GOODMAN, L.S., GILMAN, A.: The pharmacological basis of therapeutics. 3rd edition. New York: Macmillan 1965.
HORTON, E.W.: Human urinary kinin excretion. Brit. J. Pharmacol. **14**, 125—132 (1959).
— JONES, R.L.: Prostaglandins A_1, A_2 and 19-hydroxy A_1; their actions on smooth muscle and their inactivation on passage through the pulmonary and hepatic portal vascular beds. Brit. J. Pharmacol. **37**, 705—722 (1969).
— MAIN, I.H.M.: Identification of prostaglandins in central nervous tissues of the cat and chicken. Brit. J. Pharmacol. **30**, 582—602 (1967).
— THOMPSON, C.J.: Thin-layer chromatography and bioassay of prostaglandins in extracts of semen and tissues of the male reproductive tract. Brit. J. Pharmacol. **22**, 183—188 (1964).
JUORIO, A.V., VOGT, M.: Adrenaline in bird brain. J. Physiol. (Lond.) (1970) [in the press].
KEELE, C.A.: Clinical and pathological aspects of kinins in man. Proc. roy. Soc. B **173**, 361—369 (1969).
LANDE, I.S. DE LA, GLOVER, W.E.: The limit of sensitivity of bioassay of catecholamines on the perfused arterial segment. J. Pharm. Pharmacol. **18**, 324—325 (1966).
— HARVEY, J.A.: A new and sensitive bioassay for catecholamines. J. Pharm. Pharmacol. **17**, 589—593 (1965).
LAWRENCE, A.J., SCHILD, H.O., SMITH, G.M.: Extraction and assay of urogastrone. Brit. J. Pharmacol. (1970) [in the press].
RIGLER, R., HOLZBAUER, M.: Über die Natur des melanophorenexpandierenden Prinzips der Hypophyse, sein Verhalten gegen Ascorbinsäure und seine Bestimmung in biologischen Flüssigkeiten. Z. Biol. **108**, 196—209 (1956).

ROBERTS, M., ADAM, H.M.: New methods for the quantitative estimation of free and conjugated histamine in body fluids. Brit. J. Pharmacol. **5**, 526—541 (1950).
SAFFRAN, M., SCHALLY, A.V.: In vitro bioassay of corticotropin: modification and statistical treatment. Endocrinology **56**, 523—532 (1955).
SCHILD, H.O.: Automatic apparatus for pharmacological assays on isolated preparations. Brit. J. Pharmacol. **1**, 135—138 (1946).
SHARMAN, D.F.: Methods of determination of catecholamines and their metabolites. In: Methods and techniques of neuroscience. Ed. by R. FRIED. New York: Marcel Dekker Inc. (in the press).
— VOGT, M.: The noradrenaline content of the caudate nucleus of the rabbit. J. Neurochem. **12**, 62 (1965).
SMITH, G.M., LAWRENCE, A.J., COLIN-JONES, D.G., SCHILD, H.O.: The assay of gastrin using the perfused rat stomach. Brit. J. Pharmacol. **38**, 206—213 (1970).
STRAUGHAN, D.W.: Assay of acetylcholine on the rat blood pressure. J. Pharm. Pharmacol. **10**, 783—784 (1958).
SZERB, J.C.: The estimation of acetylcholine, using leech muscle in a microbath. J. Physiol. (Lond.) **158**, 8—9 P (1961).
UNGER, R.H., EISENTRAUT, A.M., MADISON, L.L.: The effect of total starvation upon the levels of circulating glucagon and insulin in man. J. clin. Invest. **42**, 1031—1039 (1963).
— — MCCALL, M.S., MADISON, L.L.: Glucagon antibodies and an immunoassay for glucagon. J. clin. Invest. **40**, 1280—1289 (1961).
VANE, J.R.: A sensitive method for the assay of 5-hydroxytryptamine. Brit. J. Pharmacol. **12**, 344—349 (1957).
— The blood-bathed isolated organ: a method of testing the circulating blood for active substances. J. Physiol. (Lond.) **143**, 75—76 P (1958).
— The release and fate of vaso-active hormones in the circulation. Brit. J. Pharmacol. **35**, 209—242 (1969).
VANOV, S., VOGT, M.: Catecholamine-containing structures in the hypogastric nerves of the dog. J. Physiol. (Lond.) **168**, 939—944 (1963).
VOGT, M.: The secretion of the denervated adrenal medulla of the cat. Brit. J. Pharmacol. **7**, 325—330 (1952).
YALOW, R.S., BERSON, S.A.: Immunoassay of endogenous plasma insulin in man. J. clin. Invest. **39**, 1157—1175 (1960).

Chapter 30

Immunoassay

S. SPECTOR

With 2 Figures

A critical consideration in the assessment of the pharmacological effects of drugs is a determination of their concentration in biological fluids or tissues. This may be a relatively minor problem if the concentrations are high; but, when the concentrations are low, extremely sensitive assays are required. Several types of highly sensitive assays have been devised and these may be divided into two groups, pharmacological and chemical. The pharmacological methods are based on quantitative differences in the effects of drugs on isolated organ preparations. Although these pharmacological methods can be very sensitive, they are not as specific as chemical methods. However, there is no chemical method with adequate specificity or sensitivity for the assay of polypeptides such as bradykinin or vasopressin or protein hormones such as insulin, growth hormone, ACTH or TSH. It was only with the introduction of immunologic methods with their sensitivity and precision that quantitative information on polypeptides and protein hormones could be obtained. Moreover, the immunologic methodology can be applied to the assay of small molecules and offers, as well, the exciting possibility of studying mechanisms and functions of small and large molecules by producing deficiencies in living animals through the use of antisera.

Those molecules capable of stimulating the production of antibody are by definition referred to as antigens. One usually thinks of antigenic substances in relation to infectious organisms; however, chemical substances also exert antigenicity. In order for a chemical to elicit an antibody response it must be of critical weight and also be foreign to the organism. Large molecules may appear unfamiliar to the body because of their amino acid sequence or their configuration.

The work of LANDSTEINER (1945) showed that small molecules, which by themselves are be incapable of eliciting an antibody response, may act as antigens when artificially incorporated into larger molecules. There are a number of procedures for the coupling of such small molecules, referred to as haptens, to large molecules to form antigens. One general procedure is to conjugate the hapten to a protein by diazotization (TABACHNICK and SABOTKA, 1959, 1960). In this method primary aromatic amines are diazotized by nitrous acid in an aqueous solution. The diazonium salt formed is very reactive and may react with any nucleophilic group in a macromolecule to form a conjugated product. The macromolecule used is generally a foreign protein in a purified form, although one may also use the serum protein of the animal to be immunized. In the latter case, the attached haptenic group will be the only determinant group that will promote the formation of antibodies.

Water soluble carbodiimides are also widely used to couple a hapten to a protein (SHEEHAN and HESS, 1955; GOODFRIEND et al., 1964). Structurally the carbodiimides are R—N=C—N—R′ (R,R′=alkyl or aryl) (KHORANA, 1953) and can form stable peptide or amide bonds to link two molecules if one contains a free carboxyl function and the other free amino group. Carbodiimides can also couple compounds containing phosphate, alcohol and thiol groups. Coupling in the presence of an agent such as N,N'-dicyclohexylcarbodiimide is rapid and occurs at room temperature. The general reaction is:

$$RCOOH + NH_2R' + C_6H_{11}N{=}C{=}NC_6H_{11} \rightarrow RCONHR' + C_6H_{11}NHCONHC_6H_{11}$$

In a typical synthesis 10 mg bovine gamma globulin is dissolved in 2 ml of 0.02 M potassium phosphate buffer, pH 7.4. To this mixture equal molar concentrations (in water) of carbodiimide reagent and the small molecule are added. The reaction mixture is stirred for 2—3 h at 20°C, and then dialyzed against 0.15 M sodium chloride-0.01 M potassium phosphate pH 7.4. This procedure was used by GOODFRIEND et al. (1964) to produce antibodies to bradykinin and angiotension in rabbits. OLIVER et al. (1968) conjugated digitoxin to a protein by the use of carbodiimide and developed rabbit antibody to digitoxin.

BUTLER and CHEN (1967) prepared rabbit antidigoxin antibodies employing another procedure to conjugate the hapten to protein. They oxidized digoxin with periodate as described by ERLANGER and BEISER (1964), so that the two vicinyl hydroxyl groups on oxidation would react with free amino groups of a protein to form an antigen. These authors found that not only could the antibodies induced by this antigen bind with digitoxin, which they anticipated because of its close chemical similarity to digoxin, but they could also react with other steroids. The authors point out that just as antibodies to steroid hormones have been reported to interfere with some physiological action of the hormones (GOODFRIEND and SEHON, 1961; NERI et al., 1964), it would be reasonable to assume that antibodies to the cardiac glycoside may interfere with its pharmacologic effects.

Although the conjugation of haptenic groups to proteins to form antigens has been extensively used to elicit the production of antibodies to such important hormones as thyroxin (CHURCHILL and TAPLEY, 1964) and progesterone (ERLANGER et al., 1959), small molecules have also been attached to synthetic polypeptides to form immunogenic macromolecules which are capable of eliciting antibodies specifically directed toward the small molecule (SELA, 1965). For example, vitamin B_6 was attached to multichain polypeptides by forming a Schiff base and then reducing it with sodium borohydride to form a stable CH_2NH link as reported by FISCHER et al. (1958). On injection of this antigen to rabbit, antibodies were obtained which were specific for pyridoxal. These antibodies now offer a great potential for elucidating the role of the vitamin in various biological systems. Obviously, studies of this kind could be extended to other vitamins, coenzymes, and drugs.

The problem of opiate tolerance and addiction is of considerable importance and despite the extensive use of opiates for centuries our understanding of these processes is very limited. Furthermore, available methods for measuring opiates in plasma and tissue fluids have either been too insensitive or non-specific to be used for routine clinical tests. Morphine specific antibodies might be an extremely useful tool 1) for measuring minute levels of the drug by an immunological assay; 2) for studying the localization of morphine either by the histochemical fluorescent antibody technique developed by COONS (1956), or by chemically coupling the antibody to ferritin (SCHICK and SINGER, 1961), an electron dense protein, so that the morphine antibody complex would be visible in electron micrographs; 3) for studying the mechanisms for the development of tolerance and physical dependence.

Antibodies directed against morphine have been produced by an antigen which was made by coupling morphine to bovine serum albumin (SPECTOR and PARKER, 1970). The coupling procedure employed was as follows: morphine free base was converted to morphyoxyacetic acid as described in Beilstein. The morphoxyacetic acid was then coupled to protein (human or bovine serum albumin) by the use of the carbodiimide method as shown in Fig. 1:

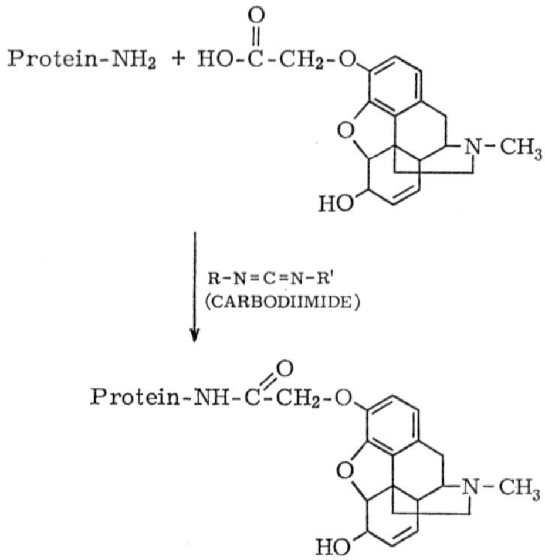

Fig. 1

Rabbits were then immunized with the morphine-protein conjugate in complete Freund's adjuvant (0.4 ml/footpad). In order to obtain a greater titer of the antibody, animals were injected with the antigenic complex in complete adjuvant every few weeks thereafter. Rabbit gamma globulin containing antimorphine antibody was purified by precipitation with 40% ammonium sulfate followed by diethylaminoethyl (DEAE) cellulose chromatography.

Several procedures can be used to demonstrate the presence of antibodies to morphine in the rabbit gamma globulin fraction. A qualitative procedure which is only indicative of the presence of the morphine antibody is the ring test. The antibody is put in a narrow test tube and the antigen is carefully layered over it. At the interface of the two solutions a precipitate will form. A modification of this test may be used to determine whether the antibodies recognize the hapten (morphine). The hapten is added to the antibody in the test tube before the antigen is introduced; its combination with the antibody prevents the formation of the antigen-antibody complex and thus no precipitate will be formed; this is referred to as hapten inhibition. Another procedure is to determine the amount of radiolabeled hapten which can be bound to the antibody. The antibody and labeled hapten are placed on either side of a semipermeable membrane and dialyzed. At equilibrium of the system the difference in the concentrations of isotope inside and outside of the bag reflects the amount bound to the antibody. It is critical to have a nonspecific gamma globulin as a control to eliminate the possibility of nonspecific binding.

An immunoassay was also developed which can be used to indicate the presence of morphine antibody or to assay morphine. The technique, first reported by YALOW and BERSON (1960), uses isotopic dilution in the presence of specific antibodies and is both specific and sensitive. It is based on the competition of labeled and unlabeled antigens or haptens for their specific antibody, i.e.:

a) Hapten* + Antibody → [Hapten* — Antibody].

b) Hapten* + Hapten + Antibody → [Hapten* — Antibody] + [Hapten — Antibody].

Unlabeled hapten whose concentration is to be determined is mixed with a known amount of labeled hapten. Antibodies directed to the hapten are added. In order to perform the assay, it is necessary that the concentration of the antibodies be the same order of magnitude as the concentration of the unlabeled hapten so that the antibody sites are saturated with the hapten. As a consequence of the competition between the unlabeled and labeled hapten the amount of the label which binds to the antibody is inversely proportional to the amount of unlabeled hapten. Alternatively, the amount of labeled hapten remaining free is proportional to the concentration of unlabeled hapten. After equilibrium is reached, the free hapten may be separated from the antibody-hapten complex by a variety of procedures. Charcoal coated with a large molecule such as albumin or dextran will adsorb the hapten, but not the antibody-hapten complex. This is, in essence, a form of instant dialysis and has been effectively used to assay for angiotensin (GOODFRIEND et al., 1968) and for insulin (HERBERT et al., 1965). Another procedure for the separation of free hapten from the antibody-hapten complex is to precipitate the antibody-hapten complex by the addition of neutral saturated ammonium sulfate. The amount of radioactivity in either the precipitate or the supernatant is determined and compared with the standards. A typical calibration curve for morphine is illustrated in Fig. 2:

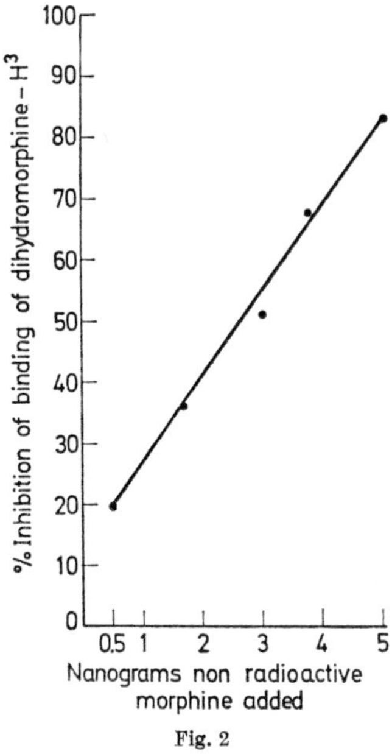

Fig. 2

A control must be run in which a nonspecific gamma globulin is substituted for the antibody to assess the amount of nonspecific binding that occurs.

Preliminary evidence obtained with C^{14}-dihydromorphine indicates that this method may detect 50 ng of morphine in serum. When the affinity constant of the antibody for the hapten is very high the sensitivity of the method may be increased by diluting the antibody preparations and by labeling the morphine with ^{131}I or ^{125}I as described by HUNTER and GREENWOOD (1962).

The widespread use of drugs today in our culture makes it of great interest to learn whether some of these compounds possess antigenic activity themselves or whether they can bind to proteins and thereby induce an immunological response.

References

Butler, V.P., Jr., Chen, J.P.: Digoxin specific antibodies. Proc. nat. Acad. Sci. (Wash.) **57**, 71—78 (1967).

Churchill, W.H., Tapley, D.F.: Antibodies specific for thyroxine and its analogues. Nature (Lond.) **202**, 29—31 (1964).

Coons, A.H.: Histochemistry with labeled antibody. Int. Rev. Cytol. **5**, 1—23 (1956).

Erlanger, B.F., Beiser, S.M.: Antibodies specific for ribonucleosides and ribonucleotides and their reaction with DNA. Proc. nat. Acad. Sci. (Wash.) **52**, 68—74 (1964).

— Borek, F., Beiser, S.M., Lieberman, S.: Steroid-protein conjugates. II. Preparation and characterization of conjugates of bovine serum albumin with progesterone, deoxycorticosterone, and estrone. J. biol. Chem. **234**, 1090—1094 (1959).

Fischer, E.H., Kent, A.K., Snyder, E.R., Krebs, E.G.: The reaction of sodium borohydride with muscle phosphorylase. J. Amer. chem. Soc. **80**, 2906—2907 (1958).

Goodfriend, T.L., Ball, D.L., Farley, D.B.: Radioimmunoassay of angiotensin. J. Lab. clin. Med. **72**, 648—662 (1968).

— Levine, L., Fassman, G.D.: Antibodies to bradykinin and angiotensin: A use of carbodiimides in immunology. Science **144**, 1344—1346 (1964).

— Sehon, A.H.: Antibodies to estrone-protein conjugates. Canad. J. Biochem. **39**, 941—960 (1961).

Herbert, V., Lau, K.S., Gottlieb, C.W., Bleicher, S.J.: Coated charcoal immunoassay of insulin. J. clin. Endocr. **25**, 1375—1384 (1965).

Hunter, W.M., Greenwood, F.C.: Preparation of iodine-131 labeled human growth hormone of high specific activity. Nature (Lond.) **194**, 495—496 (1962).

Khorana, H.G.: The chemistry of carbodiimides. Chem. Rev. **53**, 145—166 (1953).

Landsteiner, K.: Specificity of serological reactions. Cambridge: Harvard University Press 1945.

Neri, R.O., Tolkodorf, S., Beiser, S.M., Erlanger, B.F., Agate, F.S., Jr., Lieberman, S.: Further studies on the biological effects of passive immunization with antibodies to steroid-protein conjugates. Endocrinology **74**, 593—598 (1964).

Oliver, G.C., Jr., Parker, B., Brasfield, D.L., Parker, C.W.: The measurement of digitoxin in human serum by radioimmunoassay. J. clin. Invest. **47**, 1035—1042 (1968).

Schick, A.F., Singer, S.J.: On the formation of covalent linkages between two protein molecules. J. biol. Chem. **236**, 2477—2485 (1961).

Sela, M.: Advances in Immunology. Ed. by F.S. Dixon, Jr. and J.H. Humphrey. New York: Academic Press 1965.

Sheehan, J.C., Hess, G.P.: A new method fof forming peptide bonds. J. Amer. chem. Soc. **77**, 1067—1068 (1955).

Spector, S., Parker, C.W.: Radioimmunoassay for morphine. Science **168**, 1347—1348 (1970).

Tabachnick, M., Sobotka, H.: Azoproteins. I. Spectrophotometric studies of amino acid azo derivatives. J. biol. Chem. **234**, 1726—1730 (1959).

— — Azoproteins. II. A spectrophotometric study of the coupling of diazotized arsanilic acid with proteins. J. biol. Chem. **235**, 1051—1054 (1960).

Yalow, R.S., Berson, S.A.: Immunoassay of endogenous plasma insulin in man. J. clin. Invest. **39**, 1157—1175 (1960).

Chapter 31

Paper, Column and Thin Layer Chromatography, Counter-Current Distribution and Electrophoresis

Elwood O. Titus

With 1 Figure

A. Introduction

As more potent drugs are used in ever decreasing dosage, studies of drug metabolism require analytical and separatory methods of increasing sensitivity. This demand has led to the development of powerful new techniques such as gas chromatography coupled to mass spectrometry. It has also generated a formidable outpouring of papers on modifications of the more classical techniques, which are the subject of this chapter, i.e. counter-current distribution, various kinds of chromatography and electrophoresis. For the most part these techniques permit drug metabolism to be studied quite effectively with relatively simple and inexpensive apparatus. Paper and thin layer chromatography have received particular emphasis since very small amounts of material can be examined, an important consideration in studies with modern, highly potent drugs. Those separation procedures with which this chapter is primarily concerned, i.e. counter-current distribution and various kinds of chromatography, all make use of the same device, repeated partition of a substance between two phases. In counter-current distribution these phases are two immiscible liquids. In chromatography the solid absorbent may be imagined as subdivided into infinitesimal volumes so that the process may be treated as a series of repeated partitions of solute between the descending solvent and the immobilized volumes of absorbent. In partition chromatography, whether it be column, paper, or thin layer, the immobile phase is liquid retained by capillarity within a suspending solid. The absorptive properties of the suspending solid may in some cases also contribute to the equilibrium. The fractionation procedures considered here are thus basically similar. They share the advantage of providing both a means for isolation and an identifying physical constant, such as the distribution constant obtainable from counter-current data, the retention volume in liquid-liquid partition chromatography and the R_f of paper chromatography. Underlying the theoretical treatment of all three of these methods is the assumption that for any given solute the ratio of concentration in the mobile phase to that in the immobile phase is a constant. Since retention volume and R_f are derivable from this distribution constant, all three methods provide a measure of the same physical property.

Since the manner in which repeated partitions contribute to effective separation has been made particularly clear by the mathematical treatment of counter-current distribution (Stene, 1944; Craig and Craig, 1956; Hecker, 1953) this procedure has been selected as the first for discussion. The basic similarity between this and other fractionation procedures was of course recognized by these authors and has been pointed out many times (Dean, 1969). A particularly clear resume of the mathematical treatment of various procedures was included in the earlier of Stahl's (1962, 1969) two volumes on thin layer chromatography.

Much of the discussion of the relationship between solute structure and the liquid pairs suitable for distribution also applies to the selection of solvents for chromatographic procedures. Not infrequently, a liquid-liquid pair suitable for counter-current distribution of a substance will serve with very little modification for the partition or paper chromatographic isolation of the material. For substances such as quaternary ammonium compounds which are completely ionized and essentially insoluble in organic solvents, paper electrophoresis may offer advantages over chromatography or counter-current distribution.

The pharmacologist contemplating studies of drug metabolism will find abundant descriptions of the various methods together with detailed operating instructions in a number of texts. In addition to the references cited above there is a review of counter-current distribution by Titus (1960). Chromatography, including the classical procedures of column chromatography that have been used for many years, is well treated by Cassidy (1957) and Lederer and Lederer (1957). Paper chromatography and electrophoresis are discussed in great detail by Block et al. (1958) and Smith (1960). Electrophoresis is treated also in a useful book by Bier (1967) and in earlier work by Audubert and De Mende (1960). To the previously mentioned works of Stahl (1962, 1969) on thin layer chromatography may be added others by Truter (1963) and Randerath (1966). Since all these techniques are now so familiar, this chapter will deal only incidentally with operating procedures and will confine itself primarily to those features of the methods which make them applicable to drug studies. A brief but very useful discussion of the applicability of various separatory procedures to different biochemical problems has been presented by Pfleiderer (1965).

Perhaps the most commonly encountered problem in the fractionation of drug metabolites is the choice of a solvent system appropriate for the distribution or chromatography of the anticipated structure. The variety of structures examined by these methods is now so vast that one can usually find examples of the fractionation of substances with properties similar to those of the new drug under investigation. Two useful guides here are the *Analytical Review*, published annually in conjunction with the April issue of *Analytical Chemistry*, and an encyclopedic work by Clarke (1969). In the latter the structures of a large number of drugs are presented and with each is included information on fractionation methods appropriate for its purification.

B. Extraction from Tissues

The procedures for initial extraction of metabolites from tissue or body fluids will also extract minor amounts of normal constituents. The quantitative determination of metabolites in the subsequent fractionation should therefore be carried out as nearly as possible with methods that establish the relationship of the product to the parent drug. It is fortunate that radioactive labeling of drugs for metabolic studies is now widespread. Since so many drugs absorb in the ultraviolet spectrophotometric methods are also widely used. Some indication of the normal tissue constituents that absorb in the ultraviolet and that might appear when acidified or alkaline tissue homogenates are extracted with organic solvents is given in a paper by Kaempe (1969). Many drugs and their metabolites are acids or bases that are extractable into organic solvents in the nonionized form. Extraction from deproteinized tissue extracts that have made strongly acidic or alkaline is therefore a common procedure for recovering these substances.[1] The precipitation of protein which is usually necessary if emulsification is not to hinder such extractions may be done with 5% trichloracetic acid or by bringing the extract to 0.4 N in perchloric acid. Not infrequently the tissue is homogenized in 0.1 N HCl. Several extractions of the filtrates with cold peroxide-free ether will sometimes remove the trichloracetic acid remaining from the precipitation without extracting the salts of basic drugs. Precipitation of $KClO_4$ by titration with K_2CO_3 is often a good way to remove excess $HClO_4$ from deproteinized solutions. When acid is undesirable protein may be precipitated by adding 2 volumes of 0.3 N $Ba(OH)_2$ to a sample, followed by 2 volumes of 5% $ZnSO_4 \cdot 7H_2O$. After vigorous shaking the proteins and the precipitated zinc and barium salts can be filtered off (SOMOGYI, 1945).

Since hydroxylated metabolites of drugs often appear in urine as conjugates with sulfate or glucuronic acid, hydrolysis with HCl or H_2SO_4 may be required before the desired substance can be extracted into organic solvents. Sulfuric acid has the advantage of being less soluble in the extracting solvents. Autoclaving for 1 h in about 2% H_2SO_4 would be a representative procedure for glucuronide hydrolysis, whereas milder conditions, 1 M H_2SO_4 at temperatures up to 37°C for periods up to 4 days, may well be suitable for sulfate hydrolysis. Enzymatic removal of these groups is also common and a study has been made of the optimal incubation conditions for this purpose (BEYER, 1965). An excellent practical guide to the preliminary recovery of organic substances from body fluids and tissues by a variety of methods is the handbook by SCOTT (1969).

C. Counter-Current Distribution

I. Theory

Of the various methods for isolation of drugs and metabolites, counter-current distribution offers certain advantages. Since the pattern of distribution of a substance is predictable from its partition coefficient, the procedure is useful analytically. Small amounts of impurity are revealed by discrepancies between observed and predicted distribution patterns and all of the components of a mixture can usually be accounted for by evaporation of the contents of the apparatus. The process is essentially a series of single extractions. Ideally in each of these, solute distributes between the two immiscible solvents according to the Nernst relationship, i.e., K, the ratio of the concentration in the upper phase to that in the lower, remains constant despite changes in concentration or the presence of other solutes. If the volumes of the two solvent phases are identical, $K = p/q$ where p represents the fraction of a component in the upper phase and q the fraction in the lower phase and $p + q = 1$. It will be useful later to note that $p = \frac{K}{K+1}$ and $q = \frac{1}{K+1}$.

The apparatus generally used provides a series of glass tubes mounted in series on a rack and numbered 0, 1, 2 ---- r. At the beginning of the operation a fixed volume of the lower layer from a previously equilibrated pair of immiscible solvents is placed in each tube. These lower layers remain in place throughout subsequent operations. The sample is dissolved in tube 0 and a fixed volume of upper layer

1 However, drugs that are highly bound to proteins may not be freed during acidification. Under these conditions plasma and tissue homogenates must be extracted directly and then returned to an aqueous phase (see Chapter 22).

is added. After equilibration, which is achieved by rocking the whole train of tubes, the phases are allowed to settle and the apparatus is then gradually tilted so that the upper phase drains off through a side port into an adjacent reservoir tube. The latter delivers the upper layer into the next equilibration tube when the apparatus is tilted back. At each step fresh upper layer must be added to tube 0 and after each sequence of rocking and tilting all of the upper layers simultaneously move forward one position. All of these operations are mechanized in modern apparatus and trains of several hundred tubes are entirely practical. The distribution is complete when the foremost of the advancing upper layers has reached the last tube. The process may readily be visualized, using as an example a unit quantity of solute with a K of one. In this case $p = q = 0.5$ so that half of the solute originally introduced into tube 0 is taken into the upper layer at the first extraction. This half is then moved over lower 1 in the first transfer. It is easily seen that after two transfers one-fourth of the material (i.e. p^2) will be in tube 2, one half $(p \cdot q + p \cdot q)$ in tube 1 and one fourth (q^2) in tube 0. At this stage it is already apparent that as the process continues the solute will become distributed through the apparatus as a gradually broadening band. For $K = 1$ the tube or tubes of maximum concentration will always occur in the center of the band and will be in the center of the apparatus upon completion of the run. For substances of K greater than one, the fraction $\frac{K}{K+1}$, carried forward by the upper layer at each transfer will be more than one-half and the band will be displaced toward the higher numbered tubes. With a sufficient number of transfers the bands containing substances of different K can be separated completely.

Distribution data are customarily plotted with the total amount of solute in both layers as ordinate against tube number as abscissa. The tubes are numbered from 0 and the numbers increase in the direction in which the upper layer moves. Figure 1 illustrates the distribution through 50 transfers to be expected for two

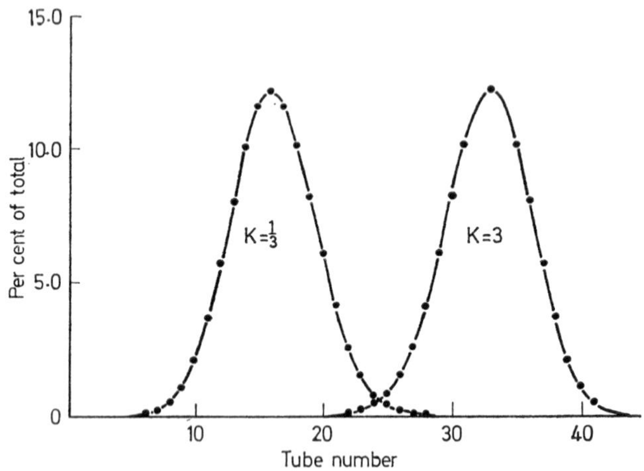

Fig. 1. The theoretical distribution of two substances of $K = {}^1/_3$ and $K = 3$ in a countercurrent distribution apparatus of 50 tubes

substances of $K = 3$ and $K = 1/3$. Readers interested in using the technique should consult the exhaustive review by its originator (CRAIG and CRAIG, 1956). Operating procedures and apparatus, including commercially available automated equipment have also been described in this and other reviews (CRAIG et al., 1951; HECKER, 1955; TITUS, 1960).

The analytical utility of the procedure derives largely from the ease with which the theoretical distribution of a pure substance can be plotted. It can readily be seen by diagramming successive steps and calculating the contents of each tube in terms of p and q that after n transfers the fraction of the total solute in any tube, r, will be given by the rth term of the binomial expansion $(q + p)^n = 1$.

Since $p = \frac{K}{K+1}$ and $q = 1 - p = \frac{1}{K+1}$ the binomial expansion becomes

$$\left(\frac{1}{K+1} + \frac{K}{K+1}\right)^n = 1$$

Theoretical curves may be plotted from the following expression which gives $T_{n,r}$, i.e. the fraction of a solute present in the rth tube after n transfers (RIETZ, 1927).

$$T_{n,r} = \frac{n!}{r!\,(n-r)!}\left(\frac{1}{K+1}\right)^n K^r$$

But there are much more convenient methods. WAY and BENNETT (1951), for example, have pointed out that solutions of this expression have been tabulated (National Bureau of Standards, 1950). In the standard table $T_{n,r}$ is treated as a function of p and q, these letters having the same significance as above, i.e., $\frac{K}{K+1}$ and $\frac{1}{K+1}$ respectively. Theoretical distribution curves may then be constructed from tabulated values once p and q have been calculated from K. A useful table of p and q values as a function of K has been included in the paper of WAY and BENNETT (1951).

It is often convenient to use the relationship between successive terms of a binominal expansion (WILLIAMSON and CRAIG, 1947).

$$\frac{T_r}{T_{(r-1)}} = \frac{K\,(n+1-r)}{r}$$

If the value of any point on the curve is known, all the other points can be calculated, providing K is known. Since the tubes near the peak of a distribution curve are most likely to contain pure solute, values from two adjacent points in this region may be used to calculate K. The latter is then used to construct a theoretical curve by calculation of values for the terms preceding and following the initially chosen points. After a theoretical curve which coincides with the largest possible number of experimental points in one band has been calculated, the difference between observed concentrations and those predicted by theory may then be plotted as a function of tube number to give the distribution of impurities. If the second pattern indicates the presence of several compounds, the process may be repeated until a curve for the distribution of each impurity has been obtained. The process must of course terminate whenever the differences to be plotted become statistically insignificant because of uncertainties in the experimental values. This kind of analytical application can be useful in such applications as assessing the radiochemical purity of isotopically labeled substances. The calculations can be computerized (POHL, 1965) and a program designed to carry out essentially the operations described above has been described by PRIORE and KIRDANI (1968) and tested in a study of the metabolites of estriol (KIRDANI and PRIORE, 1968).

II. Prediction of Separability

Distribution curves generated by the binomial expansion predict the extent to which several components of differing K are separable. See, for example, Fig. 1.

By inspection one can estimate that a mixture of four components ranging in K from 0.1—10 could be well separated by 100 transfers and partially resolved by about 25 transfers. As the number of components in a mixture increases, larger numbers of transfers are required. The bands widen as more transfers are applied but the fraction of the total tubes occupied by more than negligible amounts of a particular component lessens.

The extent to which two components of differing K are separable is predictable by mathematical procedures less cumbersome than inspection of generated curves. This is made possible by a characteristic of distribution curves pointed out by MARTIN and SYNGE (1941) and by CRAIG and CRAIG (1956). Thus curves generated in stepwise fashion by the binomial expansion assume the form of the normal curve of error as the number of transfers approaches infinity. Even at values of n as low as 25, however, curves plotted by the binomial expansion can be approximated by a normal curve of error and discrepancies between the two are usually less than the uncertainty in the analytical determinations. The treatment of counter-current data by statistical methods is thus possible and a number of useful simple expressions have been derived. In general these are applicable without important error to distributions of about 25 transfers or more if the value of K is between 0.1 and 9. The position, N, of the maximum in a distribution curve may be related to K by the expression (BOCK, 1950).

$$N = \frac{nK}{K + 1}$$

The width of a band containing 99% of a solute is approximated by the expression

$$\sqrt{nK/(K + 1)^2}$$

(CRAIG and CRAIG, 1956).

HECKER (1953) has published an exhaustive analysis of the conditions required for separation. With the aid of tables and curves from this paper, the planning of counter-current distribution separations is relatively rapid. The publication lists values for n, the number of transfers required for various degress of purification of two component mixtures. The important variables are a function α, essentially the geometric mean of the two distribution constants, and β, the ratio of the two K's. Obviously at $\beta = 1$ separation is impossible under any circumstances. For any other given value of β the separation of the two substances is optimal when the geometric mean of the distribution constants is 1. In this case the distribution curves of the two substances will lie symmetrically on either side of the middle tube of the apparatus, as in Fig. 1.

In all of the above discussion it has been assumed that the distribution ends when the first of the advancing upper layers has reached the last tube and no material leaves the apparatus. If further transfers are applied, each additional step will result in emergence of one volume of upper layer from the last unit in the train and the bands will eventually emerge from the apparatus in a manner analogous to the elution of fractions from a chromatographic column. This "single withdrawal technique" has been mechanized by the addition of a fraction collector at the end of the distribution train (CRAIG and CRAIG, 1956) and is sometimes advantageous. If, for example, the composition of the lower layer interferes with the analytical determination of the separated components, the distribution may be continued by the single withdrawal procedure until all of the desired fractions have appeared in the emergent upper layers. Enhanced resolution of slow moving bands may sometimes be obtained if faster moving material is allowed to pass out of the apparatus while many more transfers are applied to the fractions remaining within.

In graphical presentations of data obtained by the single withdrawal procedure the first sample to emerge is usually plotted furthest to the right and subsequently emerging fractions are plotted from right to left until this curve meets that representing the contents of the machine, which is plotted as usual. By this procedure the peaks representing individual components are arranged in order of increasing K. If a 100 tube apparatus is taken as an example the first fraction to emerge in a single withdrawal operation will be the 100th tube of a 100 transfer distribution. The second will be the 100th tube of a 101 transfer distribution, etc. It has been shown by STENE (1944) that the contents of the emergent fractions correspond to the terms of a Pascal distribution. GHOSH et al. (1965) have published a procedure for constructing theoretical curves from tables of probability distribution. Theoretical curves may be conveniently calculated with the expression (CRAIG and CRAIG, 1956).

$$y = \frac{1}{\sqrt{2\pi\, n/K}}\, e^{\frac{-x^2}{2n/K}}$$

Here n is the average number of transfers in the band, i.e., the tube number of the maximum of the emergent curve, y is the fraction of a solute in a given tube and x is the distance from the maximum to the tube in question. This expression is an approximation which gives good results with distributions of about 100 transfers or more.

A double withdrawal procedure (CRAIG and CRAIG, 1956) has also been described and discontinuous extraction trains permitting the transfer of either phase have been described by JANTZEN (1948), TSCHESCHE and KÖNIGE (1950) and VERZELE (1953).

III. Choice of Solvent Pairs for Counter-Current Distribution

A few practical considerations should be kept in mind in selecting solvents. Since the phases must separate quickly, systems prone to emulsification should be avoided. High boiling solvents or salt solutions may be undesirable if it is necessary to recover the solute. The distribution constant should be independent of concentration. Since solutes are diluted rapidly during distribution and quickly approach ideal behavior, deviations from a linear isotherm are a relatively rare cause of skewed distribution patterns.

For testing the homogeneity of a substance a system of two liquid phases between which the solute distributes approximately equally is advisable. Since counter-current distribution is most effective when the geometric mean of the K's for two substances is 1, minor impurities occuring before or after the main peak are most likely to be efficiently separated. For the same reason it is common practice in undertaking the counter-current distribution of an unknown mixture to select a solvent pair in which the total solutes distribute equally. Such a system is most likely to give effective resolution. When the resolution of two closely related substances is a problem, it may be worth while to try a number of solvent systems since a relatively small increase in the ratio, β, of their distribution constants can greatly lessen the transfers required for separation (HECKER, 1953, 1954).

A few simple generalizations may be useful in selecting liquid pairs for particular solutes. Lipophilic structures pass from water into hydrocarbon solvents because the CH_2 moieties of the drug associate with those of the solvent, with exclusion of the water between them; thus the aliphatic hydrocarbons provide essentially no opportunity for dipole-dipole interaction and none for hydrogen bonding. By contrast drugs with appreciable numbers of polar or polarizable groups

Table 1

Pentane	Dioxane
Isopentane	Amyl acetate
Hexane	Isopropyl acetate
Heptane	Ethyl acetate
2,2,4-Trimethylpentane	Methyl acetate
Cyclohexane	Nitrobenzene
Cyclopentane	Cyclohexanol
Thiophene	Tertiary pentanol
Benzene	Butanol
Toluene	Secondary butanol
Ethylene dichloride	Propanol
Tetrachloroethylene	Ethanol
Methylene chloride	Methanol
Carbon tetrachloride	Acetonitrile
Chloroform	Nitromethane
Pentanol	Nitroethane
α-Dichlorobenzene	Methoxyethylene glycol
Carbon disulfides	Pyridine
The higher ethers	Morpholine
Diisopropyl ether	Aniline
Diethyl ether	Phenol
Furan	Acetic acid
Furfural	Formamide
Pyridine homologs	Water
Methyl ethyl ketone	Hydrochloric acid
Methylcyclohexanone	Sulfuric acid
Acetone	Salt solutions

will tend to have partition coefficients more favorable to water than to solvents like hexane. In general, substituents such as NH_2 or OH increase the solubility of drugs in more polar liquids, the effect being largely due to hydrogen bonding between solute and solvent. Ethers, amines, aldehydes and ketones will act as proton acceptors in the formation of such bonds. The hydroxyl groups of water and alcohols can serve both as donors and acceptors. Alcohols such as butanol and its homologues, which have sufficiently large nonpolar groups so that they form a second phase with water, are thus excellent solvents for the extraction of more polar drugs.

Craig and Craig (1956) have published a very useful list of common solvents arranged in the order of increasing dielectric constants (Table 1).

In general solvents are miscible with others listed nearby but immiscible with those far removed. The list is useful in devising liquid pairs for extraction studies or for counter-current distribution. For those solvents which are insoluble in water the list indicates the order of increasing ability to remove more polar solutes from aqueous solution. Solvent combinations that have been used for a great variety of substrates have been tabulated in reviews by von Metzsch (1953, 1956) and the earlier of these reviews contains a useful table of critical solution temperatures for various solvent mixtures. Several reviews offer useful guides to the choice of solvent mixtures for drugs and natural products (Craig and Craig, 1956; Titus, 1960). Systems for phospholipids (Cole et al., 1953; Olley and Lovern, 1953; Olley, 1956) and fatty acids (Ahrens and Craig, 1952) have been published.

Sugars, glycosides and other highly hydroxylated compounds can be distributed in systems prepared from water and ethanol-chloroform or ethanol-chloroform-glycol monoether mixtures. Aqueous solutions, often containing dilute acetic acid or ammonia, may be used with butanols for the distribution of peptides and have been used for some cardiac glycosides. For extremely lipid soluble nonelectrolytes, the choice of solvent pairs is somewhat limited since these compounds are insoluble in water, often cause emulsification and may associate in nonpolar solvents. Successful systems for these usually include petroleum ether or hexane and a mixture of organic solvents just polar enough to separate as a second phase. Methanol or ethanol containing a little water, nitromethane, nitroethane, acetonitrile and methylcellosolve, have been used in various combinations as the second phase.

In general the greatest difference between partition coefficients of chemically similar solutes will be observed with solvents that differ most in polarity or the ability to form hydrogen bonds, i.e. solvents most widely separated in the list cited earlier. Systems of water plus a single organic solvent are thus theoretically advantageous and this advantage may often be exploited if the solute is an acid or base so that K is a function of the pH of the aqueous phase. In most cases only the unionized form of acidic or basic drugs is extracted into the organic layer of a liquid pair. The distribution of these substances between organic solvents and aqueous solutions is therefore very sensitive to pH. If, for example, the solute in question is an organic amine and if the pH of the aqueous phase is sufficiently acidic so that salt formation with organic base is appreciable, then at least two equilibrium conditions must both be satisfied in the final distribution of amine. The relative concentrations of free base in solvent and water must satisfy the Nernst partition constant. At the same time free base entering the aqueous phase will be protonated until the concentration of the resultant cation comes into equilibrium with the hydrogen ion and free base in the aqueous phase. If the aqueous half of a liquid-liquid pair is strongly buffered so that the concentration of hydrogen ion is not altered by small amounts of the amine to be distributed, the pH can be the most important determinant of the final distribution of drug.

The dependence of partition coefficients of bases on the pH of the aqueous phase is particularly marked at pH values below the pKa of the drug, since $K' = K/(1 + 10^{pKa-pH})$, where K' is the coefficient at any given pH and K is the coefficient of the unionized base. Buffered systems with chloroform or ethylene dichloride have been widely used for alkaloids and are useful in separating the metabolites of quinoline antimalarials.

Three component mixtures that separate into two phases are widely used. Methanol: water mixtures can be used as a second phase with chloroform for the distribution of alkaloids but at the sacrifice of the selectivity offered by the control of the pH.

For the substances of increasing polarity, butanol may often be substituted for chloroform. For basic polar substrates, butanol systems with slightly acidic buffers are often useful.

Favorable distribution coefficients can sometimes be obtained by ion pair extraction. Even at pH sufficiently acidic to ionize them, some organic bases can be extracted into organic solvents as ion pairs with certain anions. An admirably clear explanation of ion pair extraction has appeared recently. Higuchi and Michaelis (1968), Higuchi et al. (1967) have observed that the extraction of dextromethorphan from aqueous solutions of low pH into mixtures of cyclohexane and chloroform or pentanol depends on the presence of bromide ions. Extractability is ascribed to the formation of complexes between the ion pair and the polar solvent that is dissolved in cyclohexane. The data indicate that complexes containing 3—5 molecules of solvent per ion pair can be expected. The extraction of codeine, lidocaine, promazine and strychnine as ion pairs with a number of inorganic anions has been studied by Schill et al. (1965). Iodide and thiocyanate in chloroform-water systems gave useful coefficients and similar pairs with methadone, papaverine, emetine, meclizine and pyrilamine are extractable (Persson and Schill, 1966). Other publications from the same group (Gustavii and Schill, 1966a, b) will also be of interest.

Ion pair extractions of pharmaceutical amines with *p*-toluene sulfonate have been studied by Doyle and Levine (1967). This acid in butanol-water systems has been used for the distribution of the very water soluble antibiotic, streptomycin (Titus and Fried, 1948). The isolation of transfer-RNA in a system containing tri-n-butyl amine is another dramatic example of the use of ion pairs to achieve a useful distribution constant (Karau and Zachau, 1964).

At pH values low enough for significant protonation to occur, amino acids will form complexes with tetraphenyl borate that partition between ether and water with K values in the range of 5—50 (Beyermann, 1965). The well-known dye extraction methods (Brodie et al., 1947; Ballard et al., 1954; Axelrod, 1960; Schill, 1965a, b) for the estimation of organic bases in biological material use ion pair extraction (Divatia and Biles, 1961; Hull and Biles, 1964) and the literature on this subject may offer useful clues to good systems for counter-current distribution.

The formation of complexes other than ion pairs can be a means of controlling the partition ratio. Scholfield et al. (1963), have taken advantage of the preferential formation of silver complexes by the *cis* isomer of monoenoic methyl esters to separate *cis* and *trans* isomers in a hexane-90% methanol system containing 0.2 M $AgNO_3$. A mixture of methyl trienoates was also partially separated into six fractions. As might be expected, the most rapidly moving of these was all *trans* and the most retarded by its preferential solubility in the aqueous phase was all *cis* (Scholfield et al., 1966).

In applying counter-current distribution to studies of drug metabolism one should keep in mind the probability that the products of most metabolic alterations will be more polar than the parent drug. Occasionally these changes may be very dramatic. The deamidation of the insecticide, 0,0-dimethyl-S-(N-methylcarbamylmethyl) phosphorothioate, which has a K of 41.5 in chloroform-pH 7 buffer, gives a product with a K of approximately 3×10^{-3} (Knaak and O'Brien, 1960; Uchida et al., 1964). The metabolism of pentobarbital is probably more representative, however. In a butanol-0.25 M pyrophosphate system at pH 9.4, pentobarbital has a K of 12. The alcoholic and acidic metabolites, 5-ethyl-5-(3-hydroxy-1-methylbutyl) barbituric acid and 5-ethyl-5-(1-methyl-3-carboxypropyl) barbituric acid have coefficients of 0.67 and 0.15, respectively. Metabolic removal of an N-alkyl group is a common pathway. The loss of N-ethyl from the antimalarial, 4-(3-diethyl amino-2-hydroxypropylamino)-7-chlorquinoline, increased K from 1.1 to 17 in a $CHCl_3$-phosphate buffer system.

Although water is a component of most distribution systems, nonaqueous liquid pairs are occasionally useful for the further fractionation of material already partially purified. A potentially very useful application has been described by Beroza and Bowman (1965a, b) (Bowman and Beroza, 1965, 1966), who have separated trace amounts of pesticides by gas chromatography. Solvent systems used in this work were hexane with either acetonitrile or 90% dimethylsulfoxide, isoctane with dimethyl formamide or 80% octane and heptane/90% ethanol. In cases where different materials gave identical retention times or where further identification was necessary, fractions were dissolved in the upper phase of an immiscible solvent pair and shaken with the lower phase. The concentration of solute in the upper phase was determined by quantitative gas chromatography before and after extraction. For the chlorinated hydrocarbons, which can be determined by electron affinity methods, counter-current distribution can be carried out with nanogram quantities. Distribution constants for 131 pesticides have been tabulated (Bowman and Beroza, 1965).

D. Chromatography

I. The Properties of Adsorbents Used in Column Chromatography

Since drug metabolism is usually best studied by micro methods, preparative chromatography on columns has not been used as widely in this field as in the isolation of natural products or the fractionation of synthetic products. The operations of column chromatography have been familiar for many years and are well described in the texts on the subject listed in the Introduction. This section will therefore be largely devoted to the factors that govern the choice of an adsorbent appropriate to the structure of the substrate or the choice of the most suitable mode of operation, i.e., adsorption, liquid-liquid partition or reversed phase chromatography. It will be of interest to examine the contributions of various groups on drug molecules to adsorption on the more commonly used absorbents. These relationships will dictate not only the manner in which the various absorbents are used in column chromatography, but also the way they are applied in the more extensively used thin layer procedures. Not only adsorption but also liquid-liquid partition chromatography can be carried out on columns and here, too, discussion of the relative merits of the two modes of column operation will be relevant to thin layer chromatography, which can be an adsorption process, liquid-liquid partition or, as is probably most often the case, a mixture of both.

A number of adsorbents have rather limited applicability to drug metabolism. Activated carbons, e.g. Norite or Darco, have a high affinity for aromatic amines, purines etc. Adsorption of such substances from neutral aqueous solutions and their subsequent elution with alcoholic ammonia may sometimes be an effective means of recovering certain drugs from tissue extracts. Activated magnesium silicates, the Florisils, have been described in the standard texts. In the author's laboratory these have occasionally been used for the preliminary separation of steroids from crude tissue extracts before final fractionation by other techniques. By far the most useful adsorbents, however, are alumina and silica gel.

Chromatographic alumina, until recently probably the most widely used adsorbent, is prepared by dehydration of alumina trihydrate by heating at temperatures ranging from 150—700° C. The product is a mixture of γ-alumina and a little alumina monohydrate with some sodium carbonate. High temperature ignition at more than 900° C completes the dehydration and produces the less active α-alumina (Cassidy, 1957). The adsorbing power of alumina is customarily classified by the rate of movement of a series of azobenzene derivatives down a column under standardized conditions (Brockmann, 1949). The most active alumina is designated as Grade I and others are numbered in order of decreasing adsorptive power. The lower grades can be prepared from the higher by the controlled addition of small increments of water. Various grades, calibrated according to Brockmann (1949), are commercially available. A half century of chromatographic experience has produced numerous studies of the relationship between the structure of organic molecules and affinity for alumina. These have been reviewed in the standard texts. The principles of adsorption on alumina have been discussed in an informative paper by Cummings et al. (1959), which also presents experimental data on the relative strengths of binding of a number of molecular structures.

Because of the complexity of the alumina surface a variety of binding mechanisms can operate. Among the weaker, but nevertheless useful, mechanisms is the formation of complexes between alumina and the π electron systems of aromatic structures. By this mechanism polynuclear aromatic hydrocarbons are absorbed onto alumina from relatively inert solvents, such as petroleum ether, and separate according to the number of aromatic rings. As alumina is washed with aromatic solvents like benzene, which can compete for the adsorbing site, the polynuclear hydrocarbons are displaced.

The most important source of affinity of a nonionic solute for alumina is probably hydrogen bonding through a proton donor group. Hydroxylated organic substances are thus more strongly bound than aromatic hydrocarbons and will be displaced only by more polar solvents. Proton acceptor groups, such as the oxygens of carbonyl compounds or ethers, have low affinity. What adsorption they exhibit probably results from hydrogen bonding with the relatively few hydroxyls on the alumina surface serving as the proton donors.

The ability of alumina to adsorb cations is evidenced by the presence of sodium carbonate in preparations of chromatographic alumina. Ion exchange with adsorbed cations appears to be a second mechanism, since basic organic compounds can be adsorbed on alumina and their adsorption is enhanced if the alumina is treated with alkali before heat activation. Some of the data cited by CUMMINGS (1959) suggest that aromatic amines may be adsorbed as micelles and that the relative ability of individual amines to form micelles or to stack at the adsorption site will affect the extent of their binding. Ion exchange with chloride ions introduced by prior treatment of alumina with HCl appears to be a mechanism for the adsorption of acidic organic substances. Chelation with aluminum in the alumina crystal lattice is probably an additional mechanism since *o*-dihydroxy-, aminoazo- or hydroxyazo-compounds are more tightly bound than their *p*-isomers.

The manner in which alumina is used for chromatography is dictated largely by the properties enumerated above. Since the surface has several adsorptive and ion-exchanging components and since different groups in a molecule interact with the surface by qualitatively different mechanisms, binding to alumina is not likely to be describable by a simple linear adsorption isotherm. In characterizing drug metabolites, therefore, adsorption chromatography on alumina would not ordinarily be used to provide an identifying physical constant, in this case an adsorption coefficient, easily derivable from chromatographic data. Preparative separations, however, can be quite effective. Here the usual procedure is to prepare a slurry of the alumina in the least polar of the solvents which are to pass over the column. The slurry is often briefly subjected to a vacuum to remove adsorbed gases from the adsorbent surface and then poured into a column. The solvent is allowed to descend until the meniscus approaches the top of the packed adsorbent. At this point the solute, dissolved in a minimum of the first solvent, is layered on top of the column and allowed to run in. Occasionally the sample for fractionation will be only partly soluble in the first solvent to enter the column. In this case a concentrated solution of the sample in a more polar solvent is sometimes mixed into a little alumina and the moist powder is dried in vacuum, resuspended in a little of the first solvent and added to the top of the column. The mixture is now separated into bands by running the solvent through the column. A single solvent may be used, but more commonly the column is eluted with solvents of progressively greater polarity. Slow flow rates encountered with polar solvents on alumina may be increased by mixing filter aids, such as Celite or Hyflo-Super Cel, with the adsorbent. Much of what has been said concerning alumina applies equally well to chromatography on columns of silicic acid (finely powdered silica gel). This adsorbent is readily available commercially in particle sizes suitable for chromatography. It is activated by heating above 100°C, but the severe dehydration at temperatures exceeding 150°C decreases its adsorptive capacity and it may be concluded that the hydroxyl groups of silicic acid play a major role in solute retention (TRUEBLOOD and MALMBERG, 1949). As with alumina there is a long history of chromatographic applications of silicic acid, which is summarized in the numerous standard texts. The theoretical basis for adsorption of variously substituted organic compounds on silicic acid has been reviewed by SPORER and TRUEBLOOD (1959). These authors measured the relative adsorption from benzene solutions of a large series of aromatic compounds with various substituents containing *O* and *N*. The order of decreasing adsorption affinities was $—CH_2NH_2$, $—COOH$, $—CH_2OH$, $—NH_2$, $CH_3CO—$, $—OH$, $—CHO$, $—NO_2$, $—OCH_3$, an arrangement very similar to that which would be expected on alumina. Hydrogen bonding with the solute serving as proton donor to oxygens of the adsorbent is apparently an important force in the adsorption of organic molecules on silicic acid just as it is on alumina. SPORER and TRUEBLOOD (1959) point out, however, that the silanol hydroxyl groups of silicic acid can serve as proton donors to acceptors on the substrate. This would explain the stronger adsorption of more basic amines noted by ILER (1955). It is an attractive hypothesis that the significant difference between the adsorptive capacities of alumina and silicic acid lies in the ability of the latter to serve as proton donor in hydrogen bonding. The oxygen of esterified fatty acids, for example, can serve only as acceptors in hydrogen bond formation yet these and similar substances can be chromatographed quite successfully on silicic acid (HIRSCH and AHRENS, 1958). Ketones, esters and ethers may be effective as eluting agents by virtue of their ability to compete for hydrogen bonding sites on silicic acid.

Silicic acid columns are usually prepared in a manner similar to the alumina columns described above. Solutes are first adsorbed from a nonpolar solvent and then move down the column as bands and are ultimately eluted with more polar solvents. Plots of the concentration of solute in the emergent solutions as a function of the volume of eluent may be unsymmetrical and show considerable tailing if the adsorption coefficient changes appreciably as the solute is diluted by broadening of the band as it passes down the column. Indeed SPORER and TRUEBLOOD (1959) report instances in which the adsorption coefficient varies with concentration of the dissolved solute down to about 10^{-4}M. The bands may sometimes be sharpened by gradient elution procedures. In these a second, somewhat more polar solvent is continuously added to the principle eluting solvent in a mixing chamber which feeds eluent to the top of the column. With appropriate apparatus the rate of increase in the concentration of the more polar constituent can be linear or exponential. In any case, both alumina and silicic acid columns are usually eluted by a succession of solvents of increasing polarity until no further fractions emerge. There has been considerable discussion in the earlier chromatographic literature of "eluotropic series", i.e. lists of solvents arranged in order of their increasing ability to displace adsorbed solutes from columns. These are usually arrangements in the order of increasing dipole moment and the eluotropic series are usually not greatly different from the list of solvents given in the section on counter-current distribution. In view of the differences between various adsorbents noted above and the differences in the mechanism of adsorption of different molecular structure, it is clear that the eluotropic series will vary somewhat with different adsorbents. Several examples are given by LEDERER and LEDERER (1957). A list of common solvents in order of their increasing adsorbability on silica gel has been published by KNIGHT and GROENNINGS (1954): heptane, diisobutylene, benzene, isopropyl chloride, diisopropyl ether, ethyl ether, sec-butanol, ethanol, water, acetone, methanol, pyruvic acid. It is common practice with either alumina or silica gel columns to make a gradual transition from one solvent to that of the next higher polarity by eluting with a series of mixtures in which the concentration of the second solvent increases in stepwise fashion. This procedure avoids the disruptive effects of localized heating which can ensue when solvents with high heats of adsorption first encounter the adsorbent. Very modest increases in the polarity of the eluting solvent often greatly increase the mobility of adsorbed solutes.

Readers interested in using column chromatography for the isolation of drugs or metabolites should consult the texts and reviews cited earlier for detailed methods. Some idea of the types of compounds for which these methods are appropriate can be obtained from specific examples of successful applications.

Very nonpolar substances can be fractionated. TENNEY and STURGIS (1954) have observed that monoolefins can be separated from diolefins and aromatic substances on silica gel. Alumina is better for the fractionation of aromatic hydrocarbons, which are separable provided they differ in the number of aromatic nuclei.

The chromatography of steroids has been particularly successful and has been reviewed extensively (BUSH, 1954; HEFTMANN, 1955). Alumina columns eluted with mixtures of petroleum ether and benzene have been widely used for the preparation of adrenal hormones (REICHSTEIN and SHOPPEE, 1949).

The active ingredients of Cannabis are lipids with some olefinic bonds, some aromatic character and occasional hydroxyls, a combination of properties that lends itself to chromatography on columns. KORTE and SIEPER (1960) have used alumina to isolate cannabidiol from a German species of hemp. Here the eluting series was ligroin, ligroin plus ether, ether and ether plus 5% methanol. The paper of KORTE and SIEPER provides an interesting opportunity to compare the effectiveness of column chromatography and counter-current distribution since the same material was analyzed by distribution between the two phases obtained by mixing ligroin, $CHCl_3$ and water (10:9:1).

Cardiac glycosides represents an interesting class of compounds intermediate between the relatively lipid soluble steroids and the highly polar carbohydrates; they can be absorbed onto neutralized alumina, and eluted with chloroform mixed with variable amounts of methanol (SCHINDLER and REICHSTEIN, 1951a). As the glycosides become sufficiently polar to require these solvents for elution, they also become sufficiently water soluble to permit their fractionation by the liquid-liquid partition techniques to be discussed later and the excellent resolution attainable has led some workers to prefer the latter methods.

The large volume of literature on highly polar substances, such as sugars, indicate that most workers prefer partition or paper chromatographic methods of fractionation, but column chromatography has been used. With these compounds adsorption on Florex XXX, Magnesol or Silene EF is effective. A representative paper by LEW et al. (1945) describes the elution of sugars and polyhydroxy compounds with alcohols, ether, dioxane, ketones, acids, pyridine and water alone or in various mixtures. Amino sugars, uronic acids and N-acetylamino neuraminic acid can, of course, be fractionated on ion exchange columns. Although chromatography is likely to be slow, alumina can be used with carbohydrates so polar as to be elutable only with methanol or water. For example, streptomycin, a strongly basic antibiotic which is largely carbohydrate, was purified by adsorption from methanol onto acid washed alumina and elution with aqueous methanol (CARTER et al., 1945).

Nitrogenous bases and alkaloids have been chromatographed on solid adsorbents, but relatively little use of this technique has been made to study metabolites of these structures. Metabolites of mepacrine were isolated by KING et al. (1946) on alumina columns. The literature on this field is summarized in readily available texts. Alumina and silica gel as well as less powerful adsorbents may be used for organic amines and alkaloids. Solvents in the range of polarities from benzene to ether are useful eluents, the former being used in a considerable number of the alkaloid fractionations cited by LEDERER and LEDERER (1957).

Although alumina and silicic acid are among the most widely used adsorbents, they can sometimes cause undesirable secondary reactions during the adsorption of the solute. This is particularly troublesome if the substance in question is sensitive to the free alkali usually present on the surface of chromatographic alumina. Inactivation of Veratrum alkaloids (FRIED et al., 1950), migration of benzoyl groups (SCHMID and BOLLIGER, 1954), dehalogenation of tertiary halides (ZAORAL, 1953), and isomerization of Δ^5-3-keto-steroids (REICHSTEIN and SHOPPEE, 1949) are among the many effects observed. These can often be avoided by the use of neutral or acid washed alumina, but deacetylation of acetyl cardiotonic glycosides is particularly troublesome and such substances are better chromatographed on magnesium silicate rather than alumina (SCHINDLER and REICHSTEIN, 1951b). However, isomerization of unsaturated compounds can occur on silicic acid.

Occasionally the adsorptive properties can be modified or improved by incorporation of other substances into a silicic acid or alumina column. A mixed column of copper carbonate and alumina, for example, within which α-amino acids are adsorbed as their copper complexes has been used to separate these compounds from mixtures (THOMPSON et al., 1953).

Silver nitrate, as noted earlier, can form π complexes with unsaturated compounds, and incorporation of this salt into solid adsorbents has been used to enhance the retention of acetylenic and polyolefinic substances. Modified adsorbents are useful in the fractionation of contraceptive steroids (ERCOLI et al., 1964). Methyl esters of unsaturated fatty acids can be fractionated on silicic acid which has been suspended in two parts v/w of 50% aqueous $AgNO_3$, heated to 100°C, cooled, filtered and dried. The product is mixed with half its weight of Celite to improve flow rates and elution is carried out with mixtures of benzene in light petroleum ether (DE VRIES, 1963). SGOUTAS and KUMMEROW (1964) have observed an interesting isotope effect on such columns. Tritiated methyl linoleate was found to be separable from C^{14}-methyl linoleate, possibly because the bulky H^3 atoms at the double bond affected the strength of the silver-π bond complex.

Although the dextran gels used for molecular sieving are not usually considered as chromatographic absorbents, they do have a striking affinity for compounds rich in π electrons. A planar structure and an extensive system of conjugated double bonds in the solute favor adsorption. The more tightly cross linked polymers, such as Sephadex G-10 and G-15, are particularly good adsorbents. For aromatic molecules small enough to penetrate the interstices of the Sephadex, column chromatography is an excellent means of separation. Amino acids may be chromatographed, for example, on a 1.0 cm × 142 cm column of Sephadex G-10 equilibriated with 1% acetic acid. Eluting solvents are 1% acetic acid plus 2.0 M NaCl. With polypeptides of dimensions similar to those of the capillary bed in the dextrans, the molecular sieving becomes a factor as well as adsorption, and the gels are particularly useful for fractionating protein hydrolysates.

Sephadex gels always contain a small number of carboxyl groups, which lead to interesting consequences. In the tightly cross linked Sephadex polymers negatively charged substances or highly charged substances carrying around them an ionic double layer tend to be excluded from the pores and move more rapidly through the column. These ionic effects are dissipated by high ionic strength so that acidic aromatic substances tend to be more retarded in salt solutions. This phenomenon is probably responsible for the successful isolation of conjugated estrogens from urine (Beling, 1961). Twenty ml of urine were added to a Sephadex column and eluted with water. All of the estrogens appeared in a fraction of only 3 ml essentially free of other urinary constituents. The effect is probably due to the fact that the conjugate would normally move faster than low molecular weight salt, but is retarded by the effects noted above. As the salt moves down, any of the conjugated estrogen tending to remain behind is accelerated by the oncoming water and the final result is a concentration in the boundary between salt and water.

Gel chromatography on tightly cross-linked Sephadex is a promising technique. Readers interested in applying it should consult the review by Janson (1967).

II. Liquid-Liquid Partition Chromatography

In liquid-liquid partition chromatography a separation is effected by distribution of the components of a mixture between a stationary liquid phase and mobile liquid phase. The latter is allowed to percolate through a column of packed granular material which acts as a support for the stationary liquid. It is assumed in theoretical treatments of the process that the relative retention of various solutes by the column is a function only of the partition coefficient between the two solvents. The process is thus analogous to counter-current distribution and the earlier discussion of the choice of solvent systems for particular fractionation problems will apply equally to partition chromatography. It is important, of course, that the solvent system be compatible with the solid support used. The stationary phase support should be an inert, stable and porous granule that can hold over 50% of its dry weight of the polar liquid. Usually a particle size of 100—150 μ will permit adequate flow rates. The stationary liquid should be strongly adsorbed to the supporting solvent but the mobile liquid and the solutes to be separated should not. Martin and Synge (1941), who introduced the technique as a means of fractionating amino acids in protein digests, used silicic acid as a suspending medium. Deviations from the theoretically predicted elution curves were ascribed in part to adsorption of the solute on the supporting agent. Other materials such as potato starch and various forms of cellulose have also been used as supports and have also shown some adsorptive capacity. Martin (1950a, b) in reviewing this problem felt that hydrated cellulose, which was originally regarded as an inert support, might be more accurately considered as a strong polysaccharide solution or a complex gel and it may be that the limited adsorption of aromatic substances by this material occurs by the same mechanism as in dextran gels (Janson, 1967). After some controversy as to whether partition chromatography is really a liquid-liquid extraction process, it is now generally recognized that the line of demarcation between adsorption and partition chromatography is not sharp. Kay and Trueblood (1954) have observed experimentally the transition from adsorption to true liquid-liquid extraction as the water content of a silicic acid-Celite mixture is increased.

The diatomaceous filter aids, Celite and Hyflo Super Cel, are now widely used. These are described in a Technical Bulletin, No. FF221, of the Johns Mansville Company. Celite 545 with a particle diameter of 20—40 μ is probably the most generally useful (Levine, 1963a). Columns must be prepared so as to ensure that the fixed phase is stable, i.e. the amount of immobilized polar liquid does not change during passage of the other solvent. Several packing techniques have been described. The immobile phase may be added to a stirred suspension of the solid support in the mobile solvent (Haenni et al., 1953a). The immobile liquid may be added to the solid support and the thoroughly mixed, slightly moist powder is then tamped into the column (MARTIN and SYNGE, 1941). The exact amount of liquid to be used is determined empirically, but if it is enough to make the mixture sticky so that it packs into balls it is usually too much. Depending on the solvent, quantities from 1—1.28 ml/g of Celite have been found practical (LEVINE, 1961; HAENNI et al., 1953b). FISCHBACH et al. (1947) recommend the use of about 90—95% of that volume of solvent which is required to make the mixture with Celite sticky. Technical details and lists of useful references concerning column packing and the determination of optimal flow rates will be found in papers by HAENNI et al. (1953a, b) and LEVINE (1961).

Since it is impossible in a short chapter to deal with the numerous applications of partition chromatography, three examples of its use have been rather arbitrarily selected from the literature to illustrate how some of the advantages of this technique can be exploited. Certain of these advantages derive from the similarity of partition chromatography to counter-current distribution. Undesirable chemical changes in the solute catalysed by strong adsorbents may be avoided in liquid systems. The nonlinearity of adsorption isotherms makes the theoretical treatment of classical adsorption chromatography cumbersome and the susceptibility of the adsorbent to deactivation makes reproducibility a problem. Partition chromatography with its linear isotherms, i.e. constant K, is more amenable to theoretical treatment and is highly reproducible. The retention volume, i.e. that volume of effluent at which the peak in the concentration of emerging solute occurs, can thus be used as an identifying physical constant. The analytical usefulness of partition chromatography is nicely illustrated by the work of LAMBERT and PORTER (1964). These authors prepared a column of water-ethylene glycol suspended on finely ground (100—120 mesh) C-22 Silocel firebrick. The mobile phase was hexane-CCl_4. The 8 foot by one-fourth inch column was designed to be maintained under a constant pressure, which was not reduced between runs. Samples were injected into the stream of mobile solvent as it entered the column and the concentration of emergent material was monitored by a differential refractometer. Retention volumes of standard samples were reproducible for periods up to 4 years on such a column. As the authors point out, the use of a mobile solvent of constant concentration makes it possible to monitor the effluent by a universally applicable method, such as refractive index; liquid-liquid chromatography under these circumstances is thus essentially like gas-liquid chromatography with the exception that larger amounts (100—1000 mgs) can be handled. Partition chromatography therefore becomes a substitute for gas chromatography for substrates that are non-volatile or heat labile. One of the resolutions described by the authors, the separation of *cis* and *trans* crotonate derivatives of the insecticide, Phosdrin, exemplifies the advantages of this technique. The substance, although relatively non-polar, would not be volatile at ordinary temperatures and would be expected to isomerize at high temperatures or on alumina and silicic acid surfaces.

The theory of partition chromatography has been discussed by a number of authors (MARTIN and SYNGE, 1941; CASSIDY, 1957; DE VAULT, 1943; KLINKENBERG and SJENITZER, 1956; TRENNER, 1957). A linear partition isotherm is usually assumed in these treatments. MARTIN and SYNGE (1941) treat the partition column as a series of infinitesimal elements of volume, each of which is analogous to a tube of the counter-current distribution process. The curve describing the shape of a moving band of solute would thus take the form of a distribution curve and, as mentioned earlier, would approach the form of the normal curve of error as the number of transfers became very large. The latter then would be the form of the developing band in the integrated expression for what is really a continuous rather than stepwise process. These authors have provided a useful expression for the concentration, C, in the effluent as a function of the volume of the mobile phase, V, passed through the column. Their expression can be reduced to

$$C = \frac{q}{V_R}\left(\frac{r}{2\pi}\right)^{1/2} e^{\left(-\frac{r}{2}\right)\left(1 - V/V_R\right)^2}$$

where r is the number of theoretical plates in the column, q is the amount of solute originally added and V_R is the retention volume. V_R is related to the distribution constant, K, for a particular substance by the expression

$$V_R = V_M + KV_S$$

where V_M is the volume of the column occupied by the mobile phase and V_S is that volume occupied by the stationary phase.

The picture of the partition chromatographic process that emerges from the theoretical treatments may be put to use in several ways. The shape of the solute band moving down a column is adequately described by a Gaussian distribution and experimentally the elution curves of Lambert and Porter are Gaussian. Elution curves representing incomplete resolution of several components may be analysed by computer, since Stone (1962) has written a program for the resolution of curves that result from the superposition of several Gaussian curves.

The simple relationship between retention volume and K means that highly accurate values for the partition coefficients of several components of a mixture are easily obtained. Conversely, the chromatographic behavior of a mixture of components may be predicted if the individual partition coefficients are known. Some of the changes in partition coefficient as substituents are metabolically introduced into drug molecules were mentioned in an earlier section. Given this information one can calculate the volume of solvent required to elute an anticipated metabolite. The planning of partition chromatographic procedures is obviously facilitated if one can predict the change in distribution constant when a new group is introduced into a known molecule. Partition chromatography of related groups of compounds and homologous series have been carried out for this purpose (Martin, 1950b). The standard free energy change, ΔG, for the passage of a substance from one solvent to another is related to the partition coefficient, K, by

$$\ln K = -\frac{\Delta G}{RT}$$

where R is the gas constant and T is absolute temperature. If one regards the standard free energy of transfer of a molecule as simply the sum of the free energy changes of all the individual subunits of the molecule e.g. —CH_2—, —OH, etc., then the introduction of any particular group will always give the same increment to ln K and the change in partition of the molecule becomes predictable. This was, of course, recognized as an oversimplification by Martin (1950b) and better semi-empirical expressions for the relationship of ln K to the number of added groups have been derived by Pierotti et al. (1959). In practice, if one two-phase system is chosen as a standard, the change in log V_R associated with a particular molecular change will be relatively constant throughout a number of related compounds.

In all of the above applications it was necessary to keep the liquid-liquid system constant in order to obtain the advantages offered by partition chromatography. With the introduction of kieselguhrs like Celite, which support large volumes of aqueous phase and exhibit minimal adsorption, it has become practical to elute partition columns with several mobile liquids of successively greater eluting power. So long as none of the series of solvents is appreciably miscible with water, the behaviour of the column is not distorted. This type of elution has been particularly useful with steroids. The paper of Hegedus et al. (1953) is representative of a long series of studies of cardiac glycosides in Reichstein's laboratory. These authors chromatographed *strophanthus* glycosides on Hyflo Super-Cel impregnated with water and eluted with petroleum ether, benzene and chloroform in various ratios. With solvents of polarity so greatly different from water the effects of structural differences in the steroids are enhanced so that excellent resolution is achieved. The extractability of the cardiac glycosides in these solvents is not high and it was necessary to use large columns and very large volumes of eluting solvents. In a somewhat similar procedure (BANES, 1954) formamide-water was used as immobile phase and iso-octane was used to elute digitoxigenin. Digitoxin emerged in benzene-chloroform and gitoxin in chloroform. The metabolites of pentobarbital were separated by chromatography on Celite pH 10.8 buffer using chloroform and chloroform with increasing percentages of ethyl acetate as eluting solvents (PALMER et al., 1969).

Reversed phase chromatography is a third type of liquid-liquid partition fractionation that has been widely applied to lipids. In this procedure a lipophilic supporting phase is used to immobilize a nonpolar liquid and the column is eluted with aqueous buffers or other polar solvents. As with conventional partition chromatography, the method became practical with the development of adequate supporting media. Siliconized Celite or Super-Cel is now universally used and is easily prepared (HOWARD and MARTIN, 1950). Hyflo Super-Cel is dried at 100° C, then allowed to stand in a closed dessicator containing dichloro-dimethyl silane. When the reaction is complete all of the solid should float when mixed with water. The treated powder is washed thoroughly with methanol and allowed to dry. HOWARD and MARTIN used octane supported on the column and elution with methanol to separate the C_{12} to C_{18} fatty acids. The procedure is especially useful for mixtures of highly unsaturated lipids, which isomerize readily on adsorbent surfaces or at high temperatures. Polyunsaturated fatty acids were prepared in high purity using acetonitrile-methanol as a mobile phase and heptane on celite that had been treated as described above.

A few examples will illustrate the application of partition chromatography to various types of drugs. Penicillins have been separated on silicic acid columns carrying phosphate buffer, pH 6.4, by elution with ether (FISCHBACH et al., 1947). A great many basic drugs and alkaloids have been fractionated on acidic columns. Dilute acids, 0.1—0.3 M, are commonly used as are citrate or phosphate buffers of pH up to 4.5. The eluting solvent varies with the drug. Chloroform is frequently used for the more polar drugs. Hyoscine and hyoscyamine have been separated at pH 6.2 by elution with ether and chloroform (EVANS and PARTRIDGE, 1948). The water-insoluble alkaloids of ergot have been separated on Solka-Floc, using a pH 3.4 buffer and ether as the liquid phases (BRINDLE et al., 1951). Ether and pH 2.0 phosphate on Hyflo Super-Cel effectively separated a number of the opium alkaloids (LINDBLAD and AGREN, 1954). Occasionally it is advantageous to include non-ionic polar organic solvents in the bound phase. Some of the more polar adrenocortical steroids, for example, are not as water soluble as the cardiac glycosides, and do not lend themselves to procedures like that of HEGEDUS et al. (1953). They can be eluted from adsorption columns with more polar solvents, but these steroids of intermediate polarity may sometimes be best resolved by partition between ethylene glycol and toluene or petroleum ether-toluene (2+8) (MORRIS and WILLIAMS, 1953). BANES (1953) has used formamide-water (4:1) supported on Celite and elution with benzene-isooctane (3:2) to resolve 11-dehydrocorticosterone and corticosterone. For C_{19} as well as the C_{21} steroids, nitromethane is sometimes useful as the immobile solvent and elution with heptane or petroleum ether containing small percentages of chloroform is effective. See, for example, JONES and

STRITCH (1953). The extractability of ion pairs into organic solvents is useful in liquid-liquid partition chromatography as well as counter-current distribution. Simple halide salts can sometimes be used as in the separations of strychnine, dihydrocodeinone and pheniramine on Celite — 2N HCl with chloroform as the mobile solvent (LEVINE, 1963b). Sulfonic acid (0.5 M) has been used in a similar system and *p*-toluene sulfonic acid, which forms ion pairs of considerably greater solubility in organic solvents, can be used for a variety of alkaloids (LEVINE and OTTES, 1961).

Partition chromatography is a promising technique for the study of drug metabolism. It is in some respects analogous to counter-current distribution with a large number of transfers. Systems applicable to a great variety of drugs can be selected from the literature. The review by LEVINE (1963a) will be helpful here. Not infrequently the effects of expected metabolic changes, such as hydroxylation or N-dealkylation, on the partition coefficient in a given system will be predictable, so that systems likely to be useful for metabolic studies may be designed with reasonable success.

III. Paper and Thin Layer Chromatography

1. Introduction

Paper chromatography was introduced by CONSDEN et al. (1944) in order to eliminate the preparation of solid supports in partition chromatography and to reduce the quantity of materials needed. With the development of spray reagents to reveal the location of compounds, analytical methods applicable to very small amounts of drugs and radioactivity techniques, paper and thin layer chromatography have become the methods of choice in most studies of drug metabolism. Although paper was originally considered as an inert support for the aqueous portion of a developing solvent, it is now evident that adsorption and ion exchange also contribute to the retention of solutes. With the supports used in thin layer chromatography adsorption may predominate with nonpolar solvents, but partition becomes important with water or other highly polar solvents which become bound to the adsorbent. The advantages conveyed by the use of thin supports are speed, flexibility and applicability on a micro scale, but the basic principles underlying the procedures are those that have been dealt with in the preceding sections. Thus if one considers paper chromatography and thin layer chromatography on silicic acid treated with polar solvents as primarily partition chromatography, the information on use of solvents and structure-partition relationships that has been developed from counter-current distribution and from liquid-liquid partition chromatography becomes applicable to these micromethods. With nonpolar solvents the thin layer of silicic acid can be primarily an adsorbent. Here the capacity to serve as donor as well as acceptor in hydrogen bonding means that a great variety of organic structures can be adsorbed and that a number of solvents can compete for the binding sites and serve as eluents. Again the information from conventional chromatography becomes relevant. Silicic acid is by no means the only adsorbent used in thin layer procedures but the variety of ways in which it acts make chromatography with this support a remarkably flexible tool.

2. Paper Chromatography

The procedures of paper chromatography are basically simple and are described in the texts enumerated in the Introduction. A drop of solution containing the mixture is placed on a strip of filter paper near one end. In order to minimize the area occupied by the sample, the volume of transferring solvent is kept small. If the sample is not already dissolved in the solvent to be used for development, excess solvent is commonly evaporated by directing a stream of air or nitrogen across the paper surface. The end of the paper is then immersed in a developing solvent which moves along the strip by capillarity. As the moving solvent passes the point at which sample was applied, the various components begin to move in the direction of solvent flow. Usually the process is stopped before the advancing solvent front has completely traversed the paper and the location of the front is marked before the paper is dried in a hood. Separate components of the mixture may be located on the paper by spraying with colorimetric reagents, fluorescence under ultraviolet light, counting of radioactivity, etc. Since most filter papers contain minute traces of fluorescent impurities, it is sometimes possible to see ultraviolet absorbing substances as dark areas against a faint fluorescence if the chromatogram is examined under ultraviolet light in a darkroom. Transverse sections cut from the developed chromatogram can then be eluted for quantitative determination of the components.

In ascending chromatography, often the simplest procedure, the paper containing the samples may be rolled into a cylinder and held in that form by loosely sewing or stapling the vertical edges together. The two edges thus brought together must not quite touch each other since the flow of solvent would be altered in the region of contact. The paper cylinder is then set into a glass jar containing a layer of the developing solvent and the top is sealed with a flat glass plate. Paper strips may also be suspended from a framework within the jar so that the lower end dips into solvent.

Apparatus for descending chromatography is generally available from supply houses. A semicylindrical trough to hold the developing solvent is positioned at the top of a jar or tank. One end of the paper is dipped into the bottom of this trough and held in place by the weight of a glass rod in the trough. Parallel to the glass trough and usually a centimeter or two away is an antisiphoning rod, over which the paper strip passes and from which it hangs down into a jar or cabinet. The whole apparatus is sealed from the atmosphere. Samples are applied near the top of the paper, just below the point of contact with the antisiphoning rod, and descend with the solvent.

The ascending procedure is advantageous in two-dimensional chromatography. For this the sample is placed near one corner of a sheet of paper and the solvent is allowed to rise. The edge near which the sample has ascended is then placed at the bottom in a second system so that mixtures which were only partially resolved in the first solvent system may be more completely separated in the second. Alternatively, descending chromatography may be used with the second system. In this case the development of the chromatogram may be continued after the solvent front has reached the bottom edge of the filter paper. If the solvent is to be allowed to drip off the bottom edge, serration of the edge with pinking shears will prevent the temporary accumulation of excess solvent along the edge and possible distortion of the chromatogram.

Paper chromatography is always carried out in a sealed apparatus. Usually the inside of the apparatus is lined with a layer of paper moistened with the developing solvent. These procedures help to maintain a constant solvent content throughout the length of the paper and prevent distortion by localized evaporation. Temperature control is important, because the relative volumes and the composition of the phases into which the multicomponent solvent systems separate vary markedly with temperature. The area must be free of draughts and temperature gradients if reproducible results are to be obtained. Any of a variety of filter papers may be used. Whatman No. 1 or other papers of equivalent weight are commonly used.

Somewhat greater capacity may be attained with Whatman No. 3 or papers of equivalent weight, but it should be pointed out that papers of different manufacture will vary somewhat in speed and resolving power.

Paper chromatography, like counter-current distribution and partition chromatography, is used for qualitative identification as well as for quantitative analyses. The identifying physical constant is R_f, that fraction of the distance between origin and solvent front which was traveled by the solute. R_f is calculated by measuring the distance from the center of the point of application to the center of the solute spot, i.e. to the position of maximum concentration of the moving band. CONSDEN et al. (1944) showed that paper chromatography may be treated theoretically in the same manner as column partition chromatography. If partition between a mobile solvent and a fixed solvent retained on the paper is the sole determinant, R_f can be shown to equal $\frac{A_m}{A_m + KA_f}$ where A_m is the cross sectional area of the column occupied by the mobile phase, A_f is the cross sectional area occupied by the fixed solvent and K is the partition coefficient. The treatment is analogous to that mentioned earlier for counter-current distribution. Thus the development of the chromatogram may be considered as a series of stepwise equilibrations in infinitesimal elements of volume of the paper. Since the number of these elements and the numbers of transfers applied must be considered as very large, the concentration of solute plotted as a function of distance along the paper takes the shape of a band corresponding to the curve of error. As before when the number of transfers is large, the ratio of the mean distance traveled by the substance to the distance traveled by the advancing solvent is equal to the fraction of solute in the mobile phase at equilibrium. This was $\frac{K}{K+1}$ for counter-current distribution and is $\frac{A_m}{A_m + KA_f}$ for paper chromatography. R_f is thus in theory predictable from the partition coefficient between solvents if one knows the relative volume of the two solvents in a saturated paper. Whatman No. 1 paper at usual humidities has about 0.3 μl of water per mg and if equilibrated with solvents that are immiscible with water, it gains in addition about 0.9 μl of solvent per mg (DIKSTEIN, 1959). WOKSMUNDZKI and SOCZEWINSKI (1959) have calculated a formula for the R_f in terms of the ionization constant of an acid or base, partition coefficient and pH, and have used paper chromatographic data to choose systems for counter-current distribution. This kind of application, however, is very rare. R_f is sensitive to so many factors, including viscosity of the solvents, trace metals in the paper, diffusion of the advancing solute, etc., that it is better considered as an empirical constant, valid only for a particular type of paper under exactly specified conditions. The design of paper chromatographic systems for specific applications is thus an empirical process. The relationships between solute structure and partition coefficient that have been discussed earlier are usually applied more intuitively than exactly but are nevertheless useful. Paper sheets are seldom impregnated with polar phase. It is usually assumed that polar components contained in the advancing solvent will dissolve in the water bound to the paper or seek their own equilibrium with the paper. In the adaptation of solvent systems from counter-current distribution to paper chromatography, therefore, it is common practice to select the less polar phase of a liquid-liquid system as the developing solvent for paper.

Buffered systems may be used on paper for ionizable drugs and SOCZEWINSKI (1960) has derived expressions for optimizing the pH for particular separations. To separate atropine from hyoscine and brucine from strychnine CARLESS and

WOODHEAD (1951) have used butanol saturated with 1/15 M phosphate or citrate buffers (pH 5—9) and have determined R_f as a function of pH. Plots of R_f vs pH for ergot alkaloids in ether saturated with buffer were sigmoidal, essentially similar to titration curves. For these substances R_f varied from 0—1 as the pH increased. Good resolution was obtainable except that ergotoxin could not be resolved into ergocristine, ergocornine or ergokryptine.

Alkaloids and basic drugs generally are chromatographed in mixtures of butanol, acetic acid and water. In typical preparations 4—10 ml of glacial acetic acid are added to 100 ml of butanol and the mixture is saturated with water. The chromatography of a great variety of biologically and pharmacologically important bases is tabulated in BLOCK et al. (1958). As a general rule the inclusion of a little organic acid in a butanol-water system will prevent tailing and give improved resolution of organic bases. Small amounts of ammonia or simple organic amines may be similarly helpful for substances with acidic groups. Some combinations that have been successfully used for alkaloids are the upper layer from a mixture of butanol-ethanol-NH_4OH-water (90:10:1:97); butanol-formic acid-water (12:1:7) and 10% acetic acid in 5% sodium acetate, saturated with *n*-butyl ether.

A great many drugs of current interest are indoles. Both the basic derivatives such as the tryptamines and the various indole acids can be fractionated on paper with butanol-acetic acid-water (60:15:25) as the developing solvent. Butanol-pyridine-water (1:1:1) may give somewhat better resolution of acidic indoles from the neutral and basic derivatives. In either system molecules differing significantly in polarity, e.g. 5-hydroxytryptamine and 5-methoxy tryptamine, are well resolved. For more closely related substances, such as contiguous members of a homologous series like indole acetic and indole propionic acid, resolution is improved by using shorter chain length alcoholic solvents. Isopropanol-NH_4OH-water (10:1:1) has been used for these substances (STOWE and THIMANN, 1954). Solvent systems for a large number of indoles have been tabulated by BLOCK et al. (1958).

Isopropanol-ammonia systems have also been used for phenolic substances and aromatic acids but benzene-propionic-water (2:2:1) (ARMSTRONG et al., 1956) may give a wider spread of R_f values in this series.

DE ZEEUW (1969) has published an exhaustive review of paper and thin layer methods for the fractionation of a considerable number of hypnotics, sedatives, etc. that are of interest in toxicology or forensic medicine. The compounds all bear some structural resemblance to the barbiturates, the criterion for inclusion being the presence of the characteristic R—CO—NH-group or the R—O—CO—NH_2 carbamate group in the molecule. The review also includes a list of the most common pathways of metabolism of these drugs and some information on the relative rates of metabolic breakdown. Some 26 solvent mixtures for paper chromatography are listed, a number of these being mixtures of butanol with various concentrations of ammonia. A number of the derivatives, such as pyrithyldion, glutethimide, etc., that are less polar than barbiturates, moved very rapidly in these systems and for these toluene-25% ammonia (10:1) gave somewhat better resolution. Several of the systems used solvents less miscible with water than butanol, and in these instances, the paper was often saturated with a polar organic solvent before development with a less polar mobile liquid. Chloroform-benzene (1:1) used with a paper previously impregnated with 50% formamide in ethanol was one example.

Some of the difficulties in applying partition paper chromatography to steroids have been summarized by BUSH (1954). In ordinary systems, steroids tend to move either too fast or not at all. Adsorption to paper causes tailing of the hydroxylated steroids and even those derivatives with relatively large numbers of hydroxyl groups are too insoluble in aqueous solvents to partition well. Impregnation of the paper with polar organic solvents was therefore introduced by Zaffaroni et al. (1950), who found benzene-formamide or toluene-propylene glycol systems most satisfactory for the separation of adrenocortical hormones. The papers were immersed in the lower solvent phase obtained by shaking the two components of the immiscible pair. The wet paper was then placed between dry sheets of filter paper and squeezed between rollers to remove the excess of the viscous polar solvent and descending paper chromatography was carried out as usual. In order to minimize diffusion, narrow strips of paper were used. Excellent resolution was obtained, but the solutes moved so slowly that it was usually necessary to let the mobile solvent drip off the paper for several hours. Spots were identified by their mobility with respect to a standard substance rather than by R_f. The success of this technique, which has been enormously useful in studies of adrenocortical function, led to other applications. Most of the successful methods employed impregnation either with the solvents used by Zaffaroni et al. (1950) or with more volatile systems of the sort introduced by Bush (1952), who equilibrated benzene, methanol and water and impregnated the papers with the lower phase. For weakly polar steroids, methyl esters of acetylated bile acids, for example, the use of toluene and ethylene glycol monophenyl ether is recommended. Cardiac steroids can be chromatographed by procedures like that of Zaffaroni (Schindler and Reichstein, 1951c) and extremely polar members of this class can be chromatographed with butanol-water or butanol-toluene-water mixtures. In this case the paper was drawn through the lower layer before addition of the samples and developed with the upper layer as the mobile phase. The paper chromatography of steroids in general has been reviewed by Heftmann (1955) and that of cardiac steroids by Nover et al. (1968).

The catecholamines and 5-hydroxy indoles are also substances of great pharmacological interest. Paper chromatographic systems for these biogenic amines are similar to those used for other polar molecules but a few precautions should be kept in mind. The catecholamines are easily oxidized at pH above 7 and in the presence of traces of some heavy metals. They are unstable in strong ultraviolet light. The catecholamines are very water soluble, but can be extracted by butanol from tissue homogenates saturated with salt. Back extraction into a small volume of acid gives a concentrated solution (Shore, 1959). Papers for catecholamine chromatography should be washed in 0.5 N HCl followed by 0.1% Versene and water in order to remove traces of heavy metals (Goldstein and Abelin, 1956). Butanol-acetic acid-water (4:1:5) (Schayer et al., 1953) and freshly distilled phenol saturated with 0.1 N HCl or water (James, 1948) have been used as developing solvents. R_f values for a number of biogenic amines and phenolic amines on cellulose phosphate ion exchange (Whatman P-20, Reeve Angel and Co.), have been published by Roberts (1962). The eluting solvent was prepared by mixing 1 part of a 0.2 M ammonium acetate buffer, pH 6.0, with 2 parts of isopropanol.

At the other extreme from such water soluble compounds as the biogenic amines are the very nonpolar lipoidal substances, such as the higher fatty acids and their esters, some plant pigments, etc. The systematic fractionation of lipids on silicic acid (see Hirsch and Ahrens, 1958) and thin layer chromatography on silicic acid are frequently more convenient than paper chromatography for such materials, but a variety of reversed phase systems have been developed. In all of these, the filter paper is treated to make it water repellent, i.e. a nonpolar phase is immobilized on the paper. There are several methods for treating paper. It can be passed through an aqueous solution of 62% liquid latex and air dried, then washed with alcohol and stored in cartons (Ashley and Westphal, 1955). It can be siliconized by passing it through a solution of 5% Dow Corning Silicone No. 1107 in cyclohexane after which it is blotted and dried at 100°C; such paper is permanently hydrophobic even after washing with organic solvents (KRITCHEVSKY and TISELIUS, 1951). Sometimes it is simply washed thoroughly with a series of organic solvents, dehydrated in a vacuum and passed through solutions of paraffins or olive oil in ether (ASHLEY and WESTPHAL, 1955). Some representative developing systems are methanol-decalin (8:1), 78% ethanol, in acetic acid-water (9:1) and diethylene glycol-acetic acid-tetralin (60:20:11). A great number of other combinations may be found in texts on paper chromatography. Fatty acids are seldom chromatographed directly; they are usually converted to hydroxamates for good separations. Lipid separations can also be carried out on silicic acid paper made by immersing paper first in sodium silicate and then in acid after which it is washed and dried for activation. Such paper is brittle and fragile and usually offers no advantage over thin layer systems.

3. Thin Layer Chromatography

The operations of thin layer chromatography are essentially those of ascending paper chromatography except that the supporting medium is a layer of adsorbent surfaced on about 20 cms of glass or plastic plate. The sample is deposited as a droplet near the edge of the plate. The latter is then set into a developing solvent which rises through the thin film of adsorbent by capillarity. The various components travel with the advancing solvent at different rates characterized by an R_f as in paper chromatography. The process is carried out in a sealed tank or jar and a lining or wick of filter paper is usually placed inside the jar to keep the atmosphere saturated with solvent. The procedure has a number of advantages. It is fast, requiring from 15 or 20 min to periods of a few hours at the most, and it requires only minute amounts of material. Since the solid adsorbent is supported on glass the isolated fractions can be located by agents, such as sulfuric acid sprays, that would destroy a paper chromatograph. REITSEMA (1954) was among the earliest to take advantage of a thin layer supported on a glass plate by means of a binding substance. But much of the development of the method is due to STAHL, whose treatise on the subject (1969) exhaustively reviews the history and applications of the technique. The recent handbook by SCOTT (1969) is a very useful source of information about types of adsorbent, sources of commercially available equipment, and applications to biologically important separation problems. The pharmacologist will find the review of TRUHAUT et al. (1968) invaluable, since it deals extensively with the identification of drugs and their metabolites by thin layer techniques.

Thin layer plates are readily prepared. A row of 20×20 cm glass plates, carefully cleaned and free of traces of grease, is set into a flat holder on the bench top and a creamy suspension, usually of about 25 g of adsorbent thoroughly stirred with about 50 ml of water, is put into a spreader which is then drawn over the line of plates. The spreader is a metal trough with a carefully machined slit at the bottom which delivers a layer of 0.25 mm thickness onto the plate. The plates are allowed to dry slowly in air until most of the moisture has evaporated, then activated by heating at 100°C. Various adsorbents are commercially available. Most now contain $CaSO_4$ as a binder. Prolonged heating above 120°C should be avoided since excessive dehydration of the binder can loosen the adsorbent. By far the most generally used adsorbent is silicic acid (Kieselgel G of STAHL). This provides a slightly acidic surface, which has proved useful with all of the solvent systems thus far tried. Alumina has been used, especially for some acidic substances and steroids. Kieselguhr G, a standard preparation devised by STAHL, is a powdered diatomaceous earth, which provides a neutral surface and is sometimes useful when the system is acting primarily by partition between adsorbed liquids. Cellulose, cellulose acetate and various ion exchanging derivatives of cellulose have all had specialized applications. Most suppliers of chromatographic equipment now provide pre-coated plates either on glass or various inert plastics. One of the reasons for the rapid acceptance of thin layer chromatography was its applicability to lipids and this technique, together with gas chromatography, is now indispensable in lipid laboratories. As might be expected from the success of Hirsch and Ahrens (1958) in separating the various classes of lipids on columns of silicic acid, this adsorbent is usually used. Alumina has a tendency to catalyze hydrolysis and isomerization of certain lipids and is little used. Mixtures of petroleum ether with 1—5% of benzene or diethyl ether have successfully separated hydrocarbons, alkyl esters, sterol esters and polyenol esters from each other. Molecules with more polar functional groups remain at the origin in such chromatograms, but fatty alcohols and aldehydes, and mono-di-and triglycerides are separable into groups if the petroleum ether contains about 10—50% diethyl ether. If free fatty acids occur in these fractions, the tendency for tailing caused by the association of these compounds in solution may be overcome by including a little glacial acetic acid in the solvent mixtures. Lipids of considerable polarity, such as the phosphatides, are often separated with chloroform, methanol and water. A mixture in the ratio 65:25:4 gives excellent separation of the various classes of phospholipids. There is now a vast literature on lipid thin layer chromatography, well summarized by Stahl (1969). In general, chromatography of relatively non-polar substances on thin layers of silica gel separates compounds belonging to different classes but not closely related compounds; lipids that differ only in features that do not contribute to adsorption, such as the length of an alkyl side chain, are better resolved by gas chromatography. Thin layer techniques are thus often used as a preliminary to gas chromatographic resolution. One example of this type of application is the work of Brooks et al. (1967), who prepared the trimethylsilyl ethers of the steroids in pregnancy urine and subjected the product to chromatography on thin layers of silica gel with chloroform or benzene-chloroform (8:2) before final resolution by gas chromatography.

In all of these applications the thin layer was serving as adsorbent rather than as support for partition chromatography and this mode of operation has been applied extensively to drugs and their metabolites. Baumler and Ripstein (1961), for example, have recovered methaminodiazepoxide (Librium) and its metabolite, 2-amino-5-chlorobenzophenone, from biological material and separated them on silica gel, using only benzene as the solvent. Smith and Hermann (1968) have found that ethyl acetate-benzene (8:2) was useful for the separation and identification of a number of benzothiadiazine antidiuretics. Others have found that inclusion of a little alcohol improves resolution. Coutinho et al. (1969) used ethyl acetate-ethanol (95:5) and chloroform-methanol (9:1) to fractionate chlordiazepoxide and its metabolites in a study of the relationship between circulating metabolites and duration of action of the drug in mice. Pharmacologists interested in the metabolism of indoles may consult a paper by Ballin (1964) who examined the effect of systematically varying the proportions of chloroform, carbon tetrachloride and methanol on the chromatographic behaviour of a wide variety of indole drivatives. Since silica gel is slightly acidic, it is frequently used for the chromatography of basic drugs. It is a very common practice to include small amounts of an organic amine in the developing solvent as a means of altering the mobility of the drug. A good example of this technique is reported by Baumler and Ripstein (1963), who found that a number of morphine derivatives and phenothiazines could be resolved in methanol-acetone-triethanolamine (1:1:0.03) on silica. The phenothiazines have received a great deal of attention in recent years and their metabolism is now known to include sulfoxidation, N-demethylation, introduction of hydroxyl groups on aromatic rings and the formation of N-oxides (DALY and MANIAN, 1967). Examination of the literature on this class of compounds alone would provide a good sampling of the many ways in which thin layer techniques have been applied to metabolic studies. NOIRFALISE (1965) examined the chromatographic behaviour of 11 phenothiazine derivatives in 30 solvent mixtures. Since he was interested in forensic applications of thin layer techniques, he also examined the ability of his systems to separate benzedrine, codeine, morphine, strychnine and a variety of other bases. Chloroform-ethanol (1:1) and acetone-ammonia (100:1) were among the more useful solvents COCHIN and DALY (1963a) have devised systems useful for both the phenothiazines and their metabolites. Benzene-dioxane-NH_4OH (60:35:5) and (10:30:10) were used as well as an acidic system, ethanol-acetic acid-water (50:30:20), and a neutral one, methanol-butanol (60:40). Their scheme for the examination of compounds in four systems was also useful for identification of antihistamines. DALY and MANIAN (1967) used a series of very polar mixtures containing organic amines to examine the hydroxy-chlorpromazines and their metabolites. Probably the most generally useful of the more recent papers of this type is one by FIKE (1966), who examined the R_f of 140 basic drugs in five systems. As might be expected from the complexity of the interaction of silicic acid with different types of solvents, the change in R_f resulting from the introduction of a particular group on a molecule will vary with the system used. Nevertheless, the correlations between structure and R_f reported by FIKE (1966) will be useful to those contemplating work in this area. The system which gave the broadest spread of R_f values through the whole series of drugs was simply silicic acid developed with acetone. In general, those factors that most strongly influenced R_f were the degree of steric hindrance around groups that could form hydrogen bonds, basicity and the presence or absence of a pyridyl ring. COCHIN and DALY (1962) have tested thin layer systems for the identification of analgesic drugs in extracts from urine. They examined 16 basic drugs in 6 systems, which were usually rather complex solvent mixtures. Ethanol-pyridine-dioxane-water (50:20:25:5) and methanol-butanol-benzene-water (6:15:10:15) are examples. With these systems morphine could be resolved from normorphine, levorphanol from methorphan and morphine from dihydromorphinone.

Methods for the identification and isolation of barbiturates and their metabolites by thin layer chromatography have been investigated. COCHIN and DALY (1963b) examined both barbiturate and non-barbiturate hypnotics and found chloroform-acetone (9:1) and benzene-acetic acid (9:1) on silica gel to be useful. These systems were found to give good resolution of the hydroxylated metabolites from the parent drugs. DE ZEEUW's review (1969) of the barbiturates and structurally related drugs lists some 28 solvent systems that have been successfully used. These include a variety of solvent mixtures, many with 5 components.

A few examples will illustrate the types of systems that can be used for steroid and steroid-like substances. BARBIER et al. (1959) used 15—30% acetic acid in cyclohexane for a series of etianic acids and methyl etianates. The large number of variants used in this study makes it a valuable source of information on the effects of substituents on steroid chromatography. Partition methods similar to those used with the more polar steroids on paper are also useful on thin layer. In my laboratory silica gel plates are immersed in acetone containing 20% propylene glycol and hung in air for 10 min. The steroid is then placed on the adsorbent and the plate is developed in toluene saturated with propylene glycol. By minor variations in the concentration of the propylene glycol and the addition of small amounts of ethanol to the toluene the system can be adapted to various cardiac aglycones. Good resolution of closely related substances can be obtained in about 20 min. A very similar procedure is used by AGURELL et al. (1969) in an effort to study the metabolism of marijuana constituents. In this case, the plates were impregnated by immersion in 20% of dimethylformamide in acetone and developed in light petroleum ether containing 20% of diethyl ether. The method readily separates cannabidiol from cannabinol and Δ^9-tetrahydrocannabinol. Bile acids, which are difficult to separate because of their pronounced tendency toward self association, have been chromatographed by GÄNSHIRT et al. (1960) using the upper layer from a mixture of toluene-acetic acid-water (5:5:1).

Systems for thin layer chromatography of biogenic amines are not dissimilar to those used with paper. In a recent study of the metabolism of tyramine and octopamine in rat brain, for example, BREESE et al. (1969) used butanol-isopropanol-ammonia (45:35:20) to separate octopamine, its metabolite 4-hydroxyphenyl glycol, and the glucuronide of the latter on silica gel. A class of compounds rather different from the usual basic drugs has been studied by DI CARLO et al. (1969) who examined the metabolism of pentaerythritol trinitrate and pentaerythritol in dogs. Derivatives of these compounds were well resolved by toluene-ethyl acetate-butanol-water (10:5:2:0).

The adsorptive properties of silica gel can be modified by additives, exactly as for column chromatography. Impregnation with silver nitrate to enhance π complex formation is of course valuable in the examination of the ethinyl steroids and has been applied to other steroids. A good example of the technique was recently provided by LISBOA and PALMER (1967), who coated their plates with silica gel that had been impregnated with 25% silver nitrate. A series of Δ^{16} C_{11} steroids was examined in several simple solvent mixtures, perhaps the best of these being benzene-ethanol (98:2) or (95:5). Hexane-benzene (1:1) has been used in a very similar procedure for the separation of waxes (HASHIMOTO et al. 1967). One of the most interesting attempts at modification was made by BERG and LAM (1964), who fractionated a series of polycyclic aromatic hydrocarbons on alumina and silica plates that had been impregnated with a number of substances known to give stable complexes with the hydrocarbons. These included picric acid, styphnic acid, 2,4,7-trinitrofluorene and a variety of purines. Two of these combinations gave good resolution. About 7.5—15 mg of trinitrofluorene on a 20×20 cm alumina plate and 0.5 g of caffeine on a silica plate were useful. The plates were developed with petroleum ether or heptane to which was added 2—5% of pyridine if the adsorbent was silica gel or 1% of ether if the adsorbent was alumina.

Highly cross-linked Sephadex gels have been used in a variant of thin layer chromatography. Suspensions of Sephadex are spread on a glass plate to form a solid layer. Since adhesion to the glass is poor, the plates are not set into the tanks vertically but are inclined at low angles. Fractionation is by descending chromatography and the rate of flow of the solvent is regulated by the angle of inclination (WIELAND and DETERMANN, 1967).

A technique closely akin to thin layer chromatography has been used recently in some studies of drug metabolism. Sheets of woven glass fiber are impregnated with adsorbent and used as in thin layer or ascending paper chromatography. Glass paper is commercially available and the procedures are described in a recent book (HAER, 1969). PAYNE and MASON (1968) have used glass fiber impregnated with silica gel and silver nitrate to resolve Δ^4 and Δ^5 androstene diols, a difficult separation with ordinary techniques. The solvent systems here were chloroform or cyclohexane-ethyl acetate (7:1). Glass fiber chromatography with alumina as the adsorbent and a mixture of chloroform-cyclohexane-acetic acid (20:80:2) as the solvent has been used to fractionate the metabolites of radioactive phenelzine (CLINESCHMIDT and HORITA, 1969). One of these was identified as phenylacetic acid. PRESTON's (1967) study of the excretion of 3-methoxy-4-hydroxy mandelic acid is of interest as a comparison of glass fiber with conventional thin layer procedures. With the same adsorbent, silica gel, conventional thin layer chromatography in isopropanol-95% ethanol-01 N NH_4OH (5:1:1) required 2 h while comparable separation on glass fiber required only 12 min. Despite the similarity in the adsorbents, the solvent used on the thin layers was ineffective on glass. Here, a somewhat less polar combination, toluene-acetic acid-ethyl acetate (70:20:5) was successful.

E. Electrophoresis

For those substances which can acquire electrical charge by ionization, electrophoresis on a supporting medium offers a means of fractionation. This procedure has been used extensively for many years for the separation of proteins. Although it has had relatively little application to problems of drug metabolism, it is occasionally useful. The separation of small molecular weight substances is almost universally carried out on filter paper, although columns of buffer supported on inert media have been used for aniline dyes (PORATH and STÖRIKO, 1962). A concise description of the principles of electrophoresis has been published by WALDMAN-MEYER (1963). Paper electrophoretic techniques are given in great detail by BLOCK et al. (1958) and a recent book by BIER (1967) gives an excellent treatment of all aspects of electrophoresis.

The procedures are basically simple. Filter paper, moistened with a buffer in which the substrate will ionize, is suspended between two chambers, each containing the buffer. The two ends of the paper are dipped into the chambers, which contain platinum electrodes for the application of the potential gradient. In order to avoid the disruptive effects of convection and bubbling of gas near the electrodes, the chambers are usually relatively large and the point at which the paper enters the solution is separated from the electrode by a baffle plate. Since substances will migrate faster through buffer adhering to the surface of the paper than through the buffer entrapped within the interstices, it is important to avoid excess moistening of the paper. The usual technique for this is to hold the paper between two flat glass or plastic plates and to apply an even pressure during the run. Cooling is of course a problem since high voltages are applied. Approximately 2000 volts across a length of about 40 cm of paper would be a representative situation. Adequate cooling is achieved by circulating coolant through the pressure plates in contact with the paper. In another type of technique the paper is suspended in a rectangular tank filled with hexane. The bottom of the tank is divided into two chambers, each containing the buffer and an electrode and the paper is suspended in such a way that each end dips into one of the buffer reservoirs. The non-conducting hexane, which overlies the buffer reservoirs, serves as a cooling medium and may be circulated through an external heat exchange. Since the paper hangs nearly vertically from both sides of its suspending rack, gravitational flow removes any unwanted extra buffer on the surface. This technique is used for proteins and amino acids but is unsuitable for drugs with high lipid solubility that might form hexane soluble micelles in the ionized state. Hexane cooled apparatus, however, has been used for phenolic acids (STURM and SCHEJA, 1964).

Separation by electrophoresis depends on the migration of charged molecules in an electric field. The migration velocity is directly proportional to the applied voltage gradient, the physical dimensions of the electrophoretic mobility being

cm^2, sec^{-1}, V^{-1}. Although electrophoretic mobility should theoretically be a characteristic physical constant, the observed mobilities are of course dependent on a number of experimental conditions. In paper electrophoretic separations a compound is usually characterized by its relative mobility with respect to some standard substance under carefully specified conditions. The structure of filter paper alters the mobility since the migrating substance must pass through a tortuous mesh of fine capillaries on its way to the electrode. Adsorption to cellulose is sometimes a drawback to the separation of proteins on paper, but is probably not important in electrophoresis of small molecules. One complication in paper electrophoresis is electroosomosis, which can be described as a solvent flow through a capillary system brought about by the electric potential gradient. Since filter paper usually becomes negatively charged, a flow of solution to the cathode occurs on application of the current. A second complication arises from the heat developed when the current flows. This causes evaporation of the solvent from the paper; thus there is always a tendency for bulk flow of liquid from the ends of the paper toward the middle. This latter movement of the solvent is minimized by maintaining an even temperature over the whole paper. In the usual electrophoretic apparatus the only significant opportunity for evaporation occurs at the edges of the paper. If wide strips are used and the sample is applied well away from the sides, distortion of the electrophoretic pattern by edge effects is minimal. The bulk flow of liquid due to electroosmosis is usually uniform over the paper surface, and even though it contributes to the observed mobilities of charged species it can be ignored. If it is necessary to correct mobilities for electroosmotic flow, the latter can be measured by observing the rate of movement of a neutral, non-ionizable substance when the current is on.

As might be expected, paper electrophoresis has been used for the fractionation of drugs and their metabolites that are quaternary salts and thus, completely ionized. Way et al. (1963) as part of a study of the metabolism of radioactive pyridine-2-aldoxime methiodide isolated 1-methyl-2-cyano-pyridinium by paper electrophoresis in 0.05 M sodium acetate, pH 4.5. Guanethidine, by virtue of its guanidinium structure, is ionized at all but extremely high pH values. Its metabolism has been examined by McMartin (1969) who detected the formation of an N-oxide and 6-carboxyhexyl-2-imino-imidazoline by paper electrophoresis in pyridine acetate buffer, pH 6.1. Separation required 250 volts for 15 h. A number of applications of paper electrophoresis to the separation of alkaloids are summarized by Winek et al. (1963), who found that starch gels could also be used. In this case, starch was suspended in 1 N acetic acid and allowed to gel in a flat tray. Just before complete gelation paper wicks were inserted at each end and these were used to convey the electrolyte from the chamber to the gel. Paper electrophoresis has been used for the analysis of food additives (Criddle et al., 1964) and even for polycyclic aromatic hydrocarbons in the form of ionizable complexes with caffeine (Rothwell and Whitehead, 1967).

Two dimensional paper electrophoresis may be performed as in paper chromatography (Buchanan and Corfield, 1967) and electrophoresis may be combined with chromatography as in the well known "curtain electrophoresis" procedure for continuous separation. In this, a mixture of solutes is continuously delivered to a spot at the top center of a paper through which solvent descends as in the usual chromatographic procedure. Transverse application of a potential divides the descending mixture into individual streams (see Block et al., 1958). Electrophoresis may be carried out on thin layers of adsorbents similar to those used in thin layer chromatography. A number of applications have been reviewed by Criddle et al. (1964).

In applying paper electrophoresis to studies of drug metabolism, it is important to consider whether the anticipated changes in structure are likely to change the electrophoretic properties of the parent molecule. In 1% acetic acid, paper electrophoresis failed to separate imipramine from desmethylimipramine and didesmethylimipramine from iminodibenzyl (SCHNEIDER and SCHNEIDER, 1968). In pyridine-acetic acid-water (9:1:90) the relative mobilities of amphetamine and methamphetamine with respect to dopamine as a standard were 1.14 and 1.19. Hydroxylation of the latter to ephedrine changed the mobility to 1.05. Electrophoresis thus offered no advantage over chromatographic procedures in this instance (REISCH et al., 1968). For the acidic metabolites of the catecholamines, however, paper electrophoresis is quite effective (KLEIN and CHERNAIK, 1961; STURM and SCHEJA, 1964). Some of the problems in applying electrophoresis to biological problems are reviewed by CLOTTEN and CLOTTEN (1962).

References

AGURELL, S., NILSSON, I.M., OHLSSON, A., SANDBERG, F.: Elimination of tritium labelled cannabinols in the rat with special reference to the development of tests for the identification of cannabis users. Biochem. Pharmacol. **18**, 1195—1201 (1969).

AHRENS, E.H., JR., CRAIG, L.C.: The extraction and separation of bile acids. J. biol. Chem. **195**, 763—776 (1952).

ARMSTRONG, M.D., SHAW, K.N.F., WALL, P.E.: The phenolic acids of human urine. Paper chromatography of phenolic acids. J. biol. Chem. **218**, 293—303 (1956).

ASHLEY, B.D., WESTPHAL, U.: Separation of small quantities of saturated higher fatty acids by reversed-phase paper chromatography. Arch. Biochem. **56**, 1—10 (1955).

AUDUBERT, R., DE MENDE, S.: The principles of electrophoresis. Translated by A.J. POMERANS. New York: MacMillan 1960.

AXELROD, J.: The estimation of basic drugs by dye methods. In: Toxicology, mechanisms and analytical methods. Vol. 1, ed. by C.P. STEWART and A. STOLMAN. New York: Academic Press 1960.

BALLARD, C.W., ISAACS, J., SCOTT, D.G.W.: The photometric determination of quaternary ammonium salts and of certain amines by compound formation with indicators. J. Pharm. Pharmacol. **6**, 971—985 (1954).

BALLIN, G.: Dünnschichtchromatographische Trennung von Indolderivaten in neutralen Fließmitteln. J. Chromat. **16**, 152—156 (1964).

BANES, D.: The chemical assay of adrenal cortex extracts. J. pharm. Sci. **42**, 669—673 (1953).

— A new partition chromatographic procedure for the assay of pharmaceuticals. J. pharm. Sci. **43**, 580—584 (1954).

BARBIER, M., JÄGER, M., TOBIAS, H., WYSS, E.: Anwendung der Dünnschichtchromatographie auf Steroide. Helv. chim. Acta **42**, 2440—2446 (1959).

BAUMLER, J., RIPSTEIN, S.: Über den Nachweis von Methaminodiazepoxide (Librium) und seiner Metaboliten. Helv. chim. Acta **44**, 2208—2210 (1961).

— — Die Dünnschichtchromatographie als Schnellmethode zur Analyse von Arzneimitteln. Pharm. Acta Helv. **36**, 382—388 (1963).

BELING, C.G.: Purification of urinary conjugated oestrogens by gel filtration. Nature (Lond.) **192**, 326—327 (1961).

BERG, A., LAM, J.: Separation of polycyclic aromatic hydrocarbons by thin layer chromatography on impregnated layers. J. Chromat. **16**, 157—166 (1964).

BEROZA, M., BOWMAN, M.C.: Extraction of insecticides for clean up and identification. J. Ass. offic. Agr. Chem. **48**, 358—370 (1965a).

— — Identification of pesticides at nanogram level by extraction p-values. Anal. Chem. **37**, 291—292 (1965b).

BEYER, K.-H.: Zur fermentativen Aufarbeitung toxikologischen Untersuchungsmaterials. 6. Mitteilung zur Chemie und Analytik der Schlafmittel. Z. Anal. Chem. **212**, 139—145 (1965).

BEYERMANN, K.: Distribution of tetraphenyl borates of amino acids and oligopeptides between aqueous solutions and organic solvents. Z. Anal. Chem. **212**, 199—211 (1965).

BIER, M.: Electrophoresis, Vol. 2. New York: Academic Press 1967.

BLOCK, R.J., DURRUM, E.L., ZWEIG, G.: A manual of paper chromatography and paper electrophoresis, 2nd ed. New York: Academic Press 1958.

BOCK, R.M.: A derivation of the concentration distribution equation for the Craig counter current apparatus. J. Amer. chem. Soc. **72**, 4269—4270 (1950).

Bowman, M.C., Beroza, M.: Extraction p-values of pesticides and related compounds in six binary solvent systems. J. Ass. offic. Agr. Chem. **48**, 943—952 (1965).
— — Device and method for determining extraction p-values with unequilibrated solvents of unequal phase volumes. Anal. Chem. **38**, 1427—1428 (1966).
Breese, G.R., Chase, T.N., Kopin, I.J.: Metabolism of tyramine-^{3}H and octopamine-^{3}H by rat brain. Biochem. Pharmacol. **18**, 863—869 (1969).
Brindle, H., Carless, I.E., Woodhead, H.B.: The separation of alkaloids by partition paper chromatography. J. Pharm. Pharmacol. **3**, 793—814 (1951).
Brockmann, H.: Chromatography of colourless substances and the relation between constitution and adsorption affinity. Discuss. Faraday Soc. **7**, 58—64 (1949).
Brodie, B.B., Udenfriend, S., Dill, W.: The estimation of basic organic compounds in biological material. V. Estimation by salt formation with methyl orange. J. biol. Chem. **168**, 335—339 (1947).
Brooks, C.J.W., Chambaz, E., Horning, E.C.: Thin layer and column chromatographic group separations of steroids as trimethylsilyl ethers. Isolation for GLC analysis of pregnanediol and estriol in pregnancy urine. Anal. Biochem. **19**, 234—242 (1967).
Buchanan, J.H., Corfield, M.C.: An easily constructed apparatus for two dimensional paper electrophoresis. J. Chromat. **31**, 274—278 (1967).
Bush, I.E.: Methods of paper chromatography of steroids applicable to the study of steroids in mammalian blood and tissues. Biochem. J. **50**, 370—378 (1952).
— Chromatography of steroids and sterols. Brit. med. Bull. **10**, 229—236 (1954).
Carless, J.E., Woodhead, H.R.: Separation of alkaloids by paper chromatography. Nature (Lond.) **168**, 203 (1951).
Carter, H.E., Clark, R.K., Jr., Dickman, S.R., Loo, Y.H., Skell, P.S., Strong, W.A.: Isolation and purification of streptomycin. J. biol. Chem. **160**, 337—342 (1945).
Cassidy, H.G.: Fundamentals of chromatography. In: Technique of organic chemistry, vol. X. New York: Interscience Publ., Inc. 1957.
Clarke, E.G.C., ed.: Isolation and identification of drugs. London: The Pharmaceutical Press 1969.
Clineschmidt, B.V., Horita, A.: The monoamine oxidase catalyzed degradation of phenelzine-1-^{14}C′, an irreversible inhibitor of monoamine oxidase. Biochem. Pharmacol. **18**, 1021—1028 (1969).
Clotten, R., Clotten, A.: Hochspannungselektrophorese: Ihre Anwendungsmöglichkeiten für biochemische und klinisch-chemische Trennprobleme. Stuttgart: Georg Thieme 1962.
Cochin, J., Daly, J.W.: Rapid identification of analgesic drugs in urine with thin layer chromatography. Experientia (Basel) **18**, 294—295 (1962).
— — The use of thin layer chromatography for the analysis of drugs. Identification and isolation of phenothiazine tranquilizers and of antihistamines in body fluids and tissues. J. Pharmacol. exp. Ther. **139**, 160—165 (1963a).
— — The use of thin layer chromatography for the analysis of drugs. Isolation and identification of barbiturates and nonbarbiturate hypnotics from urine, blood and tissue. J. Pharmacol. exp. Ther. **139**, 154—159 (1963b).
Cole, P.G., Lathe, G.H., Ruthven, C.R.J.: Application of countercurrent methods to the fractionation of lipid material from human placenta. Biochem. J. **55**, 17—23 (1953).
Consden, R., Gordon, A.H., Martin, A.J.P.: Qualitative analysis of proteins: a partition chromatographic method using paper. Biochem. J. **38**, 224—232 (1944).
Coutinho, C.B., Cheripko, J.A., Carbone, J.J.: Relation between the duration of anticonvulsant activity of chlordiazepoxide and systemic levels of the parent compound and its major metabolites in mice. Biochem. Pharmacol. **18**, 303—316 (1969).
Craig, L.C., Craig, D.: Extraction and distribution. In: Technique of organic chemistry, Vol. 3, 2nd ed. New York: Interscience 1956.
— Hausmann, W., Ahrens, P., Harfenist, E.J.: Automatic countercurrent distribution equipment. Anal. Chem. **23**, 1236—1244 (1951).
Criddle, W.J., Moody, G.J., Thomas, J.D.R.: Electrophoresis using thin layer materials. J. chem. Educ. **41**, 609 (1964).
— — — Thin film electrophoresis. Part I. The electrophoretic behavior of coal tar food colors on paper and thin films. J. Chromat. **16**, 350—359 (1964).
Cummings, T., Garven, H.C., Giles, C.H., Rahman, S.M.K., Sneddon, J.G., Stewart, C.E.: Adsorption at inorganic surfaces. Part IV. Mechanism of adsorption of organic solutes by chromatographic alumina. J. chem. Soc. 535 (1959).
Daly, J.W., Manian, A.A.: The metabolism of hydroxy chlorpromazines by rat liver microsomes. Biochem. Pharmacol. **16**, 2131—2136 (1967).
Dean, J.A.: Chemical separation methods. New York: Van Nostrand Reinhold 1969.
De Vault, D.: The theory of chromatography. J. Amer. chem. Soc. **65**, 532—540 (1943).

De Vries, B.: Quantitative separations of higher fatty acid methyl esters by adsorption chromatography on silicic acid impregnated with silver nitrate. J. Amer. Oil Chemists Soc. **40**, 184—186 (1963).

De Zeeuw, R. A.: Paper and thin layer chromatographic techniques for separation and identification of barbiturates and related hypnotics. In: Progress in Chemical Toxicology, Vol. 4, ed. by A. Stolman. New York: Academic Press 1969.

Di Carlo, F. J., Melgar, M. D., Haynes, L. J., Gala, R. L., Crew, M. C.: Metabolism of pentaerythritol trinitrate and pentaerythritol by dogs. J. Pharmacol. exp. Ther. **168**, 235—239 (1969).

Dikstein, S.: The effect of molecular structure on the R_f value, a contribution to the theory of paper chromatography. J. Chromat. **2**, 204—300 (1959).

Divatia, G. J., Biles, J. A.: Physical chemical study of the distribution of some amine salts between immiscible solvents. J. pharm. Sci. **50**, 916—922 (1961).

Doyle, T. D., Levine, J.: Application of ion-pair extraction to partition chromatographic separation of pharmaceutical amines. Anal. Chem. **39**, 1282—1287 (1967).

Ercoli, A., Vitai, R., Gardi, R.: Adsorbents for detection isolation and evaluation of ethynyl steroids. Steroids **3**, 479—485 (1964).

Evans, R. A., Parr, W. H., Evans, W. C.: Paper partition chromatography of phenolic substances. Nature (Lond.) **164**, 674—675 (1949).

Evans, W. C., Partridge, M. W.: The partition chromatography of alkaloids — Solanaceous alkaloids. Quart. J. Pharm. **21**, 126—137 (1948).

Fike, W. W.: Structure-R_f correlations in the thin layer chromatography of some basic drugs. Anal. Chem. **38**, 1697—1702 (1966).

Fischbach, H., Eble, T. E., Mundell, M.: Separation of penicillin by partition chromatography. J. pharm. Sci. **36**, 220—223 (1947).

Fried, J., White, H. L., Wintersteiner, O.: The hypotensive principles of Veratrum viride. J. Amer. chem. Soc. **72**, 4621—4629 (1950).

Gänshirt, H., Koss, F. W., Morianz, K.: Untersuchung zur quantitativen Auswertung der Dünnschichtchromatographie. Arzneimittel-Forsch. **10**, 943—947 (1960).

Ghosh, S. B., Schaad, L. J., Bush, M. T.: Binomial probability distribution tables for the calculation of withdrawn series of counter-current distribution. Anal. Chem. **37**, 1122—1123 (1965).

Goldstein, M., Abelin, I.: Determination of catecholamines and pyrocatechols in human urine. Helv. chim. Acta **39**, 158—167 (1956).

Gustavii, K., Schill, G.: Determination of amines and quaternary ammonium ions as complexes with picrate. I. Constants needed in the calculation of extraction conditions. Acta pharm. Suec. **3**, 241—258 (1966a).

— — Determination of amines and quaternary ammonium ions as picrate complexes. II. Interference by foreign anions. Acta pharm. Suec. **3**, 259—268 (1966b).

Haenni, E. O., Carol, J., Banes, D.: Colorimetric determination of α-estradiol in estrogenic mixtures using partition chromatography. J. pharm. Sci. **42**, 162—167 (1953a).

— — — Partition chromatography of some estrogenic diols. J. pharm. Sci. **42**, 167—172 (1953b).

Haer, F. C.: An introduction to chromatography on impregnated glass fiber. Ann. Arbor, Mich.: Ann. Arbor Sci. Publ. 1969.

Hashimoto, A., Hirotani, A., Mukai, K.: Thin layer chromatography of true wax. Nippon Nogei Kagaku Kaishi **41**, 139—144 (1967).

Hecker, E.: A simple separation function for counter-current distribution and its importance in practice. Z. Naturforsch. **8b**, 77—86 (1953).

— Selection of solvent systems for multistage distribution. Chimia **8**, 229—236 (1954).

— Verteilungsverfahren im Laboratorium. Weinheim: Verlag Chemie 1955.

Heftmann, E.: Partition chromatography of steroids. Chem. Rev. **55**, 679—711 (1955).

Hegedus, H., Tamm, C., Reichstein, T.: Diglycoside von Strophantus intermedius pax. Helv. chim. Acta **36**, 357—369 (1953).

Higuchi, T., Michaelis, A. F.: Mechanism and kinetics of ion pair extraction. Rate of extraction of dextromethorphanium ion. Anal. Chem. **40**, 1925—1931 (1968).

— — Tan, T., Hurwitz, A.: Ion pair extraction of pharmaceutical amines. Role of dipolar solvating agents in extraction of dextromorphan. Anal. Chem. **39**, 974—979 (1967).

Hirsch, J., Ahrens, E. H., Jr.: Separation of complex lipid mixtures by the use of silicic acid chromatography. J. biol. Chem. **233**, 311—320 (1958).

Howard, G. A., Martin, A. J. P.: The separation of C_{12}—C_{18} fatty acids by reversal phase partition chromatography. Biochem. J. **46**, 532—538 (1950).

Hull, R. L., Biles, J. A.: Physical chemical study of the distribution of some amine salts between immiscible solvents. II. Complexation in the organic phase. J. pharm. Sci. **53**, 869—872 (1964).

ILER, R.K.: The colloid chemistry of silica and the silicates. Ithaca, N.Y.: Cornell University Press 1955.

JAMES, W.O.: Demonstration and separation of noradrenaline, adrenaline and methyladrenaline. Nature (Lond.) **161**, 851—852 (1948).

JANSON, J.-C.: Adsorption phenomena on Sephadex. J. Chromat. **28**, 12—20 (1967).

JANTZEN, E.: Das fractionierte Destillieren und das fractionierte Verteilen, Dechema, Monographic, Vol. V. No. 48. Berlin: Verlag Chemie 1948.

JONES, J.K.N., STRITCH, S.R.: The separation of ketosteroids by partition chromatography using nitromethane as stationary phase. Biochem. J. **53**, 679—684 (1953).

KAEMPE, B.: Interfering compounds and artifacts in the identification of drugs in autopsy material. In: Progress in chemical toxicology. New York-London: Academic Press 1969.

KARAU, W., ZACHAU, H.G.: Isolierung von serinspezifischen Transferribonucleinsäure-Fraktionen. Biochim. biophys. Acta (Amst.) **91**, 549—558 (1964).

KAY, L.M., TRUEBLOOD, K.N.: Immobile phase in chromatography on silicic acidcelite. Role of water in the mechanism of development. Anal. Chem. **26**, 1566—1572 (1954).

KING, E.J., GILCHRIST, M., TARNOKY, A.L.: Spectrophotometric study of the excretion products of mepacrine compared with synthetic acridine and diphenylamine derivatives. Biochem. J. **40**, 706—721 (1946).

KIRDANI, R.Y., PRIORE, R.L.: Statistical analysis of data from countercurrent distribution. II. Some applications and limitations of the method. Anal. Biochem. **24**, 377—392 (1968).

KLEIN, D., CHERNAIK, J.M.: Determination of urinary 3-methoxy-4-hydroxymandelic acid by paper electrophoresis. Clin. Chem. **7**, 257—264 (1961).

KLINKENBERG, A., SJENITZER, F.: Holding-time distributions of the Gaussian type. Chem. Engl. Sci. **5**, 258—270 (1956).

KNAAK, J.B., O'BRIEN, R.D.: Effect of EPN on in vivo metabolism of malathion by rat and dog. J. Agr. Food Chem. **8**, 198—203 (1960).

KNIGHT, H.S., GROENNINGS, S.: Indicator chromatographic analysis of organic mixtures. Anal. Chem. **26**, 1549—1553 (1954).

KORTE, F., SIEPER, H.: Isolierung von Haschisch-Inhaltsstoffen aus Cannabis sativa non indica. Justus Liebigs Ann. Chem. **630**, 71—83 (1960).

KRITCHEVSKY, T.H., TISELIUS, A.: Reversed phase partition chromatography by steroids on silicone-treated paper. Science **114**, 299—300 (1951).

LAMBERT, S.M., PORTER, P.E.: Analytical and preparative applications of liquid-liquid partition chromatography. Anal. Chem. **36**, 99—104 (1964).

LEDERER, E., LEDERER, M.: Chromatography, a review of principles and applications. Amsterdam-London-New York-Princeton: Elsevier 1957.

LEVINE, J.: Analysis of acetyl salicylic acid and acetyl salicylic acid tablets. J. pharm. Sci. **50**, 506—509 (1961).

— Column partition chromatography in pharmaceutical analysis. J. pharm. Sci. **52**, 1015—1031 (1963a).

— Determination of dihydrocodeinone in mixtures with antihistamines. J. Ass. offic. Agr. Chem. **46**, 641—642 (1963b).

— OTTES, R.T.: A new extraction procedure for alkaloids. J. pharm. Sci. **44**, 291—293 (1961).

LEW, B.W., WOLFROM, M.L., GOEPP, R.M., JR.: Chromatography of carbohydrates and some related compounds. J. Amer. chem. Soc. **67**, 1865 (1945).

LINDBALD, C.G., AGREN, A.: Stability of tetrapon (papaveret). Farm. Revy. **53**, 69—79 (1954).

LISBOA, B.P., PALMER, R.F.: Application of thin layer chromatographic techniques to the separation of Δ^{16}-C_{19} steroids and related compounds. Anal. Biochem. **20**, 77—86 (1967).

MARTIN, A.J.P.: Partition chromatography. Ann. Rev. Biochem. **19**, 517—542 (1950a).

— Some theoretical aspects of partition chromatography. Biochem. Soc. Symposia **3**, 4—20 (1950b).

— SYNGE, R.L.M.: A new form of chromatogram employing two liquid phases. A new theory of chromatography. Biochem. J. **35**, 1358—1368 (1941).

MCMARTIN, C.: The separation and detection of metabolites of guanethidine. Biochem. Pharmacol. **18**, 238—242 (1969).

MORRIS, C.J.O.R., WILLIAMS, D.C.: The polarographic estimation of steroid hormones. Biochem. J. **54**, 470—475 (1953).

National Bureau of Standards: Tables of the binomial probability distribution. Applied Mathematics series, Vol. 6, Washington, D.C., 1950.

NEHER, R., WETTSTEIN, A.: Papier-Chromatographie von schwach polaren Steroiden. Helv. chim. Acta **35**, 276—283 (1952).

NOIRFALISE, A.: Mise en évidence de quelques dérivés phénothiazines par chromatographie en couche mince de silicagel. J. Chromat. **19**, 68—74 (1965).

NOVER, L., BAUMGARTNER, G., LUCKNER, M.: Über die Beziehungen zwischen chemischer Struktur und chromatographischem Verhalten bei Herzglykosiden. J. Chromat. **32**, 93—161 (1968).

OLLEY, J.: Application of counter-current distribution to phospholipid chemistry. Chem Ind. (Lond.) p. 1120—1130 (1956).

— LOVERN, J.A.: The lipids of fish. III. Acetone-insoluble fraction of an acetone extract of the flesh of the haddock. Biochem. J. **54**, 559—569 (1953).

PALMER, K.H., FOWLER, M.S., WALL, M.E., RHODES, L.S., WADDELL, W.J., BAGGET, B.: The metabolism of R(+) and RS pentobarbital. J. Pharmacol. exp. Ther. **170**, 355—363 (1969).

PAYNE, A.H., MASON, M.: Application of glass fiber chromatography for the separation of C_{19} steroids. Anal. Biochem. **26**, 460—462 (1968).

PERSSON, B.-A., SCHILL, G.: Extraction of amines as complexes with inorganic ions. Part 2. Determination of constants when the amine is extracted as complex and base. Acta pharm. Suec. **3**, 281—302 (1966).

PFLEIDERER, G.: Möglichkeiten und Grenzen in der Anwendung moderner biochemischer Analysenverfahren. Z. Anal. Chem. **212**, 64—77 (1965).

PIEROTTI, G., DEAL, C.H., DERR, E.L.: Activity coefficients and molecular structure. Ind. Eng. Chem. **51**, 95—102 (1959).

POHL, F.A.: Comprehension and evaluation of chemical data. Z. Anal. Chem. **209**, 19—35 (1965).

PORATH, J., STÖRIKO, K.: Zonenelektrophorese in äthanolischen Pufferlösungen. J. Chromat. **7**, 385—391 (1962).

PRESTON, J.A.: 3-Methoxy-4-hydroxy mandelic acid (VMA) by microfiber chromatography. Clin. Chem. **13**, 19—25 (1967).

PRIORE, R.L., KIRDANI, R.Y.: Statistical analysis of data from counter-current distribution. I. Method for estimation of quantity and partition coefficient of each component. Anal. Biochem. **24**, 360—376 (1968).

RANDERATH, K.: Thin-layer chromatography. Transl. by D.D. LIBMAN, 2nd ed. New York: Academic Press 1966.

REICHSTEIN, T., SHOPPEE, C.W.: Chromatography of steroids and other colorless substances by the method of fractional elution. Discuss. Faraday Soc. **7**, 305—311 (1949).

REISCH, J., ALFER, H., MOELLMANN, H.: Beitrag zur Hochspannungselektrophorese einiger Phenyläthylamino-Abkömmlinge. Pharmazie **23**, 245—246 (1968).

REITSEMA, R.H.: Characterization of essential oils by chromatography. Analyt. Chem. **26**, 960—963 (1954).

RIETZ, H.L.: Mathematical statistics. La Salle, Ill.: Open Court 1927.

ROBERTS, M.: A note on the use of cellulose phosphate cation-exchange paper for the separation of catecholamines and some other biogenic amines. J. Pharm. Pharmacol. **14**, 746—749 (1962).

ROTHWELL, K., WHITEHEAD, J.K.: Polycyclic aromatic hydrocarbons — as caffeine complexes. Chem. Ind. (Lond.) 1967.

SCHAYER, R.W., KENNEDY, J., SMILEY, R.L.: Effect of dibenamine on the metabolism of radioactive adrenaline. J. biol. Chem. **202**, 39—43 (1953).

SCHILL, G.: Photometric determination of amines and quaternary ammonium compounds with bromothymol blue. Part 4. Extraction constants and calculation of extraction conditions. Acta pharm. Suec. **2**, 13—43 (1965a).

— Photometric determination of amines and quaternary ammonium compounds with bromothymol blue. Part 5. Determination of dissociation constants of amines. Acta pharm. Suec. **2**, 99—108 (1965b).

— MODIN, R., PERSSON, B-A.: Extraction of amines as complexes with inorganic anions. Acta pharm. Suec. **2**, 119—136 (1965).

SCHINDLER, O., REICHSTEIN, T.: Die Glycoside der Wurzeln von Adenium Honghel. Helv. chim. Acta **34**, 18—27 (1951a).

— — Die Glykoside der Samen von Strophanthus courmontii Sacl. Helv. chim. Acta **34**, 1732—1739 (1951b).

— — Identification and separation of digitaloid glycosides and aglucons by chromatography on impregnated filter paper. Helv. chim. Acta **34**, 108—116 (1951c).

SCHMID, M.D., BOLLIGER, H.R.: 2-Thioäthyl-D-glucose-Derivate aus dem 6-Trithyl-tetrabenzoat. Helv. chim. Acta **37**, 884—892 (1954).

SCHMIDT, B., CLINE, V., HORITA, A.: The monoamine oxidase catalyzed degradation of phenelzinc 1-^{14}C, an irreversible inhibitor of monoamine oxidase. Biochem. Pharmacol. **18**, 1011—1020 (1969).

SCHNEIDER, G., SCHNEIDER, G.: Zur papierelektrophoretischen Trennung des Psychopharmakons Tofranil und einiger seiner Metaboliten. J. Chromat. **37**, 348—349 (1968).

SCHOLFIELD, C.R., BUTTERFIELD, R.O., DUTTON, H.J.: Fractionation of geometric isomers of methyl linolenate by argentation counter-current distribution. Anal. Chem. **38**, 1694—1697 (1966).
— JONES, E.P., BUTTERFIELD, R.O., DUTTON, H.J.: Argentation in counter-current distribution to separate isologues and geometric isomers of fatty acid esters. Anal. Chem. **35**, 1588—1591 (1963).
SCOTT, R.M.: Clinical analysis by thin layer chromatography techniques. Ann. Arbor-London: Ann. Arbor-Humphrey Science Publishers 1969.
SGOUTAS, D.S., KUMMEROW, F.A.: Exposure of an isotope effect by ^{3}H labeled fatty acids on silica-silver nitrate chromatography. J. Chromat. **16**, 448—453 (1964).
SHORE, P.A.: A simple technique involving solvent extraction for estimation of noradrenaline and adrenaline in tissues. Pharmacol. Rev. **11**, 276—277 (1959).
SMITH, I.: Chromatographic and electrophoretic techniques. London: W. Heinemann Medical Books Ltd. 1960.
SMITH, P.J., HERMANN, T.S.: Separation and identification of benzothiadiazines in commercial formulations by thin layer chromatography and infra-red spectroscopy. Anal. Biochem. **22**, 134—144 (1968).
SOCZEWINSKI, E.: Efficiency of separation in buffered paper chromatography of organic electrolytes. Nature (Lond.) **188**, 391—392 (1960).
SOMOGYI, M.: Determination of blood sugar. J. biol. Chem. **160**, 69—73 (1945).
SPORER, A.H., TRUEBLOOD, K.N.: A quantitative study of the relation between molecular structure and adsorption affinity on silicic acid-celite columns. J. Chromat. **2**, 499—512 (1959).
STAHL, E.: Dünnschichtchromatographie. Berlin-Göttingen-Heidelberg: Springer 1962.
— Thin layer chromatography, a laboratory handbook, 2nd ed. translated by M.R.F. ASHWORTH. Berlin-Heidelberg-New York: Springer 1969.
STENE, S.: Theory of systemic extraction and related convection problems. Arkiv. Kemi. Mineral. Geol. A18, No. 18 (1944).
STONE, H.: Mathematical resolution of overlapping spectral lines. J. Opt. Soc. Amer. **52**, 998—1003 (1962).
STOWE, B.B., THIMANN, K.V.: The paper chromatography of indole compounds and some indole containing auxine of plant tissues. Arch. Biochem. **51**, 499—515 (1954).
STURM, A., JR., SCHEJA, H.W.: Die Trennung der Phenolsäuren mit Hilfe der Hochspannungselektrophorese. J. Chromat. **16**, 194—200 (1964).
TENNEY, H.M., STURGIS, F.E.: Separability of hydrocarbons by elution chromatography. Anal. Chem. **26**, 946—953 (1954).
THOMPSON, J.F., POLLARD, J.K., STEWARD, F.C.: γ-Aminobutyric acid in plants. A new procedure for isolating amino acids other than α-amino acids. Plant Physiol. **28**, 401—414 (1953).
TITUS, E.O.: Counter-current distribution, In: Toxicology, mechanisms and analytical methods, Vol. **1**, ed. by C.P. STEWART and A. STOLMAN. New York: Academic Press 1960.
— FRIED, J.: Counter-current distribution studies on streptomycin: The tautomerism of streptomycin. J. biol. Chem. **174**, 57—70 (1948).
TRENNER, N.R.: Column partition chromatography. Rahway, N.J.: Merck and Co. 1957.
TRUHAUT, R., BOUDENE, C., CLAUDE, J.R.: Application of thin layer chromatography to analytical toxicology. Ann. biol. Clin. **26**, 93—111 (1968).
TRUEBLOOD, K.N., MALMBERG, E.W.: Chromatographic properties of silicic acid-celite. Anal. Chem. **21**, 1056—1058 (1949).
TRUTER, E.V.: Thin layer chromatography. London: Cleaver Hume Press 1963.
TSCHESCHE, R., KÖNIGE, H.B.: Apparatus for counter-current distribution for preparative purposes. Chem.-Ing.-Tech. **22**, 214—215 (1950).
UCHIDA, T., DAUTERMAN, W.C., O'BRIEN, R.D.: The metabolism of dimethoate by vertebrate tissues. J. Agr. Food Chem. **12**, 48—52 (1964).
VERZELE, M.: A new method of separation on a preparative scale based on counter-current distribution. Bull. Soc. chim. Belges **62**, 619—639 (1953).
VON METZSCH, F.A.: The choice of solvents for the distribution between two liquid phases. Angew. Chem. **65**, 586—598 (1953).
— Anwendungsbeispiele multiplikativer Verteilungen. Angew. Chem. **68**, 323—334 (1956).
WALDMAN-MEYER, H.: Protein mobilities and ion binding constants evaluated by zone electrophoresis. Chromat. Rev. **5**, 1—45 (1963).
WAY, E.L., BENNETT, B.M.: Rapid estimation of counter-current distribution values. J. biol. Chem. **192**, 335—338 (1951).
WAY, J.L., MASTERSON, P.B., BERES, J.A.: The metabolism of C^{14}-2-PAM in the isolated perfused rat liver. III. 1-Methyl-2-cyano pyridinium ion. J. Pharmacol. exp. Ther. **140**, 117—124 (1963).

WIELAND, T., DETERMANN, H.: Some recent developments in gel chromatography with special reference to thin layers. J. Chromat. **28**, 2—11 (1967).

WILLIAMSON, B., CRAIG, L.C.: Identification of small amounts of organic compounds by distribution studies. V. Calculation of theoretical curves. J. biol. Chem. **168**, 687—697 (1947).

WINEK, C.L., BEAL, J.L., CAVA, M.P.: Gel electrophoresis of alkaloids. J. Chromat. **10**, 246—247 (1963).

WOKSMUNDZKI, A., SOCZEWINSKI, E.: A paper chromatographic method for the determination of suitable buffer systems for counter-current distribution. Nature (Lond.) **184**, 977 (1959).

ZAFFARONI, A., BURTON, R.B., KEUTMAN, E.H.: Adrenal cortical hormones. Analysis by paper partition chromatography and occurrence in the urine of normal persons. Science **111**, 6—8 (1950).

ZAORAL, M.: Dehydrohalogenation of halo compounds on activated alkaline aluminum oxide. Chem. Listy. **47**, 1872—1874 (1953).

Chapter 32

Isotope Dilution Analysis

VINCENT T. OLIVERIO and ANTHONY M. GUARINO

With 4 Figures

A. Introduction

This chapter describes the use of radioactive isotope dilution analysis in combination with various analytical separation techniques for the identification and quantitative determination of a labeled substance and its metabolite(s) in laboratory animals and man. Recent experience in studying the disposition of several drugs and other foreign compounds will serve as models to illustrate this procedure. The emphasis is on methodology and the pharmacological findings will be described only in part.

The typical drug metabolism study involves the *in vivo* administration of a compound which becomes distributed in various body fluids and tissues of the animal. The parent compound may remain unaltered, or it may undergo enzymatic changes which result in one or more new compounds, or it may be degraded to simpler compounds spontaneously even without the intervention of enzymes. The ability to detect and measure these changes, even for drugs administered at extremely low doses, is often made possible by the techniques discussed in this chapter.

B. Isotope Dilution Analysis

Radioactive isotope dilution analysis (IDA) was introduced by HEVESY and HOBBIE (1932). The basic principle is simple. It involves the homogeneous dilution of a labeled compound of known specific activity (radioactivity in counts per min or distintegration per min per unit weight) with the same unlabeled compound. The reduction in specific activity caused by this dilution may be used to calculate either the amount of labeled compound originally present or the amount of unlabeled compound which was added. Since only the value of the specific activity is needed in these calculations, it is not necessary to isolate the compound quantitatively from physiological systems, but it is necessary that the labeled compound be uniformly mixed with the unlabeled compound and that the portion which is isolated from the mixture be purified until constant specific activity is obtained.

The radioactive isotopes ordinarily used in drug metabolism studies are the weak β-emitting ^{14}C, tritium (^{3}H), and to a lesser extent, ^{35}S, and the stronger β-emitters, ^{32}P and ^{36}Cl. However, it is possible to incorporate a much higher percentage of tritium into a given organic molecule than is possible with the other isotopes named. Even though tritium is not as strong a β-emitter as ^{14}C, the improved sensitivity of recent radioisotopic instrumentation has offset this disadvantage. Since in drug metabolism studies ^{3}H and ^{14}C are used almost exclusively, the remaining discussion will mainly be concerned with drugs labeled with these isotopes. The synthesis of ^{3}H and ^{14}C labeled drugs and some general precautions to be considered in using these tracers in pharmacologic studies are reviewed in chapter 25 in this volume.

1. Direct Methods

There are two general types of IDA: these are termed *direct* and *indirect*. In the direct procedure a *known amount* of the *isotopically labeled compound* is added to a *mixture* containing an unknown amount of the same unlabeled compound. As SCHMID et al. (1969) recently pointed out, the accuracy of this method is dependent on the ratio of the quantity of labeled compound which is added to the quantity of the non-labeled compound already present in the mixture. This ratio must not exceed 2:1 to keep the margin of error $\pm 3\%$ or less. The direct IDA method is probably not convenient for assaying quantities of less than 1 mg since this entails extremely tedious and careful techniques of isolation, purification, and measurement. The equation used for direct IDA follows (GORSUCH, 1968):

Let: A_O = Original activity of labeled compound per unit time (counts per min or distintegration per min)

M_O = Original amount of labeled compound (grams, moles, millimoles, etc.)

S_O = Original specific activity of labeled compound (activity per amount of compound) i.e.,

$$S_O = \frac{A_O}{M_O} \tag{1}$$

M_U = Amount of unlabeled compound (this is unknown).

The labeled compound is added to a sample containing the unlabeled compound, thereby, diluting the labeled compound by unlabeled compound. After the diluted material is isolated from the sample and purified, the specific activity of the diluted material is determined; the amount of unlabeled compound originally present can then be calculated as follows:

The specific activity of diluted material (S_D) is given by:

$$S_D = \frac{A_O}{M_O + M_U} \tag{2}$$

Solving equation (1) for A_O, substituting this expression for A_O into equation (2), and solving for M_U gives:

$$M_U = M_O \left[\frac{S_O}{S_D} - 1 \right] \tag{3}$$

The advantage of this method is that quantitative separation of $M_O + M_U$ from the mixture is not necessary in order to measure S_D. However, purification of that portion of material separated from the mixture is mandatory.

2. Inverse Methods

The inverse IDA procedure entails the addition of a *known quantity* of *non-radioactive compound* to a *mixture* containing an unknown amount of the labeled compound, resulting in a reduction of its specific activity. The quantity of the labeled compound in the original mixture can be calculated from the expression obtained by solving equation (3) for M_O (ARONOFF, 1956):

$$M_O = \frac{M_U S_D}{S_O - S_D} \tag{4}$$

In this procedure, it is assumed that S_O of the metabolite may be calculated from the activity per mole of its precursor. In contrast to direct isotope dilution, the inverse procedure allows for the addition of a relatively large quantity of unlabeled carrier compound which facilitates isolation and purification techniques.

In fact, the inverse IDA procedure is often used in drug metabolism studies to aid in isolation procedures even when radioactive quantification is not required. The addition of large amounts of carrier compound assures against losses of very small quantities of the radioactive material which may occur during separations. Frequently, there is enough radioactive material to detect but not enough material to measure by an independent technique such as UV spectroscopy (*e.g.*, see Folic Acid Antagonist and Cyclophosphamide sections below). In order to make reliable measurements when quantification is required, the labeled compound must be present in sufficient quantity in the original mixture or have a high specific activity. It also is obvious that in either the direct or inverse IDA procedures the accuracy of the assay is affected by the purity of the compounds added or isolated, and by the accuracy of the method used to measure radioactivity. These factors will be dealt with later.

C. Modifications of Isotope Dilution Analysis

There are situations in which the direct and inverse procedures must be modified in order to deal with complex mixtures of labeled metabolites or parent compound.

In some cases it may not be possible to obtain a particular labeled carrier substance of sufficient purity for a dilution analysis. This can be dealt with by employing *derivative isotope dilution analysis* or *double isotope dilution analysis*. *Derivative isotope dilution analysis* first suggested by Keston et al. (1946) involves the conversion of a non-labeled compound to a labeled derivative with a suitable labeled reagent. The analogous non-radioactive derivative then is added to the mixture to dilute the labeled derivative, as in the usual inverse IDA method. The diluted derivative is isolated and purified to constant specific activity, its radioactivity is measured and compared to the radioactivity of the reagent. This technique requires either a quantitative reaction of the non-labeled compound with the radioactive reagent or, at least, high and reproducible yields of the labeled derivative. Since a number of labeled byproducts may also be formed, a selective isolation procedure and efficient methods of purification must be used.

Double isotope dilution analysis, first described by Block and Anker (1948), involves the formation of a derivative labeled with two different isotopes which is isolated and purified either directly or after the addition of a non-radioactive carrier derivative. An excellent discussion of several versions of the double isotope method has been published by Radin (1964).

The success of the various isotope dilution procedures in a drug metabolism study involves making an "intelligent guess" as to the molecular structure of the radioactive or non-radioactive carrier diluent which is to be added to biological fluids (urine, bile, blood, cerebrospinal fluid) and tissues or to artificial pools (extracts) of drug metabolites or degradation products. Fortunately, as mentioned above, the isotope dilution procedures do not require the quantitative isolation of substances, but it is important to select the best possible methods of isolation, purification, and measurement of radioactivity.

D. Some Analytic Techniques Used in Conjunction with Radioassay Methods

1. Conversion of Samples to a Uniform Physical State

Liquid and solid samples should not be compared in radioassays and therefore all samples to be counted should be converted to the same physical state. Although materials on chromatograms (thin-layer, paper) and frozen whole body or tissue sections may be detected by autoradiography, the radioactivity of β-emitting substances is usually measured by liquid scintillation counting procedures which have been described in detail in a number of excellent technical bulletins (RADIN, 1964; RAPKIN, 1967). Major advances in the field since 1963 have been reviewed by PARMENTIER and TENHAAF (1969).

Generally, two techniques are used to produce samples suitable for counting: digestion and combustion. Digestion involves the solubilization of samples by acids or alkali, including a number of organic amine bases. These procedures are not time-consuming and do not require elaborate equipment; they are especially convenient when they can be carried out in the counting vial and when problems of color quenching can be avoided. However, combustion is generally move satisfactory than digestion for samples containing low levels of radioactivity or for samples which are colored. This latter problem occurs frequently, especially when tissues containing large amounts of blood are digested. Solutions which absorb in the visible region, i.e., appear colored, are likely to "quench" the transfer of energy from the sample to the photomultiplier tube in the liquid scintillation spectrometer, thus interfering with the counting. RAPKIN (1967) offers a variety of solutions to this problem, *e.g.*, bleaching and ultrasonic agitation, and should be consulted if the problem occurs or is anticipated.

Combustion methods are either wet or dry. Wet combustion usually involves the use of strong oxidizing agents and is primarily applicable to ^{35}S or ^{14}C labeled compounds. Although it does not require much special glassware or equipment, it is time-consuming. The most widely used method for the preparation of biological specimens for liquid scintillation counting has been the oxygen flask combustion procedure (RAGLAND, 1966; DAVIDSON and OLIVERIO, 1968) in which the sample is simply burned in a flask filled with oxygen; the radioactive carbon dioxide or tritiated water produced is counted in a suitable absorbing solution containing scintillators.

Our modification of the method described by KELLY et al. (1961) simplifies the apparatus and takes advantage of the superior properties of phenethylamine for absorbing CO_2, as described by WOELLER (1962). Details of variations of the original SCHONIGER (1955) method have appeared in the literature (RAPKIN, 1967; RAGLAND, 1966; JEFFAY, 1962) and do not require further elaboration. Suffice to say that we have satisfactorily processed over 10,000 samples by this method in the last 7 years.

However, since the oxygen flask combustion method is still somewhat laborious and does not permit the complete work-up of more than 25—30 samples per day by one technician, we explored the possibility of constructing a device which would permit the combustion of at least 100 samples per day. Primarily through the efforts of Dr. J.I. PETERSON (see PETERSON et al., 1969; PETERSON, 1969) a simple, semi-automated combustion apparatus was developed (Fig. 1) and has completely replaced the use of the oxygen flask combustion method in our laboratory. In contrast to other combustion methods, this system offers a convenient method of sample containment and introduction, rapid and complete catalytic burning of all varieties of organic samples, and collection by a new technique which combines the scintillation absorbing solvent with the water and carbon dioxide as they are produced during combustion. Tritium in water and ^{14}C in carbon dioxide can be determined separately to achieve optimum counting efficiency, or simultaneously by a double isotope counting technique depending on the choice of two collecting devices that are available with the apparatus.

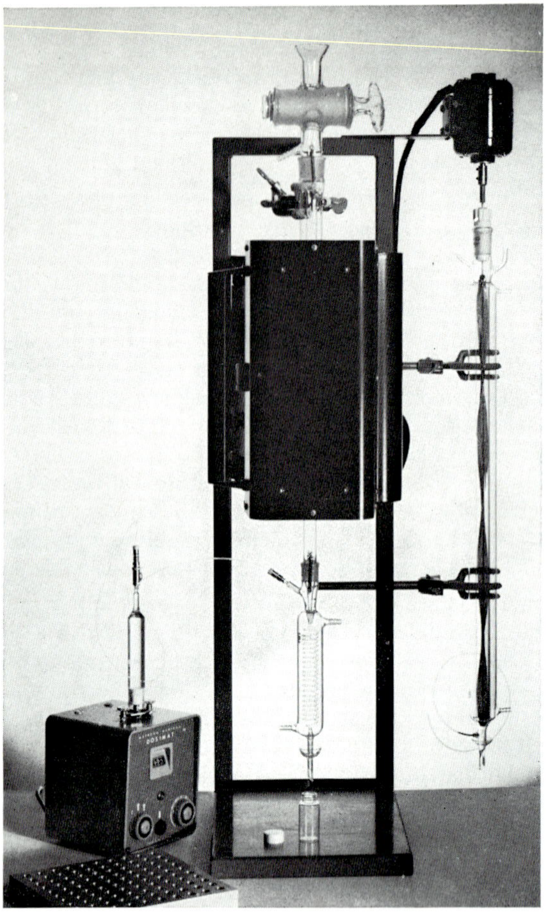

Fig. 1. The Peterson semi-automated combustion apparatus and ancillary equipment. (Photograph courtesy of Dr. J.I. Peterson, National Institutes of Health, Bethesda, Maryland)

In this procedure, whole samples or homogenates of tissues up to one-half gram in dry weight are introduced into the lower portion of a hardened gelatin capsule placed in an aluminum carrier block base (seen in Fig. 1) and evaporated by gentle heat (about 60 °C) overnight. The capsule containing the sample is then capped and dropped into the top of the apparatus; a stopcock is rotated to deliver the sample into a combustion tube containing a catalyst and housed in an oven held at 600 °C. After the sample burns in a stream of oxygen, it enters a condensing coil where it is mixed with a measured amount of scintillator absorbing solvent and delivered to a standard scintillation vial for counting. The procedure can be repeated every 3 min. Recoveries of radioactivity added to tissue blanks are essentially quantitative. Using this apparatus we have analyzed tissue homogenates and blood from animal species ranging from crayfish and sharks to mice and monkeys.

Almost simultaneously with the development of the Peterson combustion apparatus, the Packard Instrument Co. (Kaartinen, 1969) introduced a semi-automated combustion apparatus for the determination of ^{3}H and ^{14}C in biological materials. It is still too early to evaluate the performance of this instrument based on day-to-day laboratory operation, but in principle it offers the advantages found in the Peterson apparatus and a few additional conveniences. A comparison of the oxygen flask combustion technique and the two semi-automated combustion methods discussed above was made at a recent symposium on liquid scintillation counting (DAVIDSON et al., 1969).

2. Addition and Purity of Carrier Material

Inverse and direct isotope dilution techniques require the use of carrier substances of the highest purity, both chemically and radiochemically. The presence of traces of radiolabeled impurities can significantly alter the final calculated specific activity of the material being analyzed and can lead to erroneous conclusions regarding the metabolism of foreign compounds. There is also the necessity of insuring the homogenous mixing of the carrier compound with the material to be diluted. The amount of carrier substance to be added will depend both on the specific activity of the carrier or sample to be diluted and on the efficiency of the isolation and purification procedures.

3. Isolation of Drugs and Drug Metabolites

The search for a drug metabolite often begins with administration of the isotopically labeled parent compound to small animals housed in a metabolism cage (preferably constructed of glass) which is designed to separate and quantitatively collect urine and feces. Blood samples may also be withdrawn at appropriate time intervals before killing the animal. In our experience, the best assurance against cross contamination of feces and urine in mice or rats is the use of the anal cup technique (OLIVERIO and DAVIDSON, 1962).

Physiological fluids and body tissues can be prepared for liquid scintillation counting by digestion or combustion methods as described above. Aliquots of these biological samples are often subjected to such isolation procedures as solvent extraction, absorption, precipitation or partition, etc. However, in most cases solvent extraction techniques are employed. This is usually a simple extraction into an organic solvent in a separatory funnel, although the counter current distribution apparatus can be used for multiple extractions. Quite often the alert investigator will gain some insight into the possible structure of a metabolite by its solvent extraction behavior.

4. Purification of Isolated Material

Following isolation of a suspected metabolite or related compounds, various purification procedures may be required for further resolution and identification. These include any suitable procedure, such as ion-exchange, paper, thin-layer or column chromatography, gas chromatography, electrophoresis, crystallization, distillation, gel absorption or solvent partition. In some cases involving a compound difficult to purify, a derivative may have to be made and isolated to establish the identity of the compound in question. In drug metabolism research, a combination of solvent extraction methods with various chromatographic techniques is probably used most widely for isolation and purification.

Chromatographic methods offer the greatest advantage in terms of simultaneous identification and purification. For example, systemic use of spray reagents on paper or thin-layer chromatograms often allows identification of specific structural features of the metabolite from the characteristic color produced. In cases where spray reagents are not practical, radioactivity can serve as a built-in detector of the substance on the chromatogram. Then a comparison can be made between migration values (R_f) or elution characteristics of the labeled metabolite and a pure unlabeled compound suspected to be identical in structure. Identical mobility, especially in several different solvent systems, is highly indicative of identical structures. Thin-layer chromatographic techniques are especially appealing because, in addition to being relatively simple and less time-consuming than other purification methods, they do not require the isolation of a large amount of material for characterization. Often, several hundred micrograms is sufficient for the entire identification and quantification of a compound.

5. Concentration and Radioactivity Measurements

Information relating radioactivity to mass (specific activity) is quite commonly obtained by weighing the sample after crystallization and determining the radioactivity after application of any method which will convert the sample to a suitable physical state for liquid scintillation counting. For example, the oxygen-flask or semi-automated combustion methods cited earlier can be used. However, there is often not enough material to purify by crystallization. In these instances pure labeled or unlabeled carrier can be added, or chromatography combined with UV absorption spectrometry, colorimetric analysis, or fluorescence spectroscopy; gas chromatography alone or with mass spectrometry; polarography, or titrimetry can be used. Spectrometric techniques have the added advantage of allowing the assay of a substance without its destruction.

The remainder of this chapter will deal with several recent examples of the use of isotope dilution analysis in combination with a number of the isolation, separation, purification, and detection methods discussed above.

E. Applications of Isotopic Dilution Techniques

There are numerous examples of applications of isotope dilution techniques in the literature; those we have selected relate to pharmacology and typify the kinds of supportive analytic techniques which commonly are employed in conjunction with IDA.

1. Examples of Direct Methods

a) Pentobarbital

TITUS and WEISS (1955) were among the first to propose the use of radioactive tracers to guide in the isolation of sufficient material for direct chemical identification of a drug metabolite. Their study of the metabolism of pentobarbital is an excellent example of the power of appropriate analytic separation methods combined with direct isotopic dilution.

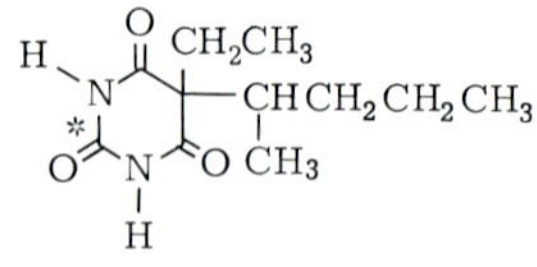

^{14}C-Pentobarbital

As mentioned above, the behavior of an unknown metabolite during extraction procedures may provide clues to its structure. Thus, these investigators observed that a urinary metabolite of pentobarbital could be quantitatively extracted into ether from solutions of pH less than 3. This fact suggested that the metabolite might be the carboxylic acid derivative of pentobarbital, 5-ethyl-5-(1-methyl-3-carboxypropyl) barbituric acid (pentobarbital carboxylic acid, PCA). Preliminary experiments showed ten radioactive spots on paper chromatograms of urine from dogs receiving 2-^{14}C-pentobarbital. Since most of these substances were readily identifiable from previous studies, TITUS and WEISS focused their attention on the then-unknown metabolite, pentobarbital carboxylic acid. In order to isolate and confirm the identity of PCA the following procedure was adopted.

The labeled acidic metabolite was added to the urine of dogs receiving large amounts of unlabeled pentobarbital. The urine at pH 7 was then extracted several times with n-butanol, the pooled extracts were evaporated *in vacuo*, and the residue subjected to a 10 transfer countercurrent system. The bulk of the radioactivity appeared in tubes 3 to 7; after concentration of the contents of these tubes, the resulting material was subjected to a 124 transfer countercurrent distribution in 25 ml layers of mutually saturated n-butanol and 0.25 M pyrophosphate buffer, pH 9.4. Paper chromatography of selected fractions from this run indicated only partial separation of the metabolites. Further resolution of the countercurrent fractions was obtained by chromatography on large sheets of Whatman No. 3 (heavy) paper. The radioactive component was located by radioautography and eluted with 85% methanol.

To obtain enough material for the isolation and characterization of the suspected PCA, a sample of the radioactive material which had been eluted only from the area of the paper chromatograms corresponding to that of PCA, was added to pooled urine from several dogs treated with a total of 50 grams of unlabeled sodium pentobarbital. In an exemplary cautious manner, which is recommended to the reader anticipating use of this procedure, TITUS and WEISS did not immediately expend their entire sample on an unproven technique. First these workers repeated the above extraction and countercurrent procedures on a pilot basis (1/100 aliquot) before the remainder of the pooled urine was passed through the same extraction and countercurrent procedures as above, and each step was monitored for radioactivity. Large quantities of the metabolite were isolated and purified in this way. The metabolite could then be definitely identified as PCA by comparing the following physical properties of the compound with those of authentic PCA: UV absorption, melting point, pKa, molecular weight, elemental analysis, partition coefficient, infrared absorption, and x-ray powder diagrams.

b) Tolbutamide

Prior to the study of THOMAS and IKEDA (1966) methods used to measure metabolites of the oral hypoglycemic agent, tolbutamide, were unable to detect the hydroxymethyl metabolite.

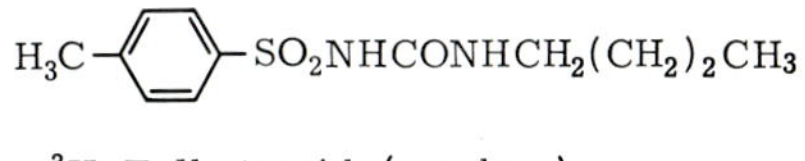

^{3}H-Tolbutamide (random)

The use of randomly tritiated tolbutamide permitted both the assay of this metabolite and its isolation in crystalline form. Rats were treated with an initial radioactive dose of tolbutamide followed by 19 non-radioactive doses and finally, a terminal radioactive dose. The 48-hr urine collections following administration of non-radioactive tolbutamide were pooled but not those following administration of the tritium-labeled drug. Paper chromatography of the initial and terminal urine samples revealed a radioactive zone having a R_f corresponding to that of the hydroxymethyl tolbutamide (HMT). The radioactive urine samples were then combined with the non-radioactive sample pool for the isolation of metabolites. Note that this dosage schedule avoids use of the isotopic compound on most days of the study, but provides a relatively large amount of material which contains a *mixture* of radioactive and non-radioactive samples, i.e., an "indicator" quantity of the desired metabolite in its labeled form and an "isolation and identification" amount of the compound in its non-labeled form. Hence, the presence of the radioactive species was used to monitor the material in collection tubes from a 200-tube Craig countercurrent distribution apparatus. Four hundred mg of crystalline material was obtained by acidification and extraction of the contents of the tubes containing the suspected HMT. The identity of this compound was established as HMT by comparison with synthetic HMT by the following techniques: melting point determination, UV, IR, and NMR spectroscopy, paper and thin-layer chromatography, and elemental analysis.

2. Examples of Indirect Methods

a) Warfarin

Whereas the above examples illustrate the use of the rather laborious countercurrent technique as a separation procedure, BARKER et al. (1970) provide a recent example of the use of thin-layer chromatography (TLC) and paper chromatography in conjunction with inverse IDA. Test compounds considered to be potential metabolites of warfarin, either obtained commerically or synthesized,

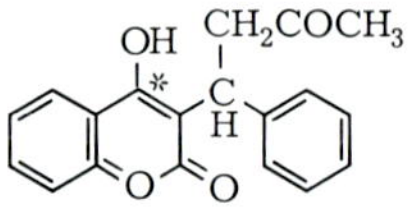

^{14}C-Warfarin

were compared chromatographically with the ^{14}C-warfarin metabolites present in ether extracts of acidified urine from rats treated with the drug. Each metabolite which migrated with the same R_f value as one of the test compounds was then examined by inverse IDA as follows: a weighed amount of the test compound was added to a small measured portion of the urine extract and was successively recrystallized from a suitable solvent. A portion of the compound from each crystallization was removed, dried to constant weight and counted. The identity of the metabolite with the added test compound was considered to be confirmed if the recrystallizations produced a material of constant specific activity which migrated as a single radioactive spot in a chromatographic system. By this use of inverse isotope dilution THOMAS and IKEDA were able to demonstrate the following substances in rat urine after treatment of the animals with 4-^{14}C-warfarin: the parent drug, 4′-, 6-, 7-, and 8-hydroxy warfarin and the interesting condensation product of warfarin, 2,3,-dihydro-2-methyl-4-phenyl-5-oxa-8 pyrano(3,2-c)-(1)benzopyran.

b) Probenecid

In the following example (GUARINO and SCHANKER, 1968) the probenecid metabolites were not identified, but the use of inverse IDA showed that little, if any, of the proposed acyl glucuronide of probenecid was excreted in rat bile.

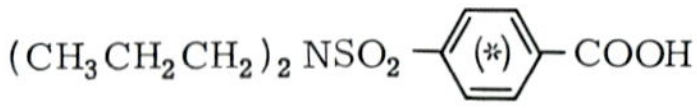

^{14}C-Probenecid (ring)

Ring labeled ^{14}C-probenecid was injected i.v. into rats with cannulated bile ducts. At a dose of 0.1 mg/kg it was found that 84% of the radioactivity in bile occurred as glucuronide conjugates. Up until this time only the acyl glucuronide

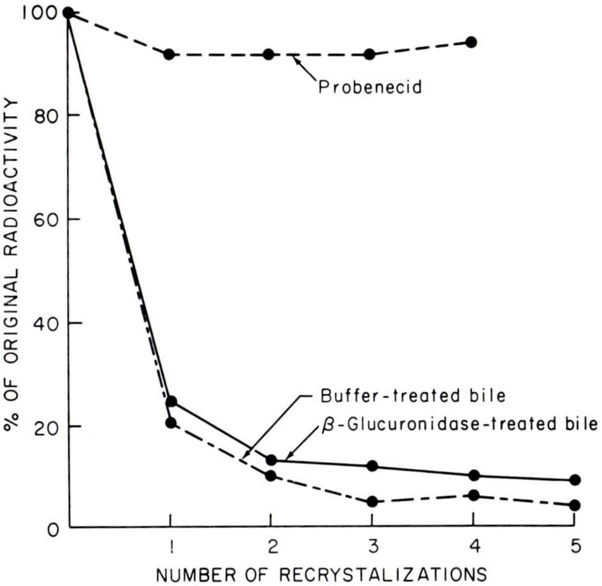

Fig. 2. Inverse isotope dilution analysis of pure ^{14}C-probenecid and of bile from rats treated with 0.1 mg/kg of ^{14}C-probenecid. Bile samples were incubated for 24 hr either with acetate buffer (0.1 M, pH 4.5) or β-glucuronidase in acetate buffer (0.1 M, pH 4.5). GUARINO and SHANKER, 1968. (Figure reproduced from *J. Pharmacol. exp. Ther.* through the courtesy of The Williams and Wilkins Company)

of the drug had been reported and hence treatment of the radioactive metabolite with β-glucuronidase would be expected to yield the parent compound. To test this, bile from rats dosed with the labeled drug was treated with buffer (control) or with β-glucuronidase and weighed amounts of non-labeled probenecid were added. The probenecid in each sample was successively recrystallized from ethanol-water. A small portion from each recrystallization was removed, dried to constant weight, and counted. Figure 2 shows that the radioactivity fell precipitously with recrystallization and leveled off at less than 10% of its initial amount by the fifth recrystallization. This figure also includes the results obtained by this procedure with a sample of pure ^{14}C-probenecid; in this case the specific activity was >95% of the original. Hence, these authors were able to conclude that most of the aglycone released after β-glucuronidase treatment was *not* probenecid and that the rat therefore excreted very little of the acyl glucuronide in the bile. It was later shown by GUARINO et al. (1969), using combination gas chromatography-mass spectrometry, that four metabolites of probenecid appear in rat bile: N-dealkylated probenecid, an ester glucuronide of a side-chain oxidized metabolite, and two ether glucuronides of the side-chain hydroxylated drug. Again, the reader is reminded that these studies were prompted by a *negative* result of inverse isotopic dilution studies, *i.e.*, the proposed metabolite was incorrect. But since it had been shown that glucuronides were present, other types of glucuronides were sought when the acyl glucuronide was eliminated, proving that even a wrong guess can be valuable.

c) *Fluroxene*

BLAKE et al. (1967) provide an example of some interesting ancillary techniques which were required in handling volatile compounds during use of the inverse IDA. In most previous studies it had been assumed that volatile anesthetics were refractory to the enzymatic alterations encountered by other drugs because most of an anesthetic dose could be recovered unchanged in the expired air. These workers showed that fluroxene (2,2,2-trifluroethyl vinyl ether) is biotrans-

$$CF_3CH_2OCH = {}^*CH_2$$

^{14}C-Fluroxene

formed to trifluoroethanol (TFE) glucuronide and trifluoroacetic acid (TFAA) which are excreted in the urine. Treatment of the urine with β-glucuronidase released TFE. However, the volatility of TFE and TFAA necessitated their conversion to the solid derivatives, the N-α-naphthylcarbamate ester of TFE (m.p. 79°) and the benzyl thiouronium salt of TFAA (m.p. 179°) by the addition of the appropriate derivatizing agents to urine samples from animals treated with the ^{14}C-labeled anesthetic. The derivatives were isolated and identified by elemental analysis and infrared spectroscopy before they were employed in the inverse isotope dilution studies. Such studies showed that 10—20% of the urinary activity was present as TFAA and 20—50% as TFE glucuronide.

d) Folic Acid Antagonists

In 1959, our laboratory began to investigate the pharmacology of the folic acid antagonists, methotrexate (MTX) and dichloromethotrexate (DCM). Both of these compounds had shown consistent antitumor effects in animals, while clinically, MTX had proven effective in the treatment of choriocarcinoma and acute lymphocytic leukemia in children. Our investigations were prompted by striking inconsistencies in earlier studies of the absorption and excretion of MTX, and a general lack of information of the possible metabolic alterations which the folic acid antagonists might undergo *in vivo*. Much of the confusion undoubtedly had arisen from the inherent impurity and instability of these drugs and from the lack of adequately sensitive and specific analytical methods for the determination of these compounds and their possible metabolites in biological media. All these problems are very common in early studies of a new drug.

As a first approach, a method was developed which permitted the quantitative separation, purification and analysis of mixtures of folic acid antagonists that differed by as little as one functional group. This was achieved by diethylaminoethyl (DEAE) ion-exchange cellulose chromatography in combination with UV spectrophotometry (OLIVERIO, 1961). Then our efforts were directed to labeling

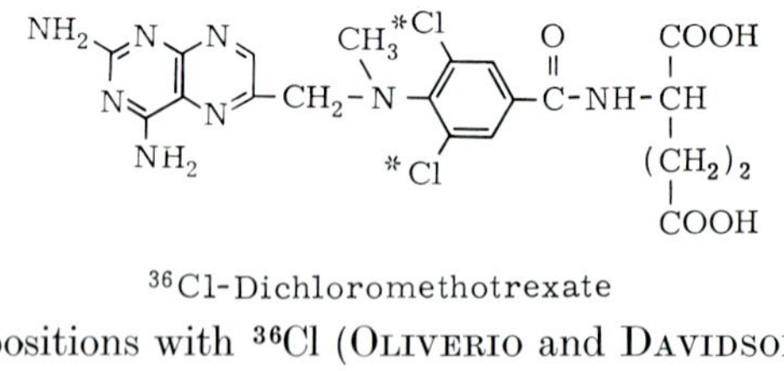

^{36}Cl-Dichloromethotrexate

DCM in the 3′,5′-positions with ^{36}Cl (OLIVERIO and DAVIDSON, 1961) by a modification of a method reported by ANGIER and CURRAN (1959) for the chlorination of MTX.

In animal (OLIVERIO and DAVIDSON, 1962) and human (DAVIDSON and OLIVERIO, 1965) studies of the physiologic disposition of ^{36}Cl-DCM, radioactivity was determined by liquid scintillation counting techniques. A typical elution pattern from a DEAE cellulose column of a bile sample from a rabbit treated with ^{36}Cl-DCM is seen in Fig. 3. Note that the addition of non-labeled carrier allowed for monitoring of the drug by UV spectroscopy at 254 mμ.

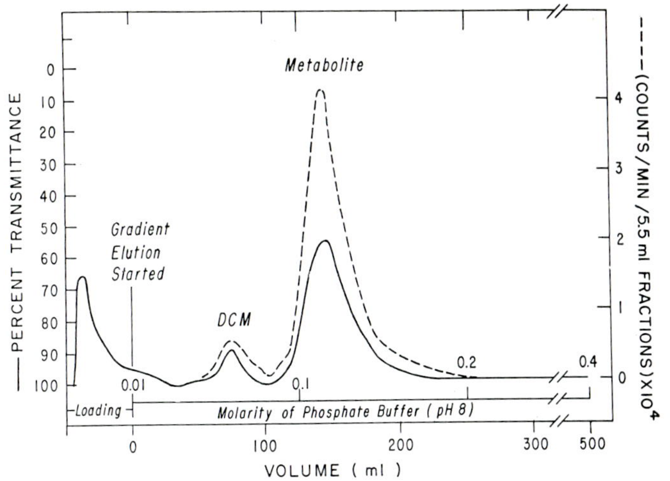

Fig. 3. DEAE cellulose chromatographic separation of 0.2 ml bile from a rabbit treated with ^{36}Cl-DCM. Note that the presence of drug was monitored by two independent methods, spectrometry at 254 mμ (—) and radioactivity (- - - -). OLIVERIO and DAVIDSON, 1962. (Figure reproduced from *J. Pharmacol. exp. Ther.* through the courtesy of The Williams and Wilkins Company)

DCM, representing 10% of the radioactive load, was eluted with uniform specific activity (counts per min per optical density unit), followed by a single peak containing the remainder of the total radioactivity and representing the metabolite, 7-hydroxy DCM. The structure of the metabolite was subsequently confirmed by LOO and ADAMSON (1965).

Studies were performed in man by JOHNS et al. (1964) where the MTX was randomly tritiated by exchange with tritiated acetic acid in the presence of platinum catalyst. The ^{3}H-MTX was purified by chromatography on DEAE cellulose columns by elution with neutral phosphate buffers. The plasma disappearance and renal excretion was measured after administration of ^{3}H-MTX to patients. Highly radioactive urines were chromatographed directly by placing an aliquot on the DEAE cellulose column and eluting with neutral phosphate buffers to separate, identify and measure the concentration (by UV spectroscopy and liquid scintillation counting) of MTX and possible metabolites. For urines low in radioactivity, inverse IDA was employed prior to extraction, concentration, chromatography and liquid scintillation counting as follows: One ml of an aqueous solution of unlabeled carrier MTX (1 mg/ml) was added to 50 ml of urine. The urine was acidified by concentrated HCl and extracted with two separate portions of liquid phenol. The combined phenol extracts were extracted with a mixture of water and ether. The ether layer was removed and the aqueous layer was extracted twice more with ether. The aqueous layer was neutralized with 0.1 N sodium hydroxide and chromatographed on a DEAE cellulose column with neutral phosphate buffers.

In the determination of the absorption, excretion, distribution, metabolism, and serum protein binding of ^{3}H-MTX in laboratory animals (HENDERSON et al., 1965a) and man (HENDERSON et al., 1965b) techniques similar to those employed by JOHNS et al. (1964) were used, except that the chromatography was modified by the use of ammonium bicarbonate buffers. A typical column chromatographic elution pattern of urine from a patient treated with an intravenous dose of

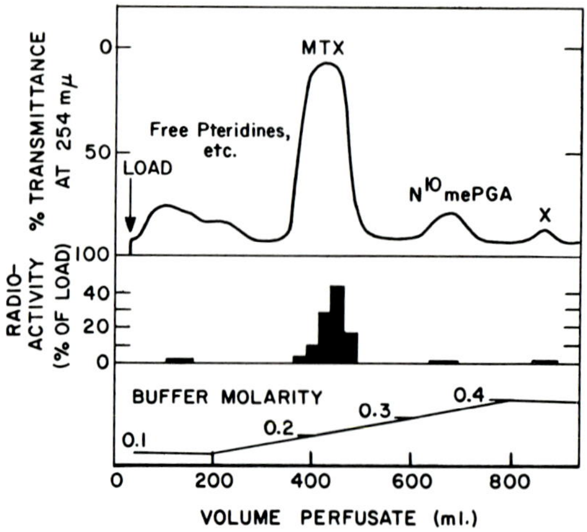

Fig. 4. DEAE cellulose chromatographic separation of urine from a patient treated with 10 mg/kg of ^{3}H-MTX. Elution was performed with ammonium bicarbonate buffer, pH 8.3 in molar concentrations as indicated. MTX and N^{10}-methylpteroylglutamic acid were identified by UV spectrometry. HENDERSON et al., 1965. (Figure reproduced from *Cancer Res.* through the courtesy of American Association for Cancer Research, Inc.)

^{3}H-MTX is shown in Fig. 4. These studies indicated that MTX, in contrast to DCM, is not significantly metabolized in the species examined.

Subsequent studies of MTX involved the use of drug specifically labeled with tritium in the 3′,5′-positions of the phenyl ring. This compound, prepared com-

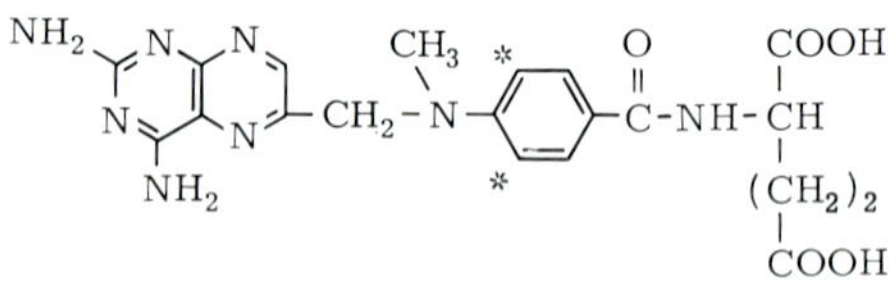

^{3}H-Methotrexate

mercially by reduction of DCM with tritium vapor, is less prone to exchange with body water since the ^{3}H-C bond is stronger than ^{3}H-N and ^{3}H-O bonds which occur in randomly labeled MTX. The stability of the tritium in MTX was especially important in studies of the transport of ^{3}H-MTX into L1210 leukemia cells (GOLDMAN et al., 1968). Specifically labeled 3′,5′-^{3}H-MTX was also employed in studies which showed that the simultaneous administration of other foreign compounds altered plasma protein binding and renal clearance of MTX in man (LIEGLER et al., 1969). More recently ZAHARKO et al. (1969) employed inverse IDA in studies of specifically labeled MTX in mice and demonstrated that the drug is metabolized by the intestinal flora and the metabolism is reduced either by treatment of mice with neomycin and sulfathioazole, or in germ-free mice. Metabolism of 3′,5′-^{3}H-MTX was also shown to occur in the gut flora of rats (ZAHARKO and OLIVERIO, 1970). Thus, while MTX does not appear to be metabolized by mammalian tissues, in some species the bacteria in the gut can effect biotransformations. This possible source of drug metabolism by intestinal microorganisms in intact animals is often ignored and should be considered in any metabolic studies which extend for more than a few hours.

e) Cyclophosphamide

Cyclophosphamide (cytoxan) is an established cancer chemotherapeutic drug which apparently exerts its carcinostatic effects after being converted to an "active form." Presumably, this is accomplished by hepatic microsomal enzymes (BROCK and HOHORST, 1963; HOHORST et al., 1965). The elucidation of the active metabolite(s) of cytoxan has been the aim of a number of comparative pharmacological studies in laboratory animals and humans.

Ring labeled ^{14}C-cytoxan has been primarily employed for tracer metabolism studies. The compound was shown to be radiochemically pure by paper and thin-layer chromatography in several separate solvent systems (MELLETT et al.,

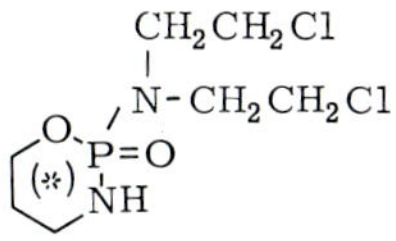

^{14} C-Cyclophosphamide (ring)

1969b). The R_f values for pure unlabeled cytoxan (detected by ninhydrin reagent) was identical to the single radioactive spot of ^{14}C-cytoxan. Throughout the metabolic studies reported by MELLETT et al. (1969a, b) and DE VITA and ADAMSON (1969) reverse IDA coupled with organic solvent extraction and liquid scintillation counting was used to determine unchanged ^{14}C-cytoxan in plasma, bile, urine, and tissue homogenates of treated animals. The biological sample was mixed with a known quantity of an unlabeled solution of cytoxan and solid NaCl; then phosphate buffer (pH 7.0) and 10% methanol in ethylene dichloride were added. A portion of the organic layer was transferred to a counting vial and after evaporation, n-amyl alcohol was added to dissolve the residue. The radioactivity of this solution was determined by liquid scintillation counting. The addition of unlabeled carrier cytoxan to the biological sample served primarily to aid in complete extraction of unchanged drug.

f) Thalidomide

Before an agent can be postulated as the mediator of a particular pharmacologic or toxic action, its presence must be demonstrated in the tissue in question. Hence, FABRO et al. (1967), using inverse IDA, found that the potent teratogen, thalidomide, as well as seven of its hydrolysis products, persist in rabbit embryos

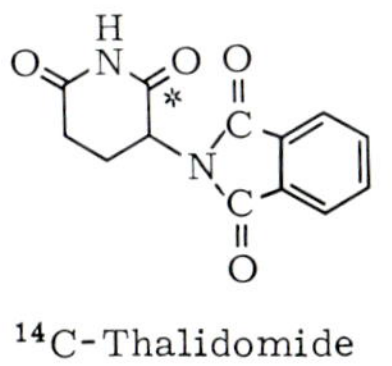

^{14}C-Thalidomide

for more than 24 hrs after dosing. This study shows that drugs in the body are altered not only enzymatically, but also by spontaneous degradation and that isotope dilution analysis can be used to identify these products as well as enzymatic metabolites.

In this study, pooled homogenized embryos or maternal blood were freeze-dried to a powder, which was extracted three times with methanol. After centrifugation, the extract was concentrated under reduced pressure and aliquots were dried as spots on paper; a solution containing 50 μg of the carrier compound was applied to the spots. This latter step exemplifies another variation of IDA where carrier is added to a paper chromatogram. The chromatograms were developed to obtain a preliminary separation. Radioactive compounds in the embryo, maternal tissues and excreta were then identified and measured by standard inverse isotope dilution techniques. It was shown that thalidomide and its hydrolysis products were more concentrated in the embryo than in the maternal plasma. This very important finding indicates that the parent compound and its breakdown products accumulate in the embryo, probably because thalidomide can readily pass the placental barrier and hydrolyze spontaneously in the fetal tissues to polar compounds. These compounds, being less lipid soluble, would not be expected to readily re-enter the maternal blood stream, where they would become available for excretion.

Pharmacologists are often called upon to study compounds other than those regarded as drugs. In the following sections, examples germane to the fields of food additives and industrial toxicology will be considered.

g) Tartrazine

Because food additives may be in the diet during most of the lifetime of a consumer, extensive metabolic and toxicologic testing must be done on these agents. In 1916 tartrazine (FD & C Yellow No. 5; Color Index No. 19140) was added to the list of food colors certified by the U.S. Department of Agriculture.

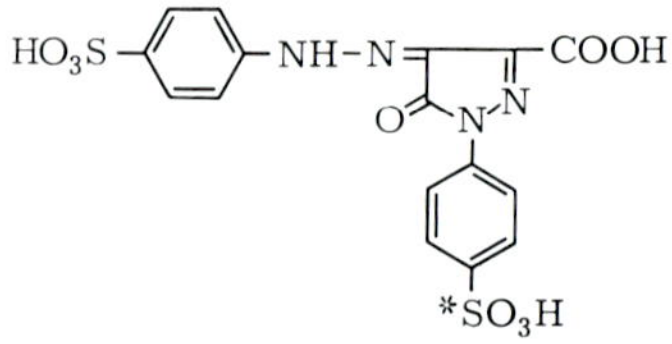

^{35}S-Tartrazine

This agent is used internationally and an Australian team led by A.J. Ryan and the late S.E. Wright has provided considerable information on its metabolism.

Ryan et al. (1969) were unable to determine the nature of the radioactivity in urine of rats dosed with tritiated tartrazine either because of the low specific activity of the dye or problems encountered in liquid scintillation counting. This latter difficulty may have been due to the high degree of quenching usually associated with the measurement of any intensely yellow material by this counting technique. To overcome these problems tartrazine was labeled with the stronger β-emitter, ^{35}S, and administered to rats. Inverse isotopic dilution studies with sulfanilic acid and 4-sulphophenylhydrazine demonstrated that these metabolites accounted for 49% and 30% respectively, of the radioactivity in 48-hr urine samples from these rats. The isolated sulfanilic acid was purified by successive recrystallization from HCl in the usual way, but the hydrazine analog posed some obstacles. Oxidation of 4-sulphophenylhydrazine was prevented by the addition of a small amount of zinc dust during the initial crystallization; however, this compound could not be recrystallized as such because when added to the solubilizer, hyamine hydroxide, products which were chemiluminescent and deeply colored were formed. Therefore the hydrazine metabolite was cyclized with ethyl acetoacetate to 1-(4-sulphophenyl)-3-methyl-5-pyrazolone and this derivative was crystallized to constant specific activity.

h) Benzene and Cyclohexane

In a single chapter, Parke (1965) has summarized the results of many experiments in which inverse IDA was the major tool in determining the metabolic fate of several industrial chemicals and solvents. For example, L-phenylmercapturic acid in rabbit urine following ^{14}C-benzene administration was identified by IDA after this compound was hydrolyzed to thiophenol and further characterized by its conversion to thiophenyl-*p*-nitrobenzoate and phenylmercuric mercaptide. The similarity of the specific radioactivities of the two latter derivatives to that of phenylmercapturic acid was used as further confirmation that the original choice of a proposed metabolite was correct.

In studies on another important industrial chemical, cyclohexane, PARKE (1965) pointed out the need for confirmation of the isotopic and chemical purity of the compounds under study. When trace amounts of labeled metabolites are found, one must establish that these arise from the compound under study and not from traces of impurities in original samples. PARKE found that isotope dilution determinations of phenol in the urine of rabbits treated with ^{14}C-cylcohexane showed that 0.5—1% of the dose appeared as phenol. However, PARKE was able to show that the original radiolabeled cyclohexane given to the animals contained about 1.5% ^{14}C-benzene and that direct hydroxylation of this compound gave rise to phenol. Accordingly, ^{14}C-cyclohexane purified by gas chro matography did not give rise to phenol when metabolized by rabbits.

PARKE (1965) presented many other examples of the use of inverse isotope dilution and this reference should be consulted by any reader contemplating use of this important method for identifying metabolites of foreign substances.

References

ANGIER, R.B., CURRAN, W.V.: The Halogenation of 4-Amino-4-deoxy-N^{10}-methylpteroylglutamic Acid (Methotrexate) and Other Pteroylglutamic Acid Derivatives. J. Amer. chem. Soc. **81**, 2814—2818 (1959).

ARONOFF, S.: Quantitization techniques in techniques of radiobiochemistry, pp. 35—64. Ames: The Iowa State College Press 1956.

BARKER, W.M., HERMODSON, M.A., LINK, K.P.: The metabolism of 4-C^{14}-warfarin sodium by the rat. J. Pharmacol. exp. Ther. **171**, 307—313 (1970).

BLAKE, D.A., ROZMAN, R.S., CASCORBI, H.F., KRANTZ, J.C.: Anesthesia LXXIV: Biotransformation of fluroxene I. Metabolism in mice and dogs *in vivo*. Biochem. Pharmacol. **16**, 1237—1248 (1967).

BLOCK, K., ANKER, H.S.: An extension of the isotope dilution method. Science **107**, 228 (1948).

BROCK, N., HOHORST, H.J.: Über die Aktivierung von Cyclophosphamide *in vivo* und *in vitro*. Arzneimittel-Forsch. **13**, 1021—1031 (1963).

COSULICH, D.B., SEEGER, D.R., FAHRENBACH, M.J., ROTH, B., MOWAT, J.H., SMITH, J.R., HULTQUIST, M.E.: Analogs of pteroylglutamic acid. VI. 3′,5′-dihalopteroyl derivatives. J. Amer. chem. Soc. **73**, 2554—2557 (1951).

DAVIDSON, J.D., OLIVERIO, V.T.: The physiologic disposition of dichloromethotrexate-Cl^{36} in man. Clin. Pharmacol. Ther. **6**, 321—327 (1965).

— — Tritium and carbon-14 by oxygen flask combustion. In: Advances in tracer methodology, Vol. 4, pp. 67—79. Ed. by S. ROTHCHILD. New York: Plenum Press 1968.

— — PETERSON, J.I.: Combustion of samples for liquid scintillation counting. In: The current status of liquid scintillation counting, pp. 222—235. Ed. by E. BRANSOME. New York: Grune and Stratton 1970.

DEVITA, V.T., ADAMSON, R.H.: The metabolism of ^{14}C-cyclophosphamide: Comparative drug metabolism studies on African and American patients with lymphosarcoma and Burkitt's tumor, pp. 218—225. Proceedings of the Sixth International Congress of Chemotherapy, Tokyo, Japan, Vol. II (1970). Tokyo: University Press, Tokyo.

FABRO, S., SMITH, R.L., WILLIAMS, R.T.: The fate of C^{14}-thalidomide in the pregnant rabbit. Biochem. J. **104**, 565—569 (1967).

GOLDMAN, I.D., LICHTENSTEIN, N.S., OLIVERIO, V.T.: Carrier-mediated transport of the folic acid analogue, methotrexate, in the L1210 leukemia cell. Biochim. biophys. Acta (Amst.) **243**, 5007—5017 (1968).

GORSUCH, T.T.: Radioactive isotope dilution analysis in Radiochemical Centre review no. 2 Amersham, The Radiochemical Centre, 1968, pp. 1—12.

GUARINO, A.M., CONWAY, W.D., FALES, H.M.: Mass spectral identification of probenecid metabolites in rat bile. Europ. J. Pharmacol. 8, 244—252 (1969).
— SCHANKER, L.S.: Biliary excretion of probenecid and its glucuronide. J. Pharmacol. exp. Ther. 164, 387—395 (1968).
HENDERSON, E.S., ADAMSON, R.H., DENHAM, C., OLIVERIO, V.T.: The metabolic fate of tritiated methotrexate. I. Absorption, excretion, and distribution in mice, rats, dogs, and monkeys. Cancer Res. 25, 1008—1017 (1965).
— — OLIVERIO, V.T.: The metabolic fate of tritiated methotrexate. II. Absorption and excretion in man. Cancer Res. 25, 1018—1024 (1965).
HEVESY, G., HOBBIE, R.: Über die Ermittlung des Bleigehaltes von Gesteinen. Z. anal. Chem. 88, 1—6 (1932).
HOHORST, H.J., ZIEMAN, A., BROCK, N.: Alkylierende Substanzen in Serum and Urin nach Injection von Cyclophosphamide. Arzneimittel-Forsch. 15, 432—434 (1965).
JEFFAY, H.: Oxidation techniques for preparation of liquid scintillation samples. Packard Technical Bulletin No. 10 (1962).
JOHNS, D.G., HOLLINGSWORTH, J.W., CASHMORE, A.R., PLENDERLEITH, I.H., BERTINO, J.R.: Methotrexate displacement in man. J. clin. Invest. 43, 621—629 (1964).
KAARTINEN, N.: A new oxidation method for the preparation of liquid scintillation samples. Packard Technical Bulletin 18, 1—9 (1969).
KELLY, R.G., PEETS, E.A., GORDON, S., BUYSKE, D.A.: Determination of C^{14} and H^3 in biological samples by Schoniger combustion and liquid scintillation techniques. Analyt. Biochem. 2, 267—273 (1961).
KESTON, A.S., UDENFRIEND, S., CANNAN, R.K.: Micro-analysis of mixtures (amino acids) in the form of isotopic derivatives. J. Amer. chem. Soc. 68, 1390 (1946).
LIEGLER, D.G., HENDERSON, E.S., HAHN, M.A., OLIVERIO, V.T.: The effect of organic acids on renal clearance of methotrexate in man. Clin. Pharmacol. Ther. 10, 849—857 (1969).
LOO, T.L., ADAMSON, R.H.: The metabolite of 3′,5′-dichloro-4-amino 4-deoxy-N^{10}-methylpteroylglutamic acid (dichloromethotrexate). J. Med. Chem. 8, 513—515 (1965).
MELLETT, L.B., EL DAREER, S.M., LUCE, J.K., FREI, E., III: Activation of cyclophosphamide metabolism in various species. Pharmacologist 11, 273 (1969a).
— — RALL, D.P., ADAMSON, R.H.: Metabolism of cyclophosphamide-C^{14} by various marine species. Arch. int. Pharmacodyn. 177, 60—70 (1969b).
OLIVERIO, V.T.: Chromatographic separation and purification of folic acid analogs. Analyt. Chem. 33, 263—265 (1961).
— DAVIDSON, J.D.: Synthesis of radioactive Cl^{36}-dichloromethotrexate. J. pharm. Sci. 50, 353—354 (1961).
— — The physiological disposition of dichloromethotrexate-Cl^{36} in animals. J. Pharmacol. exp. Ther. 137, 76—83 (1962).
PARKE, D.V.: Radioisotopes in the study of the metabolism of foreign compounds. In: Isotopes in experimental pharmacology, pp. 315—341. Ed. by L.J. ROTH. Chicago: University of Chicago Press 1965.
PARMENTIER, J.H., TENHAAF, F.E.L.: Developments in liquid scintillation counting since 1963. Int. J. appl. Radiat. 20, 305—333 (1969).
PETERSON, J.I.: A carbon dioxide collection accessory for the rapid combustion apparatus for preparation of biological samples for liquid scintillation analysis. Analyt. Biochem. 31, 204—210 (1969).
— WAGNER, F., SIEGEL, S., NIXON, W.: A system for convenient combustion preparation of tritiated biological samples for scintillation analysis. Analyt. Biochem. 31, 189—203 (1969).
RADIN, N.S.: How to use the radioisotopic derivative method in quantitative analysis. In: A collection of comprehensive scientific papers on the application and measurement of radioactivity, Nuclear Chicago Corp. 1964, pp. 9—12.
RAGLAND, J.B.: Combustion of samples for liquid scintillation counting. The Nucleus, Nuclear-Chicago Corp. 20, 1—11 (1966).
RAPKIN, E.: Laboratory Scintillator, Vol. 11, 1L—6L. New York: Picker-Nuclear White Plains 1967.
RYAN, A.J., WELLING, P.G., WRIGHT, S.E.: Further studies on the metabolism of tartrazine and related compounds in the intact rat. Fd. Cosmet. Tox. 7, 287—295 (1969).
SCHMID, K., RUSS, W., EGGER, H.P., KEBERLE, H.: Isotope dilution analysis with the aid of preparation thin-layer chromatograph. In: International conference on radioactive isotopes in pharmacology, pp. 67—82. Ed. by WASER, P.B. and B. GLASSON. New York: Wiley — Interscience 1969.
SCHONIGER, W.: Eine mikroanalytische Schnellbestimmung von Halogen in organischen Substanzen. Mikrochim. Acta 123—129 (1955).
THOMAS, R.C., IKEDA, G.G.: The metabolic fate of tolbutamide in man and in the rat. J. Med. Chem. 9, 507—510 (1966).

TITUS, E., WEISS, H.: The use of biologically prepared radioactive indicators in metabolic studies; Metabolism of pentobarbital. J. biol. Chem. **214**, 807—820 (1955).
WOELLER, F.H.: Liquid scintillation counting of $C^{14}O_2$ with phenethylamine. Analyt. Biochem. **2**, 508—511 (1962).
ZAHARKO, D.S., BRUCKNER, H., OLIVERIO, V.T.: Antibiotics alter methotrexate metabolism and excretion. Science **166**, 887—888 (1969).
— OLIVERIO, V.T.: Reinvestigation of methotrexate metabolism in rodents. Biochem. Pharmacol. (in press) (1970).

Chapter 33

Gas Chromatography-Mass Spectrometry

A.M. Guarino and H.M. Fales

With 8 Figures

A. Introduction

In choosing a method by which to identify drug metabolites, the quantity of material which is available is a prime consideration. In this regard, pharmacologists find themselves midway between natural products chemists and biochemists. Usually the former has reasonably large quantities of material available in a relatively high state of purity. The biochemist on the other hand, is usually forced to deal with submicrogram quantities; radioactivity may be the only objective evidence of the existence of a compound. This is a consequence of the biochemist's use of purified enzyme preparations which only allow for the conversion of mg quantities under the carefully controlled conditions he usually wishes to maintain. Attempts to scale up such processes may bring about a whole new set of problems. The pharmacologist interested in drug metabolism deals with enzyme systems as present in intact organs or at least parts of organs (liver slices, etc.), and in general this permits conversion of somewhat larger quantities. In fact, most drugs in use today are employed at mg rather than μg levels and so the investigation of their metabolism is at least practicable. This chapter discusses the advantages and disadvantages of mass spectrometry, especially as combined with gas chromatography, for such investigations.

At the present time, the natural products chemist fortunate enough to acquire mg quantities of material is able to utilize a broad spectrum of sophisticated instruments whose output often results in the rapid elucidation of structure. Foremost among the new techniques is nuclear magnetic resonance (nmr) (see also Chapter 9, this Volume). In this method, the material is dissolved in any one of a variety of deuterated solvents and the electronic environment of each proton in the molecule is disclosed through a displacement of signals from that of a reference material. Magnetic coupling between adjacent protons may complicate the spectrum in highly saturated compounds, but when this effect is minimal complete structural elucidation may become almost trivial. Certainly, this is the first tool to be used today when mg quantities of material are available in a reasonably pure state. When the structure proves to be exceedingly difficult, recourse may be made to X-ray crystallography by which the exact and complete position of every atom may often be ascertained. However, in order to employ this method the material must be isolated in crystalline form or converted to a crystalline derivative. With modern computational methods this process is not as difficult as in the past and there is every indication that it may even supercede all other methods for the structural analysis of crystalline compounds. If this is true, more attention will have to be paid to the fundamental problem of crystallizing drug metabolites.

At present, fractional mg quantities of material are required for nmr studies, but it now appears that pulse methods combined with Fourier transform analysis and computer signal averaging techniques may allow investigations to be carried out on μg quantities. The requirement for purity is high if a total analysis is to be performed, since all proton-bearing impurities are observed. For example, while a small quantity of hydrocarbon or butyl phthalate would not impair an ultraviolet analysis of an unsaturated steroid, it would excessively complicate its nmr spectrum.

For these reasons, structural information on submicrogram quantities of material has been obtained in the past primarily through indirect methods involving chemical reactions and chromatography. For example, a compound isolated from an ion exchange resin through the radioactivity of a given fraction is treated with a reagent capable of altering its acidic or basic nature, resulting in a change in its chromatographic behavior on the same resin. From the success or failure of this reaction, the presence or absence of a functional group such as an amine or phenol can be inferred.

Paper chromatography, gas chromatography, and thin-layer chromatography all have been key tools for such studies, along with Sephadex column, ion exchange resins and countercurrent chromatography (see also Chapter 31, this Volume). Gas chromatography (gc), while more limited in scope than the other techniques because of the requirement that the substance possess a finite vapor pressure at reasonable temperatures, is inherently a more powerful chromatographic technique since it conveys information reflecting the molecular weight. Thus the retention time allows for the presence of limited combinations of molecular weight and polarity, so that if polarity is known from other data (chromatographic tailing, solvent extractability, etc.), the molecular weight may be estimated. Again, conversion of substances at the submicrogram level with various reagents results in predictable shifts in retention time which often reveal structural features of a molecule. The basic principles involved with the use of gc in the assay of drugs has been covered in a previous chapter in this book (Chapter 27, this Volume). Some other basic references in this area are suggested: Ettre and Zlatkis (1967); McNair and Bonelli (1967). There are also available several references either in biological applications of gc or specific applications to pharmacology and toxicology: Alber (1969); Anders and Mannering (1967); Brochmann-Hanssen and Oke (1969); Dalgliesh et al. (1966); Gray (1961); Gudzinowicz (1967); Street (1969); Szymanski (1964); Woltz and Clark (1966).

The nature of pharmacological investigations is such that some knowledge of all of the above methods is essential today. Thus, μg and occasionally even mg amounts of material are available from drug metabolism studies because intact organisms are usually utilized. On the other hand, the material is often contaminated with other endogenous organic substances (see below) which make its isolation extremely difficult, time consuming, and attendant with many opportunities for loss of material. For example, Burtis and Warren (1968) using anion-exchange chromatography and other procedures identified 50 compounds in the urine of normal male subjects. Other workers have analyzed for these same substances by other methods: Dalgliesh et al. (1966) present a gas liquid chromatographic (glc) procedure which permits the separation and identification on the same chromatogram of a wide range of substances naturally occurring in urine or tissue extracts. Their procedure will detect organic compounds which are either free *or* conjugated. The method has proven satisfactory for fatty acids, carboxylic acids, hydroxy acids, keto acids, polyhydroxy compounds such as glycerol, aromatic compounds, steroids, glycine, mercapturic acids, and glucuronides. The procedure did not prove satisfactory for sulfate conjugates, imidazoles or polypeptides. The nature of all compounds was confirmed by the use of combined gc-mass spectroscopy. The authors provide data on about 100 such compounds.

The pharmacologist has an advantage in that he invariably knows the structure of the initial compound and expects only a limited number of biotransformations. In general, drug metabolites may be expected to be polar materials, at least more polar than the original drug, and appropriate measures can be taken to utilize this fact in their isolation. Drug metabolism usually involves very simple reactions such as introduction of oxygen at activated positions, dealkylation, oxidation and reduction, hydroxylation, etc. It is precisely in the investigation of such transformations that the mass spectrometer realizes its full potential. For example, the mass spectrometer easily identifies the addition of 16 mass units when a C-H bond is converted to a C-O-H linkage. Even the biotransformation of a secondary alcohol to a ketone resulting in loss of two mass units, is a trivial matter for any modern mass spectrometer. At a more sophisticated level, the high resolution mass spectrometer can allow distinction between the introduction of oxygen (15.9949) and CH_2+H_2 (16.0313). This very powerful technique is illustrated elsewhere in this volume (Chapter 34).

Concerning the requirement for purity, the presence of small amounts of material of grossly different molecular weight often does not interfere seriously with an ms analysis. Still, in order to be able to explain easily the full spectrum, it is distinctly advantageous to have confidence in the purity of a substance. Gas chromatography provides an ideal method for presenting the material to the spectrometer in a pure condition and it is the combination of these methods which is stressed here.

B. Operation of the Combined Gas Chromatograph-Mass Spectrometer

The following list of references include basic information regarding the practice and application of mass spectrometry: Beynon (1960); Beynon et al. (1968); Beynon and Williams (1963); Biemann (1962); Budzikiewicz et al. (1964, 1967); Duckworth (1953); Field and Franklin (1957); McLafferty (1963); McLafferty (1966); Silverstein and Bassler (1967); Stenhagen (1966); White (1968).

The essentials of a simple mass spectrometer system are outlined as follows: The sample, in the form of a vapor at very low pressures, is introduced to a small metal box (ion-chamber) through which a stream of electrons, produced by a heated filament, is passed. This electron stream collides with, or approaches close enough to, the vaporized sample molecules to cause an electron to be expelled from the sample by the force fields produced. As a result a positive ion is produced having the same molecular weight as the original species (less one electron). It may seem unusual to the reader that an electron is used as the bombarding particle to remove another electron. The reason for this is simply that they are convenient projectiles easily produced in large numbers by a heated filament.

Since it takes less energy to remove one electron from a bond than it does to completely break a bond, it might seem that the process could be stopped at this point providing electrons of just the minimum energy are employed. Then a series of positive ions representing the molecular weights of all compounds present in the vapor stream would be produced. This is in fact true, although because of the spread of energies of electrons coming from the hot filament, it is usually difficult to adjust the electron stream so that this condition occurs. In addition, this "threshold" energy varies for different substances, being low for aromatic, heteroatom containing species and high for simple hydrocarbons; thus the technique could be used to perform an accurate quantitative analysis only where all substances were very chemically similar. In actual practice the electron energy is maintained at a much higher level than that just required for ionization. The purpose of this is three-fold: 1) Reproducibility of the spectrum is more easily maintained. 2) Sensitivity is enhanced considerably through the action of more energetic electrons. 3) Fragmentation which results from the molecule being exposed to excessive electronic energy is often very helpful in structural elucidation (see below).

After ions corresponding to the molecular weight and fragmentation products of a molecule are produced in the ion chamber, they must be sorted according to mass and charge. In general, the problem of charge is less important since at the energies commonly used (about 70 electron volts) the majority of species are +1 in charge. Negative ions are also present and may be studied by reversing the polarity of the system, but little information has appeared on their use. Compounds which can more easily accommodate the presence of two positive charges (*e.g.*, aromatic hydrocarbons, amines, etc.) may display a considerable number of such ions in their spectrum. Structurally, their main use has been in disclosing the presence of such systems and in identifying a parent ion at $^1/_2$ of its apparent mass (see below).

After the ions have been produced, they are sorted according to their mass to charge (M/e) ratio by subjecting them to an electrostatic field which causes them to be propelled out of the ion chamber under the influence of a high voltage (2—8 KV). Then the rapidly moving particles (ions) are passed through a magnetic field where they are deflected to a degree that is inversely proportional to their mass and directly proportionally to their charge. This produces a fan of ion trajectories which may be allowed to impinge upon a photographic plate for their detection as a series of lines which are simply images of the original defining slit. Alternatively, electrical scanning of the electromagnetic field allows this series of ions to pass over a detector located at a fixed position. This detector, essentially the same sort of photomultiplier used in ultraviolet spectrophotometers, amplifies the signal which is then amplified further and finally displayed on an oscillographic light-beam recorder whose speed is some multiple of the magnetic scanning speed. The spectrum then appears as a series of peaks whose height is proportional to the number of ions produced and collected at a given mass. A magnet is not the only means by which ions may be separated; in another instrument attaining newfound popularity the ions are accelarated at a relatively low voltage and allowed to pass through a region where they are subjected to a combination of electrostatic and radiofrequency (RF) fields. The ions then travel in a cork-screw path. For a given value of the aforementioned field, ions of only one M/e ration will travel along a path of constant radius; all others will diverge and not be collected at the detector. This instrument, called the quadropole mass spectrometer, has certain advantages as well as disadvantages compared with magnetic instruments. For example, while its mass range tends to be more limited (around 400) it can produce a display of ions that is essentially linear in respect to M/e ratio. Furthermore, high voltage and hysteresis problems commonly encountered with magnetic instruments are avoided. Still another instrument operates in a pulsed mode and the flight time of the ions, which can be related to their mass, is indirectly measured. The time-of-flight mass spectrometers are capable of extraordinarily fast spectral measurements (~10,000 scans/sec) and are very useful in studying fast reactions. Their mass range, resolution and peak height accuracy is somewhat limited, however, and they are comparatively seldom used in the identification of metabolites.

One of the most striking features of mass spectra contrasted with other types of spectra is the use of recorder systems possessing 3 pens, resulting in 3 simultaneous displays of the signal at amplification factors of 1, 10, and 1000. Few other analytical instruments can boast of such a wide dynamic range (about 10^6). This wide range is useful since the production of ions within the source itself may vary over a similar range. In point of fact, a very weak peak in the high mass region of the spectrum often carries more important information than very intense peaks at lower masses.

Because of the rapid response of the multiplier, the whole mass spectrum may be scanned within a time period of 0.1—3 sec. This is particularly important when the spectrometer is coupled to a gas chromatograph where the peaks may elute in rapid succession.

It is obvious that during their trajectory through the mass spectrometer the ions must encounter no other molecules; other wise collisions will result through which the ions may be scattered. To prevent this the ms system is evacuated with a combination of high speed diffusion and roughing pumps whose main purpose is to lower the pressure to about 10^{-6} mm Hg. Under these conditions the mean free path for a molecule or an ion is of the order of meters and collisions are very infrequent. In the past, it was common practice to admit samples to the ion chamber in the form of pure gases at low pressures. Little attention was paid to the problems inherent in vaporizing compounds of higher molecular weights and greater polarity. The first breakthrough came when it was discovered that small amounts of solid or liquid material might be placed on the tip of a probe which was inserted directly into the ion-chamber itself. Under these conditions, heating the sample produced vapor directly adjacent to the electron beam so that it was no longer necessary to conduct samples through the tortuous path from an externally heated vaporization chamber. This system produced a noticeable improvement in the quality of the spectrum since sensitive materials now were not decomposed by hot chamber walls. Sensitivity also was enhanced since it was not necessary to fill the external chamber with vapor to a pressure of $\sim$1 mm Hg. Due to the probe system the spectra of very thermolabile organic materials are today obtainable at the lowest possible temperatures. This system, in fact, has been responsible, probably more than any other single development, for the rapid increase in applications to biological problems. However it must be emphasized that the probe system is poorly suited to the investigation of mixtures since it is essentially a fractional distillation assembly of one theoretical plate. Nonetheless careful perusal of successive scans during the lifetime of the sample may enable an experienced user to acquire some information regarding the components of a sample.

Since the output of a gas chromatograph consists of the vapor of a compound mixed with the vapor of the carrier gas, this apparatus especially lends itself to mass spectrometry. The mass spectrum of a carrier gas of low molecular weight would not, of itself, be a problem, but the pressure (about 1 atmosphere) at the effluent end of the gas chromatograph presents great difficulties. As was mentioned previously the ms requires pressures no larger than 10^{-6} mm Hg within the ionization chamber, a factor of $\sim 10^{-7}$ less than that of the gc eluate. One solution to this problem consists in splitting the effluent of the column with a simple T-connector, leading only a very small portion of the flow into the ionization region. The diffusion pumps attached to the ionization chamber may now be able to handle the relatively small volume of carrier gas. Unfortunately, this approach necessarily means that a correspondingly small amount of sample will be introduced. Some instrument manufacturers, even today, recommend this approach, maintaining that the sensitivity of the ion multiplier makes up for any loss so incurred. However, increased sensitivity of the detection system can only be carried to certain limits: although the photomultiplier is capable of observing even a single ion, enough ions must be present at a given M/e value to register a statistically significant signal. This is a very real problem when rapid scans are required, as is the case in gas chromatography where a peak may elute within a few seconds. For this reason some sort of device is desirable to separate the carrier gas from the sample. At the present time separators have several forms, all varying somewhat in effectiveness. The first design, proposed by Ryhage (1964), is simply a series of jets enclosed by a tube through which the carrier gas is forced to flow in its travel from the gc to the ionization chamber. For example, helium is often used as a carrier gas and, owing to its higher rate of diffusion, it moves to the outer circumference of the jet stream where it is pumped away. Because of the severe drop in pressure, the time during which the samples are exposed to the stainless steel walls of the jet is very short; in fact the jet stream must be travelling at supersonic speeds. The LKB-9000 mass spectrometer provides such a system. Ideally, a line-of-sight condition would be provided between the gc outlet tube and the ionization region but, to date, it has been necessary to add a valve at the separator end in order to allow the solvent front to be by-passed so as to prevent harm to the ion chamber and filament.

The LKB-Ryhage separator consists of two stages form aximum efficiency and the transmission of sample to the spectrometer is about 50—70%, unless the molecular weight is extremely low. In our experience, this system has proved extremely effective, especially when it is necessary to study samples of high molecular weight and complexity. Of course, it might not be as useful where one wished to study low molecular weight gases evolved by micro-organisms or metabolism of volatile anaesthetics.

In general, spectra obtained via the separator in gas liquid chromatographic systems show no more evidence of thermal decomposition than those obtained via the direct insertion probe referred to above. We have yet to observe a case wherein a peak was observed on a standard gc apparatus using an all-glass column which did not also provide a mass spectrum of usable quality after passing through the separator. Furthermore, this type of separator appears to contribute very little to the tailing or diffusion of one peak into another and the gc resolution is undiminished. In day-to-day operation we have found it necessary to maintain a relatively high ion-chamber temperature (about 300°C) and as a result the thermal degradation encountered is somewhat greater than that obtained under ideal conditions. The high temperature is required to achieve rapid elimination of the sample from the ion chamber and thus to achieve an "instantaneous view" of the eluate from the gas chromatographic column.

Much of the biologically oriented gc-ms literature appears to have resulted from the use of the Becker-Ryhage system, attesting to its success. Nonetheless, other separators are available. One used on a wide variety of mass spectrometers was designed by Biemann and Watson (1965). This device also utilizes preferential diffusion of helium and consists simply of a porous glass or ceramic tube through which the effluent is passed. The porous tube is encased in an outer tube which is open to a pump for removal of the helium as it diffuses through the inner tube. This system is relatively simple to construct and may be adopted to the inlet system of a wide variety of spectrometers. Unfortunately, the glass surfaces appear to catalyze reactions and therefore the destruction of many polar organic compounds and dehydration and irreversible adsorption are often encountered. The extent to which these effects occur seems to be extremely variable and an investigator who spends some effort properly adjusting the flow rate and temperature may be able to achieve quite satisfactory results.

A third system designed by LLEWELYN and LITTLEJOHN (1966) is the most simple device of all. A stretched thin silicone rubber disk is placed over a supporting glass frit heated to a given temperature. Under these conditions organic compounds, but not helium, are soluble in the membrane and pass through to the other side which is open to the ion chamber. Thus, the effluent from a gas chromatograph need only pass over the membrane in order to observe a signal as the sample diffuses through. As in the case of the Biemann separator, varying results have been reported with this device, but in most cases peak tailing appears to be relatively pronounced and it seems that some loss in quality of the gas chromatogram may be expected. Other modifications of these systems have been reviewed (DEJONGH, 1970).

A whole new approach has been proposed based on recent developments in chemical ionization mass spectroscopy (ci-ms) (FIELD, 1968; FALES et al., 1969) where an electron beam is passed through a relatively high pressure of a reagent gas such as methane (CH_4), under the action of electron bombardment at pressures of about 1 mm Hg, and is converted to ions such as CH_5^+ and $C_2H_5^+$. These ions undergo secondary collisions with the sample which is added to the methane at very low concentrations in a direct insertion probe. Upon collision, a proton is transferred from these methane-derived ions to the compound being studied and a new ion appears with a molecular weight of one mass unit more than that originally possessed by the molecule. Due to the excess energy contained in CH_5^+ and $C_2H_5^+$, the resulting protonated substance may also undergo fragmentation, although it is invariably less than that encountered in electron bombardment at 70 e.v. These factors tend to make ci-ms particularly valuable in studies of basic, electron rich molecules which can easily accommodate a proton. Most drugs fall into this category and this technique should be especially useful. Furthermore, in ci-ms a fairly large fraction of the effluent of a gas chromatographic column may be led directly into the ion source of a mass spectrometer. A commercial instrument for ci-ms has been produced by the Finnigan Corporation (Palo Alto, California) and Scientific Research Industries (Baltimore, Maryland). This instrument utilizes a quadropole ms which, incidentally, is especially suited for ci methods since it employs a low accelerating voltage. A separator is not necessary here, although an ideal system would undoubtedly include one so that the apparatus might be used in the usual electron impact (ei) mode as well.

C. Mass Spectral Fragmentation Processes

Many excellent references are available covering the details of the fragmentation processes observed under electron impact (BEYNON, 1960; BIEMANN, 1962; BUDZIKIEWICZ et al., 1964; FIELD and FRANKLIN, 1957; MCLAFFERTY, 1963, 1966; SILVERSTEIN, 1967; and STENHAGEN, 1966), and this subject will not be covered in detail here. However, a few simple rules will be mentioned since they pertain especially to molecules likely to be encountered in drug metabolism studies.

The first question concerns whether or not a molecular ion (molecule less one electron) will appear in the mass spectrum. This ion is by definition a free radical and therefore has a certain instability. It has been formed by rather high energy electronic processes and so contains considerable energy at the moment of its formation. This energy may be dissipated by electronic and vibrational processes in the molecule itself or it may concentrate in a bond causing the molecule to fragment. Less fragmentation will be observed when the molecule possesses a greater number of bonds, and so unsaturated systems invariably show more intense molecular ions than do saturated ones. Furthermore, if the molecule contains a ring structure, *two* bonds must be broken for fragmentation to occur. Thus, highly aromatic unsaturated ring compounds are inclined to show very large molecular ions. The presence of heteroatoms (N,O,S, etc.) in such ring systems also increases the intensity of the molecular ion by providing stable locations for the positive charge. The presence of heteroatoms in saturated systems, on the other hand, actually lowers the intensity of the molecular ion and it is often missing altogether. In such a case, the most intense peak is usually the one containing the heteroatom and an adjacent carbon atom, cleavage having occurred with concomittant charge stabilization;

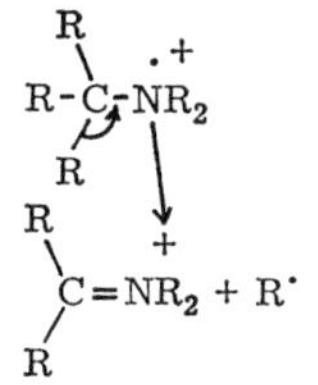

When this occurs the structure must be reconstructed from this information alone. One often sees the use of low voltage electrons (7—10 ev) recommended for the identification of a molecular ion in mass spectrometry; however it must be remembered that this technique causes *all* peaks in the spectrum to diminish in intensity and it is only the fact that the molecular ion diminishes *less rapidly* than the fragmentation peaks that makes the technique useful. If no parent ion is present at high electron voltages, none will be present at low voltages. An alternative method that is often very helpful is to insert an extremely large amount of sample, either by gc or by a direct insertion probe, into the ion chamber which thereby acquires a pressure approaching that encountered in the chemical ionization method. Under these conditions the compound itself serves as a protonating agent and a peak may appear at mol. wt. +1.

When uncertainty exists regarding the identity of a molecular ion, it may be useful to remember that ions formed by simple cleavage of the molecular ion contain an even number of electrons. Simple valence considerations then, show that when a compound has an odd number of nitrogen atoms the molecular ion will also be odd, and its fragments containing nitrogen will be even in mass. Similarly, fragment ions not containing nitrogen will be odd in mass regardless of their parent ions. Analysis of the spectrum becomes more complicated when a molecule contains three nitrogens rather than one but the same principles apply.

Rearrangement processes lead to opposite rules and unfortunately these occur with disconcerting regularity in electron impact spectroscopy. In some cases however, they can be easily identified and utilized for structural information. For example, loss of water would be expected whenever the molecule contains a hydroxyl group. The hydrogen which combines with the hydroxyl group need not be located on the adjacent carbon atom however. Carbonyl groups may also trigger loss of water. The presence of hydrogen in a position γ to the carbonyl group, wherein a six member transition state can be envisioned, facilitates cleavage and proton transfer: The event is responsible for the base peak (largest peak in the spectrum) in saturated esters and is known as the McLafferty rearrangement:

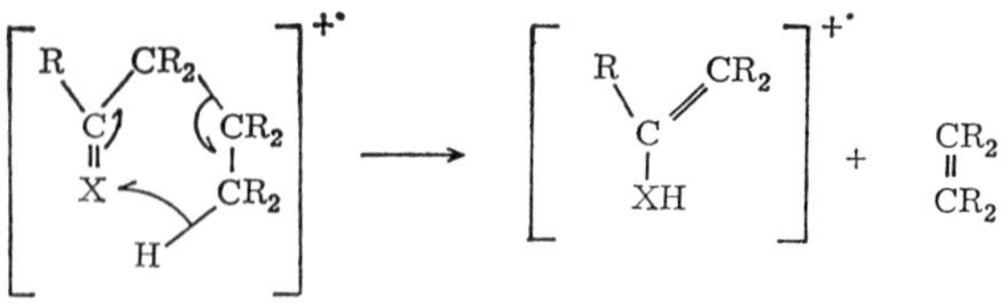

Loss of other small neutral molecules such as CO, CO_2, H_2S, SO_2, NO, NO_2, etc. is also common and the overall process somewhat resembles pyrolysis. Methoxyl groups are often lost as methanol and loss of 32 mass units is relatively diagnostic for this group. The loss of 15 mass units suggests a methyl group, although this occurs by rearrangement even in the case of benzene. Metastable ions are present in the spectrum where they appear as broad peaks at lower masses. They are evidence of a transition occurring between two ions of moderate intensity and their mass obeys the relationship: mass metastable $= \frac{M^2 \text{ fragment}}{M \text{ precursor}}$. However these ions do not imply that the species lost in the fragmentation has a single, simple structure. For example, many steroids lose the elements of CH_5O, which arises from the very rapid sequential loss of CH_3 and H_2O (SEIBL, 1968).

Carbon atoms which contain four substituents frequently undergo fragmentation owing to stabilization of the charge by the resulting tertiary carbonium ion. For the same reason, cleavage at allyl or benzyl carbon atoms is facilitated since the resulting carbonium ions contain an easily delocalized charge. In this sense, a double bond or aromatic ring can be considered to be electronically equivalent to a heteroatom.

The presence of isotopes is extremely simple to observe in mass spectrometry, especially when the natural abundances of the isotopes are comparable. Thus, the presence of chlorine which contains three times as much ^{35}Cl as ^{37}Cl is easily observed and this element provides an internal tag assuring the investigator that he is not dealing with an artifact whose fragmentation pattern might otherwise fortuitously resemble that of the drug. Simple observation of the molecule ions, or even of fragmentation ions, enables one to count the number of such heteroatoms through their characteristic pattern. For example, a molecule containing one chlorine atom (^{37}Cl), 25%; (^{35}Cl), 75%; would appear as a set of 4 lines, the minor satellites being due to the naturally occurring 1% ^{13}C.

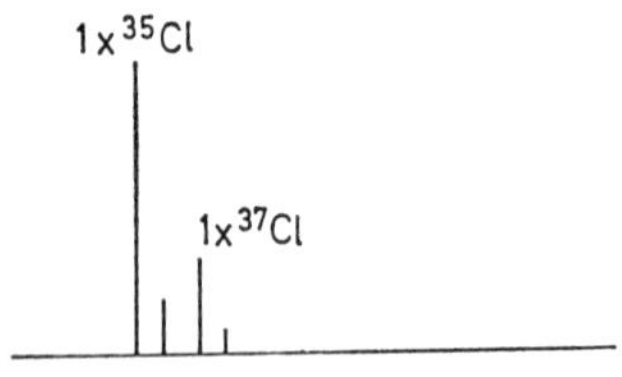

A compound containing chlorine atoms will present a more complex pattern:

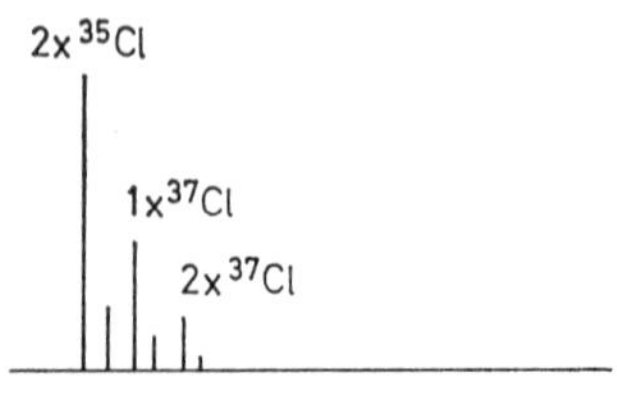

For the same reason, since there exists in nature approximately 1% ^{13}C, doublets separated by 1 mass unit can be expected for each ionic species including the molecular ion. The ratio of the intensity of the higher mass member of the doublet (Im+1) to the intensity of the lower (Im) times 100 gives directly a rough estimate of the number of carbon atoms present in the ion: i.e., ethane shows $\frac{I_{31}}{I_{30}} = 2\%$ while methane shows $\frac{I_{17}}{I_{16}} = 1\%$. Such use of relative isotope abundances to determine the chemical formula of an unknown has often been recommended, but the technique is less effective with heterocyclic or unsaturated molecules because of their tendency to acquire a proton by ion-molecule reactions, leading to an excessively high value for this ratio.

Rearrangement reactions under electron impact can be extensive and a very cautious approach must be taken toward the interpretation of such ions. Some extreme examples of this phenomenon have been observed in the case of the oft-used silyl ether derivatives. While these adducts are very useful in aiding the volatilization of a hydroxylic compound, the silyl group tends to migrate extensively and also participates in a variety of somewhat poorly defined fragmentation processes. For this reason we have always preferred methyl ethers whenever they can be prepared through simple addition of methanolic diazomethane, as is the case with phenols, carboxylic acids, imides, etc. Furthermore, methyl ethers can be easily obtained in deuterated form simply by allowing the diazomethane in ether to stir in contact with alkaline D_2O for a few minutes. The decanted diazomethane in ether is ready for use immediately and results in the incorporation of three deuterium atoms (CD_3), at all affected positions, presumably via prior exchange of the OH group. Where simple hydroxyl groups are present, recourse must be made to silyl ethers prepared with hexamethyldisilazane and trimethylchlorosilane or one of the newer silylation reagents (BSA, BTSFA, etc.), Pierce Chemical Co. (Rockford, Illinois). Alternatively, acetylation with pyridine and acetic anhydride may be employed. Both silylation and acetylation reagents are also available in deuterated forms.

D. Applications of Mass Spectrometry to the Problem of Identifying Drug Metabolites

In this section we will be using the term "drug" in its broadest sense, thus including any chemical which produces an effect on a living organism. In a recent report prepared by the National Academy of Sciences entitled "Application of Metabolic Data to the Evaluation of Drugs", it was pointed out that the amount of metabolic data required concerning a drug depends on its type, the stage of its development and its intended clinical use. This report also points out that high priority should be given to research on the application of glc, ms, nmr, and other physico-chemical techniques in studies of drug metabolism. Of these techniques, mass spectrometry stands out not only because of its ability to provide information on the structure of very small quantities of a metabolite, but also because structures can often be proposed in the absence of reference compounds. In studies of drug metabolism, one must of course differentiate between recovered parent compound and possible metabolites, and therefore early mass spectral studies involved the identification of drugs prior to their administration. Also, a knowledge of the fragmentation pathways of a given drug may be very useful in suggesting structures for its metabolite. For example, Grützmacher and Arnold (1966) provided one of the first reports concerning mass spectrometry of various barbiturates. A similar report was published by Coutts and Locock (1968). Mass

Table 1. *Classes of compounds and/or metabolites of interest to pharmacologists which have been studied by mass spectrometry*

Class	*Parent Compounds Studied*	*Biotransformation Studied*	*References*
Analgesics and Antipyretics	Aspirin	Conjugation with glycine	EMERY (1960); SCOTT et al. (1968); HORNING (1969)
	Phenacetin	O-dealkylation followed by: Ring hydroxylation followed by: Conjugation by transmethylation	BURTIS et al. (1970)
	Pyramidon	N-dealkylation followed by: Conjugation by acetylation	ARNOLD and GRÜTZMACHER (1969)
Alkaloids	Many alkaloids	—	BUDZIKIEWICZ et al. (1964)
	Morphine, Codeine, Heroin	—	AUDIER et al. (1965)
	Codeine	—	FALES et al. (1969)
	Physostigmine	—	FALES et al. (1969)
Sedatives and Hypnotics	Many barbiturates	—	COUTTS and LOCOCK (1968, 1969)
			GRÜTZMACHER and ARNOLD (1966)
		Hydroxylation of alkyl side chain	ARNOLD and GRÜTZMACHER (1969)
			PALMER et al. (1969)
	Phenobarbital	Hydroxylation of aromatic ring	HORNING et al. (1969)
	Hexobarbital	Hydroxylation of alicyclic ring followed by: Oxidation to alicyclic ketone	ARNOLD and GRÜTZMACHER (1969)
	Pentobarbital	Hydroxylation of alkyl side chain Oxidation to carboxylic acid	PALMER et al. (1969)
	Noludar	Hydroxylation of alicyclic ring	ARNOLD and GRÜTZMACHER (1969)
	Ethanol	Conjugation of hydroxy group with glucuronic acid	JAAKONMAKI et al. (1967)
Stimulants	Amphetamine	—	BECKETT et al. (1967)
	Methyl amphetamine	—	BECKETT et al. (1967); REISCH et al. (1968)
Catecholamines	Phenethylamines	—	REISCH et al. (1968)
	Epinephrine	Conjugation by transmethylation	ÄNGGÅRD and SEDVALL (1969)
	Norepinephrine	Conjugation by transmethylation	ÄNGGÅRD and SEDVALL (1969)
	Dopamine	Conjugation by transmethylation	ÄNGGÅRD and SEDVALL (1969)
	Epinephrine	Oxidative deamination to carboxylic acid	ÄNGGÅRD and SEDVALL (1969)

Table 1 (continued)

Class	Parent Compounds Studied	Biotransformation Studied	References
	Norepinephrine	Oxidative deamination to carboxylic acid	ÄNGGÅRD and SEDVALL (1969); REISCH et al. (1968)
	Dopamine	Oxidative deamination to carboxylic acid	ÄNGGÅRD and SEDVALL (1969); REISCH et al. (1968)
	3,4-dimethoxyphenethylamine	—	CREVELING and DALY (1967)
	3,4-dimethoxyphenylacetic acid	—	KUEHL et al. (1966)
Tranquilizers			
Phenothiazines	Many phenothiazines		DUFFIELD et al. (1968); GILBERT and MILLARD (1969)
	Chlorpromazine	Oxidative deamination to carboxylic acid	HAMMAR et al. (1968)
	Thiazesin	Hydroxylation of aromatic ring	DREYFUSS et al. (1968)
Benzodiazepines	Chlorodiazepoxide (Librium)	Reduction of N-oxide	SCHWARTZ et al. (1968a)
		N-dealkylation	SCHWARTZ et al. (1968a)
		Hydroxylation of aromatic ring	SCHWARTZ et al. (1968a)
		Oxidative deamination to heterocyclic ketone	SCHWARTZ et al. (1968a)
	Diazepam (Valium)	N-dealkylation	SCHWARTZ et al. (1967)
		Hydroxylation of aromatic ring	
		Hydroxylation on heterocyclic ring ($CH_2 \rightarrow CHOH$)	
	Flurazepam (Dalmane)	N- di-dealkylation	SCHWARTZ et al. (1968b)
		Hydroxylation of aromatic ring	SCHWARTZ et al. (1968b)
		Oxidative deamination of ethylamino side chain to primary alcohol followed by:	SCHWARTZ et al. (1968b)
		N-dealkylation of heterocyclic nitrogen	
Hallucinogens	LSD	—	BELLMAN (1968)
	Dimethyltryptamine	—	BUDZIKIEWICZ et al. (1964)
	Tetrahydrocannabinol	Hydroxylation of alkyl side chain	NILSSON et al. (1970)
	Tetrahydrocannabinol analogs	—	VON SPULAK et al. (1968)
	Phencyclidine	—	LINDGREN et al. (1969)

Table 1. (continued)

Class	*Parent Compounds Studied*	*Biotransformation Studied*	*References*
Antibiotics	Tetracyclines	—	HOFFMAN (1966)
	Griseofulvin	—	BALLANTINE and FENWICK (1969)
Hormones and Steroids	Many steroids	—	FRIEDLAND et al. (1959); BUDZIKIEWICZ and DJERASSI (1962)
	Stigmasterol	Reduction of ethylenic chain	ENEROTH et al. (1965)
	Estriol	—	LUUKKAINEN and ADLERCREUTZ (1967)
	Stilbesterol-hexestrol	—	ADLERCREUTZ et al. (1967)
	Prostaglandin F_2d	Oxidation of secondary alcohol to ketone	GRANSTROM and SAMUELSSON (1969)
		Reduction of Δ^{13} ethylene bond	GRANSTROM and SAMUELSSON (1969)
Vitamins	B_6 and antimetabolites	Oxidation of primary alcohol to aldehyde	DEJONGH et al. (1968)
		Conjugation of alcohol to phosphate	DEJONGH et al. (1968)
		Oxidation of aldehyde to carboxylic acid	DEJONGH et al. (1968)
		Hydroxylation of side chain to alcohol	DEJONGH et al. (1968)
	D_2	Hydroxylation of side chain to alcohol	DEJONGH et al. (1968)

spectral studies of several parent drug molecules and metabolites are listed in Table 1. Other compounds that either are drugs or resemble drugs and have been studied by ms methods appear in Tables 2 and 3.

Surprisingly, there are relatively few examples in the literature of the use of combined gc-ms in drug metabolite studies. This is true in spite of the fact that the necessary equipment is known to be available to many of the more prominent drug houses. It can only be assumed that this is due to the proprietary nature of this information and it is hoped that these groups will see fit to publish more results in the near future.

It is not absolutely necessary that gc be combined directly with ms; samples can be collected at the end of the gc column just as in liquid chromatography. We have also resorted to such techniques in order to collect sufficient material for nmr. Surprisingly, a real difficulty may be encountered with *higher* molecular weight materials since they tend to form aerosols upon being suddenly cooled at the column outlet. We have found (FALES et al., 1962) that when argon is employed as a carrier gas it can be condensed by liquid nitrogen in an open U tube as it exits from the column. In so doing, the condensing vapor phase appears to prevent aerosol formation and nearly quantitative collection becomes possible.

1. Ethanol

JAAKONMAKI et al. (1967) proved how effective the above method could be in a study of

Table 2. *Pesticides which have been studied by mass spectrometry*

Parent Compounds Studied	*Biotransformation Studied*	*References*
Many chlorinated hydrocarbons	—	JORG et al. (1966); DAMICO and BARRON (1968)
Banol	Conjugation of ring hydroxyl with glucuronic acid	FRIEDMAN and LEMIN (1967)
Bromacil	Hydroxylation of alkyl side chain to primary alcohol	GARDINER et al. (1969)
	Hydroxylation of alkyl side chain to secondary alcohol	GARDINER et al. (1969)
	Reductive dehalogenation	GARDINER et al. (1969)
2,4-D	—	JORG et al. (1966)
DDT	Dehydrohalogenation to DDE	PLIMMER et al. (1968); BIROS and WALKER (1970)
	Reductive dehalogenation to DDD	PLIMMER et al. (1968)
Dicamba	Hydroxylation of aromatic ring	BROADHURST et al. (1966)
	Demethoxylation	BROADHURST et al. (1966)
Dieldrin (Aldrin epoxide)	—	BIROS and WALKER (1970); DAMICO et al. (1968)
Heptachlor epoxide	—	DAMICO et al. (1968)
Lindane	—	DAMICO et al. (1968)
	Dehydrohalogenation	REED and FORGASH (1968)
Malathion	—	JORG et al. (1966)
Polychlorinated biphenyls	—	BAGLEY et al. (1970)
Rotenone	Hydroxylation of heterocyclic ring	FUKAMI et al. (1967)
	Oxidation of ethylenic side chain to primary alcohol	FUKAMI et al. (1967)
Siduron	Hydroxylation of aromatic ring	BELASCO et al. (1969)
	Hydroxylation of alicyclic ring	BELASCO et al. (1969)
Terbacil	Hydroxylation of side chain to primary alcohol followed by:	RHODES et al. (1969)
	Oxidation to acid	RHODES et al. (1969)
	Reductive dehalogenation	RHODES et al. (1969)

Table 3. *Miscellaneous drug or drug related compounds that have been studied by mass spectrometry*

Parent Compounds Studied	*Biotransformation Studied*	*References*
Acetylcholine	—	HAMMAR et al. (1968)
Allopurinol	Oxidation of heterocyclic ring to ketone (oxipurinol)	CHALMERS et al. (1969)
Anthranilate diuretics	N-demethylation followed by:	SMITH and GROSTIC (1967)
	Cyclization to diazepinone	
Azobicycloalkanes	Hydroxylation of alicyclic ring	JOHNSON et al. (1968)
Chloropheniramine	N-mono and di-demethylation	KABASAKALIAN et al. (1968)
Cyclopiazonic acid (like lysergamide)	—	HOLZAPFEL (1968)
Ephedrine	—	FALES et al. (1970); REISCH et al. (1968)
Esters	—	EMERY (1960)
Guanidines, N-substituted	—	BEYNON et al. (1968)
Halo acetates and benzoates	Oxidative dehalogenation to hydroxy compound (mechanism)	GOLDMAN et al. (1968); MILNE et al. (1968)
Hydrocarbons	—	STENHAGEN (1966)
Hydroxylamines, aromatic	—	COUTTS and MUKERJEE (1970)
Hypoxanthine	—	CHALMERS et al. (1969)
Isoprene	—	JANSSON and LARSSON (1969)
Limonene	Oxidation of ethylenic side chain to tertiary alcohol	WADE et al. (1966)
	Oxidation of alkyl side chain to primary alcohol	WADE et al. (1966)
Naphthaline	Hydroxylation of aromatic ring (mechanism)	HOLTZMAN et al. (1967)
Nucleosides	—	BIEMANN and MCCLOSKEY (1962)
Oxoquinazolines	—	BOGENTOFT and DANIELSSON (1969)
Phytanic acid	α-Oxidation of side chain	MIZE et al. (1969)
Probenecid	Hydroxylation of alkyl side chain to primary alcohol followed by:	GUARINO et al. (1969)
	Oxidation to carboxylic acid	GUARINO et al. (1969)
	Hydroxylation of alkyl side chain to secondary alcohol	GUARINO et al. (1969)
	N-depropylation	GUARINO et al. (1969)
Pteridine diuretic	O-demethylation of aliphatic ether side chain	SISENWINE and WALKENSTEIN (1969)
Quinine	—	FALES et al. (1970)
Quinidine	Oxidation of ring to ketone	PALMER et al. (1969)
Quinoline hydroxamic acid	—	COUTTS and HINDMARSH (1969)
Stilbene	Hydroxylation of aromatic ring	SINSHEIMER and SMITH (1968)
	Reduction of ethylenic bond to alkane	SINSHEIMER and SMITH (1968)
Tremorine	Oxidation of heterocyclic ring to ketone	KARLEN and BOGENTOFT (1969)
Triprolidine	Oxidation of alkyl side chain to primary alcohol followed by:	KUNTZMAN et al. (1968)
	Oxidation to carboxylic acid	KUNTZMAN et al. (1968)
Xanthine	—	CHALMERS et al. (1969)

the metabolism of ethanol in rats and man. The urinary acidic and neutral fractions were first extracted with ethyl acetate, and then the acids were collected by ion exchange on DEAE-Sephadex, treated with diazomethane to convert RCOOH to RCOOME, and finally silylated with hexamethyldisilazane-trimethylchlorosilane to protect any hydroxyl groups present. Under these conditions, the authors were able to identify a peak as ethyl β-D-glucosiduronic acid which was found to elute near the eicosane internal standard.

The authors first compared the retention time with authentic material which was synthesized. In order to confirm that the peak was indeed the metabolite, material was collected at the column end as described above and injected into the mass spectrograph by means of the direct insertion probe. Its mass spectral fragmentation pattern was compared to that of authentic material. In this case, the mass spectrum was used only as a fingerprint; in fact the nature of the two largest peaks at M/e 204 and 217 was not discussed. Presumably they are due to the species

$(CH_2OTmSi)_2$ (M/e 204) and

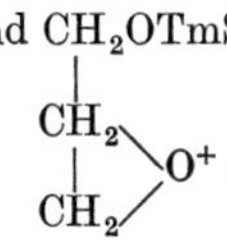

± TmSi (M/e 217)

split out from the middle of the glucuronic acid chain. This guess is based on the fact that both ions appear to contain two silicone atoms as judged by the height of the peaks at M/e 206 and 219 which are largely due to the presence of the ^{30}Si isotope (~3.1 natural abundance). In fact, by itself the mass spectrum would not have shed much light on the nature of the metabolite unless one was willing to place a great deal of confidence in the origin of the peak representing loss of 15 mass units from the molecular ion. Here, and in many other studies, structural analysis *via* details of the mass spectrum was fortunately not required.

2. Aspirin

While not dealing with the *metabolism* of aspirin and aspirin-like compounds, Scott et al. (1968) show how substitution on the aromatic ring, which might be expected from metabolism, can greatly affect the mass spectrum. Using rules derived from studies of unsubstituted salicylic acids, *e.g.*, Fig. 1, these authors were able to rationalize the fragmentation pattern of the more complicated 3-amino-5-iodo derivatives (Fig. 2). In particular, they noticed the predominance of processes involving the loss of small molecules (methanol, water, etc.) from *ortho* substituents compared to more usual processes such as loss of NO and NO_2 from nitro substituents.

3. Phenacetin

Normally, the 3-methoxy metabolite of phenacetin is not observed but Burtis et al. (1970) employed uv, ir and ms spectral analysis to show the presence of this metabolite in the urine of a patient with a neuroblastoma. After treatment of a patient with 10 g of the drug, a urine sample was subjected to a high pressure anionic exchange separation using Dowex 1-X 8. The collected fractions were lyophilized, dissolved in methanol, and subjected to the aforementioned spectral analysis. The mass spectra of phenacetin (4-ethoxyacetanilide), 4-hydroxy-acetanilide (HA) and 3-methoxy-4-hydroxyacetanalide (MHA) showed strong molecular ion peaks (M/e 179, 151, 181), and each exhibited a loss of 42 mass units. Loss of the elements of ketene results from rearrangement of a proton of the acetyl group to the benzene ring, followed by cleavage at the amide bond. By analogy with the altered metabolism of catecholamines known to occur in patients

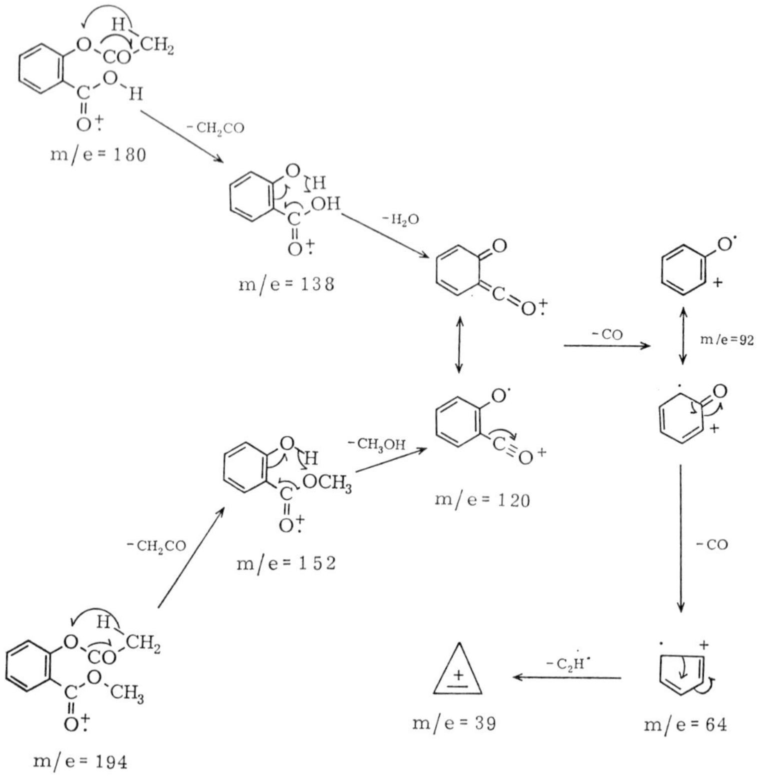

Fig. 1. Fragmentation pathways of aspirin. Reprinted with permission of SCOTT et al., 1968 and Heyden and Son, Ltd., London

with neuroblastoma, the authors argue that MHA arises from the hydroxylation and methylation of HA by the same enzymes responsible for the conversion of epinephrine to 3-methoxy-4-hydroxymandelic acid according to the following scheme:

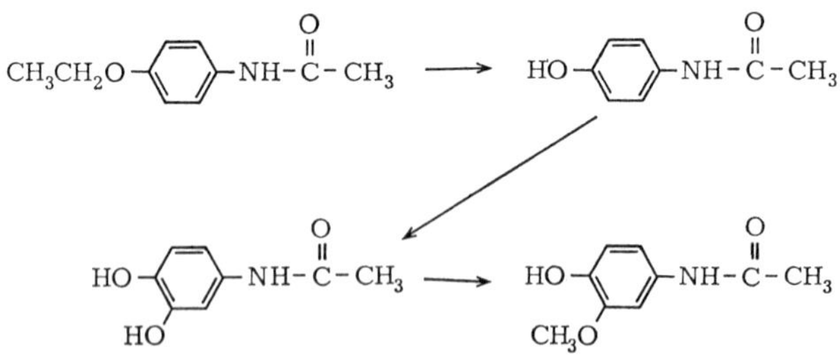

4. Tremorine

In another case concerning the metabolism of tremorine (I),

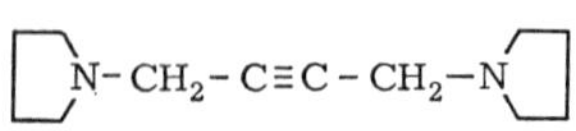

I

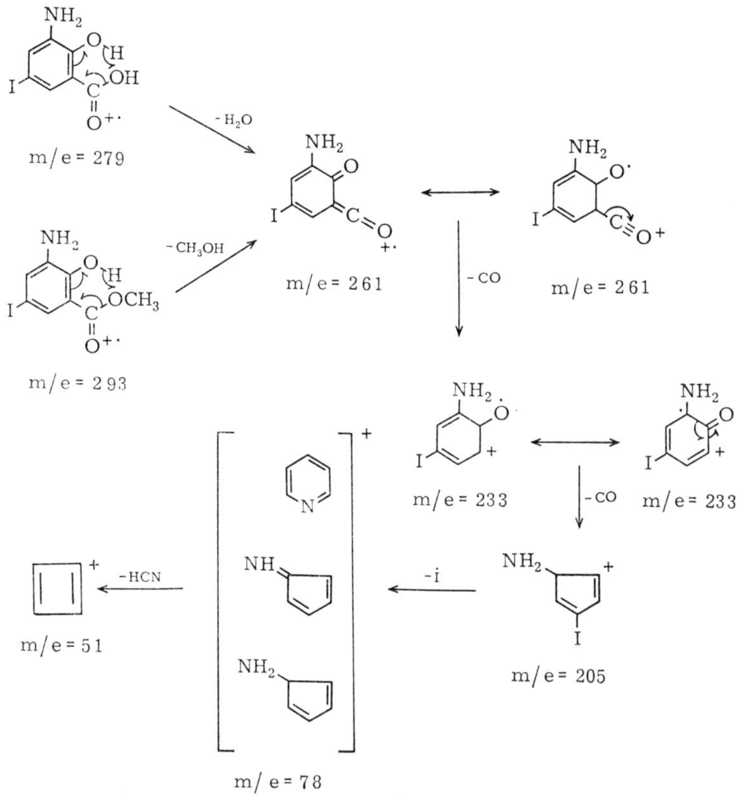

Fig. 2. Fragmentation pathways of 2-hydroxy-3-amino-5-iodobenzoic acid and 2-acetoxy-3-amino-5-iodobenzoic acid. Reprinted with permission of SCOTT et al., 1968 and Heyden and Son Ltd., London

an extensive mass spectral study of the original drug and its chemically prepared derivatives was conducted (KARLEN and BOGENTOFT, 1969). These authors noted that increasing heteroatom content in the form of oxygens adjacent to the nitrogen atom (II) enormously increased the intensity of the parent ion which was

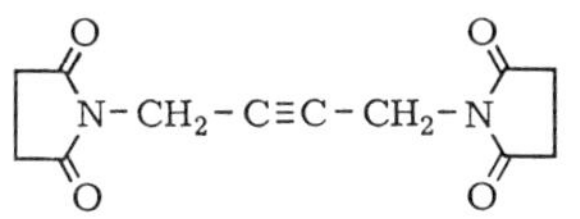

II

barely detectible with tremorine itself. This was perhaps to be expected, both due to the increased heteroatom (oxygen) content and due to suppression of hydrogen rearrangement to the pyrollidine ring, the latter being responsible for the intense pyrrolidine ion at M/e 71 in tremorine itself. Chemical ionization methods would undoubtedly have aided in this study by providing intense ions at P+1 for tremorine and its unoxygenated analogues.

5. Siduron

In a study of the metabolism of siduron (III) (BELASCO and REISER, 1969) thin layer chromatography was employed after deconjugation with β-glucuronid-

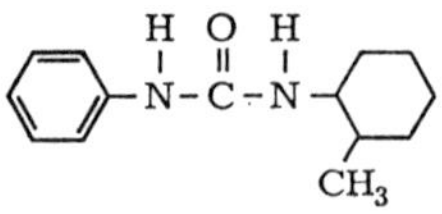

III

ase. The mass spectrum (Fig. 3) indicate in a very clear way that hydroxylation on either or both rings has occurred. The authors were also able to eliminate the possibility that hydroxylation of the aromatic ring had occurred in the *ortho* position (although the *ortho* and *para* derivatives possessed the same mass spectrum) by carefully noting the difference in volatilization temperatures of the two derivatives (85°C for the *o*-isomer, 115—120°C for the *p*-isomer). They were

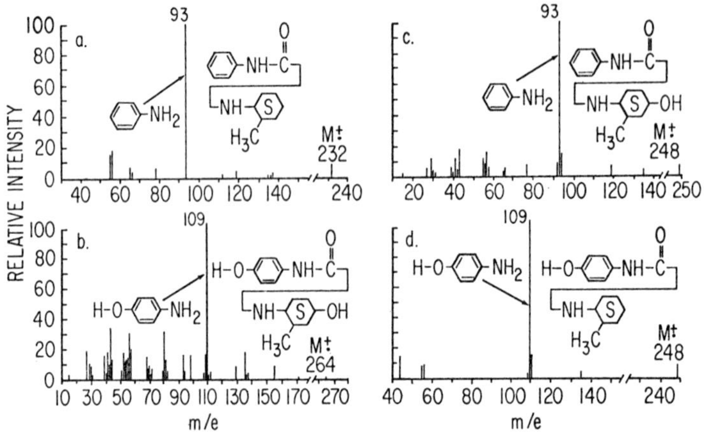

Fig. 3. Mass spectra of siduron and its metabolites. Reprinted with the permission of BELASCO and REISER, 1969 and the American Chemical Society, Washington, D.C.

fortunate in having enough metabolite to confirm the exact location of the hydroxyl group in the aliphatic ring by nmr analysis. It is interesting to note that combined gc-ms would have been useful by eliminating the need for thin layer chromatography (tlc) and in confirming the nature of the *para* hydroxy substituent, since it would surely have shown a retention time differing from that of the *ortho* isomer.

6. Naphthalene

The advantages of gc-ms are easily seen in a study on the metabolism of naphthalene (HOLTZMAN et al., 1967). Although not a drug itself, naphthalene-like nuclei are present in many drugs and these authors wished to study the exact mechanism by which rat liver microsomes catalyze incorporation of oxygen. This was accomplished by incubating the system in the presence of 77% $^{18}O_2$. The resulting naphthalene 1,2-diol (IV) contained one atom of ^{18}O and one atom of ^{16}O, presumably from water. In order to determine whether the ^{18}O atom was at the 1 or 2 position on the naphthalene nucleus, the substance was treated with

IV

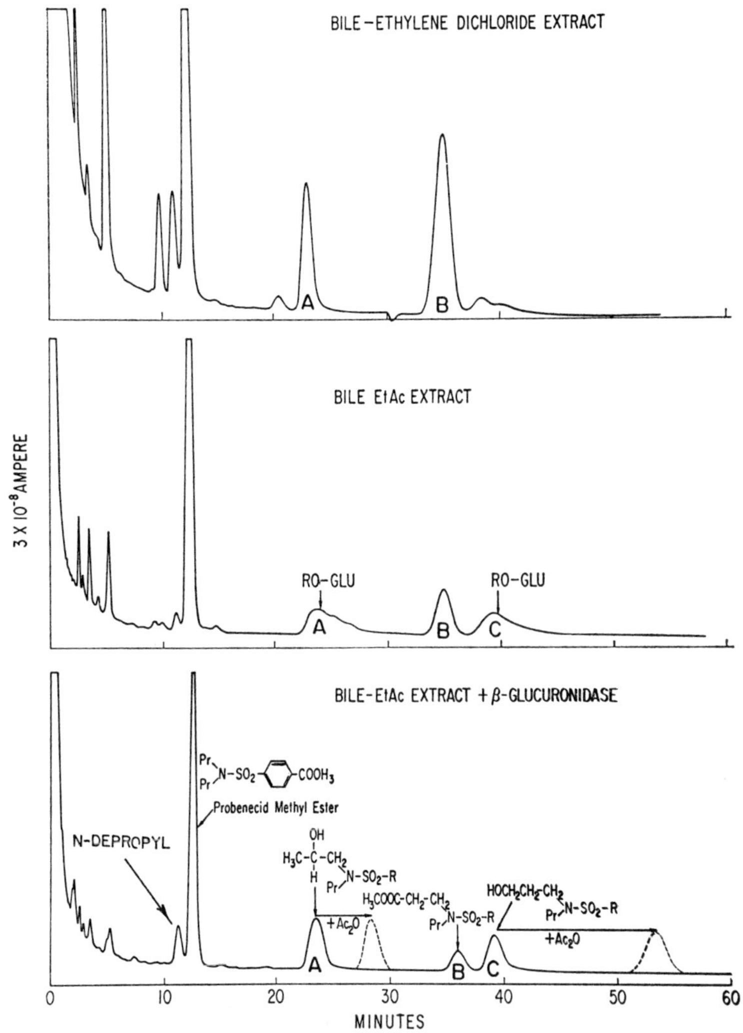

Fig. 4. Gas chromatogram of methyl esters of probenecid and its metabolites isolated from rat bile. Reprinted with permission of GUARINO et al., 1969 and North-Holland Publishing Co., Amsterdam

hydrochloric acid which dehydrated it to a mixture of 95% α- and 5% β-naphthol, as determined by gas liquid chromatography (glc) on a nonpolar liquid phase. The mixture was then silylated to improve chromatographic behavior and investigated using combined gc-ms where it was observed that the α-isomer contains all of the ^{18}O while the β-isomer contains none. Therefore the ^{18}O from $^{18}O_2$ was initially introduced at the α-position.

7. Probenecid

In a recent study of the metabolism of probenecid in the rat, we had occasion to employ most of the foregoing principles (GUARINO et al., 1969). Since probenecid is a carboxylic acid, all materials were treated with diazomethane in ether prior to gas chromatography to improve their chromatographic behaviour. Thus Fig. 4 shows the gas chromatogram of an ethylene dichloride extract of acidified bile. The large peak appearing at 13 min is unchanged probenecid while the peak immediately in front is N-depropylprobenecid, a not unexpected metabolite. Two other large peaks are seen due to metabolites A and B, are seen at 23 and 36 min respectively. When ethyl acetate was used in a second extraction, after ethylene dichloride, more polar components were extracted, and an additional peak, metabolite C, was observed on glc. It was interesting to note that peaks A and C show an extreme degree of tailing, although peak A, as obtained in the ethylene dichloride extract, was symmetrical. This suggested to us that A and C were probably glucuronide conjugates which exhibited tailing as they decomposed in the flash heater to form the free metabolites along with glucuronic acid dehydration products. This was confirmed when it was noted that β-glucuronidase treatment of the ethyl acetate extract prior to methylation gave *symmetrically shaped* peaks at A and C since they were now deconjugated. The fact that they were originally present as glucuronides suggested that peaks A and C, but not peak B, contained hydroxyl groups. Further evidence was easily obtained when the glucuronidase-treated extract was acetylated with acetic anhydride which caused both peaks to shift to longer retention times as expected when primary or secondary alcohols are converted to their acetates. With this preliminary information in hand, the gc-mass spectra of all metabolites were obtained after the mass spectrum of the methyl ester of probenecid itself was examined in some detail (Fig. 5).[1] It is apparent that the molecular ion at M/e 299 is extremely

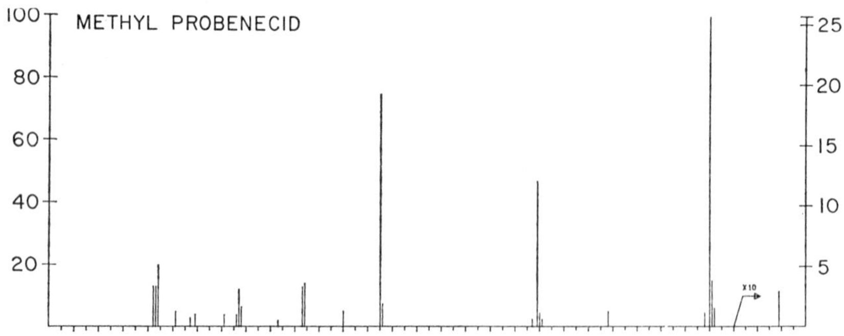

Fig. 5. Mass spectrum of methyl probenecid. Reprinted with permission of GUARINO et al., 1969 and North-Holland Publishing Co., Amsterdam

weak even when expanded by a factor of ten. This is to be expected, since the N-propyl group of a sulfonamide undergoes the beta cleavage referred to previously, losing an ethyl group in the process and giving rise to an intense ion at mass 270. If the metabolite was known to be extremely pure, it might be possible to affirm that the very weak molecular ion at mass 299 was significant. However, it might also be safely predicted that identification of molecular ions of metabolites would be difficult since such a weak peak might easily be confused with a small amount of impurity. Even when introduced by glc, one may not be assured of absolute purity, and the liquid phase "bleeding" from the gc column constitutes an additional source for error. Fortunately in this case, the use of the phenylmethylsilicone, OV-17, as the liquid phase allows the easy identification of silicone-containing ions in the spectrum because, as mentioned previously, silicone has

1 (Please note that in the original paper the mass spectra of metabolites A and C have been inadvertently interchanged. The spectrum is correct as presented here.)

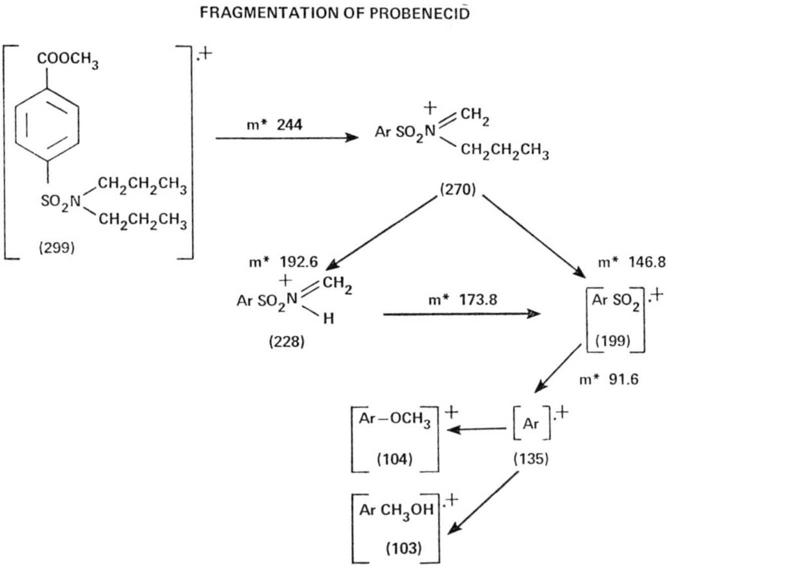

Fig. 6. Fragmentation pathways of methyl probenecid. Reprinted with permission of GUARINO et al., 1969 and North-Holland Publishing Co., Amsterdam

3.1% natural abundance of an isotope due to ^{30}Si. In the case of probenecid itself, a small metastable ion at M/e 244 supplies further evidence that the large ion at M/e 270 is *not* the molecular ion but a fragment ion and that it does indeed arise by cleavage from M/e 299 ($244 = \frac{(270)^2}{299}$.) Such metastable ions usually require that both fragment and precursor ions be present in moderate intensity. Further cleavage between the S and the N atoms in the sulfonyl group (Fig. 6) gives rise to an ion at M/e 199 which is the third most intense peak in the spectrum. Cleavage on the opposite side of the sulfonyl group gives rise to the carbomethoxyphenyl fragment of the molecule (mass 135). These three fragmentations account for most of the important features of the spectrum.

When the gc mass spectrum of metabolite A (Fig. 7) was investigated, the ions at mass 135 and 199 indicated that the carbomethyhoxphenylsulfonamide

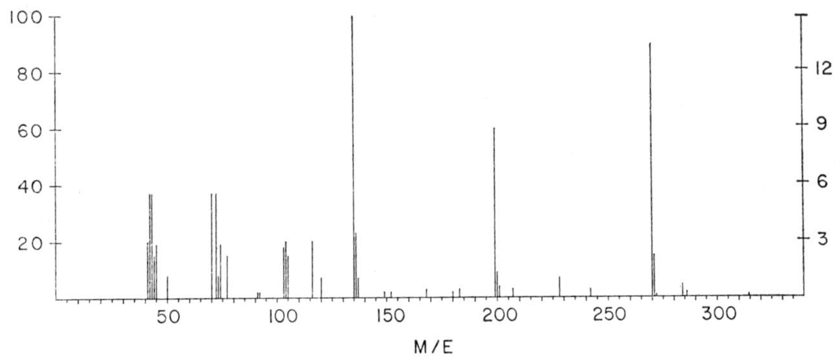

Fig. 7. Mass spectrum of metabolite A. Reprinted with permission of GUARINO et al., 1969 and North-Holland Publishing Co., Amsterdam

moiety was intact and the only question remaining was in regard to the nature of the substituents on the nitrogen atom. The ion at mass 270, by comparison with probenecid, indicated the presence of one intact propyl group and at least one CH_2 of the other side chain. At this point, knowledge of the molecular weight would have been most helpful since we had accounted for most of the molecular features. Unfortunately, the small peak at M/e 314, did not allow such a decision to be made with any confidence. The major difference between the spectrum of metabolite A and probenecid methyl ester itself was in the presence of the weak ions at mass 242 and 116 (Fig. 7). M/e 242 was, by itself, not particularly useful, although its even mass suggested that it was a fragment ion still containing nitrogen. Furthermore, the presence of sulfur was obvious in this fragment from the intensity of the ion at 244 relative to the intensity at 242 (natural abundance of $^{34}S = 4.2\%$), although this relationship is not apparent from the simplified chart of Fig. 7. M/e 242 is just 14 mass units higher than 228 and it was reasonable to think that the structure of this ion was similar to that of the ion at M/e 228 in the case of probenecid, except that it contained another CH_2 group. The ion at M/e 116, however, was extremely important since it did not contain sulfur as judged by its isotope peaks at 118. On the other hand, when 116 is added to 199, mass 315 is deduced and suggests that mass 315 is the molecular weight of the unknown metabolite. Although the structure of M/e 116 may also have been deduced by considering various combinations of C, H, N and O, in this case the formula was derived by employing high-resolution mass spectroscopy which indicated the formula to be $C_6H_{14}NO$. This formula shows that the fragment contains no unsaturated linkages but does contain an oxygen, and the only logical deduction is that a hydroxyl group is present on one of the alkyl side chains. This would be the site of the hydroxyl group previously indicated by the gc retention time shift after conversion to the acetate. Two locations are chemically possible for this hydroxyl group: β or γ to the nitrogen atom. The former was chosen as a first hypothesis because of the well-known beta oxidation of primary amines *in vivo*. Further support for this location was deduced from the fact that marked fragmentation would be expected, due to the placement of two heteroatoms on adjacent carbon atoms. When this occurs, beta cleavage is facilitated since both the positive charge and the radical are stabilized by resonance:

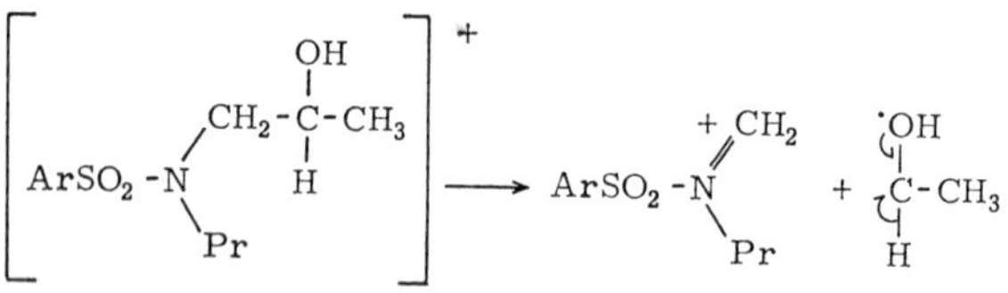

Final support for this structure was obtained through synthesis of metabolite A itself. The structures of metabolites B and C were deduced in much the same manner and the structure of B was also confirmed by synthesis.

Recently we have reinvestigated the mass spectrum of metabolite A, using the chemical ionization method with methane. Comparing Fig. 8 with 7, immediately exposes the advantages of *both* techniques. Chemical ionization clearly outlines the molecular weight by the peak at M/e 316 (M + 1) and shows a hydroxyl group to be present via the peak at M/e 298 (M + 1—18), while electron impact (Fig. 7) exhibits useful fragmentation data.

The point we wish to emphasize in this example is that success was achieved through the combination of gc-ms aided by consideration of logical metabolic

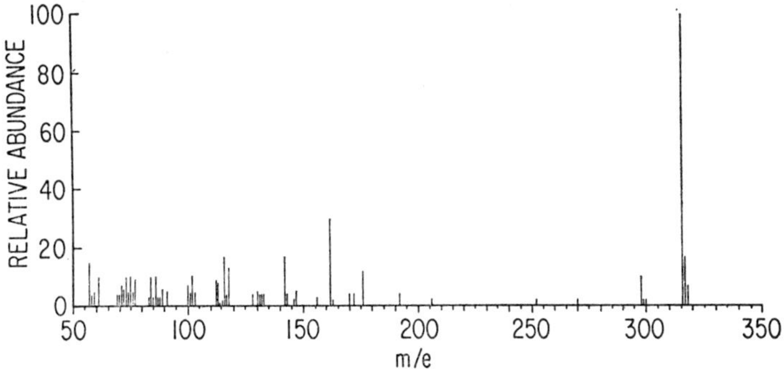

Fig. 8. Mass spectrum of metabolite A subjected to chemical ionization

processes and derivatization on a micro scale to ascertain functionality. We feel that any one of these methods by itself would not be sufficient to fully establish the structure of the metabolites. We wish further to emphasize that at no time was any of the material submitted to classical purification procedures except for selected extractions. It seems to us that isolation of metabolites in highly purified or crystalline form is seldom necessary today since the introduction of gc-ms techniques. In fact, during the early phases of these studies paper chromatographic, thin-layer chromatographic, and paper electrophoretic techniques failed to give adequate resolution of probenecid and its metabolites. For example, chromatographic and electrophoretic methods seldom gave more than two radioactive spots. Undoubtedly, the great similarities of the physical properties of these metabolites was responsible for these early observations. On the other hand, with the aid of glc the parent compound and its metabolites were easily separated. The compounds were identified readily even in the absence of some reference compounds.

The usual procedures for isolation and identification of drug metabolites from urine are hampered by: (1) problems of complete collection, and (2) the appearance of large amounts of normal excretion products which often interfere with the extraction and/or the assay of drugs and their metabolites. However, if a drug and its metabolites do appear in bile, this biological fluid is usually easier to work with than urine. Hence, by the use of renal-ligated rats one can often enhance biliary excretion and then begin isolation and identification procedures on cleaner and more concentrated biological samples than one would obtain by collecting urine samples. It is therefore proposed that during the early phases of drug development, a rapid method for approximating the quantitative and qualitative importance of drug metabolism would be gc-ms analysis of extracts of bile samples.

8. Brief Accounts of Mass Spectral Studies of Miscellaneous Compounds of Interest to Pharmacologists and Toxicologists

a) Limonene

Wade et al. (1966) solved an interesting problem which arose because a particular patient was demonstrating high "pregnanediol" values as determined by the standard clinical assay. The mass spectrum of this material showed that the high values were not due to the presence of a steroid but rather due to a monoterpene. Since there was no previous record of a monoterpene being synthesized by the human, it was an easy matter to establish that the dietary source of this compound, called uroterpene, was limonene.

b) Phytanic Acid

Various foods in the human diet contain the isoprenoid branched-chain acid, phytanic acid. MIZE et al. (1969) used gc-ms to show that animals fed this acid initially degrade the compound by alpha oxidation, with subsequent degradation steps being due to beta-oxidation. Persons with Refsum's disease lack the enzyme systems necessary for alpha oxidation and the material accumulates in their tissues.

c) Isoprene

Although the method may have limited application to drug metabolism there appears to be considerable promise in the techniques employed by JANSSON and LARSSON (1969) in identifying organic compounds in human breath by the use of gc-ms. They used an interesting collection technique involving a respiratory mask and plastic bag. Material thus collected can be easily stored or concentrated for further study. Their gc analysis of breath constituents in untreated adults confirms the presence of compounds such as methane, acetone, methanol, and ethanol previously identified by other means. These authors also reported the existence of isoprene in human breath. It seems that compounds such as volatile anaesthetics could be easily studied by this technique.

d) Acetylcholine

Acetylcholine was synthesized *in vitro* from minced ox brain but it was not found in significant amounts in freshly minced brain. Hence, HAMMAR et al. (1968) used combined gc-ms to identify acetylcholine in fresh rat brain through its N-demethylation with sodium benzenethiolate followed by gc of the resulting tertiary amine.

e) The "Pink Spot" in Urine from Schizophrenics

Mass spectrometry was used to solve an interesting problem in the area of psychopharmacology. It was reported that there occurred in the urine of schizophrenics a material providing a "pink spot" on paper chromatography. Several methods have been used in an attempt to isolate and identify the compound responsible: solvent extraction, ion exchange chromatography, paper and thin-layer chromatography, countercurrent distribution, and various color reactions, but none of these methods provided positive structural information. Although elution of this "pink spot" and subsequent thin-layer chromatography shows that there are at least seven different components, CREVELING and DALY (1967) were able to identify 3,4-dimethoxyphenethylamine by its characteristic ms fragmentation pattern. KUEHL et al. (1966) using gc-ms found that administration of 3,4-dimethoxyphenethylamine to normal and schizophrenic people did not affect the excretion of 3,4-dimethoxyphenylacetic acid in their urine, and so its biological function remains a mystery.

f) Bee Scent

In a review of the use of mass spectroscopy in the identification of hydrocarbons, STENHAGEN (1966) mentions a case where an analysis of bee scent was conducted with the use of only nine bees, the scent being identified as dihydroambrettolide and two of its analogs. In contrast BUTENANDT et al. (1959), using classical methods, had to collect about one-half million insects in order to identify the silk moth scent.

g) Trans-stilbene

SINSHEIMER and SMITH (1968) found that trans-stilbene undergoes a novel metabolic transformation for this class of compounds. Where other reports of metabolic reductions of C-C double bonds are primarily limited to Δ^4-3-keto-steroids and certain cinnamic acids, trans-stilbene forms the reduction metabolite, 4,4′-dihydroxybibenzyl by oxidation on the aromatic nucleus.

h) Pteridines

By the use of mass spectrometry alone SISENWINE and WALKENSTEIN (1969) demonstrated that the pteridine diuretic (Wy-5256) underwent a major metabolic biotransformation by the uncommon route of O-demethylation of the aliphatic ether side chain.

i) Tetracycline

Because of the large number of functional groups present in the tetracycline molecule, conventional methods of structure determination are laborious. HOFFMAN (1966), using mass spectroscopy, took advantage of the fact that the functional groups direct fragmentation along well-defined lines, so that alteration of a given group is easily disclosed.

j) Polychlorinated biphenyls (PCB's)

BAGLEY et al. (1970) used tlc and combined gc-ms to solve a very important contemporary problem in environmental toxicology. In their field studies of organochlorine pesticide residues in bald eagles they observed very complex gas chromatograms, even after preliminary zonal separation on thin-layer plates. By the time-consuming use of three different columns, most of the commonly occurring organochlorine pesticides could be identified, but there still occurred several unidentified peaks. Several of these peaks corresponded to various PCB's which are industrial compounds widely used as plasticizers. These workers also confirmed earlier reports that the gc retention times of some PCB's were in fact very close to those of nine commonly occurring organochlorine pesticides. Hence, early gc assays for these pesticides are suspect.

k) DDT

Gc-ms was found to be particularly useful by BIROS and WALTER (1970) in an analysis of pesticide residues and their metabolites where they were able to positively identify the components of a mixture without resorting to the usual time-consuming separation methods ordinarily used in these problems. Furthermore, the sensitivity was high enough to allow studies with the limited quantities of residues usually encountered in human tissues. This study is particularly relevant because it afforded a more positive means for confirming the identity of the pesticide residues.

E. Forensic Applications

Because of the great sensitivity and structural specificity of mass spectrometry, this method of analysis combined with gas chromatography and thin-layer chromatography has obvious forensic potential. The authors have applied gc-ms in solving a number of problems which have arisen from two sources: Samples from attempted suicides were obtained from a local community hospital and illicit drugs were obtained from young patients treated at a local walk-in clinic (Washington Free Clinic, Washington, D.C.). In the overdose cases, we have found that simple extraction of biological fluids, such as stomach washings or urine, with organic solvents usually provides an adequate clean-up procedure before investigation of the sample by gc-ms procedures. From consideration of the parent ion and the fragmentation patterns in conjunction with a library of reference spectra, we have usually been able to provide an identification rapidly enough to aid the physician in his treatment of such cases.

Among the compounds we have encountered from the walk-in clinic have been STP and HOG ("peace pill" PCP). The first compound is 2,5-dimethoxy-4-methylamphetamine, a hallucinogen earlier synthesized by a drug company in an experimental program. LINDGREN et al. (1969) used combined gc-ms to identify the second drug, HOG (phencyclidine, 1-(1-phenylcyclohexyl)piperidine). This compound came to the attention of these workers because earlier tests for known "street drugs" such as barbiturates, amphetamine, LSD, etc., were negative. The molecular ion and fragmentation pattern allowed its identification in a straightforward manner, and we can confirm its apparent importance in local drug traffic.

The street drugs which we have analyzed have largely borne out the deceptive practices reported by CHEEK et al. (1970). Small amounts of LSD and phencyclidine are easily analyzed by the direct insertion probe technique after ethanol extraction of the tablet or capsule. We have yet to find psilocybin or mescaline in any of the samples which we have analyzed.

References

ADLERCREUTZ, H., JOHANSSON, C.J., LUUKKAINEN, T.: Gas chromatographic and mass spectrometric studies in the influence of metabolites of bis (p-acetoxyphenyl) cyclohexylidenemethane on the estimation of estrogens in urine. Ann. Med. exp. Fenn. **45**, 269—276 (1967).

ÄNGGÅRD, E., SEDVALL, G.: Gas chromatography of catecholamine metabolites using electron capture detection and mass spectrometry. Anal. Chem. **41**, 1250—1256 (1969).

ALBER, L.L.: All-purpose gas-liquid chromatographic column for pharmaceuticals. J. Ass. Off. Anal. Chem. **52**, 1295—1300 (1969).

ANDERS, M.W., MANNERING, G.J.: Applications of gas chromatography to toxicology. Progr. chem. Tox. **3**, 121—218 (1967).

Application of Metabolic Data to the Evaluation of Drugs: A report prepared by the Committee on Problems of Drug Safety of the Drug Research Board, National Academy of Sciences — National Research Council: Clin. Pharmacol. Ther. **10**, 607—634 (1969).

ARNOLD, W., GRÜTZMACHER, W.F.: Massenspektrometrischer Nachweis von Arzneimittelmetaboliten (Barbiturate, Noludar, Pyramidon) in Rahmen der forensischen Analyse. Fresenius' Z. anal. Chem. **247**, 179—188 (1969).

AUDIER, H., FETIZON, M., GINSBURG, D., MANDELBAUM, A., RULL, T.: Mass spectrometry of morphine alkaloids. Tetrahedron Letters **1**, 13—22 (1965).

BAGLEY, G.E., REICHEL, W.L., CROMARTIE, E.: Identification of polychlorinated biphenyls in two bald eagles by combined gas-liquid chromatography-mass spectrometry. J. Ass. Off. Anal. Chem. **53**, 251—261 (1970).

BALLANTINE, J.A., FENWICK, R.G.: The mass spectra of griseofulvin analogues. Characteristic fragmentation processes in the mass spectra of spirocyclohexenones and spirocyclohexanones containing the griseofulvin skeleton. Org. Mass. Spect. **2**, 1145—1169 (1969).

BECKETT, A.H., TUCKER, G.T., MOFFAT, A.C.: Routine detection and identification in urine of stimulants and other drugs, some of which may be used to modify performance in sport. J. Pharm. Pharmacol. **19**, 273—294 (1967).

BELASCO, I.J., REISER, R.W.: Metabolic fate of siduron in the animal. J. Agr. Food Chem. **17**, 1000—1003 (1969).

BELLMAN, S.W.: Mass spectral identification of some hallucinogenic drugs. J. Ass. Off. Anal. Chem. **15**, 164—175 (1968).

BEYNON, J.H.: Mass spectrometry and its applications to organic chemistry. Amsterdam: Elsevier 1960.

— HOPKINSON, J.A., WILLIAMS, A.E.: The mass spectra of some guanidines. Org. Mass. Spect. **1**, 169—187 (1968).

— SAUNDERS, R.A., WILLIAMS, A.E.: The mass spectra of organic molecules. Amsterdam: Elsevier 1968.

— WILLIAMS, A.E.: Mass and abundance tables for use in mass spectrometry. Amsterdam: Elsevier 1963.

BIEMANN, K.: Mass spectrometry, applications to organic chemistry. New York: McGraw-Hill 1962.

BIEMANN, K., MCCLOSKEY, J.A.: Application of mass spectrometry to structural problems. VI. Nucleosides. J. Amer. chem. Soc. **84**, 2005—2007 (1962).

— WATSON, J.T.: Recording and interpretation of high resolution mass spectra of natural products as eluted from a gas chromatograph. Monatsh. Chem. **96**, 305—315 (1965).

BIROS, F.J., WALKER, A.C.: Pesticide residue analysis in human tissue by combined gas chromatography-mass spectrometry. J. Agr. Food Chem. **18**, 425—429 (1970).

BOGENTOFT, C., DANIELSSON, B.: Studies on the medicinal chemistry of oxoquinazolines. VI. Mass spectra of isomeric N- and O-alkylated 4-oxoquinazolines. Acta pharm. Suecia **6**, 589—598 (1969).

BROADHURST, N.A., MONTGOMERY, M.L., FREED, V.H.: Metabolism of 2-methoxy-3,6-dichlorobenzoic acid (dicamba) by wheat and bluegrass plants. J. Agr. Food Chem. **14**, 585—588 (1966).

BROCHMANN-HANSSEN, E., OKE, T.O.: Gas chromatography of barbiturates, phenolic alkaloids, and xanthine bases: Flash-heater methylation by means of trimethylanilinium hydroxide. J. pharm. Sci. **58**, 370—371 (1969).

BRUNNEE, C., TEN NOEVER DE BRAUW, M.C.: Z. Anal. Chem. **229**, No. 5, 321 (1967).

BUDZIKIEWICZ, H., DJERASSI, C.: Mass spectrometry in structural and stereochemical problems. I. Steroid Ketones. J. Amer. chem. Soc. **84**, 1430—1439 (1962).

— — WILLIAMS, D.H.: Interpretation of mass spectra of organic compounds. San Francisco: Holden-Day 1964.

— — — Structure elucidation of natural products by mass spectrometry. Vol. I: Alkaloids; Vol. II: Steroids, terpinoids, sugars, and miscellaneous compounds. San Francisco: Holden-Day 1964.

— — — Mass spectrometry of organic compounds. San Francisco: Holden-Day 1967.

BURTIS, C.A., BUTTS, W.C., RAINEY, W.T.: Separation of the metabolites of phenacetin in urine by high-resolution anion exchange chromatography. Amer. J. clin. Path. **53**, 769—777 (1970).

— WARREN, K.S.: Identification of urinary constituents isolated by anion-exchange chromatography. Clin. Chem. **14**, 290—301 (1968).

BUTENANDT, A. VON, ECKMAN, R.B., STAMM, D., HUCKER, E.: Über den Sexual-Lockstoff des Seidenspinners Bombyx mori. Reindarstellung und Konstitution. Z. Naturforsch. **14**b, 283—284 (1959).

CHALMERS, R.A., PARKER, R., SIMMONS, H.A., SNEDDEN, W., WATTS, R.W.E.: The conversion of 4-Hydroxypyrazolo [3,4-d] pyrimidine (Allopurinol) into 4,6-dihydroxypyrazolo [3,4-d] pyrimidine (oxipurinol) *in vivo* in the absence of xanthine-oxygen oxidoreductase. Biochem. J. **112**, 527—532 (1969).

CHEEK, F.E., NEWELL, S., JOFFE, M.: Deceptions in the illicit drug market. Science **167**, 1276 (1970).

COUTTS, R.T., HINDMARSH, K.W.: Mass spectra of some quinoline hydroxamine acids and related compounds. Org. Mass. Spect. **2**, 681—696 (1969).

— LOCOCK, R.A.: Identification of medicinal barbiturates by means of mass spectrometry. J. pharm. Sci. **57**, 2096—2100 (1968).

— — The $(M-43)^+$ ion in the mass spectra of some medicinal barbiturates. J. pharm. Sci. **58**, 775—776 (1969).

— MUKHERJEE, G.: Identification of the aromatic hydroxyamine group by mass spectrometry. Org. Mass. Spect. **3**, 63—65 (1970).

CREVELING, C.R., DALY, J.W.: Identification of 3,4-dimethoxyphenethylamine from schizophrenic urine by mass spectroscopy. Nature (Lond.) **216**, 190—191 (1967).

DALGLIESH, C.E., HORNING, E.C., HORNING, M.G., KNOX, K.L., ARGER, K.Y.: A gas-liquid-chromatographic procedure for separating a wide range of metabolites occuring in urine or tissue extracts. Biochem. J. **101**, 792—810 (1966).

DAMICO, J.N., BARRON, R.P.: The mass spectra of some chlorinated pesticidal compounds. Org. Mass. Spect. **1**, 331—342 (1968).

— CHEN, J.Y., COSTELLO, C.E., HAENNI, E.D.: Structure of Klein's metabolites of aldrin and of dieldrin. J. Ass. Off. Anal. Chem. **51**, 48—55 (1968).

DEJONGH, D.C.: Mass spectrometry, Annual Review in Analytical Chemistry. Anal. Chem. **42**, No. 5 169R—205R (1970).

— PERRICONE, S.C., GAY, M.L., KORYTNYK, W.: Mass spectrometry of vitamin B_6: Different forms of the vitamin, its metabolites, and antimetabolites, and analogs. Org. Mass. Spect. **1**, 151—166 (1968).

DREYFUSS, J., COHEN, A.I., HESS, S.M.: Metabolism of thiazesim, 5-(2-dimethylaminoethyl)-2,3-dehydro-2-phenyl-1,5-benzothiazepin-4 (SH)-one in the rat *in vivo* and *in vitro*. J. pharm. Sci. **57**, 1505—1511 (1968).

DUCKWORTH, H.E.: Mass spectrometry. London: Cambridge Univ. Press 1953.

DUFFIELD, A.M., CRAIG, J.C., KRAY, L.R.: Electron impact promoted fragmentation of some phenothiazine derivatives. Tetrahedron **24**, 4267—4276 (1968).

EMERY, E.M.: Mass spectra of aromatic esters. Anal. Chem. **32**, 1495—1506 (1960).

ENEROTH, P., HELLSTROM, K., RYHAGE, R.: Identification of two neutral metabolites of stigma sterol found in human feces. Steroids **6**, 707—719 (1965).

ETTRE, L.S., ZLATKIS, A.: The practice of gas chromatography. New York: Interscience 1967.

FALES, H.M., HAAHTI, E.O.A., LUUKKAINEN, T., VANDEN HEUVEL, W.J.A., HORNING, E.C.: Milligram-scale preparative gas chromatography of steroids and alkaloids. Anal. Biochem. **4**, 296—305 (1962).

— LLOYD, H.A., MILNE, G.W.A.: Chemical ionization mass spectrometry of complex molecules. II. Alkaloids. J. Amer. chem. Soc. **92**, 1590—1597 (1970).

— MILNE, G.W.A., VESTAL, M.C.: Chemical ionization mass spectrometry. J. Amer. chem. Soc. **91**, 3682—3685 (1969).

FIELD, F.H.: Chemical ionization mass spectrometry. Accounts Chem. Res. **1**, 42—49 (1968).

— FRANKLIN, J.L.: Electron impact phenomena. New York: Academic Press 1957.

FRIEDLAND, S.S., LANE, G.H., LONGMAN, R.T., TRAIN, K.E., O'NEAL, M.J.: Mass spectra of steroids. Anal. Chem. **31**, 169—174 (1959).

FRIEDMAN, A.R., LEMIN, A.J.: Metabolism of 2-chloro-4,5-dimethyl phenyl N-methylcarbamate in bean plants. J. Agr. Food Chem. **15**, 642—647 (1967).

FUKAMI, J.I., YAMAMOTO, I., CASIDA, J.E.: Metabolism of rotenone *in vitro* by tissue homogenates from mammals and insects. Science **155**, 713—716 (1967).

GARDINER, J.A., REISER, R.W., SHERMAN, H.: Identification of the metabolites of bromacil in rat urine. J. Agr. Food Chem. **17**, 967—973 (1969).

GILBERT, J.N.T., MILLARD, B.J.: Pharmacologically interesting compounds — I: High resolution mass spectra of phenothiazines. Org. Mass. Spect. **2**, 17—31 (1969).

GOLDMAN, P., MILNE, G.W.A., KEISTER, D.B.: Carbon-halogen bond clevage III. Studies on bacterial halidohydrolases. J. biol. Chem. **243**, 428—434 (1968).

GRANSTROM, E., SAMUELSSON, B.: The structure of the main urinary metabolite of prostaglandin $F_{2}a$ in the guinea pig. Europ. J. Biochem. **10**, 411—418 (1969).

GRAY, G.M.: Gas chromatography. In: Tools of biological research. Ed by H.J.B. ATKINS. Vol. 3, pp. 79—97 Springfield, Ill.: Thomas 1961.

GRÜTZMACHER, H.F., ARNOLD, W.: Massenspektren von Barbitursäurederivaten. Tetrahedron Letters **13**, 1365—1374 (1966).

GUARINO, A.M., CONWAY, W.D., FALES, H.M.: Mass spectral identification of probenecid metabolites in rat bile. Europ. J. Pharmacol. **8**, 244—252 (1969).

GUDZINOWICZ, B.J.: Gas chromatographic analysis of drugs and pesticides. New York: Marcel Dekker, Inc. 1967.

HAMMAR, C.G., HANIN, I., HOLMSTEDT, B., KITZ, R.J., JENDEN, D.J., KARLEN, B.: Identification of acetylcholine in fresh rat brain by combined gas chromatography-mass spectrometry. Nature (Lond.) **220**, 915—917 (1968).

— HOLMSTEDT, B., RYHAGE, R.: Mass Fragmentography. Identification of chlorpromazine and its metabolites in human blood by a new method. Anal. Biochem. **25**, 532—548 (1968).

HOFFMAN, D.R.: The mass spectra of tetracyclines. J. Org. Chem. **31**, 792—796 (1966).

HOLTZMAN, J., GILLETTE, J.R., MILNE, G.W.A.: The metabolic products of naphthalene in mammalian systems. J. Amer. chem. Soc. **89**, 6341—6344 (1967).

HOLZAPFEL, C.W.: The isolation and structure of cyclopiazonic acid, a toxic metabolite of *Penicillium Cyclopium* Westling. Tetrahedron **24**, 2101—2119 (1968).

HORNING, M.G., WATERBURY, L.D., HORNING, E.C., HILL, R.M.: Placenta; transfer of drugs: Drugs and drug metabolites in the neonate. In: The foetoplacental unit. Ed. by A. PECILE and C. FINZI, pp. 305—312. Excerpta med. (Amst.) 1969.

JAAKOMAKI, P.I., KNOX, K.L., HORNING, E.C., HORNING, M.G.: The characterization by gas-liquid chromatography of ethyl β-D-glucosiduronic acid as a metabolite of ethanol in rat and man. Europ. J. Pharmacol. **1**, 63—70 (1967).

JANSSON, B.O., LARSSON, B.T.: Analysis of organic compounds in human breath by gas chromatography-mass spectrometry. J. Lab. clin. Med. **74**, 961—966 (1969).

JOHNSON, R.A., HERR, M.E., MURRAY, H.C., REINEKE, L.M., FONKEN, G.S.: The microbiological oxygenation of some azabicycloalkanes. J. Org. Chem. **33**, 3195 (1968).

JORG, J., HOURIET, R., SPITELLER, G.: Massenspektren von Pflanzenschutzmitteln. Monatsh. Chem. **97**, 1064—1087 (1966).

KABASAKALIAN, P., TAGGART, M., TOWNLEY, E.: Urinary excretion of chloropheniramine and its N-demethylated metabolites in man. J. pharm. Sci. **57**, 856—858 (1968).

KARLEN, B., BOGENTOFT, C.: A mass spectrometric investigation of tremorine and related acetylenic amines and amides. Acta. pharm. Suecica **6**, 543—560 (1969).

KUEHL, F.A., ORMOND, R.E., VANDENHEUVEL, W.J.A.: Occurrence of 3,4-dimethoxyphenyl acetic acid in urines of normal and schizophrenic individuals. Nature (Lond.) **211**, 606—608 (1966).

KUNTZMAN, R., SERNATINGER, E., TSAI, I., KLUTCH, A.: New methodology for studies of drug metabolism. In: Importance of fundamental principles in drug evaluation Ed. by D.H. TEDESCHI and R.E. TEDESCHI, pp. 87—103. New York: Raven Press 1968.

LINDGREN, J.E., HAMMER, C.G., HESSLING, R., HOLMSTEDT, B.: The chemical identity of "Hog" — a "new" hallucinogen. Amer. J. Pharm. **141**, 86—90 (1969).

LLEWELYN, P.M., LITTLEJOHN, D.P.: Presented at the Pittsburgh Conference on analytical chemistry and applied spectroscopy, Pittsburgh, Pa. (1966); see also D.R. BLACK, R.A. FLATH and R. TERANISHI: Membrane molecular separators for gas chromatographic-mass spectrometric interfaces. J. Chromatographic Sci. **7**, 284—289 (1969).

LUUKKAINEN, T., ADLERCREUTZ, H.: Mass spectrometric studies in the specificity of estriol determination in urine by gas-liquid chromatography. Ann. Med. exp. Fenn. **45**, 264—268 (1967).

MCLAFFERTY, F.: Mass spectrometry of organic ions. New York: Academic Press 1963.

— Interpretation of mass spectra; an introduction. New York: W.A. Benjamin 1966.

MCNAIR, H.M., BONELLI, E.J.: Basic gas chromatography. Consolidated Printers for Varian Aerograph, Walnut Creek, Calf. (1967).

MILNE, G.W.A., GOLDMAN, P., HOLTZMAN, J.L.: The metabolism of 2-fluorobenzoic acid. II. Studies with $^{18}O_2$. J. biol. Chem. **243**, 5374—5376 (1968).

MIZE, C.E., AVIGAN, J., STEINBERG, D., PITTMAN, R.C., FALES, H.M., MILNE, G.W.A.: A major pathway for the mammalian oxidative degradation of phytanic acid. Biochim. biophys. Acta (Amst.) **176**, 720—739 (1969).

NILSSON, I.M., AGURELL, S., NILSSON, J.L.G., OHLSSON, A., SANDBERG, F., WAHLQVIST, M.: Δ^1-Tetrahydrocannabinol: Structure of a major metabolite. Science **168**, 1228—1229 (1970).

PALMER, K.H., FOWLER, M.S., WALL, M.E., RHODES, L.S., WADDELL, W.J., BAGGETT, B.: The metabolism of R (+)- and RS-phenobarbital. J. Pharmacol. exp. Ther. **170**, 355—363 (1969).

— MARTIN, B., BAGGETT, B., WALL, M.E.: The metabolic fate of orally administered quinidine gluconate in humans. Biochem. Pharmacol. **18**, 1845—1860 (1969).

PLIMMER, J.R., KEARNEY, P.C., VON ENDT, D.W.: Mechanism of conversion of DDT to DDD by *Aerobacter aerogenes*. J. Agr. Food Chem. **16**, 594—597 (1968).

REED, W.T., FORGASH, A.J.: Lindane: Metabolism to a new isomer of pentachlorocyclohexene. Science **160**, 1232 (1968).

REISCH, J., PAGNUCCO, R., ALFES, H., JANTOS, N., MOLLMANN, H.: Mass spectra of derivatives of phenylalkylamines. J. Pharm. Pharmacol. **20**, 81—86 (1968).

RHODES, R.C., REISER, R.W., GARDINER, J.A., SHERMAN, H.: Identification of the metabolites of terbacil in dog urine. J. Agr. Food Chem. **17**, 974—979 (1969).

RYHAGE, R.: Use of a mass spectrometer as a detector and analyses for effluents emerging from high temperature gas liquid chromatography columns. Anal. Chem. **36**, 759—764 (1964).

SCHWARTZ, M.A., BOMMER, P., VANE, F.M.: Diazepam metabolites in the rat: Characterization by high resolution mass spectrometry and nuclear magnetic resonance. Arch. Biochem. **121**, 508—516 (1967).

— VANE, F.M., POSTMA, E.: Chlordiazepoxide metabolites in the rat. Characterization by high resolution mass spectrometry. Biochem. Pharmacol. **17**, 965—974 (1968a).

— — — Urinary metabolites of 7-chloro-1-(2-diethylaminoethyl)-5-(2-flurophenyl)-1,3-dihydro-2H-1,4-benzodiazepin-2-one dihydrochloride. J. med. Chem. **11**, 770—774 (1968b).

SCOTT, W.M., WACKS, M.E., ESKELSON, C.D., TOWNE, J.C., CAZEE, C.: The elimination of small neutral molecules and fragments in mass spectra. — I. Substituted salicyclic acids and their derivatives. Org. Mass. Spect. **1**, 847—855 (1968).

SEIBL, J.: Information on metastable transitions in the mass spectra of organic compounds. Helv. chim. Acta **50**, 263—268 (1967).

SILVERSTEIN, R.M., BASSLER, G.C.: Spectrometric identification of organic compounds. 2nd Ed. New York: Wiley, 1967.

SINSHEIMER, J.E., SMITH, R.U.: 4,4'-Dihydroxybibenzyl, a reduction metabolite of *trans*-stilbene. J. pharm. Sci. **57**, 713—714 (1968).

SISENWINE, S.F., WALKENSTEIN, S.S.: The metabolic fate of the pteridine diuretic, Wy-5256. J. pharm. Sci. **58**, 867—871 (1969).

SMITH, D.L., GROSTIC, M.F.: Mass spectrometric identification of the metabolites of methyl N-(o-aminophenyl)-N-(3-dimethylaminopropyl) anthranilate. J. med. Chem. **10**, 375—379 (1967).

VON SPULAK, F., CLAUSSEN, V., FEHLHABER, H.W., KORTE, F.: Haschisch-XIX. Cannabidiolcarbonsäure-tetrahydrocannabitriol-ester, ein neuer Haschisch-Inhaltsstoff. Tetrahedron **24**, 5379—5383 (1968).

Stenhagen, E.: Mass spectrometry in biochemical research. Chimia **20**, 346—357 (1966).
Street, H. V.: Gas liquid chromatography of submicrogram amounts of drugs. IV. Identification of barbiturates, hydantoins, amides, imides, carbamates, phenylbutazone, carboxylic acids and hydrazine derivatives by direct derivative formation within the gas chromatograph. J. Chromat. **41**, 358—366 (1969).
Suda, T., DeLuca, H. F., Schnoes, H., Blunt, J. W.: 25-Hydroxyergocalciferol: A biologically active metabolite of Vitamin D_2. Biochem. biophys. Res. Commun. **35**, 182—185 (1969).
Szymanski, H. A.: Biomedical applications of gas chromatography. New York: Plenum Press 1964.
Thomas, D. W., Biemann, K.: The alkaloids of *Voacanga africina*. Lloydia **31**, 1—8 (1968).
Wade, A. P., Wilkinson, G. S., Dean, F. M., Price, A. W.: The isolation characterization and structure of uroterpenol, a monoterpene from human urine. Biochem. J. **101**, 727—734 (1966).
White, F. A.: Mass spectrometry in science and technology. New York: Wiley 1968.
Woltz, H. H., Clark, S. J.: Gas chromatography in the analysis of steroid hormones. New York: Plenum Press 1966.

Chapter 34

The Application of Various Spectroscopies to the Identification of Drug Metabolites

PETER BOMMER and FLOIE M. VANE

With 5 Figures

A. Introduction

It has long been recognized that structural elucidation of drug metabolites contributes greatly to the understanding of the mechanism of drug action. However, in the past, the difficult and expensive nature of this task restricted studies to relatively few drugs.

With the advent of sophisticated chromatographic techniques, such as gas, paper, thin layer and the newer types of countercurrent chromatography, identification of known metabolites has become an order of magnitude simpler. Distribution of the metabolite in a given countercurrent fraction or its detection or elution at a given chromatographic retention time or migration value are easily compared to similar values for reference samples (see chapters 27 and 31). Confirmation of favorable chromatographic behavior is often obtained by isotope dilution techniques (see chapter 32) or by other methods, such as infrared or ultraviolet spectroscopy. Unfortunately, reference metabolites are often not available and it is fortunate that more recent methods, such as mass and nuclear magnetic resonance spectroscopy, are able to furnish structural information on metabolites without requiring synthesis of model compounds. This success can largely bə attributed to the fact that invariably the structure of the administered drug is known and most metabolic changes are rather simple. The information obtained from the isolation is often of great assistance in determining the structure even by spectral means; *e.g.*, if the metabolite is known to be an amine and thus contains nitrogen, the mass spectrum can be more easily interpreted in this light.

The basic principles of mass, nuclear magnetic resonance, infrared, ultraviolet and optical rotatory dispersion spectroscopies will be presented along with references to books which contain detailed descriptions and further applications. As examples from the authors' laboratories, the application of mass spectrometry and nuclear magnetic resonance spectroscopy to the structure determination of the metabolites of diazepam and triprolidine will be presented. The second section of the bibliography contains selected literature references in which one or more of the spectroscopies discussed in this chapter are used for structure elucidation of drug metabolites.

This chapter does not mean to imply that pharmacologists or biochemists should become experts in the interpretation of spectral data. Although this is possible, it would, in most circumstances, be impractical. The spectral approach to the structure determination of drug metabolites will normally depend on two groups of scientists: the biochemists responsible for the drug metabolism studies and the spectroscopists who are primarily responsible for the interpretation of the spectral data. A major factor in the efficiency and success of this approach will be the communication between the two groups; this factor is directly related to each group's awareness of the other workers' techniques and procedures. The paramount challenge will be the quantity and purity of the isolated sample and this will be discussed in the next section.

B. Sample Requirements and Isolation Procedures

The approximate minimum sample size and the sample form are listed for each spectroscopy in Table 1. The minimum sample ranges from approximately 10^{-8} g for low resolution mass spectrometry to 10^{-4} g for nuclear magnetic resonance spectroscopy. These values will vary with the specific structural problem and the sensitivity of the individual instrument.

Table 1. *Approximate minimum sample required for spectroscopic analysis of drug metabolites*

	Minimum Sample (g)	Sample Form
Mass Spectrometry		Vapor Phase
Low Resolution	10^{-8}—10^{-6}	
High Resolution	10^{-7}—10^{-5}	
Ultraviolet	10^{-6}—10^{-4}	Solution
Infrared (Raman)	10^{-5} (10^{-4})	Solution or Dispersion (Solid)
ORD, CD	10^{-4}	Solution
Nuclear Magnetic Resonance		Solution
Single Scan	10^{-3}	
Signal Averaging	10^{-4}	

The spectral interference caused by various impurities in the sample will be different for each spectroscopy. Wherever possible, it is strongly recommended that "blank" or "control" samples which have undergone the same separation processes as the metabolite be submitted for analysis with each metabolite sample. This will allow the spectroscopist to determine the areas of impurity interference and will make his interpretation more meaningful.

One of the most common methods for isolation of small samples is thin layer chromatography (see chapter 31). The use of drugs labeled with radioactive isotopes contributes greatly to the success of this procedure. Contamination of the sample is very difficult to avoid, but it can be minimized by precautionary measures, such as using high purity solvents, avoiding exposure of the plates to organic compounds, and pre-washing the plates.

Another approach for isolating metabolites is the collection of samples from a gas chromatograph (see chapter 27). The tedious nature of this method has been eliminated by directly coupling the gas chromatograph to a mass spectrometer. This combination of gas chromatography and mass spectrometry is steadily increasing in popularity and is discussed in detail in chapter 33. Although combinations of gas chromatography with other spectroscopies, such as infrared spectroscopy, are becoming available, no applications of these combined methods in metabolic studies have been reported. The use of these combinations at present is limited to stable, volatile compounds usually of low molecular weight.

C. Mass Spectrometry

(Biemann, 1962; Budzikiewicz et al., 1967; McLafferty, 1967)

The application of mass spectrometry to organic compounds is limited to samples which can be volatilized in a high vacuum at temperatures below those which cause thermal decomposition. This means that a compound, when heated, must attain a vapor pressure of approximately 10^{-6} mm Hg at temperatures of about 250—300° C. Fortunately, most drugs fall into this class of compounds. Very polar compounds, such as sugars and peptides, and compounds with very high molecular weights are excluded from mass spectroscopic study by this limitation. However, the volatility of many polar compounds can be sufficiently increased by preparing derivatives. To study the structure of proteins and other large molecules, it is necessary to degrade the molecules into smaller units and to deduce the complete structure of the original molecules from the structures of these subunits.

The compound in the vapor state is bombarded by a beam of electrons supplied by a heated filament in an enclosed region of the spectrometer known as the ion chamber. The resulting ions (molecular ions) usually possess such a high excess energy that many are decomposed to form neutral and charged fragments. This fragmentation is not a random process but is related to the structure of the molecule; *e.g.* double bonds are stronger than single bonds and break less frequently.

The positively charged molecular ion and its fragments are accelerated by an electric field and then dispersed in a magnetic field according to the inverse of their mass-to-charge ratios (m/e). Since the charge on most ions is one, the m/e value will reflect the mass of the ion. The ions are collected and recorded either by a photoplate or by scanning the magnetic field and collecting the ions as they pass over an ion multiplier. From the resulting mass spectrum, the m/e values of the molecular and fragment ions as well as their relative intensities are determined.

Mass spectrometers fall into approximately three categories in regard to resolving power: "low" resolution capable of separating m/e 400 from m/e 401 with approximately 10% valley between the successive peaks, "medium" resolution capable of separating m/e 400.0 from m/e 400.4 approximately, and "high" resolution capable of separating m/e 400.00 from m/e 400.02 with the same valley. To attain medium and high resolution, it is necessary either to construct instruments with larger magnetic dispersing systems or to resort to double focusing. In double focusing systems the ion beam is first passed through an electrostatic sector whose function is to collimate the ion beam in terms of energy before it undergoes mass dispersion by the electromagnet. This is necessary because the method by which ions are produced in the ion chamber (electron impact) leads to ions containing a range of velocities after acceleration. This distribution of velocities leads to peak broadening at the recorder output. With low or even medium resolution mass spectrometers, it cannot be determined if an ion having an m/e 72 has an elemental composition of C_5H_{12} (72.094), C_4H_8O (72.057), $C_4H_{10}N$ (72.081), or whether it is a mixture of these ions. Of course, if mass 72 was the molecular ion of a compound or was known for other reasons to contain merely one species, its formula might be determined even with a low resolution mass spectrometer. Unfortunately, most commercially available low resolution mass spectrometers are not equipped with sufficiently accurate mass measurement systems to allow such measurements to be convenient. The high resolution mass spectrometer, on the other hand, is capable of resolving all such species and furthermore of measuring them accurately, either manually or by sophisticated computer systems. Generally, such measurements may be performed with an accuracy of a few parts per million and, with the more sophisticated systems, it is possible to measure all of the ions in the mass spectrum automatically. Knowledge of this myriad of elemental compositions can greatly aid in the interpretation of the spectrum although the large quantity of data is somewhat overwhelming. It must be immediately emphasized that, in the specific case of drug metabolites, it is often possible to presume a large portion of the elemental composition of a metabolite so that even low resolution systems may be quite sufficient for many studies. High resolution mass spectrometry, which determines the formulas of the ions, aids considerably in the interpretation of the mass spectrum of an unknown. In this sense, high resolution mass spectrometric data should be even more useful to the novice in the field than to the more sophisticated interpreter.

It is undeniably true, however, that the operation and maintenance of a high resolution system requires the full-time attention of dedicated personnel. This is in contrast to the operation of a low or medium resolution mass spectrometer which may often be operated and interpreted directly by pharmacologists, provided some technical support is available for maintenance purposes.

Knowledge of the molecular weight of a metabolite is usually sufficient to determine the type of metabolic process which has occurred: oxidation, reduction, hydrolysis, etc. If the drug undergoes several structural changes, elucidation of the structure of a metabolite would be difficult without the high resolution data that permit the unambiguous determination of the molecular formula. For example, addition of an oxygen atom in the hydroxylation of a drug might be confused with the combination of N-methylation and hydrogenation of a double bond; both metabolic changes correspond to the addition of 16 mass units. Of course, in the former case one would expect to observe loss of water from the molecular ion, but if the drug originally contained a hydroxyl group, the metabolic addition of a second hydroxyl group might not be easily ascertained. In general, however, depending upon the degree and type of mass spectral fragmentation, the sites of metabolic transformation can usually be allocated to a particular portion of the molecule and, in favorable cases, even to specific structural groups or atoms. An additional advantage of high resolution over low resolution mass spectrometry is that it is less sensitive to interference from impurities introduced from the isolation procedure, since they usually have molecular compositions that differ from those of the metabolite. Sometimes the same effect results from the nature of the atoms constituting the drug. For example, atoms such as chlorine, bromine, or sulfur are present naturally as mixtures of two isotopes in a ratio characteristic of the particular atom. The result is that spectra of such drugs contain characteristic groupings of peaks for each ion containing these atoms. Unfortunately, in the case of nitrogen, oxygen, and carbon, the isotopes which occur naturally are present in such low abundance ($<1\%$) that they are of little use in revealing the presence of these atoms in a molecular ion or its fragments, although it is true that by very careful measurements of intensities some useful approximations may be made.

D. Nuclear Magnetic Resonance Spectroscopy

(Bhacca and Williams, 1964; Bovey, 1969; see also chapter 9).

In nuclear magnetic resonance spectroscopy (nmr) involving protons (pmr), the protons distributed about an organic molecule are employed as magnetic probes to determine the electronic environment, hence substitution patterns, at the carbon atoms to which they are attached. Furthermore, their mutual interaction supplies evidence relating to their internuclear distance and geometry. By careful interpretation of the data, the complete carbon skeleton can often be reconstructed. To be successfully employed as a probe in this manner, an atom must possess a magnetic moment which requires that either the atomic number or the atomic mass be odd. For this reason, ^{12}C cannot be employed directly as a probe determination of the carbon skeleton. On the other hand, ^{13}C could be so utilized but its low natural abundance (1%) and the low sensitivity of existing spectrometers restrict application to metabolism studies. FOURIER transform analysis of pulsed nmr signals (FARRAR, 1970) shows great promise in overcoming these limitations and, in the near future, we shall undoubtedly see applications even to drug metabolites.

In the case of proton nmr spectroscopy, application of the technique to the identification of metabolites is also limited by low instrumental sensitivity (4—20 mg for a routine analysis) and the requisite purity of the sample, since all proton bearing species are observed. This is indeed unfortunate, since nmr is probably the most powerful tool available today for the structural elucidation of many organic compounds and drugs. One relatively simple method by which the sensitivity may be increased by factors of 10- to 50-fold involves repetitive scanning of the spectrum while accumulating the data in a relatively simple computer. By this method, the signal to noise ratio is increased by the $\sqrt{n}$, where n = number of scans. The pulse and FOURIER transform method is also applicable to proton spectra and soon may greatly increase utilization of nmr for metabolite identification.

It is worth noting that mass spectrometry is often highly complementary to nmr spectroscopy. The mass spectrum of a metabolite, particularly its high resolution spectrum, can accurately determine the number of hydrogens it contains. The same information is theoretically available from the sum of all individual band areas observed in its nmr spectrum, but in practice it is often difficult to obtain an exact value, particularly when the material is somewhat impure. On the other hand, if the total number of protons is known from the mass spectrum, allowances may often be made for such impurities and instrumental difficulties, permitting more positive assignments of areas to specific functional groups. In the reverse sense, structural information obtained from perusal of the high resolution and low resolution mass spectrum often suggests functional groups [*e.g.* $(CH_3)_2NCH_2$] which are particularly easy to confirm through observation of even a crude nmr spectrum.

The basis for observation of an nmr signal with ^1H is as follows: because the proton possesses a magnetic moment, two orientations are possible with regard to an externally applied magnetic field. If radiofrequency energy of a certain wavelength (megahertz) is supplied, transitions will occur between the two states and the radiofrequency energy absorbed or emitted may be observed in a delicately balanced bridge network. The frequency and field necessary are related by a constant for each nucleus called the magnetogyric ratio. If an organic compound is placed in such an intense magnetic field, the field actually experienced by each proton will be altered by the presence of electrons in neighboring bonds and by charges on nearby nuclei. While the absolute magnitude of such "screening" effects is very small indeed compared with that of the applied field, the electrons and adjacent nuclei are so close to the nucleus being observed that their effect is measurable. The magnitude of this effect and the sophistication of the instrumentation required may be appreciated when it is realized that the whole range of signal displacements (called the chemical shift) occupies only ~ 20 parts per million (ppm) of magnetic field. This is, in fact, the ppm scale observed on the abscissa of most nmr spectra, and important structural correlations are based on chemical shift differences of no more than 0.25 ppm. Chemical shifts are usually reported as the difference (ppm) between the absorption positions of the protons of interest and the resonance position of an added internal reference. Tetramethylsilane is usually chosen for this purpose, since its protons give a single absorption peak that is shifted from the resonance positions of most protons due to the high degree of shielding by the electron clouds around silicon.

It may be readily understood that as electrons are inductively withdrawn from a C-H bond, the hydrogen atom will acquire a greater positive charge. It is therefore reasonable to expect that the ppm scale will somewhat resemble an acidity scale. For example, alkanes are the least acidic of all organic materials, since the protons are well shielded by the electrons of the C-H bond. Such protons are therefore found near the highly shielded tetramethylsilane reference standard, being shifted downfield by about 1—2 ppm from it. Carboxylic acids, on the other hand, are found at the opposite end of the scale ($\sim$ 11 ppm), being less shielded due to the inductive effects of the carbonyl group. Protons on double bonds are more acidic than those in saturated hydrocarbons and so appear at 5 ppm. Formal positive charges or negative charges are also easily observed in nmr spectroscopy. For example, the resonance signal from an N-methyl group undergoes a similar downfield shift of about 1 ppm when it is converted to its corresponding positively charged ammonium salt by the addition of trifluoroacetic acid.

The foregoing description is something of an oversimplification. Other effects, mainly relating to the distribution of electron clouds in fixed directions about the nucleus, must also be considered. For example, alcoholic protons are obviously more acidic than olefinic protons, yet appear at relatively small chemical shifts (about 2—3 ppm). This is understandable because, although the proton is acidic due to the electron withdrawing nature of the oxygen atom nucleus, the heavy cloud of unshared electrons on oxygen act effectively to shield it from the applied field. Furthermore, the actual position of the OH resonance is dependent upon the concentration of sample in the solution. At higher concentrations there is an increase in intermolecular hydrogen bonding which results in the decreased shielding of the proton. A single broad band is observed reflecting the exchange between bonded and unbonded protons when the exchange rate is of the same order as the chemical shift difference between the two species expressed in frequency terms. Extensive listings of chemical shifts for protons in fixed environments have been prepared and reference to these lists often facilitates structural elucidation.

In contrast to the usual forms of light spectroscopies where one observes an instantaneous view of the various species responsible for absorption, the time range over which measurements are made in nmr is of the order of milliseconds so that processes which occur faster than this are observed only as a weighted average of the various species involved. This is one of the interesting facets of nmr spectroscopy, since many processes involving configurational changes take place in similar time ranges and can therefore be observed through changes in band shape with temperature and structure; for example, an NH group of an amide, RCONHR, may appear as two separate peaks at low temperature due to the two rotational isomers A and B with the area of each peak proportional to

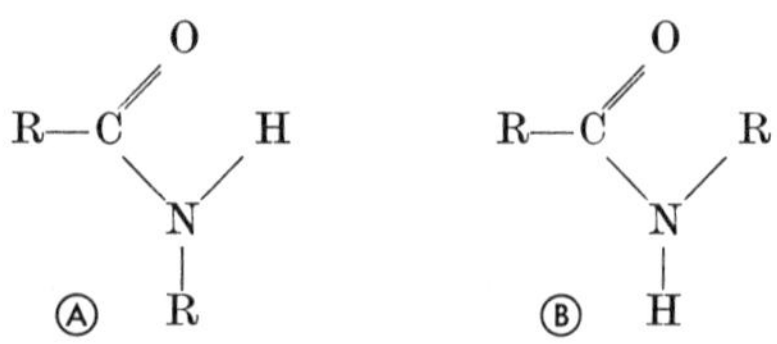

the amount of each species present. As the solution is warmed, the interconversion rate may increase so that the apparatus is no longer able to distinguish fully between the two and the valley between them will begin to diminish. Finally, at higher rates a single peak will appear due to the averaging of the fields of A and B.

As mentioned previously, the areas under the peaks are directly related to the numbers of protons responsible for absorption of a given functional group, which greatly facilitates the complete interpretation of an nmr spectrum.

One feature of nmr spectroscopy is the interaction between neighboring protons, which both aids and hinders interpretation of the spectra. Thus if a proton has a nearby neighbor whose nucleus is aligned with the externally applied field, the two fields add and it will be necessary to adjust the applied field to maintain the required resonance condition. But on the average, at room temperature, there will be almost an equal number of neighbors whose nuclei will be aligned contrary to the externally applied field, and protons experiencing this effect will require a field adjustment in the opposite direction. This results in a splitting of the signal into two bands.

It may be readily inferred that, if the number of nearby proton neighbors is large, the complexity of the splitting, or spin coupling as it is called, will become very great and the spectrum may become very difficult to interpret. Since this effect will be greatest in highly saturated compounds, it is fortunate indeed that drugs and their metabolites are usually unsaturated, often containing aromatic nuclei which serve to insulate proton resonance peaks from each other. In most cases, the nmr spectrum of a known drug can be interpreted in its entirety and so changes in structure due to metabolism stand out dramatically when spectra are compared to those of the original drug.

Another advantage of nmr spectroscopy is that a wide range of aqueous and nonaqueous solvents can be successfully utilized. The only requirement is that the solvent shall not contain protons that absorb energy in the same region as the material under investigation. Since the deuterium nucleus does not absorb in the same region as the proton, this requirement is met by various deuterated solvents, which fortunately are commercially available. It is preferable to obtain spectra of the drug and its metabolites in the same solvent. However, if this is not possible because of the increased polarity ot the metabolites, different solvents may be used and large correction factors are not needed unless an aromatic solvent is used. Furthermore, functionality of a drug metabolite can often be observed through reactions carried out directly in the nmr sample tube. For example, the presence of hydroxyl groups can be easily ascertained by simply adding a small amount of D_2O to the sample and observing disappearance of the suspected signal as ROH is converted through an exchange reaction to ROD. A great deal of additional information can be obtained through variation of instrumental parameters. For example, the spin coupling between nuclei, referred to above as a complicating factor, can be overcome through decoupling methods. In these procedures, the nucleus suspected of perturbing another is irradiated with a high intensity of radiofrequency power thus changing the nature of the magnetic environment. This removes the spin coupling effect and the spectrum is considerably simplified.

It has been recently discovered that addition of small amounts of chelates containing the rare earth element europium causes the chemical shift scale of nearby functional groups to be magnified markedly owing to the presence of the strong paramagnetic effect of the europium nucleus. Since the resulting spectrum is extraordinarily simplified, this method shows great promise (SANDERS and WILLIAMS, 1970).

E. Infrared Spectroscopy

(COLTHUP et al., 1964; HERZBERG, 1945)

As mentioned in the introduction, infrared spectroscopy has been used mainly to prove identity between a metabolite and a known compound. Because of its specificity and wealth of detail, infrared is one of the best methods for this purpose.

Absorption of infrared radiation results in transitions between vibrational or rotational energy levels of atoms or groups of atoms within the molecule. Complex molecules have many such modes and each mode gives rise to an absorption band, whose intensity depends on the change in dipole moment of the vibrating group and whose wavelength depends on the relative masses of the vibrating atoms. Roughly, an infrared spectrum can be divided into two parts: the first lying between 4000—1200 cm^{-1} and the second from 1200—$\sim$ 400 cm^{-1}.

For structure determination, the first region is of greater interest, since it contains bands more easily attributed to specific functional groups. The second region contains a complex pattern of absorption bands that arise from interactions between vibrations of the molecular skeleton and is frequently referred to as the "fingerprint" region, since it is highly sensitive to even subtle changes in molecular geometry.

The former region can give useful information about the presence or absence of groups like OH, NH, CO, CHO, COOH, COOR, $CONR_2$, and thus may be particularly helpful in elucidating metabolic changes, since changes in these types of groups are common. While the groups themselves are well delineated by this technique, the group frequencies are not particularly susceptible to the nearby environment and therefore cannot serve as effective probes for the remainder of the skeletal structure. In the past, when infrared spectroscopy was the only tool available for structural analysis, many attempts were made to take advantage of band displacements both in this region and in the fingerprint region. Considerable success was achieved in relating the frequencies of CO absorption to the presence or absence of unsaturation adjacent to the carbonyl group, and some correlations were achieved regarding the types of aromatic systems responsible for C=C absorption at 1670 cm^{-1}. A few correlations were also found relating to ether linkages (*e.g.* methylenedioxy groups) as well as aromatic substitution through the bands between 950 and 1225 cm^{-1}. But, in general, these correlations held up only in very restricted classes of compounds and many exceptions were noted. Any attempt to achieve correlations through analysis of the spectra of complex organic compounds using first principles seems hopelessly complicated. However, a new approach involving "learning machines" (WANGEN and ISENHOUR, 1970) has recently been proposed to uncover information hidden within the complex overlapping of bands. In this technique, the infrared spectra of a series of compounds, all possessing one common structural feature, are compared with a like series of spectra without this structural feature. The information in the form of band intensities and frequencies or wavelengths is entered into a computer in matrix tabulation form. The computer then repeatedly compares the two series, finding a learning surface or vector characteristic of this group, provided one is present. The method is purely empirical, and a correlation characteristic of a given learning vector may depend upon very obscure combinations of intensities and frequencies that never could be obtained by human perusal of the spectra. By its very nature, however, correlations can be built on some totally extraneous factor and therefore may be false. Nonetheless, recent results appear most promising.

Satisfactory infrared spectra are easily obtained experimentally with micro sampling accessories on even a few micrograms of material. Certainly, 100 μg of material is sufficient for a fairly routine analysis. The optics and cells of IR spectrometers are usually constructed of sodium chloride so that nonaqueous solvents must be used. In addition, it is advisable to avoid alcoholic solvents, simply because their own infrared absorption is so intense that it tends to blank out the absorption of the compound in question. This is true, even though the usual double beam principles are employed by which the solvent absorption is cancelled out, because the solvent absorbs so strongly that insufficient light penetrates either cell to give a satisfactory signal for comparison. Certain advantages are realized by the use of liquid solvents compared to mull or KBr techniques, which utilize crystalline material. For example, *d*, *l* and *dl* forms of a compound all show identical infrared spectra in solution, and one would not be misled by the different spectra sometimes observed when racemates are compared with optically active forms in the crystalline state. At the same time, group frequency correlations tend to be more strictly observed in solvents. The fingerprint region with solutions usually shows less detail, since crystal lattice interactions are missing. For this reason, similarities within a given series may be easier to observe, but two compounds differing in stereochemistry, for example, may be more easily confused than in the case of solid state spectra.

In view of the limited choice of solvents, it is fortunate that infrared spectra can be obtained on crystalline substances. In fact, next to X-ray crystallography, the infrared spectrum of a crystalline substance is probably one of its most characteristic properties. These spectra are obtained by mulling the crystalline material with a few drops of Nujol, in which case the somewhat opaque paste of mixture is spread on a rock salt window in front of the beam. Alternatively, the sample may be intimately ground with potassium bromide. The powdered mixture is then placed into a press and a clear pellet containing the sample is produced. The potassium bromide method has great advantages in economy of sample compared to the mulling technique, but the presence of hydroxyl groups is often obscured, since the potassium bromide itself can easily acquire water during improper storage or handling. The fingerprint region is usually identical in both types of spectra.

In a newer sampling procedure, the material is spread as a thin film over a special plate of infrared-transparent material, and the infrared beam passing through the edge of the plate is reflected many times from the sample film at the surface, thus increasing the total efficiency of absorption. In this method, called attenuated total reflectance, a satisfactory spectrum may be obtained from a minimum amount of sample without the intervention of solvent, and the sample may be recovered by simply rinsing the plate with the same solvent used to deposit the film. In contrast, sample recovery from potassium bromide pellets is often difficult.

Fourier transform methods also promise to increase the sensitivity and the speed with which infrared spectra may be obtained. If proper sample handling systems were available, it seems entirely reasonable to expect that infrared spectra could be obtained even on complex molecules, such as drugs and their metabolites, as they are eluted from a gas chromatograph. This would indeed be an extremely important instrumental development, since infrared is by far the best method to differentiate among the various types of carbonyl groups.

Laser Raman spectroscopy is a recent addition to the spectroscopic tools used for structure determination in organic chemistry. Raman spectroscopy is complementary to infrared spectroscopy, because it can disclose groups, such as carbon-carbon double and triple bonds, sulfur bonds, etc., which are often not detected with infrared spectroscopy. However, even in extremely small amounts, many impurities produce enough fluorescence to completely mask the RAMAN spectrum.

F. Ultraviolet Spectroscopy

(SCOTT, 1964)

Molecules which contain at least one multiple bond or a free electron pair yield a measurable ultraviolet spectrum in the region above 185 mμ. Just as in infrared spectroscopy, the absorption of ultraviolet radiation is due to transitions between different energy levels of the molecule. But, in this case, the energy levels are associated with electronic states rather than vibrational and rotational states.

Unsaturated groups such as C=C, C=O, NO_2, etc. which are responsible for electronic absorption are called chromophores. Auxochromes are groups such as OH, NH_2, Cl, etc. which can supply a free electron pair to the chromophore. Increasing the number of conjugated unsaturated groups in a chromophore, or addition of auxochromes increases the number of electronic states and decreases the energy required to cause a transition between the states. When less energy is required to cause a transition between states, a shift to longer wavelengths (lower energies) is observed. This is known as a "red shift". In a series of conjugated polyenes, the shift in frequency of light absorbed is almost proportional to the number of conjugated double bonds and therefore the extended length of the molecule.

The intensity of absorption in the ultraviolet is a function of the degree to which the excited state differs in electronic symmetry from the ground state; thus absorption of a single double bond is relatively weak, because the excited state is very similar in symmetry to the ground state as might be surmised simply from the appearance of the molecule. On the other hand, absorption of an unsaturated ketone is very strong since the excited state can involve interactions between the π orbitals of the double bond and the π orbitals of the carbonyl, a situation not as important in the ground state. In general, the greater the number of multiple bonds and/or free electron pairs in a chromophore, the greater the intensity of absorption, i.e., the extinction coefficient, and the less sample that will be required for detection.

Much of the field of analytical biochemistry has been devoted to the development of "color" reactions, even though the "color" may only be observed in the ultraviolet region of the spectrum. One of the strong points of ultraviolet spectroscopy is its extreme sensitivity; extinction coefficients tend to be large compared to other forms of spectroscopy, *i.e.* infrared, etc. A second advantage is that a wide variety of solvents, aqueous and nonaqueous, may be employed. Since most inorganic salts do not appreciably absorb ultraviolet light, buffered solutions may also be used. Naturally, when an unshared electron pair undergoes protonation, it can no longer interact as strongly with adjacent double bonds; thus highly characteristic pH dependent changes in the ultraviolet absorption of many drugs can be observed. Furthermore, since such small quantities are required, the sample is essentially at infinite dilution and BEER's law (linear variation in optical density with concentration) is usually obeyed.

Ultraviolet spectroscopy has made its greatest contribution in elucidating structural changes adjacent to a chromophore. Since aromatic rings are chromophores, this technique is particularly relevant to drugs containing such structures. Examples of biotransformations detectable by ultraviolet absorption are: hydroxylation of an aromatic ring, oxidation of a benzylic carbon to a ketone or acid, reduction of an aromatic nitro group, dealkylation of aromatic amines and ethers, and introduction of additional conjugated double bonds.

The hydroxylation of an aliphatic carbon causes only a slight increase in the absorption at very short wavelengths and is therefore usually obscured by the absorption of ultraviolet light by other chromophores. Other metabolic processes, such as dealkylation of aliphatic amines or ethers, also have little effect on the absorption spectrum.

Ultraviolet spectroscopy is usually less sensitive than infrared to impurities from thin layer chromatography isolations; however, interference is sometimes observed due to scattering by silica gel in the far ultraviolet region.

Undoubtedly, ultraviolet spectroscopy will be familiar to all pharmacologists from the time of their earliest training. Since it conveys such easily interpreted data, it will often be the first method to be used in drug metabolism studies. This is, of course, particularly true if the compound has, in fact, undergone a change in ultraviolet spectrum during metabolism, since it is likely that ultraviolet methods will be used to locate the metabolite as it is being isolated. But even when this is not the case, the failure of a drug to exhibit a change in its ultraviolet spectrum provides important information, since it reduces the need to consider a wide variety of biotransformations. Finally, ultraviolet detectors are extremely fast and spectra may be obtained very rapidly. It is surprising therefore that ultraviolet spectrometers have not been combined with gas chromatography, which would undoubtedly be of great use with complex molecules.

G. Optical Rotatory Dispersion and Circular Dichroism

(CRABBÉ, 1965; see also chapter 9, this volume)

Optically active compounds transmit right and left circularly polarized light at unequal velocities resulting in a rotation of the plane of polarization. In contrast to standard optical rotation measurements which measure the rotation at one wavelength (589 mμ, sodium D line), an optical rotatory dispersion (ORD) curve shows the rotation as a function of wavelength (185—700 mμ). For compounds which do not absorb within this range, the ORD curve will consist of a plane curve which increases in rotation with decreasing wavelength. For many compounds, this results in an increase of sensitivity of several orders of magnitude, which permits a corresponding decrease in the amount of sample required.

If a molecule contains a chromophore that interacts with the asymmetric center, measurement of the ORD will give an anomalous curve which will show a peak and a trough in the spectral region in which the chromophore absorbs. This phenomenon results from the combination of unequal absorption and unequal velocity of transmission of left and right circularly polarized light and is called a "COTTON effect." COTTON effects can be used to determine absolute configuration in some types of compounds, *e.g.*, 3-keto steroids, amino acids, etc.

Circular dichroism (CD), which measures the unequal absorption of the left and right circularly polarized light, is also used to detect molecules with optically active chromophores. CD is especially useful for molecules with multiple COTTON effects, since the curves are easier to interpret.

Many enzymatic reactions proceed stereoselectively or stereospecifically. Accordingly, ORD and CD may contribute greatly to the study of those metabolic reactions in which these phenomena are involved.

H. Diazepam Metabolites

The first metabolic application of high resolution mass spectrometry and nuclear magnetic resonance in the authors' laboratories was the study of the metabolites of diazepam (SCHWARTZ et al., 1967).

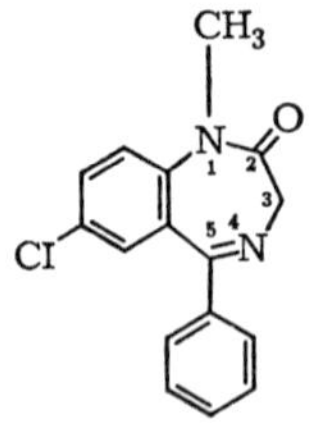

Diazepam

The intestines of a rat pretreated with 25 mg of diazepam-^{3}H intraperitoneally were extracted with ethyl acetate before and after hydrolysis of glucuronides and/or sulfates. Labeled de-esterified products were separated by thin layer chromatography; the silica gel corresponding to each band was scraped off the plate and washed with ethanol to elute the components. Radioactivity was determined in the various eluates, and the radioactive components were subjected to a second thin layer chromatographic separation by a different solvent system. The radioactive components were eluted with alcohol as described above and concentrated; portions of the sample were evaporated to dryness in capillary tubes for mass spectral analysis.

Four metabolites, A, B, C, and D, were isolated. Comparison of their molecular compositions with that of diazepam (Table 2) showed that metabolites

Table 2. *Molecular composition of diazepam metabolites as determined by high resolution mass spectrometry*

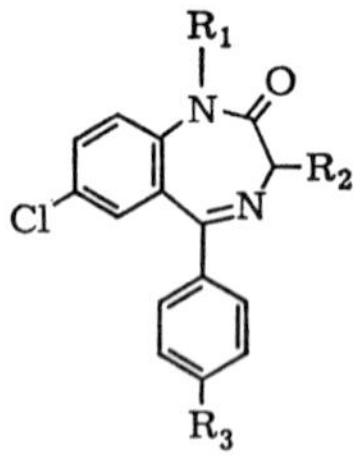

Compound	Molecular ion (m/e) Observed	Calculated	Molecular Composition C	H	N	O	Cl	Structure R_1	R_2	R_3
Diazepam		284.0716	16	13	2	1	1	CH_3	H	H
Met A	300.0685	300.0666	16	13	2	2	1	CH_3	OH	H
Met B	300.0660	300.0666	16	13	2	2	1	CH_3	H	OH
Met C	316.0616	316.0615	16	13	2	3	1	CH_3	OH	OH
Met D	286.0504	286.0509	15	11	2	2	1	H	H	OH

A and B had gained one oxygen, C had gained two oxygens, and D had gained one oxygen and lost one carbon and two hydrogens.

Although metabolites A and B had identical molecular ions, their fragmentation patterns were different. A portion of the computer printout for the high resolution mass spectrum of B is shown in Fig. 1. The absence of a fragment ion at m/e 284 (molecular ion — 16 mass units, M-16), which is a characteristic fragmentation of N-oxides, eliminates the possibility of an N-oxide structure. There is a strong fragment ion at m/e 272 (M-28), which is formed by the loss of CH_2N from the molecular ion. From mass spectral studies on diazepam-3,3-d_2 and other diazepam analogs, it is known that the loss of CH_2N involves C-3 and N-4. There-

Upper Limits of Molecular Composition

Element	*Maximum*
C	16
H	14
N	2
O	2
CL5	1
CL7	1

Mass Output Range 0.01–0.90

(CL5 → Chlorine-35; CL7 → Chlorine-37)

DENS	DIST	MASS	CALC	ERR	C/C13		H	N	O	CL5	CL7	
87	128.2730	185.1529	*									
73	142.3770	207.0329	207.0325	0.38	10	0	8	2	1	1	0	→ M–C_6H_5O
85	146.2035	213.1872	*									
87	148.6010	217.0891	217.0891	–0.04	16	0	11	1	0	0	0	Background
106	149.2165	218.0965	218.0970	–0.44	16	0	12	1	0	0	0	Background
136	149.8305	219.1039	219.1048	–0.86	16	0	13	1	0	0	0	Background
99	171.5215	256.2413	*									
114	179.7215	271.0649	271.0638	1.10	15	0	12	2	1	1	0	→ M–H, CO
232	180.2570	272.0485	272.0478	0.65	15	0	11	1	2	1	0	→ M–H, HCN
144	180.8045	273.0559	273.0557	0.26	15	0	12	1	2	1	0	
134	181.3415	274.0458	274.0449	0.96	15	0	11	1	2	0	1	
70	186.8305	284.2702	*									
166	194.5910	299.0660	299.0587	1.32	16	0	12	2	2	1	0	→ M–H
190	195.1115	300.0660	300.0666	–0.58	16	0	13	2	2	1	0	→ M^+
136	195.6250	301.0600										
100	196.1425	302.0635	302.0636	–0.10	16	0	13	2	2	0	1	

* Impurity peaks

Fig. 1. Computer printout for the high resolution mass spectrum of metabolite B. The first column, DENS, gives a value proportional to the intensity of the darkness of each line on the photoplate; DIST is the distance in mm of each line from a reference point; MASS is the mass calculated from the above distance; CALC is the calculated mass of the elemental composition given in the last columns; ERR is the difference in millimass between the determined mass (MASS) and the mass calculated from the elemental composition (CALC); the elements listed begin with the C-12 and C-13 isotopes of carbon and end with the Cl-35 and Cl-37 isotopes of chlorine. Structural information has been added to this record to aid in interpretation of the data. From SCHWARTZ et al. (1967), copyright Academic Press, Inc.

fore, the presence of the m/e 272 ion eliminates the possibility of a hydroxyl group on C-3. The weak peak at m/e 207 (M-93), which is formed by the loss of C_6H_5O (Fig. 1), suggests that in metabolite B the hydroxyl is on the 5-phenyl ring. The mass spectrum of A did not contain a peak at m/e 272, but a strong peak was observed at m/e 256 (M-CH_2NO). This observation, coupled with the absence of a M-16 peak, identifies metabolite A as 3-hydroxy diazepam.

Similar interpretation of the mass spectrum of metabolite C showed that it contained a hydroxyl group on C-3 and a second hydroxyl group on the 5-phenyl ring. Interpretation of the spectrum of metabolite D indicated that it was the desmethyl analog of metabolite B.

It is very difficult to determine aromatic substitution patterns by mass spectrometry. Therefore, the position of the hydroxyl group on the 5-phenyl ring (*ortho*, *meta*, or *para*) could not be determined from the mass spectra of metabolites B, C, and D.

Nmr, however, readily distinguishes *ortho*, *meta* and *para* disubstituted benzenes. For example, the nmr spectrum of the aromatic protons of metabolite B shows the protons of the 5-phenyl ring (2′, 3′, 5′, 6′) as two distorted doublets (∼ 6.8, 7.4 ppm) with each doublet corresponding to two protons (Fig. 2). This

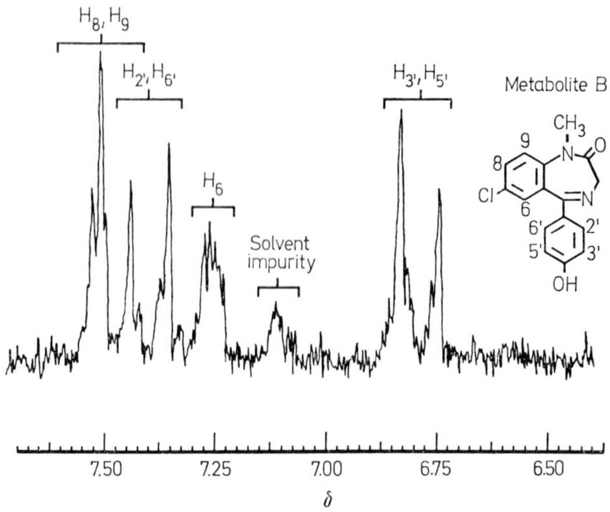

Fig. 2. Nmr spectrum of the aromatic protons of diazepam metabolite B. The spectrum was obtained by signal averaging ~420 μg of metabolite B dissolved in acetone-d_6. From SCHWARTZ et al. (1967), copyright Academic Press, Inc.

pattern is characteristic of a *para* substituted benzene. Similar studies indicated that the structures of the other metabolites are as shown in Table 2.

I. Triprolidine Metabolites

Two metabolites of triprolidine were isolated from *in vitro* studies with the

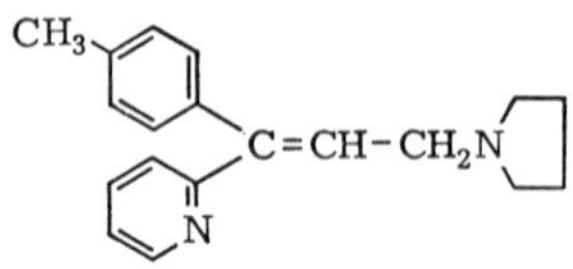

Triprolidine

enzymes of guinea pig liver (KUNTZMAN et al., 1968). Incubation of triprolidine with the liver microsomes and a NADPH-generating system produced metabolite I which still possessed basic properties, while incubation with the 9,000 × *g* supernatant fraction afforded a very polar metabolite, II. Metabolite I could be converted to metabolite II by incubation with the 100,000 × *g* soluble fraction of the guinea pig liver. The samples for spectral analysis were isolated by procedures similar to those described for the diazepam metabolites.

The pertinent ions in the mass spectra of triprolidine, metabolite I and metabolite II are summarized in Table 3. Reasonable bond cleavages that would lead to the observed fragment ions are illustrated in Fig. 3. Study of the mass spectrum of triprolidine revealed that all of the pertinent ions listed in Table 3 contain the tolyl group.

The mass spectrum of metabolite I showed a molecular ion at m/e 294.1734 which corresponded to the addition of one oxygen atom to triprolidine. The molecular composition of metabolite II revealed that the metabolic change involved the addition of two oxygen atoms and the loss of two hydrogen atoms. The mass spectral fragmentation patterns of the two metabolites were very

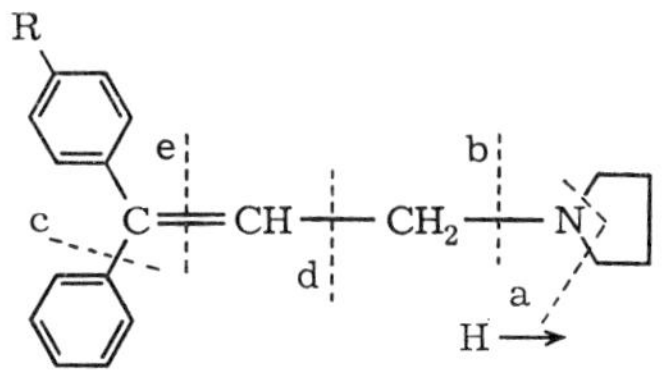

Fig. 3. Mass spectral fragmentations of triprolidine (R=CH_3) and metabolite I (R=CH_2OH) and metabolite II (R=CO_2H). The elemental compositions and masses of the ions are listed in Table 3

similar to that of triprolidine. In fact, all the pertinent ions in triprolidine were observed in the spectrum of metabolite I; however, they appeared at m/e values that were approximately 15.995 amu (equivalent to the mass of one oxygen) higher than the corresponding ions in the triprolidine spectrum. Similarly, the ions in the spectrum of metabolite II were shifted by approximately 29.974 amu (equivalent to two oxygens minus two hydrogens). This means that the metabolic changes in the two metabolites must have occurred in the portion of the molecule that is common to all the ions, namely, the tolyl group. The most reasonable explanation for the data would be the oxidation of the methyl group of triprolidine to CH_2OH (metabolite I) followed by further oxidation to CO_2H (metabolite II). Confirmation was obtained by an nmr spectrum of metabolite I.

The nmr spectra of triprolidine and metabolite I are shown in Fig. 4. The signals at 0.5—1.7 ppm in the spectrum of metabolite I are due to impurities incorporated during the isolation procedure and the signal at ~7.3 ppm is due to undeuterated chloroform in the deuterochloroform solvent. The methyl peak at 2.38 ppm (relative area = three protons) in the spectrum of triprolidine is not present in the spectrum of metabolite I. There is a new singlet at 4.75 ppm which has a relative area of two protons. This evidence, along with the fact that triprolidine and metabolite I have identical ultraviolet spectra, is compatible with the oxidation of the CH_3 to

Table 3. *Pertinent mass spectral data of triprolidine, metabolites I and II*

Ion	Structure[a]	Triprolidine DETM[b]	CALC[c]	C	H	N	Metabolite I DETM	CALC	C	H	N	O	Metabolite II DETM	CALC	C	H	N	O
Molecular ion (M)		278.1758	278.1783	19	22	2	294.1734	294.1732	19	22	2	1	308.1506	308.1525	19	20	2	2
M-H_2O							276.1618	276.1626	19	20	2	0						
M-C_4H_9	a	221.1074	221.1079	15	13	2	237.1055	237.1028	15	13	2	1	251.0860	251.0820	15	11	2	2
M-C_4H_8N	b	208.1143	208.1126	15	14	1	224.1092	224.1075	15	14	1	1	238.0863	238.0868	15	12	1	2
M-C_5H_4N	c	200.1447	200.1439	14	18	1	216.1391	216.1388	14	18	1	1	230.1181	230.1181	14	16	1	2
M-$C_5H_{10}N$	d	194.0939	194.0925	14	12	1	210.0922	210.0919	14	12	1	1	224.0720	224.0712	14	10	1	2
M-C_4H_8N,H_2O							206.0953	206.0970	15	12	1	0						
M-$C_6H_{11}N$	e	181.0902	181.0891	13	11	1	197.0839	197.0841	13	11	1	1	211.0657	211.0633	13	9	1	2

[a] Probable bond cleavages leading to these ions are given in Fig. 3.
[b] DETM is the mass determined from the observed data.
[c] CALC is the calculated mass of the combination of elements which are given in the next column.

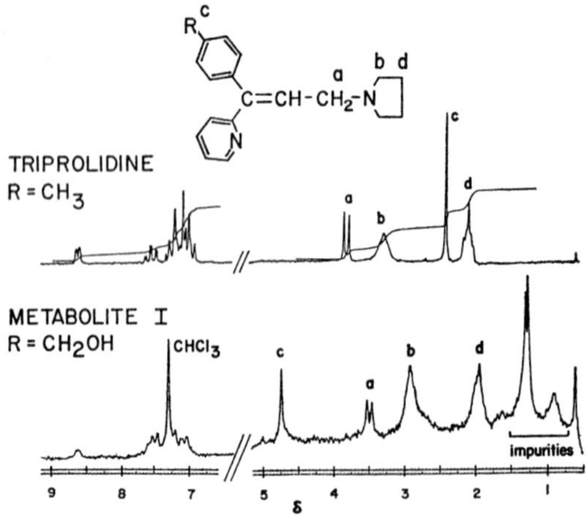

Fig. 4. The nmr spectra of triprolidine and metabolite I. The spectrum of metabolite I was obtained by averaging 25 scans of ~200 μg dissolved in deuterochloroform

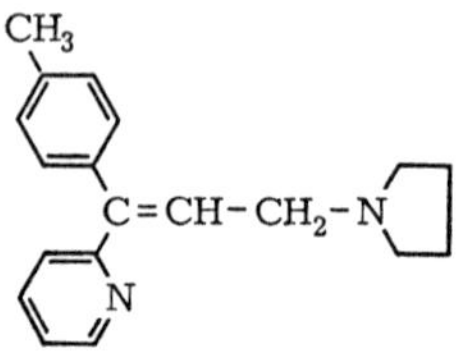

Triprolidine

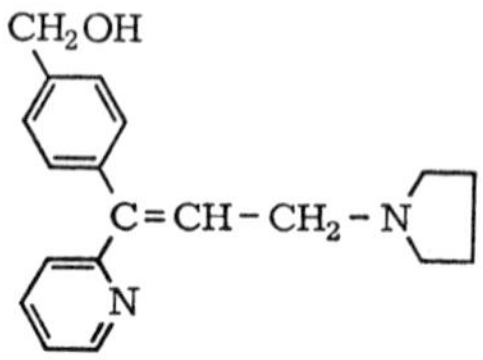

Metabolite I

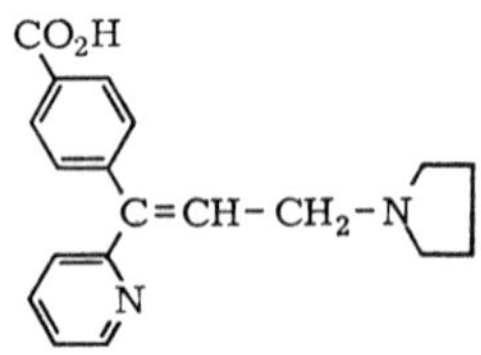

Metabolite II

Fig. 5. Structure of triprolidine and metabolites

CH_2OH. Further oxidation of the CH_2OH to a COOH would lead to metabolite II. The structures are summarized in Fig. 5.

References

Bhacca, N.S., Williams, D.H.: Applications of nmr spectroscopy in organic chemistry. Illustrations from the steroid field. San Francisco-London-Amsterdam: Holden-Day, Inc. 1964.

Biemann, K.: Mass spectrometry. Organic chemical applications. New York-San Francisco-Toronto-London: McGraw-Hill Book Company, Inc. 1962.

Bovey, F.A.: Nuclear magnetic resonance spectroscopy. New York: Academic Press 1969.

Budzikiewicz, H., Djerassi, C., Williams, D.H.: Mass spectrometry of organic compounds. San Francisco-Cambridge-London-Amsterdam: Holden-Day, Inc. 1967.

Colthup, N.B., Daly, L.H., Wiberley, S.E.: Introduction to infrared and Raman spectroscopy. New York-London: Academic Press 1964.

Crabbé, P.: Optical rotatory dispersion and circular dichroism in organic chemistry. San Francisco-London-Amsterdam: Holden-Day, Inc. 1965.

HERZBERG, G.: Molecular spectra and molecular structure, II: Infrared and RAMAN spectra of polyatomic molecules. Princeton-Toronto-New York-London: D. Van Nostrand Company, Inc. 1945.

KUNTZMAN, R., SERNATINGER, E., TSAI, I., KLUTCH, A.: New methodology for studies of drug metabolism. In: Importance of fundamental principles in drug evaluation. New York: Raven Press 1968.

McLAFFERTY, F.W.: Interpretation of mass spectra. New York-Amsterdam: W.A. Benjamin, Inc. 1967.

SANDERS, J.K.M., WILLIAMS, D.H.: A shift reagent for use in nuclear magnetic resonance spectroscopy. A first-order spectrum of n-hexanol. Chem. Comm. **7**, 422 (1970).

SCHWARTZ, M.A., BOMMER, P., VANE, F.M.: Diazepam metabolites in the rat: characterization by high resolution mass spectrometry and nuclear magnetic resonance. Arch. Biochem. **121**, 508—516 (1967).

SCOTT, A.I.: Interpretation of the ultraviolet spectra of natural products. New York: Pergamon Press 1964.

WANGEN, L.E., ISENHOUR, T.L.: Semiquantitative analysis of mixed gamma-ray spectra by computerized learning machines. Anal. Chem. **42**, 737—743 (1970).

Selected references to additional studies using spectroscopic methods for structure determination of drug metabolites

ARNOLD, W., GRÜTZMACHER, H.F.: Die Identifizierung von Barbituratmetaboliten mittels Massenspecktrometrie und Infrarot-Spektrum. Arch. Toxikol. **25**, 200—215 (1969).

CHANG, T., SAVORY, A., GLAZKO, A.J.: A new metabolite of 5,5-diphenylhydantoin (Dilantin). Biochem. biophys. Res. Commun. **38**, 444—449 (1970).

DREYFUSS, J., COHEN, A.I., HESS, S.M.: Metabolism of thiazesim, 5-(2-dimethyl-aminoethyl)-2,3-dihydro-2-phenyl-1,5-benzothiazepin-4(5H)-one, in the rat *in vivo* and *in vitro*. J. pharm. Sci. **57**, 1505—1511 (1968).

GALPIN, D.R., COCHRAN, T.G., HUITRIC, A.C.: Application of nuclear magnetic resonance and optical rotatory dispersion to studies in drug metabolism-stereoselectivity in the metabolism of *trans*-2-*p*-tolyl-cyclohexanol and *trans*-2-*o*-tolylcyclohexanol in the rat. Biochem. Pharmacol. **18**, 979—991 (1969).

PALMER, K.H., FOWLER, M.S., WALL, M.E., RHODES, L.S., WADDELL, W.J., BAGGETT, B.: The metabolism of R(+)- and RS-pentobarbital. J. Pharmacol. exp. Ther. **170**, 355—363 (1969).

SCHWARTZ, M.A., VANE, F.M., POSTMA, E.: Chlordiazepoxide metabolites in the rat. Characterization by high resolution mass spectrometry. Biochem. Pharmacol. **17**, 965—974 (1968).

— — — Urinary metabolites of 7-chloro-1-(2-diethylaminoethyl)-5-(2-fluorophenyl)-1,3-dihydro-2H-1,4-benzodiazepin-2-one dihydrochloride. J. med. Chem. **11**, 770—774 (1968).

SMITH, D.L., GROSTIC, M.F.: Mass spectrometric identification of the metabolites of methyl N-(*o*-aminophenyl)-N-(3-dimethylaminopropyl) anthranilate. J. med. Chem. **10**, 375—379 (1967).

Section Five: Sites of Drug Metabolism

Chapter 35

Introduction: Pathways of Drug Metabolism

R.T. WILLIAMS

When drugs enter the body, the majority of them are metabolized and transformed partly or wholly into other substances. These transformations are catalysed by enzymes which are found mainly in the liver, although they are also found in lesser amounts in other tissues such as intestine, kidney and lung. Although the majority of drugs are metabolized in the body there are some which are not metabolized at all and are excreted unchanged, whereas there are others which change spontaneously into other substances without the participation of enzymes. From the point of view of their fate in the body drugs can therefore be divided broadly into three types as follows:

a) drugs which undergo enzyme catalysed transformations

b) drugs which are not metabolized and are excreted unchanged

c) drugs which undergo spontaneous reactions when given the appropriate physical conditions such as pH or when they contact a suitable physiological compound with which they can react.

The majority of drugs belong to type *a*, but some drugs can undergo a combination of enzyme catalysed and spontaneous reactions. Although enzyme catalysed reactions are carried out by the tissues of the body, it is now becoming clear that some transformations of drugs can also be carried out by the gut flora (SCHELINE, 1968).

A. The Biphasic Metabolism of Drugs

The reactions which drugs undergo can be classified as oxidations, reductions, hydrolyses and syntheses. Because of the nature of these reactions and the biological activity of the products, it is convenient to regard the metabolism of drugs as occurring generally in two phases (WILLIAMS, 1959). The oxidations, reductions and hydrolyses occur in the first phase and can result in

1. the inactivation of a drug
2. the conversion of an initially inactive compound into an active drug
3. the conversion of an active drug into another active drug.

The second phase of drug metabolism consists of synthetic reactions, most of which convert active compounds into inactive excretory products. This concept of drug metabolism can be represented as follows:

Drug	Phase I ——————→ activation or inactivation	Oxidation reduction and/or hydrolysis products	Phase II ——————→ inactivation	synthetic or conjugation products

Phase I reactions usually introduce into the drug molecule groups such as OH, COOH and NH_2 which enable the phase I products to undergo the synthetic reactions frequently referred to as conjugations. If the drug already contains any of the above groups, e.g. phenol, then it can undergo conjugation directly without the intervention of a phase I reaction. Sometimes, a drug may undergo only phase I reactions as in the case of ethanol, which is oxidized mainly to CO_2.

In both phases the polarity of the drug is usually increased; the products of phase II are strong organic acids and, occasionally, strong organic bases, which are readily excreted. To illustrate let us consider the metabolism of the well-known antipyretic and analgesic drug, phenacetin (SMITH and WILLIAMS, 1949). This drug is a neutral lipid-soluble compound which is oxidatively de-ethylated in the first phase of its metabolism to the weak acid, *p*-acetamidophenol, which has a pKa of about 10. In the second phase, *p*-acetamidophenol is conjugated mainly with glucuronic acid to give *p*-acetamidophenylglucuronide which is a strong acid with a pKa of about 3.5. At the pH of the blood this glucuronide is virtually completely ionized, highly water-soluble and readily excreted by the kidney.

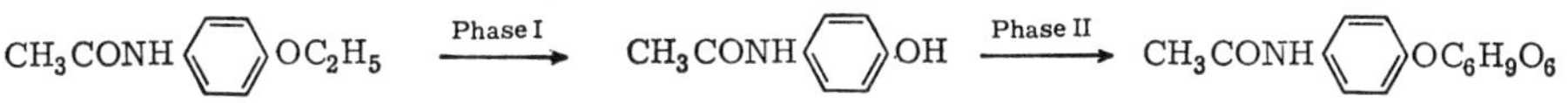

Phenacetin neutral | (ionization at pH 7.4) | *p*-acetamidophenol pKa ca. 10, ca. 0.25% | *p*-acetamidophenylglucuronide pKa ca. 3.5, 99.99%

It appears, therefore, that drugs are metabolized in the body along pathways which tend to lead to the formation of water-soluble, polar compounds which are readily excreted. Both phenacetin and its phase I metabolite, *p*-acetamidophenol, are active drugs but the activity of phenacetin is largely due to this metabolite. The phase II metabolite, *p*-acetamidophenylglucuronide, is an inactive excretory product and its formation terminates the activity of phenacetin.

B. Phase I Reactions

The reactions of drugs which can be classified as oxidations, reductions and hydrolyses are carried out by enzymes which occur predominantly in the liver, although some metabolizing activity is also to be found in extrahepatic tissues such as the kidney and intestinal tissue and to a lesser extent in the lungs, adrenals and blood. The majority of these reactions are carried out by enzymes located in the endoplasmic reticulum of the hepatic cells (BRODIE et al., 1955; GILLETTE, 1963). On homogenization of the liver, the endoplasmic reticulum is disrupted, giving rise to small vesicles which can be separated from the homogenate by high-speed centrifugation to give the fraction called microsomes. Many of the reactions of drugs can be carried out *in vitro* with the microsomes and suitable co-factors, particularly reduced nicotinamide-adenine dinucleotide phosphate (NADPH).

The oxidative reactions carried out by the microsomes have been extensively studied (GILLETTE, 1963, 1966) and it has been shown that the oxidizing system contains at least two catalysts, namely the NADPH-oxidizing flavoprotein, known as NADPH-cytochrome c reductase and a CO-binding haemoprotein called cytochrome P-450 (see chapter 38, this volume). Microsomal oxidation of drugs has a specific requirement for NADPH and molecular oxygen and the system fits into the category of mixed-function oxidases. Detailed accounts of the microsomal and nonmicrosomal enzyme systems are given in the succeeding chapters. What follows is a brief account of the main pathways of drug metabolism.

I. Oxidative Reactions

The oxidative reactions carried out by the liver microsomes are many and varied and they include the following types.

1. The Oxidation of Aromatic Rings

Aromatic rings are oxidized to produce phenols (see chapter 39). This reaction is usually referred to as aromatic hydroxylation and is one of the most intensely studied of microsomal reactions. It occurs with carbocyclic and heterocyclic aromatic systems and the main site of oxidation is usually, but not always, that of highest electron density; consequently the oxidation is orientated. The oxidation may occur at more than one site so that more than one monophenol and some polyphenols may be produced. Aniline, for example, gives rise to two monophenols and is hydroxylated *in vivo* in both the *ortho* and *para* positions thus:

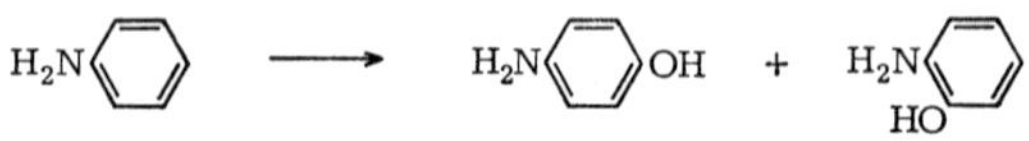

Benzene is hydroxylated mainly to phenol and to a lesser exent to the polyphenols, catechol, quinol and hydroxyquinol:

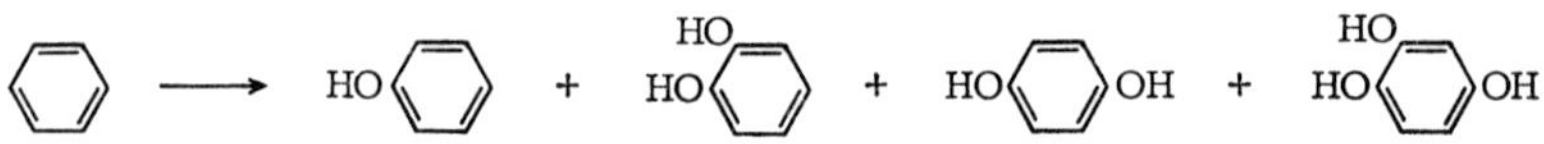

2. The Oxidation of Alkyl Chains

Compounds containing alkyl chains can be oxidized in the body with the production of primary, secondary or tertiary alcohols, the nature of the alcohol produced depending upon the location of the oxidation in the alkyl chain and upon the nature of the alkyl group. Oxidation usually occurs at the ω or (ω-1) carbon atom. If the attack occurs at the ω position of a chain, then further oxidation to a carboxylic acid can occur. These reactions can be summarized as follows:

a) $RCH_2CH_3 \longrightarrow RCH_2CH_2OH \longrightarrow RCH_2COOH$ (ω oxidation)
b) $RCH_2CH_3 \longrightarrow RCHOHCH_3$ ((ω-1) oxidation)
c) $RR'R''CH \longrightarrow RR'R''COH$ (tertiary alcohol formation)

where R, R′, R″ are alkyl groups.

d) Oxidation of compounds containing cycloalkane rings, the products in this case being secondary alcohols.

Examples of the above reactions are given below.

a) ω Oxidation: 5-Ethyl-5-hydroxyethylbarbituric acid is a minor metabolite of barbital (B = barbiturate ring system).

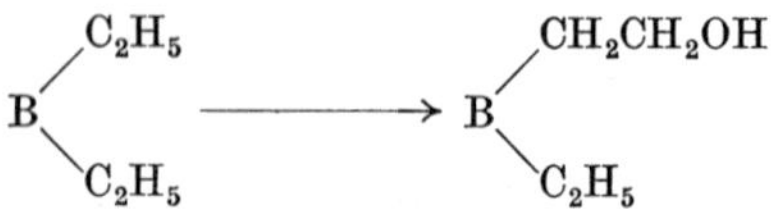

b) (ω-1) Oxidation: 5-Ethyl-5(3′-hydroxy-1′-methylbutyl)barbituric acid is a metabolite of pentobarbital.

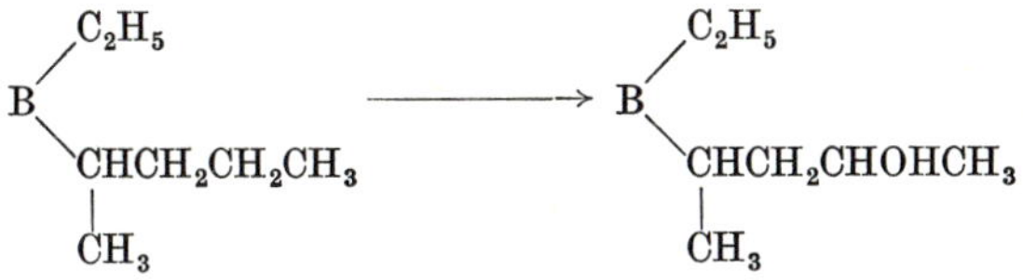

c) *Tertiary alcohol formation:* 5-Ethyl-5-(3′-hydroxyisoamyl)barbituric acid is a metabolite of amobarbital.

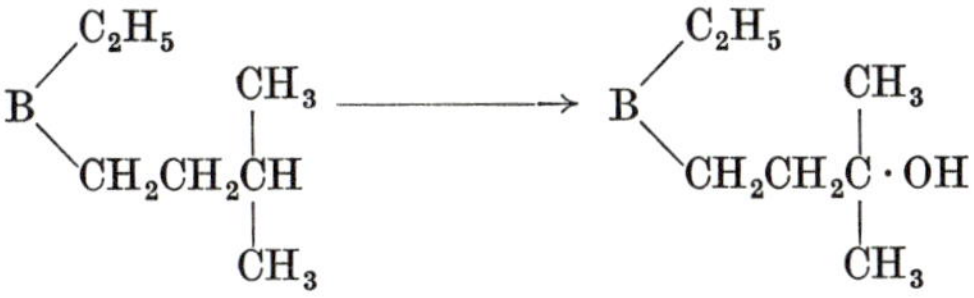

d) *Cycloalkane oxidation:* Cyclohexanol is a metabolite of cyclohexane.

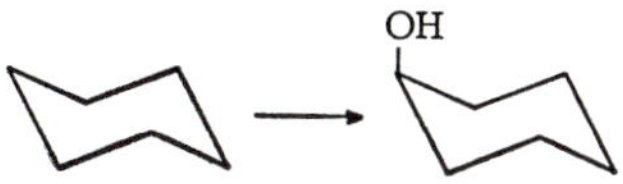

3. Oxidative Dealkylation

Alkyl groups, particularly methyl groups, can be oxidatively removed by liver microsomes when they are attached through oxygen (*O*-methyl), nitrogen (*N*-methyl) or sulphur (*S*-methyl) (see chapter 41). The reactions can be represented as follows:

$$ROCH_3 \longrightarrow ROCH_2OH \longrightarrow ROH + HCHO$$
$$RR'NCH_3 \longrightarrow RR'NCH_2OH \longrightarrow RR'NH + HCHO$$

where R′ = H or CH_3.

The initial step is apparently the oxidation of the methyl group to hydroxymethyl which is then lost as formaldehyde and eventually oxidized to CO_2. Ethyl groups can be oxidized in a similar manner, and released as acetaldehyde which is then metabolized *via* acetate mainly to CO_2. Examples of these reactions are the *O*-demethylation of codeine (3-methylmorphine) to morphine, the *N*-demethylation of imipramine to desmethylimipramine (desipramine) and the *O*-de-ethylation of phenacetin to *p*-acetamidophenol. *S*-Demethylation ($—S\ CH_3 \longrightarrow —SH$) also occurs, possibly by a similar mechanism, an example being the demethylation of 4-methylmercaptopurine to 4-thiopurine.

4. N-Oxidation

Primary, secondary and tertiary amines are oxidized in the body and these reactions can be carried out by liver microsomes (see chapter 40). The primary and secondary amines give rise to hydroxylamines and the tertiary amines to amine oxides:

a) $RNH_2 \longrightarrow RNHOH$
b) $RR'NH \longrightarrow RR'NOH$
c) $RR'R''N \longrightarrow RR'R''NO$

where R, R′, and R″ are usually alkyl groups although one of them can be an aryl group (see below).

The first reaction (a) occurs frequently with arylamines such as aniline, *p*-chloraniline and *p*-phenetidine and carcinogenic amines such as 2-naphthylamine, 4-aminobiphenyl and 4-aminostilbene. The second reaction (b) has been found with *N*-methylaniline and its ethyl and butyl homologues and the third (c) with trimethylamine, chlorpromazine and *N*,*N*-dimethyltryptamine.

N-Hydroxylation has also been found to occur with urethane ($EtOCONH_2$) and also with the carcinogen acetamidofluorene, an acetylated primary amine; thus the following reactions can be added to a—c above:

d) $ROCONH_2 \longrightarrow ROCONHOH$
e) $ArNHCOCH_3 \longrightarrow ArN(OH)COCH_3$

5. Sulphoxidation

This reaction consists of the oxidation by microsomes of divalent sulphur, especially in a heterocyclic system, to the sulphoxide and sometimes to the sulphone.

$$>S \longrightarrow >SO \longrightarrow >SO_2$$

Examples are chlorpromazine and other phenothiazines which are oxidized to the corresponding 5-oxides and in some cases to the sulphones.

6. Replacement of S by O

This reaction, which is carried out by the liver microsomes, is of considerable importance in the activity of some types of organo-phosphorus insecticides (see chapter 43). It also occurs to some extent during the metabolism of certain thiobarbiturates which are partly converted to the corresponding oxybarbiturates. There are therefore at least two kinds of reactions under this heading, namely the conversion of P=S to P=O and of C=S to C=O.

For the organo-phosphorus insecticides the reaction is

$$R'O-P(OR)_2{=}S \longrightarrow R'O-P(OR)_2{=}O$$

an example being the conversion of parathion (R = Et; R′ = $C_6H_4NO_2$) to paraoxon which is an active metabolite. A thiobarbiturate which undergoes the reaction C=S ⟶ C=O is thiopental, which is partly converted *in vivo* to pentobarbital.

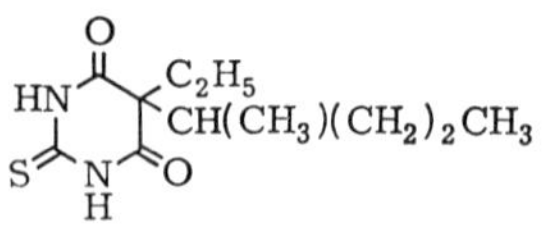

Thiopental

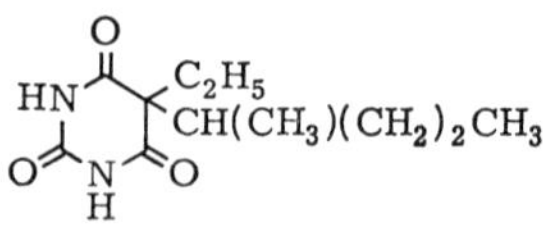

Pentobarbital

7. Epoxidation

This reaction consists of the enzymic addition of oxygen across a double bond (see chapter 39). It has been found to occur with aromatic compounds such as naphthalene and probably benzene and certain organo-chlorine insecticides such as heptachlor and aldrin. The reaction, which is carried out by liver microsomes in the presence of molecular oxygen and NADPH, is as follows:

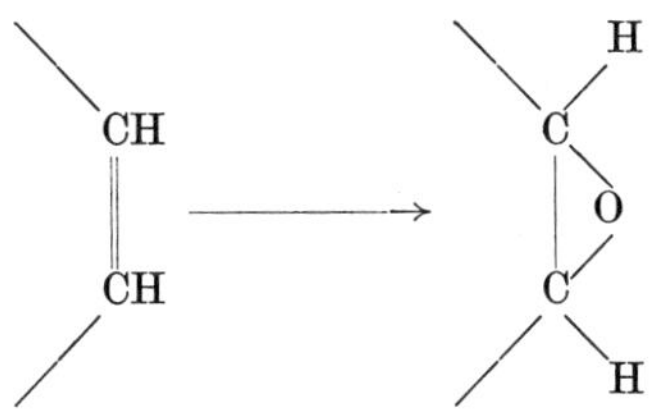

It is probably the initial method of oxidative attack on an aromatic system, since the epoxide can give rise to a phenol by rearrangement, to a dihydrodiol by the enzymic addition of water, and to a glutathione conjugate by reaction with glutathione in the presence of a suitable enzyme (see JERINA et al., 1968).

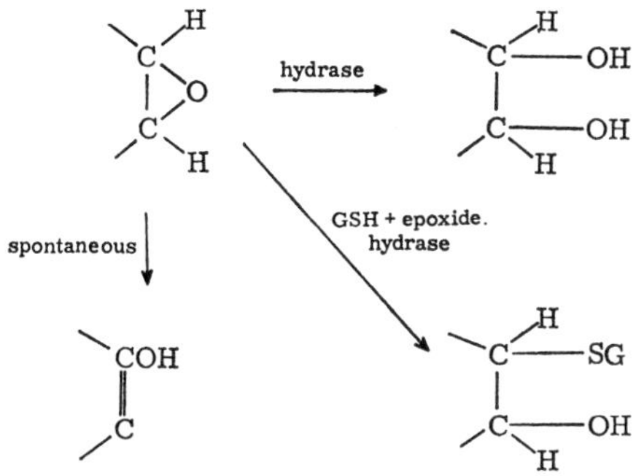

II. Reductions

Several types of reductive reactions of drugs are now known to occur in the body, some of which are now being intensively studied (GILLETTE, 1966) and are described in detail in chapter 42. The reactions which are most frequently encountered are the following:

a) The reduction of nitro compounds to amines, which occurs in several steps
$RNO_2 \longrightarrow RNO \longrightarrow RNHOH \longrightarrow RNH_2$

b) The reduction of azo compounds to amines
$RN:NR' \longrightarrow RNHNHR' \longrightarrow RNH_2 + R'NH_2$

c) The reduction of ketones to secondary alcohols
$RCOR' \longrightarrow RCHOHR'$

Examples of the above reactions are (a) the reduction of aromatic nitro compounds such as chloramphenicol, nitrobenzene, 2,4,6-trinitrotoluene and *p*-nitrobenzoic acid. The reduction of nitro compounds is partly carried out by liver microsomes which contain an enzyme system called nitro-reductase. Both 4-hydroxylamino- and 4-amino-2,6-dinitrotoluene have been shown to be urinary metabolites of T.N.T. (CHANNON et al., 1944).

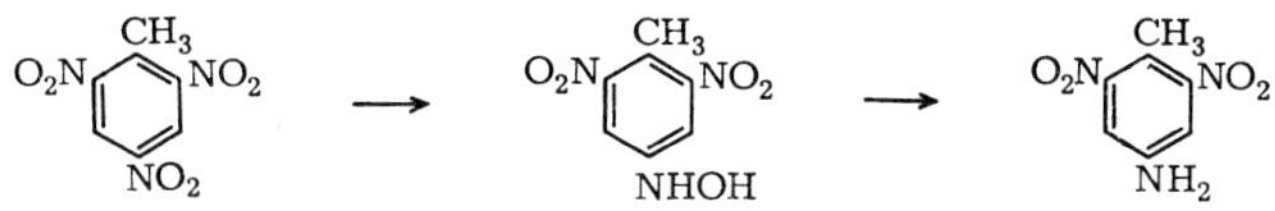

TNT

b) The reduction of drugs such as Prontosil and Neoprontosil to sulphanilamide which is responsible for the antibacterial activity of the parent drugs. Liver microsomes contain the enzyme azoreductase which reduces these drugs, but there is now evidence that these azo drugs and azo dyes used for food colouring can also be reduced by the gut flora.

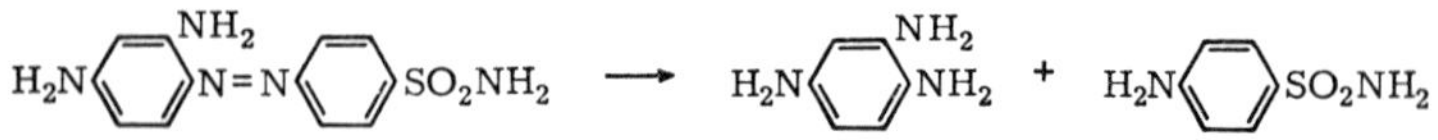

Prontosil Sulphanilamide

c) Ketones such as acetophenone and propiophenone are readily reduced in the body to the corresponding secondary alcohol, methyl phenyl carbinol and ethyl phenyl carbinol, respectively. The reduction is asymmetric since only one optical form of the secondary alcohol is produced.

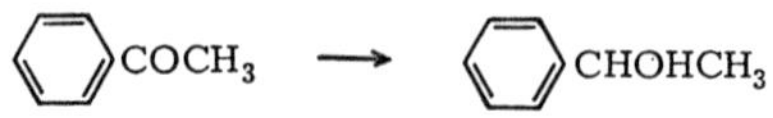

Acetophenone (-)Methyl phenyl carbinol

In addition to these, other reductive reactions are seen less frequently; for example, some aldehydes are reduced to primary alcohols, a well-known case being the conversion of chloral hydrate to trichloroethanol; occasionally double bonds are reduced; pentavalent arsenicals are reduced to the trivalent forms; and compounds containing disulphide links are reduced to the corresponding sulphydryl derivatives:

d) $RCHO \longrightarrow RCH_2OH$
e) $RCH{:}CHR' \longrightarrow RCH_2CH_2R'$
f) $R \cdot AsO(OH)_2 \longrightarrow RAsO$
g) $RS \cdot SR' \longrightarrow RSH + R'SH$

III. Hydrolyses

The commonest types of hydrolyses which occur in the body are those of esters and amides (see chapter 50).

a) $ROCOR' \longrightarrow ROH + R'COOH$
b) $RCONH_2 \longrightarrow RCOOH + NH_3$

A large number of drugs are esters of various kinds and many are hydrolysed in the body to yield phenols, alcohols and carboxylic acids. The enzymes which carry out these reactions are widely distributed, occurring not only in liver microsomes but also in the plasma and other tissues. Furthermore these enzymes vary widely from tissue to tissue and with species and strain. The variation in their occurrence in different species has been of value in the design of insecticides and their variation within a species is of considerable interest in pharmacogenetics.

C. Conjugations or Phase II Reactions

Foreign compounds containing suitable chemical groups such as OH, NH_2 and COOH, phase I metabolites of drugs and many natural metabolites of the body can undergo synthetic reactions called conjugations (WILLIAMS, 1967a) which usually result in their detoxication. Conjugation means the union or coupling of two substances in the body and detoxication implies that the toxicity of a compound has been reduced or abolished. The conjugation product is thus made up of two parts, one the foreign compound or its phase I metabolite and the other a compound provided by the organism and referred to as a conjugating agent. The conjugating agents are derived mainly from the body's carbohydrate and protein sources. For example *p*-acetamidophenol, the phase I active metabolite of phenacetin, is converted in the body by synthesis into *p*-acetamidophenylglucuronide. The conjugating agent in this case is glucuronic acid which is provided by the body *via* glucose from its carbohydrate sources. The conjugation product, *p*-acetamidophenylglucuronide, is readily excreted and shows no pharmacological activity. There are ten major conjugation reactions and all of these except two occur in man.

I. Types of Conjugation Reactions

1. Glucuronic Acid Conjugation

This reaction is the most widespread of the conjugation reactions and can occur with compounds containing all the commonly reactive groups, that is OH, COOH, NH_2 and SH (DUTTON, 1966, see also chapter 45). These compounds include alcohols, phenols, carboxylic acids (mainly aromatic), amines, amides, certain sulphonimides (—SO_2NH—), thiols and dithioic acids (CSSH). The products are *β*-D-glucuronides of the general structure

RX·CH(CHOH)$_3$CHCOOH (ring: —O— linking the two CH)

where X is O, —N(|), —NH or S.

2. Glucoside Conjugation

This occurs mainly in insects (SMITH, 1968) with compounds containing OH groups, the conjugates being *β*-glucosides of the structure

RO·CH(CHOH)$_3$CHCH$_2$OH (ring: —O— linking the two CH)

3. Hippuric Acid Synthesis

The conjugating agent in this reaction is glycine and the synthesis occurs mainly with aromatic acids which form conjugates of the general structure, RCONHCH$_2$COOH; the simplest example is the conversion of benzoic acid to hippuric acid

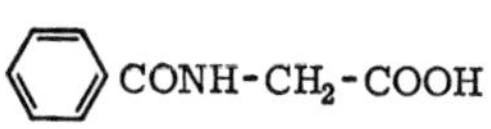

4. Mercapturic Acid Synthesis

Mercapturic acids (BOYLAND and CHASSEAUD, 1969, see also chapter 55) are derivatives of *N*-acetylcysteine, R · S CH$_2$CH(NHCOCH$_3$)COOH, the cysteine moiety being derived from glutathione. The formation of mercapturic acid has now been found to occur with a wide variety of foreign compounds which include aromatic hydrocarbons, arylamines, aryl, alkyl and aralkyl halides, aryl and alkyl nitro compounds, certain phenols, esters, unsaturated carboxylic acids, etc. In most cases, these compounds react with glutathione under the influence of one of the many *S*-glutathione transferases to give a glutathione conjugate which is converted in a series of enzymically controlled reactions to a cysteine derivative, R · S CH$_2$CH(NH$_2$)COOH. The final step involves the acetylation of the cysteine derivative to the mercapturic acid.

5. Ornithuric Acid Synthesis

When benzoic acid is given to hens it appears in the urine mainly as *N*,*N'*-dibenzoylornithine,

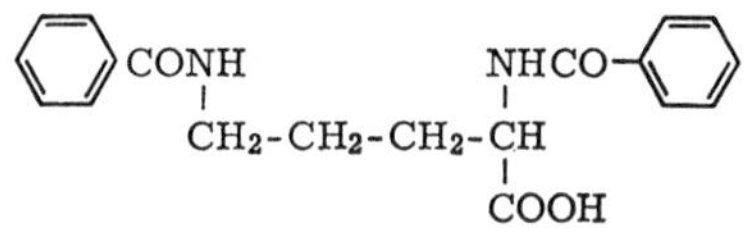

and not as hippuric acid as found in mammals. The reaction occurs with aromatic acids in certain birds and reptiles, but not in pigeons and doves which conjugate aromatic acids with glycine as do mammals (BALDWIN et al., 1960).

6. Glutamine Conjugation

This conjugation is also peculiar to certain species and occurs only with certain compounds; for example, the main metabolite of phenylacetic acid in man is phenacetylglutamine:

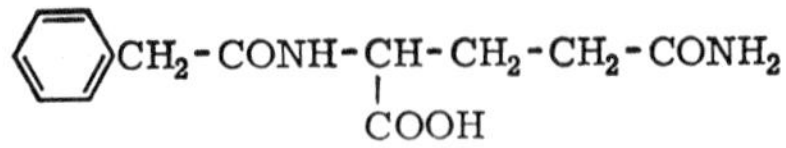

It has been found to occur in Old and New World monkeys, but not in any other species lower on the evolutionary scale. Whilst man and the Old World monkeys conjugate phenylacetic acid only with glutamine, it has been found recently in the author's laboratory that New World monkeys may conjugate the acid with both glutamine and glycine, producing both phenacetylglutamine and phenaceturic acid, whereas lower animals conjugate it only with glycine. Glutamine conjugation has been found so far to occur only with phenylacetic acid, indolyl-3-acetic acid, diphenylmethoxyacetic acid (a metabolite of diphenylhydramine in the rhesus monkey) and 3,4-dihydroxy-5-methoxyphenylacetic acid (a metabolite of mescaline in man).

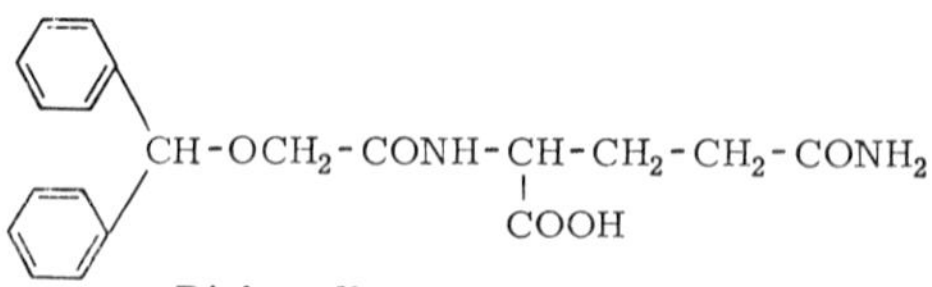

Diphenylhydramine metabolite

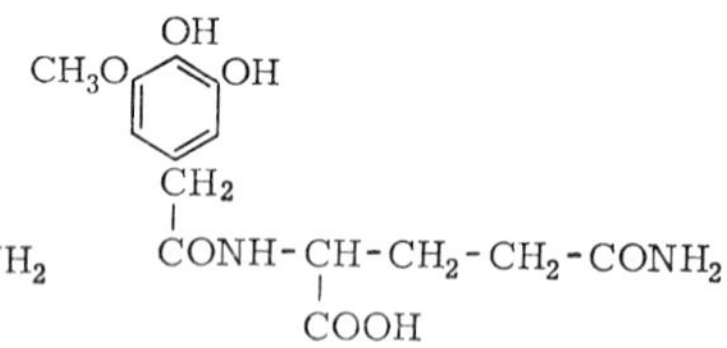

Mescaline metabolite

7. Ethereal Sulphate Synthesis

This reaction consists of the conjugation of a hydroxy compound with sulphate to produce an acid ester of sulphuric acid (see chapter 53). It is largely a reaction of phenols:

$$ArOH + SO_4^{2-} \longrightarrow ArOSO_3H$$

However it has been found also to be a minor reaction of some aliphatic alcohols and aromatic amines, the latter being converted into sulphamates:

$$ArNH_2 \longrightarrow ArNHSO_3H$$

It is a reaction which is widespread among species, except the pig and possibly the hamster.

8. The Cyanide Detoxication

Most conjugation reactions occur either with several types of compounds, e.g. glucuronic conjugation, or with several compounds of the same type, e.g. glutamine conjugation. The conjugation of cyanide to form thiocyanate, however, is limited to the cyanide ion alone, i.e. $CN^- \rightarrow SCN^-$. The reaction is enzymic, the donor of sulphur being thiosulphate and the enzyme, thiosulphate sulphurtransferase (rhodanese). The reaction is widespread among species and the conversion of cyanide to thiocyanate involves a 200-fold reduction in toxicity. Despite this, the process must be inefficient since cyanide is a highly toxic compound.

9. Methylation

Several types of compounds can be methylated in the body (see chapter 56). These compounds, however, must contain OH, SH and NH_2 or substituted NH_2 groups. The nitrogen atom in aromatic nitrogen heterocycles can also be methylated *in vivo*, to give rise to a quaternary nitrogen cation. The methylation of free or substituted amino groups has been observed mainly with endogenous amines containing aliphatic groups. Methylation of aromatic amines may not occur. Examples of these methylations are the conversion of the primary amine, noradrenaline to adrenaline, of the secondary amine, guanidoacetic acid to creatine and of the tertiary amine, dimethylaminoethanol to the quaternary base, choline. These reactions can be written in the general form:

$$\begin{aligned} RNH_2 &\longrightarrow RNHCH_3 \\ RR'NH &\longrightarrow RR'NCH_3 \\ RR'R''N &\longrightarrow RR'R''\overset{+}{N}CH_3 \end{aligned}$$

Methylation of heterocyclic nitrogen is a minor reaction of pyridine, quinoline and isoquinoline which are converted in the corresponding *N*-methyl quaternary bases.

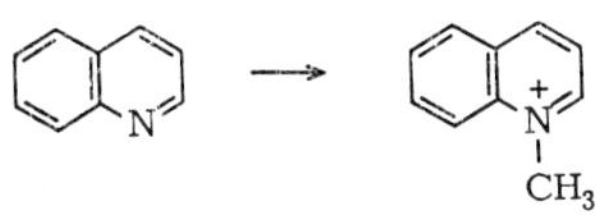

The hydroxy compounds which are methylated *in vivo* are usually phenols. However, the methylation of monophenols is relatively rare, examples being the conversion of *N*-acetylserotonin to melatonin and of 4-hydroxy-3,5-diiodobenzoic acid to the corresponding 4-methoxy acid in man. Methylation is more characteristic of polyphenols, provided at least two of the hydroxyl groups are vicinal.

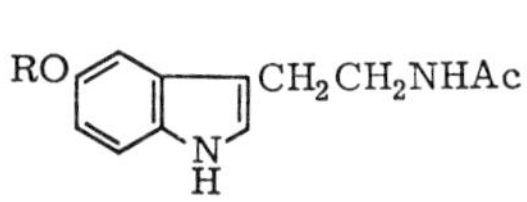

N-Acetylserotonin (R=H)
Melatonin ($R=CH_3$)

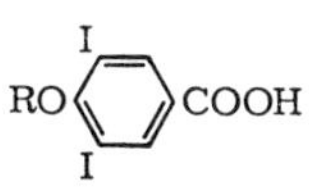

4-Hydroxy-3,5-diiodo-benzoic acid (R=H)
4-Methoxy metabolite ($R=CH_3$)

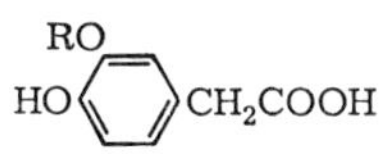

Homoprotocatechuic acid (R=H)
Homovanillic acid ($R=CH_3$)

O-Methylation is therefore a reaction of catechols, but only one hydroxyl is methylated, usually the one which is *meta* to a substituent. Well-known examples are the methylation of adrenaline to metanephrine and of homoprotocatechuic acid to homovanillic acid. In some instances, methylation of the *para* hydroxyl group occurs to a minor extent since homoisovanillic acid is a minor metabolite of homoprotocatechuic acid.

Sulphydryl groups are also potentially capable of being methylated *in vivo*. Thus thiouracil is converted *in vivo* to *S*-methylthiouracil to a small extent; there is evidence that ethylmercaptan is also methylated *in vivo* since ethyl methyl sulphone is a metabolite of diethyldisulphide (see below).

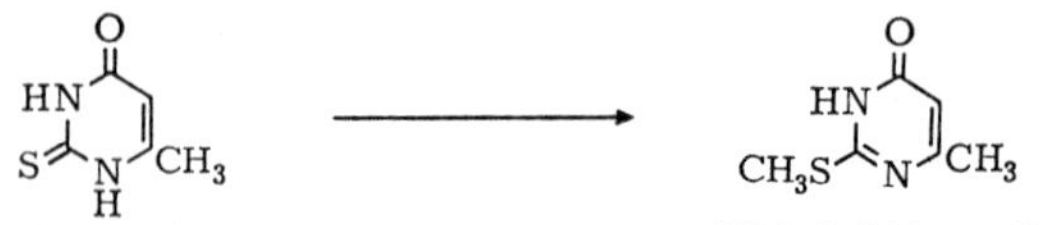

Thiouracil → S-Methylthiouracil

$C_2H_5SSC_2H_5$ Diethyldisulphide → C_2H_5SH Ethylthiol → $C_2H_5SCH_3$ Ethylmethyl sulphide → $C_2H_5SOCH_3$ Ethylmethyl sulphoxide → $C_2H_5SO_2CH_3$ Ethyl methyl sulphone

These methylations are catalysed by specific methyl transferases which determine to which acceptor molecule the methyl group is transferred. The methyl donor, *S*-adenosylmethionine, appears to be common to all methylations.

10. Acetylation

Acetylation is mainly a reaction of NH_2 groups (see chapter 54). The acetylation of OH and SH groups in specific compounds is known, but it is not a general reaction of such groups; the known instances of *O*- and *S*-acetylation are the conversion of choline to acetylcholine and of CoA to acetyl-CoA, respectively.

There are at least five types of NH_2 groups which can be acetylated *in vivo* and these are listed as follows.

a) Aliphatic Amine (RNH_2 where R = alkyl group). An example is histamine which is partly converted into acetylhistamine in the body:

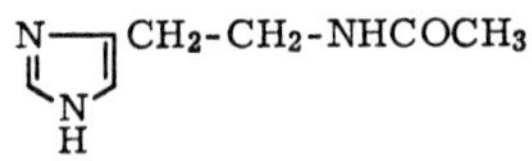

b) Certain Amino Acids (—$CH(NH_2)COOH$). *S*-Phenylcysteine is acetylated in the body to give phenylmercapturic acid or *N*-acetyl-*S*-phenylcysteine. The guinea pig appears to be defective in this reaction.

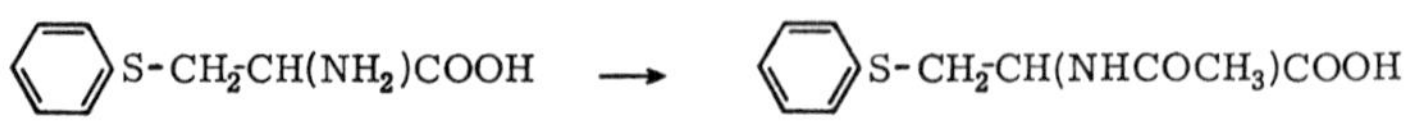

c) Aromatic Amines (Ar NH_2). The best known example of this reaction is the conversion of sulphanilamide to N^4-acetylsulphanilamide. Almost all the sulphonamide drugs undergo acetylation in most animal species except the dog.

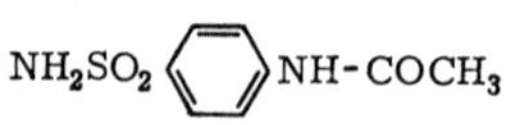

N^4-Acetylsulphanilamide

d) Sulphonamide (—SO_2NH_2). Sulphanilamide has been shown to be acetylated not only in the N^4-position but also to a lesser extent in the N^1-position to form sulphacetamide. This reaction also occurs in the dog (see above).

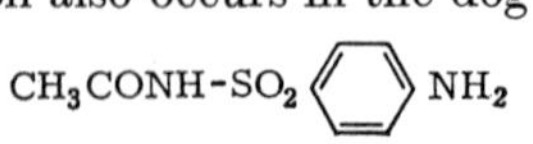

N^1-Acetylsulphanilamide

In a number of species including man, but not the dog, sulphanilamide gives rise to three acetyl derivatives, namely N^1-monoacetyl-, N^4-monoacetyl- and N^1,N^4-diacetyl-sulphanilamide.

e) Hydrazine and Hydrazide (—$NHNH_2$ and —$CONHNH_2$). Hydrazine is acetylated in the body to 1,2-diacetylhydrazine and since monoacetylhydrazine is also converted to diacetylhydrazine *in vivo*, the monoacetyl derivative is probably formed first.

$$NH_2NH_2 \longrightarrow NH_2NHCOCH_3 \longrightarrow CH_3CONHNHCOCH_3$$

Hydrazides, such as isoniazid are also acetylated. This reaction occurs in man and in rabbits, but not in the dog which is thus unable to acetylate hydrazides or aromatic amines.

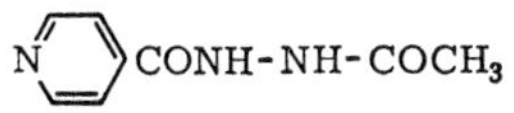

Isoniazid metabolite

Species variations in acetylation indicate that there are several transacetylases. In all these reactions the donor of the acetyl group is acetyl-CoA.

Other forms of biological acylation, namely formylation and succinylation, have now been observed but these are usually minor and rare reactions. 2-Formamido-1-naphthyl hydrogen sulphate has been detected as a minor metabolite of 2-naphthylamine (Boyland and Manson, 1965) and *N*-(*p*-chloro-*a*-methylphenacyl)succinamic acid as a metabolite of 4′-chloro-2-ethylaminopropiophenone in the urine of rats and dogs (Weinstock et al., 1969).

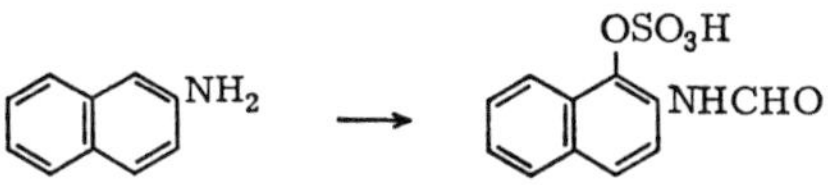

2-Naphthylamine 2-Formamido-1-naphthyl hydrogen sulphate

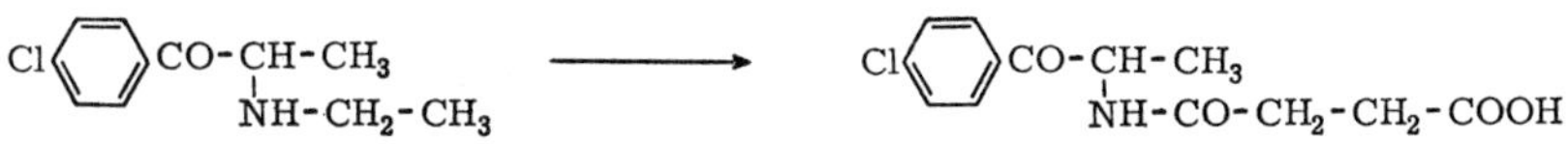

4′-Chloro-2-ethylaminopropiophenone N-(*p*-Chloro-*a*-methylphenacyl) succinamic acid

II. Mechanism of Conjugation

Since conjugations are synthetic reactions they require a source of energy which is usually supplied *via* adenosine triphosphate (ATP). With the exception of mercapturic acid formation these reactions are characterised by the formation of an activated nucleotide as an intermediate and a transferring enzyme which catalyses the final step between the nucleotide and the conjugation product. The activated nucleotide, however, can be a derivative of either the conjugating agent or the foreign compound, so that there are two kinds of conjugation reactions which can be represented approximately as follows:

(a) Conjugating agent —energy→ conjugating agent nucleotide —foreign compound / + transferase→ conjugated product

(b) Foreign compound —energy→ foreign compound nucleotide —conjugating agent / + transferase→ conjugated product

Defects in conjugation reactions can arise as a result of an inability to form the intermediate nucleotide or of faulty production of the transferase. Glucuronic acid and glucoside conjugations, ethereal sulphate synthesis, methylation and acetylation belong to category (a) and hippuric acid and ornithuric acid syntheses and glutamine conjugation belong to category (b).

Mercapturic acid synthesis, however, seems not to belong to either of these categories and sometimes depends upon an initial microsomal oxidation of the foreign compound to a reactive product which tends to combine spontaneously, but nevertheless with enzyme assistance, with glutathione. The conversion of cyanide to thiocyanate seems to be a simple reaction between cyanide and thiosulphate catalysed by the enzyme, rhodanese.

An example of (a), the first type of conjugation, is glucuronide synthesis and of (b), the second type, hippuric acid synthesis; the relevent steps in these reactions with phenol and benzoic acid as examples of foreign compounds, are as follows:

	series of reactions		phenol +	
Glucose	⟶	uridine diphosphate glucuronic acid	⟶	phenyl-glucuronide
	involving ATP		glucuronyl transferase	

	series of reactions		glycine +	
Benzoic acid	⟶	Benzoyl-CoA	⟶	hippuric acid
	involving ATP		glycine *N*-acylase	

The intermediate nucleotides for various conjugation reactions are uridine diphosphate glucuronic acid for glucuronic acid conjugation, uridine diphosphate glucose for glucose conjugation, aryl-CoA for hippuric acid and ornithine conjugation, arylacetyl-CoA for glutamine conjugation, phosphoadenosinephosphosulphate for sulphate synthesis, *S*-adenosylmethionine for methylation and acetyl-CoA for acetylation.

There also appears to be a difference in tissue distribution of type (a) and (b) conjugations. Although the liver is the main organ for conjugations, type (a) may also occur in other tissues such as the kidney, intestine and lung and in some cases in the spleen, brain, pancreas and blood, but type (b) seems to be confined to the liver and kidney.

D. Compounds which are not Metabolized

The majority of foreign compounds can be metabolized in the body, but there are some which appear to resist metabolism and are excreted unchanged. However, several compounds which, in the past, were reported to be completely inert metabolically have now been found, by modern techniques, to be metabolized to a very minor extent. Compounds which are not readily metabolized could be dangerous, because, as already pointed out, phase I and phase II reactions tend to make compounds more polar so that they can be readily excreted; if this does not occur the compound could accumulate in the body to toxic proportions and possibly circulate for a prolonged period.

There are two kinds of compounds which appear to resist metabolism, highly polar compounds and certain apparently non-polar compounds whose resistance to metabolic change is not readily explained. In addition, there are certain compounds which are not absorbed from the alimentary tract and certain volatile compounds whose contact with metabolizing tissues is so short that they appear resistant to metabolism.

Since the apparent objective of metabolism is to increase the polarity of a compound it is reasonable to expect that an already highly polar compound will be excreted without further change. In fact, a polar compound may not readily penetrate to the sites in the cell where it can be metabolized and, in any case, further metabolism may not increase its polarity and thus would not be of any advantage to the organism. Examples of this type of compound are strong organic acids such as arsanilic acid (MOODY and WILLIAMS, 1964) and 5,5'-methylenedisalicylic acid (DAVISON and WILLIAMS, 1968) both of which are used in medicated feeds for swine and poultry, and strong organic bases such as guanidine and the neuromuscular blocking agent, hexamethonium and its analogues.

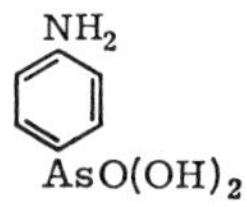

Arsanilic acid
(pKa 4.1)

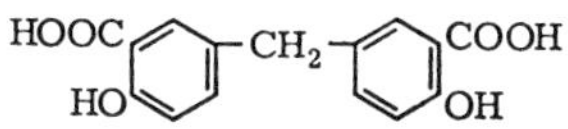

Methylenedisalicylic acid
(pKa 3.5)

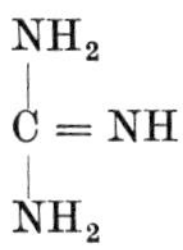

Guanidine
(pKa 13.6)

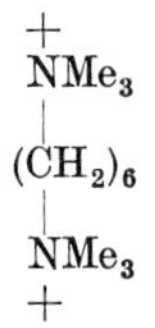

Hexamethonium
(very strong base)

These compounds are virtually completely ionized at pH 7.4 and are, in effect, excreted entirely unchanged.

The other type includes compounds such as the drug, barbital, hexachlorobenzene, a fungicide, and anaesthetics such as ether and halothane. Barbital is a long duration hypnotic, which is metabolized to the extent of about 5% in rats (GOLDSCHMIDT and WEHR, 1957) but is mainly excreted unchanged at a very slow rate; its long duration of action is, no doubt, associated with its slow excretion and relatively slow metabolism.

In the case of ether ($C_2H_5OC_2H_5$; b.p. 34.6°) and halothane ($CF_3CHClBr$; b.p. 50.2°) and similar anaesthetics, it is probable that because of their volatility their contact with metabolizing tissues is so short that little metabolism can occur. However, evidence has been obtained that they are metabolized to a slight extent, ether to CO_2 *via* ethanol and acetaldehyde and halothane to trifluoroacetic acid and chloride and bromide ions (see VAN DYKE and CHENOWETH, 1965 see also chapter 44).

E. Spontaneous Reactions

Although most foreign compounds which enter the body are metabolized enzymically, there are some which will react without the intervention of an enzyme, given the appropriate physical conditions or contact with a suitable physiological compound (which may be a simple molecule or a macromolecule). It is also possible that some compounds are metabolized by both non-enzymic and enzymic processes. There appear to be three kinds of reactions which can be considered under this heading.

a) Spontaneous reactions which occur given the right physical conditions such as pH or reactive groupings in body constituents.

b) Spontaneous reactions which can be enzyme assisted. These reactions are thermodynamically favoured and proceed at measurable rates non-enzymically.

c) Spontaneous reactions which give rise to products which are then further metabolized by enzymic means, or *vice versa*, enzymic reactions giving products which are then changed spontaneously.

A striking example of a compound undergoing the first type of reaction in the body is thalidomide. At pH 7.4 thalidomide breaks down spontaneously to twelve other compounds. The spontaneous hydrolysis of thalidomide is pH dependent, for the half-life of the drug is 24 hours at pH 6, 11 hours at 7.0, 5 hours at 7.4 and 1.25 hours at pH 8.0. Thalidomide contains four substituted amide bonds (a, b, c, d) (see below) all of which are unstable especially above pH 7.0 (SCHUMACHER et al., 1965).

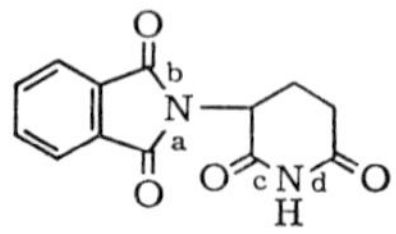

Thalidomide

The bonds a and b are equivalent and are more readily broken by hydrolysis than c and d. None of the breakdown products of thalidomide are teratogenic, and it appears probable that the teratogenicity of the drug is related to its ability to react with various tissue components spontaneously (see WILLIAMS, 1968).

The second type of spontaneous reactions are those involving, for the most part, compounds which react with sulphydryl compounds such as glutathione and give rise to mercapturic acids. Boyland distinguishes three types of these reactions:

a) Those which only proceed spontaneously (but also can be enzyme assisted) following an initial oxidative reaction in which the compound is converted enzymically to a metabolite which can then react spontaneously. Compounds undergoing this type of reaction include the monohalogen benzenes, naphthalene and phenanthrene. The general pattern is as follows:

$$X \xrightarrow{\text{microsomal oxidation}} \text{X-epoxide} \xrightarrow{\text{spontaneous reaction}} \text{X-glutathione conjugate}$$

Chloro-, bromo- and iodo-benzenes, naphthalene and phenanthrene (X, see above) are believed to be converted to epoxides enzymically by the hepatic microsomes. The epoxides can then react spontaneously with glutathione although this conjugation can be assisted by glutathione *S*-epoxide-tranferase which is found in the liver.

b) Those which proceed quite rapidly spontaneously but whose rate is further increased by the presence of the enzyme. Compounds undergo this type of reaction are benzyl chloride, alkyl bromides and sulphabromophthalein.

c) Those which proceed very slowly in the absence of the enzyme, in this case a glutathione *S*-aryltransferase. The spontaneous reaction depends upon pH as does also the enzymic reaction. Examples of compounds undergoing this type of reaction are 2,4-dichloronitrobenzene and 2,3,5,6-tetrachloronitrobenzene, the 2-chloro group being replaced by glutathione in the first compound and the nitro group in the second.

F. The Excretion of Foreign Compounds

As a result of the transformations of foreign compounds either enzymically or nonenzymically, three types of compounds may be eliminated from the body:

a) the original compound unchanged, b) phase I metabolites, i.e. oxidation, reduction and hydrolysis products and c) phase II metabolites or conjugation products. The relative amounts of these three types of products depend upon a number of factors including the tissue distribution of the compound, route of administration and dosage schedule of the compound; the species, age, sex and strain of the animal; and environmental factors such as temperature, stress, the presence of other chemicals, season, time of day etc.

The main channel of elimination for the majority of compounds is the urine, although some compounds may be eliminated partly or almost entirely in the faeces (see chapters 18 and 19). However, in the case of certain compounds, both urinary and faecal excretion may be preceded by biliary excretion which depends upon species and upon the molecular weight and polarity of the compound or its metabolites (Millburn et al., 1967; Abou-El-Makarem et al., 1967). Biliary excretion of a compound could involve it in an enterohepatic circulation.

Other channels of the elimination of foreign compounds and their metabolites can be of considerable importance in some cases. The air expired through the lungs is an important route for the excretion of volatile compounds such as benzene, ether, halothane and carbon tetrachloride, and for volatile metabolites such as CO_2 (often a product of demethylation), dimethyl sulphide (a minor metabolite of dimethylsulphoxide), and acetone (a metabolite of isopropanol). Foreign compounds and their metabolites can also be eliminated through the skin and appear in the sweat, hair and nails, and some are known to be secreted in the saliva and milk (see Williams, 1967b).

References

Since this chapter is an introduction to the several succeeding chapters, only a limited number of references are given here. A more detailed bibliography will be found in those chapters.

Abou-El-Makarem, M.M., Millburn, P., Smith, R.L., Williams, R.T.: Biliary excretion of foreign compounds. Species differences in biliary excretion. Biochem. J. **105**, 1289—1293 (1967).

Baldwin, B.C., Robinson, D., Williams, R.T.: The fate of benzoic acid in some domestic and other birds. Biochem. J. **76**, 595—600 (1960).

Boyland, E., Chasseaud, L.F.: The role of glutathione and glutathione S-transferases in mercapturic acid biosynthesis. Advanc. Enzymol. **32**, 173—219 (1969).

— Manson, D.: 2-Formamido-1-naphthyl hydrogen sulphate; a metabolite of 2-naphthylamine. Biochem. J. **95**, 7P (1965).

Brodie, B.B., Axelrod, J., Cooper, J.R., Gaudette, L., La du, B.N., Mitoma, C., Udenfriend, S.: Detoxication of drugs and other foreign compounds by liver microsomes. Science **121**, 603—604 (1955).

Channon, H.J., Mills, G.T., Williams, R.T.: The metabolism of 2,4,6-trinitrotoluene (α-T.N.T.) Biochem. J. **38**, 70—85 (1944).

Davison, C., Williams, R.T.: The metabolism of 5,5′-methylenedisalicylic acid in various species. J. Pharm. Pharmacol. **20**, 12—18 (1968).

Dutton, G.J.: Ed. Glucuronic Acid, Free and Combined. New York and London: Academic Press 1966.

Gillette, J.R.: Metabolism of drugs and other foreign compounds by enzymatic mechanisms. Progr. Drug Res. **6**, 11—73 (1963).

— Biochemistry of drug oxidation and reduction by enzymes in hepatic endoplasmic reticulum. Advanc. Pharmacol. **4**, 219—261 (1966).

Goldschmidt, S., Wehr, R.: Der Metabolismus von Veronal. Z. physiol. Chem. **308**, 9—19 (1957).

Jerina, D.M., Daly, J.W., Witkop, B., Zaltzman-Nirenberg, P., Udenfriend, S.: The role of arene oxide-oxepin systems in the metabolism of aromatic substrates. III. Formation of 1,2-naphthalene oxide from naphthalene by liver microsomes. J. Amer. chem. Soc. **90**, 6525—6527 (1968).

MILLBURN, P., SMITH, R. L., WILLIAMS, R. T.: Biliary excretion of foreign compounds. Biphenyl, stilboestrol and phenol in the rat. Molecular weight, polarity and metabolism as factors in biliary excretion. Biochem. J. **105**, 1275—1281 (1967).

MOODY, J. P., WILLIAMS, R. T.: The fate of arsanilic acid and acetylarsanilic acid in hens. Fd. Cosmet. Toxicol. **2**, 687—693 (1964).

SCHELINE, R. R.: Drug metabolism by intestinal microorganisms. J. pharm. Sci **57**, 2021 to 2037 (1968).

SCHUMACHER, H., SMITH, R. L., WILLIAMS, R. T.: The metabolism of thalidomide. The spontaneous hydrolysis of thalidomide in solution. Brit. J. Pharmacol. **25**, 324—372 (1965).

SMITH, J. N.: The comparative metabolism of xenobiotics. Advanc. comp. Physiol. Biochem. **3**, 173—232 (1968).

— WILLIAMS, R. T.: The metabolism of phenacetin in the rabbit. Biochem. J. **44**, 239—242 (1949).

VAN DYKE, R. A., CHENOWETH, M. B.: Metabolism of volatile anesthetics. Anesthesiology **26**, 348—357 (1965).

WEINSTOCK, J., PARKER, S. E., LUCYSZYN, G. W., INTOCCIA, A. P.: N-(p-chloro-α-methylphenyl)succinamic acid, a succinic acid conjugate of an α-aminoketone. Pharmacologist **11**, 240 (1969).

WILLIAMS, R. T.: Detoxication Mechanisms, 2nd ed. London: Chapman and Hall 1959.

— The biogenesis of conjugation and detoxication products. Chapt. 9 in Biogenesis of Natural Compounds. 2nd. ed., pp. 589—639. Ed. by P. BERNFELD. Oxford: Pergamon Press 1967a.

— Patterns of excretion of drugs in man and other species. In: Drug Responses in Man, pp. 71—82. Ed. by G. E. W. WOLSTENHOLME and R. PORTER. London: Churchill 1967b.

— Thalidomide. A study of biochemical teratology. Arch. environm. Hlth **16**, 493—502 (1968).

Subsection A: Microsomal Enzymes

Chapter 36

Some Morphological Characteristics of Hepatocyte Endoplasmic Reticulum and Some Relationships between Endoplasmic Reticulum, Microsomes, and Drug Metabolism

J.R. Fouts[1]

I. Some Morphological Considerations

Some very fine reviews of the morphology and function of hepatocellular endoplasmic reticulum (ER) have been published in the last few years. Any of the newer textbooks of histology or cytology will list these in profusion and the reader is referred to such standard texts if "endoplasmic reticulum" is a new encounter for him. It would be presumptious of me to do more in this area than point out a few characteristics of ER of particular concern to those interested in drug metabolism and pharmacology.

The liver is historically the organ associated with foreign chemical disposition. Nothing we know at this time suggests that our preoccupation with this organ has led us to overlook sites of more general importance in drug metabolism. However, it must be emphasized that for a particular drug, or a particular route of administration, other organs may be more important in that drug's metabolism than is the liver.

It is also important to remember that the liver is not an aggregation of identical cells. Histologically, the liver is composed of several different cell groupings. Most mammalian liver has more than one lobe and the blood supply, etc. of these lobes can be different. At the cellular level there are different types such as Kupfer cells, parenchymal cells, and bile duct cells. Even within a given cell type there can be variations in richness of cytoplasm. In many of our own studies we have been impressed by variation in amount of endoplasmic reticulum in different hepatocytes from the same lobe of liver — particularly the amount and arrangement of smooth-surfaced endoplasmic reticulum (SER). Also, Loud (1968) has pointed out that the SER of parenchymal cells is much more abundant in centrilobular cells than in midzonal and peripheral regions of the hepatic lobule. On the other hand, he found that the rough-surfaced endoplasmic reticulum (RER) was dispersed fairly uniformly in all parts of the lobule (Loud, 1968). I am merely stating here what has been said many times before by others: these variations in cell arrangement, blood flow, cell type, cytoplasmic richness, are either known to be or suspected of being reflected in variations in function. We might, therefore, expect that different types of liver cells would have different functions in drug metabolism.

It is relatively hard to separate the Kupfer cells from parenchymal cells and from bile duct cells. Relatively pure preparations of Kupfer cells have been made

1 National Institute of Environmental Health Sciences, National Institutes of Health, USPHS, Research Triangle Park, North Carolina 27709.

and some kinds of drug metabolism appear to be carried on here. Thus, GOVIER (1965) has shown that acetylation of sulfanilamide and *p*-aminobenzoic acid occurs in reticuloendothelial cells from liver, but not in parenchymal cells. To my knowledge, no one has studied the Kupfer vs. parenchymal cell for other types of drug metabolism carried on by the liver — e.g., glucuronide conjugation, mixed function oxidations, reductions, or hydrolytic reactions.

Even within a given hepatic cell type we have little information as to variations in drug-metabolizing enzyme activity. Is mixed function oxidase or glucuronidation activity uniformly distributed throughout the liver lobule ? One way to answer this question might be the use of histochemical techniques and WATTENBERG and LEONG (1962) have done this. Using several species including rat, mouse, hamster, monkey and man, these workers showed that an enzyme system capable of metabolizing several polycyclic hydrocarbons was not evenly distributed throughout the hepatic lobule, but was instead concentrated in the central portion. If the polycyclic hydrocarbon metabolizing systems are the same as the mixed-function oxidases, then we could expect most microsomal oxidative drug metabolisms to be unevenly distributed in the liver lobule. This enzyme similarity is a reasonable assumption to make in light of much recent evidence, but the reader should be aware that it is only an assumption. We are still left with questions about other types of drug metabolism — e.g., glucuronidation, hydrolysis. Information about these pathways is not available to my knowledge. Histochemical demonstrations of these enzymes will be complicated by the fact that the products of these reactions are usually very water-soluble and this makes localization (diffusion) artifacts probable.

This particular chapter is to deal only with microsomes and drug metabolism and so some disclaimers should be made. Other parts of the hepatic cell contain enzymes capable of metabolically altering drugs — e.g., nuclei and mitochondria; or may contain enzymes similar to those in microsomes — e.g., hydrolases. The main considerations in this chapter will be the microsomal oxidative, reductive or glucuronidating enzymes — other authors will deal with other types of drug metabolism or other localizations of drug metabolism. It would be expected that non-uniform distribution of these enzymes amongst different types of hepatic cells and from one area of the liver lobule to another would also occur.

These non-uniform microsomal and extra-microsomal enzyme distributions may be quite important in understanding why some drug metabolisms are affected by a given treatment while other metabolisms are unchanged, or why hepatotoxins whose action depends on metabolism frequently affect certain hepatic cells or areas of the liver much more than others. This is an area of structure-function relationships that should receive much more attention than it is now getting. A major drawback to such attention is the time-consuming nature of the studies needed. Histochemistry and electron microscopy are not often capable of routine or mass application in drug metabolism studies.

CLAUDE has written a fine review of the relationships between the ER and microsomes in various cell types with particular reference to drug metabolism (CLAUDE, 1969). There is little I can add to what is included there and the reader is urged to refer to that chapter. For purposes of the present discussion, it is necessary only to restate some points made by CLAUDE and various other authors:

a) Microsomes result from the fragmentation of both SER and RER and associated structures during homogenization of liver cells.

b) Microsomes are therefore a very heterogeneous fraction; microsomes contain membrane fragments of quite different size, chemical and physical properties.

c) Yields and compositions of "microsomes" from a given amount of liver tissue will depend on techniques of homogenization, centrifugation, washing etc. as well as on the functional state of the ER in the liver cell before homogenization (hyper- or hypoplasia, etc.).

d) The origin of rough-surfaced microsomes is more certain (coming from RER) than the source of smooth-surfaced microsomes (can come from SER, Golgi, etc.).

e) In the intact liver cell, RER and SER are often located in quite different parts of the cytoplasm with only very few places of actual physical continuity between them. The configuration and arrangement of RER in the cytoplasm is quite different from that of SER in the intact liver cell. In an homogenate, and especially in the microsomal fraction as isolated by differential centrifugation, both rough and smooth-surfaced microsomes are vesicular and placed in what may be quite unnatural relationships one to the other. What this means in terms of what we measure as microsomal drug metabolizing-enzyme activity is unknown. It would be expected that some artifacts would result, but investigations of these possibilities have not been made to my knowledge. If any of these drug-metabolizing enzymes are allosteric or have reactive sites affected by membrane structure, it is possible that enzymes in a vesicular membrane (*in vitro* as microsomes) might be quite different from those in a membrane arranged as a long tube or sheet (*in vivo*, as ER).

The purpose of this part of the discussion is to point out that drug metabolizing enzyme activity in microsomes may be quite different from drug metabolizing enzyme activity, substrate-cytochrome interactions, etc. as they occur in the intact cell. Again, the plea is for caution and restraint in interpretation of results or proposals of molecular mechanisms of enzyme action, construction of model systems etc. Coupled with this conservatism is the hope that more correlative studies will be made using histochemistry, electron microscopy etc., so that we can get at least some idea of how microsomal enzyme behavior compares with the *in vivo* systems in hepatocellular ER.

II. Some Structure-activity Correlations

Since microsomes are derived from hepatic ER (and perhaps some associated structures such as the Golgi apparatus and the outer nuclear envelope), it is reasonable to ask whether marked changes in ER structure, arrangement or amount, are reflected in changes in enzyme activity of the microsomal fraction? A number of studies have been made which suggest that in some cases, the reflection is a good one, whereas in others it gets pretty muddy. The best correlations are seen when ER increases; microsomal enzyme activity often increases in such cases. Marked proliferation of ER often involves only one kind of ER — the SER. Marked increases in amount of RER to the extent seen with SER after certain drug exposures (e.g. phenobarbital) are not known to me. Changes in amount of SER can best be observed when there are increases since the normal liver cell does not have easily visible and large amounts of SER. Destruction of this normally rather inconspicuous organelle would have to be proportionately extensive to be readily observed and believed. Damage to SER by drug, etc. pretreatment of animals is also harder to document than with RER. Damage to RER can take the form of vesiculation or loss of attached ribosomes. A change from a laminar arrangement of tubules studded with particles to vesicles is not too difficult to recognize. A change from a system of random tubules and vesicles to a system of vesicles is somewhat harder to see. Realization of such a change is complicated by the fact that it can occur during sample preparation rather than be due to an *in vivo* action of some drug, physiological or pathological process. Even when SER vesiculation is accompanied by swelling, the observer is confronted with the many possibilities that he is looking at a preparation artifact rather than an effect which occurred prior to the animal's death. CLAUDE spends some time discussing this property of sensitivity of the ER (CLAUDE, 1969, p. 7—8), a property which makes damage to ER especially hard to document.

Studies of whether hepatic RER or SER is more easily damaged by a given treatment or chemical substance are few in number. My own laboratory has shown that several drug-metabolizing enzymes in smooth-surfaced microsomes from rat liver are more labile to preincubation in buffer than these enzymes in rough-surfaced microsomes from the same liver. This differential lability is seen with rat liver, but not with rabbit liver (GRAM et al., 1967; FOUTS et al., 1966). We know virtually nothing about whether SER and RER differ in susceptibility to injury, or whether this may depend on type of injury, type of animal species, extent of injury, time between injury and sample preparation, etc. Also complicating such studies is the possibility that the injurious chemical may be concentrated to different extents in RER vs. SER. A chemical with high affinity for constituents of RNA would be more likely to affect RER than SER due to the large differences in RNA concentration. Differences in lipid composition of RER and SER are inferred from studies on smooth vs. rough-surfaced microsomes and such differences in lipid composition (GLAUMANN and DALLNER, 1968; DALLNER and ERNSTER, 1968) could lead to differences in sequestration of lipid-soluble drugs and chemicals having injurious properties. Finally, differences in enzyme composition of SER and RER may mean different metabolisms of a given chemical to its active or inactive forms, or different sites of attack in RER vs. SER.

Thus, the available literature best correlates ER structure with ER enzyme activity in cases where ER increases in amount. The best known of such correlations also relate increases in amount of SER with increases in microsomal constituents (e.g. cytochrome P-450) or enzyme activities (mixed-function oxidases).

REMMER and MERKER (1963) were among the first to report that phenobarbital treatment of animals resulted in a massive proliferation of hepatic SER along with increases in several hepatic microsomal enzyme activities. There are now known to be several hundred drugs and chemicals which when administered to animals will result in increased hepatic microsomal enzyme activity (see review by CONNEY, 1967, for a listing of some of these). Only a few of these have been investigated for their effects on hepatic ER (or SER) structure.

Attempts have been made to classify chemicals which stimulate or induce hepatic microsomal enzyme activity in terms of their mechanism of action. Ultimately we will be interested in knowing which of the many steps in enzyme synthesis are affected by which inducer, and by what mechanisms enzyme activation or modulation can occur. At present, the best correlations between hepatic microsomal enzyme activity and amount of ER occur with those chemicals or drugs which apparently increase enzyme activity by causing increased amounts of the enzyme to be accumulated. And this enzyme, by tests now available to us, appears to be the same as or very similar to that in the untreated (control animal) — i.e. its cytochrome P-450 has the same ethyl isocyanide and substrate-induced difference spectra and its enzyme kinetics are the same as in the control animal (Km is the same). This class of hepatic microsomal enzyme inducers includes most barbiturates, and chlorinated hydrocarbon insecticides. Here, increased hepatic microsomal enzyme activity is associated with easily-documented proliferation of SER in most parenchymal cells (see examples in REMMER and MERKER, 1963; FOUTS and ROGERS, 1965; ORTEGA, 1966).

Correlations of ER structure with hepatic microsomal enzyme activity have generally been unavailable with chemicals and drugs which appear to increase enzyme activity by mechanisms different from those set in motion by the phenobarbital-insecticide class. Thus, we were unable to document any massive proliferation of ER (SER) following treatment of rats with 3-methylcholanthrene or 3,4-benzpyrene (FOUTS and ROGERS, 1965). These polycyclic hydrocarbons produce marked increases in some hepatic microsomal enzyme activities and changes in microsomal cytochrome P-450, but current evidence favors a different mechanism of action than with phenobarbital or chlordane (see SLADEK and MANNERING, 1969a, b for examples). Studies of effects of anabolic steroids on hepatic cell ER and correlation with effects of these steroids on microsomal drug metabolism have not been reported to my knowledge.

III. Some Problems in Correlating ER Structure and Microsomal Enzyme Activity

The time-course of increase in microsomal enzyme activity does not exactly coincide with the time course of increase in SER following phenobarbital treatment of rats (REMMER and MERKER, 1965). Both drug-metabolizing enzyme activity and microsomal P-450 can be shown to increase before increases in amount of SER can be observed with the electron microscope. Similarly when the enzyme inducer (phenobarbital) is withdrawn, there is a more rapid fall-off in hepatic microsomal enzyme activity than decrease in amount of SER (ERNSTER and ORRENIUS, 1965). This latter situation therefore results in a hypertrophic, but hypoactive SER — large numbers of membranes, but normal or subnormal amounts of microsomal drug-metabolizing enzymes. Such a result seems also to occur when some hepatic microsomal drug metabolizing enzyme inducers are given repeatedly. Thus, HUTTERER et al. (1968) have reported that repeated large doses of dieldrin given to rats resulted in a liver having large amounts of SER, elevated cytochrome P-450 levels, but reduced activity of several drug-metabolizing enzymes. These authors have also reported that patients having alcoholic hepatitis have excess amounts of SER, but less than normal drug-metabolizing enzyme activities (HUTTERER et al., 1968).

Such results appear to indicate that SER increases caused by acute administration of hepatic microsomal drug metabolizing enzyme inducers will be accompanied by corresponding changes in microsomal enzyme activity, but that prolonged exposure to such inducers (particularly at high doses) can lead to a state where structure and function no longer correlate — where SER is still proliferated, but enzyme activity has returned to normal or subnormal levels. Before this is accepted as a generality, it should be pointed out that it may apply only to some inducers and only at high doses of inducers. Thus, prolonged exposure to moderate doses of phenobarbital (WILSON and FOUTS, 1966) or dieldrin (HUTTERER et al., 1968) results in an SER which is both structurally and functionally hyperactive. The situation is also complicated by the fact that high doses of some inducers can be inhibitors of hepatic microsomal drug metabolizing enzyme activities. Directly added to *in vitro* incubation mixtures, many inducers of microsomal enzymes can become inhibitors. Thus, high doses of inducers administered *in vivo* may cause an enhanced enzyme activity that will be masked *in vitro* and *in vivo* by the inducer acting as an inhibitor. Such situations might be clarified if hepatic microsomal enzyme activity were measured at various times after the last dose of inducer, or if one could set up an enzyme system known to be free of inducer or metabolities (e.g. by using washed microsomes from inducer-pretreated animals, plus drug substrate, plus TPNH). These situations have usually not been met in papers where it is claimed that a given treatment has resulted in proliferated hepatic cell SER which is not matched by increased microsomal drug-metabolizing enzyme activity, and so the question is not yet answered to everyone's satisfaction.

Then too it has been reported in various meetings that certain inhibitors of protein synthesis can have effects on enzyme activity which appear to allow dissociation of ER structure and function. Thus, an inhibitor administered simultaneously with an inducer may lead to a proliferation of hepatic SER without altering enzymatic activity. Again this evidence suggests a hypertrophic, hypoactive ER. A few observations need recall, however. Most of these inhibitors of enzyme synthesis (ethionine, actinomycin D, puromycin, etc.) are either substrates or inhibitors of hepatic microsomal drug-metabolizing enzyme activities — an effect that is dose-related and quite apart from any action as an anti-inducer. These alternative substrate-inhibitor actions of these antimetabolites on hepatic microsomal enzyme activities can be easily demonstrated in a variety of systems ranging from intact animal to isolated incubation mixtures. These effects should not be overlooked particularly when there is evidence that induced enzymes may be more sensitive to inhibitors than control enzymes (see Table 2, page 112 of article by Wada et al., 1968). Finally, a recent paper by Lowe et al. (1968) is particularly interesting since it suggests that antimetabolite-pretreated animals can have an ER that rearranges spontaneously. This might mean that hepatic SER is normal in amount in anti-metabolite pretreated animals as long as the animal is living, but that somewhere between sacrifice and the electron microscope, conditions could exist (especially during fixation and embedding) allowing rearrangement of membranes to produce massive complexes of SER in the cytoplasm. No such post-mortem membrane conversion to SER was seen in control liver — only in rats pretreated with actinomycin C (Lowe et al., 1968).

IV. Localization of Drug Metabolizing Enzymes in Submicrosomal Fractions

From all the previous discussions and the many symposia, etc. devoted to the question, it would seem possible that the morphological heterogeneity of the microsomal fraction might be reflected in chemical and biochemical heterogeneities. The microsomal fraction can be subdivided by various processes based on the fact that the different membrane components of the fraction have different sizes, different weights and/or different metal-binding properties. A very comprehensive review of some of the major considerations in subfractionations of hepatic microsomes has recently appeared (Dallner and Ernster, 1968).

Studies have been made by several laboratories of the submicrosomal distributions of a number of hepatic drug-metabolizing enzymes or components of such enzyme systems. Different methods of fractionation have been used, different animal species have been tested, different enzymes etc. have been measured. It is therefore not too surprising that different results have been obtained. I have discussed some of the reasons why results may differ in two recently published articles (Fouts and Gram, 1969; Fouts et al., 1966). Some of the conclusions of our work might be repeated, but one of the most important still seems to be — it is not necessary to choose up sides over whether smooth or rough-surfaced microsomes contain more of the drug-metabolizing enzymes of the whole microsomal fraction. So far there is more than enough evidence to suggest that results can be markedly affected by the animal species used, pretreatment or environment of animal prior to sacrifice, method of subfractionation employed, and finally, which enzyme systems one studies. The importance of methodology cannot be overestimated in my opinion. A recent paper by BERGSTRAND and DALLNER (1969) emphasizes that even the centrifuge and especially the type of centrifuge head used in the fractionation can be critical. In my own laboratory we have begun studies on enzyme composition of microsomal subfractions prepared using a zonal rotor. Perhaps this technique coupled with discontinuous gradients will allow preparation of subfractions in amounts and purity not available heretofore.

In light of some of our recent studies on the effects of Mg^{+2} on microsomal drug-metabolizing enzymes and electron transport systems (PETERS and FOUTS, 1970) it will be interesting to see how microsomal subfractions might differ in metal binding as related to metal-enzyme interactions Such studies only typify the rationale behind separation of microsomal subfractions. We expect to find different enzymes, different effects of inhibition, different effects of inducers etc. in different microsomal fractions. Such subfractionation should also allow a closer look at the relationships between ER structure in intact cells and enzyme activity in different microsomal subfractions. That such relationships exist and have practical importance in understanding drug action, toxicity, species differences in drug action and toxicity, organ damage specificity by drugs and chemicals, etc., is a hypothesis governing much of our work.

Acknowledgments

Research work in the author's laboratory as cited in this paper was supported by grants from the National Institutes of Health, National Institute of General Medical Sciences, especially GM 12675.

References

BERGSTRAND, A., DALLNER, G.: Isolation of rough and smooth microsomes from rat liver by means of a commercially available centrifuge. Analyt. Biochem. **29**, 351—356 (1969).

CLAUDE, A.: Microsomes, endoplasmic reticulum and interactions of cytoplasmic membranes. In: Microsomes and Drug Oxidations. New York: Academic Press 1969.

CONNEY, A.H.: Pharmacological implications of microsomal enzyme induction. Pharmacol. Rev. **19**, 317—366 (1967).

DALLNER, G., ERNSTER, L.: Subfractionation and composition of microsomal membranes: a review. J. Histochem. Cytochem. **16**, 611—632 (1968).

ERNSTER, L., ORRENIUS, S.: Substrate-induced synthesis of the hydroxylating enzyme system of liver microsomes. Fed. Proc. **24**, 1190—1199 (1965).

FOUTS, J.R., GRAM, T.E.: The metabolism of drugs by subfractions of hepatic microsomes. The case for microsomal heterogeneity. In: Microsomes and drug oxidations. New York: Academic Press 1969.

— ROGERS, L.A.: Morphological changes in the liver accompanying stimulation of microsomal drug metabolizing enzyme activity by phenobarbital, chlordane, benzpyrene, or methylcholanthrene in rats. J. Pharmacol. exp. Ther. **147**, 112—119 (1965).

— — GRAM, T.E.: The metabolism of drugs by hepatic microsomal enzymes. Studies on intramicrosomal distribution of enzymes and relationships between enzyme activity and structure of the hepatic endoplasmic reticulum. Exp. molec. Path. **5**, 475—490 (1966).

GLAUMANN, H., DALLNER, G.: Lipid composition and turnover of rough and smooth microsomal membranes in rat liver. J. Lipid Res. **9**, 720—729 (1968).

GOVIER, W.C.: Reticuloendothelial cells as the site of sulfanilamide acetylation in the rabbit. J. Pharmacol. exp. Ther. **150**, 305—308 (1965).

GRAM, T.E., ROGERS, L.A., FOUTS, J.R.: Further studies on the metabolism of drugs by subfractions of hepatic microsomes. J. Pharmacol. exp. Ther. **155**, 479—493 (1967).

HUTTERER, F., SCHAFFNER, F., KLION, F.M., POPPER, H.: Hypertrophic, hypoactive smooth endoplasmic reticulum. A sensitive indicator of hepatotoxicity exemplified by dieldrin. Science **161**, 1017—1019 (1968).

LOUD, A.V.: A quantitative stereological description of the ultrastructure of normal rat liver parenchymal cells. J. Cell Biol. **37**, 27—46 (1968).

Lowe, H., Grunewald, I., Zeidler, H.: Zur Bildung endoplasmatischer Membranen in der Leberparenchymzelle *in vitro*. III. Die Bildung von agranularen Membrankomplexen *in vitro* nach Vorbehandlung mit Aktinomyzin C. Acta biol. med. germ. **20**, 393—408 (1968).
Ortega, P.: Light and electron microscopy of dichlorodiphenyltrichloroethane (DDT) poisoning in the rat liver. Lab. Invest. **15**, 657—679 (1966).
Peters, M. A., Fouts, J. R.: The influence of magnesium and some other divalent cations on hepatic microsomal drug metabolism *in vitro*. Biochem. Pharmacol. **19**, 533—544 (1970).
Remmer, H., Merker, H. J.: Enzyminduktion und Vermehrung von endoplasmatischen Reticulum in der Leberzelle während der Behandlung mit Phenobarbital (Luminal). Klin. Wschr. **41**, 276—283 (1963).
— — Effect of drugs on the formation of smooth endoplasmic reticulum and drug metabolizing enzymes. Ann. N.Y. Acad. Sci. **123**, 79—97 (1965).
Sladek, N. E., Mannering, G. J.: Induction of drug metabolism. I. Differences in the mechanisms by which polycyclic hydrocarbons and phenobarbital produce their inductive effects on microsomal N-demethylating systems. Molec. Pharmacol. **5**, 174—185 (1969a).
— — Induction of drug metabolism. II. Qualitative differences in the microsomal N-demethylating systems stimulated by polycyclic hydrocarbons and by phenobarbital. Molec. Pharmacol. **5**, 186—199 (1969b).
Wada, F., Shimakawa, H., Takasugi, M., Kotake, T., Sakamoto, Y.: Effects of steroid hormones on drug-metabolizing enzyme systems in liver microsomes. J. Biochem. (Tokyo) **64**, 109—113 (1968).
Wattenberg, L. W., Leong, J. L.: Histochemical demonstration of reduced pyridine nucleotide dependent polycyclic hydrocarbon metabolizing systems. J. Histochem. Cytochem. **10**, 412—420 (1962).
Wilson, J. T., Fouts, J. R.: The effect of chronic phenobarbital administration on some hepatic drug-metabolizing enzyme activities in the rat. Biochem. Pharmacol. **15**, 1238—1241 (1966).

Chapter 37

Model Systems in Studies of the Chemistry and the Enzymatic Activation of Oxygen

V. ULLRICH and HJ. STAUDINGER

With 9 Figures

A. Introduction

In 1955 it was first established by isotope experiments with ^{18}O labeled oxygen that the oxygen molecule does not only serve as an electron acceptor in biological oxidations, but is also used by special enzymes for a direct oxygenation of organic compounds (MASON et al., 1955). If both oxygen atoms of the molecule are introduced into the substrate the enzymes are termed dioxygenases (HAYAISHI, 1962). The more important group of the oxygenases uses one atom of oxygen for the oxygenation of the substrate and therefore, these enzymes are called monooxygenases according to the terminology of HAYAISHI (1968). These enzymes are more commonly known as mixed function oxidases (MASON, 1957) or mixed function oxygenases since they have a second function as oxidases when reducing the second oxygen atom to water according to the equation:

$$RH + O_2 + DH_2 = ROH + H_2O + D$$

DH_2 as an external electron donor is an essential cofactor for these enzymatic reactions.

The chemical mechanism of oxygen activation and the reaction of the active oxygen species with the substrate is still unknown. So far all attempts have failed to demonstrate the reactive species directly by physical methods. Therefore chemical models have been investigated in order to understand the mechanisms of oxygen activation and hydroxylation.

In 1954 UDENFRIEND and his coworkers (UDENFRIEND et al., 1954; BRODIE et al., 1954) first described a nonenzymatic system which was able to hydroxylate organic compounds; since then a variety of similar systems have been described. Most of them have been suggested as model systems for monooxygenases. However, knowing more about the chemical properties of these enzymes today, only a few of them can be accepted as true models for monooxygenases. These models must have an absolute requirement for molecular oxygen which is reduced by two electrons to an active oxygen species having chemical properties very similar to or identical with the enzymatically formed active oxygen. However, it cannot be expected that a model system will exhibit the same substrate specificity or specificity with regard to the CH-bond attacked. These are for the most part steric effects in the enzymatic reaction due to the special configuration of the protein moiety.

During the last decade many data on the chemical properties of the active oxygen of monooxygenases have been reported which are summarized and discussed in section B. Considerations on the nature of the active oxygen together with model reactions are presented in section C. In the last part of this article the known hydroxylating systems will be critically discussed with regard to the hydroxylation mechanisms involved and their significance as model systems for monooxygenases.

B. Chemical Properties of the Active Oxygen in Enzymatic Monooxygenations

I. Hydroxylations of Aliphatic CH-Bonds

Most of the physiological substrates for monooxygenases are attacked at a saturated carbon atom and hydroxylated to the corresponding alcohol. This is observed with steroids where the hydroxylation occurs at the secondary CH-bonds of the aliphatic ring or at methyl groups (HAYANO, 1962). Long chain fatty acids are hydroxylated at the ω and ω-1 position (PREISS, 1964). The preference for the saturated carbon atom in hydroxylation is also seen in the nonspecific monooxygenation systems of liver microsomes. These monooxygenases exhibit several fold higher specific activities towards aliphatic compounds like cyclohexane (ULLRICH, 1969a) or isopentane (FROMMER, 1970) than towards to aromatic compounds. In a study of the hydroxylation of aliphatic compounds by liver microsomes (Table 1) we observed a rather constant difference in the formation of primary, secondary and tertiary alcohols (FROMMER, 1970). An increase in strength of the CH-bond leads to a decrease in attack which is a common feature of a selective substitution mechanism. The pattern of alcohols derived from one hydrocarbon molecule remained constant when competitive inhibitors were added. It is unlikely, therefore, that various enzymes are involved in the hydroxylation of the different positions:

Table 1. *Hydroxylation of aliphatic compounds by rat liver microsomes*[a]

Substrate	% Hydroxylation/CH-bond prim.	sec.	tert.	Ratio sec./prim.	tert./sec.
2-Methylbutane					
$H_3C-CH(CH_3)-CH_2-CH_3$ Rat[a)]	0.8	11.9	87.3	15.4	7.3
Rabbit[b)]					
Methylcyclohexane					
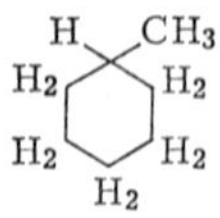	0.5	49.3[b]	50.2	53	3.3
Butane					
$H_3C-CH_2-CH_2-CH_3$	<0.4	>99.6	—	>100	—

[a] average of 9 preparations
[b] average of total ring hydroxylation

We are instead dealing with one nonspecific monooxygenase system which involves a selectively attacking active oxygen species.

As a special feature of steroid hydroxylations it was found that the configuration at the carbon atom is retained (HAYANO et al., 1958), a course reminiscent of electrophilic displacement reactions. The rapid exchange of deuterium or tritium with the medium makes it difficult to prove experimentally whether the oxygen is introduced into the organic molecule by a displacement or an insertion reaction. The rather weak CH-bonds adjacent to heteroatoms like nitrogen, oxygen or sulfur are very easily attacked by the active oxygen of the monooxygenase system in liver leading to dealkylation (BRODIE et al., 1958). The oxygen atom is found in the resulting aldehyde (RENSON et al., 1965) indicating that C-hydroxylation at the α-carbon atom occurs first yielding a semiacetal as an unstable intermediate:

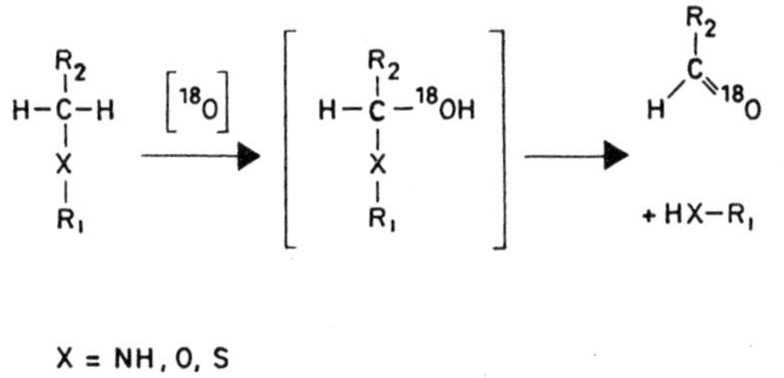

Fig. 1. Mechanism of dealkylation by liver microsomes

II. Monooxygenation of the Isolated Double Bond

Compounds with isolated carbon-carbon double bonds are epoxidised by the active oxygen of the microsomal monooxygenation system (WONG and TERRIERE, 1965). BLOOM and SHULL (1955) described an interesting experiment with a steroid hydroxylating system which introduces an axial hydroxyl group at the 11-carbon atom. When a steroid with a double bond at this carbon atom was used as a substrate, the epoxide was formed, also axial to the carbon atom. Obviously the active oxygen undergoes electrophilic addition to the π-electron system if the axial CH-bond is not available. With some unsaturated molecules it may happen that the epoxide is not stable enough and is further converted chemically or by an enzymatic system. Thus, in liver microsomes epoxides can be converted enzymatically to the dihydrodiol compound by addition of water (JERINA et al., 1968). Similarly conjugation with glutathione can occur :

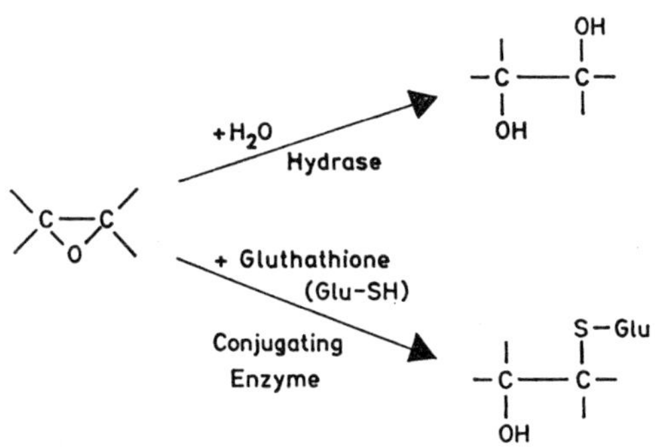

Fig. 2. Formation of dihydrodiols and premercapturic acids from epoxides

When trichloroethylene is used as a substrate for the microsomal system chloral hydrate is found as the main metabolite (BYINGTON and LEIBMAN, 1965). The following mechanism via a rearrangement of an epoxide intermediate has been proposed:

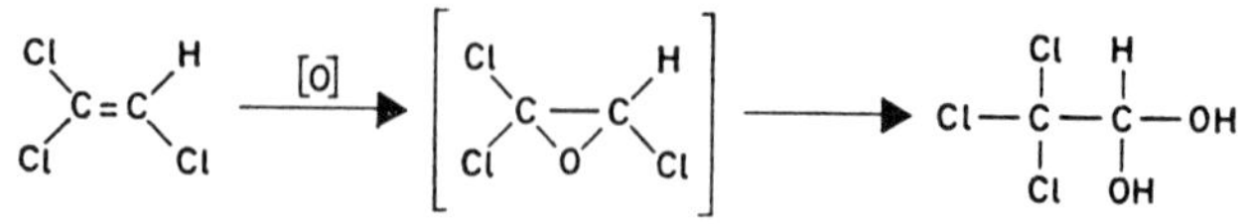

Fig. 3. Hypothetical scheme for the formation of chloral hydrate from trichloroethylene

The migration of the chlorine atom during the course of this monooxygenation is now well understood by the finding of the "NIH-shift" in aromatic systems which will be discussed in the next section.

III. Monooxygenation of Aromatic Systems

Hydroxylations at the aromatic nucleus are important pathways in the metabolism of phenylalanine and tryptophane. These monooxygenations are catalysed by specific enzymes and only one carbon atom at the aromatic ring is hydroxylated. In contrast, the liver microsomal monooxygenases are rather nonspecific with regard to substrates and the position of the hydroxylated carbon atom. Table 2 gives the distribution of the phenolic products of some monoaromatic compounds obtained by the microsomal monooxygenation:

Table 2. *Hydroxylation of monosubstituted aromatic compounds in liver microsomes*

Substrate	% Hydroxylation at position ortho	meta	para	Ratio meta/para	References
Aniline	15	n. d.	85	<0.01	POSNER et al. (1956)
Acetanilide	5	1	94	0.01	ULLRICH et al. (1968)
Toluene	59	13	28	0.47	ULLRICH (1969b)
Anisol	11	0	89	0	ULLRICH and STAUDINGER (1968)
Benzonitril	n. d.	n. d.	n. d.	n. d.	ULLRICH (unpublished), JERINA (personal communication)
Nitrobenzene	n. d.	n. d.	n. d.	n. d.	ULLRICH (unpublished)

n. d. = not detectable

For all substrates with electron releasing substituents at the nucleus very low meta/para ratios are found. This is a characteristic feature of an electrophilic substitution mechanism. In agreement with an electrophilic attack by the active oxygen no detectable hydroxylation is observed when aromatic compounds with electron attracting substituents are used as substrates. The rather low attack of the ortho-position indicates the existence of steric effects in the course of hydroxylation.

From the electrophilic nature of the active oxygen it was suggested that addition to the aromatic π-electron system occurs (ULLRICH and STAUDINGER, 1968) forming arene oxide-oxepines as intermediates in aromatic hydroxylation (JERINA et al., 1968). This hypothesis is supported by two important findings. The naphthalene molecule containes a 10 π-electron system with a high degree of double bond character in one ring. The monooxygenase system in liver microsomes converts naphthalene into the 1,2-dihydrodiol compound (BOYLAND and WILTSHIRE, 1953). A mechanism via an epoxide intermediate was suggested very early by BOYLAND and BOOTH (1962):

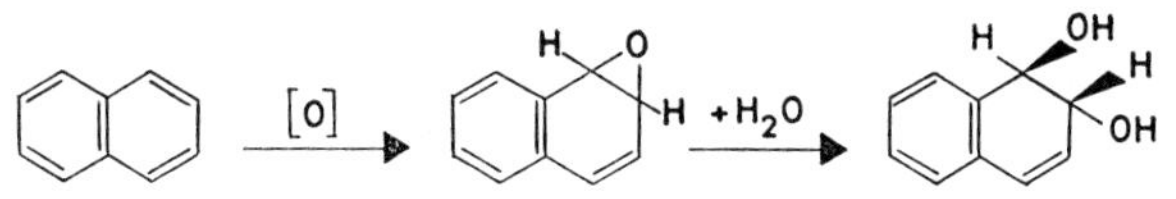

Fig. 4. Mechanism of naphthalene–1,2-dihydrodiol formation

This scheme was established recently by the isolation of the naphthalene 1,2-oxide from incubation mixtures (JERINA et al., 1968). Epoxide intermediates can also explain the phenomenon of migration of substituents during aromatic hydroxylation:

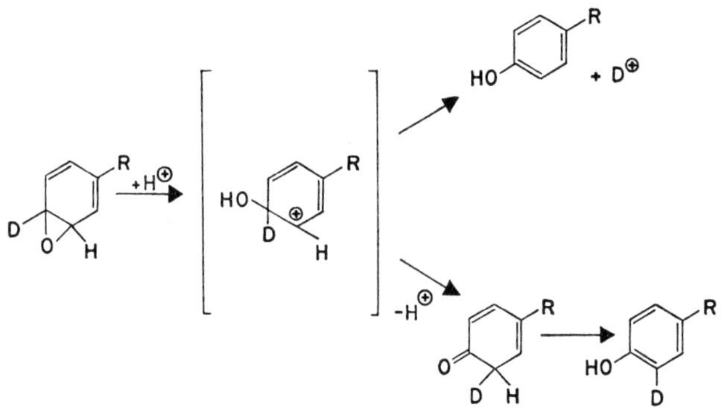

Fig. 5. Proposed scheme for the migration of substituents via arene oxides

This rearrangement of the monooxygenated molecule was termed "NIH-shift" (GUROFF et al., 1967) and is similar to the formation of chloral hydrate from trichloroethylene.

IV. Monooxygenation at Heteroatoms

Lipophilic secondary or tertiary amines and thioether compounds usually are metabolized by the microsomal system yielding the corresponding oxides (BAKER and CHAYKIN, 1962; KAMM and GILLETTE, 1958). The oxygen atom is derived from the oxygen molecule indicating that the oxidation at sulfur or nitrogen atoms are also characteristic for the active oxygen species of monooxygenase reactions.

C. Model Reactions for the Enzymatic Active Oxygen

As was previously pointed out the monooxygenase reactions seem to be compatible with the assumption of an electrophilic oxygen species as the active agent.

Neither oxygen itself nor hydrogen peroxide are activated enough to react in this way. Of the two possible radical states of oxygen the O_2H-radical has been shown to posses only weak oxidizing properties and is unable to hydroxylate organic compounds (NORMAN and LINDSAY SMITH, 1965).

The OH-radical as the second radical species is well known to hydroxylate aromatic compounds by an electrophilic addition mechanism (DORFMAN et al., 1962; DIXON and NORMAN, 1963). However, the formation of epoxides and dihydrodiols, the NIH-shift and the stoichiometry of monooxygenations are not in accordance with the OH-radical as active oxygen species.

Reactions very similar to the enzymatic monooxygenations are observed when hydrogen peroxide is activated in the presence of boron trifluoride (MCCLURE and WILLIAMS, 1952) or by acylation with trifluoroacetic acid (CHAMBERS et al., 1959). In both cases a strong polarization of the O-O bond occurs which allows the formation of an OH^+-ion in the transition state (IBNE RASA and EDWARDS, 1962):

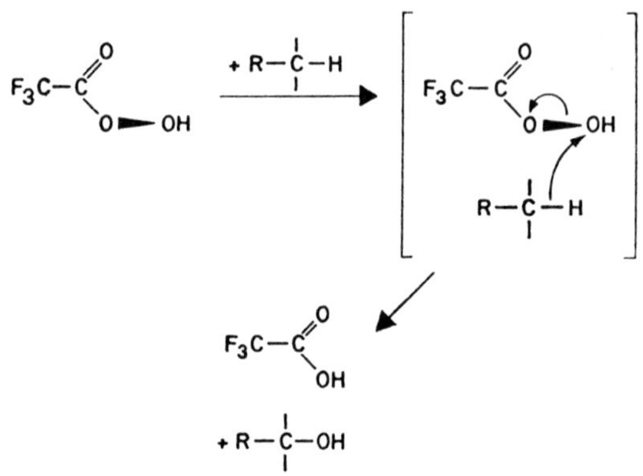

Fig. 6. Mechanism of hydroxylation by trifluoroperacetic acid

Aliphatic and electrophilic aromatic hydroxylations (NORMAN and LINDSAY SMITH, 1965), epoxidations and the NIH-shift (GUROFF et al., 1967; ULLRICH et al., 1968) are catalysed by these peracids. However, all of these oxidations proceed under unphysiological conditions, usually in nonaqueous medium and in the presence of strong acids. Therefore, the use of peracids as models for the active oxygen in monooxygenation has been questioned.

In order to avoid the postulation of an OH^+-ion, a model was sought that generated an uncharged oxygen atom, which is called "oxene" analogous to the carbene species to which it is isoelectronic. A common source of oxene is the photolysis of N_2O in the gas phase (YAMAZAKI and CVETANOVIC, 1964).

Studies on aliphatic hydroxylation in this system have revealed that the oxene exists mainly in the singlet state which is far more reactive than the electrophilic enzymatic active oxygen. These difficulties can be overcome by working with organic N-oxides in solution. During the photolysis of pyridine-N-oxide STREITH et al. (1967) obtained phenol when using benzene as a solvent. Similar results have been reported with pyrazine-N-oxide and toluene (IGETA et al., 1968). In the case of organic molecules with carbon-carbon double bonds the corresponding epoxides were found under these conditions (TSUCHIYA et al., 1969). The NIH-shift also has been observed during the photolysis of pyridine-N-oxide which is in accordance with the assumption that oxepines are intermediates in the hydroxylation mechanism (JERINA, personal communication). Obviously the results obtained by the photolysis of N-oxides correspond exactly to the results with peracids.

In Table 3 the chemical features of several known oxygen species are summarized and compared with the chemical properties of the enzymatic monooxygenation reaction:

Table 3. *Reactions of active oxygen species in comparison to monooxygenase reactions*

Active Oxygen	Source	Aromatic Hydroxylation	Aliphatic Hydroxylation	Epoxidation	Migration of Substituents
H_2O_2	3% Solution	—	—	—	—
$.O_2H$	H_2O_2 + Ce(IV)	—	—	—	—
.OH	H_2O_2 + Fe(II)EDTA	+ electrophilic	only tertiary CH-bonds	—	—
OH^+	Trifluoroperacetic acid	+ electrophilic	+ selective	+	+
O	$N_2O + h \cdot \nu$ (gas phase)	—	+ unselective	—	—
[O]	N-oxides $+ h : \nu$	+ electrophilic	+ selective	+	+
Monooxygenases		+ electrophilic	+ selective	+	+

By this comparison it becomes evident that the enzymatically formed active oxygen probably reacts by a mechanism very similar to the peracid oxidations or the oxidations during photolysis of N-oxides. These mechanisms involve a rather selective and strongly electrophilic oxygen species. For peracids this species is most probably the OH^+-ion (the protonated oxygen atom) which is formed in the transition state of the reaction, whereas the photolysis of N-oxides should give rise to a species of atomic oxygen. This mechanism resembles strongly the "carbenoid" reactions. These are defined by their tendency to addition and displacement reactions in contrast to the reactions of free carbenes (CLOSS and MOSS, 1964). The selectivity of a carbenoid mechanism is influenced by the nature of the leaving groups in the transition state (KIRMSE, 1969). Similar conditions also apply for the peracid oxidations or the light-induced oxidations by N-oxides which then also can be regarded as "oxenoid" reactions. Therefore, based on the similarity of these chemical and enzymatic reactions, we would like to suggest that the active oxygen species in enzymatic monooxygenations also has oxenoid character.

D. Model Systems for Oxygen Activation by Monooxygenases

Although there is strong indication for the oxenoid nature of the active oxygen in monooxygenase reactions, one has to prove how such a species can be formed by a transfer of two electrons to the oxygen molecule.

Hydrogen peroxide is the stable end product of a two-electron reduction of oxygen but it is ineffective in supporting hydroxylations. It was first pointed out by GEORGE (1965) that the energetics of the oxygen reduction are favorable enough to allow the formation of an oxygen atom and water instead of hydrogen peroxide:

$$O_2 + H_2 \begin{cases} \nearrow H_2O_2 & \Delta F° = -45.9 \text{ kcal/Mole} \\ \searrow O + H_2O & \Delta F° = -10.8 \text{ kcal/Mole} \end{cases}$$

(Aqueous solution, $[H^+] = 1$, $T = 298°$ K)

Therefore, considerable efforts have been devoted in the past decade to prove this hypothesis experimentally and to find a model system for the activation of oxygen.

All investigations on model systems started out with the early observation of UDENFRIEND and his group (1954), who discovered that a mixture of ferrous iron, EDTA, ascorbate and oxygen in an aqueous solution is able to hydroxylate aromatic compounds. The mechanism of these hydroxylations was studied by BRESLOW and LUKENS (1960). Their results indicated that the hydroxylations proceed by OH-radicals as in the Fenton-System (BARB et al., 1951).

Since OH-radicals cannot be considered as the active oxygen in enzymatic monooxygenations, the Udenfriend system became less interesting until NORMAN and RADDA (1962) and STAUDINGER and ULLRICH (1964a, b) discovered that hydroxylation by OH-radicals was not the only mechanism for the formation of phenols in this system. The new hydroxylation mechanism turned out to involve a highly reactive species which was also found to occur as the only active oxygen in an aqueous system of stannous phosphate complex and oxygen (ULLRICH et al., 1967; ULLRICH and STAUDINGER, 1969).

The chemical properties of the new species of active oxygen compared with OH-radicals can be seen from Table 4:

Table 4. *Hydroxylation by OH-radicals and in the stannous phosphate-oxygen system*

	System Fe^{2+} / EDTA / Ascorbic Acid / H_2O_2 / N_2	System Sn^{2+} / HPO_4^{2-} / O_2
Acetanilide	% OH — Actanilide 46.5 o / 2.5 m / 51.0 p	% OH — Acetanilide 34 o / 44 m / 22 p
Anisol	% OH — Anisol 66 o / 0 m / 34 p	% OH — Anisol 36 o / 47 m / 17 p
Toluene	% Cresol 59 o / 10 m / 31 p	% Cresol 46 o / 37 m / 17 p
Cyclohexane	—	Cyclohexanol
2-Methylbutane	2-Methylbutanol-2 (trace)	all isomeric alcohols prim. : sec. : tert. CH-bond 1.2 : 1.0 : 2.8

Most important and characteristic for the new mechanism is the unselective formation of alcohols from aliphatic compounds which does not occur with OH-radicals.

The oxygen atom of the hydroxyl group formed is derived from molecular oxygen and the stoichiometry of the hydroxylation is according to the equation:

$$Sn^{2+} + {}^{18}O_2 + RH \xrightarrow{+ H^{\oplus}} Sn^{4+} + R\,{}^{18}OH + OH^-$$

Therefore, this system can very well be regarded as a model for the two-electron activation of oxygen although the chemical reactivity of the active oxygen formed is much higher than in monooxygenase reactions.

In order to obtain a better model it was obviously important to look for systems in which the oxygen reduction and activation was mediated by ferrous and cuprous complexes, as in the enzymatic reaction. HAMILTON (1964) proposed a system of ferrous iron, ascorbate and oxygen which should hydroxylate and epoxidate by the following concerted mechanism:

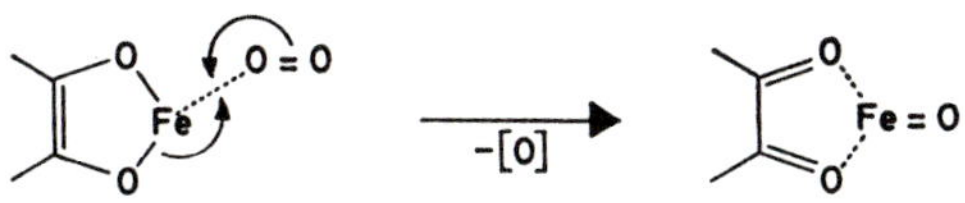

Fig. 7. Oxenoid hydroxylation mechanism by iron-endiole complexes and oxygen

However, using ascorbate, we did not find a hydroxylation activity in this system (ULLRICH and AMADORI, unpublished).

Following the idea of a concerted two electron transfer to oxygen, ULLRICH (1969) described a system in which oxygen was reduced by a ferrous-2-mercapto-benzoic acid complex. The thiol group was chosen as a redoxactive ligand in order to provide a two-electron donating entity. The chemical properties of this system are summarized in Table 5 and compared to the non-specific monooxygenations in liver microsomes.

Obviously the active oxygen species has electrophilic character and an oxenoid structure as indicated by its ability to form the dihydrodiol compound from naphthalene. Studies with ^{18}O revealed that all oxygen of the hydroxyl groups is derived from molecular oxygen (FROMMER, 1970). Although no migration of substituents during hydroxylation has been detected (FROMMER, 1970), this system may be regarded as the best model for studying the oxygen activation in monooxygenase reactions.

It seems very likely that the iron atom participates in the reaction. Two hypothetical mechanisms can be discussed:

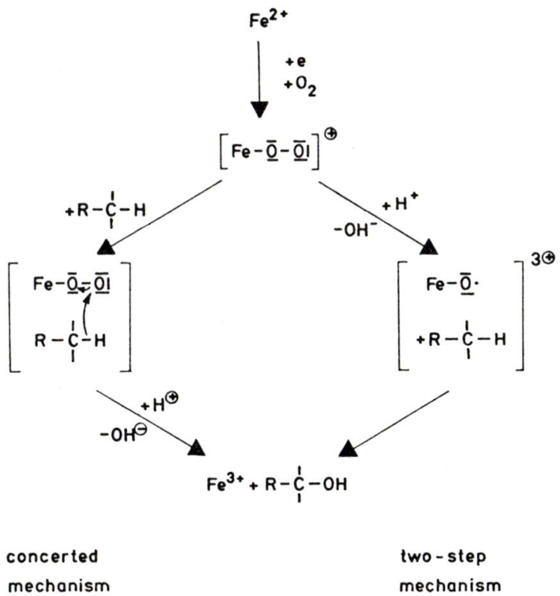

Fig. 8. Possible hydroxylation mechanisms by iron-thiol complexes and oxygen

Table 5. *Monooxygenation by liver microsomes and the iron(II)-2-mercaptobenzoic acid complex*

Substrate	Rat Liver Microsomes / NADPH / O_2	Fe^{2+} / 2-Mercaptobenzoic Acid / O_2
Cyclohexane	Cyclohexanol	Cyclohexanol
2-Methylbutane	Activity prim. : sec. : tert. CH-bond = 1: 14.8 : 109	Activity prim. : sec. : tert. CH-bond = 1: 2 : 12.4
N-Acetylphenetidin % Hydroxylation (ring) : % Dealkylation	2 : 98	43 : 57
Acetanilide % o- : % m- : % p- OH-Acetanilide	12 : 3 : 85	57 : 3 : 40
Toluene % o- : % m- : % p- Cresol	59 : 13 : 28	61 : 13 : 26
Naphthalene % (1+2)-Naphthol : % 1.2-Dihydrodiol	20 : 80	20 : 80

As an alternative active oxygen complex the ferrylion

$$Fe^{2\oplus} - \overline{\underline{O}} \quad \text{or} \quad Fe^{4\oplus} - \overline{\underline{O}} - H$$

is proposed by several authors (INGRAHAM, 1962; SIH, 1969). However, this species has been identified as the active intermediate in peroxidase reactions in which no hydroxylation of organic compounds can be observed.

In some of the well investigated monooxygenase systems like the non-specific monooxygenases in liver, the steroid 11β- and 21-hydroxylase, or the camphor-hydroxylating system from *pseudomonas putida*, cytochrome P-450 has been shown to function in the activation of oxygen (COOPER et al., 1967; ESTABROOK et al., 1963; COOPER et al., 1965; GUNSALUS, 1968). Evidence accumulates that the unusual properties of this cytochrome may be caused by the participation of sulfur in the coordination sphere of the heme-iron (NARASIMHULU et al., 1964; MASON et al., 1965). A thiol group would be a suitable donor for the second electron. The unusual anisotropic low-spin EPR-signal of cytochrome P-450 (MIYAKE et al., 1968) would be in accordance with this assumption since the EPR-spectra of heme complexes with thiol groups as ligands are almost identical (RÖDER and BAYER, 1969; JEFCOATE and GAYLOR, 1969) (Fig. 9).

A thiol group also could be responsible for the low potential of the cytochrome (WILLIAMS, R.J.P., personal communication).

If the participation of a thiol group can be established for cytochrome P-450, the hydroxylating systems containing ferrous iron and sulfhydryl compounds can be regarded as true models for the oxygen activation by this cytochrome and probably for monooxygenases in general. It would then be promising to study the mechanism of oxygen activation by direct investigation of these model systems.

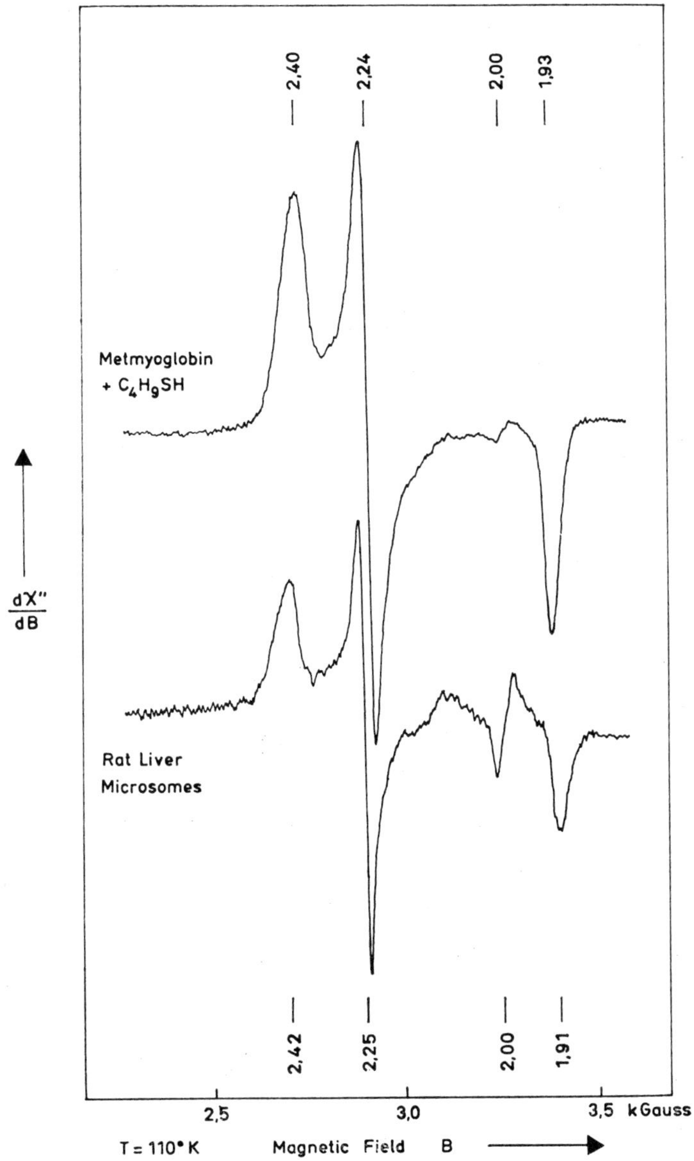

Fig. 9. EPR-spectra of cytochrome P-450 and the myoglobin-n-butyl mercaptane complex (H. Ruf, unpublished)

References

Baker, J.R., Chaykin, S.: The biosynthesis of trimethylamine — N-oxide. J. biol. Chem. **237**, 1309—1313 (1962).

Barb, W.G., Baxendale, J.H., George, P., Hargrave, K.R.: Reactions of ferrous and ferric ions with hydrogen peroxide. Part I. The ferrous ion reaction. Trans. Faraday Soc. **47**, 462—500 (1951).

Bayer, E., Hill, H.A.O., Röder, A., Williams, R.J.P.: The interaction between haem-iron and thiols. Chem. Commun. **1969**, 109.

BLOOM, B.M., SHULL, G.M.: Epoxidation of unsaturated steroids by microorganisms. J. Amer. chem. Soc. **77**, 5767—5768 (1955).
BOYLAND, E., BOOTH, J.: The metabolic fate and excretion of drugs. Ann. Rev. Pharmacol. **2**, 129—242 (1962).
— WILTSHIRE, G.H.: Metabolism of naphthalene by liver slices. Biochem. J. **53**, 424—426 (1953).
BRESLOW, R., LUKENS, L.N.: On the mechanism of action of an ascorbic acid-dependent nonenzymatic hydroxylating system. J. biol. Chem. **235**, 292—296 (1960).
BRODIE, B.B., AXELROD, J., SHORE, P.A., UDENFRIEND, S.: Ascorbic acid in aromatic hydroxylation. II. Products formed by reaction of substrates with ascorbic acid, ferrous ion, and oxygen. J. biol. Chem. **208**, 741—750 (1954).
— GILLETTE, J.R., LADU, B.N.: Enzymatic metabolism of drugs and other foreign compounds. Ann. Rev. Biochem. **27**, 427—453 (1958).
BYINGTON, K.H., LEIBMAN, K.C.: Metabolism of trichloroethylene in liver microsomes. II. Identification of the reaction product as chloral hydrate. Molec. Pharmacol. **1**, 247—251 (1965).
CHAMBERS, R.D., GOGGIN, P., MUSGRAVE, W.K.R.: The oxidation of aromatic hydrocarbons and phenols by trifluoroperoxyacetic acid. J. chem. Soc. 1804—1807 (1959).
CLOSS, G.L., MOSS, R.A.: Carbenoid formation of arylcyclopropanes from olefins, benzal bromides, and organolithium compounds and from photolysis of aryl diazomethanes. J. Amer. chem. Soc. **86**, 4042—4053 (1964).
COOPER, D.Y., LEVIN, S., NARASIMHULU, S., ROSENTHAL, O., ESTABROOK, R.W.: Photochemical action spectrum of the terminal oxidase of mixed function oxidase systems. Science **147**, 400—402 (1965).
— NOVACK, B., FOROFF, O., SLADE, A., SAUNDERS, E., NARASIMHULU, S., ROSENTHAL, O.: Photochemical action spectrum of reconstituted steroid 11β-hydroxylase of bovine adrenal mitochondria. Fed. Proc. **26**, 341 Abstr. 478 (1967).
DIXON, W.T., NORMAN, R.O.C.: An intermediate in homolytic aromatic substitution. Proc. chem. Soc. 97—99 (1963).
DORFMAN, L.M., TAUB, A., BÜCHLER, R.E.: Pulse radiolysis studies. I. Transient spectra and reaction-rate constants in irradiated aqueous solutions of benzene. J. chem. Physics **36**, 3051—3061 (1962).
ESTABROOK, R.W., COOPER, D.Y., ROSENTHAL, O.: The light reversible carbon monoxide inhibition of the steroid C 21 — hydroxylase system of the adrenal cortex. Biochem. Z. **338**, 741—755 (1963).
FROMMER, U.: Dissertation, Gießen (1970).
GEORGE, P.: The fitness of oxygen. In: Oxidases and Related Redox Systems. Ed. by KING, MASON and MORRISON. New York-London-Sydney: Wiley 1965.
GUNSALUS, I.C.: A soluble methylene hydroxylase system: structure and role of cytochrome P-450 and iron-sulfur protein components. Hoppe-Seylers Z. physiol. Chem. **349**, 1610—1613 (1968).
GUROFF, G., DALY, J.W., JERINA, D.M., RENSON, J., WITKOP, B., UDENFRIEND, S.: Hydroxylation-induced migrations: The NIH-shift. Science **158**, 1524 (1967).
HAMILTON, G.H.: Oxidation by molecular oxygen. II. The oxygen atom transfer mechanism for mixed-function oxidases and the model for mixed-function oxidases. J. Amer. chem. Soc. **86**, 3391—3392 (1964).
HAYAISHI, O.: Oxygenases. New York-London: Academic Press 1962.
— Oxygenases. In: Biochemie des Sauerstoffs. Ed. by B. HESS and HJ. STAUDINGER. Berlin-Heidelberg-New York: Springer 1968.
HAYANO, M.: Oxygenases in lipid and steroid metabolism. In: HAYAISHI, O.: Oxygenases. New York-London: Academic Press 1962.
— GUT, M., DORFMAN, R.I., SEBEK, O.K., PETERSON, D.H.: Steric considerations in the enzymatic course of the hydroxylation of steroids. J. Amer. chem. Soc. **80**, 2336—2337 (1958).
IBNE-RASA, K.M., EDWARDS, J.: The mechanism of the oxidation of some aromatic amines by peroxyacetic acid. J. Amer. chem. Soc. **84**, 763 (1962).
IGETA, H., TSUCHIYA, T., YAMADA, M., ARAI, H.: Photo-induced oxygenation by pyrazine N-oxides. I. Chem. pharm. Bull. **16**, 767 (1968).
INGRAHAM, L.L.: Biochemical mechanisms. New York-London: Wiley 1962.
JEFCOATE, C.R.E., GAYLOR, J.L.: Ligand interactions with haemoprotein P-450. II. Influence of phenobarbital and methylcholanthrene induction processes on P-450 spectra. Biochemistry **8**, 3464—3472 (1969).
JERINA, D.M., DALY, W., J., WITKOP, B., ZALTZMAN-NIRENBERG, P., UDENFRIEND, S.: Role of arene oxide-oxepine system in the metabolism of aromatic substrates. I. In vitro conversion of benzene oxide to a premercapturic acid and a dihydrodiol. Arch. Biochem. **128**, 176—183 (1968).

JERINA, D.M., DALY, J.W., WITKOP, B., ZALTZMAN-NIRENBERG, P., UDENFRIEND., S.: The role of orene oxide-oxepine systems in the metabolism of aromatic substrates. III. Formation of 1.2-naphthalene oxide from naphthalene by liver microsomes. J. Amer. chem. Soc. **90**, 6525—6527 (1968).

KAMM, J.J., GILLETTE, J.R., BRODIE, B.B.: Metabolism of chlorpromazine to chlorpromazine sulfoxide by liver microsomes. Fed. Proc. **17**, 382 (1958).

KIRMSE, W.: Carbene, Carbenoide und Carbenanaloge. Weinheim: Verlag Chemie 1969.

MASON, H.S.: Mechanisms of oxygen metabolism. Advanc. Enzymol. **19**, 79—233 (1957).

— FOWLKS, W.L., PETERSON, E.: Oxygen transfer and electron transport by the phenolase comxple. J. Amer. chem. Soc. **77**, 2914—2915 (1955).

— NORTH, J.C., VANNESTE, M.: Microsomal mixed function oxidations: the metabolism of xenobiotics. Fed. Proc. **24**, 1172—1180 (1965).

MCCLURE, J.D., WILLIAMS, P.H.: Hydrogen peroxide-boron trifluoride etherate, a new oxidizing agent. J. org. Chem. **27**, 24—26 (1952).

MIYAKE, Y., GAYLOR, J.L., MASON, H.S.: Properties of a submicrosomal particle containing P 450 and flavoprotein. J. biol. Chem. **24**, 5788—5797 (1968).

NARASIMHULU, S., COOPER, D.Y., ROSENTHAL, O.: Function of sulfur groups in aerobic hydroxylases. 148th Natl. Meeting Amer. Chem. Soc., Sept., Abstr. 41 (1964).

NORMAN, R.O.C., LINDSAY SMITH, J.R.: Mechanisms of aromatic hydroxylation and ring-opening reactions. In: Oxidases Related Redox Systems (Vol. I). Ed. by KING, MASON and MORRISON. New York-London-Sydney: Wiley 1965.

— RADDA, G.K.: Aromatic hydroxylation: the electrophilic character of the hydroxyl radical, and its significance in biological hydroxylation. Proc. chem. Soc. **1962**, 138.

POSNER, H.S., MITOMA, C., UDENFRIEND, S.: Enzymatic hydroxylation of aromatic compounds. Arch. Biochem. **61**, 431—441 (1956).

PREISS, B., BLOCH, K.: ω-Oxidation of long chain fatty acids in rat liver. J. biol. Chem. **239**, 85—88 (1964).

RENSON, J., WEISSBACH, W., UDENFRIEND, S.: On the mechanisms of oxidative cleavage of aryl-alkyl ethers by liver microsomes. Molec. Pharmacol. **1**, 145—147 (1965).

RODER, A., BAYER, E.: Elektronenspinvesonanz-Untersuchungen an Hamin-Meraptan-Complexen. Europ. J. Biochem. **11**, 89—92 (1969).

SIH, C.J.: Enzymatic mechanism of steroid hydroxylation. Science **163**, 1297—1300 (1969).

STAUDINGER, HJ., ULLRICH, V.: Zum Reaktionsmechanismus der nichtenzymatischen Hydroxylierung. Zugleich Untersuchungen über die Aktivierung von Sauerstoff. Z. Naturforsch. **19**b, 409—413 (1964a).

— — Über die Existenz des Perhydroxylradicals in wäßrigen Lösungen und seine Bedeutung bei Oxydationsreaktionen. Z. Naturforsch. **19**b, 877—882 (1964b).

STREITH, J., DANNER, B., SIGWALT, C.: Photochemistry of pyridine oxides: atomic oxygen transfer in solution; a new synthesis of phenol. Chem. Commun. 979—980 (1967).

TSUCHIYA, T., ARAI, H., IGETA, H.: Photo-induced oxygenation by pyrazine N-oxides. II. Formation of epoxides from ethylenic compounds. Tetrahedron Letters **32**, 2747—2750 (1969).

UDENFRIEND, S., CLARK, C.T., AXELROD, J., BRODIE, B.B.: Ascorbic acid in aromatic hydroxylation. I. A model system for aromatic hydroxylation. J. biol. Chem. **208**, 731—740 (1954).

ULLRICH, V.: On the hydroxylation of cyclohexane in rat liver microsomes. Hoppe-Seylers Z. physiol. Chem. **350**, 357—365 (1969a).

— Oxygen activation by the iron(II)-2-mercaptobenzoic acid complex. A model for microsomal mixed function oxygenases. Z. Naturforsch. **24**b, 699—704 (1969b).

— AMADORI, E., STAUDINGER, HJ.: Zum Mechanismus der Hydroxylierung bei der Autoxidation von Zinn(II)phosphat-Lösungen. Z. Naturforsch. **22**b, 226 (1967).

— STAUDINGER, HJ.: Aktivierung von Sauerstoff in Modellsystemen. In: Biochemie des Sauerstoffs. Ed. by B. HESS and HJ. STAUDINGER. Berlin-Heidelberg-New York: Springer 1968.

— — Zum Mechanismus der Hydroxylierungen mit molekularem Sauerstoff und Zinn(II)-Komplexen. Z. Naturforsch. **24**b, 583—588 (1969).

— WOLF, J., AMADORI, E., STAUDINGER, HJ.: The mixed function oxygenation of 4-halogeno-acetanilides in rat liver microsomes and model systems. Hoppe-Seylers Z. physiol. Chem. **349**, 85—94 (1968).

WONG, D.T., TERRIERE, L.C.: Epoxidation of aldrin, isodrin, and heptachlor by rat liver microsomes. Biochem. Pharmacol. **14**, 375—377 (1965).

YAMAZAKI, H., CVETANOVIC, K.J.: Collisional deactivation of excited singlet oxygen atoms and their insertion into the CH-bonds of propane. J. chem. Phys. **41**, 3703—3710 (1964).

Chapter 38

Cytochrome P-450 – Its Function in the Oxidative Metabolism of Drugs[1]

RONALD W. ESTABROOK

With 23 Figures

The oxidative transformation of a large variety of compounds of pharmacological interest is known to occur primarily in the liver. The participation in these reactions of an enzyme complex associated with the disrupted endoplasmic reticulum (microsomal fraction) of liver was established in the mid-1950's by the group at the National Institutes of Health under the direction of B.B. BRODIE (BRODIE, 1955; COOPER and BRODIE, 1955). Indeed, this laboratory has served as the major source of investigators and ideas for the work which has led to our present understanding of the multitude of parameters modifying drug metabolism. Biochemical studies on drug metabolism gained their initial impetus from the studies of R.T. WILLIAMS and his collaborators (1959), who identified many of the products formed in the body and characterized the major pathways of detoxification. Parallel to the studies by BRODIE and his group were a number of other investigations directly related to the biochemical mechanism of such oxidative reactions. Studies of the metabolic pathways for steroids (SAMUELS, 1961), the use of oxygen-18 to assess the role of molecular oxygen (HAYANO et al., 1955; MASON, 1957; HAYAISHI, 1962), the spectrophotometric study of microsomal pigments (KLINGENBERG, 1958), and the detailed investigation by pharmacologists of "drug tolerance" (CONNEY et al., 1956, 1960; BURNS et al., 1955; REMMER, 1959), all came to the forefront at about the same time. Examination of each of these facets of the problem added to our present understanding of the mechanism of drug hydroxylation reactions, reactions that are now classified as mixed function oxidation (MASON, 1957) or monooxygenase (HAYAISHI, 1962) type reactions. Since many of the earlier studies have been well covered in extensive reviews, the present article is concerned only with the discovery and characterization of cytochrome P-450, a microsomal pigment now accepted as the terminal oxidase for "oxygen activation" in many drug degrading reactions (COOPER et al., 1965a).

I. Discovery of Cytochrome P-450

DAVID KEILIN, during his productive career, recognized that some tissues, in particular liver and kidney, contained an additional pigment which obscured the characteristic absorption bands of reduced cytochromes *b* and *c*, known to be localized in the mitochondria (KEILIN and HARTREE, 1940). It was not recognized that this additional pigment — now termed cytochrome b_5 (PAPPENHEIMER and WILLIAMS, 1954) — was associated with the microsomal fraction of some cell

1 Supported in part by a United States Public Health Service Research Grant, GM 16488.

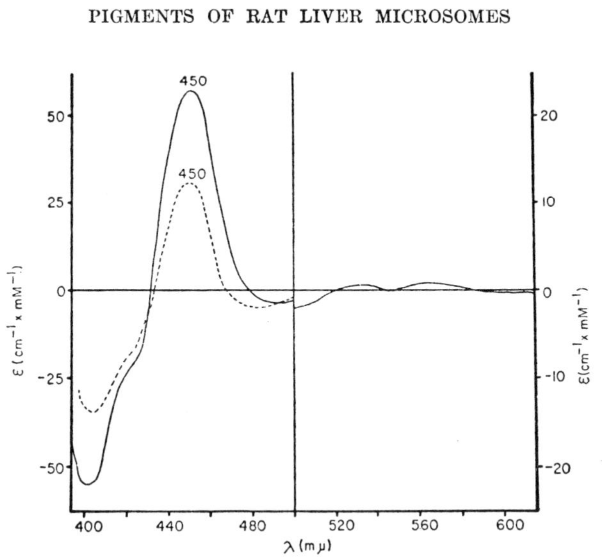

Fig. 1. The first report on the spectral properties of the carbon monoxide complex of reduced cytochrome P-450. The dotted curve represents the difference spectrum obtained with DPNH reduction in the presence of CO; the solid line curve represents the difference spectrum observed after sodium dithionite reduction in the presence of CO. The millimolar extinction coefficients refer to the cytochrome b_5 present in the liver microsomes. From KLINGENBERG (1958)

types until the studies by STRITTMATTER and BALL (1952). The limits of spectrophotometric instrumentation available in the early 1950's led STRITTMATTER and BALL (1952) to employ a detergent, sodium deoxycholate, to clarify their samples for accurate measurements of spectra. It was later disovered (KLINGENBERG, 1958) that this treatment destroys the cytochrome P-450 associated with the microsomes — a result which delayed the first report of a carbon monoxide binding pigment in microsomes by nearly 6 years and which misled RYAN and ENGEL (1957) who observed the carbon monoxide inhibition of a steroid hydroxylation reaction catalyzed by adrenal cortex microsomes.

The mid-1950's was a period of significant advancement in the application of the rapid and sensitive spectrophotometric techniques developed by CHANCE (1957) for the examination of turbid biological samples. A frequent visitor to CHANCE's laboratory during that time was A.M. PAPPENHEIMER, who was interested in a cytochrome pigment found in the mid-gut of the *Cecropia* larvae (CHANCE and PAPPENHEIMER, 1954). These studies prompted another member of the laboratory, G.R. WILLIAMS, to study further the reactions of cytochrome b_5 of liver microsomes. These investigations revealed that more reduced diphosphopyridine nucleotide was required to reduce cytochrome b_5 than was theoretically necessary, leading CHANCE and WILLIAMS (1954) to postulate that an additional electron accepting component, other than cytochrome b_5, was present in microsomes. Although not reported in the original article by CHANCE and WILLIAMS (1954), G.R. WILLIAMS in his systematic study of microsomal pigments recognized the presence of a carbon monoxide binding pigment. It was not until 1958 that KLINGENBERG (1958), at that time a postdoctoral fellow at the Johnson Research Foundation, first reported the spectral details (Fig. 1) of a microsomal hemoprotein which reacts with carbon monoxide forming a rather broad absorption band with a maximum at 450 mμ. The lability of this carbon monoxide-binding pigment to detergents, such as cholate and deoxycholate, as well as to acid pH, has often been observed since the first report by Klingenberg on the "great instability of the CO addition compound".

Although Klingenberg had surmised from the imbalance of total heme content of microsomes to the content of cytochrome b_5 that the CO-binding pigment was indeed a hemoprotein, the subsequent studies of Garfinkel (1958) suggested an opposite conclusion. As stated by Garfinkel, referring to the CO-binding pigment of liver microsomes, "It is suggested that this pigment contains some sort of a metal ion in view of its complexing properties. Since there is no photochemical effect on the CO complex, and, also, only the one peak (a careful search for α and β peaks like those of hemoproteins having been unsuccessful) it is probably not an iron hemoprotein. The fact that this pigment is destroyed by digestion and by exposure to low pH suggests that the same lipids which hold together the microsomal particle also are involved in its structure."

It was not until 1962 that a preliminary communication appeared from the laboratory of Omura and Sato (1962) reaffirming the earlier conclusion of Klingenberg (1958) that the microsomal fraction of liver did contain a hemoprotein other than cytochrome b_5. The data published in this initial brief note by Omura and Sato (1962) and subsequently published in detail (1964a, b), reinitiated interest in the chemistry of cytochrome P-450 and its degradation product P-420. The observation that the reduced form of cytochrome P-450 combines with carbon monoxide, as well as ethyl isocyanide (Fig. 2), has served as one of the

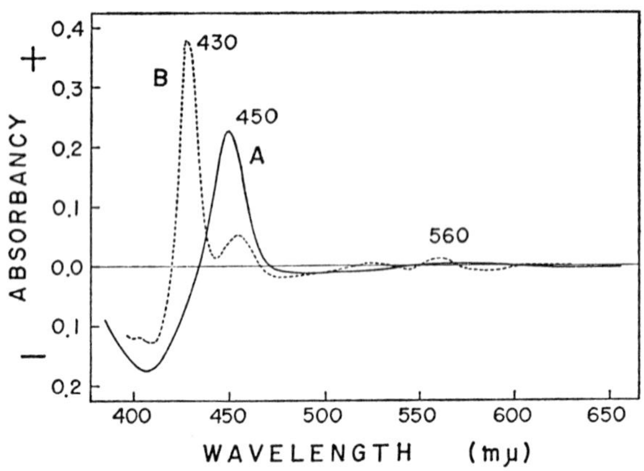

Fig. 2. The spectral properties of the carbon monoxide and ethyl isocyanide derivative of reduced cytochrome P-450 of liver microsomes. Microsomes were suspended to 2 mg protein per ml in 0.1 M phosphate buffer, pH 7.0 and reduced with sodium dithionite. The solid line curve represents the difference spectrum observed in the presence of CO while the dashed line curve represents the difference spectrum obtained on addition of ethyl isocyanide (final concentration, 1 mM). From Omura and Sato (1962)

major factors in further research on the identity of various types of cytochrome P-450 as observed with liver microsomes from animals treated with different "inducing compounds" (Sladek and Mannering, 1969). The studies of Omura and Sato (1964b) characterized P-420 (Fig. 3) and described the isolation and purification of this pigment. Although it is frequently considered that P-420 is the consequence of an irreversible destruction of cytochrome P-450, it is interesting to note that Omura and Sato (1962) claimed that P-420 in lipase-digested micro-

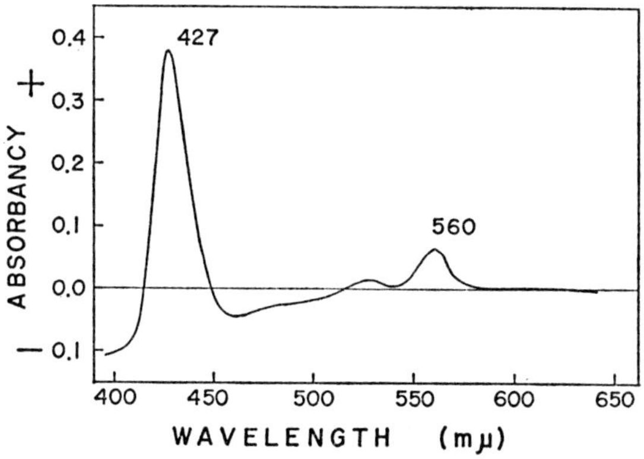

Fig. 3. The reduced minus oxidized difference spectrum of P-420. Venom digested liver microsomes were placed in special Thunberg-type cells and reduced with sodium dithionite under anaerobic conditions. The contents of the reference cuvettes were reduced with DPNH (0.1 mM) under aerobic conditions. The content of microsomal protein was 3 mg per ml in 0.1 M phosphate buffer, pH 7.0. From Omura and Sato (1962)

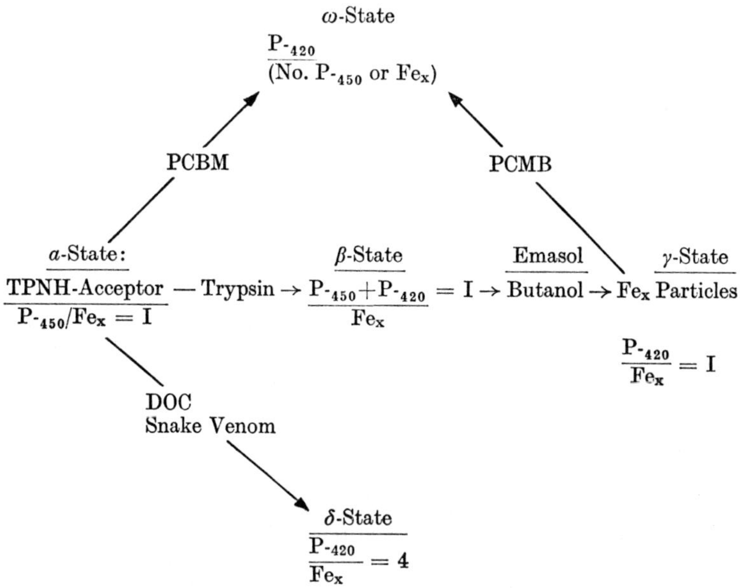

Fig. 4. Various stages of degradative changes of cytochrome P-450 as proposed by Mason et al. (1965a). The various states of modification on treatment of microsomes with deoxycholate (DOC), crude lipase (snake venom), a mercurial (parachloromercuribenzoate, PCMB), a proteolytic enzyme (trypsin) and detergent mixture (Emasol) are indicated. The concentration of the hemoproteins determined by spectral analysis or electron paramagnetic resonance (FeX) in the different forms are indicated by the ratios. From Mason et al. (1965a)

somes is enzymatically reducible by DPNH or TPNH under appropriate conditions. This observation has never been confirmed although it does open the possibility of a reversible interconversion between cytochrome P-450 and P-420. As summarized by Mason et al. (1965a) (Fig. 4), the conversion of cytochrome P-450 to P-420 can involve a very complex series of reactions. There is no doubt that the lability of P-420 to sodium dithionite reduction in the presence of oxygen

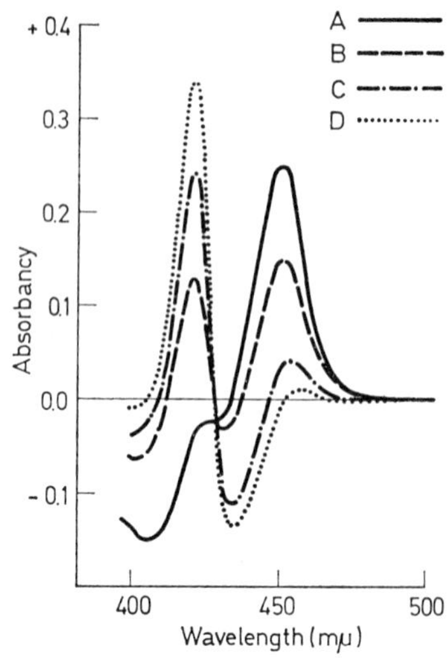

Fig. 5. Changes in the carbon monoxide binding pigments of liver microsomes during digestion by snake venom lipase. Liver microsomes (2 mg protein per ml) were suspended in 0.1 M tris-acetate buffer, pH 8.5, and digested with 0.05% (final concentration) of heat-treated snake venom at 0° under pure N_2. At the times indicated a sample of the digest was withdrawn and after addition of sodium dithionite and carbon monoxide the difference spectrum was recorded. Curve A, 1 min after addition of heated venom; Curve B, 5 min; Curve C, 20 min; Curve D, 60 min. From Omura and Sato (1964)

(presumably the consequence of hydrogen peroxide generated as a product of the reaction) has led to considerable confusion in the further elucidation of P-420 as it relates to cytochrome P-450. However, the refractory nature of membrane-bound cytochrome P-450 to isolation and purification will require an even more detailed evaluation of this pigment in order to gain further information on the chemical nature of cytochrome P-450. As first indicated by Klingenberg (1958), and later described in detail by Omura and Sato (1964a), it is possible (Fig. 5) to stoichiometrically convert P-450 to P-420 under appropriate conditions.

The cytochrome P-420 isolated by Sato and Omura (1964b) possesses a number of interesting properties. In their original description of this pigment, Omura and Sato (1964b) noted its ability to undergo aggregation at pH values more acid than 7.5. This phenomena has recently been confirmed by Shoeman et al. (1969b), who have shown, by electron microscopic examination, the formation of long membranous tubules when P-420 molecules associate. The question remains, however, whether this aggregation is a consequence of interaction of P-420 molecules or due to adventitious structural protein molecules associated with the P-420. The P-420 isolated by Omura and Sato (1964b) contains about 7 mμmoles of heme per milligram of protein. Cytochrome P-450 isolated by Katagiri et al. (1968) from *Pseudomonas putida* has a molecular weight of about 40,000—50,000 per heme. This is equivalent to about 25 mμmoles of heme per milligram of protein. If mammalian cytochrome *P*-450 resembles the bacterial cytochrome P-450, the P-420 isolated by Omura and Sato (1964b) is therefore only 35—40% pure. Furthermore, the influence of pH on the spectral properties of P-420 (Fig. 6), presumably reflecting changes associated with aggregation, can easily lead to confusion in interpreting ligand induced spectral changes of P-420 as a model for reactions of cytochrome P-450.

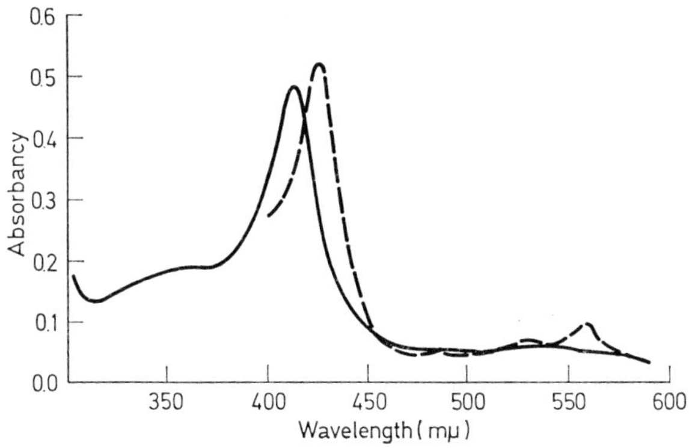

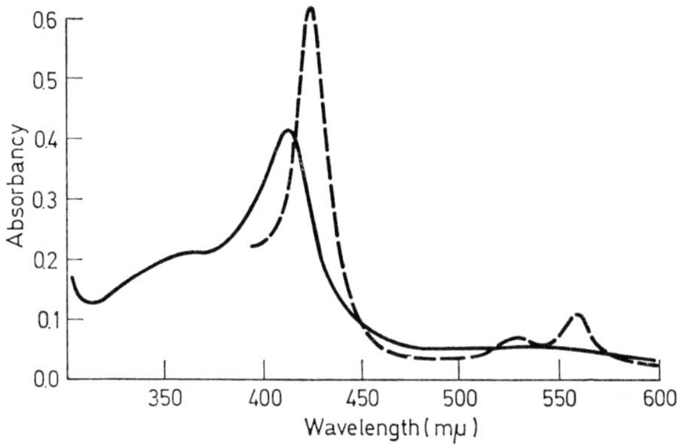

Fig. 6. The influence of pH on the absorption spectra of isolated P-420. The solid line curves represent the spectra of the oxidized hemoprotein; the dashed curves represent the spectra obtained after addition of sodium dithionite. The reaction cuvettes contained the equivalent of 3.7 mμmole of protoheme per ml dissolved in 0.1 M phosphate buffer, pH 7.0 (upper figure) or 0.1 M tris-acetate buffer, pH 9.0 (lower figure). From OMURA and SATO (1964)

II. Function of Cytochrome P-450

About 1960, a fruitful collaboration was established between DAVID COOPER and OTTO ROSENTHAL of the Harrison Department of Surgical Research, University of Pennsylvania, and the author while he was associated with the Johnson Research Foundation. Dr. COOPER, a surgeon, was investigating the influence of various steroids on hypertension. These studies led COOPER to question the control mechanism of steroid hydroxylation reactions catalyzed by enzymes present in the adrenal cortex. At that time, ESTABROOK was concerned with mitochondrial oxidation-reduction reactions, particularly as they reflect energy conservation. COOPER's knowledge of the steroid metabolism literature together with ESTABROOK's availability to the sophisticated instrumentation developed by BRITTON CHANCE, set the stage for the unraveling of a fascinating series of studies describing the role of cytochrome P-450 as the long-sought pigment necessary to activate oxygen in drug and steroid metabolism (ESTABROOK et al., 1963; OMURA et al., 1965). It is fair to say that much that is known today about the mechanism of liver microsomal oxidative metabolism of drugs is derived from observations made with the steroid hydroxylating system of the adrenal cortex.

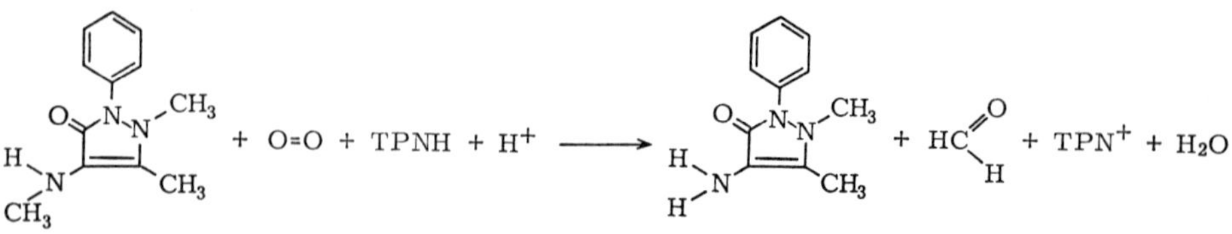

Fig. 7. An example of the proposed stoichiometry for mixed function oxidation reactions. The N-demethylation of monomethyl-4-aminoantipyrine to formaldehyde and 4-aminoantipyrine concomitant with the oxidation of TPNH and reduction of atmospheric oxygen is shown

At first it was apparent that there was no direct experimental evidence to show that the stoichiometry (Fig. 7) proposed by MASON (1957) for a mixed function oxidation reaction was applicable to microsome catalyzed hydroxylation reactions. By a combination of techniques, such as a sensitive polarographic method for measuring oxygen utilization, a fluorometic method for measuring reduced pyridine nucleotide oxidation, and a chemical method for measuring

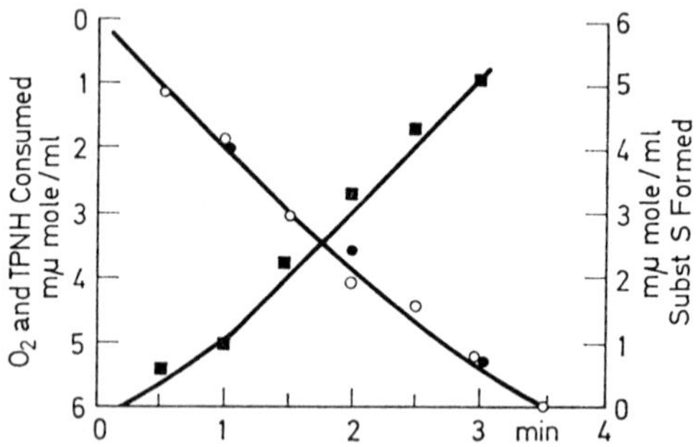

Fig. 8. The stoichiometry of TPNH oxidation, oxygen utilization and substance S formation during the adrenal cortex microsomes catalyzed hydroxylation of 17-hydroxyprogesterone. Three parallel experiments were carried out with the same preparation of adrenal cortex microsomes. The increase in rate of oxygen utilization (open circles) was determined polarographically after addition of 17-hydroxyprogesterone to a mixture of microsomes fortified with TPNH and a TPNH generating system containing glucose-6-phosphate and glucose-6-phosphate dehydrogenase. A similar experiment was carried out to measure fluorometrically the increase in the rate of TPNH oxidation (solid circles) but in the absence of the TPNH generating system. Samples were removed at the times indicated to determine colorimetrically the amount of product (cortexalone) formation (solid squares). From COOPER et al. (1962)

steroid product formation, the validity of MASON's hypothesis (1957) was established (COOPER et al., 1962). The result of this first series of experiments which measured the TPNH dependent 21-hydroxylation of 17-hydroxyprogesterone as catalyzed by adrenal cortex microsomes is shown in Fig. 8. Unraveling the details of the reaction system now became a challenge. How is oxygen activated so that one atom of molecular oxygen is incorporated into the product and the other atom reduced to water?

The observation that microsome-catalyzed hydroxylation reactions are inhibited by carbon monoxide was established by RYAN and ENGEL (1957) for a steroid substrate and by CONNEY et al. (1957) for a carcinogenic compound. The role of cytochrome P-450 as the site of inhibition by carbon monoxide, as well as the role of the cytochrome in "oxygen activation" for hydroxylation reactions, has been described in detail in a recent review (ESTABROOK et al., 1969). Briefly, the application of the photochemical action spectrum technique developed by WARBURG (1949) permitted the identification of cytochrome P-450 as the key component in many microsomal catalyzed reactions (ESTABROOK et al., 1963).

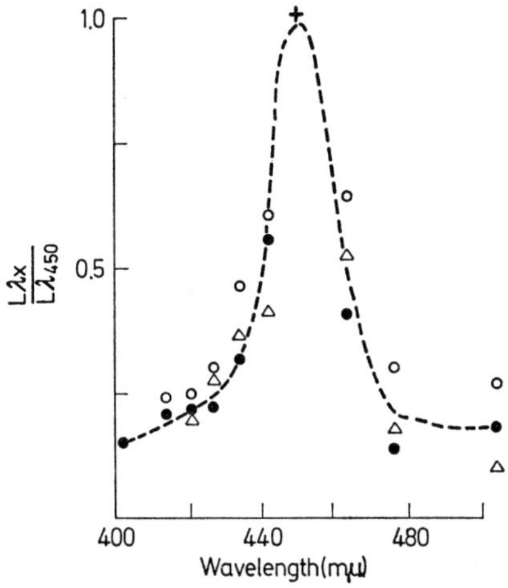

Fig. 9. The photochemical action spectra for the carbon monoxide inhibition of hepatic microsomal mixed-function oxidation reactions. Liver microsomes (3 mg of protein per 2.5 ml of reaction mixture) were incubated in tris-phosphate buffer, pH 7.4; containing $MgCl_2$, TPNH, glucose-6-phosphate, and glucose-6-phosphate dehydrogenase and codeine (solid circles), monomethyl 4-aminoantipyrine (open circles), or acetanilide (triangles). Control samples were incubated under an atmosphere of CO/O_2 or N_2/O_2 for 10 min in the dark at 25°C to determine the extent of inhibition of the reaction. Experimental samples were incubated under similar conditions but irradiated with a constant light energy of varying wavelengths obtained from a 1500 watt Xenon lamp with appropriate interference filters and neutral density filters. The light sensitivity for reversal of CO inhibition expresses the extent of activity determined upon irradiation of the sample with specific wavelengths of light after normalization to the maximal activity observed with light of 450 mμ. From COOPER et al. (1965a)

The extension of these observations on the role of cytochrome P-450 in steroid hydroxylation reactions to a number of similar reactions catalyzed by liver microsomes during drug metabolism was readily accomplished (COOPER et al., 1965a). The result of one series of such experiments is shown in Fig. 9. Thus, within a brief span of 5 years, a new respiratory pigment has been recognized (KLINGENBERG, 1958), much of its chemistry defined (OMURA and SATO, 1962, 1964a, b) and its biological function established (COOPER et al., 1965a; ESTABROOK et al., 1963). The last 8 years, since the original definition of the role of cytochrome P-450 in drug and steroid metabolism, have seen a profusion of interest in further elaborating the parameters modifying the function of cytochrome P-450.

III. How Does Cytochrome P-450 Function?

Parallel with the studies on the carbon monoxide inhibition of cytochrome P-450-catalyzed reactions, was a series of electron paramagnetic resonance studies emanating from the laboratory of HOWARD MASON (HASHIMOTO et al., 1962). These investigations described the properties of a low spin hemoprotein compound present in the microsomal fraction of liver. This component, originally designated as FeX by MASON, is now recognized as cytochrome P-450 (MASON, 1965b). The correlation of electron paramagnetic resonance with spectrophotometric studies has extended our understanding of how cytochrome P-450 functions.

Another major advance in our knowledge of cytochrome P-450 relevant to drug metabolism originated from studies on the interaction of steroids with the cytochrome P-450 of adrenal cortex microsomes. NARASIMHULU et al. (1965) observed that the addition of 17-hydroxyprogesterone to adrenal cortex microsomes resulted in a small but significant spectral change (Fig. 10). The magnitude

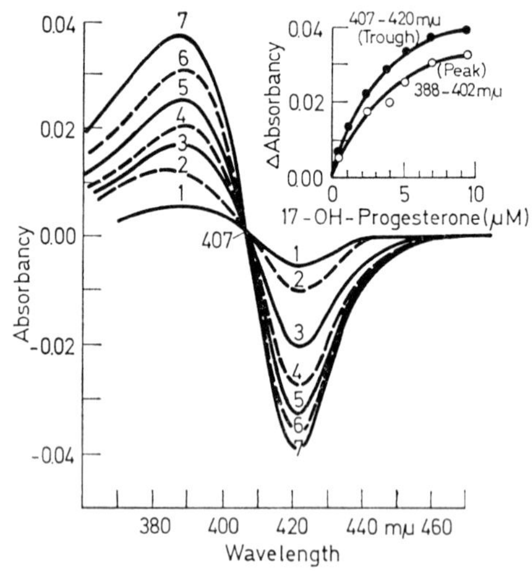

Fig. 10. The steroid induced spectral change observed with a Triton clarified preparation of adrenal cortex microsomes. Microsomes from beef adrenal cortex were isolated and clarified with Triton N-101 as described by NARASIMHULU et al. (1965). The difference spectra were obtained in a Cary Model 14 spectrophotometer after addition of various concentrations of 17-hydroxyprogesterone. The insert (upper right) indicates the magnitude of spectral change observed at 420 mμ (trough) or 388 mμ (peak) relative to the isosbestic point (407 mμ) with the indicated concentrations of 17-hydroxyprogesterone. From NARASIMHULU et al. (1965)

of this spectral change was dependent (Fig. 11) on the concentration of steroid added, as well as on the concentration of cytochrome P-450 in the reaction vessel, suggesting a direct binding of the substrate to an "active site" on the hydroxylating enzyme complex (COOPER et al., 1965b). As interest developed in the role of cytochrome P-450 in drug metabolism by liver microsomes, it was apparent that similar experiments should be carried out with this system. Preliminary experiments showed that such spectral changes could be observed when hexobarbital was added to a suspension of liver microsomes. In an exciting few days of experimentation combining the talents of GILLETTE, REMMER, and their coworkers, the groundwork was established providing evidence that the first step

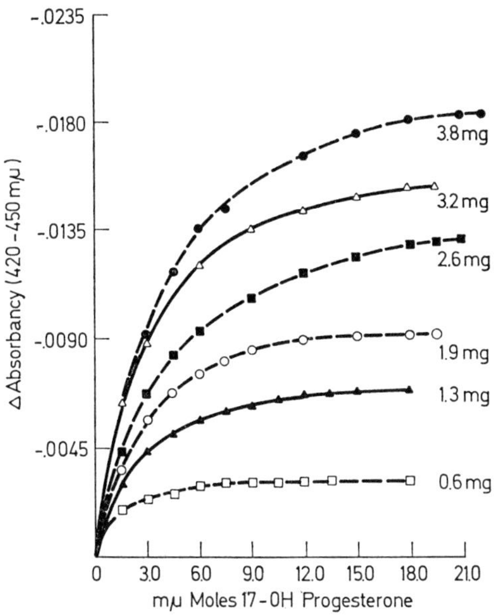

Fig. 11. The spectral titration of cytochrome P-450 of adrenal cortex microsomes with 17-hydroxyprogesterone. Beef adrenal cortex microsomes were suspended in a tris-phosphate, glycylglycine buffer mixture and the magnitude of spectral change at 420 mμ relative to 450 mμ determined after addition of varying aliquots of 17-hydroxyprogesterone. The experiment was repeated at varying protein concentrations (0.6—3.8 mg/ml) as indicated. From Cooper et al. (1965b)

in drug oxidative metabolism was the formation of a complex between the drug substrate and oxidized cytochrome P-450 (Remmer et al., 1966). Furthermore, it was determined that substrates could be divided into two groups, according to the type of spectral change observed (Remmer et al., 1966; Schenkman et al., 1967). These were named Type I and Type II classes of substrates (Fig. 12). The former (Type I) includes a great variety of compounds ranging from simple alkanes to complex heterocyclic chemicals. The second group (Type II) appears restricted to certain nitrogenous aromatic compounds. Shortly after the initial publication on substrate interaction with liver microsomal cytochrome P-450, Imai and Sato (1966) published similar results confirming and extending these observations.

During the 5 years that have intervened since these original observations on substrate-induced spectral changes with cytochrome P-450, our knowledge of the detailed nature of the reactions has been woefully lacking. Using electron spin resonance to study the perturbation of the 3d electrons associated with the paramagnetic iron of oxidized cytochrome P-450, Cammer et al. (1968) showed electron delocalizations on addition of substrates (Fig. 13). Whether this change in electron density is a primary or secondary effect on the ligand interactions of oxidized cytochrome P-450 remains to be seen. The restoration of the spectral properties of oxidized cytochrome P-450, after removal of substrate by centrifugation, shows that substrate binding is reversible and suggests that no major modification of the heme ligands has occurred (Schenkman et al., 1967). Moreover, the change in oxidized cytochrome P-450 (Fig. 14) elicited by the interaction of Type II compounds suggests that there is only one binding site for these sub-

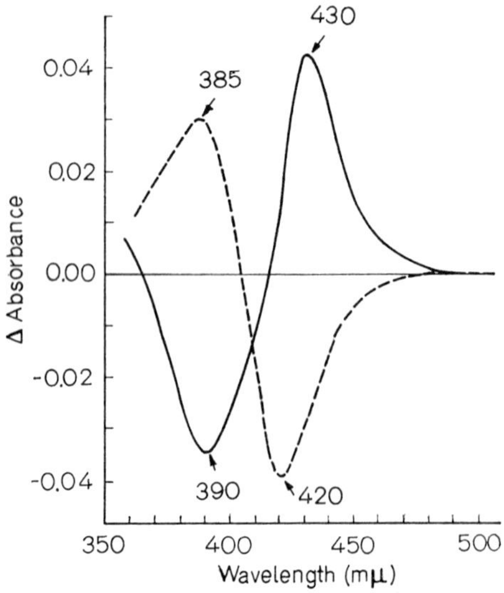

Fig. 12. The two types of spectral interaction observed on addition of substrates to liver microsomes. Liver microsomes prepared from phenobarbital treated male rats were diluted to 6.0 ml with 50 mM tris-chloride buffer, pH 7.4. In separate experiments the spectral changes observed on addition of 18 mM aniline (solid line curve) or 5 mM hexobarbital (dashed curve) were recorded

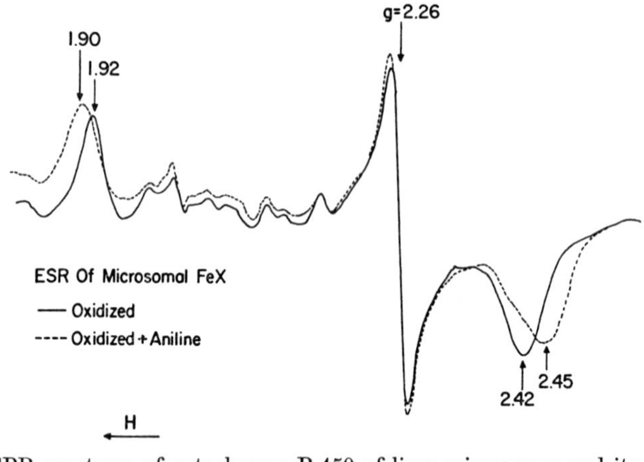

Fig. 13. The EPR spectrum of cytochrome P-450 of liver microsomes and its complex with aniline. Liver microsomes were obtained from rats pretreated by daily intraperitoneal injections of phenobarbital. The microsomes were suspended in 0.2 M tris-chloride buffer, pH 7.4, to a protein concentration of 38 mg/ml. A 1.0 ml aliquot of microsomal suspension was placed in a 3 mm (O.D) quartz, EPR tube and frozen in liquid nitrogen. The first derivative spectra were determined with a Varian Model 4500-10A EPR spectrometer. The solid line represents the spectrum obtained with untreated microsomes while dashed line represents the spectrum of a sample of microsomes in the presence of 5 mM aniline. From CAMMER et al. (1968)

strates on the cytochrome P-450 (LEIBMAN et al., 1969). The question of whether there are single or multiple sites for Type I compounds still cannot be resolved since complex effects observed with Type I substrates and the effect of Type II compounds on Type I-induced spectral changes (Fig. 15) cannot yet be explained.

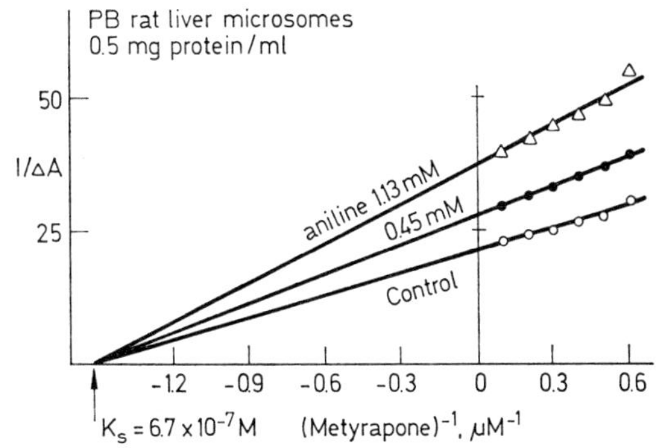

Fig. 14. The effect of aniline on the difference spectra produced by metyrapone. Liver microsomes were diluted to a protein concentration of 0.5 mg per ml in the presence of 0.45 mM or 1.13 mM aniline. The magnitude of the absorbance change at about 430 mμ relative to 470 mμ was determined spectrophotometrically after addition of various aliquots of 1 mM metyrapone. From LEIBMAN et al. (1969)

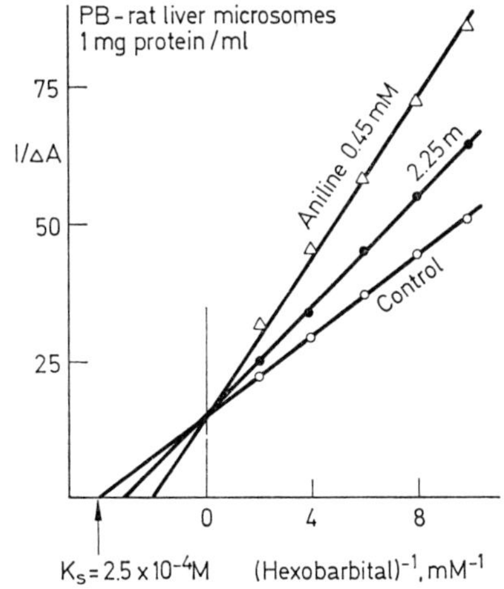

Fig. 15. The effect of aniline upon the difference spectra produced by hexobarbital addition to liver microsomes. Rat liver microsomes were diluted with tris-chloride buffer, pH 7.4, containing the indicated concentrations of aniline to a final protein concentration of 1 mg per ml. The contents of the sample cuvette were then titrated with aliquots of 50 mM hexobarbital and the spectral change at 420 mμ relative to 470 mμ determined. From LEIBMAN et al. (1969)

IV. Cytochrome P-450: Monomorphous or Polymorphous ?

The pharmacologist has long been faced with the dilemma of how to explain the great variability in rates of drug metabolism observed with different species, different sexes, or even different strains of animals. Initially the discovery of cytochrome P-450 offered hope that a basic mechanism for drug oxidative detoxification would be disclosed. It soon became apparent, however, that these differences could not be ascribed solely to cytochrome P-450. This has led to a continuing search for the existence of multiple types or forms of cytochrome P-450.

The initial studies by REMMER et al. (1966) showed that the Type I- induced spectral change was enhanced in liver microsomes isolated from animals pretreated with phenobarbital but diminished in those from animals pretreated with

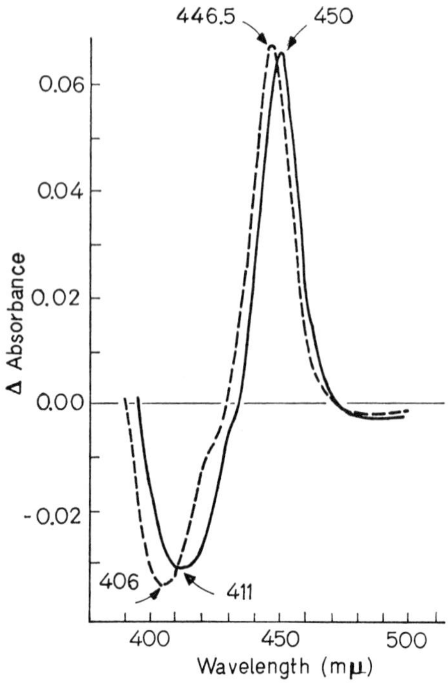

Fig. 16. The spectral properties of the CO complex of reduced cytochrome P-450 associated with microsomes from animals pretreated with phenobarbital or 3-methylcholanthrene. Young male rabbits were injected intraperitoneally with either phenobarbital or 3-methylcholanthrene and microsomes were isolated from the perfused livers. Aliquots of the two types of microsomes were diluted in 0.1 M phosphate buffer, pH 7.4, and the pigments reduced with sodium dithionite. The contents of one cuvette were gassed for 1 min with carbon monoxide and the resulting difference spectrum recorded. The solid line curve represents the difference spectrum for the CO complex of reduced cytochrome P-450 associated with microsomes from phenobarbital treated animals. The dashed curve represents a comparable experiment with microsomes from 3-methylcholanthrene treated animals. The protein concentration in the reaction mixture was adjusted so the absorbance maxima at 450 mμ and 446.5 mμ for the two spectra are nearly identical. From HILDEBRANDT et al. (1969)

3,4-benzpyrene. These studies have been extended and confirmed by the recent studies of SHOEMAN et al. (1969a). Studies on the differences in overall oxidative activity (CONNEY et al., 1960), changes in rate of turnover of the heme of cytochrome P-450 (LEVIN and KUNTZMAN, 1969a, b), and, in particular, differences in reactivity of reduced cytochrome P-450 with ethyl isocyanide (SLADEK and MANNERING, 1966) all lead to the conclusion that multiple forms of cytochrome P-450 exist in liver. Perhaps most indicative that there is more than one form of cytochrome P-450 are the small but real differences observed in the spectral properties (Fig. 16) of the CO complex of reduced cytochrome P-450, i.e. the appearance of an absorbance band at 446—448 mμ with microsomes from animals pretreated with polycyclic hydrocarbons (ALVARES et al., 1967; HILDEBRANDT et al., 1969). Even stronger evidence emerges from spectral studies where the "apparent absolute absorption spectrum" of cytochrome P-450 can be recorded (Fig. 17). In these studies HILDEBRANDT et al. (1969) demonstrated a marked spectral difference between the pigment induced by phenobarbital and that induced by the carcinogenic compound 3-methylcholanthrene, indicating without a doubt that a major modification of cytochrome P-450 had occurred. These

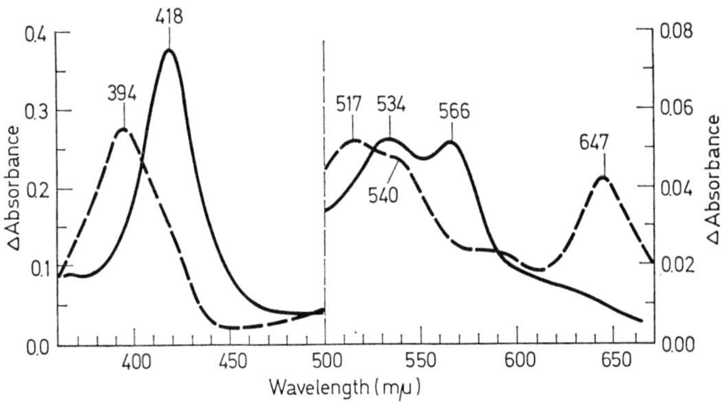

Fig. 17. The apparent absolute absorption spectrum of the two forms of cytochrome P-450 obtained on induction with phenobarbital or 3-methylcholanthrene. Microsomes from livers of control, phenobarbital or 3-methylcholanthrene treated rabbits were examined spectrophotometrically to determine the content of cytochrome b_5. The spectrum of the additional pigment associated with microsomes from phenobarbital treated rabbits (solid line curve) was determined by recording the spectral difference between a cuvette containing liver microsomes from phenobarbital treated rabbits (2.2 mg protein per ml, 0.73 mμmoles cytochrome b_5 per mg, 2.92 mμmoles hemin per mg) minus a cuvette containing liver microsomes from a saline treated control rabbit (3.0 mg protein per ml, 0.51 mμmoles cytochrome b_5 per mg, 1.44 mμmoles hemin per mg). The additional pigment associated with microsomes from 3-methylcholanthrene treated rabbits (dashed line curve) was determined in a similar manner by recording the spectral difference between a cuvette containing liver microsomes from 3-methylcholanthrene treated rabbits (3.0 mg protein per ml, 0.79 mμmoles cytochrome b_5 per mg, 2.5 mμmoles hemin per mg) minus a cuvette containing liver microsomes from a corn oil treated control rabbit (3.0 mg protein per ml, 0.78 mμmoles cytochrome b_5 per mg, 1.6 mμmoles hemin per mg). Microsomes were diluted in 50 mM tris buffer, pH 7.5, containing 15 mM KCl to the protein concentrations indicated. Temperature, 25°C. From HILDEBRANDT et al. (1969)

workers also showed that two spectrally identifiable forms of cytochrome P-450 could be partially interconverted by the addition of Type I or Type II substrates, lending credence to the hypothesis that the differences observed upon induction may reflect in part the formation of incompetent complexes. The understanding of these differences in cytochrome P-450 remains as one of the major challenges for the immediate future. The answer to this question should open new vistas for resolving observed differences in the rate of metabolism of various drugs.

V. The Enzymatic Reduction of Cytochrome P-450

An examination of the overall reaction for cytochrome P-450 catalyzed mixed-function oxidation reactions points to the fact that the reaction requires a two electron transfer system in order to complete a cycle of cytochrome P-450 oxidation and reduction (ESTABROOK et al., 1969). The anaerobic titration of the pigments of microsomes (Fig. 18) with reduced pyridine nucleotide has yielded evidence that cytochrome P-450 is a single electron acceptor (ULLRICH et al., 1968). Recent studies by WATERMAN and MASON (1970) on the oxidation-reduction potential of cytochrome P-450 reaffirms the conclusion that only a single electron is required for the reduction of the oxidized form. It is now well established that the flavoprotein, TPNH-cytochrome c-reductase, is a necessary component in the flow of reducing equivalents from TPNH to cytochrome P-450 (ORRENIUS and ERNSTER, 1964). In addition it has been suggested that a further component, X (Fig. 19), is required to bridge electron transport from the flavoprotein reductase to the hemoprotein (ESTABROOK et al., 1969; DALLNER et al., 1966). Only

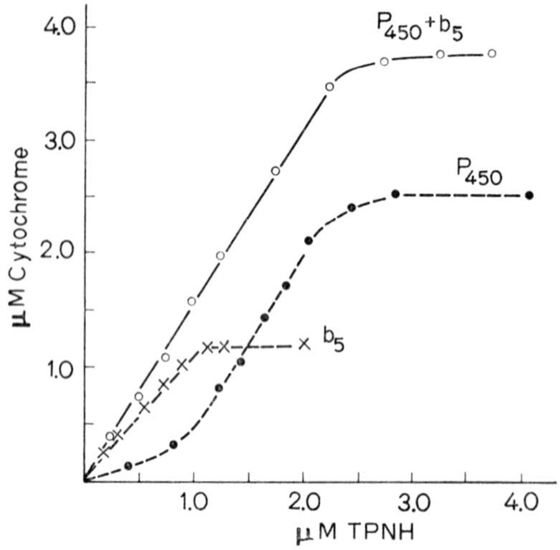

Fig. 18. The anaerobic titration of microsomal hemoproteins with TPNH. Each sample contained microsomes from the liver of an induced rabbit (1.5 mg/ml), ETP (0.8 mg/ml), Tris-chloride buffer, 50 mM (pH 7.5), $MgCl_2$, 5m M, and succinate, 7.5 mM. The extent of hemoprotein reduction was calculated from the difference in absorption of two samples, one of which had been reduced anaerobically with TPNH. Anaerobiosis was achieved by bubbling with deoxygenated gas for 3 min in airtight cuvettes supplied by Aminco. CO and helium were used for the determination of cytochrome P-450 (solid circles) and cytochrome b_5 reduction (crosses) respectively. Additions of TPNH were made anaerobically by means of a plunger unit incorporated into the cuvette, using known volumes of a standard TPNH solution. From ULLRICH et al. (1968)

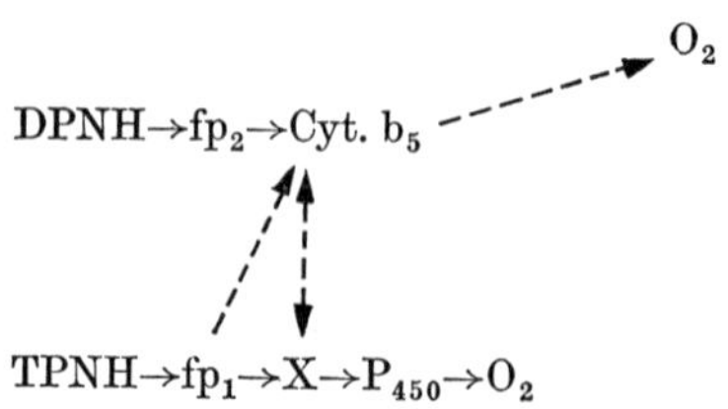

Fig. 19. One proposed pathway of electron transport associated with microsomes. TPNH-cytochrome c reductase is indicated by f_{p1}, while DPNH-cytochrome b_5 reductase is indicated by f_{p2}. The factor X is unknown, but is considered an obligatory intermediate in electron transport to cytochrome P-450. From ESTABROOK et al. (1969)

recently has evidence accumulated that the rate limiting step in the flow of reducing equivalents from reduced pyridine nucleotide to cytochrome P-450 may be altered by addition of mono and divalent ions without alteration in the amount of the enzymes present (HILDEBRANDT et al., 1970a).

The reduction of cytochrome P-450 can be readily measured by determining, under anaerobic conditions, the rate of formation of the reduced cytochrome P-450-CO complex (COOPER et al., 1965b; GIGON et al., 1969). The finding of GIGON et al. (1969) that the oxidized cytochrome P-450-substrate complex is more rapidly reduced than the uncomplexed form of oxidized cytochrome P-450 favors the hypothetical scheme postulated in Fig. 20. These observations, however, still do not explain how two electrons interact in the overall reaction. Two hyoptheses are currently under consideration. The first suggests the presence of a second electron acceptor associated with cytochrome P-450, such as a sulfhydryl group (COOPER et al., 1965b). The addition of mercurials, such as mersalyl, in

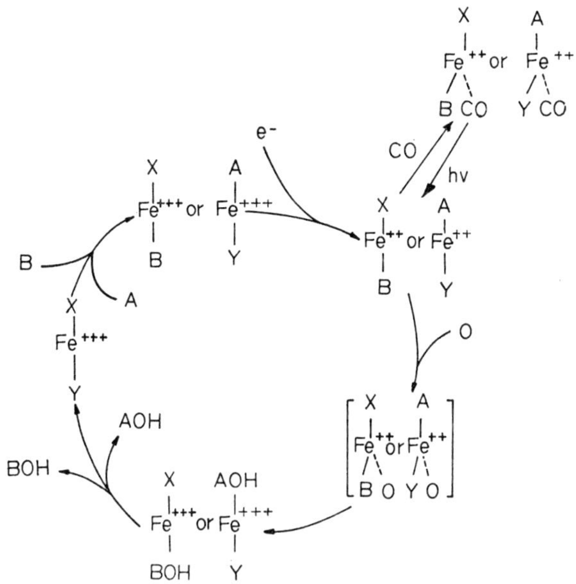

Fig. 20. A proposed scheme illustrating the types of substrate interaction which might occur during the oxidation-reduction cycle for cytochrome P-450 function. The compounds X and Y represent two types of natural ligands of the heme of cytochrome P-450. The compounds A and B represent the two classes of substrates giving the Type I or Type II binding spectrum with oxidized cytochrome P-450 (Fe^{+++}). The interaction of oxygen (O), carbon monoxide (CO) and reducing equivalents (e) are indicated

rather high concentrations can cause a marked modification in the spectral properties of cytochrome P-450 (Fig. 21), generally resulting in its conversion to P-420. Although the inclusion of a sulfhydryl group as a second electron acceptor is intellectually interesting and appears most reasonable when considering the "paper chemistry" of the system, the multitudinous sites of interaction of mercurials must make one skeptical of accepting such results as direct evidence for a primary role of sulfhydryl groups as electron acceptors during the function of cytochrome P-450.

The second hypothesis (Fig. 22) suggests a role for cytochrome b_5 as a donor of the second electron (ESTABROOK et al., 1969). In this case it is proposed that reduced cytochrome b_5 reacts with an oxygenated form of reduced cytochrome P-450. In particular, recent studies by HILDEBRANDT et al. (1970b) on changes in the steady state reduction of cytochrome b_5 during drug metabolism, together with evidence for a new spectral species of cytochrome P-450 present during the steady state (ESTABROOK et al., 1970), lends strength to the postulated role for cytochrome b_5 in this reaction. The synergistic effect of DPNH on TPNH catalyzed reactions also points to a potential role for cytochrome b_5 (ESTABROOK and COHEN, 1969). At the present time, evidence is still accumulating supporting this hypothesis, but it is far from proven. Hopefully in the near future this question will be resolved.

VI. The Organization of the Microsomal Electron Transport Chain

The above discussion has centered on the chemistry and properties of cytochrome P-450 as it functions in drug oxidative metabolism. It should not be forgotten, indeed any investigator who has attempted to purify cytochrome

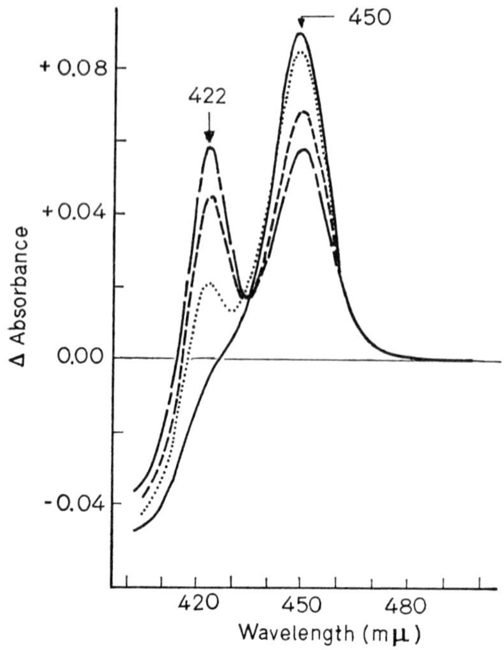

Fig. 21. The effect of mercurials on the conversion of microsomal cytochrome P-450 to P-420. Microsomes from rat liver were diluted in 0.1 M phosphate buffer, pH 7.4, and divided equally into two cuvettes. Sodium dithionite was added to the contents of each cuvette to reduce the microsomal hemoproteins and then the contents of one cuvette was gassed with carbon monoxide. At zero time 0.1 mM p-CMB was added to the cuvette containing CO. The time course of conversion of P-450 to P-420 was then determined by recording the difference spectra at the times indicated. From COOPER et al. (1965b) p. 876

P-450 can never forget, that the enzyme complex is an intregal part of a membrane system. Calculations have been presented elsewhere (ESTABROOK et al., 1969) to show that cytochrome P-450 is the major constituent of microsomes, composing as much as 20% of the protein of the membrane.

A challenge to our understanding of cytochrome P-450 function is the spatial organization — the topography — of the enzyme complex within the membrane. It is not generally appreciated that the reaction components which function in cytochrome P-450 catalyzed mixed function oxidation reactions are not in a simple 1:1 stoichiometric ratio. As shown in Table 1, analytical studies indicate that only one molecule of the flavoprotein (TPNH-cytochrome c reductase) is present for about 20 molecules of cytochrome P-450. Thus, a single flavoprotein must be encircled by cytochrome P-450 molecules in the nearly monomolecular anatomy of the membrane. One such visualization of the molecular architecture of these molecules in the membrane is shown in Fig. 23. Included in this schematic representation is a consideration of cytochrome b_5 and its associated flavoprotein, DPNH-cytochrome b_5 reductase. Alternatively, one could visualize the unknown component, X, as a mobile carrier shuttling from a single flavoprotein dehydrogenase to the various cytochrome P-450 molecules in the membrane.

Summary

As in much of science, the advances produced to date regarding our understanding of the role of cytochrome P-450 in drug oxidative metabolism have

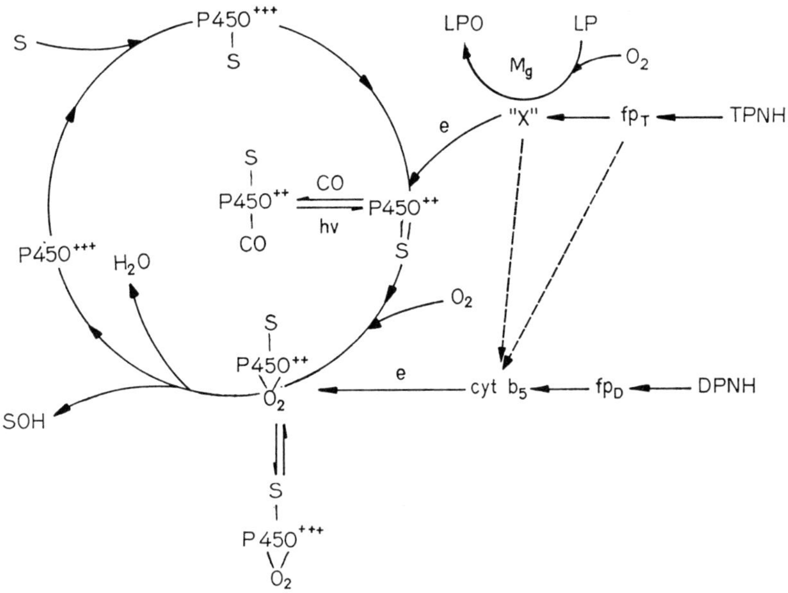

Fig. 22. A proposed reaction scheme including a function for cytochrome b_5 during the oxidation and reduction of cytochrome P-450. The substrate to be hydroxylated is indicated by (S). The flavoproteins TPNH-cytochrome c reductase and DPNH-cytochrome b_5 reductase are indicated by f_{pt} and f_{pd} respectively. The pathway of lipid peroxidation is indicated by LP to LPO

Table 1. *Pigment content of rat liver microsomes*

	Control	Phenobarbital Induced
Cytochrome b_5	0.35 (12)	0.73 (6)
Cytochrome P-450.	0.57 (20)	2.35 (20)
Flavoprotein (TPNH-cytochrome c) . .	0.03 (1)	0.12 (1)

The concentrations of hemoproteins in liver microsomes from control or phenobarbital treated male rats were determined spectrophotometrically. The content of the flavoprotein, TPNH-cytochrome c reductase, was estimated from activity measurements with microsomes and related to comparable studies with the isolated, purified flavoprotein. Concentrations are expressed as mμmoles per mg protein. The numbers in brackets refer to the ratio of hemoprotein concentration to flavoprotein concentration within the same sample of microsomes.

resulted from a dialectic discourse between many scientists. It is generally recognized that cytochrome P-450 is not the panacea for all problems of drug metabolism by liver microsomes. It is firmly established, however, that cytochrome P-450 is a unique and interesting pigment which does participate in a multitude of different reactions in a manner not yet fully understood. Many challenges remain as the chemistry of this hemoprotein and the control of its function are gradually unraveled. The last 10 years have seen rapid advances in our understanding of mixed function oxidation reactions. Those investigators intimately involved in drug metabolism must be greatly indebted to the pioneers in the field

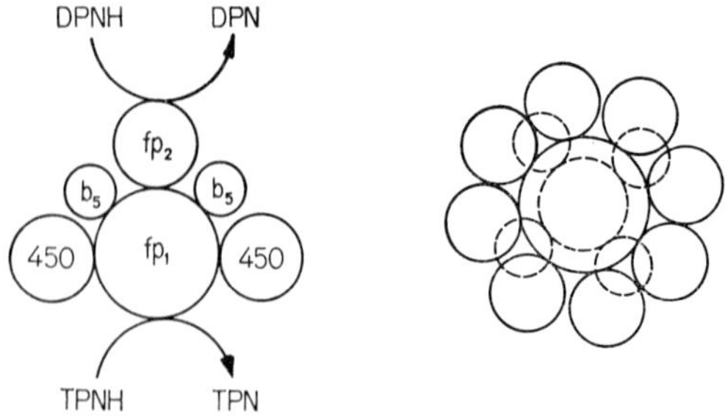

Fig. 23. A visualization of the molecular arrangement of cytochromes and flavoproteins in the microsomal membrane. The figure on the left represents a cross-section through the membrane while the figure on the right represents a view on to the plane of the membrane sheet. The flavoproteins TPNH-cytochrome c reductase and DPNH-cytochrome b_5 reductase are indicated by f_{p1} and f_{p2} respectively. It is suggested that the inside-outside polarity of the membrane would be represented by the bottom and top of the left hand figure

such as BRODIE, WILLIAMS, MASON, ERNSTER, STAUDINGER, SATO etc. for providing us with a cornucopia of ideas and observations which will lead to future insights into this potentially major advancement in our understanding of the maintance of homeostasis. In this era of the liberal use of drugs, insecticides, artificial steroids, potential carcinogenic compounds, as well as man's immersion in an environment of pollutants, the role of the defense mechanisms for detoxification loom with increasing importance through the darkness of ignorance.

Addendum

A review of this nature cannot encompass all the evidence presented from many laboratories, evidence which contributes to our present concepts of microsomal drug oxidation reactions. This is due in large part to the myopia of the author who has developed his own interpretation of our present day understanding of the system under discussion. The author asks the forbearance of many of his contemporaries for not including their contributions. This has not been done because of a prejudgement on the relative importance of these studies, many of which are excellent, but because of the pressing limitations of time and space.

References

ALVARES, A.P., SCHILLING, G., LEVIN, W., KUNTZMAN, R.: Studies on the Induction of CO-Binding Pigments in Liver Microsomes by Phenobarbital and 3-Methylcholanthrene. Biochem. biophys. Res. Commun. **29**, 521—526 (1967).

BRODIE, B.B.: Detoxication of Drugs and Other Foreign Compounds by Liver Microsomes. Science **121**, 603 (1955).

BURNS, J.J., ROSE, K., GOODWIN, S., REICHENTHOL, J., HORNING, E.C., BRODIE, B.B.: Metabolic Fate of Phenylbutazone in Man. Amer. J. Pharm. **113**, 481—489 (1955).

CAMMER, W., SCHENKMAN, J.B., ESTABROOK, R.W.: EPR Measurements of Substrate Interaction with Cytochrome P-450. Biochem. biophys. Res. Commun. **23**, 264—268 (1968).

CHANCE, B.: Techniques for the Assay of the Respiratory Enzymes. In: Methods in Enzymology, *Vol. IV*, pp. 273—329. Ed. by S.P. COLOWICK, and N.O. KAPLAN. New York: Academic Press 1957.

— PAPPENHEIMER, A.M., JR.: Kinetic and Spectrophotometric Studies of Cytochrome b_5 in Midgut Homogenates of *Cecropia*. J. biol. Chem. **209**, 931—944 (1954).

— WILLIAMS, G.R.: Kinetics of Cytochrome b_5 in Rat Liver Microsomes. J. biol. Chem. **209**, 945—951 (1954).

CONNEY, A.H., BROWN, R.R., MILLER, J.A., MILLER, E.C.: The Metabolism of Methylated Aminoazo Dyes. VI. Intracellular Distribution and Properties of the Demethylase System. Cancer Res. **17**, 628—634 (1957).

CONNEY, A.H., DAVISON, C., GASTEL, R., BURNS, J.J.: Adaptive Increases in Drug Metabolizing Enzymes Induced by Phenobarbital and other Drugs. J. Pharmacol. exp. Ther. **130**, 1—8 (1960).

— MILLER, E.C,, MILLER, J.A.: The Metabolism of Methylated Aminoazo Dyes. V. Evidence for Induction of Enzyme Synthesis in the Rat by 3-Methylcholanthrene. Cancer Res. **16**, 450—459 (1956).

COOPER, D.Y., ESTABROOK, R.W., ROSENTHAL, O.: The Stoichiometry of C_{21} Hydroxylation of Steroids by Adrenocortical Microsomes. J. biol. Chem. **238**, 1320—1323 (1962).

— LEVINE, S., NARASHIMHULU, S., ROSENTHAL, O., ESTABROOK, R.W.: Photochemical Action Spectrum of the Terminal Oxidase of Mixed Function Oxidase Systems. Science **147**, 400—402 (1965a).

— NARASHIMHULU, S., ROSENTHAL, O., ESTABROOK, R.W.: Spectral and Kinetic Studies of Microsomal Pigments. In: Oxidases and Related Redox Systems, pp. 838—860. Ed. by T.E. KING, H.S. MASON and M. MORRISON. New York: Wiley 1965b.

COOPER, J.R., BRODIE, B.B.: The Enzymatic Metabolism of Hexobarbital (Evipal). J. Pharmacol. exp. Ther. **114**, 409—417 (1955).

DALLNER, G., SIEKEVITZ, P., PALADE, G.E.: Biogenesis ofEndoplasmicReticulumMembranes. II. Synthesis of Ceris Titertive Microsomal Enzymes in Developing Rat Hepatocytes. J. Cell Biol. **30**, 97—117 (1966).

ESTABROOK, R.W., COHEN, B.: Organization of the Microsomal Electron Transport System. In: Microsomes and Drug Oxidation, pp. 95—105. Ed. by J. GILLETTE et al. New York: Academic Press 1969.

— COOPER, D.Y., ROSENTHAL, O.: The Light reversible Carbon Monoxide Inhibition of the Steroid C-21-Hydroxylase System of Adrenal Cortex. Biochem. Z. **338**, 741—755 (1963).

— HILDEBRANDT, A., REMMER, H., SCHENKMAN, J.B., ROSENTHAL, O., COOPER, D.Y.: The Role of Cytochrome P-450 in Microsomal Mixed Function Oxidation Reactions. In: The 19 Colloquium der Gesellschaft für Biologische Chemie, pp. 142—177. Ed. by B. HESS and H.J. STAUDINGER. Berlin-Heidelberg-New York: Springer 1969.

— NETTER, K., PAWAR, S., HILDEBRANDT, A., LEIBMAN, K.: Steady State of Cytochrome P-450 of Liver Microsomes During Drug Hydroxylation Reactions. Fed. Proc. **29**, 874 (1970).

GARFINKEL, D.: Studies on Pig Liver Microsomes I. Enzymic and Pigment Composition of Different Microsomal Fractions. Arch. Biochem. **77**, 493—509 (1958).

GIGON, P.L., GRAM, T.E., GILLETTE, J.R.: Studies on the Rate of Reduction of Hepatic Microsomal Cytochrome P-450 by Reduced Nicotinamide Adenine Dinucleotide Phosphate: Effect of Drug Substrates. Molec. Pharmacol. **5**, 109—122 (1969).

HASHIMOTO, Y., YAMANO, T., MASON, H.S.: An Electron Spin Resonance Study of Microsomal Electron Transport. J. biol. Chem. **237**, 3843—3844 (1962).

HAYAISHI, O.: *Oxygenases*. New York: Academic Press 1962.

HAYANO, M., LINDBERG, M.D., DORFMAN, R.I., HANCOCK, J.E.H., VON DOERING, E.W.: On the Mechanisms of the C-11β-Hydroxylation of Steroids; with H_2O^2 and $O_2{}^{18}$. Arch. Biochem. **59**, 529—532 (1955).

HILDEBRANDT, A., ESTABROOK, R.W.: DPNH and Ionic Strength as Positive Effectors of Microsomal Mixed Function Oxidations. Fed. Proc. **29**, 738 (1970a).

— — unpublished results (1970b).

— REMMER, H., ESTABROOK, R.W.: Cytochrome P-450 of Liver Microsomes — One Pigment or Many. Biochem. biophys. Res. Commun. **30**, 607—612 (1969).

IMAI, Y., SATO, R.: Substrate Interaction with Hydroxylase System in Liver Microsomes. Biochem. biophys. Res. Commun. **22**, 620—626 (1966).

KATAGIRI, M., GANGULI, B.N., GUNSALUS, I.C.: A Soluble Cytochrome P-450 Functional in Methylene Hydroxylation. J. biol. Chem. **243**, 3543—3545 (1968).

KEILIN, D., HARTREE, E.F.: Succinic Dehydrogenous-Cytochrome System of Cells. Proc. roy. Soc. B **129**, 277—306 (1940).

KLINGENBERG, M.: Pigments of Rat Liver Microsomes. Arch. Biochem. **75**, 379—386 (1958).

LEIBMAN, K.C., HILDEBRANDT, A.G., ESTABROOK, R.W.: Spectrophotometric Studies of Interaction Between Various Substrates in Their Binding to Microsomal Cytochrome P-450. Biochem biophys. Res. Commun. **36**, 789—794 (1969).

LEVIN, W., KUNTZMAN, R.: Biphasic Decrease of Radioactive Hemoprotein from Liver Microsomal CO-Binding Particles. Effect of 3-Methylcholanthrene. J. biol. Chem. **244**, 3671—3684 (1969a).

— — Biphasic Decrease of Radioactive Hemoprotein from Liver Microsomal CO-Binding Particles. Effect of Phenobarbital and Chlordane. Molec. Pharmacol. **5**, 499—506 (1969b).

MASON, H.S.: Mechanism of Oxygen Metabolism. In: Advances in Enzymology. Vol. XIX. Ed. by F.F. NORD. New York: Chider Science Publ., Inc. 1957.

Mason, H. S., North, J. C., Vanneste, M.: Microsomal Mixed Function Oxidations, The Metabolism of Xenobiotics. Symposium on Electron Transport Systems in Microsomes. Fed. Proc. **24**, 1172—1180 (1965a).
— Yamano, T., North, J. C., Hashmoto, Y., Sakagishi, P.: The Structure and Oxidase Function of Liver Microsomes. In: Oxidases and Related Redox Systems, pp. 879—899. Ed. by T. E. King, H. S. Mason and M. Morrison. New York: Wiley 1965b.
Narasimhulu, S., Cooper, D. Y., Rosenthal, O.: Spectrophotometric Properties of a Trition Clarified Steroid 21-Hydroxylase System of Adrenocortical Microsomes. Life Sci. **4**, 2101—2107 (1965).
Omura, T., Sato, R.: A New Cytochrome in Liver Microsomes. J. biol. Chem. **237**, 1375 to 1381 (1962).
— — The Carbon Monoxide-Binding Pigment of Liver Microsomes. I. Evidence for Its Hemoprotein Nature. J. biol. Chem. **239**, 2370—2378 (1964a).
— — The Carbon Monoxide-Binding Pigment of Liver Microsomes. II. Solubilization, Purification and Properties. J. biol. Chem. **239**, 2379—2385 (1964b).
— — Cooper, D. Y., Rosenthal, O., Estabrook, R. W.: Functions of Cytochrome P-450 of Microsomes. Symposium on Electron Transport System in Microsomes. Fed. Proc. **24**, 1181—1189 (1965).
Orrenius, S., Ernster, L.: Phenobarbital-induced Synthesis of the Oxidative Demethylating Enzymes of Rat Liver Microsomes. Biochem. biophys. Res. Commun. **16**, 60—65 (1964).
Pappenheimer, A. M., Jr., Williams, C. M.: Cytochrome b_5 and the Dihydrocoenzyme Oxidase System in the Cecropia Silkworm. J. biol. Chem. **209**, 915—929 (1954).
Remmer, H.: Der beschleunigte Abbau von Pharmaka in den Lebermicrosomen unter dem Einfluß von Luminal. Naunyn-Schmiedeberg's Arch. exp. Path. Parmak. **235**, 279—290 (1959).
— Schenkman, J. B., Estabrook, R. W., Sasame, H., Gillette, J., Narashimhulu, S., Cooper, D. Y., Rosenthal, O.: Drug Interaction with Hepatic Microsomal Cytochrome. Molec. Pharmacol. **2**, 187—190 (1966).
Ryan, K. G., Engel, L.: Hydroxylation of Steroids at Carbon 21. J. biol. Chem. **225**, 103—114 (1957).
Samuels, L. T.: Metabolism of Steroid Hormones. In: Metabolic Pathways, Vol. I, pp. 431 to 438. Ed. by D. M. Greenberg. New York: Academic Press 1961.
Schenkman, J. B., Remmer., H., Estabrook, R. W.: Spectral Studies of Drug Interaction with Hepatic Microsomal Cytochrome. Molec. Pharmacol. **3**, 113—123 (1967).
Shoeman, D. W., Chaplin, M. D., Mannering, G. J.: Induction of Drug Metabolism. III. Further Evidence for the Formation of a New P-450 Hemoprotein After Treatment of Rats with 3-Methylcholanthrene. Molec. Pharmacol. **5**, 412—419 (1969a).
— White, J. G., Mannering, G. J.: Cytochrome P-450: Tubular Aggregates from Hepatic Microsomes. Science **165**, 1371—1372 (1969b).
Sladek, N. E., Mannering, G. J.: Evidence for a New P-450 Hemoprotein in Hepatic Microsomes from Methylcholanthrene Treated Rats. Biochem. biophys. Res. Commun. **24**, 668—674 (1966).
Strittmatter, C. F., Ball, E. G.: A Hemochromogen Component of Liver Microsomes. Proc. nat. Acad. Sci. (Wash.) **38**, 19—37 (1952).
Ullrich, V., Cohen, B., Cooper, D. Y., Estabrook, R. W.: Reactions of Hemoprotein P-450. In: Structure and Function of Cytochromes, pp. 649—655. Ed. by K. Okunuki, M. D. Kamen and I. Sekuzu. University of Tokyo Press 1968.
Warburg, O.: Heavy Metal Prosthetic Groups and Enzyme Action. London and New York: Oxford University Press (Clarendon) 1949.
Waterman, M., Mason, H. S.: The Redox Potential of Liver Cytochrome P-450. Biochem. biophys. Res. Commun. **39**, 450—454 (1970).
Williams, R. T.: Detoxication Mechanisms, 2nd Ed. London: Chapman and Hall 1959.

Chapter 39

Enzymatic Oxidation at Carbon

J. Daly

A. Introduction

The enzymatic oxidation of organic substrates at carbon includes such reactions as aliphatic hydroxylation, conversion of ketones to esters or lactones, peroxidation, epoxidation, aromatic hydroxylation, and dehydrogenation. In mammals, such oxidative metabolism of drugs and other foreign substances is, to a great extent, catalyzed by hepatic enzymes that are associated with the reticuloendothelial system. This drug-metabolizing system appears in the microsomal fraction of liver homogenates. It accepts a wide range of substrates and may convert one substrate to a variety of oxidized products by attack at heteroatoms and at aliphatic, aromatic and olefinic positions. The same hepatic system catalyzes the oxidation of many endogenous substrates, such as fatty acids and steroids (Chapter 46). The enzyme(s) concerned with binding and oxidation of the organic substrate are usually hemoprotein(s) referred to as cytochrome P-450. The present chapter will attempt to delineate the current knowledge on mechanism and preferred route of oxidative metabolism at carbon.

B. Aliphatic Hydroxylation

I. Hydroxylation at the Terminal Methyl Group

Aliphatic moieties in both foreign compounds and endogenous substrates are typically oxidized at the terminal methyl group. This metabolic route is frequently referred to as ω-oxidation. The initial product is a primary alcohol, which is usually further metabolized to aldehyde and acid by the action of soluble dehydrogenases. The reaction occurs with many straight and branched chain fatty acids (Table 1).

Table 1. *Aliphatic hydroxylation: compounds undergoing hydroxylation at the terminal methyl group*

Lauric acid, stearic acid, palmitic acid, oleic acid, and myristic acid	Preiss and Bloch (1964)
Decanoic acid	Ichihara et al. (1969a)
2,2-Dimethylstearic acid	Bergstrom et al. (1954)
3,6-Dimethyloctanoic acid	Stokke et al. (1967)
Sorbic acid amide	Wakabayashi and Shimazono (1963)
Dodecyl sulfate	Denner et al. (1969)
Thiopental and pentobarbital	Cooper and Brodie (1955)
Secobarbital	Tsukamoto et al. (1963)
5,5-Diethylbarbituric acid	Goldschmidt and Wehr (1957)
Hexane, octane, decane and hexadecane	Ichihara et al. (1969b) Kusunose et al. (1969) McCarthy (1964), Das et al. (1968)
sec-Butylaniline	Alexander et al. (1968)
Propylbenzene	El Masry et al. (1956)

Phytanic acid, however, is instead converted by α-hydroxylation to pristanic acid (MIZE et al., 1969). Hydroxylation of the ω-methyl group also occurs with many xenobiotic compounds (Table 1). Hydroxylation at a ω-methyl group and subsequent β-oxidative degradation appears involved in the metabolism of endogenous fatty acids and tocopherol (SIMON et al., 1956) and in the conversion of cholesterol to cholic acid (BERGSTROM et al., 1957). The major metabolite of prostaglandin E_2 in humans has undergone ω-hydroxylation (HAMBERG and SAMUELSSON, 1969).

The hepatic enzyme system which catalyzes the ω-hydroxylation of fatty acids has been solubilized (LU et al., 1969a). Further investigation revealed the non-specificity of this system which also catalyzes the oxidation (allylic hydroxylation, and N- and O- dealkylation) of a variety of drugs (LU et al., 1969b).

II. Hydroxylation at the Penultimate Methylene Group

In addition to oxidation of the terminal methyl group, alkyl moieties are also commonly oxidized at the ω-1 methylene position. Frequently, this metabolism is favored over ω-oxidation, as in the examples given in Table 2. Metabolism of fatty acids such as stearic acid also involves ω-1 oxidation (PREISS and BLOCH, 1964). In this case, terminal methyl oxidation is favored by a 3:1 ratio.

Table 2. *Aliphatic hydroxylation: compounds undergoing hydroxylation at the penultimate methylene group*

Amobarbital	MAYNERT (1952b)
Hexethal	MAYNERT (1965)
Butethal	MAYNERT (1952a)
Methithural	PREUSS and KOPSCH (1966)
1-Hexyl-3,7-dimethylxanthine	MOHLER et al. (1966a
Meprobamate	LUDWIG et al. (1961)
Mebutamate	DOUGLAS et al. (1962)
Butylbenzene	EL MASRY et al. (1956)

III. Hydroxylation at the Benzylic Position

Many methylated aromatic or heterocyclic substrates are metabolized by hydroxylation of the methyl substituent (Table 3). The initial product, a primary alcohol, may then be dehydrogenated to aldehyde and acid by soluble dehydrogenases. Hydroxylation at a benzylic position may also occur (Table 3) with the ethyl, propyl or butyl substituents or in fused ring systems as in the stereoselective formation of S(+)-1-indanol from the indane (BILLINGS et al., 1970).

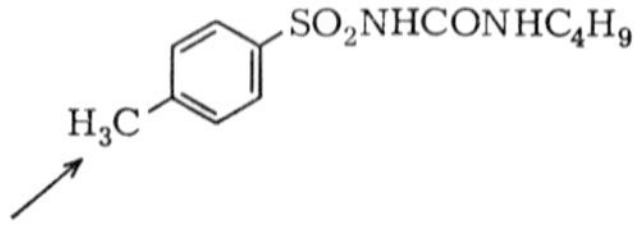

a

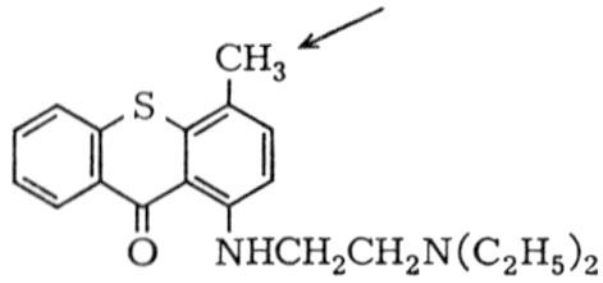

b

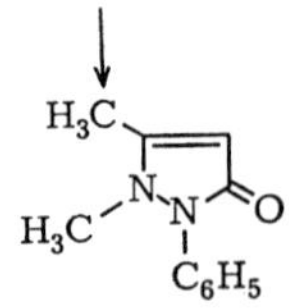

c

(1(

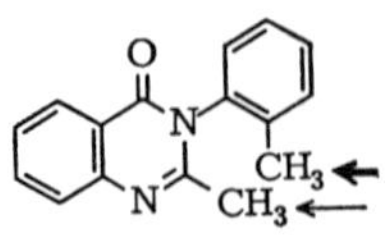

d

Table 3. *Aliphatic hydroxylation: compounds undergoing hydroxylation at the benzylic position*

Tolbutamide [1a]	TAGG et al. (1967), McDANIEL et al. (1969)
1-Diethylaminoethylamine-4-methylthiazanthone [1b]	ROSI et al. (1965)
Antipyrine [1c]	YOSHIMURA et al. (1968)
Nalidixic acid	McCHESNEY et al. (1964)
Metronidazole	STAMBAUGH et al. (1967)
3,5-Dimethylpyrazole	SMITH et al. (1965)
Metaxalone	BRUCE et al. (1966)
Methaqualon [1d]	PREUSS et al. (1966), NOWAK et al. (1966)
4-Nitrotoluene	GILLETTE (1959)
p-Xylene	BRAY et al. (1949a)
p-Cresol	BRAY et al. (1950)
4-Methylphenylurea,3-methylphenylurea	BRAY et al. (1949b)
4-Methylacetanilide,3-methylacetanilide	BRAY and THORPE (1948), DALY et al. (1968b)
Ethylbenzene, propylbenzene and butylbenzene	EL MASRY et al. (1956)
4-Ethylacetanilide	DALY et al. (1968b)
Tetralin	PARKE (1965), ELLIOTT and HANAM (1968)
Imipramine [10f]	CRAMMER and SCOTT (1966)
Amitryptyline	ESCHENHOF and RIEDER (1969)
Nortriptyline	McMAHON et al. (1963)
Noxiptilin	DUHM et al. (1969)
Indane	BILLINGS et al. (1970)

Steric factors would appear to influence whether metabolism of a methylbenzene proceeds by benzylic oxidation or by other routes. Thus, *para*-substituted methylbenzenes are metabolized mainly by benzylic hydroxylation, as for example with *trans*-2-*para*-tolylcyclohexane (2a) (GALPIN et al., 1969) and 4-methylanisole (2c) (DALY, 1970b). *Ortho*-substituted methylbenzenes, on the other hand, are usually metabolized by routes other than benzylic oxidation, as in the case of *trans*-2-*ortho*-tolylcyclohexane (2b) (GALPIN et al., 1969), and 2-methylanisole (2d) (DALY, 1970b). *Meta*-substituted methylbenzenes usually undergo less benzylic oxidation than the *para*-substituted isomers, as for example, with 3-methylanisole (2e) (DALY, 1970b).

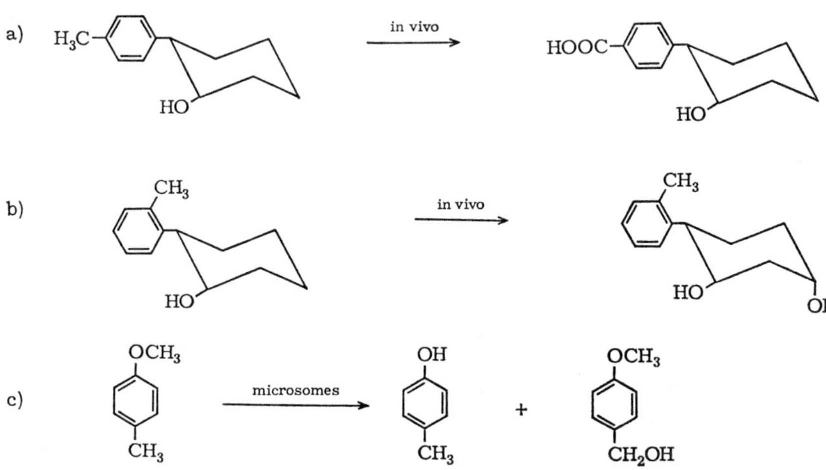

(2)

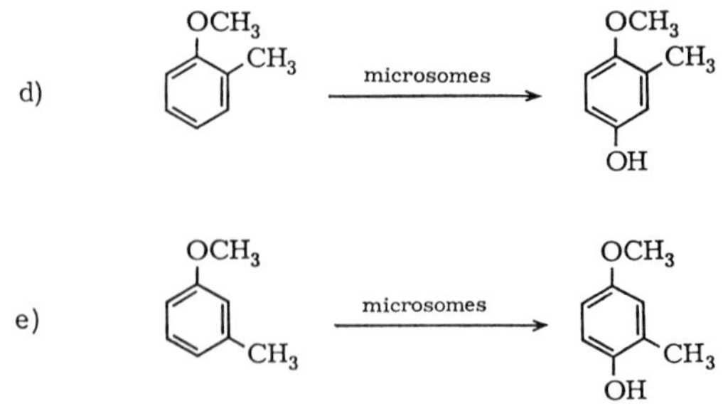

(2)

The enzyme, dopamine-β-hydroxylase, hydroxylates a variety of phenethylamines in the benzylic position to form phenethanol amines (VAN DER SCHOOT and CREVELING, 1964). The metabolism of certain phenethylamine drugs such as amphetamine, ephedrine, α-methyl-dopamine, and α-methyl-*m*-tyramine involves oxidation by this relatively specific enzyme. Alkylbenzenes other than phenethylamines do not undergo benzylic hydroxylation with dopamine-β-hydroxylase (CREVELING et al., 1962).

IV. Hydroxylation at the Allylic Position

The allylic position, like the benzylic position, appears activated toward enzymatic hydroxylation. A few examples of drugs that are metabolized by allylic

Table 4. *Aliphatic hydroxylation: compounds undergoing hydroxylation at the allylic position*

Hexobarbital (3a)	TOKI et al. (1962)
3-Phenyl-3-cyclohex-1-enyl-glutarimide	TSUKAMOTO and YOSHIMURA (1961)
p-Ionone	PARKE (1968)
5-Ethyl-5-crotylbarbituric acid	LEDVINA and BALADOVÁ (1966)
3-Methyl-4-phenyl-3-butenamide (3b)	CANONICA et al. (1968)
Methyprylon	BÖSCHE (1969)
Pentazocine (3c)	PITTMAN et al. (1969)

oxidation are given in Table 4. With pentazocine (3c), the ratio of oxidation at *cis* and *trans*-methyl groups varies from a ratio (*cis*/*trans*) of 2—3 with rat microsomes to approximately 1 with monkey (PITTMAN et al., 1969).

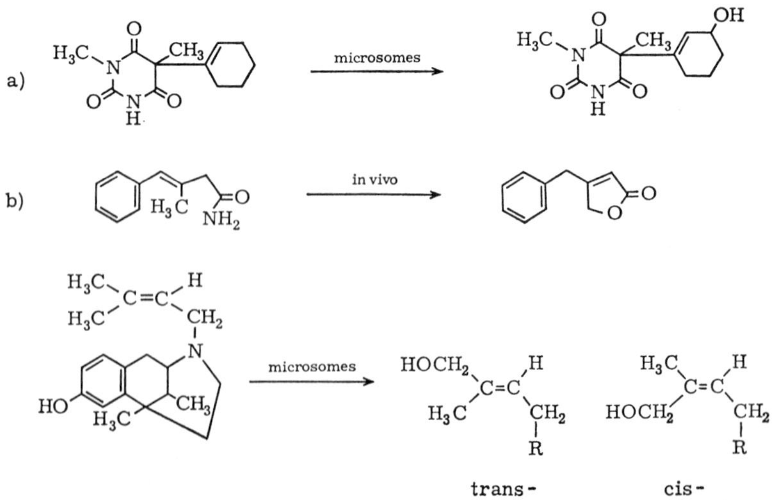

(3)

Hydroxylation at a position α- to an acetylenic group occurs in the metabolism of methohexital (1-methyl-5-allyl-5-(1-methyl-2-pentynyl)barbituricacid) (WELLES et al., 1963). This metabolism might also be considered an example of ω-1 hydroxylation.

The rate of allylic hydroxylation of hexobarbital (3a) with rat liver microsomes is markedly influenced by steric factors. The dextrorotamer is metabolized at a rate 1.6 times that of the levorotamer with microsomes from normal rats and at 2.2 times the rate with microsomes from phenobarbital-induced rats (DEGKWITZ et al., 1969; see also FURNER et al., 1969).

V. Hydroxylation of Alicyclic Rings

Cyclohexane is oxidized to cyclohexanol *in vivo* (ELLIOTT et al., 1959) and *in vitro* (ULLRICH, 1969). *In vivo*, (±)*trans*-cyclohexane-1,2-diol is also formed. With a bulky substituent in the cyclohexane ring, as in *trans*-2-*ortho*-tolylcyclohexanol [2b] (GALPIN et al., 1969), hydroxylation (axial) occurs primarily at the position furthest from this (tolyl) group. With a less bulky substituent, as in methylcyclohexane, equal amounts of 3- and 4-hydroxylated products are formed (ELLIOTT et al., 1965). Equilibration of alcohols *via* the corresponding ketones prevents an assessment of the stereochemical course of hydroxylation with methylcyclohexane. It would, however, appear that the hydroxyl group in the 3-position is introduced axially. With ethinamate (carbamic acid 1-ethynylcyclohexyl ester) and the corresponding 1-ethylcyclohexanol, hydroxylation occurs at both the 3- and 4-positions of the cyclohexyl ring (MCMAHON, 1959; PREUSS et al., 1963). The major urinary products contain a 4-equatorial hydroxyl or a 3-axial hydroxyl group. Metabolism of acetohexamide (N-(4-acetylphenylsulfonyl)N′-cyclohexylurea) affords mixtures of 3- and 4-hydroxylated products, with the relative amounts and stereochemistry dependent on the species (MCMAHON et al., 1965). Camphor and camphane are hydroxylated (axial) to a mixture of endo alcohols (3- and 5-, and 2- and 3-, resp.) (ROBERTSON and HUSSAIN, 1969). *Trans*-decalin is metabolized to (±)*trans-cis*-2-decalol (equatorial hydroxyl) while *cis*-decalin forms (±)*cis-cis*-2-decalol (axial hydroxyl) (ELLIOTT et al., 1966). Metabolism of tetralin leads to β-tetralol as a minor product with benzylic hydroxylation to α-tetralol the major metabolism (ELLIOTT and HANAM, 1968; PARKE, 1968).

An apparent tendency for alicyclic compounds to undergo axial hydroxylation may be related to similar axial hydroxylations (2β, 6β, 7α, 11β and 16α), noted in microsomal metabolism of steroids (GILLETTE, 1966). In the unnatural 9β-, 10α-testosterone, the usual hydroxylation at the 16α-axial position is unaffected, 11β-hydroxylation is reduced and no hydroxylation is observed at the 6β-position, which is now equatorial (BREUER and KNUPPEN, 1969).

Microbial metabolism of steroids by 11-β-hydroxylation appears to be sterically blocked by the presence of an 18-ethyl substituent, while metabolism by 9α- and 14α-hydroxylation is blocked by the presence of a 5α-bromo substituent (KIESLICH et al., 1969a,b).

VI. Hydroxylation on Carbon α- to a Heteroatom

A major metabolism for many drugs is the dealkylation of various N, O and S-alkyl moieties (Chapter 41). It would appear that this reaction proceeds *via* initial hydroxylation α- to the heteroatom to form an unstable hydroxylated derivative. In certain instances these derivatives are stable enough to be detected ((4a), GORROD and TEMPLE, 1969; and (4b), HODGSON and CASIDA, 1961) or to be conjugated *in vivo* with glucuronic acid (SULLIVAN et al., 1968; KEBERLE et al., 1963b).

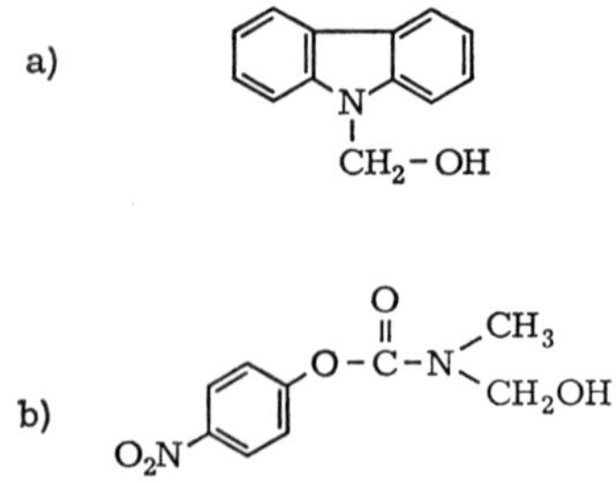

(4)

Initial hydroxylation α- to a nitrogen in a cyclic amine followed by dehydrogenation of the intermediate carbinol amine or aldehyde can lead to the formation of lactams or amino acids; i.e., nicotine to cotinine (HUCKER et al., 1960), tremorine to oxotremorine (CHO et al., 1961) or guanethidine to 2-(6-carboxyhexylamino)-ethylguanidine (ABRAMSON et al., 1969).

Steric factors influence the oxidative conversion of amphetamine and ephedrine to phenylacetone by microsomal preparations; i.e., the levorotamer is metabolized at 4—10 times the rate of the dextrorotamer (AXELROD, 1955). The N-demethylation of many drugs (AXELROD, 1956; TAKEMORI and MANNERING, 1958; SMITH et al., 1963) is also influenced by steric factors.

VII. Hydroxylation at Carbon α- or β- to a Carbonyl Group

Oxidative attack at a position α- to a carbonyl function is not a common pathway for drug metabolism. Certain acetanilides are converted to glycolanilides (KIESE and LENK, 1969). This minor metabolic pathway is favored in acetanilides in which hydroxylation at the *para*-position of the aromatic ring is blocked by the presence of a 4-chloro, bromo or propionyl-substituent. The methyl of the aceto group of the fungicide, dehydroacetic acid, is hydroxylated (BARMAN et al., 1963). The dextrorotamer of 3-ethyl-3-phenylglutarimide is hydroxylated α- to a carbonyl [5a] while the levorotamer is hydroxylated in the side chain β- to the other carbonyl of the molecule [5b] (KEBERLE et al., 1963a).

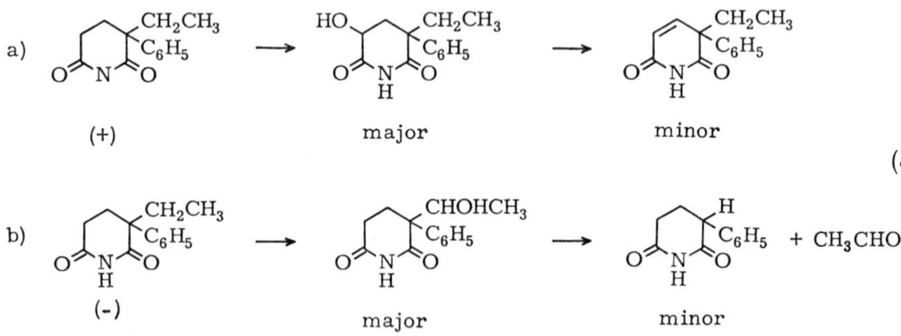

(5)

In the case of α-hydroxylation, a minor metabolite is formed by dehydration (5a), while with β-hydroxylation, dealkylation *via* a reverse aldol condensation forms 3-phenylglutarimide (5b). Hydroxylation β- to a carbonyl group and subsequent dealkylation also occurs during the metabolism of 5,5-diethylbarbituric acid (GOLDSCHMIDT and WEHR, 1957) and presumably in the dealkylation of secobarbital (WADDEL, 1963). These dealkylations are reminiscent of the oxidative 4-demethylations which occur during the conversion of lanosterol to cholesterol. This steroid-4-demethylase system does not appear to involve cytochrome P-450 (GAYLOR and MASON, 1968).

The mechanisms for the removal of the 5-vinyl group from 5-vinyl-5-(1′-methylbutyl)-barbituric acid (GELDMACHER et al., 1968; PREUSS and MULLER, 1968) and 5-ethyl-5-vinyl-barbituric acid (GOLDSCHMIDT and WEHR, 1957), or the 17α-ethynyl group from the steroid, norethindrone (PALMER et al., 1969) are unknown. Loss of vinyl substituents might involve an initial hydration of the double bond followed by a reverse aldol condensation.

As yet, no examples of oxidative attack *at a carbonyl group* to yield a lactone or ester (Baeyer-Villiger oxidation) have been reported in mammalian drug metabolism. Such reactions occur in microorganisms, as in steroid lactonizations (PRAIRIE and TALALAY, 1963) and side chain cleavages (RAHIM and SIH, 1966), in the conversion of camphor to a lactone (CONRAD et al., 1965) and in oxidation of aliphatic methyl ketones to esters (FORNEY and MARKOVETZ, 1969).

VIII. Mechanistic Studies

Aliphatic hydroxylation proceeds without inversion during microbial oxidation of steroids at 11α- and 11β-positions (HAYANO et al., 1958; COREY et al., 1958). *In vivo* in rats, 7α-hydroxylation of cholesterol-7α-^{3}H proceeds with loss of label and hence without inversion (BERGSTROM et al., 1958). Conversion of *trans*-4-^{3}H proline to *trans*-4-hydroxyproline and tritiated water with proline hydroxylase proceeds without inversion (FUJITA et al., 1964). Enzymatic hydroxylation (allylic) at an enolizable position in androstene-3,17-dione-6α-^{3}H forms the 6β-hydroxy compound with retention of label and hence configuration (BABA et al., 1963). From these examples of monooxygenase catalyzed aliphatic hydroxylations, it appears that the process is stereospecific and proceeds with retention of configuration. This has now been confirmed for the microsomal conversion of ethylbenzene to methylphenylcarbinol. Ethylbenzene is oxidized *in vitro* with microsomes to a mixture of 4 parts of R(+) and 1 part of S(—)methylphenylcarbinol (MCMAHON and SULLIVAN, 1966). The stereoselectivity of this hydroxylation of ethylbenzene is largely lost in microsomes of rats that have been pretreated with phenobarbital (MCMAHON et al., 1969; MCMAHON and SULLIVAN, 1966). When S(+)-α-^{2}H-ethylbenzene (6) was incubated with normal rat microsomes, the product consisted of

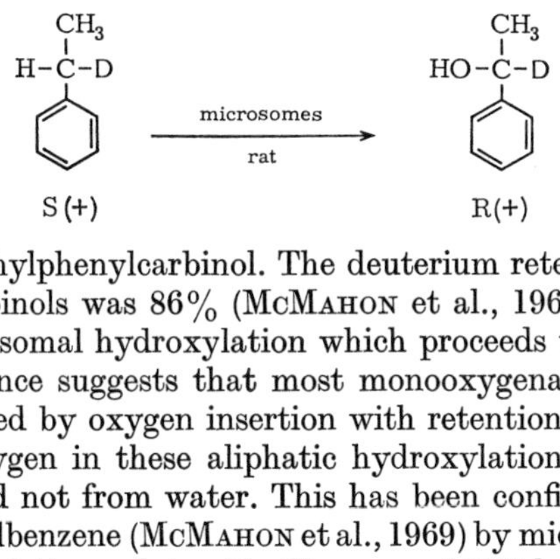

(6)

92% R(+)-α-^{2}H-methylphenylcarbinol. The deuterium retention for the mixture of entantiomeric carbinols was 86% (MCMAHON et al., 1969). This result clearly demonstrates a microsomal hydroxylation which proceeds with retention of configuration. The evidence suggests that most monooxygenase-catalyzed aliphatic hydroxylations proceed by oxygen insertion with retention of configuration.

The source of oxygen in these aliphatic hydroxylations is presumably from molecular oxygen and not from water. This has been confirmed for the benzylic hydroxylation of ethylbenzene (MCMAHON et al., 1969) by microsomal preparations. The aliphatic hydroxylations of steroids (TALALAY, 1965) by various enzymes and of phenethylamine by dopamine-β-hydroxylase (KAUFMAN et al., 1962), also proceed with utilization of molecular oxygen.

Aliphatic hydroxylation by an insertion reaction would be expected to show an isotope effect, if this step in the reaction sequence is rate-limiting. The benzylic hydroxylation of ethylbenzene to methylphenylcarbinol with microsomes shows an isotope effect (K_H/K_D) of 1.8 (MCMAHON et al., 1969), while corresponding benzylic hydroxylation of tolbutamide (1a) does not (LEMIEUX et al., 1961; TAGG et al., 1967). The conversion of tyramine to octopamine by dopamine-β-hydroxylase shows an isotope effect (K_H/K_D) of 1.6 (CREVELING et al., 1970). O-Dealkylation of 4-nitroanisole shows an isotope effect (K_H/K_D) of 2 (MITOMA et al., 1967), and N-dealkylation of morphine shows an effect (K_H/K_D) of 1.4 (ELISON et al., 1961). The ω-1 hydroxylation of 5-ethyl-5-butyl-3′-$^2H_2$-barbituric acid shows an isotope effect (K_H/K_D) of 1.6 (TANABE et al., 1969). The hydroxylation of cyclohexane to cyclohexanol (ULLRICH, 1969), and the hydroxylation of proline (PROCKOP et al., 1964) do not show an isotope effect. It is apparent that in many examples of aliphatic hydroxylation, the rate-limiting step is not insertion of oxygen into the carbon hydrogen bond.

C. Peroxidation

The peroxidation of unsaturated lipids in microsomal preparations leads to the uptake of oxygen and to the formation of malonaldehyde (ERNSTER and NORDENBRAND, 1967). Generation of hydrogen peroxide as an initiator for free radical chain reaction has been suggested. A cofactor, NADPH, and nonheme iron are necessary for lipid peroxidation (ERNSTER et al., 1968; WILLS, 1969a, b). Carbon monoxide does not inhibit lipid peroxidation so that cytochrome P-450 does not appear to be involved (NILSSON et al., 1964). In the presence of metabolizable drugs, peroxidation of lipids is inhibited (ORRENIUS et al., 1964; GOTTO et al., 1965; WILLS, 1969c; LEWIS et al., 1967). On this basis, it has been proposed that a common electron transport system is involved in lipid peroxidation and drug metabolism. Correlations of extent of drug metabolism with extent of inhibition of lipid peroxidation are, however, quite poor.

Recently, the formation of tetralin hydroperoxide (CHEN and LIN, 1968) and fluorene hydroperoxide (CHEN and LIN, 1969) during microsomal oxidation of tetralin and fluorene have been reported. The compounds were suggested as possible intermediates in the conversion of the hydrocarbons to α-tetralol and fluorenol, respectively. Peroxides have also been suggested as intermediates in hydroxylation reactions catalyzed by proline hydroxylase, γ-butyrobetaine hydroxylase, and phenylpyruvic acid hydroxylase (LINDBLAD et al., 1969).

D. Epoxidation

I. Epoxidation of Conjugated and Unconjugated Olefins

The conversion of double bond to an epoxide is now recognized as a normal process for the metabolism of foreign compounds. The epoxidation of unconjugated double bonds has been demonstrated with microsomal systems in the conversion of 1-octene and 4-octene to 1-octene epoxide and 4-octene epoxide (WATABE and MAYNERT, 1968), $\Delta^{1,3,5(10),16}$-estratetraene-3-ol to the 16α,17α-epoxide (BREUER and KNUPPEN, 1961), squalene to squalene oxide (VAN TAMELEN et al., 1966; COREY et al., 1966) and the insecticides, aldrin, isodrin and heptachlor, to their respective epoxides (WONG and TERRIERE, 1965; NAKATSUGAWA et al., 1965). 1,4-Epoxy-1,4-dihydronaphthalene is converted to the 2,3-epoxy derivative *in vivo* in rats (SIMS, 1965). The microsomal formation of styrene oxide from styrene is an example of the epoxidation of a conjugated double bond (LEIBMAN and ORTIZ, 1968a).

The *direct* conversion of an olefin to a ketone has apparently not been reported. Formation of ketones from olefins as in the metabolism of 5-allyl-5-(2-bromoallyl)barbituric acid to 5-acetonyl-5-(2′bromoallyl)barbituric acid (KEDING and SCHMIDT, 1969) could involve either direct oxidation to the ketone or hydration followed by dehydrogenation of the intermediate alcohol.

In the metabolism of steroids with microorganisms and with mammalian preparations, it has been noted that systems which catalyze aliphatic hydroxylation at the 11α, 11β, 14α, or 16α position in saturated steroids, catalyze the formation from the appropriate unsaturated steroid of an epoxy steroid with the same stereochemistry (BLOOM and SHULL, 1955; KUROSAWA et al., 1961; BREUER and KNUPPEN, 1961). Microsomal metabolism of aldrin yields the 6,7 epoxide, dieldrin (WONG and TERRIERE, 1965), while the saturated derivative, dihydroaldrin, undergoes aliphatic hydroxylation at the same position to give a mixture of 6-exo and 6-endo alcohols (BROOKS and HARRISON, 1969). These studies suggest that the enzyme-bound "active oxygen" which is inserted into a carbon-hydrogen bond will also undergo addition reactions with an unsaturated bond. In biosynthesis of cyclopenol by a mold, the oxygen of the epoxide moiety is derived from molecular oxygen (NOVER and LUCKNER, 1969).

II. Epoxidation of Aromatic Double Bonds

The conversion of aromatic substrates to arene oxides by the addition of an oxygen atom to one of the formal double bonds of the aromatic ring has often been proposed to account for dihydrodiol, catechol and premercapturic acid metabolites. An arene oxide, 1,2-naphthalene oxide, has now been identified in a biological system as the obligatory intermediate in the formation of naphthols, 1,2-dihydro-1,2-dihydroxynaphthalene, and mercapturic acid precursors from naphthalene (JERINA et al., 1968c, 1970b). The formation and metabolism of arene oxides will be discussed in detail below.

III. Epoxide Hydrase

Many epoxides, formed during metabolism of drugs, are not detected because of further metabolism by glutathione-epoxide conjugase to glutathione conjugates (Chapter 55) or by epoxide hydrase to 1,2 diols. The hepatic epoxide hydrase catalyzes the hydration of octene oxides (WATABE and MAYNERT, 1968), styrene oxide, indene oxide, cyclohexene oxide and benzene oxide (JERINA et al., 1968b), both the 16α-17α- and 16β,17β-epoxides of $\Delta^{1,3,5(10),16}$ estratetraene-3-ol (BREUER and KNUPPEN, 1961) and certain insecticide epoxides (BROOKS et al., 1968). The epoxides formed from aldrin, heptachlor and isodrin appear to be poor substrates for the hepatic epoxide hydrase. Arene oxides and epoxides of conjugated olefins are much better substrates for this enzyme than simple epoxides such as cyclohexene oxide (JERINA et al., 1968b).

The stereochemical course of hydration of a number of epoxides has been investigated. With oxides derived from cyclic olefins such as indene oxide (LEIBMAN and ORTIZ, 1968b) enzymatic hydration results in the formation of *trans*-1,2-diols. The 16α,17α-epoxide of estratetraene-3-ol forms 16,17-epiestriol by attack of water at the 17β-position (7a) while in the 16β,17β-epoxide isomer, the mixture of estriol and 16,17-epiestriol results by attack of water in both the 16α- and 17α-positions

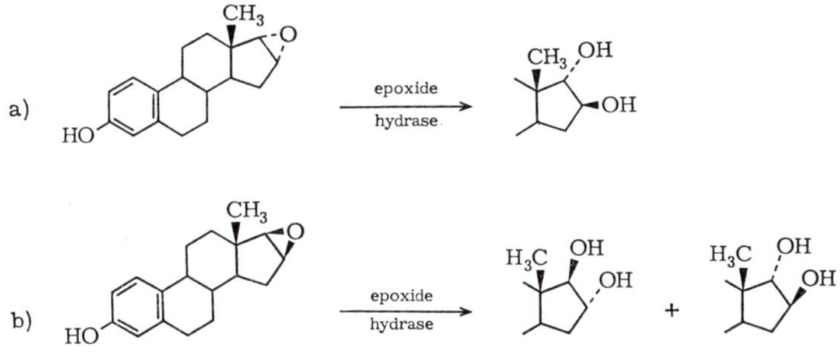

(7)

(BREUER and KNUPPEN, 1961). Steric effects due to the bridgehead methyl group would cause these differences. Styrene oxide is enzymatically hydrated by β-attack (JERINA et al., 1970c) and naphthalene oxide by attack at the 2-position (21) (JERINA et al., 1968c). The optical activity of diols obtained by enzymatic hydration of synthetic cyclohexene oxide, styrene oxide, benzene oxide, 1,2-naphthalene oxide and 9,10-phenanthrene oxide have been examined (JERINA et al., 1970c). The major enantiomere produced from cyclohexene oxide (8), benzene oxide (20) and

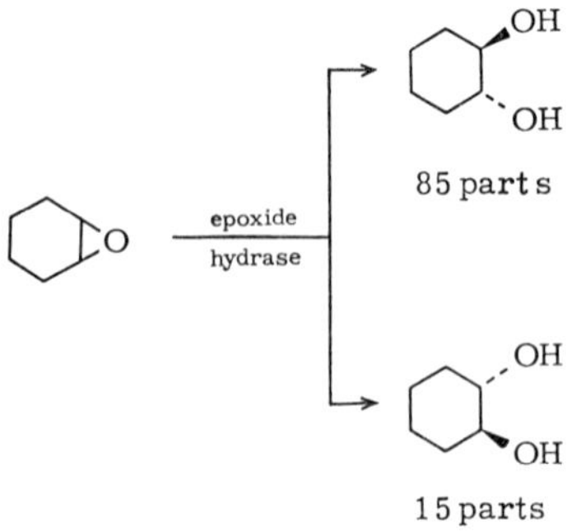

(8)

1,2-naphthalene oxide (21) has the *trans*-(1R, 2R) configuration at the carbinol atoms, while the predominate diol from 9,10-phenanthrene oxide has the *trans*-(9S, 10S) configuration. Styrene oxide forms diol with less than 1% optical purity. The products from the hydration of insecticide epoxides are optically active (BROOKS et al., 1968; KORTE and ARENT, 1965). A mechanistically interesting 1,6-hydration of an arene oxide occurs with microsomes and indene 8,9-oxide (8a) (DALY et al., 1970). It is noteworthy that nonenzymatic hydration of arene oxides has, as yet, not been accomplished.

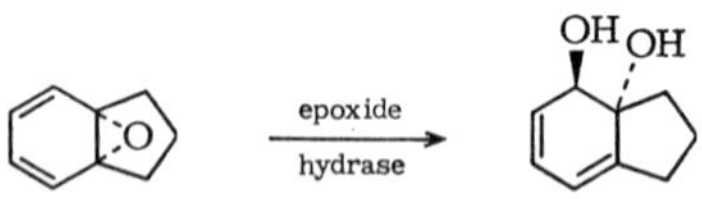

(8a)

Microsomal epoxide hydrase activity measured with styrene oxide as substrate is found to be enhanced after pretreatment of rats with phenobarbital or 3-methylcholanthrene (OESCH et al., 1970). The relationship of epoxide hydrase activity to that of another hepatic enzyme, squalene-oxidocyclase (DEAN et al., 1967) deserves investigation.

Thus, it appears certain that olefins are converted to 1,2-diols both *in vitro* and *in vivo* by the enzymatic hydration of intermediate epoxides; as, for example, in the conversion of indene and styrene to diols *in vitro* (LEIBMAN and ORTIZ, 1968b, 1969) and in the conversion of secobarbital (WADDEL, 1963), N,N-diallylmelamine (ZINS et al., 1968) and dihydronaphthalene (BOYLAND and SIMS, 1960) to diols *in vivo*. Dihydrodiols are formed from aromatic substrates *in vivo* by the action of epoxide hydrase on an intermediate arene oxide (see below).

E. Aromatic Oxidation

I. Hydroxylation of Substituted Benzenes

Microsomal hydroxylation of aromatic substrates proceeds in a manner reminiscent of electrophilic substitution reactions. Activated (electron-rich) aromatic rings are readily hydroxylated, while deactivated (electron-poor) aromatic rings are hydroxylated slowly or not at all. In addition, hydroxylation occurs at the same positions in which electrophilic substitution (bromination, etc.) takes place, i.e., in *ortho-* and *para*-positions in activated rings (aniline, anisole, acetanilide, toluene, biphenyl) (Daly et al., 1968c; Mitoma et al., 1956) and in the *meta*-position in (certain) deactivated rings (benzamide, benzoic acid) (Daly et al., 1968c).

Steric effects, however, play an important role in determining the course of microsomal hydroxylation. The most notable steric effect is the marked tendency for mono-substituted benzenes to undergo hydroxylation in the *para*-position (Table 5). The ratio of *ortho-* to *para-hydroxylation* with simple model compounds

Table 5. *Aromatic hydroxylation: compounds undergoing para-hydroxylation*

Phenobarbital	Butler (1956)
Diphenylhydantoin	Maynert (1960)
Phenformin	Hall et al. (1968)
3-Methyl-4-phenyl-3-butenamide	Canonica et al. (1968)
Phenacetylurea	Tatsumi et al. (1969)
Cincophen	Terho and Hartiala (1967)
Aniline, acetanilide, anisole, phenylthiourea, phenylhydrazine, isopropylbenzene and biphenyl	Daly (1968c), Parke (1968)
trans-Stilbene	Sinsheimer and Smith (1969)
Diphenylamine	Alexander et al. (1965)

often varies with species and with pretreatment of animals with polycyclic inducing agents. This suggests the presence of cytochrome P-450's with differing specificities. *Para*-hydroxylation is a significant metabolism even with certain substrates such as nitrobenzene and benzonitrile, which contain *meta*-directing substituents (Daly et al., 1968c; Mitoma et al., 1956; Parke, 1965). All three isomeric phenols are formed during microsomal oxidation of the deactivated rings of fluoro, chloro or bromobenzene (*ortho-*, *para*-directing) (Daly et al., 1968c). The *para*-halophenol is the major product *in vivo.*

In di- and trisubstituted aromatic substrates, the position of hydroxylation appears predictable from a consideration of the electron-donating properties of the substituents and the inherent tendency for microsomal hydroxylation to occur, if possible (see below), *para-* rather than *ortho-* to a substituent. Thus, in kynurenine (Kido et al., 1968) (9a) 3-methoxytyramine (Benington and Morin, 1968; *cf.* tyramine → dopamine, Axelrod, 1963; Lemberger et al., 1965) (9b) drazoxolon (Daniel, 1969) (9c) and 3-substituted acetanilides (9d) (Daly et al., 1968b;

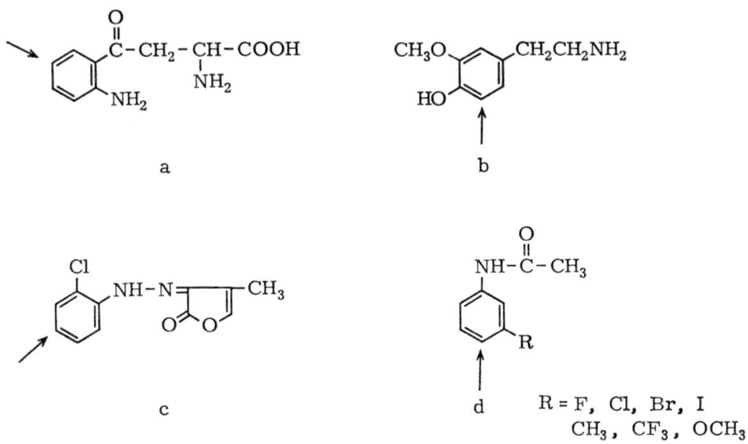

(9)

Daly, 1970b), the favored position for microsomal hydroxylation is as indicated by the arrow.

Aromatic hydroxylation at the preferred *para*-ring position is usually greatly reduced or completely blocked by the presence of a methyl, chloro, bromo, or trifluoromethyl substituent (DALY et al., 1968b; DALY, 1970b). An example of this phenomenon in drug metabolism is with phenobarbitals (SWINYARD et al., 1963) where the 4-chloro derivative has a longer biological half-life than the parent compound.

Enzymatic hydroxylation of aromatic rings occurs with introduction of oxygen from molecular oxygen. This has been shown for phenylalanine hydroxylase with phenylalanine as substrate (KAUFMAN et al., 1962), for microsomes with acetanilide as substrate (POSNER et al., 1961) and for mitochondrial kynurenine-3-hydroxylase with kynurenine as substrate (SAITO et al., 1957). The effect of deuterium on the rate of aromatic hydroxylation has been investigated in acetanilide-2,3,4,5-$^2H_5$ (TANABE et al., 1967), phenylalanine-4-^2H (GUROFF and DALY, 1967), phenobarbital-4′-^2H (PEREL et al., 1967) and anisole-2-^2H (DALY and JERINA, 1969). In all of these examples of aromatic hydroxylation, *there was no primary isotope effect*; *i.e.*, the rate of aromatic hydroxylation is not affected by the presence of deuterium rather than hydrogen at the point of hydroxylation.

II. Hydroxylation of Bicyclic and Polycyclic Aromatic Compounds

Prediction of the position of preferred metabolism in bicyclic and polycyclic aromatic substrates is more difficult. Often a number of isomeric phenols are formed. The course of hydroxylation appears to be dependent on *both* steric and electronic effects. The preferred position of hydroxylation is indicated by an arrow for a few bicyclic substrates, skatole (10a) (HORNING et al., 1959), coumarin (10b) (KAIGHEN and WILLIAMS, 1961), zoxazolamine (10c) (CONNEY et al., 1960), propranolol (10d) (BOND, 1967) and pronethalol (10e) (BOND and HOWE, 1967), and a tricyclic substance, imipramine (10f) (CRAMMER and SCOTT, 1966; *cf.*, chlorpromazine → 7-hydroxychlorpromazine; FISHMAN and GOLDENBERG, 1963). The formation of oxidized products from polycyclic hydrocarbons has been reviewed (WILLIAMS, 1959).

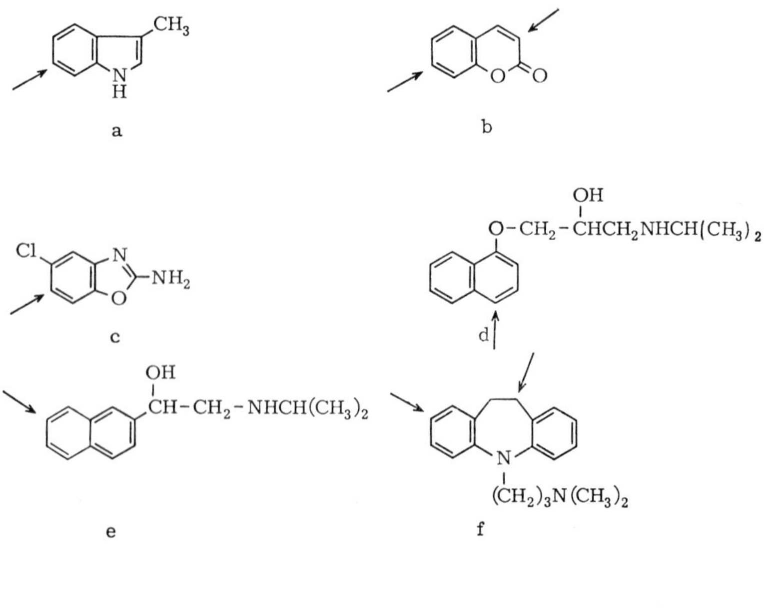

(10)

III. The NIH Shift

During investigations on the enzymatic hydroxylation of specifically tritiated and deuterated aromatic substrates, it was discovered that the substituent initially present at the point of substitution by oxygen frequently migrates during hydroxylation to an adjacent position on the aromatic ring (GUROFF et al., 1966b, c; UDENFRIEND et al., 1967) (11). The phenomenon of intramolecular migration of a ring substituent during aromatic hydroxylation has been termed the NIH Shift (GUROFF et al., 1967; DALY et al., 1968a; JERINA et al., 1970a). Isotopic label is not

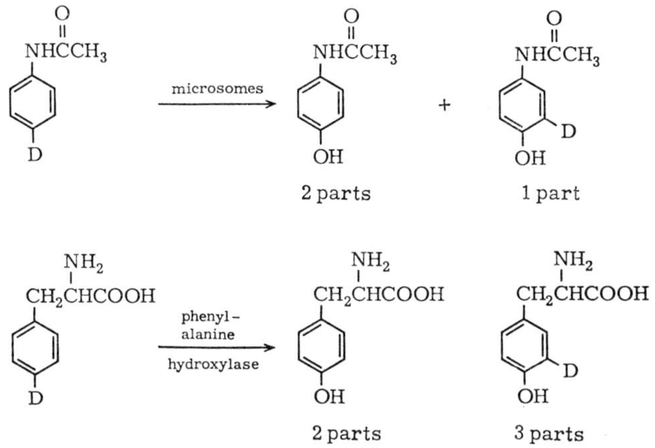

(11)

lost to a significant extent from positions adjacent to the hydroxylated carbon (12). Conversion of cinnamic acid-3-^{3}H into certain alkaloids has, however, been reported to result in significant loss of 3-^{3}H during 4-hydroxylation (BOWMAN et al., 1969).

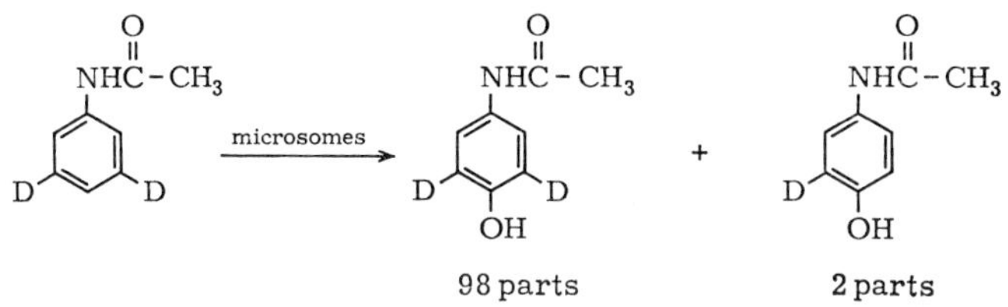

(12)

The NIH Shift was soon found to be an ubiquitous phenomenon, associated with aryl hydroxylation by monooxygenases from plant, bacterial and animal sources. The sole exception to this statement is aerobic hydroxylation of aromatic substrates such as acetanilide-4-^{2}H and anisole-4-^{2}H with peroxidase in the presence of dihydroxyfumaric acid as a reducing agent. Presumably the lack of migration of deuterium in this case is a reflection of the free radical nature of this enzymatic aryl hydroxylation. Studies on model hydroxylating systems have shown that free radical hydroxylation of aromatic rings (Fenton reagent, Udenfriend system) does not lead to migration of substituents (JERINA et al., 1967a).

Further studies on the NIH Shift revealed that the extent of migrations seen during hydroxylation is dependent on the nature of the substrate. Alkylsubstituted benzenes such as amphetamine-4-^{3}H (DALY et al., 1967), phenylalanine-4-^{3}H or 4-^{2}H (GUROFF and DALY, 1967; GUROFF et al., 1966b, c) or toluene-4-^{2}H (DALY et al., 1968c) display high retention of either deuterium (60—70%) or tritium ($> 90\%$). Phenolic substrates, such as tyrosine-3,5-$^3H_2$ and N-acetyltyramine-3,5-$^3H_2$ (DALY et al., 1967), show low migration and retention of $< 5\%$ of tritium.

Benzenesulfonanilide-4′-^{3}H or 4′-^{2}H, whose pK_a is equivalent to phenols, also shows a low retention of either deuterium or trititum (1—2%) (DALY et al., 1968c; DALY, 1970a). Less acidic acylanilines, such as acetanilide-4-^{2}H, show higher retentions of deuterium (26—55%). In the latter case, the retention of deuterium is dependent on pH, and the species of animal used as a source of microsomes. The retention with this substrate is higher with microsomes from phenobarbital-induced animals and lower with microsomes from 3-methylcholanthrene-induced animals (DALY et al., 1969). The near stoichiometric release of tritium from tyrosine-3,5-$^3H_2$ or from benzenesulphonanilide-4′-^{3}H are the basis for assays of tyrosine hydroxylase (NAGATSU et al., 1964) and microsomal hydroxylases (DALY, 1970a), respectively.

When substrates are unsymmetrical with regard to the point of substitution by oxygen, the heavy isotope may migrate preferentially in one direction. Examples of selective migration are the conversion of tryptophan to 5-hydroxytryptophan-4-^{3}H by tryptophan hydroxylase (RENSON et al., 1966) and the *in vivo* conversion of 3-desoxyestrone-3-^{2}H to estrone-2-^{2}H and 4-^{2}H (13) (NAMBARA et al., 1970).

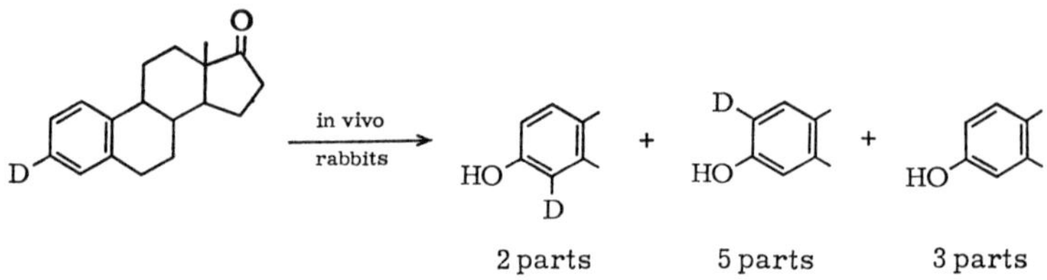

(13)

Hydroxylation-induced migration of hydrogen, deuterium, tritium, methyl, chloro and bromo substituents have been observed. Chloro, bromo or methyl groups migrate from the 4 to the 3 position during hydroxylation of 4-substituted phenylalanines with phenylalanine hydroxylase (GUROFF et al., 1966a; DALY and GUROFF, 1968). 4-Fluoro or 4-iodophenylalanine yield tyrosine as the sole product (KAUFMAN, 1961; COUNSELL, 1969). The migration of halogen occurs during the metabolism of the herbicide, 2,4-dichlorophenoxyacetic acid by fungi and plants (THOMAS et al., 1964; FAULKNER and WOODCOCK, 1965). Hydroxylation of 4-chloro- and 4-bromo-acetanilide leads to halogen migration as a minor metabolism with hepatic microsomes from benzypyrene-induced rats (ULLRICH et al., 1968) (14). With microsomes from rabbit liver, migration does not occur, and the major metabolite is hydroxyacetanilide (DALY et al., 1968b). Fluorine is lost during hydroxylation of 4-fluoroacetanilide (DALY et al., 1968b; ULLRICH et al., 1968) and 4-fluoroaniline (DALY et al., 1968b; RENSON and BOURDON, 1968). *In vivo* metab-

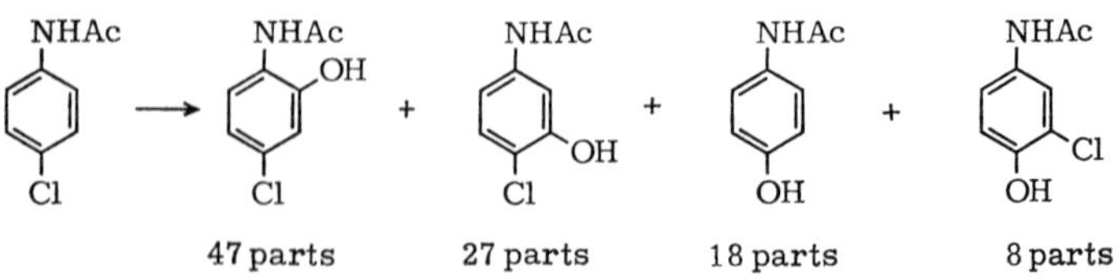

(14)

olism of the antiinflammatory agent, 2-(4-chlorophenyl)-thiazol-4-ylacetic acid provides an example of halogen migration during drug metabolism (15) (FOULKES, 1969). Loss of halogen in these metabolisms presumably occurs by a reductive loss from an intermediate oxygenated species (*cf.* KAUFMAN, 1961).

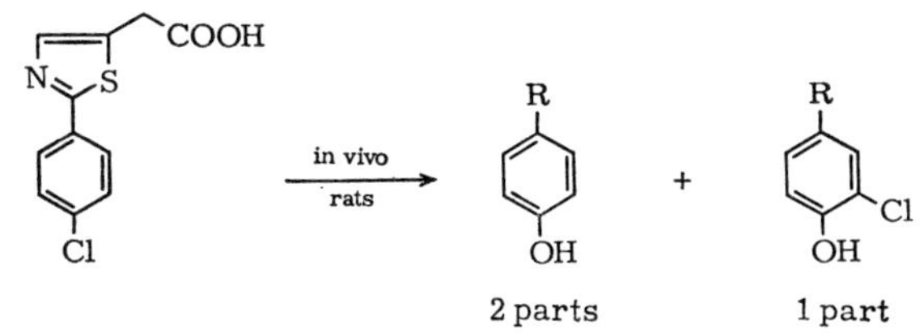

(15)

No example of methyl migration during oxidative metabolism by liver microsomal system has been reported. Instead, with *para*-substituted methylbenzenes, metabolism proceeds by hydroxylation of the methyl group. This occurs as a major metabolism with 4-methylacetanilide (DALY et al., 1968b) and 4-methylanisole (DALY, 1970b).

Probably the earliest example of the NIH Shift is the conversion of 4-hydroxyphenylpyruvic acid to homogentisic acid with the enzyme, phenylpyruvic acid oxidase (SHEPARTZ and GURIN, 1949). Ring hydroxylation, migration of the side chain and oxidative decarboxylation occur with 4-hydroxyphenylpyruvic acid, phenylpyruvic acid (KINDL, 1969) and 4-fluorophenylpyruvic acid (TANIGUCHI et al., 1964) as substrates. This enzyme is not a typical monooxygenase since it incorporates both atoms of the oxygen molecule into the substrate (LINDBLAD et al., 1969) in a reaction probably involving an intermediate cyclic peroxide.

The occurrence and magnitude of the NIH Shift has been rationalized in terms of cationoid intermediates (16) (DALY et al., 1968c). Group I substrates contain substituents without an ionizable hydrogen adjacent to the aromatic ring and exhibit relatively high retentions. Group II substrates which are capable of stabilizing the intermediate cationoid species by loss of a proton from a heteroatom adjacent to the aromatic ring show low retentions. The retention in Group II substrates decreases as the ability (reflected in increasing acidity) of the substituent XH to donate electrons increases. The retentions observed for Group II substrates (acetanilide, benzanilide) are affected by pH as predicted from the proposed mechanism (16). The effect of the source of microsomal preparations and induction with phenobarbital or 3-methylcholanthrene on retention of deuterium during hydroxylation of acetanilide-4-^{2}H has been interpreted in terms of ionization of the amide group as affected by binding and oxidation at hydrophobic and hydrophilic sites on cytochrome P-450 (DALY et al., 1969). For a thorough discussion of the

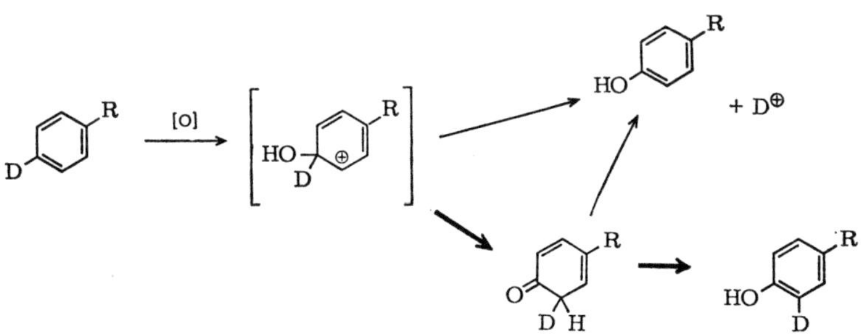

(16)

R =	OCH_3	$NCH_3SO_2C_6H_5$	CH_3	C_6H_5	C≡N	$\overset{O}{\parallel}$ C−NH_2	NO_2	Cl	Br	F
% retention =	60	53	54	64	41	42	40	54	40	47

GROUP I

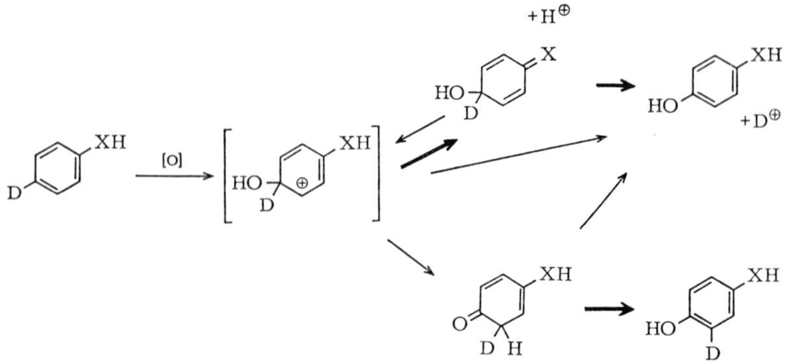

(16)

X =	O	$NSO_2C_6H_5$	NH	$\overset{O}{\overset{\Vert}{N}}CH$	$N\overset{O}{\overset{\Vert}{C}}C_6H_5$	$N\overset{O}{\overset{\Vert}{C}}CH_3$
% retention =	0	1	6	19	21	30

GROUP II

role of cationoid species and arene oxides in the NIH Shift, the reader is referred to the review by JERINA et al. (1970a).

Migrations of deuterium also occur during hydroxylation *ortho*- and *meta*- to a substituent (DALY and JERINA, 1969). The migration and retention after hydroxylation *ortho*- to a methyl group or methoxy group is similar to that observed during hydroxylation *para*- to the same substituent, despite the fact that, in *ortho*- hydroxylation there is only one ring position to which deuterium can migrate and be retained. As mentioned before, isotope is lost during hydroxylation *ortho*- or *para*- to phenols. In the two reported examples (17) (DALY and JERINA, 1969; NOVER and LUCKNER, 1969) of hydroxylation at a position *meta*- to a substituent, the retentions are markedly lower than in hydroxylation *para*- to the same substituent.

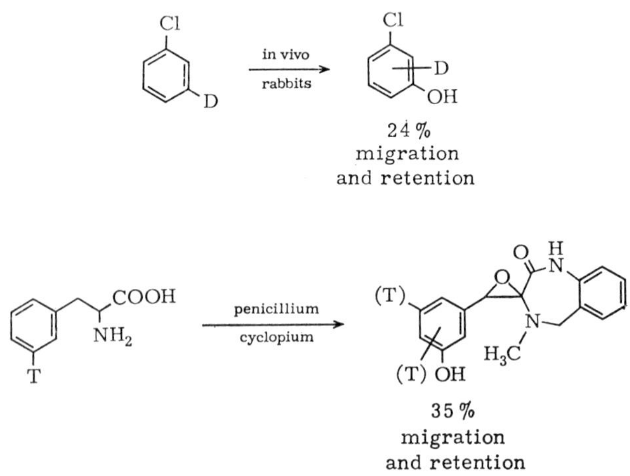

(17)

Cationoid intermediates might be formed directly by attack of "active oxygen" as depicted in [16] or indirectly as the result of the rearrangement of an arene oxide intermediate. When 3,4-toluene-4-^{2}H oxide isomerizes to 4-hydroxytoluene (18), deuterium migrates and is retained (JERINA et al., 1968a) to a degree similar to that observed for microsomal hydroxylation of toluene-4-^{2}H.

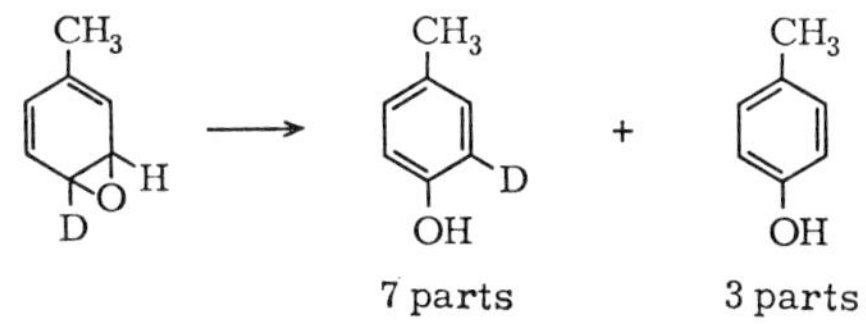

(18)

IV. Arene Oxides

Arene oxides have been frequently suggested as intermediates in the formation of dihydrodiols and premercapturic acids from aromatic substrates. It has now been demonstrated that arene oxides such as benzene oxide (JERINA et al., 1968b) and naphthalene oxide (JERINA et al., 1968c, 1970b) are converted to dihydrodiols by a hepatic epoxide hydrase and to mercapturic acid precursors in the presence of glutathione and hepatic glutathione-epoxide conjugase. The dihydrodiols and mercapturic acid precursors formed from the aromatic substrates, benzene and naphthalene, *via* oxidative pathways are identical in all respects to the same products as produced directly from the arene oxides. The arene oxides also rearrange nonenzymatically to phenols. This rearrangement is catalyzed by acid and by proteins, simple peptides and acetamide.

There would now appear to be little doubt that arene oxides are intermediates in the formation of dihydrodiol and premercapturic acid metabolites of aromatic substrates by mammalian drug metabolizing systems. Catechols are formed from aromatic substrates principally by dehydrogenation of intermediate dihydrodiol rather than by *ortho*-hydroxylation of an intermediate phenol. Thus, catechols and their O-methylated derivatives also arise from aromatic drugs by way of arene oxide formation. Further evidence that catechols do not arise from aromatic substrates via phenolic intermediates was obtained during studies of the NIH Shift in the *in vivo* metabolism of chlorobenzene-4-^{2}H (JERINA et al., 1967b) (19). The

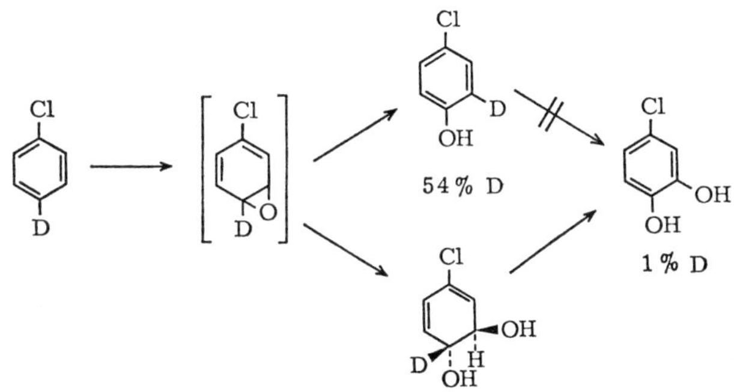

(19)

4-chlorocatechol contained only 1% D, so that it must have arisen almost exclusively by dehydrogenation of the dihydrodiol. Hydroxylation of the 4-hydroxy-3-deuterophenol would have led to 4-chlorocatechol containing 27% D (one-half of 54%). It is noteworthy that the 4-chlorobenzene-1,2-dihydrodiol is a trace metabolite in the urine of rabbits receiving chlorobenzene, but that the catechols and O-methylated catechols derived from this dihydrodiol are *the major urinary metabolites*. Thus, in the metabolism of chlorobenzene, the 3,4-oxide is the key intermediate which leads to all of the observed metabolites, including in all likelihood 4-chlorophenol by nonenzymatic rearrangement.

The enantiomeric dihydrodiols formed by the action of epoxide hydrase on benzene oxide and other arene oxides are, as mentioned above, dehydrogenated by a soluble hepatic enzyme (AYENGAR et al., 1959) to catechols. Surprisingly, the major isomer produced by enzymatic hydration of the arene oxide, is dehydrogenated more slowly than the minor isomer (20) (JERINA et al., 1970c).

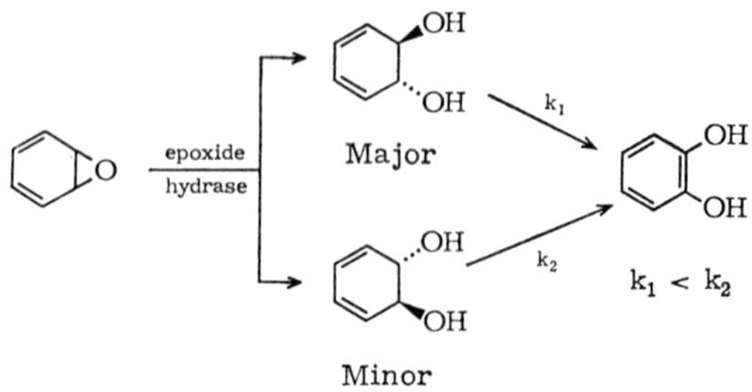

(20)

In the case of the *in vitro* metabolism of naphthalene, it has been demonstrated that 1,2-naphthalene oxide is formed, and is the obligatory intermediate in the formation of 1-naphthol, *trans*-1,2-dihydroxydihydronaphthalene and S-(1,2-dihydro-2-hydroxynaphthyl)glutathione (21) (JERINA et al., 1968c, 1970b). The 1,2-naphthalene oxide was isolated by counter current distribution and identified by color reactions, R_f on thin-layer chromatography and isomerization to α-naphthol. Naphthalene oxide appeared to be the obligatory intermediate in the formation of both naphthol and dihydrodiol; i.e., when metabolism with epoxide hydrase was blocked by a competitive substrate, styrene oxide, there was a

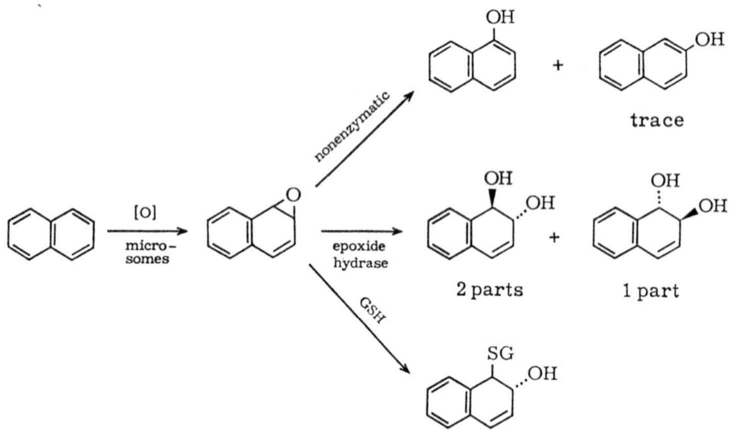

(21)

decrease in dihydrodiol formation and a concomitant increase in α-naphthol formation. Similarly the addition of glutathione-epoxide conjugase and increasing amounts of glutathione led to enhanced formation of the mercapturic acid precursor at the expense of both naphthol and dihydrodiol.

The oxygen in the 1-position of the dihydrodiol is derived from molecular oxygen (HOLTZMAN et al., 1967) and in the 2-position from water (JERINA et al., 1968c, 1970b).

The absence of dihydrodiols, catechols and mercapturic acids as metabolites of a particular aromatic compound does not, however, prove that an arene oxide is not an intermediate. In many cases, arene oxides rearrange rapidly to phenols in the presence of protein, thus preventing enzymatic hydration and conjugation with glutathione. For example, toluene 3,4-oxide rearranges very rapidly to *para*-cresol in the presence of microsomes and no dihydrodiol hydration product can be detected (JERINA et al., 1968a).

Further investigation will be required to ascertain whether arene oxides are, indeed, ubiquitous products formed in nature by the action of aryl hydroxylases. If such is the case, these enzymes should be renamed aryl oxygenases. Arene oxide intermediates have been suggested for the reactions catalyzed by the specific enzyme, tyrosine hydroxylase, in order to account for the formation of a *meta*-hydroxylated product from the normal substrate, tyrosine, and a *para*-hydroxylated product from phenylalanine (DALY et al., 1968d).

F. Summary

Present data indicate that both electronic and steric effects influence the course of aliphatic, olefinic and aromatic oxidation at carbon. "Active oxygen" appears to have electrophilic character and can undergo both insertion and addition reactions. Aliphatic hydroxylation occurs at ω- and ω-1 positions, probably due to steric factors, while benzylic and allylic hydroxylation, and hydroxylation α- to heteroatoms probably reflect the reactivity of these positions. Epoxidation of olefins has as yet not been studied in sufficient detail to define the parameters which affect this reaction. Preliminary studies have been reported on factors influencing the enzymatic hydration of epoxides. Aromatic oxidation either proceeds by arene oxide formation or by direct hydroxylation to phenols. Further investigation on the relative significance of these two alternate pathways is needed. Intermediate arene oxides rearrange to phenols, and are enzymatically converted to dihydrodiols and mercapturic acid precursors. The dihydrodiols are further metabolized to catechols and O-methylated catechols. The phenolic products obtained by enzymatic oxidation of aromatic substrates reflect attack at electron-rich positions of the aromatic nucleus, with steric effects usually directing the attack to the *para*-position. Arene oxides could be expected to isomerize to the same phenolic products that are predicted from electrophilic attack on the aromatic nucleus.

References

ABRAMSON, F.B., FURST, C.I., McMARTIN, C., WADE, R.: The isolation, identification, and synthesis of two metabolites of quanethidine formed in pig and rabbit liver homogenates. Biochem. J. **113**, 143—156 (1969).

ALEXANDER, W.E., RYAN, J., WRIGHT, S.E.: The metabolism of N-*sec*-butylaniline in the rat. Canad. J. pharm. Sci. **3**, 20—23 (1968).

— — — Metabolism of diphenylamine in the rat, rabbit and man. Food Cosmet. Toxicol. **3**, 571—579 (1965).

AXELROD, J.: The enzymatic deamination of amphetamine (benzedrine). J. biol. Chem. **214**, 753—763 (1955).

— The enzymatic N-demethylation of narcotic drugs. J. Pharmacol. exp. Ther. **117**, 322—330 (1956).

— Enzymatic formation of adrenaline and other catechols from monophenols. Science **140**, 499—500 (1963).

AYENGAR, P.K., HAYAISHI, O., NAKAJIMA, M., TOMIDA, I.: Enzymic aromatization of 3,5-cyclohexadiene-1,2-diol. Biochim. biophys. Acta (Amst.) **33**, 111—121 (1959).

BABA, S., BRODIE, H.J., HAYANO, M., PETERSON, D.H., SEBEK, O.K.: The mechanism of enzymatic hydroxylation at an enolizable position. Steroids **1**, 151—156 (1963).

BARMAN, T.E., PARKE, D.V., WILLIAMS, R.T.: The metabolism of dehydroacetic acid (DHA). Toxicol. appl. Pharmacol. **5**, 545—568 (1963).

BENINGTON, F., MORIN, R.D.: Enzymatic 5-hydroxylation of 3-methoxytyramine. Experientia (Basel) **24**, 33—34 (1968).

BERGSTROM, S., BORGSTROM, B., TRYDING, N., WESTOO, G.: Intestinal absorption and metabolism of 2:2-dimethylstearic acid in the rat. Biochem. J. **58**, 604—608 (1954).
— BRIDGWATER, R.J., GLOOR, U.: On the conversion of 3α, 7α, 12α-trihydroxycoprostanic acid to cholic acid in rat liver homogenates. Acta chem. Scand. **11**, 836—842 (1957).
— LINDSTREDT, S., SAMUELSON, B., COREY, E.J., GREGORIOU, G.A.: The stereochemistry of 7α-hydroxylation in the biosynthesis of cholic acid from cholesterol. J. Amer. chem. Soc. **80**, 2337—2338 (1958).
BILLINGS, R.E., SULLIVAN, H.R., MCMAHON, R.E.: Oxidation of indan to indanol and indanone by the hepatic microsomal system. Biochemistry **9**, 1256—1260 (1970).
BLOOM, B.M., SHULL, G.M.: Epoxidation of unsaturated steroids by microorganisms. J. Amer. chem. Soc. **77**, 5767—5768 (1955).
BOND, P.A.: Metabolism of propranolol (Internal), a potent, specific β-adrenergic receptor blocking agent. Nature (Lond.) **213**, 721—722 (1967).
— HOWE, R.: The metabolism of pronethalol. Biochem. Pharmacol. **16**, 1261—1269 (1967).
BÖSCHE, J.: Konzentrationen von Methypyrlon und dessen Metaboliten im Harn bei Vergiftungsfällen. Arzneimittel-Forsch. **19**, 123—125 (1969).
BOWMAN, W.R., BRUCE, I.T., KIRBY, G.W.: Biosynthetic incorporation of [β-^{14}C:3,5-$^{2}H_2$:4^{3}-H] cinnamic acid into capsaicin and norpluviine; lack of an apparent isotope effect following an NIH shift. J. chem. Soc. D. 1075—1076 (1969).
BOYLAND, E., SIMS, P.: Metabolism of polycyclic compounds. 16. The metabolism of 1:2-dihydronaphthalene and 1:2-epoxy-1:2:3:4-tetrahydronaphthalene. Biochem. J. **77**, 175—181 (1960).
BRAY, H.G., HUMPHRIS, B.G., THORPE, W.V.: Metabolism of derivatives of toluene 3. *o*-, *m*- and *p*-xylenes. Biochem. J. **45**, 241—244 (1949a).
— LAKE, H.J., THORPE, W.V.: Metabolism of derivatives of toluene. 2. Nuclear methyl-substituted derivatives of N-phenylurea. Biochem. J. **44**, 136—140 (1949b).
— THORPE, W.V.: Metabolism of derivatives of toluene. 1. The metabolism of acetotoludides in the rabbit. Biochem. J. **43**, 211—216 (1948).
— — WHITE, K.: Metabolism of derivatives of toluene. 4. Cresols. Biochem. J. **46**, 275—278 (1950).
BREUER, H., KNUPPEN, R.: Stoffwechsel von 9β. 10α-Testosteron in Gewebepräparation der Rattenleber und der Nebenniere des Rindes. Hoppe-Seylers Z. physiol. Chem. **350**, 581—590 (1969).
— — The formation and hydrolysis of 16α.17α-epoxyoestratriene-3-ol by rat-liver tissue. Biochim. biophys. Acta (Amst.) **49**, 620—621 (1961).
BROOKS, G.T., HARRISON, A.: The oxidative metabolism of aldrin and dihydroaldrin by houseflies, housefly microsomes and pig liver microsomes and the effect of inhibitors. Biochem. Pharmacol. **18**, 557—568 (1969).
— LEWIS, S.E., HARRISON, A.: Selective metabolism of cyclodiene insecticide enantiomers by pig liver microsomal enzymes. Nature (Lond.) **220**, 1034—1035 (1968).
BRUCE, R.B., TURNBULL, L., NEWMAN, J., PITTS, J.: Metabolism of metaxalone. J. med. pharm. Chem. **9**, 286—293 (1966).
BUTLER, T.C.: The metabolic hydroxylation of phenobarbital. J. Pharmacol. exp. Ther. **116**, 326—336 (1956).
CANONICA, L., MANITTO, P., VALCAVI, U., BOLEGO, N.Z.: Metabolism of 3-methyl-4-phenyl-3-butenamide. J. biol. Chem. **243**, 1645—1648 (1968).
CHEN, C., LIN, C.C.: Mechanism of aliphatic hydroxylation. Tetralin hydroperoxide as an intermediate in the hydroxylation of tetralin in rat liver homogenate. Biochim. biophys. Acta (Amst.) **170**, 366—374 (1968).
— — [9-^{14}C] Fluorene hydroperoxide as a possible intermediate in the hydroxylation of [9-^{14}C] fluorene by rat liver homogenate. Biochim. biophys. Acta (Amst.) **184**, 634—640 (1969).
CHO, A.K., HASLETT, W.L., JENDEN, D.J.: The identification of an active metabolite of tremorine. Biochem. biophys. Res. Commun. **5**, 276—279 (1961).
CONNEY, A.H., TROUSOF, M., BURNS, J.J.: The metabolic fate of zoxazolamine (flexin) in man. J. Pharmacol. exp. Ther. **128**, 333—340 (1960).
CONRAD, H.E., DUBUS, R., NAMTVEDT, M.J., GUNSALUS, J.C.: Mixed function oxidation. II. Separation and properties of the enzymes catalyzing camphor lactonization. J. biol. Chem. **240**, 495—503 (1965).
COOPER, J.R., BRODIE, B.B.: Enzymatic oxidation of pentobarbital and thiopental. J. Pharmacol. exp. Ther. **120**, 75—87 (1955).
COREY, E.J., GREGORIOU, G.A., PETERSON, D.H.: The stereochemistry of 11α-hydroxylation of steroids. J. Amer. chem. Soc. **80**, 2338 (1958).
— RUSSEY, W.E., ORTIZ DE MONTELLANO, P.R.: 2,3-Oxidosqualene, an intermediate in the biological synthesis of sterols from squalene. J. Amer. chem. Soc. **88**, 4750—4751 (1966).

COUNSELL, R. E.: Personal communication (1969).
CRAMMER, J. L., SCOTT, B.: New metabolites of imipramine. Psychopharmacologia (Berl.) **8**, 461—468 (1966).
CREVELING, C. R., DALY, J. W., KANAOKA, Y., KUNIEDA, T., WITKOP, B.: Hydroxylation of deuterated and tritiated tyramines: An assay for dopamine-β-hydroxylase (1970) [in preparation].
— — WITKOP, B., UDENFRIEND, S.: Substrates and inhibitors of dopamine-β-oxidase. Biochim. biophys. Acta (Amst.) **64**, 125—134 (1962).
DALY, J. W.: A simple radiometric assay for microsomal aryl hydroxylase activity. Analyt. Biochem. **33**, 286—296 (1970a).
— The metabolism of acetanilides and anisoles with rat liver microsomes. Biochem. Pharmacol. (1970b) [in press].
— GUROFF, G.: Production of *m*-methyltyrosine and *p*-hydroxymethylphenylalanine from *p*-methylphenylalanine by phenylalanine hydroxylase. Arch. Biochem. **125**, 136—141 (1968).
— — JERINA, D., UDENFRIEND, S., WITKOP, B.: Intramolecular migrations during hydroxylation of aromatic compounds. The NIH Shift. Advances in Chemistry Series, American Chemical Society, Oxidation of organic compounds III, **77**, 279—289 (1968a).
— — UDENFRIEND, S., WITKOP, B.: Hydroxylation of alkyl and halogen-substituted anilines and acetanilides by microsomal hydroxylases. Biochem. Pharmacol. **17**, 31—37 (1968b).
— — — — Hydroxylation-induced migrations of tritium in several substrates of liver aryl hydroxylases. Arch. Biochem. **122**, 218—223 (1967).
— JERINA, D.: Migration of deuterium during aryl hydroxylation. III. Effect of ortho- and meta-substituents. Arch. Biochem. **134**, 266—269 (1969).
— — FARNSWORTH, J., GUROFF, G.: The migration of deuterium during aryl hydroxylation. II. The effect of induction of microsomal hydroxylases with pentobarbital or polycyclic aromatic hydrocarbons. Arch. Biochem. **131**, 238—244 (1969).
— — WITKOP, B.: Migration of deuterium during hydroxylation of aromatic substrates by liver microsomes. I. Influence of ring substituents. Arch. Biochem. **128**, 517—527 (1968c).
— — ZIFFER, H., KLARNER, F. G., VOGEL, E., WITKOP, B.: The role of arene oxide-oxepin systems in the metabolism of aromatic substrates. VI. Homoallylic addition of water to indane 8,9-oxide. J. Amer. chem. Soc. **92**, 702—703 (1970).
— LEVITT, M., GUROFF, G., UDENFRIEND, S.: Isotope studies on the mechanism of action of adrenal tyrosine hydroxylase. Arch. Biochem. **126**, 593—598 (1968d).
DANIEL, J. W.: The metabolism of arylazoisoxazolones by rats and dogs. Biochem. J. **111**, 695—702 (1969).
DAS, M. L., ORRENIUS, S., ERNSTER, L.: On the fatty acid and hydrocarbon hydroxylation in rat liver microsomes. Europ. J. Biochem. **4**, 519—523 (1968).
DEAN, P. D. G., ORTIZ DE MONTELLANO, P. R., BLOCH, K., COREY, E. J.: A soluble 2,3-oxidosqualene sterol cyclase. J. biol. Chem. **242**, 3014—3015 (1967).
DEGKWITZ, E., ULLRICH, V., STAUDINGER, H., RUMMEL, W.: Metabolism and cytochrome P-450 binding spectra of (+) and (—) hexobarbital in rat liver microsomes. Hoppe-Seylers Z. physiol. Chem. **350**, 547—553 (1969).
DENNER, W. H. B., OLAVESEN, A. H., POWELL, G. M., DODGSON, K. S.: The metabolism of potassium dodecyl [^{35}S]. Biochem. J. **111**, 43—51 (1969).
DOUGLAS, J. F., LUDWIG, B. J., GINSBERG, T., BERGER, F. M.: The metabolic fate of mebutamate (Capla). J. Pharmacol. exp. Ther. **136**, 5—9 (1962).
DUHM, B., MAUL, W., MEDENWALD, H., PATZSCHKE, K., WEGNER, L.: Untersuchungen mit ^{14}C-markiertem Noxiptilin. Arzneimittel-Forsch. **19**, 858—870 (1969).
ELISON, C., ELLIOTT, H. W., LOOK, M., RAPOPORT, H.: Some aspects of the fate and relationship of morphine to its pharmacological activity. J. med. pharm. Chem. **6**, 237—248 (1963).
— RAPOPORT, H., LAURSEN, R., ELLIOTT, H. W.: Effect of deuteration of N—CH_3 group on potency and enzymatic N-demethylation of morphine. Science **134**, 1079—1080 (1961).
ELLIOTT, T. H., HANAM, J.: The metabolism of tetralin. Biochem. J. **108**, 551—559 (1968).
— PARKE, D. V., WILLIAMS, R. T.: Studies in detoxification 79. The metabolism of cyclo [^{14}C] hexane and its derivatives. Biochem. J. **72**, 193—200 (1959).
— ROBERTSON, J. S., WILLIAMS, R. T.: The metabolism of *cis*- and *trans*-decalin. Biochem. J. **100**, 403—406 (1966).
— TAO, R. C. C., WILLIAMS, R. T.: The metabolism of methylcyclohexane. Biochem. J. **95**, 70—76 (1965).
EL MASRY, A. M., SMITH, J. N., WILLIAMS, R. T.: Studies in detoxification 69. The metabolism of alkylbenzenes. Biochem. J. **64**, 50—56 (1956).
ERNSTER, L., NORDENBRAND, K.: Microsomal lipid peroxidation. Methods. Enzymologia **10**, 574—580 (1967).
— — ORRENIUS, S., LALDAS, M.: Microsomal lipid peroxidation. Hoppe-Seylers Z. physiol. Chem. **349**, 1604—1605 (1968).

Eschenhof, E., Rieder, J.: Untersuchungen über das Schicksal des Antidepressivums Amitryptylin im Organismus der Ratte und des Menschen. Arzneimittel-Forsch. **19**, 957—966 (1969).
Faulkner, J.K., Woodcock, D.: Fungal detoxication. Part VII. Metabolism of 2,4-dichlorophenoxyacetic and 4-chloro-2-methylphenoxyacetic acids by *Aspergillus niger*. J. chem. Soc. 1187—1191 (1965).
Fishman, V., Goldenberg, H.: Metabolism of chloropromazine. IV. Identification of 7-hydroxychlorpromazine and its sulfoxide and desmethyl derivatives. Proc. Soc. exp. Biol. (N.Y.) **112**, 501—506 (1963).
Forney, F.W., Markovetz, A.J.: An enzyme system for aliphatic methyl ketone oxidation. Biochem. biophys. Res. Commun. **37**, 31—38 (1969).
Foulkes, D.M.: Metabolism of thiazole acetic acid derivatives and the NIH Shift. Nature (Lond.) **221**, 582 (1969).
Fujita, Y., Gottlieb, A., Peterkofsky, B., Udenfriend, S., Witkop, B.: The preparation of *cis*- and *trans*-4-H^3-*L*-prolines and their use in studying the mechanism of enzymatic hydroxylation in chick embryos. J. Amer. chem. Soc. **86**, 4709—4716 (1964).
Furner, R.L., McCarthy, J.S., Stitzel, R.E., Anders, M.W.: Stereoselective metabolism of the enantiomers of hexobarbital. J. Pharmacol. exp. Ther. **169**, 153—158 (1969).
Galpin, D.R., Cochran, R.G., Huitric, A.C.: Application of nuclear magnetic resonance and optical rotatory dispersion to studies in drug metabolism-stereoselectivity in the metabolism of *trans*-2-*p*-tolylcyclohexanol and *trans*-2-*o*-tolylcyclohexanol in the rat. Biochem. Pharmacol. **18**, 979—991 (1969).
Gaylor, J.R., Mason, H.S.: Investigation of the component reactions of oxidative sterol demethylation. J. biol. Chem. **243**, 4966—4972 (1968).
Geldmacher, M., Mallinkrodt, V., Machbert, G., Geldmacher, J.: Zum Stoffwechsel der 5-vinyl-5-(1′-methylbutyl) barbitursäure beim Menschen. 1. Mitteilung: 5-(1′-Methylbutyl) barbitursäure. Arzneimittel-Forsch. **18**, 350—353 (1968).
Gillette, J.R.: Side chain oxidation of alkyl substituted ring compounds. I. Enzymatic oxidation of *p*-nitrotoluene. J. biol. Chem. **234**, 139—143 (1959).
— Biochemistry of drug oxidation and reduction by enzymes in the hepatic endoplasmic reticulum. Advanc. Pharmacol. **4**, 219—261 (1966).
Goldschmidt, S., Wehr, R.: Über Barbiturate. III. Mitteilung. Der Metabolismus von Veronal. Hoppe-Seylers Z. physiol. Chem. **308**, 9—19 (1957).
Gorrod, J.W., Temple, D.J.: The metabolism of N-methylcarbazole by hepatic microsomes. International Symposium on Microsomes and Drug Oxidations. Tübingen, Germany, July 19—22 (1969).
Gotto, A.M., Hatson, R.M., Meikle, A.W., Touster, O.: Spectrophotometric and manometric studies of NADPH and NADH oxidase activities of rat liver microsomes. Effects of drugs and adenine nucleotides. Biochem. Pharmacol. **14**, 989—1002 (1965).
Guroff, G., Daly, J.W.: Quantitative studies on the hydroxylation-induced migration of deuterium and tritium during phenylalanine hydroxylation. Arch. Biochem. **122**, 218—223 (1967).
— — Jerina, D., Renson, J., Udenfriend, S., Witkop, B.: Hydroxylation-induced intramolecular migrations: The NIH Shift. Science **157**, 1524—1530 (1967).
— Kondo, K., Daly, J.W.: The production of *meta*-chlorotyrosine from *para*-chlorophenylalanine by phenylalanine hydroxylase. Biochem. biophys. Res. Commun. **25**, 622—628 (1966a).
— Levitt, M., Daly, J.W., Udenfriend, S.: The production of *meta*-tritiotyrosine from *p*-tritiophenylalanine by phenylalanine hydroxylase. Biochem. biophys. Res. Commun. **25**, 253—259 (1966b).
— Reifsnyder, C.A., Daly, J.W.: Retention of deuterium in *p*-tyrosine formed enzymatically from *p*-deuterophenylalanine. Biochem. biophys. Res. Commun. **24**, 720—724 (1966c).
Hall, H., Ramachander, G., Glassman, J.M.: Tissue distribution and excretion of phenformin in normal and diabetic animals. Ann. N.Y. Acad. Sci. **148**, 601—611 (1968).
Hamberg, M., Samuelsson, B.: Structure of the major urinary metabolite of prostaglandin E_2 in man. J. Amer. chem. Soc. **91**, 2177—2178 (1969).
Hayano, M., Gut, M., Dorfman, R.I., Sebek, O.K., Peterson, D.H.: Steric considerations in the enzymatic course of the hydroxylation of steroids. J. Amer. chem. Soc. **80**, 2336—2337 (1958).
Hodgson, E., Casida, J.E.: Metabolism of N:N-dialkyl carbamates and related compounds by rat liver. Biochem. Pharmacol. **8**, 179—191 (1961).
Holtzman, J., Gillette, J.R., Milne, G.W.A.: The metabolic products of naphthalene in mammalian systems. J. Amer. chem. Soc. **89**, 6341—6344 (1967).
Horning, E.C., Sweeley, C.C., Dalgliesh, C.E., Kelly, W.: Mammalian hydroxylation in the 6-position of the indole ring. Biochim. biophys. Acta (Amst.) **32**, 566—567 (1959).

HUCKER, H.B., GILLETTE, J.R., BRODIE, B.B.: Enzymatic pathway for the formation of cotinine, a major metabolite of nicotine in rabbit liver. J. Pharmacol. exp. Ther. **129**, 94—100 (1960).

ICHIHARA, K., KUSUNOSE, E., KUSUNOSE, M.: Some properties and distribution of the W-hydroxylation system of medium-chain fatty acids. Biochim. biophys. Acta (Amst.) **176**, 704—712 (1969a).

— — — Microsomal hydroxylation of decane. Biochim. biophys. Acta (Amst.) **176**, 713—719 (1969b).

JERINA, D., DALY, J.W., LANDIS, W., WITKOP, B., UDENFRIEND, S.: Intramolecular migration of tritium and deuterium during nonenzymatic aromatic hydroxylation. J. Amer. chem. Soc. **89**, 3347—3349 (1967a).

— — WITKOP, B.: Deuterium migration during the acid-catalyzed dehydration of 6-deutero-5,6-dihydroxy-3-chloro-1,3-cyclohexadiene, a nonenzymatic model for the NIH Shift. J. Amer. chem. Soc. **89**, 5488—5489 (1967b).

— — — The role of arene oxide-oxepin systems in the metabolism of aromatic substrates. II. Synthesis of 3,4-toluene-4-^{2}H-oxide and subsequent "NIH Shift" to 4-hydroxytoluene-3-^{2}H. J. Amer. chem. Soc. **90**, 6523—6525 (1968a).

— — — The "NIH Shift" and a mechanism of enzymatic oxygenation. In: The role of biogenic amines and physiological membranes in modern drug therapy. Ed. by J. BIEL. New York: Marcel Dekker 1970a (in press).

— — — ZALTZMAN-NIRENBERG, P., UDENFRIEND, S.: The role of arene oxide-oxepin system in the metabolism of aromatic substrates. V. 1,2-Naphthalene oxide, product of microsomal metabolism of naphthalene. Biochemistry **9**, 147—156 (1970b).

— — — — — The role of the arene oxide-oxepin system in the metabolism of aromatic substrates. I. *In vitro* conversion of benzene oxide to a premercapturic acid and a dihydrodiol. Arch. Biochem. **128**, 176—183 (1968b).

— — — — — The role of arene oxide-oxepin systems in the metabolism of aromatic substrates. III. Formation of 1,2-naphthalene oxide from naphthalene by liver microsomes. J. Amer. chem. Soc. **90**, 6525—6527 (1968c).

— ZIFFER, H., DALY, J.W.: The role of the arene oxide-oxepin system in the metabolism of aromatic substrates. IV. Stereochemical considerations of dihydrodiol formation and dehydrogenation. J. Amer. chem. Soc. **91**, 1056—1061 (1970c).

KAIGHEN, M., WILLIAMS, R.T.: The metabolism of [3-^{14}C] coumarin. J. med. pharm. Chem. **3**, 25—43 (1961).

KAUFMAN, S.: The enzymic conversion of 4-fluorophenylalanine to tyrosine. Biochim. biophys. Acta (Amst.) **51**, 619—621 (1961).

— BRIDGERS, W.F., EISENBERG, F., FRIEDMAN, S.: The source of oxygen in phenylalanine hydroxylase and dopamine-β-hydroxylase catalyzed reactions. Biochem. biophys. Res. Commun. **9**, 497—502 (1962).

KEBERLE, H., RIESS, W., HOFFMAN, K.: Über den stereospezifischen Metabolismus der optischen Antipoden von α-Phenyl-α-äthyl-glutarimid (Doriden). Arch. int. Pharmacodyn. **142**, 117—124 (1963a).

— — SCHMID, K., HOFFMAN, K.: Über den Mechanismus der biologischen N-Desalkylierung. Arch. int. Pharmacodyn. **142**, 125—140 (1963b).

KEDING, H., SCHMIDT, G.: Isolierung und Identifizierung von Brallobarbital-Metaboliten. Arzneimittel-Forsch. **19**, 342—347 (1969).

KIDO, R., NOGUCHI, T., KASEDA, H., KAWAMOTO, M., MATSUMURA, Y.: Formation of 5-hydroxy-L-kynureine from L-kynureinine by hen liver microsomes. Arch. Biochem. **125**, 1030—1031 (1968).

KIESE, M., LENK, W.: Oxidation of acetanilides to glycolanilides and oxanilic acids in rabbits. Biochem. Pharmacol. **18**, 1324—1334 (1969).

KIESLICH, K., BERNDT, H.-D., WIECHERT, R., KERB, U., SCHULZAND, G., KOCH, H.-J.: Blockierung der mikrobiologischen 11β-Hydroxylierung von Steroiden durch 18-Methyl-Substitution. Justus Liebigs Ann. Chem. **726**, 161—167 (1969a).

— PETZOLDT, K., KOSMOL, H., KOCH, W.: Darstellung von 6α-Fluor-16α-Methyl-11, 21-Dihydroxy-1,4-Pregnadien-3,20-Dion (Fluocortolon) über eine Substrat-Struktur-gelenkte spezifische 11β-Hydroxylierung mit Curvularia lunatu. Justus Liebigs Ann. Chem. **726**, 168—176 (1969b).

KINDL, H.: Biosynthesis and metabolism of hydroxyphenylacetic acids in higher plants. Europ. J. Biochem. **7**, 340—347 (1969).

KORTE, F., ARENT, H.: Metabolism of insecticides. IX (1). Isolation and identification of dieldrin metabolites from urine of rabbits after oral administration of dieldrin-^{14}C. Life Sci. **4**, 2017—2025 (1965).

KUROSAWA, Y., HAYANO, M., BLOOM, B.M.: The epoxidation of unsaturated steroids. Agr. biol. Chem. **25**, 838—843 (1961).

KUSUNOSE, M., ICHIHARA, K., KUSUNOSE, E.: Oxidation of n-hexadecane by mouse liver microsomal fraction. Biochim. biophys. Acta (Amst.) **176**, 679—681 (1969).
LEDVINA, M., BALADOVA, D.: Über Metaboliten des Kalypnons. Pharmazie **21**, 227—229 (1966).
LEIBMAN, K.C., ORTIZ, E.: Styrene epoxide — an intermediate in microsomal oxidation of styrene to its glycol. Pharmacologist **10**, 203 (1968a).
— — Oxidation of indene in liver microsomes. Molec. Pharmacol. **4**, 201—207 (1968b).
— — Oxidation of styrene in liver microsomes. Biochem. Pharmacol. **18**, 552—554 (1969).
LEMBERGER, L., KUNTZMAN, R., CONNEY, A.H., BURNS, J.J.: Metabolism of tyramine to dopamine by liver microsomes. J. Pharmacol. exp. Ther. **150**, 292—297 (1965).
LEMIEUX, R.U., SPOREK, K.F., O'REILLY, I., NELSON, E.: The oxidation of N-*p*-benzotrideuteridesulfonyl N'-*n*-butylurea (tolbutamide-D_3) by man. Biochem. Pharmacol. **7**, 31—34 (1961).
LEWIS, S.E., WILKINSON, C.F., RAY, J.W.: The relationship between microsomal epoxidation and lipid peroxidation in houseflies and pig liver, and the inhibitory effect of derivatives of 1,3-benzodioxole. Biochem. Pharmacol. **16**, 1195—1210 (1967).
LINDBLAD, B., LINDSTEDT, G., TOFFT, M., LINDSTEDT, S.: The mechanism of α-ketoglutarate oxidation in coupled enzymatic oxygenations. J. Amer. chem. Soc. **91**, 4604—4606 (1969).
LU, A.Y.H., JUNK, K.W., COON, M.J.: Resolution of the cytochrome P-450-containing ω-hydroxylation system of liver microsomes into three components. J. biol. Chem. **244**, 3714—3721 (1969a).
— STROBEL, H.W., COON, M.J.: Hydroxylation of benzphetamine and other drugs by a solubilized form of cytochrome P-450 from liver microsomes: lipid requirement for drug demethylation. Biochem. biophys. Res. Commun. **36**, 545—551 (1969b).
LUDWIG, B.J., DOUGLAS, J.F., POWELL, L.S., MEYER, M., BERGER, F.M.: Structures of the major metabolites of meprobamate. J. med. pharm. Chem. **3**, 53—64 (1961).
MAYNERT, E.W.: Ethyl-(3-hydroxybutyl)-barbituric acid as a metabolite of neonal. J. biol. Chem. **195**, 403—406 (1952a).
— Ethyl-(3-hydroxyisoamyl)-barbituric acid as the principal metabolite of amytal. J. biol. Chem. **195**, 397—402 (1952b).
— Metabolic fate of diphenylhydantoin. J. Pharmacol. exp. Ther. **130**, 275—284 (1960).
— On the specificity of penultimate oxidation. The fate of 5-ethyl-5-hexyl-barbituric acid. J. Pharmacol. exp. Ther. **150**, 476—483 (1965).
MCCARTHY, R.D.: Mammalian metabolism of straight-chain saturated hydrocarbons. Biochim. biophys. Acta (Amst.) **84**, 74—79 (1964).
MCCHESNEY, E.W., FROELICH, E.J., LESHER, G.Y., CRAIN, A.V.R., ROSI, D.: Absorption, excretion and metabolism of a new antibacterial agent, nalidixic acid. Toxicol. appl. Pharmacol. **6**, 292—309 (1964).
MCDANIEL, G.H., PODGAINY, H., BRESSLER, R.: The metabolism of tolbutamide in rat liver. J. Pharmacol. exp. Ther. **167**, 91—97 (1969).
MCMAHON, R.E.: In vivo hydroxylation of 1-ethylcyclohexylcarbamate. II. The orientation of hydroxylation. J. org. Chem. **24**, 1834—1836 (1959).
— MARSHALL, F.J., CULP, H.W.: The nature of the metabolites of acetohexamide in the rat and in the human. J. Pharmacol. exp. Ther. **149**, 272—279 (1965).
— — — MILLER, W.M.: The metabolism of nortriptyline-N-methyl-^{14}C in rats. Biochem. Pharmacol. **12**, 1207—1217 (1963).
— SULLIVAN, H.R.: Microsomal hydroxylation of ethylbenzene, stereospecificity and the effect of phenobarbital induction. Life Sci. **5**, 921—926 (1966).
— — CRAIG, J.C., PEREIRA, W.E. JR.: The microsomal oxygenation of ethylbenzene: isotopic, stereochemical and induction studies. Arch. Biochem. **132**, 575—577 (1969).
MITOMA, C., POSNER, H.S., REITZ, H.C., UDENFRIEND, S.: Enzymatic hydroxylation of aromatic compounds. Arch. Biochem. **61**, 431—441 (1956).
— YASUDA, D.M., TAGG, J., TANABE, M.: Effect of deuteration of the O—CH_3 group on the enzymic demethylation of 0-nitroanisole. Biochim. biophys. Acta (Amst.) **136**, 566—567 (1967).
MIZE, C.E., AVIGAN, J., STEINBERG, D., PITTMAN, R.C., FALES, H.M., MILNE, G.W.A.: A major pathway for the mammalian oxidative degradation of phytanic acid. Biochim. biophys. Acta (Amst.) **176**, 720—739 (1969).
MOHLER, W., BLOTZ, I., REISER, M.: Die Struktur von Ausscheidungsprodukten des 1-Hexyl-3,7-dimethylxanthin. Arch. Pharmaz. **299**, 448—456 (1966).
NAGATSU, T., LEVITT, M., UDENFRIEND, S.: A rapid and simple radioassay for tyrosine hydroxylase activity. Analyt. Biochem. **9**, 122—126 (1964).
NAKATSUGAWA, T., ISHIDA, M., DAHM, P.A.: Microsomal expoxidation of cyclodiene insecticides. Biochem. Pharmacol. **14**, 1853—1865 (1965).
NAMBARA, T., NUMAZAWA, M., AKIYAMA, S.: Occurrence of "NIH Shift" during hydroxylation of aromatic steroid. Chem. pharm. Bull. **17**, 2394—2395 (1970).

NILSSON, R., ORRENIUS, S., ERNSTER, L.: The TPNH-dependent oxidation of luminol catalyzed by rat liver microsomes. Biochem. biophys. Res. Commun. **17**, 303—309 (1964).
NOVER, L., LUCKNER, M.: Mixed functional oxygenations during the biosynthesis of cyclopenin and cyclopenol, benzodiazepine alkaloids of *Penicillium Cyclopium* westling. FEBS Letters **3**, 292—296 (1969).
NOWAK, H., SHORRE, G., STRULLER, R.: Untersuchungen zum Metabolismus von Methaqualon. Arzneimittel-Forsch. **16**, 407—411 (1966).
OESCH, F., CREVELING, C.R., JERINA, D., DALY, J.W.: Purification and properties of a hepatic epoxide hydrase. Fed. Proc. **29**, 473 (1970).
ORRENIUS, S., DALLNER, G., ERNSTER, L.: Inhibition of the TPNH-linked lipid peroxidation of liver microsomes by drugs undergoing oxidative demethylation. Biochem. biophys. Res. Commun. **14**, 329—334 (1964).
PALMER, K.H., FEIERABEND, J.F., BAGGETT, B., WALL, M.E.: Metabolic removal of a 17*a*-ethynyl group from the antifertility steroid, norethindrone. J. Pharmacol. exp. Ther. **167**, 217—221 (1969).
PARKE, D.V.: In: Isotopes in Experimental Pharmacology, ed. by L.J. ROTH, pp. 315—342. Chicago/Ill.: University of Chicago Press 1965.
— The Biochemistry of Foreign Compounds. London: Pergamon Press 1968.
PEREL, J.M., DAYTON, P.G., TAURIELLO, C.L., BRAND, L., MARK, L.C.: Metabolic studies with deuterated phenobarbital. J. med. pharm. Chem. **10**, 371—373 (1967).
PITTMAN, K.A., ROSI, D., CHERNIAK, R., MEROLA, A.J., CONWAY, W.D.: Metabolism *in vitro* and *in vivo* of pentazocine. Biochem. Pharmacol. **18**, 1673—1678 (1969).
POSNER, H.W., MITOMA, C., ROTHBERG, S., UDENFRIEND, S.: Enzymatic hydroxylation of aromatic compounds. III. Studies on the mechanism of microsomal hydroxylation. Arch. Biochem. **94**, 280—290 (1961).
PRAIRIE, R.L., TALALAY, P.: Enzymatic formation of testoloacetone. Biochem. J. **2**, 203—208 (1963).
PREISS, B., BLOCH, K.: ω-oxidation of long-chain fatty acids in rat liver. J. biol. Chem. **239**, 85—88 (1964).
PREUSS, F.R., WILLIG, G., FRIEBOLIN, H.: Zur Konfiguration und Konformation renaler Ausscheidungsprodukte von 1-Äthinylcyclohexanol-(1). Arch. Pharmazie **296**, 157—168 (1963).
PREUSS, R., HASSLER, H.M., KOPF, R.: Zur Biotransformation des 2-Methyl-3-*o*-tolyl-4(3H)-chinazolinon (methaqualon). Arzneimittel-Forsch. **16**, 395—401 (1966).
— KOPSCH, H.W.: Zum Abbau des Methitural im tierischen Organismus. Arzneimittel-Forsch. **16**, 858—859 (1966).
PREUSS, V.F.R., MULLER, D.: Untersuchungen zur Biotransformation von 5-(1′-methyl-*n*-butyl)-5-vinylbarbitursäure. Arzneimittel-Forsch. **18**, 412—416 (1968).
PROCKOP, D.J., EBERT, P.S., SHAPIRO, B.M.: Studies with proline-3,4-H^3 on the hydroxylation of proline during collagen synthesis in chick embryos. Arch. Biochem. **106**, 112—122 (1964).
RAHIM, M.A., SIH, C.J.: Mechanisms of steroid oxidation by microorganisms. XI. Enzymatic cleavage of the pregnane side chain. J. biol. Chem. **241**, 3615—3623 (1966).
RENSON, J., BOURDON, V.: Hydroxylation et defluorination des derives fluores de l'aniline. Arch. int. Pharmacodyn. **171**, 240—242 (1968).
— DALY, J.W., WEISSBACH, H., WITKOP, B., UDENFRIEND, S.: Enzymatic conversion of 5-tritiotryptophan to 4-tritio-5-hydroxytryptophan. Biochem. biophys. Res. Commun. **25**, 504—513 (1966).
ROBERTSON, J.W., HUSSAIN, M.: Metabolism of camphors and related compounds. Biochem. J. **113**, 57—65 (1969).
ROSI, D., PERUZZOTTI, G., DENNIS, E.W., BERBERIAN, D.A., FREELE, H., ARCHER, S.: A new, active metabolite of 'miracil D'. Nature (Lond.) **208**, 1005—1006 (1965).
SAITO, Y., HAYAISHI, O., ROTHBERG, S.: Studies on oxyganeses; enzymatic formation of 3-hydroxy-*L*-kynurenine from *L*-kynurenine. J. biol. Chem. **229**, 921—934 (1957).
SHEPARTZ, B., GURIN, S.: The intermediary metabolism of phenylalanine labeled with radioactive carbon. J. biol. Chem. **180**, 663—673 (1949).
SIMON, E.J., EISENGART, A., SUNDHEIM, L., MILHORAT, A.T.: The metabolism of vitamin E. II. Purification and characterization of urinary metabolites of *a*-tocopherol. J. biol. Chem. **221**, 807—817 (1956).
SIMS, P.: Metabolism of polycyclic compounds. The metabolism of 1,4-epoxy-1,4-dihydronaphthalene in rats. Biochem. J. **95**, 608—611 (1965).
SINSHEIMER, J.E., SMITH, R.V.: Metabolic hydroxylations of *trans*-stilbene. Biochem. J. **111**, 35—41 (1969).
SMITH, A.J., WADDELL, W.J., BUTLER, T.C.: Demethylation of N-methyl derivatives of barbituric acid, hydantion, and 2,4-oxazolidinedione by rat liver microsomes. Life Sci. **7**, 486—492 (1963).

SMITH, D.L., FORIST, A.A., GERRITSEN, G.C.: Metabolism of 3,5-dimethylpyrazole-C^{14} in the rat. J. Pharmacol. exp. Ther. **150**, 316—321 (1965).
STAMBAUGH, J.E., FEO, L.G., MANTHEI, R.W.: Isolation and identification of the major urinary metabolite of metronidazole. Life Sci. **6**, 1811—1819 (1967).
STOKKE, O., TRY, D., ELDJARN, L.: α-Oxidation as an alternative pathway for the degradation of branched-chain fatty acids in man and its failure in patients with Refsum's Disease. Biochim. biophys. Acta (Amst.) **144**, 271—284 (1967).
SULLIVAN, H.R., R.E. BILLINGS, MCMAHON, R.E.: Demethylation studies. The *in vivo* and *in vitro* demethylation of N,N-dimethyl-3,5,7-trimethyladamantene-1-carboxamide. J. med. pharm. Chem. **11**, 250—254 (1968).
SWINYARD, E.A., MIYAHARA, J.T., GOODMAN, L.S.: Effect of chlorination on the anticonvalescent activity of phenobarbital. J. pharm. Sci. **52**, 463—465 (1963).
TAGG, J., YASUDA, D.M., TANABE, M., MITOMA, C.: Metabolic studies of tolbutamide in the rat. Biochem. Pharmacol. **16**, 143—153 (1967).
TAKEMORI, A.E., MANNERING, G.J.: Metabolic N- and O-demethylation of morphine and morphinan type analgesics. J. Pharmacol. exp. Ther. **123**, 171—179 (1958).
TALALAY, P.: Enzymatic mechanisms in steroid biochemistry. Ann. Rev. Biochem. **34**, 347—380 (1965).
TANABE, M., YASUDA, D., LEVALLEY, S., MITOMA, C.: The pharmacological effect of deuterium substitution on 5-*n*-butyl-5-ethylbarbituric acid. Life Sci. **8**, 1123—1128 (1969).
— — TAGG, J., MITOMA, C.: Absence of isotope effects in the microsomal hydroxylation of acetanilide. Biochem. Pharmacol. **16**, 2230—2233 (1967).
TANIGUCHI, K., KAPPE, T., ARMSTRONG, M.D.: Further studies on phenylpyruvate oxidase. J. biol. Chem. **239**, 3389—3395 (1964).
TATSUMI, K., YOSHIHARA, S., YOSHIMURA, H., TSUKAMOTO, H.: Metabolism of drugs. LXIII. The metabolic fate of ^{14}C-phenacetylurea (phenurone) in mice. Biochem. Pharmacol. **18**, 365—372 (1969).
TERHO, T., HARTIALA, K.: Hydroxylation of cinchophen by microsomal enzymes. Biochem. Pharmacol. **16**, 598—600 (1967).
THOMAS, E.W., LOUGHMAN, B.C., POWELL, R.G.: Metabolic fate of 2,4-dichlorophenoxyacetic acid in the stem tissue of *Phaseolus vulgaris*. Nature (Lond.) **204**, 884—885 (1964).
TOKI, S., TOKI, K., TSUKAMOTO, H.: Metabolism of drugs. XXXI. Metabolic fate of methyl hexabital. Chem. pharm. Bull. **10**, 708—714 (1962).
TSUKAMOTO, H., YOSHIMURA, M.: Metabolism of drugs. XXV. Biotransformations of drugs having cyclohexene ring. (2) Metabolic fate of 2-substituted cyclohexenylglutarimides. Chem. pharm. Bull. **9**, 584—587 (1961).
— — IDO, H.: Metabolism of drugs. XXXII. The metabolic fate of secobarbital [5-allyl-S-(1-methylbutyl)-barbituric acid]. Chem. pharm. Bull. **11**, 9—13 (1963).
UDENFRIEND, S., ZALTZMAN-NIRENBERG, P., DALY, J.W., GUROFF, G., CHIDSEY, C., WITKOP, B.: Intramolecular migration of deuterium and tritium during enzymatic hydroxylation of *p*-deutero- and *p*-tritio acetanilide. Arch. Biochem. **120**, 413—419 (1967).
ULLRICH, V.: On the hydroxylation of cyclohexane in rat liver microsomes. Hoppe-Seylers Z. physiol. Chem. **350**, 357—365 (1969).
— WOLFE, J., AMADORI, E., STAUDINGER, H.: The mixed function oxygenation of 4-haloacetanilides in rat liver microsomes and model systems. Hoppe-Seylers Z. physiol. Chem. **349**, 85—94 (1968).
VAN DER SCHOOT, J.B., CREVELING, C.R.: Substrates and inhibitors of dopamine-β-hydroxylase. Advanc. Drug. Res. **2**, 47—87 (1964).
VAN TAMELEN, E.E., WILLETT, J.D., CLAYTON, R.B., LORD, K.E.: Enzymic conversion of squalene 2,3-oxide to lanosterol and cholesterol. J. Amer. chem. Soc. **88**, 4752—4754 (1966).
WADDEL, W.J.: The metabolic conversion of secobarbital to 5-(1-methylbutyl)-barbituric acid and to 5-(2,3-dihydroxypropyl)-5-(1-methylbutyl)-barbituric acid. Fed. Proc. **22**, 480 (1963).
WAKABAYASHI, K., SHIMAZONO, M.: Studies of ω-oxidation of fatty acids *in vitro*. I. Overall reaction and intermediate. Biochim. biophys. Acta (Amst.) **70**, 132—142 (1963).
WATABE, T., MAYNERT, E.W.: Role of epoxides in the metabolism of olefins. Pharmacologist **10**, 203 (1968).
WELLES, J.S., MCMAHON, R.E., DORAN, W.J.: The metabolism and excretion of methohexital in the rat and dog. J. Pharmacol. exp. Ther. **139**, 166—171 (1963).
WILLIAMS, R.T.: Detoxification mechanisms. London: Chapman and Hall 1959.
WILLS, E.D.: Lipid peroxide formation in microsomes. General considerations. Biochem. J. **113**, 315—324 (1969a).
— Lipid peroxide formation in microsomes. The role of non-haem iron. Biochem. J. **113**, 324—332 (1969b).
— Lipid peroxide formation in microsomes. Relationship of hydroxylation to lipid peroxide formation. Biochem. J. **113**, 333—341 (1969c).

Wong, D.T., Terriere, L.C.: Epoxidation of aldrin, isodrin and heptachlor by rat liver microsomes. Biochem. Pharmacol. **14**, 375—377 (1965).

Yoshimura, H., Shimeno, H., Tsukamoto, H.: Metabolism of drugs. LIX. A new metabolite of antipyrine. Biochem. Pharmacol. **17**, 1511—1516 (1968).

Zins, G.R., Emmert, D.E., Walk, R.A.: Hypotensive metabolite production and sequential metabolism of N,N-diallylmelamine in rats, dogs, and man. J. Pharmacol. exp. Ther. **159**, 194—205 (1968).

Chapter 40

N-Oxidation Enzymes

John H. Weisburger and Elizabeth K. Weisburger[1]

With 2 Figures

I. Introduction

N-Hydroxylation, particularly of arylamine derivatives, is an unusual biochemical reaction, in which one of the hydrogens of a primary or secondary aromatic amine is replaced by a hydroxy group. The hydroxy group can then undergo the usual conjugation reactions with glucuronic, sulfuric or possibly phosphoric acid:

$$\text{Ar-NH R} \rightarrow \text{Ar-N(OH)R} \rightarrow \text{Ar-N(O R')R}$$

In contrast to many such reactions which lead to less toxic, readily excreted products, *N*-hydroxylation generally leads to intermediates of high chemical reactivity, which are often more toxic than the parent compound. In view of its importance, it is surprising that the exact nature of this reaction was unknown until recently, although this may be partially due to the fact that *N*-hydroxy derivatives tend to be highly active and even unstable and therefore difficult to detect.

There are a number of leads in the older literature. For example, methemoglobinemia was ascribed to metabolites of aromatic amines such as aniline. Because this blood disorder was noted in animals treated with *p*-chloro- or 2,6-dichloroaniline, which should resist ring hydroxylation, Heubner (1913) questioned whether this condition could be ascribed to a *p*- or an *o*-aminophenol and suggested that the intermediate responsible was an *N*-hydroxy derivative. Subsequently, a number of *N*-hydroxy derivatives of several different aromatic amines were supposedly identified in blood or urine. However, later developments disproved these reports. Useful reviews by Uehleke (1964a) and by Kiese (1966) detail these historic aspects.

A definitive and unambiguous demonstration that aromatic amines were converted *in vivo* to *N*-hydroxy derivatives came from two entirely different approaches.

Kiese (1959) and his group reinvestigated methemoglobin formation in animals injected with aromatic amines. In a series of important studies Kiese and Uehleke (*see* reviews above) applied a new colorimetric procedure (Herr and Kiese, 1959) to assay arylhydroxylamines and arylnitroso derivatives in blood, urine or tissues after treatment of a number of animal species with arylamines. Substitution of aniline with groups which decreased ring hydroxylation, e.g. some toluidines and *p*-chloraniline, often increased the percentage of *N*-hydroxy derivatives. Moreover, nitrosobenzene was found to be a product of the biochemical oxidation of *N*-alkylanilines.

The second advance came almost simultaneously from studies on the urinary metabolites of the carcinogen, *N*-2-fluorenylacetamide (2-acetylaminofluorene).

1 With the capable secretarial assistance of Mrs. Frances M. Williams.

Although significant amounts of several ring-hydroxylated derivatives of this carcinogen were identified in a number of species receiving a single dose (WEISBURGER and WEISBURGER, 1958), there was some reservation that any of these metabolites were related to the carcinogenicity of the agent. Indeed, chronic tests in animals showed that the ring-hydroxylated products were less carcinogenic than the parent compound. In particular, these results cast doubt on the importance of the *o*-aminohydroxy compounds, at that time prime candidates for the active intermediates (GUTMANN et al., 1958; NAGASAWA and GUTMANN, 1959; CLAYSON, 1962; BOYLAND, 1963).

By means of the chromatographic procedures developed by WEISBURGER et al. (1956), it was discovered in the laboratories of the MILLERS that after continued feeding of rats with *N*-2-fluorenylacetamide, in contrast to a single dose, a new urinary metabolite appeared which was found to be a glucuronide (CRAMER et al., 1960). After enzymic hydrolysis, the resulting product had a mobility like *N*-(1-hydroxy-2-fluorenyl)acetamide. However, detailed examination indicated that the new metabolite actually had a slightly faster mobility than the 1-hydroxy derivative, and unlike the latter, failed to form a red color when coupled with a diazonium salt; instead it yielded a yellow stain which progressively intensified when subjected to acidified *p*-dimethylaminobenzaldehyde. Careful isolation of the metabolite by paper and column techniques eventually yielded crystals of an alkali-soluble compound. On the basis of color reactions and spectral characteristics, it was suspected that the new metabolite was an *N*-hydroxy derivative. Attempts to synthesize this compound by accepted classic procedures, involving hydrogen sulfide reduction of 2-nitrofluorene, were not successful. Eventually, a selective catalytic reduction and simultaneous acetylation gave a synthetic material with the same melting point and other physical properties as the material isolated from rat urine.

The importance of this newly discovered metabolite was soon realized, since in rats it reproduced all the physiologic and pathologic effects of the parent *N*-2-fluorenylacetamide, and more (E.C. MILLER et al., 1961). The *N*-hydroxy derivative not only yielded more tumors in organs normally affected by the parent compound, but it also induced tumors at the point of injection. This observation was convincing evidence that the *N*-hydroxy derivative was closer to the proximate, actual carcinogen than the parent compound. In contrast, the various ring-hydroxylated phenolic derivatives were all either inactive or much less active than the parent compound and thus could be considered detoxification products.

These historic developments mainly involved arylamines and derivatives and this review will emphasize these compounds. Nonetheless, similar reactions, relatively little studied, lead to *N*-oxy derivatives of aliphatic amines, and certain amino heterocyclic structures. However, present information on underlying mechanism fails to establish clearly whether the biochemical systems responsible for these reactions are related. Thus, *N*-hydroxylation of aliphatic amines and the production of *N*-oxides will be alluded to only where appropriate. Also, the formation of hydroxylamino derivatives by reduction of nitro compounds will be discussed briefly.

II. *N*-Hydroxylation *in Vitro*

The first study of the *in vitro* formation of *N*-hydroxy derivatives of arylamines demonstrated that this conversion can be carried out by the microsome fraction of rat liver in the presence of NADPH (KIESE and UEHLEKE, 1961a; UEHLEKE, 1961a). However, the soluble fraction of rat liver contains a reductase

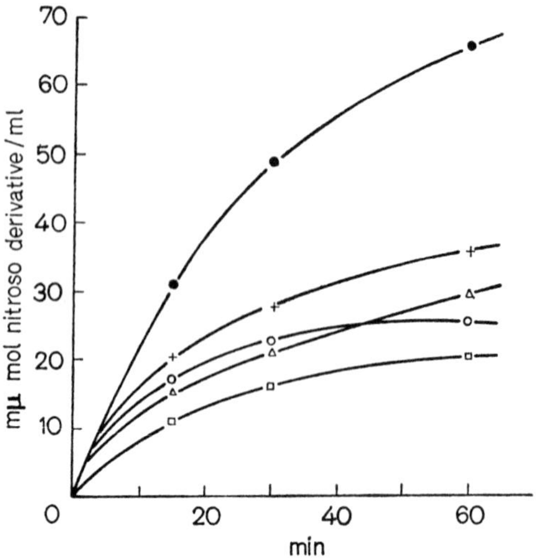

Fig. 1. *N*-Oxidation of carcinogenic amines with isolated liver microsomes from rats in the presence of NADPH. Aniline △, 2-naphthylamine ○, 2-aminofluorene +, 4-aminostilbene □, 4-aminobiphenyl ●. (From UEHLEKE, 1963a)

which reduces nitroso derivatives or arylhydroxylamines to arylamines. Thus UEHLEKE emphasizes that in order to demonstrate *N*-hydroxylation with microsome fractions, it is often imperative to remove the soluble fraction as completely as possible, by resuspending and washing the microsome fraction at least twice in the buffer system.

A series of *p*-substituted anilines were all *N*-hydroxylated faster than aniline itself, in the order: *p*-aminopropiophenone, *p*-phenetidine, *p*-chloroaniline and *p*-toluidine. With these compounds, methemoglobin formation in the cat followed a parallel course (UEHLEKE, 1962). With some carcinogenic aromatic amines, the formation of nitroso derivatives by microsomes of rat livers decreased in the order: 4-aminodiphenyl, 2-aminofluorene, aniline almost identical with 2-naphthylamine, and 4-aminostilbene (UEHLEKE, 1963a) (Fig. 1). Methemoglobin formation in the cat was again roughly proportional to the rate of oxidation (Fig. 2).

IRVING (1962, 1964) reported that microsomes from rabbit liver could convert *N*-2-fluorenylacetamide to the *N*-hydroxy derivative. The enzyme system from rabbit or hamster liver appeared to be reasonably stable, since microsomes from frozen or perfused livers, or microsomes aged up to 13 days at 0° had unchanged *N*-hydroxylase activity (IRVING, 1964; LOTLIKAR et al., 1967)[2]. The *N*-hydroxylation of *N*-2-fluorenylacetamide required NADPH or an NADPH-generating system, while NADH was not effective. The substrate was also hydroxylated in the fluorene ring, mainly at the 7-, but sometimes (depending on species) at the 3- and 5-positions as well (IRVING, 1964; BOOTH and BOYLAND, 1964; LOTLIKAR et al., 1967). Blocking the main ring position with halogen, as in *N*-(7-fluoro-2-fluorenyl)acetamide, increased the formation of the *N*-hydroxy metabolite approximately 3-fold (IRVING, 1964). 2-Fluorenamine and azoxyfluorene were

2 Parenthetically, BAUER and KIESE (1964) also found that storage of a rabbit microsome system at 2—3° did not affect its ability to convert aniline to *p*-aminophenol, but decreased its ability to form the *o*-aminophenol; they took this as evidence for a multiplicity of hydroxylating enzyme systems.

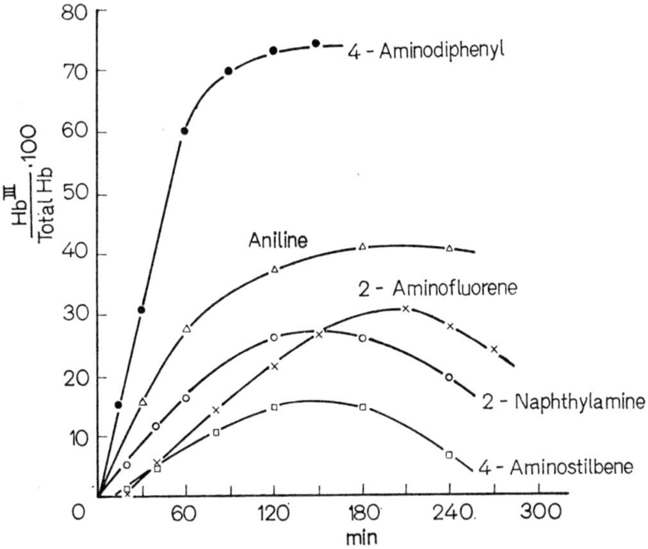

Fig. 2. Methemoglobin formation in the cat following injection of 0.5 mmole/kg amine intraperitoneally. Aniline △, 2-naphthylamine ○, 2-aminofluorene +, 4-aminostilbene □, 4-aminobiphenyl ●. (From UEHLEKE, 1963a)

also formed, indicating that deacetylation was a side reaction (however, see YOST, 1969). This was decreased by the presence of 0.1 M fluoride, without inhibiting *N*-hydroxylation.

Since UEHLEKE and BRILL (1968) noted that dogs pretreated with phenobarbital excreted much larger amounts of 2-naphthylhydroxylamine after intake of 2-naphthylamine, *N*-hydroxylation of this substance was investigated *in vitro* with microsomes from the livers of rabbits pretreated with phenobarbital (UEHLEKE, 1969b). Phenobarbital proved to be a most effective stimulator of microsomal *N*-hydroxylation. In microsomes from pretreated animals 2-naphthylamine was converted rapidly and in high yield to the corresponding *N*-hydroxy derivative. However, only traces of the nitroso compound were noted when 1-naphthylamine was used as substrate. The failure to detect *N*-hydroxylation with the 1-isomer was not due to loss of this material, for incubation of synthetic 1-naphthylhydroxylamine with the microsome system led to 92—95% recovery. Also, whereas 2-naphthylamine gave the typical type II absorption change in a suspension of microsomes, the 1-isomer did not. Thus, the question of *N*-hydroxylation of isomeric aromatic amines requires additional study to support the present concept that little or no *N*-hydroxylation takes place in *ortho*-substituted aromatic amines such as 1-naphthylamine, 1- and 4-fluorenylacetamide, 2-biphenylamine, and the like (WEISBURGER and WEISBURGER, 1966).

THAUER et al. (1965a) demonstrated that the important drug sulfanilamide not only underwent ring-hydroxylation, but was also converted to the hydroxylamino and nitroso derivatives with a 9,000 *g* supernatant or a microsome fraction of rat or human liver. The production of the hydroxylamino compounds was detected, in this case, by the *in vitro* methemoglobin production in added bovine red cells. Of the possible metabolites of sulfanilamide, only the hydroxylamine and nitroso derivatives or large amounts of 3-hydroxysulfanilamide formed oxidized hemoglobin. By thin layer chromatography the formation of the *N*-oxidation products of the sulfonamide was also demonstrated. In a parallel contribution, THAUER et al. (1965b) studied in detail methemoglobin formation with sulfanilamide and demonstrated that maximal methemoglobin was produced with 5 micromole/ml of substrate, and 0.5 micromole/ml NADPH. Although a number of other sulfonamides gave rise to methemoglobin under the same conditions, 4,4′-diaminodiphenylsulfone was most active in this respect. HJELM and DE VERDIER (1965) also noted that rat liver microsomes incubated with 4,4′-diaminodiphenylsulfone, cofactors, and red cells produced methemoglobin. This drug was about twice as active in this regard as aniline. That a metabolite was responsible for the oxidized hemoglobin can be inferred from the fact that incubation of human red cells with normal plasma had no effect, but incubation with the plasma of men given the drug produced methemoglobin.

N-Hydroxylation of *N*-2-fluorenylacetamide by rat liver microsomes was affected only slightly by pretreatment of the rats with 3-methylcholanthrene. On the other hand, a sizable increase in formation of *N*-hydroxy compound was seen with hamster, mouse and rabbit liver microsomes. Enzyme induction was partially inhibited by puromycin which operates at the level of message translation, and by actinomycin D, which affects the transcription of genetic information (LOTLIKAR et al., 1967).

Microsomes from hamster and dog liver and, to a lesser degree, cat and chicken liver gave measurable amounts of the *N*-hydroxy derivative of *N*-2-fluorenylacetamide in the presence of a NADPH generating system (IRVING, 1964). When NADPH was used, somewhat higher *N*-hydroxylating activity was noted; under these conditions rat and mouse liver microsomes also were active, but microsomes from guinea pigs and from one human liver were not. Subsequently, ENOMOTO and SATO (1967), examining *N*-hydroxylation with microsomes from a number of humans, found highly variable responses: from undetectable in patients with liver disease to as much as 32 μg/g liver per hour.

In contrast to the experiments of IRVING (1964) and LOTLIKAR et al. (1967) who failed to detect *N*-hydroxylation of *N*-2-fluorenylacetamide, KIESE et al. (1966) reported that microsomes from guinea pig liver could produce 2-nitrosofluorene with 2-aminofluorene as substrate, and other nitroso compounds with aniline and other aromatic amines. Also, KIESE and associates spectrophotometrically identified the unstable fluorenylhydroxylamine as 2-nitrosofluorene in the urine of guinea pigs injected intraperitoneally with a relatively large dose of 2-fluorenamine. The highest concentration of the material, 16 μg/ml, was noted in the first 4 h. In some tests incubation with β-glucuronidase increased the amount of 2-fluorenylhydroxylamine.

LOTLIKAR et al. (1967) found minimal *N*-hydroxylation of *N*-2-fluorenylacetamide in rat and increasing levels in rabbit, mouse and hamster, in that order. No *N*-hydroxylation was detected with once-washed microsomes from guinea pig in contrast to the data of KIESE who used twice-washed (by resuspension) microsomal preparations. It could be that slightly rinsed microsomal systems contain some reductive activity towards the *N*-hydroxy product formed. On the other hand, this explanation is not fully convincing and additional effort is required to resolve the discrepancy.

DEBACKERE and UEHLEKE (1964), using *p*-chloroaniline as substrate, showed that the guinea pig microsomes were most active compared to those from several other species in the formation of *p*-chlorophenylhydroxylamine (Table 1). They emphasized that various species exhibited different maximal reaction rates which were not necessarily related to total conversion per hour, since the rates were not linear over 60-min-periods; deviation of the reaction rate from linearity depended

Table 1. *N-hydroxylation of p-chloraniline by liver microsomes* (From DEBACKERE and UEHLEKE, 1964)

	A V max calc. mμmole/mg/min	B mμmole/mg 60 min	ratio A/B
Mouse	5.6	7.3	0.77
Rat	1.1	16.6	0.066
Guinea pig . .	6.5	21.2	0.33
Rabbit . . .	2.0	12.3	0.16
Pig	0.7	13.1	0.05
Cat	1.0	8.2	0.12
Chicken . . .	2.7	17.6	0.15

on the source of the preparation. With *p*-chloroaniline as substrate, relatively little difference was found in *N*-hydroxylation capability of microsomes from adult rats, young rats, rabbits and cats (less than 10 days old) (UEHLEKE, 1964b).

The formation of the *N*-hydroxy derivative of 4-biphenylamine with guinea pig liver microsomes was reported to be stimulated by previous treatment of the animals with phenobarbital (UEHLEKE, 1969c). The discrepancy between the results of KIESE et al. and UEHLEKE mentioned above and the American groups in respect to the presence of *N*-hydroxylation systems in guinea pigs requires resolution. Could it be that microsomes from guinea pig livers can *N*-hydroxylate arylamines, but not the *N*-acetyl derivatives?

Rabbit liver microsomes were more effective than those from kidney in *N*-hydroxylation of *p*-phenetidine. The interesting observation was made that methemoglobin formation with bovine erythrocytes *in vitro* was enhanced considerably by the presence of a microsomal system including NADPH and *p*-phenetidine, even though the product, *p*-nitrosophenetol, had much less activity than nitrosobenzene (UEHLEKE, 1969a). Certain pathologic reactions due to phenacetin or phenetidine may be a consequence of the formation of reactive metabolites *in situ*. Also, on the basis of methemoglobin formation in bovine erythrocytes incubated with mucosa from pig bladder, UEHLEKE (1967a) detected the *N*-oxidation, in decreasing order, of *p*-chloroaniline, 4-aminobiphenyl, 2-naphthylamine, aniline and 2-fluorenamine. The reaction of 4-aminobiphenyl or 4-chloroaniline also occurred with bladder mucosa alone. With *p*-chloroaniline as substrate the bladder of guinea pig had higher activity than that of pig, but the bladder of rat was less effective.

BOOTH and BOYLAND (1964) described *N*-hydroxylation of 4-acetamidobiphenyl, 4-aminobiphenyl, *N*-2-fluorenylacetamide, and *N*-acetylbenzidine with microsomes from rat or rabbit liver, but acetanilide and 2-acetamidonaphthalene failed to yield the corresponding *N*-hydroxy derivatives. The reaction was favored by inclusion of potassium fluoride which inhibited *N*-deacylation. NADPH or a system generating the nucleotide *in situ* was required. In the presence of NADPH, NADH appeared to have an enhancing effect, but by itself NADH was ineffective.

UEHLEKE and NESTEL (1967) and UEHLEKE (1968) also found that washed microsomes from rat liver converted 4-aminobiphenyl to the nitroso derivative; rabbit liver was even more active. However, some reaction was also noted with kidney, lung and small intestine. The potency of liver and kidney was increased considerably by pretreatment of rabbits for 7 days with phenobarbital. The increased activity was not necessarily proportional to the yield of microsomes per gram of organ, but there seemed to be a relationship to the level of cytochrome P-450.

Perfusion of aromatic amines, such as aniline, *N*-methyl- or *N*-ethylaniline, through the lung or liver of cats decreased the levels of the amines or the *N*-alkylanilines and increased the levels of nitroso derivatives; *N*-alkylanilines yielded both nitrosobenzene and aniline (KIESE and UEHLEKE, 1961a). Rat liver slices or homogenates fortified with NADPH were also capable of producing aniline and nitrosobenzene. Although the reaction was enhanced by the presence of erythrocytes, the microsome fraction was the active entity which formed aniline and nitrosobenzene from *N*-methylaniline (KIESE and UEHLEKE, 1961b). 2,4-Dichlorophenol inhibited the formation of aniline and enhanced that of nitrosobenzene. However, the *N*-hydroxylated products, nitrosobenzene or phenylhydroxylamine, were not converted to aniline by microsomes. In contrast, a soluble fraction of the rat liver readily reduced phenylhydroxylamine to aniline and this reaction was not inhibited by 2,4-dichlorophenol (*see* KIESE et al., 1961). Therefore, the formation of arylhydroxylamines from *N*-alkylanilines probably involves enzyme systems different from those that convert arylamines or *N*-acetylarylamines to the corresponding *N*-hydroxy derivatives. Nonetheless, some aspects of this conversion will be discussed briefly in relation to the *N*-hydroxylation of arylamines.

Decreasing yields of nitrosobenzene were obtained with rat liver microsomes in the order: *N*-methyl-, *N*-ethyl-, *N*-butylaniline, aniline itself, and N, *N*-dimethylaniline, which gave only traces (KIESE and UEHLEKE, 1961a).

Employing rat liver microsomes and *N*-alkylanilines or *N*-methylaniline as substrate, UEHLEKE (1961b, 1962) found no inhibition of nitrosobenzene formation after SKF 525A, *a,a*-dipyridyl, cyanide, hydrogen peroxide, catalase or ascorbic acid. 2,4-Dichlorophenol again increased and *p*-chloromercuribenzoate and cytochrome C inhibited the reaction. On the other hand, *a,a*-dipyridyl and acetone increased *p*-hydroxylation of aniline (ANDERS, 1969).

In a series of important papers, KAMPFFMEYER and KIESE (1963, 1964a, b, c), examined a number of factors affecting *N*-hydroxylation, using mainly microsome preparations of rabbit liver. Dog liver microsomes gave similar results but were less active than those of rabbit liver. The conversion of aniline to nitrosobenzene, or *p*-chloroaniline to the corresponding nitroso compound, increased to a maximum with increasing substrate concentration. The rate of the reaction was greatest above pH 7. In contrast, the formation of nitrosobenzene from *N*-ethylaniline decreased at pH values over 6.5. The formation of nitrosobenzene from aniline or *N*-ethylaniline was not favored by magnesium ions, but the conversion of *N*-alkylaniline to aniline was stimulated by 60 mM magnesium chloride.

2,4-Dichlorophenol did not affect the formation of nitrosobenzene from aniline but inhibited ring-hydroxylation. On the other hand, the yield of nitrosobenzene from *N*-ethylaniline was increased by 2×10^{-3} M dichlorophenol, with a coincident decrease in aniline formation. *N*-Hydroxylation of aniline was lowered severely by iproniazid and 8-hydroxyquinoline. SKF 525A or triparanol reduced the reaction slightly but ATP, semicarbazide, or *a,a*-dipyridyl had virtually no effect (Tables 2 and 3). These substances influenced the microsomal oxidation of *N*-alkylanilines differently (see below), giving further support to the view that the formation of nitrosobenzene derivatives from these substrates and aniline are carried out by different enzyme systems. Additionally, there was a difference in the rates of *N*-hydroxylation of aniline and that of *N*-ethylaniline as a function of partial oxygen pressure. Rates of the former reaction were higher at lower pressures. Moreover, the *N*-hydroxylation of aniline with rabbit liver microsomes also differs from C-hydroxylation in that *N*-hydroxylation of aniline

Table 2. *The effect of various substances upon the rate of the N-hydroxylation of p-aminopropiophenone, p-chloroaniline, and N-methyl-p-chloroaniline by rabbit liver microsomes* (From KAMPFFMEYER and KIESE, 1964a)

The data are the means and standard errors of 4 experiments. The concentration of the substrates was 1 mM. The figures in the second column indicate the concentration of nitrosocompound found after 40 min incubation. The figures in the other columns indicate the % change in activity caused by the substance quoted at the top of the column

Substrate	Nitroso-compound 10^{-5}M	Iproniazid 10^{-3}M	Triparanol 10^{-3}M	8-Hydroxy-quinoline 10^{-3}M	2,4-Dichloro-phenol $2 \cdot 10^{-3}$M	p-Chloromer-curibenzoate 10^{-3}M	N-Ethyl-maleimide $5 \cdot 10^{-3}$M	Semicarb-azide 10^{-2}M
p-Aminopropiophenone . . .	7.1	— 64 ± 3	— 17	— 88 ± 5	— 46 ± 5	— 67 ± 6	— 87 ± 4	+ 21 ± 4
p-Chloroaniline.	6.1	— 63 ± 5	— 4	— 79 ± 4	— 64 ± 4	— 89 ± 2	— 63 ± 3	+ 9 ± 5
N-Methyl-p-chloroaniline . .	3.6				+ 36 ± 9	+ 34 ± 10	+ 14 ± 7	+ 14 ± 4

Table 3. *The effect of some substances upon the N- and C-hydroxylation of aniline and N-ethylaniline, upon the N-hydroxylation of p-aminopropiophenone, and upon the dealkylation of N-ethylaniline by dog liver microsomes* (From KAMPFFMEYER and KIESE, 1964a)

The figures indicate the means of the concentrations of reaction products and effects observed after 40 min incubation in 5 experiments

	Substrate	Aniline 1 mM		N-Ethylaniline 1 mM		p-Aminopropiophenone 1 mM
	Reaction product	Nitrosobenzene	p-Aminophenol	Nitrosobenzene	Aniline	p-Nitrosopropiophenone
	μg/ml	0.8	1.2	3.0	2.0	2.8
	10^{-5}M	0.7	1.1	2.8	1.8	1.7
p-Chloromercuribenzoate . . .	10^{-3}M	— 47%	— 31%	— 70%	— 37%	— 57%
N-Ethylmaleimide	$5 \cdot 10^{-3}$M	+ 10	— 37	— 7	— 48	— 33
2,4-Dichlorophenol	$2 \cdot 10^{-3}$M	+ 8	— 44	+ 78	— 46	— 55
Semicarbazide	10^{-2}M	+ 51	— 10	— 3	— 10	+ 45
Iproniazid	10^{-3}M	— 49				— 47
Triparanol	10^{-3}M	— 43				— 6
8-Hydroxyquinoline	10^{-3}M	— 47				— 29

did not seem to be inhibited by the presence of carbon monoxide, whereas the *p*-hydroxylation of *N*-methylaniline or the formation of aniline from the latter substrate were inhibited (KAMPFFMEYER and KIESE, 1965).

APPEL et al. (1965) studied a number of other inhibitors of *N*-hydroxylation by microsomes from rabbits, cats and guinea pigs. They confirmed that the formation of nitrosobenzene from aniline was not affected by 2,4-dichlorophenol with microsomes from rabbit or guinea pig, but was slightly increased with microsomes from cat. Semicarbazide stimulated the reaction slightly with rabbit, strongly with cat, and inhibited it slightly with guinea pig. On the other hand, 8-hydroxyquinoline uniformly depressed *N*-hydroxylation with microsomes from all three species.

UEHLEKE (1967b, 1968) and LANGE (1967, 1968) examined in detail the important problem of enzyme induction by several agents in their studies of the *N*-hydroxylation of *p*-chloroaniline, aniline, *N*-alkylanilines, the *C*-hydroxylation of *N*-alkylanilines, and the *N*- and *O*-dealkylation of appropriate substrates. UEHLEKE judiciously reasoned that *p*-blocked anilines, like *p*-chloroaniline, would be most suitable for studies of *N*-hydroxylation, while longer chain *N*-alkyl derivatives, like butyl, would serve best for studies of ring-hydroxylation, and small *N*-alkyl derivatives, such as methyl or ethyl, would be best for *N*- or *O*-dealkylation studies. UEHLEKE noted that *N*-hydroxylation of *p*-chloroaniline with liver microsomes was increased most by methylcholanthrene, slightly by phenobarbital and not at all by DDT when the inducers were given separately or as mixtures to young female rats. The effect seen with the mixtures reflected that of the individual components, although DDT seemed to lower the action of phenobarbital. UEHLEKE selected conditions under which the individual inducers would exert less than maximal stimulation so as to detect any additive or synergistic effect. In contrast to the effect on *N*-hydroxylation of *p*-chloroaniline, a different response to the inducers was seen with ring-hydroxylation and *N*-dealkylation, and, of particular note, with the formation of nitrosobenzene from *N*-alkylaniline; in the last case all three inducers lowered the amount of product. Under all these conditions the relative liver weights and the microsomal content increased significantly. Chronic administration of phenobarbital increased the yield of microsomes from livers of young rats or rabbits still more, but no significant changes were noted with kidneys (rats and rabbits), or lungs, brain, small intestine (rabbits) or bladder (pig) (UEHLEKE, 1968). Nonetheless, with rabbit kidneys, repeated treatment with phenobarbital increased the *N*-hydroxylation of 4-biphenylamine, and also the 4-hydroxylation and *N*-dealkylation of *N*-methylaniline, as well as the amounts of cytochromes P-450 and b_5. On the other hand, using microsomes from rabbit liver, LANGE (1967) observed marked stimulation of the *N*-hydroxylation of aniline by rabbit liver microsomes with four large doses of DDT. This induction could be blocked by pretreatment with ethionine. A 16- to 19-fold increase in hydroxylating potency was noted after pretreatment with phenobarbital for 5 or 8 days. The phenobarbital stimulation was prevented by pretreatment with actinomycin D or partly prevented by chloramphenicol. With short incubation periods and an adequate NADPH generating system, the reaction proceeded equally well with or without nicotinamide. However, with a 40 min incubation time, the reaction was depressed approximately 60% in the absence of nicotinamide, probably because NADP was lost as a result of side reactions in the microsomal preparation.

LANGE (1968) reported on the mechanism of induction of the enzyme that catalyzes the *N*-hydroxylation of aniline in washed microsomes from rabbit liver. Considerable stimulation of *N*-hydroxylation by pretreatment with phenobarbital was accompanied by coincident increases in cytochrome P-450 and the ethyl isocyanide compound 455, whereas cytochrome b_5 showed only small changes. On the other hand, with methylaniline as substrate, cytochrome b_5 increased in proportion to the increase in ring-hydroxylation and cytochrome P-450 was also increased, but the rate of formation of nitrosobenzene was not affected. LANGE concluded that the *N*-hydroxylation of aniline may proceed without involvement of cytochrome P-450.

Recent *in vitro* experiments have taken advantage of the high level of *N*-hydroxylation of *N*-2-fluorenylacetamide obtained by methylcholanthrene induction in the hamster to examine the nature of *N*-hydroxylation in comparison to ring-hydroxylation (MATSUSHIMA and WEISBURGER, unpublished). Presently, it is considered that aromatic ring-hydroxylation consists of a series of coupled sequences ultimately involving the hemoprotein enzyme P-450, which can be determined spectrophotometrically. Cytochrome P-450 is characteristically inhibited by carbon monoxide and a number of other agents such as SKF 525A which interfere with biochemical hydroxylation. A preliminary comparative test of *N*- and ring-hydroxylation of *N*-2-fluorenylacetamide with a purified microsome preparation from hamsters pretreated with methylcholanthrene has revealed that under conditions where carbon monoxide inhibited ring-hydroxylation by 30—50%, *N*-hydroxylation was not affected. If further data bear out these results, it can be concluded that *N*-hydroxylation of arylamines may operate *via* intermediates other than the hemoprotein cycle. Further investigation in this area is most desirable, especially with respect to the specificities and the underlying mechanisms of the enzyme systems which convert aromatic amines and their derivatives into *N*-hydroxylated metabolites.

Summary: *N*-Hydroxylation of aromatic amines occurs in the microsomal fraction of tissues in the presence of NADPH or an NADPH generating system (generally less effective). The pH optimum is approximately 7.5—8 in a suitable buffer such as *tris* or phosphate. Microsomes of livers from hamsters or rabbits appear to be most active; somewhat less so are those of dogs, chickens, pigs, mice, rats, cats, and oxen. Several groups of investigators reported good activity in guinea pig liver microsomes with some substrates, but other investigators, using other substrates, found none. Microsomes from human livers appeared to be highly variable, depending on various factors. Although the liver is the most active source, *N*-hydroxylation has been detected with microsomes of kidney, lung, bladder, and small intestine, in decreasing order of effectiveness, depending also on the species. A microsome preparation appeared to retain *N*-hydroxylation capability upon storage at low temperature for some time. The reaction was not inhibited appreciably by carbon monoxide, SKF 525A, or by 2,4-dichlorophenol. On the other hand, 8-hydroxyquinoline, and iproniazid were potent inhibitors, and a number of other materials, such as *a*, *a*-dipyridyl, penicillamine, cupric chloride, or *p*-chloromercuribenzoate, had a relatively minor effect. Phenobarbital, particularly when given repeatedly, stimulated *N*-hydroxylation by liver microsomes from rat, dog, cat, but especially in rabbit. With some *N*-acylarylamines, *N*-hydroxylation *in vitro* was more difficult to demonstrate. Even with arylamines, differences in substrate susceptibility were apparent, since amines with a blocked *para* position were usually more likely to undergo *N*-hydroxylation.

While *N*-hydroxylation and ring or side chain hydroxylation are similar in some aspects, such as tissue localization, species variations, and hormonal effects, other factors, such as inhibitor specificity, relative enzyme stability, and the effect of various enzyme inducers, suggest that these reactions may involve different enzyme systems. Several of the cytochromes known to be involved in biochemical hydroxylation do not seem to participate to the same extent in *N*-hydroxylation. Thus cytochrome b_5, and possibly even cytochrome P-450, may not take part in *N*-hydroxylation. Other explanations for these differences have been offered in terms of the conformation of the membranes of the endoplasmic reticulum. A definitive answer to whether systems leading to *C*- and *N*-hydroxylated amines are identical or not requires further investigation.

III. Formation of *N*-Hydroxy Derivatives by Biochemical Reduction

While this article deals mainly with *N*-oxidation of aromatic amines, other ways of obtaining the same derivatives will be briefly discussed.

Nitrobenzene derivatives, as well as the corresponding aromatic amines, lead to disturbances of hematopoiesis in man and animals. It has been assumed that these disturbances are activated by an amino residue. However, newer concepts now suggest that the active entity is actually an arylhydroxylamine. Experimental evidence has shown that nitro compounds are reduced sequentially to arylamines *via* nitroso and hydroxylamino derivatives. Furthermore, the nitro analogs of the carcinogenic aromatic amines are also carcinogens, often exhibiting about the same organotropism and effects as the amines. When fed to rodents the nitro compounds yield tumors of the forestomach, suggesting that reduction to active intermediates can occur in the gastric mucosa. In addition, reduction of aromatic nitro compounds by microorganisms in the gut has also been demonstrated, although this subject has not received the attention it deserves (Scheline, 1968).

Williams (1959) reviewed the scant early work on the identification of arylhydroxylamines or nitroso derivatives resulting from the *in vivo* reduction of aromatic nitro compounds. Often the documentation hinged on the presence of further transformation products. Direct evidence was obtained by Uehleke (1964c) who showed that nitrosobenzene was present in the blood of some, but not all, cats given large or lethal doses of nitrobenzene. Success resulted from the realization that nitroso, and perhaps hydroxylamino, intermediate stages were seen only in the first few hours after injection of the nitro compound. Accordingly, *in vitro* reduction with a soluble fraction of rat liver in the presence of riboflavine-5-phosphate (FMN) gave measurable amounts of phenylhydroxylamine; the maximum concentration of this compound appeared in the first 10—13 min, whereas the amount of aniline formed continued to increase for about 30 min (Uehleke, 1963b). Although nitroso compounds are rarely excreted in appreciable amounts in urine, Parke (1961) found *m*-nitrosonitrobenzene and the hydroxylamine in urine of rabbits given *m*-dinitrobenzene.

Under anaerobic conditions, a soluble fraction from rat liver rapidly reduced 4-nitrobiphenyl to the corresponding amine in the presence of NADPH and FMN. Nitrosobiphenyl was reduced even more rapidly, but the conversion of 2-nitrofluorene to 2-fluorenamine was rather slow (Uehleke and Nestel, 1967). Lotlikar et al. (1965) found no 2-fluorenamine at all with a rat liver homogenate. It is to be noted that Sugimura et al. (1966) isolated an enzyme from the soluble fraction of rat liver similar to the DT diaphorase of Ernster et al. (1962), which could reduce 4-nitroquinoline-*N*-oxide, but not 4-nitroquinoline, to the corresponding hydroxylamine; it failed, however, to further reduce the hydroxylamine to the amine.

Older work suggested that the enzyme activity that converted nitrobenzene derivatives to arylamines was located in the soluble fraction of a rat liver homogenate. However, subsequent developments revealed that this reduction involved at least a two-step sequence (FOUTS and BRODIE, 1957; SUGIMURA et al., 1966; GILLETTE et al., 1968; KATO et al., 1969, 1970; JUCHAU, 1969).

Because of the ease of analysis many studies on nitro reductase use *p*-nitrobenzoic acid as a substrate. However, this compound is a fairly strong acid with a low pK_a and is fully ionized at pH 7.4. Thus, diffusion of the substrate into liver microsomes may limit the reduction of this substrate to a greater extent than it does that of less polar nitro compounds (PAUL and HARRINGTON, 1967).

In model systems, rat liver microsomes, in the presence of appreciable amounts of NADPH, reduced *p*-nitrobenzoic acid to *p*-hydroxylaminobenzoic acid and also to *p*-aminobenzoic acid (KATO et al., 1969). The time course of the reactions clearly indicated that the hydroxylamino derivative was an intermediate. This reaction was stimulated strongly by the addition of flavine mononucleotide (FMN), but inhibited severely by oxygen. When the cofactor was NADH, little reduction of the nitro compound was noted with microsomes, but when the hydroxylamino compound was used as substrate, *p*-aminobenzoic acid was formed. In the latter reaction FMN had relatively little effect.

With the soluble fraction of rat liver and either NADPH or NADH as cofactors, the reduction of *p*-nitrobenzoic acid led to *p*-hydroxylaminobenzoic acid but little aminobenzoic acid. This reduction was enhanced by FMN, but unlike the microsomal reaction, oxygen was not inhibitory.

The microsomal NADPH-mediated reduction of both hydroxylamino and amino derivatives is significantly enhanced by phenobarbital or methylcholanthrene pretreatment. On the other hand, the reduction effected by NADH and microsomes or by supernatant fractions containing either cofactor was not stimulated by such pretreatment. With a 9000 *g* supernatant, containing microsomes and supernatant, the sum of both factors was generally seen.

GILLETTE et al. (1968) (see also GILLETTE and GRAM, 1969), using different techniques, also saw a multi-step reduction from nitro derivatives to the amines. They provided evidence that cytochrome P-450 is involved, since carbon monoxide inhibited the reaction with microsomes from mouse, rat or rabbit liver. Earlier, GRAM et al. (1967a, b) reported that the activity was associated predominantly with the smooth- rather than rough-surfaced microsomes. On the other hand, it is possible that NADPH-cytochrome c reductase, in the presence of sizable amounts of flavine and NADPH, catalyzes the reduction of flavine, which in turn serves as the reducing agent. Evidence for the operation of the latter pathway in the reduction of *p*-nitrobenzoate was produced by FOUTS and BRODIE (1957) in rat livers, by JUCHAU (1969) in human and rodent placental homogenates, and by ADAMSON et al. (1965) in different strains of mice and a variety of fish, reptiles, birds and mammals. Further support comes from the fact that stimulation of mammalian nitro reductase systems by DDT is seen only when adequate amounts of NADP and tissue homogenate or soluble fraction are used (PETERS and FOUTS, 1968). Of interest is the recent finding that some unsaturated fatty acids stimulate the reduction (AUGUSTINE and FOUTS, 1969), although it is not known whether this phenomenon applies to the nitro-to-hydroxylamino step.

The carcinogen, 4-nitroquinoline-*N*-oxide, also undergoes reduction to a hydroxylamino derivative which is probably the active carcinogenic intermediate, followed by further reduction to the amine (SUGIMURA et al., 1966; KATO et al., 1970). The factors which operate for model compounds like nitrobenzoic acid also control the reduction of this carcinogen. However, a system with the properties of liver DT-diaphorase, present mainly in supernatant fractions (see also ERNSTER et al., 1962), can also reduce this compound.

There is little information available on the biochemical reduction of aliphatic nitro compounds, but there is no doubt that these materials can undergo such reactions by steps analogous to those found with aryl compounds. Also, there may be a connection to the well-known inorganic nitrogen cycle between nitrate, nitrite, hydroxylamine, and ammonia, which has been most widely studied in microbiologic systems.

IV. Formation and Reactions of Tertiary Amine and Heterocyclic *N*-Oxides

OCHIAI (1967) has summarized the synthesis and chemical, physical, and pharmacological properties of aromatic *N*-oxides with emphasis on heterocyclic *N*-oxides. In addition, BICKEL (1969) has reviewed the biochemistry of naturally occurring *N*-oxides, the pharmacology and toxicology of *N*-oxides, the formation of such compounds during drug metabolism, and the various processes involved in metabolism of *N*-oxide drugs.

Although *N*-oxidation of certain important heterocyclic drugs and alkaloids has been reported, no concerted study in this area has been made (*see* MCMAHON, 1966). In some cases, *N*-oxides were postulated as intermediates in the dealkylation of *N*, *N*-dialkylarylamines, but this concept appears untenable. Chlorpromazine *N*-oxide has been noted in urine of men given chlorpromazine. Moreover, rat liver microsomes convert this drug to the *N*-oxide in sizable quantities in the presence of optimal amounts of NADP, glucose-6-phosphate, magnesium chloride, nicotinamide, and glucose-6-phosphate dehydrogenase (BECKETT and HEWICK, 1967; FISHMAN et al., 1962). The LD_{50} of the alkaloid lasiocarpine is considerably lower than that of the corresponding *N*-oxide (BULL et al., 1958), but the chronic effects of small doses of these compounds were similar (BULL and DICK, 1959). On the other hand, BARNES et al. (1964) reported that effects of the alkaloid fulvine and its *N*-oxide are similar whether they are given in toxic or in small chronic doses.

BROWN (1968) has made important studies of purine *N*-oxides. Synthesized initially as agents for use in cancer chemotherapy (cf. SARTORELLI et al., 1964; ITAI et al., 1969), a number of these compounds have exhibited lower toxicity than the corresponding purine antimetabolites. However, the *N*-oxides were no more effective against model tumor systems than the corresponding parent compounds. It was suggested that their activity is really due to their reduction to the parent compound *in vivo*, probably by xanthine oxidase.

In the presence of a reducing agent, xanthine oxidase under anaerobic conditions converts a variety of purine *N*-oxides to their parent compounds. NADH is a less efficient electron donor than xanthine itself. Furthermore, the *N*-oxide itself can act as an electron donor if one is not added. The pH optimum is quite broad with a maximum at approximately 6.2. Conversely, in the presence of air or oxygen, xanthine oxidase can oxidize *N*-oxides; for example, guanine-3-oxide is oxidized to 8-hydroxyguanine-3-oxide. The pH optimum for this reaction is about 6.9 (STÖHRER and BROWN, 1969a).

Interestingly enough, a number of the purine *N*-oxides injected subcutaneously can induce tumors. Most potent was 3-hydroxyxanthine, which caused tumors in rats both at the point of injection and in the liver. Male rats were more susceptible than females. Guanine-3-oxide was also carcinogenic, as were 1-hydroxyxanthine and 6-mercaptopurine-3-oxide, but to a lesser extent. On the other hand, 6-mercaptopurine, 6-hydroxyaminopurine, 2-aminopurine, xanthine, guanine, and adenine were not active at the site of injection or in other tissues (TELLER et al., 1970; SUGIURA et al., 1970).

Extensive studies on the metabolism of several of these purine *N*-oxides revealed that they are converted to many products (MYLES and BROWN, 1969; STÖHRER and BROWN, 1969a, b), mainly by the action of xanthine oxidase. Such studies have provided a better understanding of the mechanism of carcinogenicity. For example, they revealed 8-chloroxanthine and 8-methylmercaptoxanthine were metabolites of the carcinogenic 3-hydroxyxanthine. These metabolites could also be obtained chemically by the reaction of synthetic 3-acetoxyxanthine with chloride ion or methionine (WÖLCKE et al., 1969; STÖHRER and BROWN, 1970). Thus certain *N*-oxides are converted to the same active intermediates that are formed from carcinogenic aromatic amines by *N*-oxidation followed by esterification. A radical mechanism has also been proposed for the formation of these intermediates and cannot be excluded (cf. KAWAZOE and ARAKI, 1967).

In studying the biological effects of heterocyclic *N*-oxides synthesized by OCHIAI and his associates, NAKAHARA discovered that 4-nitroquinoline *N*-oxide and related compounds were potent carcinogens (NAKAHARA, 1964; KAWAZOE et al., 1967; LACASSAGNE et al., 1966). Whereas it had been assumed for some time that the carcinogenicity of such substances depended on the reactivity of the nitro group *para* to the *N*-oxide function, later studies suggested that the underlying mechanism actually depended on reduction of the nitro group to yield hydroxylamino derivatives (ENDO and KUME, 1963; SHIRASU, 1965; MORI and OHTA, 1967). This reduction occurs not only in liver but also in other tissues, including the subcutaneous tissue of the rat (MATSUSHIMA et al., 1968). Certain bacteria can also reduce the nitro group to an intermediate hydroxylamine derivative, and then to 4-aminoquinoline *N*-oxide and even to 4-aminoquinoline. *A. niger*, which is most sensitive to 4-nitroquinoline *N*-oxide, reduced this compound only to the hydroxylamino intermediate, whereas other less sensitive strains of bacteria, for example, *E.coli* and *Ps.aerogenosa*, produced additional metabolites. This pathway probably accounts for the fact that hydroxylamino derivatives are not only carcinogenic in several mammalian species but also mutagenic (OKABAYASHI et al., 1965; ISHIZAWA and ENDO, 1967; KAMAHORA and KAKUNAGA, 1967; KUROKI and SATO, 1968; EPSTEIN and ST. PIERRE, 1969), since many studies have shown that the intermediates react with cellular macromolecules including DNA (MATSUSHIMA et al., 1967; TADA et al., 1967; OKANO and UEKAMA, 1967; OKANO et al., 1968; HOZUMI, 1968; TANOOKA et al., 1969). The reactive intermediate may be an ester of the hydroxylamino derivative, as is true for *N*-oxy derivatives of aromatic amines (KAWAZOE and ARAKI, 1967; ENOMOTO et al., 1968), although KATAOKA et al. (1967) have evidence for a free radical derived from 4-hydroxylaminoquinoline *N*-oxide.

ZIEGLER and associates (ZIEGLER and PETTIT, 1964, 1966; MACHINIST et al., 1966, 1968) have described a microsomal liver preparation, requiring NADPH and oxygen, which oxidized dialkylarylamines to the corresponding *N*-oxides. They have proposed *N*-oxides as intermediaries in the *N*-dealkylation of such compounds. In rats, most of the enzyme activity was concentrated in liver, but in pigs some activity was also present in kidney and lung. *N*-oxidase activity was also demonstrated in the livers of calf, rabbit, cat, bat, armadillo, brown squirrel, opossum, racoons, and a number of reptiles and birds, but several types of fish, frogs, and the English sparrow exhibited much lower activity. Cytochrome P-450 content of various tissues and species did not correlate with the extent of *N*-oxide formation. After injection of *N*, *N*-dimethylaniline or *N*, *N*-dimethyloctylamine into rats, about 5—6% and 17—19% of the dose was recovered in urine (DEHNER et al., 1968). Prior treatment with SKF 525A more than doubled the urinary *N*-oxides. These data suggest that although SKF 525A does not seem to affect the *N*-oxidation *in vitro* and *in vivo*, it does block the subsequent *N*-dealkylation step, thus allowing the *N*-oxides to accumulate. However, SKF 525A failed to alter the amount of *N*-oxides in urine when the *N*-oxides themselves were injected, suggesting that SKF 525A may increase *N*-oxide formation by blocking an alternate pathway of metabolism.

ZIEGLER et al. (1969) have partially purified the N-oxidase system from pork liver microsomes by Triton extraction, protamine precipitation of contaminating proteins, ammonium sulfate precipitation steps, and finally a Sephadex column fractionation, yielding an overall concentration factor of 60 with respect to microsomes and 1,000 with respect to liver. The oxidase is a flavoprotein, FAD being the prosthetic group. Cytochrome P-450 and monoamine oxidase activity appear absent, and the cytochrome b_5 content is apparently small, variable and of uncertain specificity. NADPH and oxygen are required. On the basis of substrate specificity and other properties, ZIEGLER et al. believe that this enzyme is related to, or even identical with, trimethylamine oxidase (BAKER and CHAYKIN, 1962). However, whether or not this system is analogous to the enzymes required for *N*-hydroxylation of primary or secondary arylamines or amides, is not clear at this time.

KIESE et al. (1966) detected the presence of *N,N*-dimethylaniline *N*-oxide and diethylaniline *N*-oxide, as well as methemoglobin formation, after intravenous injection of the corresponding parent amines in dogs. However, *in vitro* methemoglobin formation with dimethylaniline *N*-oxide occurred very slowly and the diethyl analog was even less potent. Thus, it would appear that the methemoglobin formation was not due to the *N*-oxides, but rather to other metabolites of *N,N*-dimethylaniline, probably the corresponding *p*-dimethylaminophenol, a highly active compound (*see* also KIESE, 1967).

Along these lines, HLAVICA and KIESE (1969) observed that microsomes of pig liver are much more active than those of rabbit liver in reacting with *N,N*-dimethylaniline *N*-oxide and yielding an equivalent amount of formaldehyde. However, the reaction was quite slow, presumably ruling out the *N*-oxide as an intermediate in the dealkylation of dialkylanilines (Table 4) (*see* also GILLETTE, 1963).

Table 4. *The effect of some substances on the N-oxygenation of aniline and N-alkylanilines by rabbit liver microsomes* (From HLAVICA and KIESE, 1969)

		Phenylhydroxylamine from aniline	Phenylhydroxylamine from *N*-ethylaniline	*N,N*-Dimethylaniline-*N*-oxide from *N,N*-dimethylaniline	P
p-Chloromercuribenzoate	10^{-3}M	-43 ± 5.1	$+21 \pm 6.5$	-48 ± 3.9	0.001
N-Ethylmaleimide	5×10^{-3}M	-48 ± 3.8	$+22 \pm 5.5$	-12.4 ± 2.2	0.0027
8-Hydroxyquinoline	10^{-3}M	-51 ± 3.5	-15 ± 3.5	-0.6 ± 1.0	0.01
2,4-Dichlorophenol	2×10^{-3}M	-17 ± 0.9	$+30 \pm 6.8$	$+8.9 \pm 2.9$	0.05
Semicarbazide	10^{-2}M	-31.6 ± 3.2	-40.6 ± 2.3	-41 ± 4.3	0.475
o-Phenanthroline	10^{-3}M	-53.5 ± 2.4	-8.2 ± 6.3	$+2.1 \pm 2.9$	0.10

The figures, which are the means of three to five experiments, show percent change in activity caused by the substance added. P indicates the probability of the *N*-oxygenation of *N*-ethylaniline and *N,N*-dimethylaniline being equally affected by a substance.

The conversion of *N,N*-dimethylaniline to the *N*-oxide was also documented by UEHLEKE and STAHN (1966) and ARCHAKOV et al. (1969). This *N*-oxide, as well as the more active 4-dimethylaminoazobenzene *N*-oxide, could produce methemoglobinemia, but it was felt that these *N*-oxides were not present in sufficient amounts to account for the methemoglobin levels seen in cats treated with dimethylaniline. Moreover, formaldehyde was produced in the iron-ascorbate system of UDENFRIEND et al. (1954) and BRODIE et al. (1954) by the dealkylation and rearrangement of the *N*-oxide. In comparative studies formaldehyde was also produced from the azo dye *N*-oxide, as well as from *N*,*N*-dimethylaniline *N*-oxide, in rat liver microsomes in the presence of an NADPH generating system. Erythrocytes rapidly reduced the azo dye *N*-oxide to *N*,*N*-dimethylaminoazobenzene and demethylated products. 4-Dimethylaminoazobenzene itself fails to react with erythrocytes so that the *N*-oxide participates in the dealkylation. It would seem that methemoglobinemia is related to the appearance of the demethylated azo dye and not the methyl or *N*-oxide derivatives. Possibly a hydroxylamino compound is actually involved.

A detailed comparison between the reactivity of the carcinogenic azo dye, 4-dimethylaminoazobenzene, and its *N*-oxide, both *in vitro* and *in vivo*, was made by TERAYAMA and ORII (1963) (*see* also TERAYAMA, 1967). Considerably more bound dye was found at the injection site after intramuscular injection of the *N*-oxide than after injection of the parent dye, whereas in liver the reverse was found. Likewise in guinea pigs, which are insensitive to the carcinogenicity of the azo dye, the *N*-oxide produced much more binding at the injection site than did the parent dye; virtually no binding was detected in the liver with either agent. On the other hand, intragastric administration of the compounds produced similar levels of bound dye in the liver. Curiously, the LD_{50} in mice and rats after intragastric administration was higher with the *N*-oxide than with the azo dye, but after intraperitoneal injection the *N*-oxide was much more toxic. Both agents exhibited a similar order of carcinogenicity upon long term administration. Apparently the *N*-oxide is not a key intermediate in respect to the carcinogenicity of these azo dyes. Current views point to monoalkyl *N*-oxy derivatives as the active carcinogens, as discussed elsewhere in this review.

ARRHENIUS (1968) studied the mechanism of activation of carcinogenic aromatic amines in a model system involving the conversion of *N*,*N*-dimethylaniline to the corresponding *N*-oxide. The rate of this conversion was higher in microsomes from vitamin E deficient rats and in 2-fluorenamine-pretreated animals than in controls, but lower in vitamin E-supplemented animals. Depletion of vitamin E plus treatment with 2-fluorenamine give a lower activity than treatment with 2-fluorenamine alone. Also, a protein free diet slightly increased the yield of *N*,*N*-dimethylaniline-*N*-oxide. Microsomes from guinea pig livers were more active than those from rats in producing formaldehyde from *N*,*N*-dimethylaniline, but less active in forming the *N*-oxide. The authors suggested that vitamin E protects liver from damage by toxic agents, such as 2-fluorenamine, by affecting *N*-oxidation. Data by MARGRETH et al. (1964) support the view that hepatotoxic agents increase the excretion of *N*-hydroxylated derivatives of some aromatic amine compounds, and SHIRASU et al. (1966) report that hormonal factors decreased the reduction of *N*-hydroxy derivatives (see also WILSON, 1968a, b). The data of ARRHENIUS are consistent with these findings. Even so, more evidence is required to prove that *N*-oxidation of tertiary amines is directly analogous to *N*-hydroxylation of secondary and primary amines or amides.

Recently ARRHENIUS (1970a) showed that *N*-oxidation of *N*,*N*-dimethylaniline by liver microsomes proceeded more rapidly in 0.2 M potassium phosphate buffer, pH 7.5 than in tris buffer, and that the rate remained constant for a longer time. In tris buffer addition of ADP increased the activity. In phosphate buffer the yield of *N*-oxy products depended on the substrate used. Sonication of liver microsomes for 4 min or addition of approximately 0.25 mg cholate per mg microsomal protein enhanced activity but long sonication or higher levels of cholate decreased the activity. Moreover, 0.1 mM phenylmercuridicyandiamide or *p*-chloromercuriphenylsulfonic acid, or 3 mM *N*-ethylmaleimide likewise increased the yield of *N*-oxy compound. The data support the view that the level of NADPH available controls the rate of *N*-oxidation. In a companion paper, ARRHENIUS (1970b) reported that microsomes from guinea pig liver had substantially lower *N*-oxidation capability compared to those from rat liver. Also 2-fluorenamine depressed the activity of microsomes from guinea pig liver more than it did those from rat liver when incubated simultaneously with substrate or prior to the addition of substrate. *N*-Acetoxy-N-2-fluorenylacetamide has a similar effect.

Also, two groups (SPARTHAN and CHAYKIN, 1969; CHAMBON et al., 1969) have developed assays for nicotinamide *N*-oxide and related compounds and have established that the *N*-oxide is formed *in vitro* and *in vivo* in several species, including man, on ordinary diets as well as after loading doses of nicotinamide. CHAYKIN's group had already shown that the aliphatic trimethylamine derived from choline undergoes *N*-oxidation *in vitro* in a number of animal and plant systems (BAKER and CHAYKIN, 1962; BAKER et al., 1963).

V. Conclusions

Detailed investigations on the occurrence, formation and properties of compounds containing the *N*-hydroxy group, mainly derivatives of aromatic or heterocyclic amines, have only been undertaken relatively recently. One reason is that the arylhydroxylamines are reactive compounds which precluded their easy recognition and detection. Also, toxic conditions resulting from their presence were often ascribed to other materials, thus obscuring a search for the true cause of the disease. Almost simultaneously, blood disorders such as methemoglobinemia, and carcinogenesis by aromatic nitro and amino compounds were traced to the corresponding arylhydroxylamino compounds as the responsible intermediate agents. Because of the specific interest of investigators in these two areas, research was initially directed towards the mode of formation and properties of arylhydroxylamines and arylhydroxamic acids.

Arylhydroxylamines are usually synthesized chemically by reduction of the corresponding nitro derivatives. Likewise, after intake of nitro compounds by animals or humans, the hydroxylamines are formed by reduction, or by biochemical oxidation of amines. Additional work is needed, however, to determine the exact nature of the enzyme system capable of *N*-hydroxylating arylamines and amides. Of primary interest is the identity with or divergence from the mixed function oxidases, or systems producing *N*-oxides of tertiary amines, or enzymes hydroxylating alkylamines. There is experimental support for either view. Of practical concern is the discovery of the means for lowering the activity of such enzyme systems, or of increasing the removal of arylhydroxylamines or hydroxamic acids, for most of these materials exhibit deleterious effects.

References

ADAMSON, R.H., DIXON, R.L., FRANCIS, F.L., RALL, D.P.: Comparative biochemistry of drug metabolism by azo and nitro reductase. Proc. nat. Acad. Sci. (Wash.) **54**, 1386—1391 (1965).

ANDERS, M.W.: Stimulation *in vitro* of microsomal aniline hydroxylation by 2,2′-bipyridine. Biochem. Pharmacol. **18**, 2561—2565 (1969).

Appel, W., Graffe, W., Kampffmeyer, H., Kiese, M.: Species differences in the hydroxylation of aniline and *N*-ethylaniline by liver microsomes. Naunyn-Schmiedeberg's Arch. exp. Path. Pharmak. **251**, 88—94 (1965).

Archakov, A.I., Panchenko, L.E., Karuzina, I.I., Alexandrova, T.A.: On the localization of the reactions *N*- and *C*-oxidation of dimethylaniline and peroxidation of unsaturated fatty acids in the $NADPH_2$ oxygenation system of microsomes. Dokl. Akad. Nauk SSSR, Otd. Biokh. **187**, 1415—1418 (1969).

Arrhenius, E.: Effects on hepatic microsomal *N*- and *C*-oxygenation of aromatic amines by *in vivo* corticosteroid or aminofluorene treatment, diet or stress. Cancer Res. **28**, 264—273 (1968).

— Effects of various *in vitro* conditions on hepatic microsomal *N*- and *C*-oxygenation of aromatic amines. Chem.-Biol. Interactions **1**, 361—380 (1970a).

— Effect *in vitro* of 2-aminofluorene or electrophilic agents on hepatic microsomal *N*- and *C*-oxygenation of aromatic amines. Chem.-Biol. Interactions **1**, 381—393 (1970b).

Augustine, R.P. di, Fouts, J.R.: The effects of unsaturated fatty acids on hepatic microsomal drug metabolism and cytochrome P-450. Biochem. J. **115**, 547—554 (1969).

Baker, J.R., Chaykin, S.: The biosynthesis of trimethylamine-*N*-oxide. J. biol. Chem. **237**, 1309—1313 (1962).

— Struempler, A., Chaykin, S.: A comparative study of trimethylamine-*N*-oxide biosynthesis. Biochim. biophys. Acta (Amst.) **71**, 58—64 (1963).

Barnes, J.M., Magee, P.N., Schoental, R.: Lesions in the lungs and liver of rats poisoned with the pyrrolizidine alkaloid fulvine and its *N*-oxide. J. Path. Bact. **88**, 521—531 (1964).

Bauer, S., Kiese, M.: Heterogeneousness of the microsomal enzymes effecting the *o*- and *p*-hydroxylation of aniline. Naunyn-Schmiedeberg's Arch. exp. Path. Pharmak. **247**, 144—148 (1964).

Beckett, A.H., Hewick, D.S.: The *N*-oxidation of chlorpromazine *in vitro* — the major metabolic route using rat liver microsomes. J. Pharm. Pharmacol. **19**, 134—136 (1967).

Bickel, M.H.: The pharmacology and biochemistry of *N*-oxides. Pharmacol. Rev. **21**, 325 to 355 (1969).

Booth, J., Boyland, E.: The biochemistry of aromatic amines. 10. Enzymic *N*-hydroxylation of arylamines and conversion of arylhydroxylamines into *o*-aminophenols. Biochem. J. **91**, 362—369 (1964).

Boyland, E.: The biochemistry of bladder cancer. Springfield/Ill.: Charles C. Thomas 1963.

Brodie, B.B., Axelrod, J., Shore, P.A., Udenfriend, S.: Ascorbic acid in aromatic hydroxylation. II. Products formed by reaction of substrates with ascorbic acid, ferrous ion, and oxygen. J. biol. Chem. **208**, 741—750 (1954).

Brown, G.B.: Purine *N*-oxides as antimetabolites and oncogens. In: Frontiers of Biology, Vol. 10, pp. 237—259. Amsterdam: North-Holland Publ. Co. 1968.

Bull, L.B., Dick, A.T.: The chronic pathological effects on the liver of the rat of the pyrrolizidine alkaloids heliotrine, lasiocarpine, and their *N*-oxides. J. Path. Bact. **78**, 483—502 (1959).

— — McKenzie, J.S.: The acute toxic effects of heliotrine and lasiocarpine, and their *N*-oxides on the rat. J. Path. Bact. **75**, 17—25 (1958).

Chambon, P., Chambon-Mougenot, R., Guilluy, R.: Recherches sur les metabolites à fonction *N*-Oxyde: analyse du *N*-Oxyde de *N,N*-diethylnicotinamide (Coramine *N*-Oxyde) par spectrographie de masse et par resonance magnetique nucleaire. C. R. Acad. Sci. (Paris) **269**, D 523—526 (1969).

Clayson, D.B.: Chemical Carcinogenesis. Boston: Little, Brown and Co. 1962.

Cramer, J.W., Miller, J.A., Miller, E.C.: *N*-Hydroxylation: a new metabolic reaction observed in the rat with the carcinogen 2-acetylaminofluorene. J. biol. Chem. **235**, 885 to 888 (1960).

Debackere, M., Uehleke, H.: *C*- and *N*-hydroxylation of aromatic amines by isolated liver microsomes of different species. Proc. Europ. Soc. Study Drug Toxicity **4**, 40—44 (1964).

Dehner, E.W., Machinist, J.M., Ziegler, D.M.: Effect of SKF 525-A on the excretion of amine oxides by the rat. Life Sci. **7**, 1135—1146 (1968).

Endo, H., Kume, F.: Comparative studies on the biological actions of 4-nitroquinoline 1-oxide and its reduced compound, 4-hydroxyaminoquinoline 1-oxide. Gann **54**, 443—453 (1963).

Enomoto, M., Sato, K.: *N*-Hydroxylation of the carcinogen 2-acetylaminofluorene by human liver tissue *in vitro*. Life Sci. **6**, 881—887 (1967).

— — Miller, E.C., Miller, J.A.: Reactivity of the diacetyl derivative of the carcinogen 4-hydroxylaminoquinoline 1-oxide with DNA, RNA, and other nucleophiles. Life Sci. **7**, 1025—1032 (1968).

Epstein, S.S., St. Pierre, J.A.: Mutagenicity in yeast of nitroquinolines and related compounds. Toxicol. appl. Pharmacol. **15**, 451—460 (1969).

Ernster, L., Danielson, L., Ljunggren, M.: DT Diaphorase. I. Purification from the soluble fractions of rat-liver cytoplasm, and properties. Biochim. biophys. Acta (Amst.) **58**, 171—188 (1962).
Fishman, V., Heaton, A., Goldenberg, H.: Metabolism of chlorpromazine. III. Isolation and identification of chlorpromazine-N-oxide. Proc. Soc. exp. Biol. (N.Y.) **109**, 548—552 (1962).
Fouts, J. R., Brodie, B. B.: The enzymatic reduction of chloramphenicol, p-nitrobenzoic acid and other aromatic nitro compounds in mammals. J. Pharmacol. exp. Ther. **119**, 197—207 (1957).
Gillette, J. R.: Metabolism of drugs and other foreign compounds by enzymatic mechanisms. Fortschr. Arzneimittelforsch. **6**, 11—73 (1963).
— Gram, T. E.: Cytochrome P-450 reduction in liver microsomes and its relationship to drug metabolism. In: Microsomes and Drug Oxidations, pp. 133—148. New York: Academic Press 1969.
— Kamm, J. J., Sasame, H. A.: Mechanism of p-nitrobenzoate reduction in liver: the possible role of cytochrome P-450 in liver microsomes. Molec. Pharmacol. **4**, 541—548 (1968).
Gram, T. E., Rogers, L. A., Fouts, J. R.: Effect of pretreatment of rabbits with phenobarbital or 3-methylcholanthrene on the distribution of drug-metabolizing enzyme activity in subfractions of hepatic microsomes. J. Pharmacol. exp. Ther. **157**, 435—445 (1967a).
— — — Further studies on the metabolism of drugs by subfractions of hepatic microsomes. J. Pharmacol. exp. Ther. **155**, 479—493 (1967b).
Gutmann, H. R., Burtle, J. G., Nagasawa, H. T.: Protein binding of model quinone imides. I. The synthesis of some fluorenoquinone imides. J. Amer. chem. Soc. **80**, 5551—5555 (1958).
Herr, F., Kiese, M.: Bestimmung von Nitrosobenzol im Blute. Naunyn-Schmiedeberg's Arch. exp. Path. Pharmak. **235**, 351—353 (1959).
Heubner, W.: Studien über Methämoglobinbildung. Naunyn-Schmiedeberg's Arch. exp. Path. Pharmak. **72**, 241—280 (1913).
Hjelm, M., Verdier, C.-H., de: Biochemical effects of aromatic amines. I. Methaemoglobinaemia, haemolysis and Heinz-body formation induced by 4,4'-diaminodiphenylsulphone. Biochem. Pharmacol. **14**, 1119—1128 (1965).
Hlavica, P., Kiese, M.: N-Oxygenation of N-alkyl- and N,N-dialkylanilines by rabbit liver microsomes. Biochem. Pharmacol. **18**, 1501—1509 (1969).
Hozumi, M.: Reaction of the carcinogen 4-hydroxyaminoquinoline 1-oxide with sulfhydryl groups of proteins. Biochem. Pharmacol. **17**, 765—777 (1968).
Irving, C. C.: N-hydroxylation of the carcinogen 2-acetylaminofluorene by rabbit-liver microsomes. Biochim. biophys. Acta (Amst.) **65**, 564—566 (1962).
— Enzymatic N-hydroxylation of the carcinogen 2-acetylaminofluorene and the metabolism of N-hydroxy-2-acetylaminofluorene-9-C^{14} *in vitro*. J. biol. Chem. **239**, 1589—1596 (1964).
Ishizawa, M., Endo, H.: On the mode of action of a potent carcinogen, 4-hydroxylaminoquinoline 1-oxide on bacteriophage T4. Biochem. Pharmacol. **16**, 637—646 (1967).
Itai, T., Sueyoshi, S., Nato, K., Mizuno, D.: Potential anti-cancer agents. XV. Synthesis of substituted styrylpyridazine N-oxides and their anti-cancer activity. J. pharm. Soc. Japan **89**, 132—134 (1969).
Juchau, M. R.: Studies on the reduction of aromatic nitro groups in human and rodent placental homogenates. J. Pharmacol. exp. Ther. **165**, 1—8 (1969).
Kamahora, J., Kakunaga, T.: Malignant transformation of hamster embryonic cells *in vitro* by 4-nitroquinoline 1-oxide. Biken's J. **10**, 219—242 (1967).
Kampffmeyer, H., Kiese, M.: Einige Eigenschaften der Anilin-hydroxylierenden Enzyme in Mikrosomen. Naunyn-Schmiedeberg's Arch. exp. Path. Pharmak. **244**, 375—386 (1963).
— — Further factors affecting the hydroxylation of aniline and some of its derivatives by liver microsomes. Naunyn-Schmiedeberg's Arch. exp. Path. Pharmak. **246**, 397—412 (1964a).
— — The hydroxylation of aniline and N-ethylaniline by microsomal enzymes at low oxygen pressures. Biochem. Z. **339**, 454—459 (1964b).
— — Hydroxylierung von Anilin und N-Äthylanilin durch Leber-Mikrosomen bei niedrigen Sauerstoffdrucken und unter Kohlenoxyd. Naunyn-Schmiedeberg's Arch. exp. Path. Pharmak. **247**, 374—375 (1964c).
— — The effect of carbon monoxide on the hydroxylation of aniline and N-ethylaniline by microsomal enzymes. Naunyn-Schmiedeberg's Arch. exp. Path. Pharmak. **250**, 1—8 (1965).
Kataoka, N., Imamura, A., Kawazoe, Y., Chihara, G., Nagata, C.: The structure of the free radical produced from carcinogenic 4-hydroxyaminoquinoline 1-oxide. Bull. chem. Soc. Japan **40**, 62—68 (1967).
Kato, R., Oshima, T., Takanaka, A.: Studies on the mechanism of nitro reduction by rat liver. Molec. Pharmacol. **5**, 487—498 (1969).
— Takahashi, A., Oshima, T.: Characteristics of nitro reduction of the carcinogenic agent, 4-nitroquinoline N-oxide. Biochem. Pharmacol. **19**, 45—55 (1970).

KAWAZOE, Y., ARAKI, M.: Studies on chemical carcinogens. V. O,O'-Diacetyl-4-hydroxyaminoquinoline 1-oxide. Gann **58**, 485—487 (1967).
— TACHIBANA, M., AOKI, K., NAKAHARA, W.: The structure-carcinogenicity relationship among derivatives of 4-nitro and 4-hydroxylaminoquinoline 1-oxides. Biochem. Pharmacol. **16**, 631—636 (1967).
KIESE, M.: Die Bedeutung der Oxydation von Anilin zu Nitrosobenzol für die Hämoglobinbildung nach Aufnahme von Anilin in den Organismus. Naunyn-Schmiedeberg's Arch. exp. Path. Pharmak. **235**, 360—364 (1959).
— The biochemical production of ferrihemoglobin-forming derivatives from aromatic amines, and mechanisms of ferrihemoglobin formation. Pharmacol. Rev. **18**, 1091—1161 (1966).
— Reactions of *N,N*-dimethylaniline-*N*-oxide with hemoglobin. Molec. Pharmacol. **3**, 9—14 (1967).
— RAUSCHER, E., WEGER, N.: The role of *N,N*-dimethylaniline-*N*-oxide in the formation of hemiglobin following the absorption of *N,N*-dimethylaniline. Naunyn-Schmiedeberg's Arch. exp. Path. Pharmak. **254**, 253—260 (1966).
— UEHLEKE, H.: Der Ort der *N*-Oxydation des Anilins im höheren Tier. Naunyn-Schmiedeberg's Arch. exp. Path. Pharmak. **242**, 117—129 (1961a).
— — Zwei Wege der Entmethylierung von *N*-Methylanilin durch Mikrosomen aus Rattenlebern. Naturwissenschaften **48**, 379—380 (1961b).
— — WEGER, N.: Extraerythrocytäre Einflüsse auf Hämoglobinbildung durch Phenylhydroxylamin und Nitrosobenzol in roten Zellen. Naunyn-Schmiedeberg's Arch. exp. Path. Pharmak. **242**, 130—133 (1961).
KUROKI, T., SATO, H.: Transformation and neoplastic development *in vitro* of hamster embryonic cells by 4-nitroquinoline-1-oxide and its derivatives. J. nat. Cancer Inst. **41**, 53—71 (1968).
LACASSAGNE, A., BUU-HOI, N.P., ZAJDELA, F., HOEFFINGER, J.P., JACQUIGNON, P.: Structure and carcinogenicity in some derivatives of 4-nitroquinoline *N*-oxide. Life Sci. **5**, 1945 to 1947 (1966).
LANGE, G.: Verschiedene Induktion der mikrosomalen *N*- und *p*-Hydroxylierung von Anilin und N-Äthylanilin bei Kaninchen. Naunyn-Schmiedeberg's Arch. exp. Path. Pharmak. **257**, 230—256 (1967).
— Hydroxylase-Aktivität und Hämoprotein-Gehalt von Mikrosomen aus Kaninchenleber. Naunyn-Schmiedeberg's Arch. exp. Path. Pharmak. **259**, 221—238 (1968).
LOTLIKAR, P.D., ENOMOTO, M., MILLER, J.A., MILLER, E.C.: Species variations in the *N*- and ring-hydroxylation of 2-acetylaminofluorene and effects of 3-methylcholanthrene pretreatment. Proc. Soc. exp. Biol. (N.Y.) **125**, 341—346 (1967).
— MILLER, E.C., MILLER, J.A., MARGRETH, A.: The enzymatic reduction of the *N*-hydroxy derivative of 2-acetylaminofluorene and related carcinogens by tissue preparations. Cancer Res. **25**, 1743—1752 (1965).
MACHINIST, J.M., DEHNER, E.W., ZIEGLER, D.M.: Microsomal oxidases. III. Comparison of species and organ distribution of dialkylarylamine N-oxide dealkylase and dialkylarylamine *N*-oxidase. Arch. Biochem. **125**, 858—864 (1968).
— ORME-JOHNSON, W.H., ZIEGLER, D.M.: Microsomal oxidases. II. Properties of a pork liver microsomal *N*-oxide dealkylase. Biochemistry **5**, 2939—2943 (1966).
MARGRETH, A., LOTLIKAR, P.D., MILLER, E.C., MILLER, J.A.: The effects of hepatotoxic agents and of liver growth on the urinary excretion of the *N*-hydroxy metabolite of 2-acetaminofluorene by rats. Cancer Res. **24**, 920—925 (1964).
MATSUSHIMA, T., KOBUNA, I., FUKUOKA, F., SUGIMURA, T.: Metabolism of 4-nitroquinoline 1-oxide. IV. Quantitative determination of *in vivo* conversion of 4-nitroquinoline 1-oxide in subcutaneous tissue of rat. Gann **59**, 247—250 (1968).
— — SUGIMURA, T.: *In vivo* interaction of 4-nitroquinoline-1-oxide and its derivatives with DNA. Nature (Lond.) **216**, 508 (1967).
MCMAHON, R.E.: Microsomal dealkylation of drugs. Substrate specificity and mechanism. J. pharm. Sci. **55**, 457—466 (1966).
MILLER, E.C., MILLER, J.A., HARTMANN, H.A.: *N*-Hydroxy-2-acetylaminofluorene: A metabolite of 2-acetylaminofluorene with increased activity in the rat. Cancer Res. **21**, 815—824 (1961).
MORI, K., OHTA, A.: Carcinoma of the glandular stomach of mice by 4-hydroxyaminoquinoline 1-oxide. Gann **58**, 551—554 (1967).
MYLES, A., BROWN, G.B.: Purine *N*-oxides. XXX. Biochemical studies of the oncogen 3-hydroxyxanthine. J. biol. Chem. **244**, 4072—4076 (1969).
NAGASAWA, H.T., GUTMANN, H.R.: The oxidation of *o*-aminophenols by cytochrome C and cytochrome oxidase. I. Enzymatic oxidations and binding of oxidation products to bovine serum albumin. J. biol. Chem. **234**, 1593—1599 (1959).

NAKAHARA, W.: Newer studies on the carcinogenic action of quinoline N-oxide derivatives. Arzneimittel-Forsch. **14**, 842—844 (1964).
OCHIAI, E.: Aromatic amine oxides. Amsterdam: Elsevier 1967.
OKABAYASHI, T., IDE, M., YOSHIMOTO, A., OTSUBO, M.: Mutagenic activity of 4-nitroquinoline 1-oxide and 4-hydroxyaminoquinoline 1-oxide on bacteria. Chem. pharm. Bull. **13**, 610 to 611 (1965).
OKANO, T., TAKENAKA, S., SATO, Y.: Interaction of the carcinogen 4-nitroquinoline 1-oxide with protein and aromatic amino acids. Chem. pharm. Bull **16**, 556—558 (1968).
— UEKAMA, K.: On the stoichiometric interactions between 4-nitroquinoline 1-oxide and deoxyribonucleosides, with special reference to the mode of binding of the carcinogen to DNA. Chem. pharm. Bull. **15**, 1812—1815 (1967).
PARKE, D.V.: Studies in detoxication. 85. The metabolism of *m*-dinitro[^{14}C] benzene in the rabbit. Biochem. J. **78**, 262—271 (1961).
PAUL, M.F., HARRINGTON, C.: Nitrofurans and enzyme systems of the neonatal animal. Biochem. Pharmacol. **16**, 2457—2460 (1967).
PETERS, M.A., FOUTS, J.R.: An evaluation of two procedures used in the study of *p*-nitrobenzoic acid metabolism by rat liver. Toxicol. appl. Pharmacol. **12**, 242—248 (1968).
SARTORELLI, A.C., BIEBER, A.L., CHANG, P.K., FISCHER, G.A.: Some inhibitory properties of 6-N-hydroxylaminopurine: an analog of adenine and hypoxanthine. Biochem.Pharmacol. **13**, 507—515 (1964).
SCHELINE, R.R.: Drug metabolism by intestinal microorganisms. J. pharm. Sci. **57**, 2021 to 2037 (1968).
SHIRASU, Y.: Comparative carcinogenicity of 4-nitroquinoline 1-oxide and 4-hydroxyaminoquinoline 1-oxide in 3 strains of mice. Proc. Soc. exp. Biol. (N.Y.) **118**, 812—914 (1965).
— GRANTHAM, P.H., YAMAMOTO, R.S., WEISBURGER, J.H.: Effects of pituitary hormones and prefeeding N-hydroxy-N-2-fluorenylacetamide on the metabolism of this carcinogen and on physiologic parameters. Cancer Res. **26**, 600—606 (1966).
SPARTHAN, M., CHAYKIN, S.: Determination of nicotinamide N-oxide — a human excretory product. Anal. Biochem. **31**, 286—295 (1969).
STÖHRER, G., BROWN, G.B.: Purine N-oxides. XXVIII. The reduction of purine N-oxides by xanthine oxidase. J. biol. Chem. **244**, 2498—2502 (1969a).
— — Purine N-oxides. XXVII. The metabolism of guanine 3-oxide by the rat. J. biol. Chem. **244**, 2494—2497 (1969b).
— — Oncogenic purine derivatives: evidence for a possible proximate oncogen. Science **167**, 1622—1624 (1970).
SUGIMURA, T., OKABE, K., NAGAO, M.: The metabolism of 4-nitroquinoline-1-oxide, a carcinogen. III. An enzyme catalyzing the conversion of 4-nitroquinoline-1-oxide to 4-hydroxyaminoquinoline-1-oxide in rat liver and hepatomas. Cancer Res. **26**, 1717—1721 (1966).
SUGIURA, K., TELLER, M.N., PARHAM, J.C., BROWN, G.B.: A comparison of the oncogenicities of 3-hydroxyxanthine, guanine 3-N-oxide, and some related compounds. Cancer Res. **30**, 184—188 (1970).
TADA, M., TADA, M., TAKAHASHI, T.: Interaction of a carcinogen, 4-hydroxyaminoquinoline-1-oxide with nucleic acids. Biochem. biophys. Res. Commun. **29**, 469—477 (1967).
TANOOKA, H., KAWAZOE, Y., ARAKI, M.: Reaction mechanism of 4-hydroxyaminoquinoline 1-oxide and related compounds in inactivation of the transforming activity of deoxyribonucleic acid. Gann **60**, 537—543 (1969).
TELLER, M.N., STOHR, G., DIENST, H.: Studies on the oncogenicity of 3-hydroxyxanthine. Cancer Res. **30**, 179—183 (1970).
TERAYAMA, H.: Aminoazo carcinogenesis — methods and biochemical problems. Meth. Cancer Res. **1**, 399—449 (1967).
— ORII, H.: Dye-protein binding in the animals administered with 4-dimethylaminoazobenzene amine-N-oxide and the toxicology of 4-dimethylaminoazobenzene amine-N-oxide. Gann **54**, 455—464 (1963).
THAUER, R.K., MEIFORTH, A., UEHLEKE, H.: Methämoglobinbildung durch Sulfonamide im System Leberhomogenat, Erythrocyten, NADPH und Sauerstoff. Naunyn-Schmiedeberg's Arch. exp. Path. Pharmak. **252**, 291—296 (1965b).
— STÖFFLER, G., UEHLEKE, H.: N-Hydroxylierung von Sulfanilamid zu *p*-Hydroxylaminobenzolsulfonamid durch Lebermikrosomen. Naunyn-Schmiedeberg's Arch. exp. Path. Pharmak. **252**, 32—42 (1965a).
UDENFRIEND, S., CLARK, C.T., AXELROD, J., BRODIE, B.B.: Ascorbic acid in aromatic hydroxylation. I. A model system for aromatic hydroxylation. J. biol. Chem. **208**, 731—739 (1954).
UEHLEKE, H.: N-Hydroxylierung von 2-Aminofluoren durch Lebermikrosomen. Experientia (Basel) **17**, 557 (1961a).

UEHLEKE, H.: N-Oxydation von N-alkylierten Anilinen durch isolierte Organe, Zellen und Zellbestandteile. Naunyn-Schmiedeberg's Arch. exp. Path. Pharmak. **241**, 150 (1961b).

— Relations between structure, velocity of biological N-hydroxylation and toxicity of aromatic amines. Proc. First Intern. Pharmacol. Meeting **6**, 31—37. Oxford: Pergamon Press 1962.

— N-Hydroxylation of carcinogenic amines *in vivo* and *in vitro* with liver microsomes. Biochem. Pharmacol. **12**, 219—221 (1963a).

— Nitrosobenzol und Phenylhydroxylamine als Zwischenstoffe der biologischen Reduktion von Nitrobenzol. Naturwissenschaften **50**, 335—336 (1963b).

— Biologische Oxydation und Reduktion am Stickstoff aromatischer Amino- und Nitroderivative und ihre Folgen für den Organismus. Fortschr. Arzneimittel-Forsch. **8**, 195—260 (1964a).

— Age dependent N-hydroxylation of aromatic amines and toxicity. Proc. Europ. Soc. Study Drug Toxicity **4**, 140—144 (1964b).

— Nitrosobenzol in Blute von Katzen nach Verabreichung von Nitrobenzol. Naunyn-Schmiedeberg's Arch. exp. Path. Pharmak. **247**, 412—418 (1964c).

— N-Hydroxylation of carcinogenic amines by bladder mucosa. In: Bladder Cancer, a Symposium, pp. 98—106. Birmingham: Aesculapius Publ. Co. 1967a.

— Stimulierung einiger mikrosomaler Fremdstoff-Oxydationen durch Phenobarbital, Methylcholanthren und Chlorphenothan, einzeln und in Kombinationen. Naunyn-Schmiedeberg's Arch. exp. Path. Pharmak. **259**, 66—90 (1967b).

— Extrahepatic microsomal drug metabolism. Proc. Europ. Soc. Study Drug Toxicity, Xth Mtg., 94—100 (1968).

— N-Hydroxylierung von p-Phenetidin *in vivo* und durch isolierte Mikrosomen aus Lebern und Nieren: Stimulierung durch Phenobarbital-Vorbehandlung. Naunyn-Schmiedeberg's Arch. exp. Path. Pharmak. **264**, 434—461 (1969a).

— Untersuchungen über die N-Hydroxylierung aromatischer Amine und ihre Bedeutung für die Entstehung von Harnblasentumoren. Arzneimittel-Forsch. **19**, 1033—1039 (1969b).

— Toxikologische Aspekte der N-Hydroxylierung aromatischer Amine. Naunyn-Schmiedeberg's Arch. exp. Path. Pharmak. **263**, 106—120 (1969c).

— BRILL, E.: Increased metabolic N-oxidation of 2-naphthylamine in dogs after phenobarbital pretreatment. Biochem. Pharmacol. **17**, 1459—1461 (1968).

— NESTEL, K.: Hydroxylamino- und Nitrosobiphenyl: biologische Oxydationsprodukte von 4-Aminobiphenyl und Zwischenprodukte der Reduktion von 4-Nitrobiphenyl. Naunyn-Schmiedeberg's Arch. exp. Path. Pharmak. **257**, 151—171 (1967).

— STAHN, V.: Zur biologischen Bildung von N,N-Dimethylanilin-N-Oxyd und N,N-Dimethylaminoazobenzol-N_4-Oxyd aus den Aminen sowie ihre Reaktionen mit Hämoglobin und mit Lebermikrosomen. Naunyn-Schmiedeberg's Arch. exp. Path. Pharmak. **255**, 287—300 (1966).

WEISBURGER, E.K., WEISBURGER, J.H.: Chemistry, carcinogenicity, and metabolism of 2-fluorenamine and related compounds. Advanc. Cancer Res. **5**, 331—431 (1958).

WEISBURGER, J.H., WEISBURGER, E.K.: Chemicals as causes of cancer. Chem. Engineering News **43**, 124—142 (1966).

— — MORRIS, H.P., SOBER, H.A.: Chromatographic separation of some metabolites of the carcinogen N-2-fluorenylacetamide. J. nat. Cancer Inst. **17**, 363—374 (1956).

WILLIAMS, R.T.: Detoxication Mechanisms. 2nd ed., p. 428. New York: John Wiley and Sons 1959.

WILSON, J.T.: The effect of a pituitary mammotropic tumor on hepatic microsomal drug metabolism in the rat. Biochem. Pharmacol. **17**, 1449—1457 (1968a).

— An investigation of the decrease in the metabolism of hexobarbital, aminopyrine, and *p*-nitrobenzoic acid by liver from rats bearing a pituitary mammotropic tumor. J. Pharmacol. exp. Ther. **160**, 179—188 (1968b).

WÖLCKE, U., BIRDSALL, N.J.M., BROWN, G.B.: Purine N-oxides. XXIV. The preparation of 8-substituted xanthines and guanines by a nucleophilic displacement of a 3-substituent. Tetrahedron Letters 785—788 (1969).

YOST, Y.: Oxidation of fluorenamines and preparation of 2,2′- and 4,4′-azofluorene. J. med. Chem. **12**, 961 (1969).

ZIEGLER, D.M., MITCHELL, C.H., JOLLOW, D.: The properties of a purified hepatic microsomal mixed function amine oxidase. In: Microsomes and Drug Oxidations, pp. 173—187. New York: Academic Press 1969.

— PETTIT, F.H.: Formation of an intermediate N-oxide in the oxidative demethylation of N,N-dimethylaniline catalyzed by liver microsomes. Biochem. biophys. Res. Commun. **15**, 188—193 (1964).

— — Microsomal oxidases. I. The isolation and dialkylarylamine oxygenase activity of pork liver microsomes. Biochemistry **5**, 2932—2938 (1966).

Chapter 41

Enzymatic N-, O-, and S-Dealkylation of Foreign Compounds by Hepatic Microsomes

TH. E. GRAM

With 4 Figures

A wide variety of drugs and other foreign compounds are dealkylated by enzyme systems localized in the microsomal fraction of liver and to lesser degrees, in kidney, lung, and other organs including placenta. During an investigation of the metabolism of a series of chemical carcinogens, MILLER et al. (1952) observed that after the intraperitoneal administration of 3′-methyl-4-dimethyl-^{14}C-aminoazobenzene to rats, a significant amount of $^{14}CO_2$ was recoverable from the expired air. Subsequent work (MUELLER and MILLER, 1953) revealed the presence of an enzyme system in rat liver which catalyzed the demethylation of a number of secondary amines with the liberation of formaldehyde and primary amine.

In 1955 LA DU et al. (1955) described an enzyme in mammalian liver that catalyzed the N-demethylation of aminopyrine (N,N-dimethyl-4-aminoantipyrine) with the formation of formaldehyde and 4-aminoantipyrine (Fig. 1). The

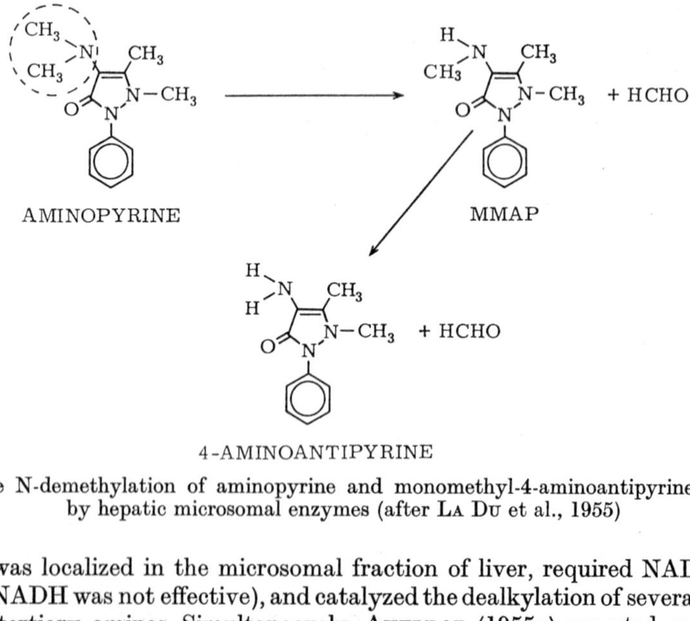

Fig. 1. The N-demethylation of aminopyrine and monomethyl-4-aminoantipyrine (MMAP) by hepatic microsomal enzymes (after LA DU et al., 1955)

enzyme was localized in the microsomal fraction of liver, required NADPH and oxygen (NADH was not effective), and catalyzed the dealkylation of several secondary and tertiary amines. Simultaneously, AXELROD (1955a) reported an enzyme in rabbit liver microsomes requiring NADPH and oxygen that catalyzed the deamination of amphetamine and a host of chemical congeners.

Table 1. *Some biological N-dealkylation reactions*

N-alkyl group cleaved	Compound	Reference
CH_3-	Aminopyrine	LA DU et al. (1955)
	Ephedrine	AXELROD (1955b)
	Morphine	AXELROD (1956b)
	Meperidine	AXELROD (1956b)
	Chlorpromazine	BECKETT et al. (1963)
	Imipramine	DINGELL et al. (1964)
	Puromycin	MAZEL et al. (1966)
	Chlorpheniramine	KAMM et al. (1969)
	Chlorcyclizine	KUNTZMAN et al. (1965)
	N-methylbarbital	MCMAHON (1963)
	Trimethadione	BUTLER et al. (1965)
	Erythromycin	MAO and TARDREW (1965)
	Chlordiazepoxide	SCHWARTZ and POSTMA (1966)
	Diazepam	SCHWARTZ et al. (1965)
	Orphenadrine	HESPE et al. (1965)
CH_3—CH_2—	3-ethylnirvanol	BUTLER and WADDELL (1959)
	N-ethylbenzilamide	ALBERT et al. (1961)
	N,N-diethyl-4-aminoantipyrine	LA DU et al. (1955)
	Benzquinamide	KOE and PINSON (1964)
	SKF 525-A	GAUDETTE and BRODIE (1959), ANDERS et al. (1966)
	Diethylpropion	SCHREIBER et al. (1968)
CH_3—CH_2—CH_2—	trifluralin	EMMERSON and ANDERSON (1966)
	N-propyl-4-bromobenzene-sulfonamide	SMITH et al. (1965)
	Chlorpropamide	WELLES et al. (1959)
	Probenecid	GUARINO et al. (1969)
CH_3 >CH— CH_3	N-isopropylamphetamine	VREE and VAN ROSSUM (1970)
	N-isopropylmethoxamine	KLUTCH and BORDUN (1967)
	N-isopropyl-4-bromobenzene-sulfonamide	SMITH et al. (1965)
CH_2 = CH—CH_2—	Nalorphine	AXELROD and COCHIN (1957), LEADSEATER and DAVIES (1964)
	Levallophan	MANNERING and SCHANKER (1958)
	N,N-diallylmelamine	ZINS (1965)
CH_3—CH_2—CH_2—CH_2—	Butamoxane; [2-(N,N-dibutyl-aminomethyl)-1,4-benzodioxane]	MCMAHON (1959)
	Ethoxybutamoxane	MCMAHON et al. (1960)
	N,N-dibutyl-4-aminoantipyrine	LA DU et al. (1955)
	N-butyl-4-bromobenzen-sulfonamide	SMITH et al. (1965)
CH_3—C(CH_3)(CH_3)—	t-butylnorchlorcyclizine	KUNTZMAN et al. (1967)
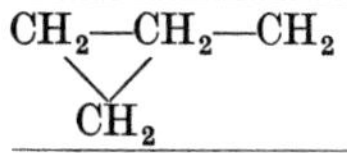	cyclazocine	MULE et al. (1968)
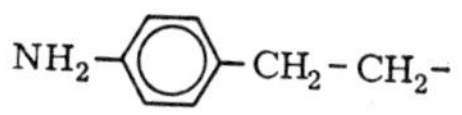	anileridine	LIN and WAY (1965)
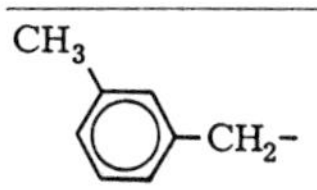	meclizine	NARROD et al. (1965)

A. N-Dealkylation

N-Dealkylation is a common metabolic pathway for the transformation of foreign compounds in man and other mammals (BRODIE et al., 1958), in birds (BRODIE and MAICKEL, 1962), fish (BUHLER and RASMUSSON, 1968; DEWAIDE and HENDERSON, 1968; CREAVEN et al., 1967), reptiles (BRODIE and MAICKEL, 1962), and insects (SMITH, 1962; CHAKRABORTY and SMITH, 1967). A recent report (FREAR, 1968) described an NADPH and oxygen dependent microsomal enzyme in the leaves of the cotton plant that catalyzes the N-demethylation of Monuron, a herbicidal compound. A partial list of biological N-dealkylation reactions is found in Table 1.

The microsomal system, compared with enzymes of intermediary carbohydrate metabolism or nucleic acid biosynthesis, has a broad substrate spectrum. A large number of chemically unrelated but generally lipophilic compounds serve as substrates for the microsomal system; carbon-nitrogen bond cleavage occurs whether nitrogen has the form of amine (secondary or tertiary), amide, carbamate, or sulfonamide (McMAHON, 1966).

I. Relationship of the N-Alkyl Substituent to the Rate of Dealkylation

Although the removal of short-chain substituents (methyl, ethyl) is most commonly encountered in pharmacology, cleavage of rather complex and bulky groups has also been described (Table 1). In a group of aminopyrine homologues in which the alkyl chain length varied from methyl to n-butyl, the rate of N-dealkylation decreased as chain length increased (LA DU et al., 1955) (Table 2). Similarly,

Table 2. *N-dealkylation of analogues of aminopyrine by rabbit liver in vitro*

Substrate	4-Aminoantipyrine formed	% of substrate dealkylated
Monomethyl-4-aminoantipyrine	1.93	36
Dimethyl-4-aminoantipyrine (aminopyrine)	0.62	11
Monoethyl-4-aminoantipyrine	0.60	11
Diethyl-4-aminoantipyrine	0.29	6
Monobutyl-4-aminoantipyrine	0.56	9
Dibutyl-4-aminoantipyrine	0.10	1

Data from LA DU et al. (1955)

SMITH et al. (1965) reported that the dealkylation rate progressively decreased as the N-alkyl substituent increased from methyl through ethyl, allyl, isopropyl, n-propyl, and n-butyl.

II. Relative Rates of N-Dealkylation of Secondary and Tertiary Amines

1. *In Vivo*

DINGELL, GILLETTE and coworkers reported that following the administration of the tertiary amine imipramine to rats, its monodemethylated metabolite desmethylimipramine (DMI) accumulated in several tissues including brain (GILLETTE et al., 1961; DINGELL et al., 1964). Very little of the primary amine des-dimethylimipramine was detected. A significant proportion of the pharmacologic effect of the parent drug was shown to be due to the formation of DMI *in vivo*. Similarly, in a series of tertiary amine methadol congeners, McMahon et al. (1965) found that the first methyl group was removed about 3 to 4 times as rapidly as the second and as a result secondary amines accumulated in tissues. Studying the metabolism of N,N-dimethylamphetamine in man, Vree and Van Rossum (1970) found that the conversion of tertiary amine to secondary amine occurred readily but further metabolism to the primary amine was very slow. Thus, about 17% of a dose of N,N-dimethylamphetamine was excreted in the urine as N-monomethylamphetamine but only about 1.5% as amphetamine.

2. *In Vitro*

Since many of the rates of dealkylation reported in the literature are not maximum velocities (V_{max}), it is hazardous to undertake a discussion of relative rates of metabolism. However, it is generally held that tertiary amines are dealkylated more rapidly than the corresponding secondary amines (Table 3).

Table 3. *Relative rates of N-demethylation of some secondary and tertiary amine pairs by hepatic microsomes*

Compound	Type of amine	Source of microsomes	Relative rate	Reference
Amitriptyline	Tert.	rat	0.79	McMahon et al.
Nortriptyline	Sec.		0.05	(1963b)
N,N-dimethylbarbital	Tert.	rat	155	McMahon (1963)
N-methylbarbital	Sec.		28	
N,N-dimethylbarbital	Tert.	rabbit	314	McMahon (1963)
N-methylbarbital	Sec.		63	
N,N-dimethyldiphenylacetamide	Tert.	rabbit	128	McMahon (1963)
N-methyldiphenylacetamide	Sec.		23	
2,4-dichloro-6-phenylphenoxy dimethylamine (Lilly 18947)	Tert.	rat	108	McMahon (1962)
2,4-dichloro-6-phenylphenoxy monomethylamine	Sec.		27	
N,N-dimethylaniline	Tert.	rat	84	McMahon (1962)
N-monomethylaniline	Sec.		50	
Methadol	Tert.	rat	2.15	McMahon et al.
Normethadol	Sec.		0.95	(1965)
10 Tricyclic anti-depressant	Tert.	rat	16—69% [a]	Bickel et al.
compounds	Sec.		5—15%	(1967)

[a] Per cent of the substrate demethylated.

McMahon (1964) pointed out three general metabolic differences among pairs of homologous secondary and tertiary amines (Table 4):

a) Demethylation of tertiary amines was slightly more sensitive to microsomal enzyme inhibitors such as SKF 525-A and DPEA.

b) Tertiary amines had consistently higher V_{max} and K_m values.

c) Pretreatment of rats with phenobarbital produced a marked stimulation (100—300% increase) in the demethylation of tertiary amines but a relatively minor effect (10—60% increase) on metabolism of the secondary amines.

One might assume that during the demethylation of a tertiary amine by microsomal enzymes, the required stoichiometry would be two moles of formaldehyde liberated for each mole of primary amine formed. However, the results of Dingell

Table 4. *Comparison of the demethylation of some pairs of secondary and tertiary amines by hepatic microsomes*

Substrate	Type of amine	Effect of SKF 525-A[a] (% inhibition)	Kinetic constants V_{max}	Kinetic constants K_m	Response to phenobarbital pretreatment[b] Control	Response to phenobarbital pretreatment[b] Phenobarbital treated
l-ephedrine	Sec.	6	79	0.20	1.0	1.6
N-methyl-*l*-ephedrine	Tert.	15	208	0.45	1.6	6.7
Nortriptyline	Sec.	0	—	—	0.7	0.8
Amitriptyline	Tert.	20	—	—	4.7	8.9
p-chlorophenylpropylmethyl-amine	Sec.	16	147	0.55	2.5	2.8
p-chlorophenylpropyldimethyl-amine	Tert.	30	460	1.4	3.8	12.5

[a] Substrate concentration in all cases was 2 mM, the inhibitor concentration was 0.05 mM.
[b] Values represent μmoles of formaldehyde formed per gram liver per hour.
Data were assembled from McMAHON (1964).

and D'ENCARNACAO (1966) and of GRAM et al. (1968) indicate the following metabolic pattern *in vitro:*

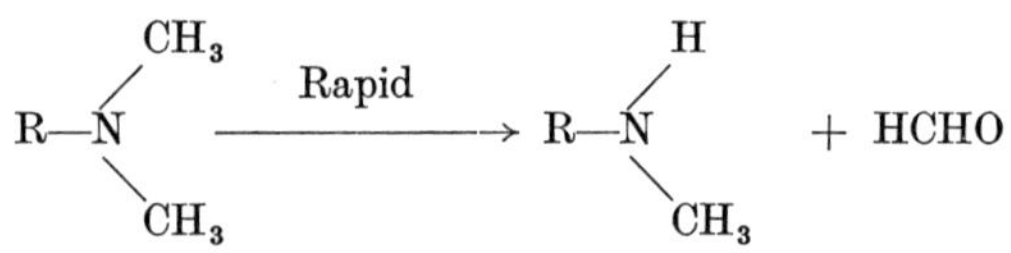

(1)

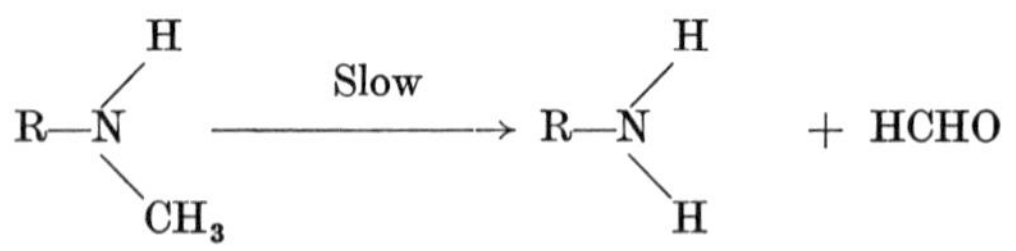

(2)

Incubation of microsomes with a tertiary amine gives rise to equivalent amounts of formaldehyde and secondary amine (Reaction 1). However, further metabolism of the secondary amine to the primary amine (Reaction 2) does not occur readily thus resulting in the formation of disproportionately large amounts of formaldehyde relative to primary amine (Table 5). The low yield of primary amine is not

Table 5. *Metabolism of some secondary and tertiary amines by rat liver microsomes*

Substrate	Type of amine	Formaldehyde formed	Primary amine formed
Aminopyrine	Tertiary	0.71	0.04
Monomethyl-4-aminoantipyrine . . .	Secondary	0.62	0.56
N,N-dimethylaniline	Tertiary	1.13	0.08
N-methylaniline	Secondary	0.46	0.45

Data from DINGELL and D'ENCARNACAO (1966) and DINGELL (1970)

due to further metabolism of the primary amine (GRAM et al., 1968). In addition to the different velocities for reactions 1 and 2 noted above, it has also been shown that tertiary amines inhibit Reaction 2, demethylation of the secondary amine,

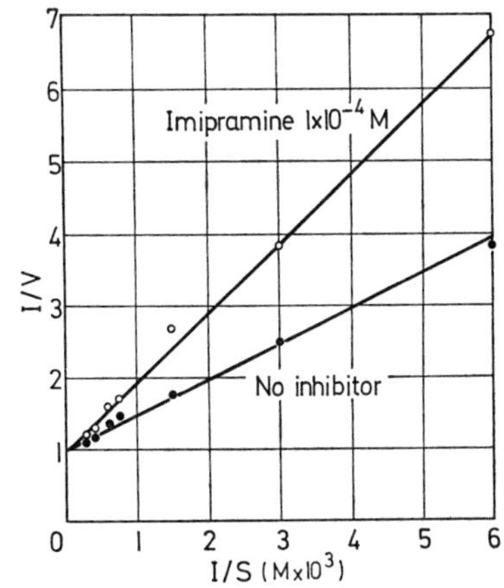

Fig. 2. Inhibition by imipramine of the demethylation of N-methylaniline by rat liver microsomes. The inhibition is competitive in nature. Similar experiments indicated that N,N-dimethylaniline competitively inhibits the demethylation of N-methylaniline (DINGELL and D'ENCARNACAO, 1966; DINGELL, 1970)

by a competitive mechanism (DINGELL, 1970; GRAM et al., 1968) (Fig. 2). These factors, in concert, create conditions under which Reaction 1 proceeds rapidly while Reaction 2 is very slow thus yielding large amounts of formaldehyde and very little primary amine.

Substrate inhibition has been reported for several drugs which undergo N-demethylation. Among these are aminopyrine (GRAM et al., 1968; DEWAIDE and HENDERSON, 1968), *l*-propoxphene (MCMAHON and SULLIVAN, 1964), meperidine (MCMAHON, 1962), and codeine (ELISON and ELLIOT, 1964). The significance of these findings is, at present, unknown. It is interesting, however, that each of these substrates is known to undergo two distinct metabolic conversions in the presence of microsomes and NADPH; aminopyrine and *l*-propoxyphene are tertiary amines and therefore undergo sequential demethylation, meperidine undergoes N-demethylation and de-esterification, and codeine both N- and O-demethylation.

III. Multiple Microsomal N-Demethylases

It should not be inferred that hepatic microsomes contain a single N-demethylase which exhibits a unified response to all environmental manipulations. For example, in rats the magnitude of the sex difference in the microsomal N-demethylation of aminopyrine or ethylmorphine is of the order of 200—300% (KATO and GILLETTE, 1965; DAVIES et al., 1968) but is only about 40% for the N-demethylation of N-methylaniline (KATO and GILLETTE, 1965). Similarly, marked species differences exist in rates of demethylation of several amines (TAKEMORI and MANNERING, 1958). Finally, the induction of microsomal N-demethylases is markedly dependent upon the substrate investigated. For example, the N-demethylation of ethylmorphine and aminopyrine, is increased several fold by treatment of animals with phenobarbital but is unaffected or decreased by treatment with 3-methylcholanthrene. Conversely, the N-demethylation of 3'-methyl-4-methylaminoazobenzene is stimulated by treatment with either 3-methylcholanthrene or phenobarbital (CONNEY, 1967; SLADEK and MANNERING, 1969). These findings suggest the possible existence of multiple N-demethylases in hepatic microsomes; the number of demethylases and their molecular differentiation is at present unknown.

IV. Mechanism of Microsomal N-Dealkylation

1. Cytochrome P-450

The central role of cytochrome P-450 in microsomal drug metabolism is well established and is described elsewhere in this volume (see Chapter 38). Briefly, carbon monoxide (CO) inhibits the N-demethylation of monomethyl-4-aminoantipyrine, the O-demethylation of codeine, and the metabolism of many other foreign compounds by enzymes in hepatic microsomes. This inhibition can be partially reversed by monochromatic light; maximum reversal is produced by light of 450 nm wavelength. The CO complex of reduced cytochrome P-450 has an intense absorption maximum at 450 nm. Accordingly, reversal of the CO-inhibition of microsomal enzymes by light at 450 nm is thought to result from photo-dissociation of the cytochrome P-450-CO complex (COOPER et al., 1965). Recently, the microsomal system of rabbit liver was solubilized and resolved into 3 components, one of which is cytochrome P-450 (LU et al., 1969). Reconstitution of the system revealed an absolute requirement for cytochrome P-450.

A current conception of electron transfer in hepatic microsomes appears in Fig. 3.

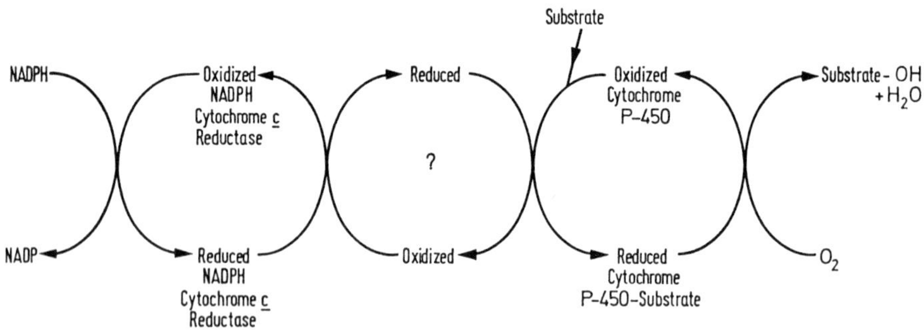

Fig. 3. A schematic representation of the electron transport chain in hepatic microsomes

2. N-Oxide Formation

Many nitrogenous drugs undergo N-oxidation. For example, N-oxides of the following compounds have been isolated and characterized; chlorpromazine (FISHMAN et al., 1962; COCCIA and WESTERFELD, 1967), chlorcyclizine (KUNTZMAN et al., 1967), imipramine (FISHMAN and GOLDENBERG, 1962; BICKEL and BAGGIOLINI, 1966), nicotinamide (CHAYKIN et al., 1965), guanethidine (ABRAMSON et al., 1969), N,N-dimethylaniline (ZIEGLER and PETTIT, 1964), and trimethylamine (BAKER and CHAYKIN, 1962). The biochemistry and pharmacology of N-oxides has been recently reviewed by BICKEL (1969).

ZIEGLER and PETTIT (1964) proposed that N,N-dimethylaniline-N-oxide was an intermediate in the conversion of N,N-dimethylaniline to monomethylaniline by microsomal enzymes. This proposal was based on the finding that the rate of demethylation (formaldehyde liberation) of the N-oxide was greater than that of

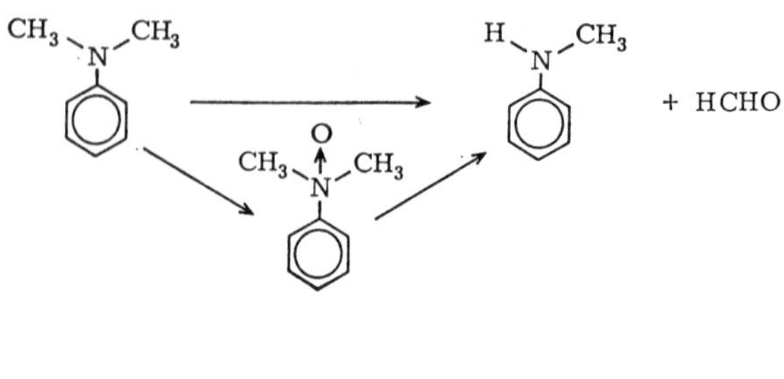

N,N-dimethylaniline (PETTIT and ZIEGLER, 1963). Subsequently it was recognized that the reaction had two distinct components (ZIEGLER and PETTIT, 1966; MACHINIST et al., 1966):

1. N,N-dimethylanine → N,N-dimethylaniline-N-oxide
2. N,N-dimethylaniline-N-oxide → N-methylaniline + HCHO

For example, reaction 2 requires NADPH while reaction 1 proceeds as readily with NADH. Reaction 2 is strongly inhibited by CO, suggesting the participation of cytochrome P-450, whereas reaction 1 is unaffected by CO. Finally, reaction 2 is very sensitive to detergents, sonication, and SKF 525-A whereas reaction 1 is resistant to these treatments.

There is considerable doubt as to the general applicability of the proposal that N-oxides are intermediates in microsomal N-dealkylation. Although ZIEGLER and PETTIT (1964) found that the rat liver microsomes demethylate N,N-dimethylaniline-N-oxide more rapidly than N,N-dimethylaniline, GILLETTE (1966) found the reverse to be the case with rabbit liver microsomes, i.e., the N-oxide was demethylated relatively slowly. Similarly, McMAHON and SULLIVAN (1964) found that the rate of demethylation of *l*-propoxyphene was one to two orders of magnitude greater than that of *l*-propoxyphene-N-oxide. In a highly definitive experiment, McMAHON and SULLIVAN (1964) incubated *l*-propoxyphene (N-methyl-^{14}C) with microsomes, NADPH, and excess nonradioactive *l*-propoxyphene-N-oxide; essentially no radioactivity was incorporated into the N-oxide pool despite extensive demethylation of ^{14}C-*l*-propoxyphene thus ruling out the intermediacy of an N-oxide in the demethylation of this substrate. Therefore, in sum, although N-oxides are undoubtedly involved in the total metabolic fate of many drugs, they are not obligatory intermediates in microsomal N-dealkylation reactions (McMAHON et al., 1969).

3. Isotope Effects on Microsomal Dealkylation

In an effort to obtain information on the chemical nature of enzymic demethylation, investigators have sought possible isotope effects. For example, ELISON et al. (1961, 1963) compared the rates of demethylation of morphine (R—NH—CH_3) and trideuterio-N-methyl morphine (R—NH—CD_3) by rat liver microsomes. The rate of demethylation of the deuterated substrate was slightly less than that of the hydrogenated material; the ratio of the rates (H/D) (V_{max}) was 1.4. The apparent K_m for the demethylation of morphine was 0.39 mM while that for deuterio-morphine was 0.57 mM implying that the deuterated compound had about 40% less affinity for enzyme. MITOMA et al. (1967) studied the relative rates of O-demethylation of o-nitroanisole and its deuterated analogue by rabbit liver microsomes and found that deuteration reduced the rate of O-demethylation by about 50%. In contrast to the findings of ELISON et al. (1961, 1963), however, deuteration of o-nitroanisole appeared to increase the affinity of enzyme for substrate by approxomately 60%. Finally, FOREMAN et al. (1969) compared the rates of deamination of *l*-amphetamine and deuterio-*l*-amphetamine by rabbit liver microsomes and found that deuterium decreased the rate of deamination (H/D = 1.9). Taken together, the data indicate that the presence of deuterium in the substrate reduces the rate of metabolism (H/D morphine = 1.4; o-nitroanisole = 2.0; *l*-amphetamine = 1.9). However, in no case did the magnitude of the isotope effect approach 6.9, the maximum value of the deuterium isotope effect (WIBERG, 1955) indicating that rupture of the C-H (C-D) bond is not the rate-limiting step in microsomal dealkylation reactions.

V. Stereospecificity in N-Dealkylation

The N-dealkylation of foreign compounds by microsomal enzymes is attended by significant stereospecificity which is rather surprising in view of the general lack of specificity of the microsomal system. In general, *l*-isomers are the preferred substrates (Table 6). Curiously, this stereospecificity is reversed in the case of hexobarbital metabolism by rat liver microsomes (DEGKWITZ et al., 1969), and the *d*-isomer is metabolized about twice as rapidly as the *l*-isomer. FURNER et al. (1969) confirmed this finding in microsomes from male rats but found no corresponding stereospecificity in microsomes from female rats.

Table 6. *Stereospecificity of hepatic microsomal enzymes*

Compound	Microsomal source	Relative activity	Reference
l-ephedrine	rabbit	150	AXELROD (1955a)
d-ephedrine	rabbit	11	—
l-amphetamine	rabbit	100	AXELROD (1955a)
d-amphetamine	rabbit	27	—
l-3-hydroxy-N-methylmorphinan	rat	75	AXELROD (1956b)
d-3-hydroxy-N-methylmorphinan	rat	25	—
l-3-methoxy-N-methylmorphinan	rat	280	AXELROD (1956b)
d-3-methoxy-N-methylmorphinan	rat	160	—
l-methadone	rat	130	AXELROD (1956b)
d-methadone	rat	60	—
l-3-methoxy-N-methylmorphinan	mouse	206	TAKEMORI and MANNERING (1958)
d-3-methoxy-N-methylmorphinan	mouse	102	
l-(—)-hexobarbital	rat	4	DEGKWITZ et al. (1969)
d-(+)-hexobarbital	rat	8	

VI. Fate of Aldehydes Formed during Metabolic Dealkylation of Drugs

A general reaction for dealkylations may be written as:

$$R—X—CH_2—R' \rightarrow R—X + R'—CHO$$

If X represents N or O, the amines and alcohols produced are readily cleared from the animal body, either in the free or conjugated state.

MILLER et al. (1952) observed that following administration of 3'-methyl-4-dimethyl-^{14}C-aminoazobenzene (3'-methyl-DAB) to rats, about 60% of the radioactivity was expired as $^{14}CO_2$. More recently, NEELY (1964) showed that following the administration of formaldehyde-^{14}C to rats, about 82% of the dose was excreted in the expired air as $^{14}CO_2$. Radioactivity also appeared in urine as methionine-^{14}C and serine-^{14}C. It is of interest in this regard that MILLER et al. (1952) reported long-term retention of about 10% of the total radioactivity after administering 3'-methyl-DAB-^{14}C to rats. Total body analysis revealed that the residual radioactivity was localized in the β carbon atom of serine and the trimethylamine portion of choline. If rats were made folic acid deficient, the incorporation of radioactivity from 3'-methyl-DAB-^{14}C into endogenous serine and choline was markedly depressed. These findings suggest that one-carbon fragments formed during the demethylation of foreign compounds *in vivo* may enter the endogenous one-carbon fragment pool to be utilized in the biosynthesis of serine, choline, methionine and purines through the participation of folic acid and presumably vitamin B_{12}.

B. O-Dealkylation

The metabolic O-dealkylation of foreign compounds in intact rats and by homogenates of rat liver and kidney was reported by HUGGINS et al. in 1948. Subsequently, a significant number of drugs have been shown to undergo O-dealkylation (Table 7). AXELROD (1956a) showed metabolic O-dealkylation to be localized in the microsomal fraction of mammalian liver, to require NADPH and oxygen, and to possess a broad substrate spectrum.

Table 7. *Drugs which undergo metabolic O-dealkylation*

Compound	Reference
Codeine	AXELROD (1955c)
Norcodeine	AXELROD (1955c)
Thebaine	AXELROD (1955c)
Phenacetin (p-ethoxyacetanilide)	AXELROD (1956a)
p-methoxyacetanilide	AXELROD (1956a)
Griseofulvin	SYMCHOWICZ and WONG (1966a, b)
Dextromethorphan	TAKEMORI and MANNERING (1958) KAMM et al. (1967)
p-nitroanisole	HUGGINS et al. (1948), NETTER and SEIDEL (1964)

I. Relationship of the O-Alkyl Substituent to the Rate of Dealkylation

As was the case for N-dealkylation, the rate of O-dealkylation in a homologous series is inversely proportional to the length of the alkyl group removed. For example, MCMAHON et al. (1963a) showed that the rate of O-dealkylation (V_{max}) by rat liver microsomes was highest for the methyl derivative and decreased through the ethyl, n-propyl, and n-butyl analogues (Table 8). The apparent K_m in this series decreased in proportion to increasing length of the alkyl group (Table 8) which is what one would predict if lipid solubility were a major determinant in the affinity of substrate for the microsomal enzyme. CREAVEN and associates (CREAVEN et al., 1967; DAVIES and CREAVEN, 1967) studying a series of substituted hydroxybiphenyl derivatives, showed progressively decreasing rates of microsomal O-dealkylation as the alkyl substituent was increased from methyl through n-butyl.

Table 8. *Kinetics of the O-dealkylation of some p-nitrophenyl ethers by rat liver microsomes*

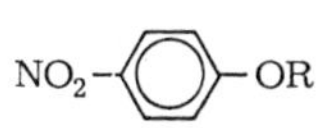

R	V_{max} (nmoles/min/g liver)	K_m (mM)
Methyl	143	16.7
Ethyl	72	0.7
n-propyl	34	0.6
n-butyl	8	0.4

Data from MCMAHON et al. (1963a)

II. Mechanism of Microsomal O-Dealkylation

The role of cytochrome P-450 in O-dealkylation was alluded to above and will not be discussed further here.

In the presence of NADPH and oxygen, hepatic microsomes catalyze O-dealkylation of ethers such as p-methoxyacetanilide (Fig. 4) (AXELROD, 1956a). RENSON et al. (1965) suggested that this reaction could be envisioned either as a cleavage of the oxygen-methyl bond (Fig. 4) (at 1) or displacement of the entire

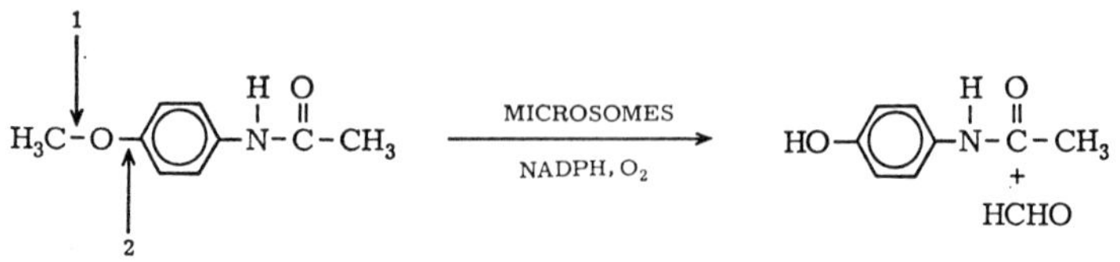

Fig. 4. O-demethylation of p-methoxyacetanilide by microsomal enzymes. RENSON et al. (1965) proposed that demethylation could occur either through cleavage of the oxygen-methyl carbon bond (at 1) or by displacement of the entire methoxy group by an incoming hydroxylating species (at 2). The data indicate that the microsomal attack occurs at position 1

methoxy group by an incoming hydroxylating species (at 2). To resolve this question, they studied the microsomal O-demethylase reaction in the presence of $^{18}O_2$ or $H_2{}^{18}O$ with regard to isotope incorporation into the metabolic product p-hydroxyacetanilide. Insignificant ^{18}O incorporation occurred in the presence of either $^{18}O_2$ or $H_2{}^{18}O$. By contrast, incubation of acetanilide with $^{18}O_2$, microsomes, and NADPH led to extensive labeling (95% of theoretical) of the product p-hydroxyacetanilide. Thus, microsomal O-demethylation was not accompanied by displacement of the intact methoxy group by an incoming oxygen species but rather by direct oxidative attack upon the methyl group (Fig. 4, at 1).

C. S-Dealkylation

The literature on metabolic S-dealkylation of foreign compounds is extremely limited. 6-Methylmercaptopurine was reported to be S-demethylated by intact rats in 1960 (SARCIONE and STUTZMAN, 1960). Subsequently, MAZEL and coworkers (1964) demonstrated that S-demethylases were localized in the microsomal fraction of liver, required NADPH and oxygen and lacked substrate specificity. 6-Methylthiopurine, methylthiopseudourea, methylmercaptan, and methylthiobenzothiazole were shown to undergo S-demethylation *in vitro*. Microsomal S-demethylases are thought to be somewhat unique in their requirement for hepatic soluble fraction; this requirement cannot be fulfilled by a NADPH-generating system (MAZEL, 1969).

D. Summary

An enormous amount of information has accumulated in the past 15 years dealing with the metabolism of exogenous compounds by hepatic microsomal enzymes. In addition to direct contributions to pharmacology, such as the characterization of factors which terminate drug action, drug interactions, and evaluation of chronic toxicity studies, research in drug metabolism has exerted important influences in related areas such as the mechanism of biological hydroxylation and the biosynthesis of intracellular membranes. It is hoped that future work in drug metabolism will have even broader relevance to pharmacology, biochemistry, physiology and cell biology.

References

Abramson, F.B., Furst, C.I., McMartin, C., Wade, R.: The isolation, identification and synthesis of two metabolites of guanethidine formed in pig and rabbit liver homogenates. Biochem. J. **113**, 143—156 (1969).

Adler, T.K.: Studies on morphine tolerance in mice. I. *In vivo* N-demethylation of morphine and N- and O- demethylation of codeine. J. Pharmacol. exp. Ther. **156**, 585—590 (1967).

Albert, J.R., Boxill, G.C., Weikel, J.H.: Anticonvulsant and toxicologic properties of some benzilic amides and the physiological disposition of the N-ethyl derivative. J. Pharmacol. exp. Ther. **131**, 85—90 (1961).

Anders, M.W., Alvares, A.P., Mannering, G.J.: Inhibition of drug metabolism. II. Metabolism of 2-diethylaminoethyl 2,2-diphenylvalerate HCl (SKF 525-A). Molec. Pharmacol. **2**, 328—334 (1966).

Axelrod, J.: The enzymatic deamination of amphetamine (Benzedrine). J. biol. Chem. **214**, 753—763 (1955a).

— The enzymatic demethylation of ephedrine. J. Pharmacol. exp. Ther. **114**, 430—438 (1955b).

— The enzymatic conversion of codeine to morphine. J. Pharmacol. exp. Ther. **115**, 259—267 (1955c).

— The enzymic cleavage of aromatic ethers. Biochem. J. **63**, 634—639 (1956a).

— The enzymatic N-demethylation of narcotic drugs. J. Pharmacol. exp. Ther. **117**, 322—330 (1956b).

— Cochin, J.: The inhibitory action of nalorphine on the enzymatic N-demethylation of narcotic drugs. J. Pharmacol. exp. Ther. **121**, 107—112 (1957).

Baker, J.R., Chaykin, S.: The biosynthesis of trimethylamine-N-oxide. J. biol. Chem. **237**, 1309—1313 (1962).

Beckett, A.H., Beaven, M.A., Robinson, A.E.: Metabolism of chlorpromazine in humans. Biochem. Pharmacol. **12**, 779—794 (1963).

Bickel, M.H.: The pharmacology and biochemistry of N-oxides. Pharmacol. Rev. **21**, 325—355 (1969).

— Baggiolini, M., The metabolism of imipramine and its metabolites by rat liver microsomes. Biochem. Pharmacol. **15**, 1155—1169 (1966).

— Flückinger, M., Baggiolini, M.: Vergleichende Demethylierung von tricyclischen Psychopharmaka durch Rattenlebermikrosomen. Naunyn-Schmiedebergs Arch. exp. Path. Pharmak. **256**, 360—366 (1967).

Brodie, B.B., Gillette, J.R., La Du, B.N.: Enzymatic metabolism of drugs and other foreign compounds. Ann. Rev. Biochem. **27**, 427—454 (1958).

— Maickel, R.P.: Comparative biochemistry of drug metabolism. In: Proceedings of the First International Pharmacological Meeting. Ed. by B.B. Brodie and E. G. Erdos. Vol. 6, pp. 299—324. New York: MacMillan 1962.

Buhler, D.R., Rasmusson, M.E.: The oxidation of drugs by fishes. Comp. Biochem. Physiol. **25**, 223—239 (1968).

Butler, T.C., Waddell, W.J.: The metabolic fate of 5-ethyl-1-methyl-5-phenyl hydantoin (1-methylnirvanol) and that of 3,5-diethyl-5-phenyl hydantoin (3-ethylnirvanol). J. Pharmacol. exp. Ther. **127**, 171—174 (1959).

— — Poole, D.T.: Demethylation of trimethadione and metharbital by rat liver microsomal enzymes. Biochem. Pharmacol. **14**, 937—942 (1965).

Chakraborty, J., Smith, J.N.: Enzymic oxidation of some alkylbenzenes in insects and vertebrates. Biochem. J. **102**, 498—503 (1967).

Chaykin, S., Dagani, M., Johnson, L., Samli, M.: The fate of nicotinamide in the mouse: urinary metabolites. J. biol. Chem. **240**, 932—938 (1965).

Coccia, P.F., Westerfeld, W.W.: The metabolism of chlorpromazine by liver microsomal enzyme systems. J. Pharmacol. exp. Ther. **157**, 446—458 (1967).

Conney, A.H.: Pharmacological implications of microsomal enzyme induction. Pharmacol. Rev. **19**, 317—366 (1967).

Cooper, D.Y., Levin, S., Narasimhulu, S., Rosenthal, O., Estabrook, R.W.: Photochemical action spectrum of the terminal oxidase of mixed function oxidase systems. Science **147**, 400—402 (1965).

Creaven, P.J., Davies, W.H., Williams, R.T.: Dealkylation of alkoxybiphenyls by trout and frog liver preparations. Life Sci. **6**, 105—111 (1967).

Davies, D.S., Gigon, P.L., Gillette, J.R.: Sex differences in the kinetic constants for the N-demethylation of ethylmorphine by rat liver microsomes. Biochem. Pharmacol. **17**, 1865—1872 (1968).

Davies, W.H., Creaven, P.J.: The effect of carcinogenic and noncarcinogenic compounds on the O-dealkylating activity of the hepatic microsomal enzyme system of the rat. Biochem. Pharmacol. **16**, 1839—1845 (1967).

DEGKWITZ, E., ULLRICH, V., STAUDINGER HJ.: Metabolism and cytochrome P-450 binding spectra of (+) and (—) hexobarbital in rat liver microsomes. Hoppe-Seylers Z. physiol. Chem. **350**, 547—553 (1969).
DEWAIDE, J. H., HENDERSON, P. T.: Hepatic N-demethylation of aminopyrine in rat and trout. Biochem. Pharmacol. **17**, 1901—1907 (1968).
DINGELL, J. V.: Personal communication (1970).
— D'ENCARNACAO, P. W.: Studies on the demethylation of secondary and tertiary amines. Pharmacologist **8**, 181 (1966).
— SULSER, F., GILLETTE, J.R.: Species differences in metabolism of impramine and desmethylimipramine. J. Pharmacol. exp. Ther. **143**, 14—22 (1964).
ELISON, C., ELLIOT, H.W.: Studies on the enzymatic N- and O-demethylation of narcotic analogesics and evidence for the formation of codeine from morphine in rats and dogs. J. Pharmacol. exp. Ther. **144**, 265—275 (1964).
— — LOOK, M., RAPOPORT, H.: Some aspects of the fate and relationship of the N-methyl group of morphine to its pharmacological activity. J. med. pharm. Chem. **6**, 237—246 (1963).
— RAPAPORT, H., LAURSEN, R., ELLIOT, H.W.: Effect of deuteration of N-CH_3 group on potency and enzymatic N-demethylation of morphine. Science **134**, 1078—1079 (1961).
EMMERSON, J. L., ANDERSON, R. C.: Metabolism of trifluralin in the rat and dog. Toxicol. appl. Pharmacol. **9**, 84—97 (1966).
FISHMAN, V., GOLDENBERG, H.: Identification of a new metabolite of imipramine. Proc. Soc. exp. Biol. (N.Y.) **110**, 187—190 (1962).
— HEATON, A., GOLDENBERG, H.: Metabolism of chlorpromazine. III. Isolation and identification of chlorpromazine-N-oxide. Proc. Soc. exp. Biol. (N.Y.) **109**, 548—552 (1962).
FOREMAN, R. L. SIEGEL F. P., MRTEK, R. G.: Synthesis of deuterio-*l*-amphetamine, *d*, sulfate. J. pharm. Sci. **58**, 189—192 (1969).
FREAR, D. S.: Microsomal N-demethylation, by a cotton leaf oxidase system, of 3-(4′-chlorophenyl)-1,1-dimethylurea (Monuron). Science **162**, 674—675 (1968).
FURNER, R. L., MCCARTHY, J. S., STITZEL, R. E., ANDERS, M. W.: Stereoselective metabolism of the enantiomers of hexobarbital. J. Pharmacol. exp. Ther. **169**, 153—158 (1969).
GAUDETTE, L. E., BRODIE, B. B.: Relationship between the lipid solubility of drugs and their oxidation by liver microsomes. Biochem. Pharmacol. **2**, 89—96 (1959).
GILLETTE, J. R.: Biochemistry of drug oxidation and reduction by enzymes in hepatic endoplasmic reticulum. In: Advances in Pharmacology, vol. 4, pp. 219—261. Ed. by S. GARATTINI and P. A. SHORE. New York: Academic Press 1966.
— DINGELL, J. V., SULSER, F., KUNTZMAN, R., BRODIE, B. B.: Isolation from rat brain of a metabolic product, desmethylimipramine, that mediates the antidepressant activity of imipramine. Experientia (Basel) **17**, 377—381 (1961).
GRAM, T. E., WILSON, J. T., FOUTS, J. R.: Some characteristics of hepatic microsomal systems which metabolize aminopyrine in the rat and rabbit. J. Pharmacol. exp. Ther. **159**, 172—181 (1968).
GUARINO, A. M., CONWAY, W. D., FALES, H. M.: Mass spectral identification of probenecid metabolites in rat bile. Europ. J. Pharmacol. **8**, 244—252 (1969).
HENDERSON, J. F., MAZEL, P.: Studies of the induction of microsomal S-, N-, and O-demethylases. Biochem. Pharmacol. **13**, 1471—1474 (1964).
HESPE, W., DE ROOS, A. M., NAUTA, W. T.: Investigation into the metabolic fate of orphenadrene hydrochloride after oral administration to male rats. Arch. int. Pharmacodyn. **156**, 180—200 (1965).
HUGGINS, C., JENSEN, E. V., CLEVELAND, A. S.: On phenyletherase. Proc. Soc. exp. Biol. (N.Y.) **68**, 477—480 (1948).
KAMM, J. J., FERULLO, C. R., MILLER, D., VAN LOON, E. J.: Metabolism of chlorpheniramine-^3H by the rat and dog. Biochem. Pharmacol. **18**, 659—671 (1969).
— TADDEO, A. B., VAN LOON, E. J.: Metabolism and excretion of tritiated dextromethorphan by the rat. J. Pharmacol. exp. Ther. **158**, 437—444 (1967).
KATO, R., GILLETTE, J. R.: Effect of starvation on NADPH-dependent enzymes in liver microsomes of male and female rats. J. Pharmacol. exp. Ther. **150**, 279—284 (1965).
KLUTCH, A., BORDUN, M.: Metabolic fate of methoxamine and N-isopropylmethoxamine. J. med. pharm. Chem. **10**, 860—863 (1967).
KOE, B. K., PINSON, R.: Isolation and characterization of urinary metabolites of benzquinamide and benzquinamide alcohol. J. med. pharm. Chem. **7**, 635—640 (1964).
KRATZ, F., STAUDINGER, HJ.: Zur Frage der Induzierbarkeit mikrosomaler Enzyme am Beispiel der Cumarinhydroxylierung in der Kaninchenleber. Hoppe-Seylers Z. physiol. Chem. **348**, 568—574 (1967).
KUNTZMAN, R., KLUTCH, A., TSAI, I., BURNS, J. J.: Physiological distribution and metabolic inactivation of chlorcyclizine and cyclizine. J. Pharmacol. exp. Ther. **149**, 29—35 (1965).

KUNTZMANN, R., PHILLIPS, A., TSAI, I., KLUTCH, A., BURNS, J.J.: N-Oxide formation: A new route for inactivation of the antihistaminic chlorcyclizine. J. Pharmacol. exp. Ther. **155**, 337—344 (1967).

LA DU, B.N., GAUDETTE, L., TROUSOF, N., BRODIE, B.B.: Enzymatic dealkylation of aminopyrine (Pyramidon) and other alkylamines. J. biol. Chem. **214**, 741—752 (1955).

LEADSEATER, L., DAVIES, D.R.: The inhibition of the liver microsomal N-demethylation of morphine by N-allylnormorphine and its pharmacological implications. Biochem. Pharmacol. **13**, 1569—1576 (1964).

LIN, S.C.C., WAY, E.L.: N-dealkylation of anileridine to normeperidine. J. Pharmacol. exp. Ther. **150**, 309—315 (1965).

LU, A.Y.H., JUNK, K.W., COON, M.J.: Resolution of the cytochrome P-450 containing ω-hydroxylation system of liver microsomes into three components. J. biol. Chem. **244**, 3714—3721 (1969).

MACHINIST, J.M., ORME-JOHNSON, W.H., ZIEGLER, D.M.: Microsomal oxidases. II. Properties of a pork liver microsomal N-oxide dealkylase. Biochemistry **5**, 2939—2943 (1966).

MANNERING, G.J., SCHANKER, L.S.: Metabolic fate of levo-3-hydroxy-N-alkylmorphinan (levallophan). J. Pharmacol. exp. Ther. **124**, 296—304 (1958).

MAO, J.C.H., TARDREW, P.L.: Demethylation of erythromycins by rabbit tissue *in vitro*. Biochem. Pharmacol. **14**, 1049—1058 (1965).

MAZEL, P.: Personal communication (1969).

— HENDERSON, J.F., AXELROD, J.: S-demethylation by microsomal enzymes. J. Pharmacol. exp. Ther. **143**, 1—6 (1964).

— KERZA-KWIATECKI, A., SIMANIS, J.: Studies on the demethylation of puromycin and related compounds by liver microsomal enzymes. Biochim. biophys. Acta (Amst.) **114**, 72—82 (1966).

MCMAHON, R.E.: The metabolism of 2-(butylaminomethyl)-1,4-benzodioxane-^{14}C. J. Amer. chem. Soc. **81**, 5199—5201 (1959).

— The metabolism of chlorethoxybutamoxane-^{14}C. J. Pharmacol. exp. Ther. **130**, 383—388 (1960).

— The competitive inhibition of the N-demethylation of butynamine by 2,4-dichloro-6-phenylphenoxyethylamine (DPEA). J. Pharmacol. exp. Ther. **138**, 382—386 (1962).

— The demethylation *in vitro* of N-methyl barbiturates and related compounds by mammalian liver microsomes. Biochem. Pharmacol. **12**, 1225—1228 (1963).

— Some observations on the *in vitro* demethylation of secondary N-methyl amines by liver microsomes. Life Sci. **3**, 235—241 (1964).

— Microsomal dealkylation of drugs: substrate specificity and mechanism. J. pharm. Sci. **55**, 457—466 (1966).

— CULP, H.W., MARSHALL, F.J.: The metabolism of *a-dl*-acetylmethadol in the rat. The identification of the probable active metabolite. J. Pharmacol. exp. Ther. **149**, 436—445 (1965).

— — MILLS, J., MARSHALL, F.J.: Demethylation studies. IV. The *in vitro* and *in vivo* cleavage of alkyl and arylalkyl-p-nitrophenyl ethers. J. med. pharm. Chem. **6**, 343—346 (1963a).

— — OCCOLOWITZ, J.C.: Studies on the hepatic microsomal N-dealkylation reaction. Molecular oxygen as the source of the oxygen atom. J. Amer. chem. Soc. **91**, 3389—3390 (1969).

— MARSHALL, F.J., CULP, H.W., MILLER, W.M.: The metabolism of nortriptyline-N-methyl-^{14}C in rats. Biochem. Pharmacol. **12**, 1207—1217 (1963b).

— SULLIVAN, H.R.: The oxidative demethylation of *l*-propoxyphene and *l*-propoxyphene-N-oxide by rat liver microsomes. Life Sci. **3**, 1167—1174 (1964).

— WELLES, J.S., LEE, H.M.: The metabolism of benzodioxane derivatives. II. Ethoxybutamoxane-^{14}C. J. Amer. chem. Soc. **82**, 2864—2866 (1960).

MILLER, E.C., PLESCIA, A.M., MILLER, J.A., HEIDELBERGER, C.: The metabolism of methylated aminoazo dyes. I. The demethylation of 3′-methyl-4-dimethyl-^{14}C-aminoazobenzene *in vivo*. J. biol. Chem. **196**, 863—874 (1952).

MITOMA, C., YASUDA, D.M., TAGG, J., TANABE, M.: Effect of deuteration of the O-CH_3 group on the enzymic demethylation of o-nitroanisole. Biochim. biophys. Acta (Amst.) **136**, 566—567 (1967).

MUELLER, G.C., MILLER, J.A.: The metabolism of methylated aminoazo dyes. II. Oxidative demethylation by rat liver homogenates. J. biol. Chem. **202**, 579—587 (1953).

MULE, S.J., CLEMENTS, T.H., GORODETZKY, C.W.: The metabolic fate of ^{3}H-cyclazocine in dogs. J. Pharmacol. exp. Ther. **160**, 387—396 (1968).

NARROD, S.A., WILK, A.L., KING, C.T.G.: Metabolism of meclizine in the rat. J. Pharmacol. exp. Ther. **147**, 380—384 (1965).

NEELY, W.B.: The metabolic fate of formaldehyde-^{14}C intraperitoneally administered to the rat. Biochem. Pharmacol. **13**, 1137—1142 (1964).

NETTER, K.J., SEIDEL, G.: An adaptively stimulated O-demethylating system in rat liver microsomes and its kinetic properties. J. Pharmacol. exp. Ther. **146**, 61—65 (1964).
PETTIT, F.H., ZIEGLER, D.M.: The catalytic demethylation of N,N-dimethylaniline-N-oxide by liver microsomes. Biochem. biophys. Res. Commun. **13**, 193—197 (1963).
RENSON, J., WEISSBACH, H., UDENFRIEND, S.: On the mechanism of oxidative cleavage of aryl-alkyl ethers by liver microsomes. Molec. Pharmacol. **1**, 145—148 (1965).
SARCIONE, E.J., STUTZMAN, L.: A comparison of the metabolism of 6-mercaptopurine and its 6-methyl analog in the rat. Cancer Res. **20**, 387—392 (1960).
SCHENKMAN, J.B., FREY, I., REMMER, H., ESTABROOK, R.W.: Sex differences in drug metabolism by rat liver microsomes. Molec. Pharmacol. **3**, 516—525 (1967).
SCHREIBER, E.C., MIN, B.H., ZEIGER, A.V., LONG, J.F.: Metabolism of diethylpropion-1-^{14}C hydrochloride by the human. J. Pharmacol. exp. Ther. **159**, 372—378 (1968).
SCHWARTZ, M.A., KOECHLIN, B.A., POSTMA, E., PALMER, S., KROL, G.: Metabolism of diazepam in rat, dog, and man. J. Pharmacol. exp. Ther. **149**, 423—435 (1965).
— POSTMA, E.: Metabolic N-demethylation of chlordiazepoxide. J. pharm. Sci. **55**, 1358—1362 (1966).
SLADEK, N.E., MANNERING, G.J.: Induction of drug metabolism. Molec. Pharmacol. **5**, 174—185 (1969).
SMITH, D.L., KEASLING, H.H., FORIST, A.A.: The metabolism of N-alkyl-4-bromobenzene-sulfonamides in the mouse. J. med. pharm. Chem. **8**, 520—524 (1965).
SMITH, J.N.: Detoxication mechanisms. Ann. Rev. Entomol. **7**, 465—480 (1962).
SYMCHOWICZ, S., WONG, K.K.: Metabolism of griseofulvin-^{14}C; studies *in vivo*. Biochem. Pharmacol. **15**, 1595—1600 (1966a).
— — Metabolism griseofulvin-^{14}C; studies *in vitro*. Biochem. Pharmacol. **15**, 1601—1606 (1966b).
TAKEMORI, A.E., MANNERING, G.J.: Metabolic N- and O-demethylation of morphine- and morphinan-type analgesics. J. Pharmacol. exp. Ther. **123**, 171—179 (1958).
VREE, T.B., VAN ROSSUM, J.M.: Kinetics of metabolism and excretion of amphetamines in man. In: International Symposium on Amphetamines and Related Compounds. Eds. E. COSTA and S. GARATTINI, pp. 165—190. New York: Raven Press 1970.
WELLES, J.S., ROOT, M.A., ANDERSON, R.C.: Urinary metabolites of chlorpropamide in dogs, rabbits and man. Proc. Soc. exp. Biol. (N.Y.) **101**, 668—671 (1959).
WIBERG, K.B.: The deuterium isotope effect. Chem. Rev. **55**, 713—743 (1955).
ZIEGLER, D.M., PETTIT, F.H.: Formation of an intermediate N-oxide in the oxidative demethylation of N,N-dimethylaniline catalyzed by liver microsomes. Biochem. biophys. Res. Commun. **15**, 188—193 (1964).
— — Microsomal oxidases. I. The isolation and dialkylarylamine oxygenase activity of pork liver microsomes. Biochemistry **5**, 2932—2938 (1966).
ZINS, G.R.: The *in vivo* production of a potent long-acting hypotensive metabolite from diallylmelamine. J. Pharmacol. exp. Ther. **150**, 109—117 (1965).

Chapter 42

Reductive Enzymes

JAMES R. GILLETTE

With 6 Figures

A. Introduction

Studies on the fate of azo and nitro compounds in the body have had a profound influence on the fields of chemotherapy, toxicology, and drug metabolism. For example, recognition that Prontosil was reductively cleaved to sulfanilamide in the body (TRÉFOUËL et al., 1935) led to the development of a large series of sulfa drugs, as well as to the realization that substances which possess little biological activity *in vitro* may be transformed in the body to substances which exert potent therapeutic effects. Drugs may also undergo biotransformation to toxic derivatives. For example, it is now accepted that methemoglobinemia caused by certain aromatic nitro compounds and aromatic amines arises from the corresponding phenylhydroxy and nitroso compounds formed by the reduction of the nitro compounds or the *N*-hydroxylation of the amines. It is also now believed that the hepatomas caused by various azo dyes, including butter yellow, are mediated by *N*-hydroxylated metabolites.

Despite the importance of azo and nitro reduction, the nature of these processes remains controversial. It should be recognized, however, that studies of these processes incur problems which ordinarily do not arise with other pathways of drug metabolism. Some azo and nitro compounds may be nonenzymatically reduced to amines by biological reducing agents, such as NADPH, NADH, and reduced flavins. Other azo and nitro compounds are reduced to primary amines by way of intermediates which are autooxidized, and formation of the primary amine metabolites is thus blocked by the presence of oxygen. Azo and nitro compounds may also be reduced by a variety of enzyme systems; some of these compounds are reduced by gut bacteria but not by mammalian enzymes. The interplay among the various enzyme systems and between the relative rates of reduction and reoxidation of the intermediates has thus made it difficult to determine which mechanisms are important in living animals.

B. Reduction of Nitro Compounds

I. Enzymatic Mechanisms in Liver

FOUTS and BRODIE (1957) reported the presence of enzyme systems in liver that convert aromatic nitro compounds, such as chloramphenicol, *p*-nitrobenzoate and nitrobenzene, to the corresponding amines. These reactions, which utilize NADH or NADPH, presumably occur as shown in Fig. 1. These authors reported, however, that the reaction readily occurred under anaerobic conditions, but was inhibited by oxygen. At least a part of the sensitivity to oxygen is due to autooxidation of the phenylhydroxylamine derivatives to nitroso derivatives. The nitroso derivatives may be reduced again to the corresponding phenylhydroxylamine

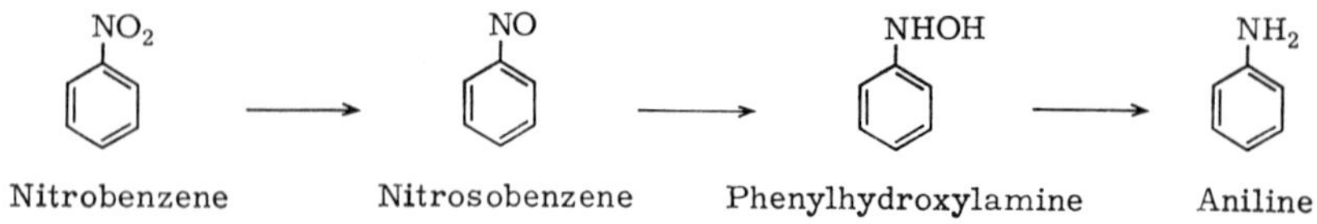

Fig. 1. Pathway of nitrobenzene reduction to aniline

enzymatically (KIESE, 1965) and nonenzymatically, the relative rates depending on the concentration of NADPH (GILLETTE, 1965). This cyclic process of oxidation and reduction presumably leads to the intracellular depletion of NADPH when the NADPH-generating systems are inadequate to maintain the cofactor in its reduced form.

FOUTS and BRODIE (1957) originally reported that the NADPH-dependent nitro reductase activity was distributed about equally between the soluble and microsomal fractions. Subsequently, GILLETTE et al. (1968) showed that formation of the primary amine from *p*-nitrobenzoate occurred almost exclusively in the microsomal fraction. The reaction was found to be catalyzed by the carbon monoxide (CO) sensitive hemoprotein, cytochrome P-450 (GILLETTE et al., 1968). This conclusion was based on the following evidence: a) CO blocks the formation of *p*-aminobenzoate in proportion to the amount of cytochrome P-450 bound as the CO complex; in addition CO blocks the oxidation of NADPH elicited by *p*-nitrobenzoic acid under anaerobic conditions. b) Changes in the rate of *p*-aminobenzoic acid formation are proportional to the increase in cytochrome P-450 content after prior treatment with phenobarbital and to the decrease in cytochrome P-450 content after prior treatment with CCl_4. c) Substances, such as SKF 525-A, hexobarbital and ethylmorphine, that combine with cytochrome P-450 to cause type I spectral changes (see Chapter 38) and stimulate cytochrome P-450 reduction (GIGON et al., 1969) also enhance the reduction of *p*-nitrobenzoic acid (SASAME and GILLETTE, 1969); whereas substances, such as SKF 26754-A and DPEA (Fig. 2), that cause type II spectral changes with cytochrome P-450 and slow the rate of cytochrome P-450 reduction (GIGON et al., 1969) decrease the rate of *p*-nitrobenzoic acid reduction (SASAME and GILLETTE, 1969). Moreover, the inhibition constants for the reduction of *p*-nitrobenzoate by the various type II substances are almost identical to the dissociation constants of their cytochrome P-450 complexes as measured spectrophotometrically (SASAME and GILLETTE, 1969).

Although cytochrome P-450 can mediate the reduction of *p*-nitrobenzoate *in vitro*, it would be rather inefficient as a nitro reductase in living animals, since in air only about 10% is present in the reduced form. It may be inferred, therefore, that the oxygen sensitivity of *p*-nitrobenzoate reduction by liver microsomes is largely due to a competition between oxygen and nitro compounds for the reduced form of cytochrome P-450. Since the affinity of cytochrome P-450 for oxygen is very high ($K_m < 0.1\ \mu M$) even trace amounts of oxygen would be expected to inhibit *p*-nitrobenzoate reduction by liver microsomes. Indeed, the delay in the appearance of *p*-aminobenzoate and the requirement for a relatively high enzyme concentration (rates are nonlinear below 1 mg microsomal protein/ml; GILLETTE et al., 1968) may be due to the time for residual amounts of oxygen, which remain after the usual gassing techniques, to be oxidized by NADPH-oxidase.

Recently, KATO et al. (1969) reported that the soluble fraction of liver contains an enzyme that reduces *p*-nitrobenzoate to *p*-hydroxyaminobenzoate, but not to *p*-aminobenzoate. This enzyme utilizes NADPH or NADH, but its identity is still obscure. It cannot be xanthine oxidase, an enzyme known to catalyze the reduction of a number of other nitro compounds; MORITA et al. (1970) has shown

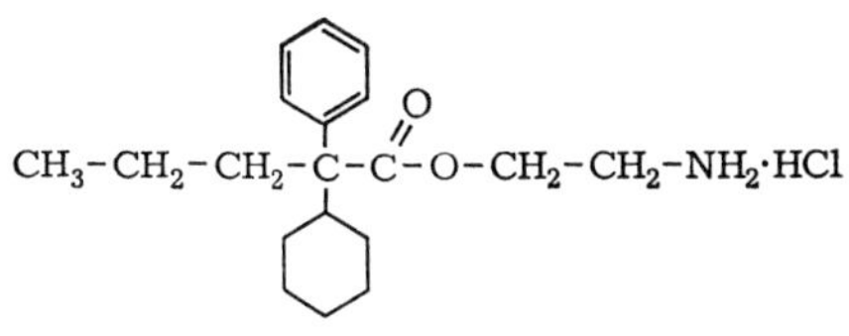

SKF-26754A

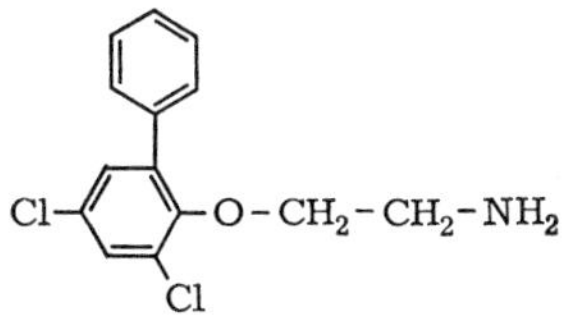

DPEA

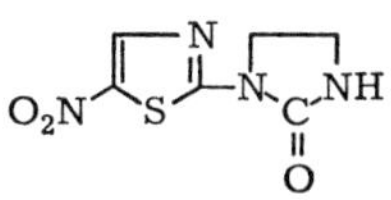

Niridazole

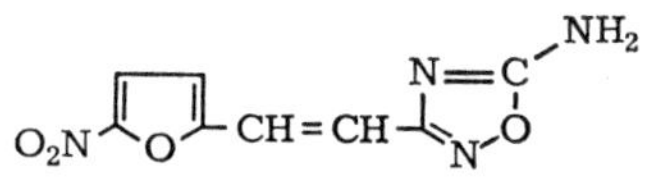

SQ 18, 506

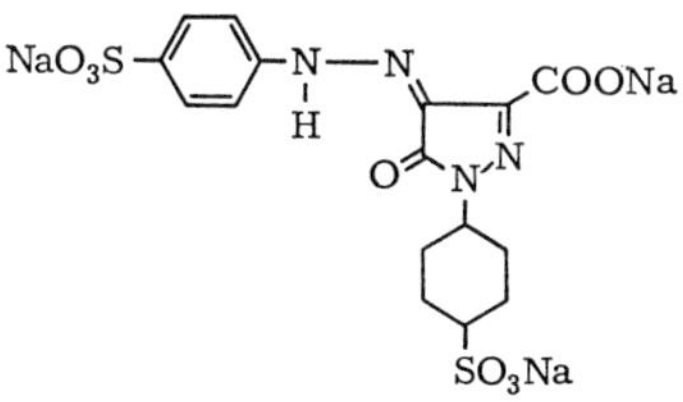

Tartrazine

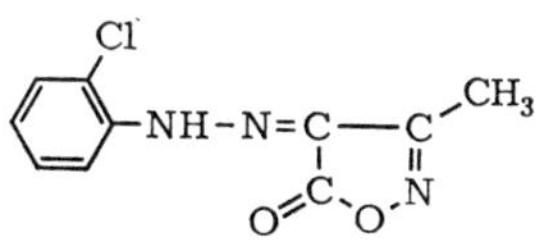

Drazoxolon

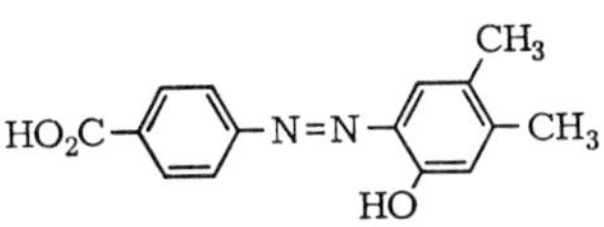

CPA

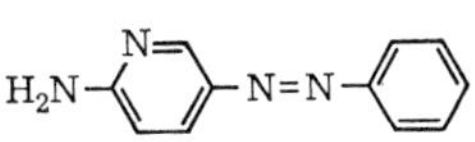

Phenylazopyridine

Fig. 2. Formulae of various compounds

that liver xanthine oxidase does not reduce *p*-nitrobenzoate, as measured by the oxidation of hypoxanthine to uric acid under anaerobic conditions. Nor can the enzyme be the diaphorase isolated by ERNSTER et al. (1962), because KATO et al. (1970) showed that dicoumarol, which inhibits this diaphorase, only partially inhibits *p*-nitrobenzoate reduction. The diaphorase, however, may catalyze the reduction of 4-nitroquinoline *N*-oxide.

Table 1. *Reduction of nitro compounds by partially purified NADPH-cytochrome c reductase*

Nitro compound	Rate of reduction (Δ OD_{400}/mg protein/min) $\times 10^3$
Niridazole	88
Nitrofurazone	421
Furazoline	542
SQ-18, 506	911

Data from FELLER et al. (1969).

Even though the soluble enzyme system represents only about one-third of the total *p*-nitrobenzoate reductase activity in liver, it may be more important than cytochrome P-450 in living animals because of its relatively low sensitivity to oxygen. According to KATO et al. (1969) oxygen blocks the formation of *p*-hydroxy-aminobenzoate by liver microsomes by about 80%, but the soluble enzyme by only about 45%. The soluble system may, therefore, catalyze the *in vivo* formation of hydroxyamino derivatives which mediate the methemoglobinemia and perhaps the hemolytic anemia caused by nitrobenzene derivatives.

Cytochrome P-450 is not the only enzyme in liver microsomes that catalyzes the reduction of nitro compounds. Recently, FELLER et al. (1970) showed that niridazole is reduced to its hydroxyamino derivative by a CO insensitive microsomal enzyme, probably NADPH-cytochrome *c* reductase. This enzyme is not readily autooxidized, but the product is readily reoxidized in air back to niridazole rather than to its nitroso analogue. Thus niridazole promotes NADPH-oxidation by liver microsomes in air even though it does not appear to be reduced under these conditions. Other nitro compounds that are reduced by NADPH-cytochrome *c* reductase and not by cytochrome P-450 are listed in Table 1 (FELLER et al., 1969).

It should be pointed out, however, that xanthine oxidase in milk and in the soluble fraction of liver catalyzes the reduction of a number of nitro compounds and nitrogen *N*-oxides, including niridazole (MORITA et al., 1970), nitrofurans

Table 2. *Effect of various nitro compounds on the uric acid formation from hypoxanthine in a partially purified rat liver xanthine oxidase*

Nitro compound	Uric acid formation Aerobic	Anaerobic
	nmoles/mg protein/min	
None	4.4	0.0
Niridazole	9.4	15.8
Nithiazide	4.2	1.3
2-Amino-5-nitrothiazole	4.1	0.6
Nitrofurazone	10.6	13.5
Nifuraldezone	9.1	7.4
Nifuroxime	11.1	14.7
Nihydrazone	11.4	11.0
Furazolidone	9.8	10.9
SQ-18, 506	6.5	8.7
p-Nitrophenol	4.5	0.0
p-Nitrobenzoate	4.5	0.0
Chloramphenicol	3.8	0.0

Data from MORITA et al. (1970).

(Taylor et al., 1951), trinitrotoluene (Bueding and Jolliffe, 1946), 2,4-dinitrophenol (Kielly, 1955), nicotinamide *N*-oxide (Murray and Chaykin, 1966) and purine *N*-oxide (Stohrer and Brown, 1969). Strangely, this enzyme can accept electrons from not only xanthine, as its name suggests, but also hypoxanthine, various aldehydes and NADH (DeRenzo, 1956; Bray, 1963). The relative rates of reduction of various nitro compounds is given in Table 2 (Morita et al., 1970).

Thus there are at least four mechanisms for the reduction of nitro compounds in liver: cytochrome P-450 and NADPH-cytochrome *c* reductase in liver microsomes, and xanthine oxidase and an unidentified *p*-nitrobenzoate reductase in the soluble fraction. Owing to the oxygen sensitivity of the intermediates of most nitro compounds and the partial pressure of oxygen in liver, it is questionable whether nitro compounds are readily converted to primary amines in this tissue, although the soluble enzymes and NADPH-cytochrome *c* reductase may be important in the formation of toxic hydroxyamine and nitroso intermediates.

II. Enzymatic Reduction of Nitro Compounds in Other Mammalian Tissues

Fouts and Brodie (1957) showed that *p*-nitrobenzoate was reduced not only by liver, but also by kidney, and to a lesser extent by lung, heart and brain. Unfortunately, the mechanisms of these enzyme systems have not been fully studied.

Recently, Juchau (1969) demonstrated that *p*-nitrobenzoate is reduced by placenta of mice and rats, but not by that of humans unless stimulated by flavins. The unstimulated mouse system is unusual in that it is heat stable; boiling the enzyme preparations for 5 min did not affect the rate of *p*-nitrobenzoate reduction. Moreover, these authors were unable to detect the presence of cytochrome P-450 even though CO almost completely blocked the reaction. Although the mechanism of *p*-nitrobenzoate reduction by this preparation remains obscure, these studies illustrate that CO inhibition does not necessarily implicate cytochrome P-450 in an enzyme reaction. As pointed out by Gillette et al. (1968) corroborative evidence is essential before cytochrome P-450 can be implicated in a reaction, because CO is also known to block other metallo-enzymes, such as glutamic dehydrogenase (Adelstein and Vallee, 1958), tyrosinase (Keilin and Mann, 1938) and β-phenethylamine hydroxylase (Friedman and Kaufman, 1965).

III. Nitro Reduction by Bacterial Enzymes

Owing to the anaerobic conditions that exist in the gut, it is possible that bacterial flora play an important role in the conversion of nitro compounds to aromatic amines in animals receiving nitro compounds orally. The importance of bacterial enzymes has not been completely evaluated, but Saz and coworkers (Saz and Marmur, 1953; Saz and Slie, 1954a, b) demonstrated that *E. coli* reduced the nitro groups of chloramphenicol, *p*-nitrobenzoate and other aromatic nitro compounds. The bacterial enzyme system requires DPN, Mn^{++} and either cysteine or glutathione and is blocked by azide, EDTA and low concentrations of aureomycin, which forms chelates with Mn^{++}. It seems likely that other nitro reductases exist in other species of bacteria.

IV. Semi-nonenzymatic Reactions

In attempting to prove that nitro reductase in liver was a flavoprotein, Fouts and Brodie (1957) observed that high concentrations ($> 10^{-5}$M) of FAD, FMN and riboflavin stimulated the reduction of *p*-nitrobenzoate by liver preparations, but that the maximal stimulatory effect was not obtained until the concentrations of these flavins reached 10^{-3}M. Although these authors suggested that the free forms of the flavins might act as artificial electron carriers between NADPH and the substrate, the mechanism was not proved until KAMM and GILLETTE (1963) showed that purified NADPH-cytochrome *c* reductase catalyzed the reduction of FAD under anaerobic conditions. On boiling the enzyme system after FAD reduction was complete and then adding *p*-nitrobenzoate, we found that the reduced FAD was reoxidized as it nonenzymatically reduced *p*-nitrobenzoate to *p*-aminobenzoate. On the basis of these results we suggested that any enzyme which reduced FAD could serve as a flavin-dependent nitro reductase.

It seems unlikely, however, that this mechanism has any functional role in living animals. Carbon monoxide does not affect the reduction of *p*-nitrobenzoate by purified NADPH-cytochrome *c* reductase and flavins, but as mentioned above, it almost completely blocks the reduction of this substrate by liver microsomes. Moreover, animal tissues contain only about 2.5×10^{-5}M of flavins (LONG, 1961) and liver microsomal fractions contain considerably less (about 0.4 ng/mg protein; SHARGELL, 1969). At these flavin concentrations nitro reductase is stimulated by less than 30%. The finding that enzymes in tissues catalyze the reduction of nitro compounds in the presence, but not in the absence, of high concentrations of flavins should, therefore, not be accepted as evidence for functional nitro reductases in those tissues. Thus it seems doubtful that parathion is reduced by liver microsomal enzymes as implied by HITCHCOCK and MURPHY (1967), who found that liver microsomes reduced this insecticide only in the presence of high flavin concentrations. Moreover, *p*-nitrobenzoate is probably not reduced by enzymes in human placenta, since the studies of JUCHAU (1969) showed that this system also required high flavin concentrations. Indeed, in a later study JUCHAU et al. (1970) pointed out that the *p*-nitrobenzoate reduction catalyzed by mouse placenta is probably not mediated by flavins, since these preparations do not contain enough flavin to account for the nitro reductase activity. Thus systems augmented by the addition of large amounts of flavins should be considered biochemical curiosities having little or no relevance to nitro reduction in living animals.

C. Azo Reduction

I. Azo Reduction in Liver

Studies by MUELLER and MILLER (1949, 1950) revealed that butter yellow and related dyes are reductively cleaved by NADPH-dependent enzymes in liver microsomes under anaerobic conditions. These studies were extended by FOUTS et al. (1957), who showed that rabbit liver 9,000 × g supernatant fraction, which contain microsomes, could also reductively cleave a large number of other azo dyes, including Prontosil, Neoprontosil, Orange III, Orange IV and even azobenzene.

Presumably, the splitting of the azo groups in these reactions takes place in two steps: first the formation of a hydrazo intermediate and then the reductive cleavage of the N-N bond (Fig. 3). In accord with this view, BRAY et al. (1951)

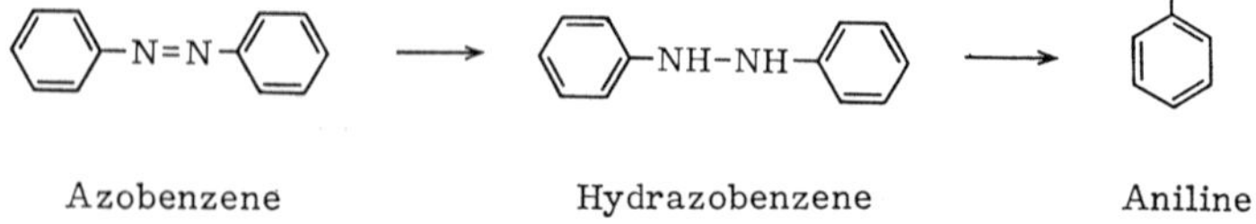

Fig. 3. Pathway of azobenzene reduction to aniline

demonstrated the presence of hydrazobenzene in urine of rabbits receiving azobenzene, and FOUTS (1957) observed that acidification of the incubation mixtures containing azobenzene led to the formation of benzidine, which could only have come from hydrazobenzene by way of the well known benzidine rearrangement.

HERNANDEZ et al. (1967a) reported that high concentrations of NADPH ($> 10^{-4}$M) reduced Neoprontosil nonenzymatically and thus recommended that studies on azo reductase be carried out at low concentrations of the cofactor and that the apparent reductase activity be corrected for the nonenzymatic reduction. Curiously, the microsomal activity did not reach the values obtained with the whole homogenate until the microsomal incubation system was supplemented with either EDTA (ethylenediamine tetracetic acid) or boiled soluble fraction, but the mechanism of this activation is not understood.

Using Neoprontosil as a substrate, HERNANDEZ et al. (1967a) found that treatment of rat liver microsomes with steapsin overnight under nitrogen provided a solubilized preparation that contained both azo reductase (Neoprontosil reductase) and NADPH-cytochrome *c* reductase activities. Although the ratio of azo reductase to cytochrome *c* reductase activities was decreased by treatment with steapsin, further purification of the enzyme did not alter the ratio of the activities. These findings led to the conclusion that NADPH-cytochrome *c* reductase could serve as an azo reductase.

A number of facts, however, indicate that NADPH-cytochrome *c* reductase does not account for all the Neoprontosil reductase activity in liver microsomes. Solubilization decreases Neoprontosil reductase activity, but stimulates NADPH-cytochrome *c* reductase activity (HERNANDEZ et al., 1967a). Treatment of rats with 3-methylcholanthrene increases azo reductase activity (CONNEY et al., 1956; HERNANDEZ et al., 1967b), but does not alter NADPH-cytochrome *c* reductase activity (VON DER DECKEN and HULTIN, 1960; HERNANDEZ et al., 1967b). Carbon monoxide inhibits Neoprontosil reduction by rat liver microsomes by about 30—40% (WRIGHT and GILLETTE, 1964; HERNANDEZ et al., 1967b), but does not inhibit Neoprontosil reduction by purified NADPH-cytochrome *c* reductase (HERNANDEZ et al., 1967b). The finding that CO partially inhibits Neoprontosil reduction by liver microsomes raised the possibility that a part of the azo reductase activity is mediated by cytochrome P-450 (see Chapter 38). In accord with this view, HERNANDEZ et al. (1967b) found that the CO sensitive portion of Neoprontosil reduction in liver microsoms from phenobarbital treated rats was proportional to the cytochrome P-450 content (Table 3). Although 3-methylcholanthrene treatment altered the ratio of the CO sensitive azo reductase to cytochrome P-450 content, this may be due to the formation of a different kind of cytochrome P-450 (see Chapter 38). However, Neoprontosil reduction is still not fully explained by NADPH-cytochrome *c* reductase and cytochrome P-450; the rate of CO insensitive Neoprontosil reduction was not proportional to the activity of NADPH-cytochrome *c* reductase in intact liver microsomes, although these activities were closely related in the solubilized microsomes in which cytochrome P-450 and perhaps other enzymes are inactivated (Table 3).

In an effort to clarify the kinetics of Neoprontosil reduction, SASAME (1969), in my laboratory, compared the disappearance of various concentrations of the azo dye in N_2 or CO (Fig. 4). At high concentrations of CO (about 6.8×10^{-4}M), Neoprontosil reduction was almost completely blocked at low substrate concentrations (< 0.03 mM), but was only partially blocked at high substrate concentrations (3.3 mM). Thus the reduction of Neoprontosil by cytochrome P-450 has a lower K_m than the reduction by the CO insensitive reaction. On subtracting the rates of Neoprontosil reduction in CO from the rates in N_2 and replotting the data, SASAME

Table 3. *Relationships between CO sensitive and insensitive Neoprontosil reduction and cytochrome P-450 and NADPH-cytochrome c reductase in rat liver microsomes*

Enzyme and Treatment	Sulfanilamide formed nmoles/30 min/mg protein N_2	CO	Cyto-chrome P-450 nmoles/mg	$\frac{N_2\text{-CO}}{\text{P-450}}$	Cyto-chrome *c* Reductase nmoles/ 30 min/ mg protein	$\frac{\text{CO} \times 100}{\text{Cytochrome } c \text{ Reductase}}$
Microsomes						
Phenobarbital	398	143	2.22	115	6630	2.16
Saline	210	134	0.65	117	3780	3.54
Microsomes						
3-Methylcholanthrene	264	172	1.75	52	3000	5.73
Corn oil	195	108	0.64	136	3510	3.08
Solubilized						
Phenobarbital	128	123	—	—	17820	0.69
Saline	68	62	—	—	9300	0.67
Solubilized						
3-Methylcholanthrene	72	69	—	—	10170	0.68
Corn oil	69	72	—	—	8820	0.82

Data from HERNANDEZ et al. (1967b).

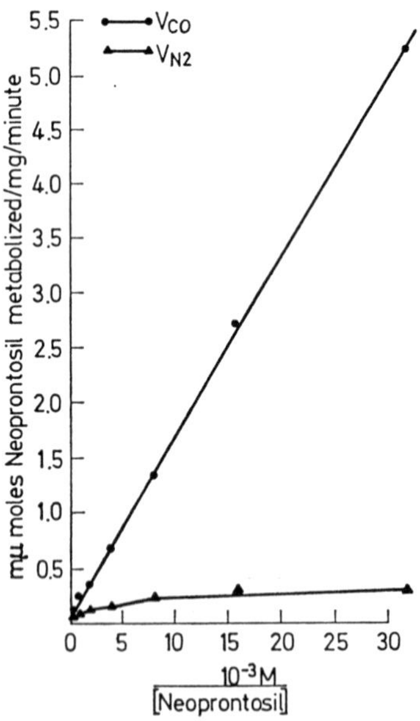

Fig. 4. Neoprontosil reduction by mouse liver microsomes under N_2 and CO

obtained a curved Lineweaver-Burk plot (Fig. 5). Although such data with particulate enzymes cannot be interpreted unequivocally, they suggest the presence of two or more CO insensitive enzymes.

SASAME (1969) also studied the mechanism by which CO inhibited the reduction of Neoprontosil. On addition of various amounts of CO to incubation mix-

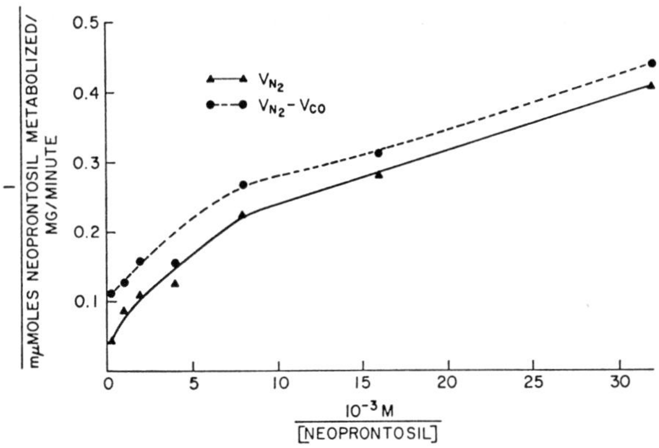

Fig. 5. Carbon monoxide insensitive reduction of Neoprontosil

tures, the inhibition appeared to be noncompetitive even when the data were corrected for the amount of CO bound to cytochrome P-450 (Fig. 6). These findings thus precluded the possibility that Neoprontosil was reduced by the transfer of

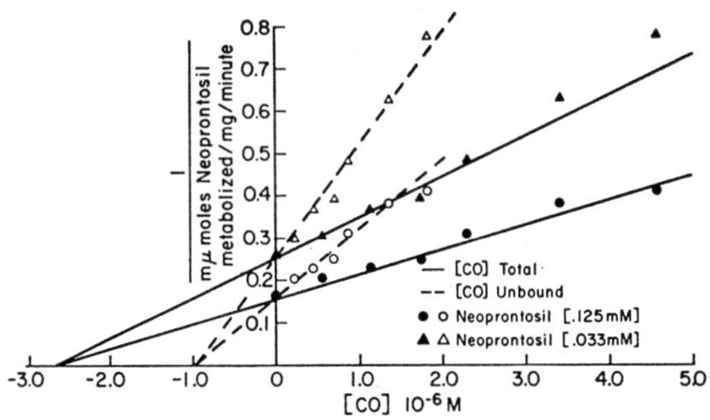

Fig. 6. Dixon plot of carbon monoxide inhibition of Neoprontosil reduction

electrons directly from the heme iron in cytochrome P-450 to the substrate. Thus the mechanism of Neoprontosil reduction by cytochrome P-450 remains obscure.

Not all azo dyes reduced by liver microsomes are mediated by cytochrome P-450. As shown in Table 4, the relative importance of the CO sensitive and CO insensitive mechanisms depends on the substrate (SHARGEL, 1969). At one extreme,

Table 4. *Effect of CO on the reduction of various azo dyes by rat liver microsomes*

Substrate	N_2	CO	Inhibition
	nmoles/30 min/250 mg liver		%
Neoprontosil.	1.93	1.43	26
Prontosil	0.41	0.30	27
Phenylazopyridine . .	0.43	0.43	0
CPA[a]	0.20	0.05	75
p-Phenylazophenol . .	2.34	1.75	25

Data from SHARGELL (1969).

[a] CPA is 1,2-dimethyl-4-(p-carboxyphenyazo)-5-hydroxyazobenzene.

CO blocks the reduction of CPA (1,2-dimethyl-4-(p-carboxyphenylazo)-5-hydroxy-azobenzene) (Fig. 2), by 75%; at the other extreme, it does not affect the reduction of phenylazopyridine (Fig. 2) at all. Unfortunately, these studies were carried out at only one substrate concentration, and thus it is impossible to determine whether these findings are due to differences in the K_m values or in the V_{max} values of the CO sensitive and CO insensitive systems.

An enzyme in the soluble fraction of liver catalyzes the reductive cleavage of the nitrogen-nitrogen bond of drazoxolon (Fig. 2) to form α-chloroaniline (DANIEL, 1969). The enzyme is insensitive to oxygen and can use either NADH or NADPH as the electron donor. Strangely the system was induced by treatment of rats with 3-methylcholanthrene but not by treatment with phenobarbital. The finding that dicoumarol blocked the reductase led DANIEL (1969) to suggest that the enzyme was similar to the diaphorase previously isolated by ERNSTER et al. (1962). Whether this enzyme participates in the reduction of other azo compounds, however, is not known.

II. Semi-nonenzymatic Reactions

FOUTS et al. (1957) found that high concentrations (10^{-5}—10^{-3}M) of riboflavin, FMN and FAD markedly enhance the reduction of Prontosil. Using Neoprontosil as the substrate, SHARGELL (1969) also found that FMN increased azo reduction to about the same extent whether liver microsomes were incubated in nitrogen or CO, indicating that the flavins exerted most of their effect on the cytochrome *c* reductase mediated azo reduction. Accordingly, flavins also stimulated Neoprontosil reduction by purified cytochrome *c* reductase.

Whether stimulation by flavins is operative *in vivo* is difficult to evaluate. As mentioned above, the total concentration of riboflavin in liver is about 25 μM (LONG, 1961; SHARGELL, 1969); at this concentration of FMN, the microsomal system was stimulated by about 50%. However, the microsomal concentration of flavins are only about 0.4 nmole/mg protein (SHARGELL, 1969). Thus, the effect would be of borderline significance and may not be operative at all.

III. Azo Reduction in Other Mammalian Tissues

Although FOUTS et al. (1957) reported the slow reduction of Prontosil by homogenates of kidney, lung, heart and brain, the enzymes catalyzing the reaction in these tissues have not been characterized. Moreover, the soluble fraction of human placenta was recently shown to reduce Neoprontosil by systems which can use either NADH or NADPH (JUCHAU et al., 1968). Although the system was not completely characterized, it differed from the liver system in that it was not stimulated by riboflavin, FMN and FAD (JUCHAU et al., 1968).

IV. Bacterial Enzymes

Intestinal bacteria from rats are known to reductively cleave a number of azo dyes, especially Neoprontosil, methyl orange and amaranth and to a lesser extent tartrazine, yellow 2 G and fast yellow (ROXAN et al., 1967a). One of the species shown to reduce tartrazine under anaerobic conditions is *Proteus vulgaris*, commonly found in human and rat intestinal flora (ROXAN et al., 1966, 1967b). Aging of the *Proteus vulgaris* cultures increases the activity of the azo reductase, and associated with this increased activity is an increase in the concentration of riboflavin in the culture medium (ROXAN et al., 1967b). Addition of FMN or riboflavin up to a concentration of 16 μM to dialyzed cell-free systems also increases the rate of reduction, thus suggesting a role of flavins similar to that in liver microsomal systems. Air prevents the reduction of tartrazine, but whether this is due to a rapid reoxidation of the hydrazo intermediate, to reoxidation of the reduced flavin or to a direct inhibition of the enzyme is not known.

V. Relative Importance of Azo Reductases

As with nitro reductases, the relative importance of the enzyme involved in azo reduction in living animals depends not only on the relative activities of the enzymes in the body and bacterial flora, but also on the rates of reoxidation of the hydrazo intermediates and thus indirectly on the partial pressure of oxygen in the tissues. Moreover, the rate of adsorption of the azo dye from the gut may influence the relative importance of the various azo reductase mechanisms. The observation that aromatic amines are excreted in urine when tartrazine was administered orally, but not when injected intraperitoneally, led to the conclusion that this azo dye was metabolized by intestinal flora, but not by mammalian azo reductase. At first it was considered that tartrazine was not a substrate for the azo reductases in liver (Ryan, Sivayavirojana and Wright cited in Jones et al., 1964). However, Daniel (1967) showed that under strictly anaerobic conditions, the compound was slowly reduced by liver 9,000 $\times$ g supernatant of rat liver, but that the reduction was completely blocked in air. It is, therefore, possible that the relatively high oxygen tension in the liver compared with that in the intestine might affect the rate of tartrazine metabolism *in vivo*.

Even Prontosil and Neoprontosil, which are among the best known substrates of liver azo reductase, may be reductively cleaved to a greater extent by bacterial flora than by liver. Gingell et al. (1969) have found that antibiotics which destroy intestinal bacteria markedly decreased the formation of sulfanilamide from Prontosil and Neoprontosil and that the effect of the antibiotics was greater with Neoprontosil than with Prontosil. Since Neoprontosil is less lipid soluble than Prontosil and is excreted more rapidly in bile, the authors suggested that differences in the rates of adsorption of these drugs from the intestine and their biliary excretion play an important role in determining the relative importance of bacterial flora and liver in azo reduction.

The classical studies of Tréfouël et al. (1935) on the conversion of Prontosil to sulfanilamide in the body illustrated the importance of drug metabolism in therapy and thus provided an impetus to studies of the biotransformation of foreign compounds in mammalian tissues. It seems ironic, therefore, that much of the sulfanilamide may have been formed by bacteria as well as by mammalian tissues. It seems even more ironic that liver azo reductases account for relatively little of the reduction of Neoprontosil in living animals even though this drug is frequently used to assay azo reductase activity in this tissue.

References

Adelstein, S.J., Vallee, B.L.: Zinc in beef liver glutamic dehydrogenase. J. biol. Chem. **233**, 589—593 (1958).

Bray, H.C., Clowes, R.C., Thorpe, W.V.: The metabolism of azobenzene and p-hydroxyazobenzene in the rabbit. Biochem. J. **49**, LXV (1951).

Bray, R.C.: Xanthine oxidase. In: The Enzymes, vol. 7, ed. by P.O. Boyer, H. Lardy and K. Myrback, pp. 533—556. New York: Academic Press 1963.

Bueding, F., Jolliffe, N.: Metabolism of trinitrotoluene (TNT) *in vitro*. J. Pharmacol. exp. Ther. **88**, 300—312 (1946).

Conney, A.H., Miller, E.C., Miller, J.A.: The metabolism of methylated amino azo dyes. V. Evidence for induction of enzyme synthesis in the rat by 3-methylcholanthrene. Cancer Res. **16**, 450—459 (1956).

DANIEL, J.W.: Enzymatic reduction of azo food colourings. Food Cosmet. Toxicol. **5**, 533—534 (1967).
— A soluble aerobic reduced nicotinamideadenenine dinucleotide (phosphate) azo reductase. Biochem. J. **111**, 19p (1969).
DERENZO, E.C.: Chemistry and biochemistry of xanthine oxidase. Advanc. Enzymol. **17**, 293—328 (1956).
ERNSTER, L., DANIELSON, L., LJUNNGVEN, M.: DT diaphorase. I. Purification from the soluble fraction of rat-liver cytoplasm and properties. Biochim. biophys. Acta (Amst.) **58**, 171—188 (1962).
FELLER, D.R., MORITA, M., GILLETTE, J.R.: Unpublished results, 1969.
— — — Enzymatic reduction of niridazole by rat liver microsomes. Biochem. Pharmacol. (1970) (in press).
FIESER, L.F., FIESER, M.: Organic Chemistry, 3rd edition. Boston: D.C. Heath and Co. 1956.
FOUTS, J.R.: Personal communication (1957).
— BRODIE, B.B.: The enzymatic reduction of chloramphenicol, *p*-nitrobenzoic acid and other aromatic nitro compounds in mammals. J. Pharmacol. exp. Ther. **119**, 197—207 (1957).
— KAMM, J.J., BRODIE, B.B.: Enzymatic reduction of Prontosil and other azo dyes. J. Pharmacol. exp. Ther. **120**, 291—300 (1957).
FRIEDMAN, S., KAUFMAN, S.: 3,4-Dihydroxyphenylethylamine β-hydroxylase. J. biol. Chem. **240**, 4763—4773 (1965).
GIGON, P.L., GRAM, T.E., GILLETTE, J.R.: Studies on the rate of reduction of hepatic microsomal cytochrome P-450 by reduced nicotinamide adenine dinucleotide phosphate. Effect of drug substrates. Molec. Pharmacol. **5**, 109—122 (1969).
GILLETTE, J.R.: Comment to the paper of KIESE (1965). Ann. N.Y. Acad. Sci. **123**, 154 (1965).
— KAMM, J.J., SASAME, H.A.: Mechanism of *p*-nitrobenzoate reduction in liver. The possible role of cytochrome P-450 in liver microsomes. Molec. Pharmacol. **4**, 541—548 (1968).
GINGELL, R., BRIDGES, J.W., WILLIAMS, R.T.: Gut flora and the metabolism of Prontosils in the rat. Biochem. J. **114**, 5—6 (1969).
HERNANDEZ, P.H., GILLETTE, J.R., MAZEL, P.: Studies on the mechanism of action of mammalian hepatic azoreductase. I. Azoreductase activity of reduced nicotinamide adenine dinucleotide phosphate-cytochrome *c* reductase. Biochem. Pharmacol. **16**, 1859—1876 (1967a).
— MAZEL, P., GILLETTE, J.R.: Studies on the mechanism of action of mammalian hepatic azoreductase. II. The effects of phenobarbital and 3-methylcholanthrene on carbon monoxide sensitive and insensitive azoreductase activities. Biochem. Pharmacol. **16**, 1877—1888 (1967b).
HITCHCOCK, M., MURPHY, S.D.: Enzymatic reduction of *O,O*-(4-nitrophenyl) phosphate, and *O*-ethyl *O*-(4-nitrophenyl) benzene thiophosphonate by tissues from mammals, birds and fishes. Biochem. Pharmacol. **16**, 1801—1811 (1967).
JONES, R., RYAN, A.J., WRIGHT, S.E.: The metabolism and excretion of tartrazine in rat, rabbit and man. Food Cosmet. Toxicol. **2**, 447—452 (1964).
JUCHAU, M.R.: Studies on the reduction of aromatic nitro groups in human and rodent placental homogenates. J. Pharmacol. exp. Ther. **165**, 1—8 (1969).
— KRASNER, J., YAFFE, S.J.: Studies on reduction of azo-linkages in human placental homogenates. Biochem. Pharmacol. **17**, 1969—1979 (1968).
— — — Model systems for aromatic nitro group reduction — Relationships to tissue catalyzed reagents. Biochem. Pharmacol. **19**, 443—453 (1970).
KAMM, J.J., GILLETTE, J.R.: Mechanism of stimulation of mammalian nitro reductase by flavins. Life Sci. 254—260 (1963).
KATO, R., OSHIMA, T., TAKANAKA, A.: Studies on the mechanism of nitro reduction by rat liver. Molec. Pharmacol. **5**, 487—498 (1969).
— TAKAHASHI, A., OSHIMA, T.: Characteristics of nitro reduction of the carcinogenic agent, 4-nitroquinolone N-oxide. Biochem. Pharmacol. **19**, 45—55 (1970).
KEILIN, D., MANN, T.: Polyphenol oxidase. Purification, nature and properties. Proc. roy. Soc. B **125**, 187—204 (1938).
KIELLY, R.K.: Purification of liver xanthine oxidase. J. biol. Chem. **216**, 405—412 (1955).
KIESE, M.: Relationship of drug metabolism to methemoglobin formation. Ann. N.Y. Acad. Sci. **123**, 141—154 (1965).
LONG, C.: Biochemists' handbook, p. 683. Princeton, N.J.: D. Van Nostrand Co. Inc. 1961.
MORITA, M., FELLER, D.R., GILLETTE, J.R.: Reduction of niridazole by rat liver xanthine oxidase. Biochem. Pharmacol. (1970) (in press).
MUELLER, G.C., MILLER, J.A.: The reductive cleavage of 4-dimethylaminoazobenzene by rat liver: The intracellular distribution of the enzyme system and its requirements for triphosphopyridine nucleotide. J. biol. Chem. **180**, 1125—1136 (1949).

MUELLER, G. C., MILLER, J. A.: The reductive cleavage of 4-dimethylaminoazobenzene by rat liver: Reactivation of carbon dioxide treated homogenates by riboflavin-adenine dinucleotide. J. biol. Chem. **185**, 145—154 (1950).
MURRAY, K. N., CHAYKIN, S.: The reduction of nicotinamide N-oxide by xanthine oxidase. J. biol. Chem. **241**, 3468—3473 (1966).
ROXAN, J. J., RYAN, A. J., WRIGHT, S. E.: Reduction of tartrazine by a *Proteus* species isolated from rats. Food Cosmet. Toxicol. **4**, 419—426 (1966).
— — — Reduction of water soluble azo dyes by intestinal bacteria. Food Cosmet. Toxicol. **4**, 367—369 (1967a).
— — — Enzymatic reduction of tartrazine by *Proteus vulgaris* from rats. Food Cosmet. Toxicol. **5**, 645—656 (1967b).
SASAME, H. A.: Unpublished results, 1969.
— GILLETTE, J. R.: Studies on the relationship between the effects of various substances on adsorption spectrum of cytochrome P-450 and the reduction of p-nitrobenzoate by mouse liver microsomes. Molec. Pharmacol. **5**, 123—130 (1969).
SAZ, A. K., MARMUR, J.: The inhibition of organic nitro-reductase by aureomycin in cell-free extracts. Proc. Soc. exp. Biol. (N.Y.) **82**, 783—784 (1953).
— SLIE, R. B.: The inhibition of organic nitro reductase by aureomycin in cell-free extracts. II. Cofactor requirements for the nitro reductase enzyme complex. Arch. Biochem. **51**, 5—16 (1954a).
— — Reversal of aureomycin inhibition of bacterial cell-free nitro reductase by manganese. J. biol. Chem. **210**, 407—412 (1954b).
SHARGELL, L. D.: Thesis. Influence of electron carrier systems in microsomal metabolism of drugs. Department of Pharmacology, George Washington University, Washington, D.C. (1969).
STOHRER, G., BROWN, G. B.: Purine N-oxides XXVIII. The reduction of purine N-oxides by xanthine oxidase. J. biol. Chem. **244**, 2498—2502 (1969).
TAYLOR, J. D., PAUL, H. E., PAUL, M. F.: Metabolism of nitrofurans. III. Studies with xanthine oxidase *in vitro*. J. biol. Chem. **191**, 223—231 (1951).
TRÉFOUËL, J., TRÉFOUËL, J., NITTI, F., BOVET, D.: Activité du p-aminophényl sulfamide sur les infections streptococciques expérimentales de la souris et du lapin. C.R. Soc. Biol. (Paris) **120**, 756—758 (1935).
VON DER DECKEN, A., HULTIN, T.: Inductive effects of 3-methylcholanthrene on enzyme activities and amino acid incorporation capacity of rat liver microsomes. Arch. Biochem. **90**, 201—207 (1960).
WRIGHT, S. E., GILLETTE, J. R.: Unpublished results, 1964.

Chapter 43

Oxidative Desulfuration and Dearylation of Selected Organophosphate Insecticides[1]

Paul A. Dahm

Desulfuration enzymes create powerful anticholinesterase metabolites of phosphorothionate $[(RO)_2\overset{S}{\overset{\|}{P}}OX]$, phosphonothionate $[(RO)(Y)\overset{S}{\overset{\|}{P}}OX]$, and phosphorodithioate $[(RO)_2\overset{S}{\overset{\|}{P}}SX]$ insecticides (Heath, 1961; O'Brien, 1960). In these formulae, "R" stands for an alkyl group such as methyl or ethyl, "X" stands for an alkyl or aryl group, and "Y" stands for a phenyl group (specifically for EPN, *O*-ethyl *O*-*p*-nitrophenyl phenylthiophosphonate). These three groups of organophosphorus compounds include several dozen compounds either being used for the management of insect-pest populations or in some stage of development for this purpose. The most comprehensive references to organophosphorus insecticides are those by Heath (1961) and O'Brien (1960). Proceedings of a conference on enzymatic oxidations of toxicants, which includes much information on drug and insecticide metabolism, was edited by Hodgson (1968). O'Brien (1962) has specifically discussed desulfuration reactions, with emphasis on the conversion of phosphorothionates to phosphates.

Diggle and Gage (1951) were the first to report the conversion of a phosphorothionate compound, parathion (*O,O*-diethyl *O*-*p*-nitrophenyl phosphorothionate), which possesses little anticholinesterase activity, to a strong anticholinesterase metabolite. This activation reaction was accomplished with rat liver slices or homogenates; heparinized rat whole blood was used as an indicator of cholinesterase inhibition. The *in vivo* conversion of parathion, and in some instances derivatives of phosphorothioic acid, to active metabolites was confirmed by Aldridge and Barnes (1952), Metcalf and March (1953), and Myers et al. (1952). Although there was strong circumstantial evidence from these workers for *in vivo* conversion of parathion to its P=O analog, paraoxon (diethyl *p*-nitrophenyl phosphate), the first definitive identification of paraoxon as the principal anticholinesterase metabolite of parathion was described by Gage (1953). He extracted paraoxon from livers of parathion-treated rats and isolated the metabolite by column chromatography. Identity of the metabolite with paraoxon was indicated by a comparison of the anticholinesterase activities, UV spectra, hydrolysis constants, and paper chromatography data of the metabolite with the authentic compound.

By differential centrifugation of rat liver homogenates, Davison (1955) showed that conversion of parathion to paraoxon occurred principally in a fraction

1 Journal Paper No. J-6584 of the Iowa Agriculture and Home Economics Experiment Station, Ames, Iowa 50010, USA. Projects No. 1351, 1435, and 1686. Preparation of this manuscript was supported by Public Health Service Research Grant ES-00205 from the Division of Environmental Health Sciences and North Central Regional Project NC-85.

containing both microsomes and the supernatant fraction. He also suggested that the microsomal enzyme system responsible for parathion metabolism was part of a metabolic system capable of acting on a variety of substrates. Evidence that reduced nicotinamide adenine dinucleotide, NADH, is required for the *in vitro* activation reaction was provided by metabolism studies of malathion, *S*-[1,2-bis(ethoxycarbonyl)ethyl] *O*,*O*-dimethyl phosphorodithioate, and its thiolphosphate analogue, malaoxon, with mice and American cockroaches (O'Brien, 1957). O'Brien (1959) also showed that either NADH or reduced nicotinamide adenine dinucleotide phosphate, NADPH, is necessary for the *in vitro* activation of several phosphorothionates [parathion; diazinon, *O*,*O*-diethyl *O*-(2-*iso*propyl-4-methyl-6-pyrimidyl) phosphorothionate; coumaphos, *O*,*O*-diethyl *O*-(3-chloro-4-methyl-2-oxo-2*H*-1-benzopyram-7-yl) phosphorothionate; ronnel, *O*,*O*-dimethyl *O*-2,4,5-trichlorophenyl phosphorothionate; and Potasan, *O*,*O*-diethyl *O*-(4-methyl-2-oxo-2*H*-1-benzopyran-7-yl) phosphorothionate], a phosphonothionate [EPN], and two phosphorodithioates [malathion and azinphosmethyl, *O*,*O*-dimethyl *S*(4-oxo-1,2,3-benzotriazin-3-4*H*-ylmethyl) phosphorodithioate]. NADPH was at least as good a cofactor as NADH in reaction studies with parathion.

Thus, from these studies and many later studies with organophosphate insecticides (Heath, 1961; O'Brien, 1960) it became clear that microsomal enzymes that catalyze the activation of organophosphate insecticides are similar to those enzymes capable of metabolizing various foreign substrates, including drugs, and some endogenous substrates, such as steroids. NADPH and oxygen seem essential for maximum reaction rates *in vitro*; magnesium and nicotinamide have often been used in reaction mixtures. The conversion of P=S organophosphates to P=O analogues greatly enhances reactivity with cholinesterases, because =O is more electrophilic than =S. The sulfur atom detached in the activation reaction *in vitro* is bound to microsomes; the final form of the detached sulfur *in vivo* is inorganic sulfate (Nakatsugawa and Dahm, 1967; Nakatsugawa et al., 1969c).

Many studies of the hydrolytic stability and anticholinesterase action of organophosphorus triesters have revealed that hydrolysis occurs quite readily at the aryl-phosphate (acid anhydride) bond, especially with P=O esters. Most workers have ascribed this hydrolytic pathway to phosphatase action at $>\overset{\text{O (or S)}}{\overset{\|}{\text{P}}}\text{—O—C}$ or $>\overset{\text{O (or S)}}{\overset{\|}{\text{P}}}\text{—S—C}$ linkages. The enzymes have sometimes been named after their substrates although specificity for the substrate has not always been proved. Mammalian liver contains phosphatases, but the spleen, serum, and other sources also have enzymes capable of this type of degradative hydrolysis (Heath, 1961; Kojima and O'Brien, 1968; O'Brien, 1960, 1963).

It has also been established that oxidative dearylation of insecticidal organophosphorus triesters occurs in mammals and insects. Nakatsugawa and Dahm (1967) found that rabbit liver microsomes not only activate parathion to paraoxon but also degrade parathion by splitting it at the aryl phosphate bond to give diethyl phosphorothioic acid (DEPTA) and *p*-nitrophenol (PNP). Both activation and degradation by microsomes required NADPH and oxygen and were inhibited by SKF 525-A (2-diethylamino diphenylpropyl acetate) and several insecticide synergists (including four 1,3-benzodioxole-containing compounds). The system was specific to parathion and did not degrade paraoxon. The degradation was also demonstrated with microsomes from rat liver and American cockroach fat body. In similar studies with parathion, NEAL (1967a), using microsomes from rats, mice, and guinea pigs, showed the formation of DEPTA and PNP as well as paraoxon. NADPH and oxygen were necessary for both oxidative desulfuration and dearylation reactions. NEAL (1967b) investigated the effects of various inhibitors and activators on rat microsomal enzymes, again by using parathion as a substrate. Metabolism was affected by the inhibitors in a manner typical of mixed-function oxidase systems. With inhibitors like SKF 525-A, *p*-chloromercuribenzoate, Cu^{2+}, and 8-hydroxyquinoline, the conversion of parathion into DEPTA was less inhibited than its conversion to paraoxon. Compounds containing reduced sulfur, such as dithiothreitol, mercaptoethanol, and 1-phenylthiourea, stimulated the overall metabolism of parathion; conversion of parathion into DEPTA, however, was stimulated more than its activation to paraoxon. The results of these detailed studies were discussed in terms of either two separate microsomal enzyme systems metabolizing parathion to DEPTA and PNP and activating parathion to paraoxon or two different binding sites for parathion that share a common electron-transport pathway.

Using microsomes from rat and rabbit livers and from house fly abdomens, NAKATSUGAWA et al. (1968) examined the *in vitro* metabolism of several organophosphorus insecticides containing substituted or unsubstituted 4-nitrophenyl ester structures. Compounds studied included parathion; the methyl, *n*-propyl, and *iso*propyl analogs of parathion; dicapthon (*O,O*-dimethyl *O*-2-chloro-4-nitrophenyl phosphorothionate); Sumithion (*O,O*-dimethyl *O*-3-methyl-4-nitrophenyl phosphorothionate); Chlorthion (*O,O*-dimethyl *O*-3-chloro-4-nitrophenyl phosphorothionate); EPN; and the P=O analogs of these eight compounds. All the P=S compounds were metabolized by two oxidative pathways, activation to P=O analogs and oxidative degradation at the aryl phosphate bond. The reactions occurred only in the presence of NADPH and oxygen. Oxidative dearylation also occurred with one P=O analog, *n*-propyl paraoxon. Similar results were obtained with diazinon and malathion with rat liver microsomes (NAKATSUGAWA et al., 1969a), indicating that oxidative dearylation is not limited to 4-nitrophenyl analogs of parathion and suggesting that it may occur with many phosphorothionate and phosphorodithioate insecticides. The importance of oxidative desulfuration and dearylation of parathion in the house fly has also been shown (NAKATSUGAWA et al., 1969b).

WOLCOTT and NEAL (1969) studied the formation of *O,O*-diethyl-*O*-phenyl phosphates and DEPTA in a series of *O,O*-diethyl-*O*-phenyl phosphorothionates with ring substituents having strong electron-withdrawing to strong electron-donating properties. After incubation of the phosphorothionates with rabbit liver microsomes and NADPH, the amount of the two types of metabolites formed from each of the original substrates was estimated, and relationships were examined between both the Michaelis-Menten constant, K_m, and V_{max} versus the Hammett substituent constant, σ. Comparisons of the $-\log V_{max}$ versus σ data showed that the unsubstituted phenyl group was the best substrate for the formation of the P=O analog and the worst substrate for formation of DEPTA. The metabolite data also suggested a biphasic response of the enzyme systems to the various substrates.

Because earlier work suggested three possible mechanisms for dearylation of organophosphate insecticides (oxidation by microsomal enzymes; hydrolysis by esterases or phosphatases; and hydrolysis by enzymes in the supernatant fractions of rat liver homogenates, presumably in the presence of reduced glutathione, GSH), NAKATSUGAWA et al. (1969c) reexamined the metabolism of parathion in the rat. Evaluation of urinary metabolites of orally administered ^{32}P- and ^{35}S-

parathion confirmed that initial metabolism of parathion involved both activation to paraoxon and degradation to DEPTA. Sulfur detached in the activation reaction was excreted as inorganic sulfate. Experiments *in vitro* with ^{35}S-parathion indicated that the aryl-phosphate cleavage of parathion was largely carried out by liver microsomal oxidases; a minor portion was catalyzed by nonoxidative soluble enzymes requiring GSH.

FUKAMI and SHISHIDO (1963, 1966), HOLLINGWORTH (1969a, 1969b), KOJIMA and O'BRIEN (1968), PLAPP and CASIDA (1958), and SHISHIDO and FUKAMI (1963), have shown that *O*-dealkylation is another important degradation route for organophosphates. Enzymes for *O*-dealkylation seem to be associated with soluble enzymes in liver. However, there is at least one report of *O*-dealkylation of chlorfenvinphos [2-chloro-1-(2',4'-dichlorophenyl)vinyl diethyl phosphate] to 2-chloro-1-(2',4'-dichlorophenyl)vinyl ethyl hydrogen phosphate by rabbit liver microsomes (DONNINGER et al., 1967). In this case production of acetaldehyde, rather than ethanol, suggested C-O bond cleavage. The reaction occurred only in the presence of NADPH and oxygen. Thus, *O*-dealkylation by microsomal enzymes may be a possible degradation mechanism for organophosphate insecticides. HOLLINGWORTH (1969a) found that GSH had little effect on the degradation of chlorfenvinphos when it was incubated with mouse liver supernatant, which may be indirect evidence for microsomal dealkylation of this vinyl phosphate.

In summary, the metabolism of insecticidal organophosphorus triesters is accomplished mainly by microsomal and soluble liver enzymes. Microsomal enzymes are responsible for oxidative desulfuration, oxidative dearylation, and, in at least one instance, *O*-dealkylation. The mechanisms of these microsomal oxidations are not completely known but require NADPH and oxygen. The soluble enzymes are responsible, in most cases, for *O*-dealkylation. Phosphatases capable of dearylating organophosphate insecticides seem to be more ubiquitous in their intra- and extracellular distribution than are the other degradative enzymes discussed in this section.

References

ALDRIDGE, W.N., BARNES, J.M.: Some problems in assessing the toxicity of the "organophosphorus" insecticides toward mammals. Nature (Lond.) **169**, 345—347 (1952).

DAVISON, A.N.: The conversion of schradan (OMPA) and parathion into inhibitors of cholinesterase by mammalian liver. Biochem. J. **61**, 203—209 (1955).

DIGGLE, W.M., GAGE, J.C.: Cholinesterase inhibition by parathion *in vivo*. Nature (Lond.) **168**, 998 (1951).

DONNINGER, C., HUTSON, D.H., PICKERING, B.A.: Oxidative cleavage of phosphoric acid triesters to diesters. Biochem. J. **102**, 26P—27P (1967).

FUKAMI, J., SHISHIDO, T.: Studies on the selective toxicities of organic phosphorus insecticides (III), the characters of enzyme system in cleavage of methyl parathion to desmethyl parathion in the supernatant of several species of homogenates (Part I). Botyu-Kagaku **28**, 77—81 (1963).

— — Nature of a soluble, glutathione-dependent enzyme system active in cleavage of methyl parathion to desmethyl parathion. J. Econ. Entomol. **59**, 1338—1346 (1966).

GAGE, J.C.: A cholinesterase inhibitor derived from *O,O*-diethyl *O-p*-nitrophenyl thiophosphate *in vivo*. Biochem. J. **54**, 426—430 (1953).

HEATH, D.F.: Organophosphorus poisons. New York-Oxford-London-Paris: Pergamon Press 1961.

HODGSON, E.: Enzymatic oxidations of toxicants. Raleigh, North Carolina: North Carolina State University 1968.

HOLLINGWORTH, R.M.: Dealkylation of organophosphorus esters by mouse liver enzymes *in vitro* and *in vivo*. J. Agr. Food Chem. **17**, 987—996 (1969a).

— The cleavage of organophosphorus triesters by liver enzymes. From Metabolism, Degradation and Mode of Action, Biochemical Toxicology of Insecticide Action. Tokyo, Japan: U.S.-Japan Seminar 1969b.

Kojima, K., O'Brien, R. D.: Paraoxon hydrolyzing enzymes in rat liver. J. Agr. Food Chem. **16**, 574—584 (1968).
Metcalf, R. L., March, R. B.: Further studies on the mode of action of organic thionophosphate insecticides. Ann. Entomol. Soc. Amer. **46**, 63—74 (1953).
Myers, D. K., Mendel, B., Gersmann, H. R., Ketelaar, J. A. A.: Oxidation of thiophosphate insecticides in the rat. Nature (Lond.) **170**, 805—807 (1952).
Nakatsugawa, T. N., Dahm, P. A.: Microsomal metabolism of parathion. Biochem. Pharmacol. **16**, 25—38 (1967).
— Tolman, N. M., Dahm, P. A.: Degradation and activation of parathion analogs by microsomal enzymes. Biochem. Pharmacol. **17**, 1517—1528 (1968).
— — — Oxidative degradation of diazinon by rat liver microsomes. Biochem. Pharmacol. **18**, 685—688 (1969a).
— — — Metabolism of S^{35}-parathion in the house fly. J. Econ. Entomol. **62**, 408—411 (1969b).
— — — Degradation of parathion in the rat. Biochem. Pharmacol. **18**, 1103—1114 (1969c).
Neal, R. A.: Studies on the metabolism of diethyl 4-nitrophenyl phosphorothionate (parathion) *in vitro*. Biochem. J. **103**, 183—191 (1967a).
— Studies of the enzymic mechanism of the metabolism of diethyl 4-nitrophenyl phosphorothionate (parathion) by rat liver microsomes. Biochem. J. **105**, 289—297 (1967b).
O'Brien, R. D.: Properties and metabolism in the cockroach and mouse of malathion and malaoxon. J. Econ. Entomol. **50**, 159—164 (1957).
— Activation of thionophosphates by liver microsomes. Nature (Lond.) **183**, 121—122 (1959).
— Toxic phosphorus esters. New York-London: Academic Press 1960.
— Desulfuration. Proc. First Intern. Pharmacol. Mtg. **6**, 111—119 (1962).
— Organophosphates and carbamates. Chap. 25, pages 205—241 in Metabolic Inhibitors, Vol. II. Hochster, R. M. and J. H. Quastel, Editors. New York: Academic Press 1963.
Plapp, F. W., Casida, J. E.: Hydrolysis of the alkyl-phosphate bond in certain dialkyl aryl phosphorothioate insecticides by rats, cockroaches, and alkali. J. Econ. Entomol. **51**, 800—803 (1958).
Shishido, T., Fukami, J.: Studies on the selective toxicities of organic phosphorus insecticides (II), the degradation of ethyl parathion, methyl parathion, methyl paraoxon and sumithion in mammal, insect and plant. Botyu-Kagaku **28**, 69—76 (1963).
Wolcott, M., Neal, R. A.: Effect of structure on the metabolism of dialkylarylphosphorothionates by rabbit liver microsomes. Toxicol. appl. Pharmacol. **14**, 644 (1969).

Chapter 44

Metabolism of Halogenated Compounds

EDWARD A. SMUCKLER[1]

With 7 Figures

Introduction

Halogenated aliphatic and aromatic compounds have come to play a constantly increasing role in our environment. A number of halogenated compounds are used medicinally as anaesthetics, antihistamines, diuretics, antihypertensives, antidiabetic agents, tranquilizers, antibiotics and antimalarials. Large amounts of halogenated compounds are used as insecticides, pesticides and as industrial solvents.

Most halogenated compounds are metabolized along pathways that do not involve the loss of halogen. For example, chlorpromazine is metabolized by N-dealkylation, aromatic hydroxylation and sulfoxidation; halogenated benzenes are converted to a variety of metabolites including their respective glucuronides and mercapturates; chlorohydrate is converted to trichloroacetic acid. In fact the substitution of a halogen for a hydrogen or a methyl group that is rapidly metabolized often leads to an analogue which is slowly metabolized. For example, chlorpropamide is metabolized more slowly than tolbutamide and fluorocitrate more slowly than citric acid.

Nevertheless a variety of substances are dehalogenated in the body, sometimes yielding active intermediates. The following is a brief review of the nature of the metabolism of halogenated organic compounds.

I. General Consideration of the Halogen-Carbon Bond

Since the stability of halogenated compounds varies widely, the chemistry of the halogen-carbon bond will be considered. Halogens form strong acids because the attraction of electrons by the halogen nucleus is considerably greater than the attraction by hydrogen ions. This strong attraction of electrons also occurs when the halogens are covalently bound to carbon and thus the electrons which form the bond are closer to the halogen nucleus than they are to the carbon nucleus. The magnitude of these inductive effects depend on the ionic radius and nuclear configuration and are greatest with F followed by Cl, Br and I (PAULING, 1960; KETELAAR, 1958; COTTRELL, 1954). This property of halogen-substituted alkyl and aryl compounds is manifested by significant dipole moment, electron negativity, bond distance and ionicity (Tables 1, 2, 3, 4). Further modifications are induced by the second, third or fourth halogen atom of the parent molecule. Generalizations derived from physical chemical studies on halogenated compounds include:

1 University of Washington, School of Medicine, Department of Pathology, Seattle, Washington 98105.

Table 4. *Electric dipole moments of alkyl or aryl derivatives*[a]

Halogen (X)	R-X	Ar-X
—Cl	2.14	1.56
—Br	2.15	1.54
—I	2.13	1.38

[a] From PAULING, L. C.: The Nature of the Chemical Bond, Ithaca, New York: Cornell University Press 1960.

B) Electrons in neighboring groups that are attached to the carbon atom that is bound to the halogen atom are drawn toward the induced partial positive charge on the carbon atom. For this reason, trichloracetic acid (pKa, 0.7) is a stronger acid than dichloracetic acid (pKa, 1.3) followed by monochloracetic acid (pKa, 2.8) and acetic acid (pKa, 4.7).

C) This polarization decreases as the distance from the primary dipole increases. For this reason β-chloroproprionic acid is a weaker acid (pKa, 4.1) than α-chloroacetic acid (pKa, 2.8).

D) A C-X bond adjacent to unsaturated bonds, including an aromatic ring, causes a delocalization of the electron field of the unsaturated system which reduces the effective C-X dipole. Thus the dipole moment of chlorobenzene is less than the dipole moment of methyl chloride.

E) The effectiveness of the halogen in producing electronic polarization is related to the inductive effect of its nucleus, F>Cl>Br>I. For this reason the C-X bond energies decrease in that order. Hence iodoacetate can alkylate SH groups, but fluoroacetate cannot.

F) The carbon-halogen bond has some characteristics of a double bond in that the bond distances are shorter than C-C bonds and delocalization of the electric field can occur.

As one would expect from these considerations of C-X bonds, the chemical reactivity of aliphatic halides is different from that of aromatic halides, and the reactivity of substances containing several halogen atoms is different from those containing one halogen atom.

1. Chemical Reactivity of Aromatic Halogen Derivatives

In these substances, two opposing factors are brought into play: (1) The halogen atom tends to withdraw electrons from the aromatic ring resulting in the formation of a dipole. (2) The halogen atom tends to form a double bond with the carbon atom, resulting in a number of resonance forms (Fig. 1).

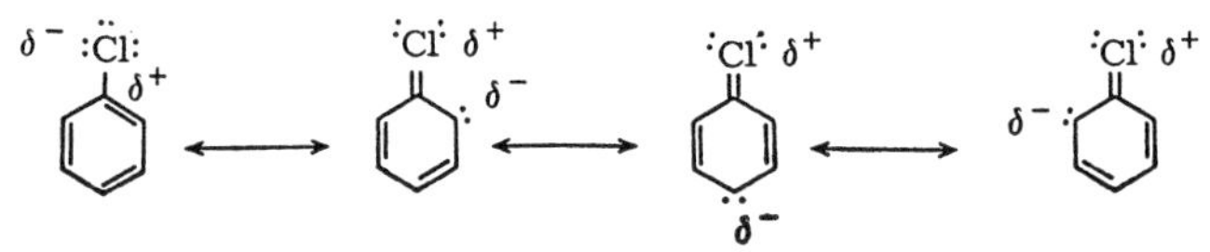

Fig. 1

The first factor makes the aromatic ring relatively resistant as compared with benzene to substitution by positively charged reagents, such as NO_2^+, SO_3H^+, and by halogens. The second permits the ring to be substituted preferentially in the ortho and para positions.

Hydrolysis of mono halobenzenes occurs only under extreme conditions because the $[(C_6H_5(Cl)(OH)]^-$ intermediate requisite to hydrolysis is not easily formed. When another electron withdrawing group, such as a nitro group, is present in the ortho or para position, however, substitution of the halogen by an electron donor occurs more easily, because the electron withdrawing group stabilizes the intermediate by delocalization of the π orbital (Fig. 2).

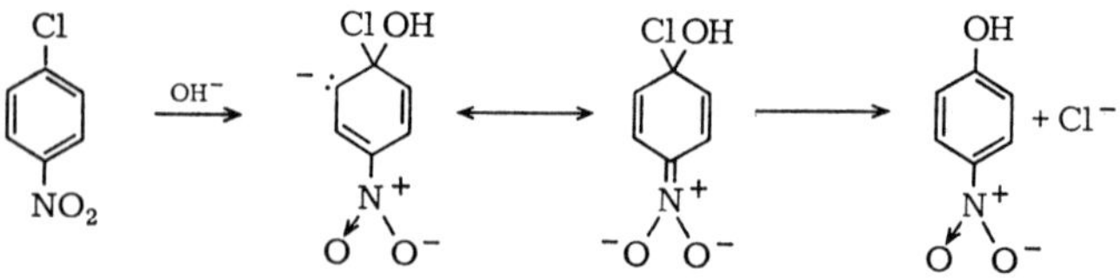

Fig. 2

Substitution occurs especially easily when both the ortho and the para positions are occupied by electron withdrawing groups. Thus 2,4-dinitrofluorobenzene rapidly reacts with the electron donors such as the unionized amino groups of amino acids (Fig. 3).

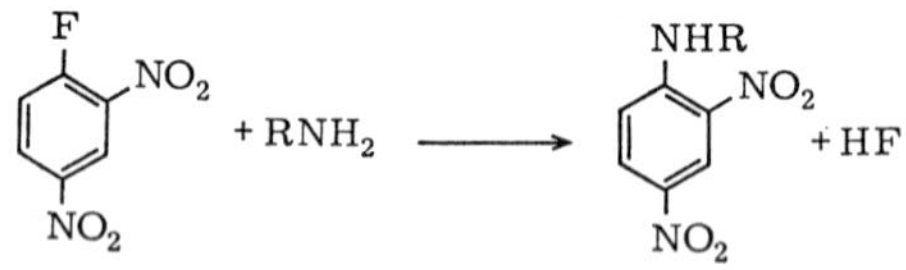

Fig. 3

However, a nitro group in the meta position does not stabilize the intermediate and thus replacement of the halogen by an electron donor does not readily occur.

Since the rate controlling step in these reactions is the formation of the intermediates, the relative rates of dehalogenation are not necessarily in the order of the bond energies of the carbon-halogen bonds. Thus 2,4-dinitrofluorobenzene reacts with electron donors more rapidly than does 2,4-dinitrochlorobenzene, even though the carbon-fluorine bond is stronger than the carbon-chlorine bond.

2. Chemical Reactivity of Aliphatic Halogen Derivatives

In saturated aliphatic halogen derivatives, the electron withdrawing effect of the halogen atom is not counterbalanced by the electron delocalization that occurs in halogenated aromatic compounds; hence the polarization of the carbon-halogen bond is fully expressed in saturated aliphatic halogen compounds. In unsaturated aliphatic halogenated compounds, the electron-delocalization effect occurs to varying extents depending on the position of the unsaturated bond.

The replacement of halogens by electron donating groups, such as hydroxyl ions, may be catalyzed by either acids or bases. In the base catalyzed reaction, the hydroxyl ion attacks the carbon on the side directly opposite to the C-X bond to form a complex which decomposes with the release of the halide ion (Fig. 4).

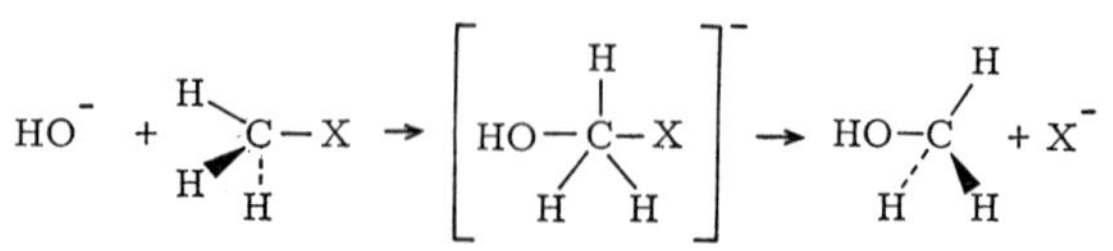

Fig. 4

With optically active substances the mechanism results in an inversion of the configuration called a Walden inversion. This kind of reaction, however, usually does not occur with groups containing three or four halogen atoms owing to the steric hinderance of the halogens and the decrease in the ionicity of the C-X bonds. Thus the haloforms and the carbon tetrahalides are more stable than the methyl halides.

In an acid catalyzed reaction, the hydrogen ion removes the halogen from the compound leaving a carbonium ion which in turn reacts with the electron donating group.

$$(CH_3)_3 - C - X + H^+ \rightarrow (CH_3)_3 - C^+ + HCl$$
$$(CH_3)_3 - C^+ + HOH \rightarrow (CH_3)_3 - COH + H^+$$

In this type of reaction the configuration is retained. Again, however, the trihalo and tetrahalo-substituted substances react slowly with electron donors, owing to the decrease in ionicity of the C-X bonds.

A variety of alkyl halides can undergo homolytic cleavage with the formation of free radicals.

$$CCl_3\,Br \xrightarrow{h\nu} CCl_3\cdot + Br\cdot$$

Although this type of reaction is usually initiated by light, BUTLER (1961) has suggested that free radicals of carbon tetrachloride may occur in liver.

II. Metabolism of Halogenated Aromatic Hydrocarbons

In his book, WILLIAMS (1959) pointed out that mono-, di- and polyhalogenated benzene derivatives are rarely metabolized in the body by dehalogenation reactions. Instead these substances are converted to phenols, catechols, glucuronides, mercapturic acids, and probably dihydro-diol derivatives. Fluoro-, bromo- and iodo-benzene are converted mainly to glucuronides of catechols and to mercapturic acids. Dichloro-, trichloro- and pentachloro-benzene derivatives are metabolized mainly to phenols.

It is possible that the mixed function oxidase in liver microsomes converts all of these substances to epoxide derivatives which in turn are converted to the various products, the relative proportions of which depend on the stability of the epoxide derivative and the activities of the epoxide hydrases and glutathione transferases. (Fig. 5). (See Chapters 55 and 39).

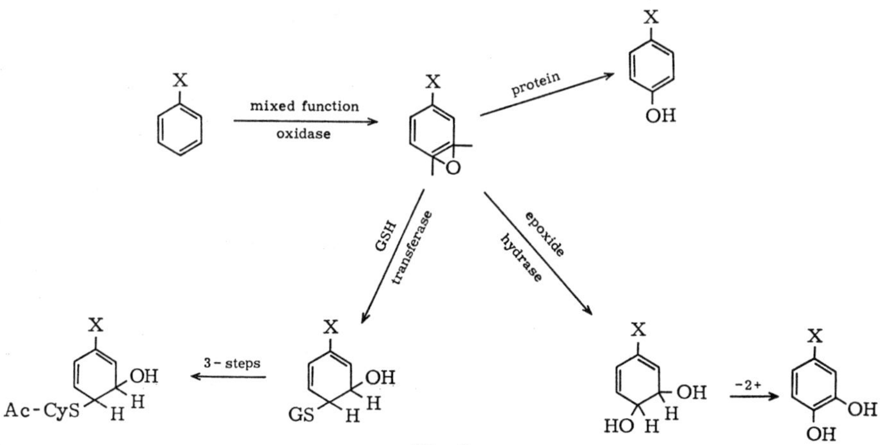

Fig. 5

In contrast, halogenated nitrobenzenes are converted to mercapturic acids by replacement of the halogen or the nitro group by glutathione. In these reactions, the halogenated nitrobenzenes need not be activated by the mixed function oxidase in liver microsomes, but are converted directly to their glutathione derivatives by the action of glutathione transferases. (See Chapter 55) (Fig. 6).

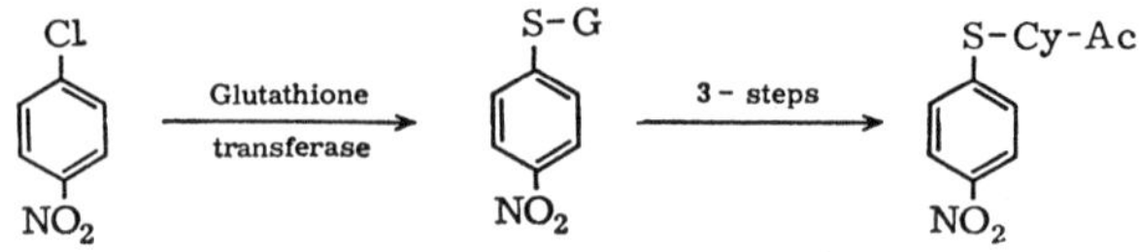

Fig. 6

Interestingly, *m*-monohalonitrobenzenes are not converted to mercapturic acids, but form hydroxylated metabolites in which the hydroxyl group is ortho and para to the halogen. As pointed out above, the nitro group in the meta position does not interfere with the delocalization of the π orbital and thus does not stabilize the intermediates formed during the replacement of halogens by electron donors such as hydroxyl ions.

In the metabolism of acetylated *p*-fluoro- and *p*-chloro-aniline derivatives by rabbit liver microsomes, however, the halogens are replaced by hydroxyl groups and thus form *p*-hydroxyacetanilide (RENSON, 1964; DALY et al., 1968). Since the microsomal system that catalyzes these reactions requires NADPH and molecular oxygen, it presumably is the same system that catalyzes the hydroxylation of acetanilide. When *p*-tritium acetanilide is used as a substrate, some of the tritium is relased as $^3H^+$ and some is transferred to the meta position. However, this transfer, called the NIH shift, apparently does not occur during the metabolism of *p*-halo-acetanilides by liver microsomes.

Another type of dehalogenation occurs with *o*-fluorobenzoic acid in bacteria (MILNE et al., 1968). In this reaction the acid is converted to an intermediate peroxide which is reduced by NADPH and then decomposes to form catechol, fluoride and carbon dioxide.

III. Metabolism of Aliphatic Halogenated Compounds

There is increasing evidence for at least two types of mechanisms for the metabolism of aliphatic halogenated compounds: one is associated with C-X bond rupture followed by the addition of a hydroxyl ion or a thio group such as glutathione, the other involves the translocation of the halide within the molecule.

The demonstration of dehalogenation *in vivo* came from the observation that inorganic bromide was found in blood and urine after administration of methyl bromide or bromochloromethane to mammals (IRISH et al., 1941; SVIRBELY et al., 1947). Comcomitantly, an explanation for the toxicity of various halogenated aliphatic compounds on the basis of the released halide was suggested (MILLER and HAGGARD, 1943). Later, HEPPEL and PORTERFIELD (1948) were able to demonstrate that slices of rat liver, kidney and spleen catalyzed the formation of bromide ions from monochloromonobromomethane, but the heart, diaphragm and brain were relatively inactive. They further demonstrated that homogenates of liver were active, but homogenates of kidney showed little or no activity. The dehalogenation demonstrated by these investigators was more rapid anaerobically than aerobically, and was inhibited by mercuric salts and sodium fluoride. Less rapid dehalogenation was found with dibromomethane and dichloromethane. Chloroform was dehalogenated slowly, and bromoform was not cleaved at all. Monobromoethane, dibromoethane, monobromomonochloroethane, and dichloromethane were cleaved. Interestingly, these investigators found that prior exposure of male rats to monochloromonobromomethane stimulated dehalogenation and suggested the presence of other enzymes (HEPPEL and PORTERFIELD, 1948).

In 1966, JOHNSON described an enzymatic dehalogenating system in rat liver that required reduced glutathione and thus is presumably a glutathione transferase (See Chapter 55). The preparation was active against monohalomethanes, particularly against iodomethane, and was significantly less active with halopropane and haloethane. It was shown that the halide ion was released during the rupture of the carbon-halogen bond. In these studies, most of the interest was placed on the utilization of glutathione during dehalogenation, less in the mechanisms involved in the dehalogenation (JOHNSON, 1966). In fact, the analysis of the activity of these enzymes against halogen-substituted alkanes was based in large part upon decrease of liver glutathione concentrations. Subsequently, an extensive study of the metabolism of 1-bromobutane in living rabbits and rats (JAMES et al., 1968), revealed the formation of conjugates with glutathione, cysteinylglycine and cysteine. Presumably these reactions are catalyzed by glutathione transferase, glutathionase and a peptidase which lead to the formation of mercapturic acid (Chapter 55).

Trichloroethylene undergoes transhalogenation in mammals and is excreted into urine as trichloroacetic acid and the glucuronide conjugate of trichloroethanol (DEFALQUE, 1961). Since these products are also formed from chloralhydrate in man, BUTLER (1949) suggested that chloralhydrate was an intermediate in the metabolism of trichloroethylene. LEIBMAN (1965) and BYINGTON and LEIBMAN (1965) confirmed this by showing that an NADPH and oxygen dependent enzyme in liver microsomes from rat and rabbit converts trichloroethylene to chloralhydrate and that enzymes in the soluble fraction convert chloralhydrate to trichloroacetic acid and trichloroethanol. Thus the microsomal enzyme system that catalyzes the transhalogenation of trichloroethylene is similar to the enzyme system that forms hydroxylated foreign compounds (See Chapter 39), and epoxides of aromatic hydrocarbons (BOYLAND and SIMS, 1965) and chlorinated hydrocarbon insecticides, such as hepatachlor and isodrin (WONG and TERRIERE, 1965). It seems possible that the metabolism of trichloroethylene proceeds along one of the following pathways (BYINGTON and LEIBMAN, 1965) (Fig. 7).

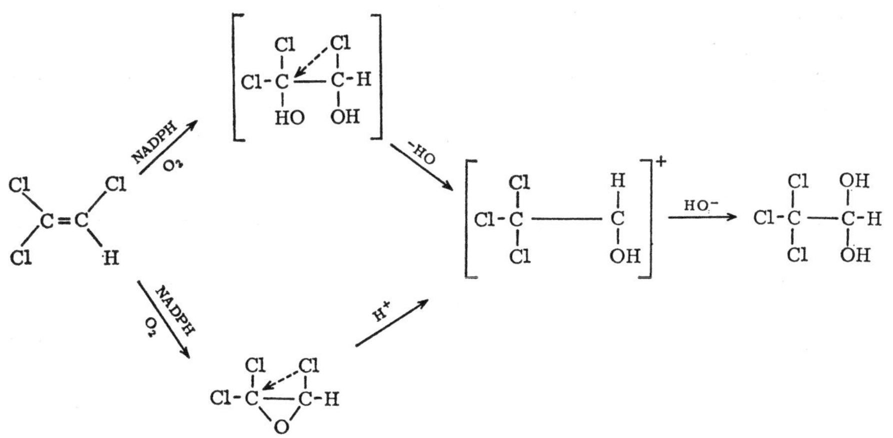

Fig. 7

These mechanisms are thus analogous to the "NIH Shift" of tritium in the hydroxylation of N-acetyl-p-^{3}H anilide (GUROFF et al., 1967).

Metabolism of CCl_4 has probably received more study than any other aliphatic halogenated compound. BUTLER (1961), McCOLLISTER et al. (1951), RUBINSTEIN and KANICS (1964), and PAUL and RUBINSTEIN (1963) have all demonstrated that CCl_4 is dehalogenated by mammalian systems. The most extensive studies of the metabolism of CCl_4 were those of BUTLER (1961) and PAUL and RUBINSTEIN (1963). They found that the system that metabolized CCl_4 was even more active against $CHCl_3$. The quantity of the haloalkanes metabolized by the mammalian system was relatively small, approximately 5% of the administered dose was converted to carbon dioxide. With CCl_4 the steps involve a progressive and apparently stepwise dehalogenation, but it should be pointed out that the intermediates have not been identified. The final conversion to CO_2 occurs in the liver and the kidney. Adipose tissue, blood and muscle have little or no capacity to dehalogenate CCl_4. It was also shown that on homogenization of liver slices the rate of dechlorination is decreased to less than $^1/_{16}$ that of the intact organ. It was also determined that the dehalogenation of $CHCl_3$ or CCl_4 was carried out by cell free systems, with a broad pH optimum (RUBINSTEIN and KANICS, 1964), and required NAD, NADH and NADP. Certain purine nucleotide analogues augmented CO_2 formation from CCl_4 and $CHCl_3$. Unfortunately, attempts to measure the loss of CCl_4 or $CHCl_3$ with reduced pyridine nucleotide or a regeneration system were not made, and indeed comparable studies using NADPH were not undertaken. This may partially explain the apparent necessity for supernatant as well as microsomes in carrying out the dehalogenation at an optimum rate.

The effect of added ATP and glutathione was measured in a cell free system and the production of CO_2 from $CHCl_3$ or CCl_4 was assayed. It was found that glutathione, in the presence of NAD or NADPH, stimulates the production of CO_2, while ATP has no effect. Similarly, FAD and folate have little effect in the absence of nucleotides. These studies suggest that microsomes, in the presence of supernatant, are able to carry out the dehalogenation of $CHCl_3$ and probably of CCl_4. However, confusion exists concerning the mechanisms of dehalogenation of these compounds. It is not clear whether NADPH or NADH is the preferred source of electrons, as no information concerning electron transport systems exists. The inhibitory effects of various substances, including parachloromercuribenzoate, may be related more to restoration of reduced nucleotides than to a direct effect on the dehalogenation itself. Present evidence does not permit the selection of the mechanisms of dehalogenation, i.e., whether this represents the formation of an intermediate phosgene, as suggested by BUTLER (1961), or a progressive dehalogenation with the formation of formaldehyde, as suggested by HEPPEL and PORTERFIELD (1948). Furthermore, the data do not permit selection of heterolytic (ionic) or homolytic (free radical) mechanisms. More recent studies by McLEAN and McLEAN (1966) have indicated that the dehalogenation of CCl_4 can be modified by stimulation of drug-metabolizing enzymes by phenobarbital treatment. These studies suggest that dehalogenation, in this instance, is carried out by enzymes in the endoplasmic reticulum which are similar to drug-metabolizing or xenobiotic enzymes. Modulation of the CCl_4-induced injury by adrenalectomy, stress, and drug suppression support this notion (McLEAN and McLEAN, 1969; SMUCKLER and HULTIN, 1966).

BUTLER (1961) initially suggested that dehalogenation of CCl_4 proceeded by homolytic cleavage. This hypothesis would necessarily result in the formation of a "neutral" halogen atom, possessing one unpaired electron. Attempts to detect this entity by electron spin resonance, however, have been unsuccessful (DANIELS, 1966; SMUCKLER, 1966; SLATER, 1967). It is possible that the quantity of radical formed is so small and its half-life so short that detection is not possible (see RECKNAGEL, 1967). On the other hand, SLATER (1968) has suggested the formation of peroxide during CCl_4 metabolism.

The metabolism of other halogenated aliphatics, including the anesthetics, has not been studied as extensively. However, there is suggestive evidence that chlorinated and brominated anesthetics are metabolized by NADPH and oxygen-requiring systems in the liver, with the release of the respective halides. In particular, halothane (1,1,1-trifluoro-2-bromo-2-chloroethane) and methoxylfluorine are dechlorinated and debrominated by mammalian liver. Both reactions require O_2 and reduced NADP, suggesting the involvement of the mixed function oxidase (VAN DYKE, 1968).

IV. Indirect Tests of Dehalogenation

There is abundant evidence indicating that many halogenated aliphatic and aromatic compounds produce significant tissue damage in mammalian species. Extensive studies with CCl_4 have indicated that the tetrasubstituted methane is not the direct toxin, but that metabolism of the parent material is requisite to the toxic action (SMUCKLER, 1966; SMUCKLER and HULTIN, 1966; MCLEAN and MCLEAN, 1966; SEAWRIGHT and MCLEAN, 1967; GARNER and MCLEAN, 1969). Utilizing the toxic action of CCl_4 as a guide, a number of investigators have assayed the toxic effects of a variety of aliphatic halogen derivatives as an indirect measure of metabolism. These analyses have included trichloromethane (chloroform) (SLATER, 1965), dichloromethane, diiodomethane, tribromomethane, triiodomethane (iodoform), carbon tetrabromide, carbon tetraiodide, 1,2-dichloroethane, 1,1,1-trichloroethane, 1,1,2,2-tetrachloroethane, pentachloroethane, halothane and 1,1,1-trifluoro-2-chloro-2-bromo-ethane (REYNOLDS and YEE, 1968). Although the results of these studies are intriguing, and demonstrate rather clearly a relationship between lability of the halogen-carbon bond and the potential of the compounds to form free radicals, certain problems have become apparent. Among these problems is the fact that tetraiodomethane, the most readily metabolized compound in the series, does not produce the morphological changes observed with CCl_4. Since these studies provide indirect evidence at best, the relationship of toxicity to dehalogenation and the problems of relative solubilities of compounds both in aqueous and nonaqueous portions of the mammalian cells makes their interpretation difficult.

V. Dehalogenation of Insecticides

Recent interest in the effects of DDT, its prolonged lifetime and its possible deleterious effect on our ecosystem has caused considerable interest in the metabolism of DDT, both in mammals and lower organisms. It was recently shown that a variety of microorganisms dechlorinate DDT (CHACKO and LOCKWOOD, 1966), but the mechanisms were not established. Furthermore, there is recent evidence that some insecticides are metabolized by a NADPH-requiring cytochrome P_{450}, involving epoxidation systems similar to that suggested above for halogen transfer. In fact, very recently it has been shown that the avian liver is capable of dechlorinating DDT.

Summary and Conclusions

The molecular mechanisms involved in biological dehalogenation are not known. On the basis of the chemistry of the halogen-carbon bond, and on the variance induced in the carbon-halogen bond by the rest of the molecule, one might expect different mechanisms to operate in aliphatic and aromatic compounds. Evidence is available indicating that dehalogenation of aromatic compounds depends upon halogen substitution and the nature of the aromatic bond. For example, there is an obvious difference in the mechanisms of the dehalogenation of aliphatic and aromatic compounds. It has been proposed that two mechanisms can be used describe the nature of the reactive product. These include dehydrochlorination, in which both hydrogen and chlorine are extracted from the molecule with the resultant formation of a double bond, and hydrolytic dehalogenation, in which a hydroxyl group or an HS-group replaces the halogen molecule. Until we are more certain of the active mechanisms involved, it is premature to make such a categorical distinction. The separation of reductive dehalogenation, utilizing reduced NADP and molecular oxygen, and peroxide-linked dehalogenation is apparently warranted in mammalian liver for a number of aliphatic halogenated materials. In these instances, the dehalogenation system appears to be part of the broader group of mixed-function oxidases present in the endoplasmic reticulum of the mammalian liver. Reevaluation of the studies on dehalogenation of other compounds might also indicate that they belong in this category. The relationship of peroxidation to dehalogenation has been suggested for bacterial systems. A mechanism whereby peroxidation and dehalogenation are coupled in the mammalian systems has been proposed by SLATER (1968). The dehalogenation and the peroxidation in this proposal are separate, but coupled by a mistake of nature. In fact, this anomalous coupling provides a possible basis for the observed production of peroxides in CCl_4 intoxication. It is intriguing to speculate that this mechanism may provide the basis for the dehalogenation itself, representing not an adventitious use of electron flow, but the prime means of handling halide bonds.

References

BOYLAND, E., SIMS, P.: Metabolism of polycyclic compounds. The metabolism of 9,10 epoxy 9,10 dihydrophenanthracene. Biochem. J. **95**, 788—790 (1965).

BUTLER, T.C.: Metabolic transformation of trichloroethylene. J. Pharmacol. exp. Ther. **97**, 84—92 (1949).

— Reduction of carbon tetrachloride in vivo and reduction of carbon tetrachloride and chloroform in vitro by tissues and tissue constituents. J. Pharmacol. exp. Ther. **134**, 311—319 (1961).

BYINGTON, K.H., LEIBMAN, K.C.: Metabolism of trichloroethylene in liver microsomes. II. Identification of the reaction product as chloral hydrate. Molec. Pharmacol. **1**, 247—254 (1965).

CHACKO, E.I., LOCKWOOD, J.L.: Chlorinated hydrocarbon pesticides: Degradation by microbes. Science **154**, 893—895 (1966).

COTTRELL, T.L.: The strengths of chemical bonds. New York: Academic Press 1954.

DALY, J.W., SUROFF, G., UDENFRIEND, S., WITKOP, B.: Hydroxylation of alkyl and halogen substituted anilines and acetanilides by microsomal hydroxylases. Biochem. Pharmacol. **17**, 31—36 (1968).

DANIELS, T.: Personal comment, 1966.

DEFALQUE, R.J.: Pharmacology and toxicology of trichloroethylene. A critical view of the world literature. Clin. Pharmacol. Ther. **2**, 665—688 (1961).

GARNER, R.C., McLEAN, A.E.M.: Increased susceptibility to carbon tetrachloride poisoning in the rat after pretreatment with oral phenobarbitone. Biochem. Pharmacol. **18**, 645—650 (1969).

GUROFF, G., DALY, J., JERINA, D., RENSON, J., UDENFRIEND, S.: Hydroxylation-induced migration: The NIH Shift. Science **157**, 1524—1530 (1967).

HEPPEL, L.A., PORTERFIELD, V.T.: Enzymatic dehalogenation of certain brominated and chlorinated compounds. J. biol. Chem. **176**, 763—769 (1948).

IRISH, D.D., ADAMS, E.M., SPENCER, H.C., ROWE, V.K.: Chemical changes of methyl bromide in the animal body in relation to its physiological effects. J. Ind. Hyg. Toxicol. **23**, 408—411 (1941).

JAMES, S.P., JEFFREY, D.A., WARING, R.H., WOOD, P.B.: Some metabolites of 1-bromobutane in the rabbit and the rat. Biochem. J. **109**, 727—736 (1968).
JOHNSON, M.K.: Studies on glutathione S-alkyltransferase of the rat. Biochem. J. **98**, 44—56 (1966).
KETELAAR, J.A.A.: Chemical constitution, an introduction of the theory of the chemical bond, 2nd ed. Amsterdam-London-New York-Princeton: Elsevier Publ. Co. 1958.
LEIBMAN, K.C.: Metabolism of trichloroethylene in liver microsomes. I. Characteristics of the reaction. Molec. Pharmacol. **1**, 239—246 (1965).
McCOLLISTER, D.D., BEAMER, W.H., ATCHISON, G.J., SPENCER, H.C.: The absorption, distribution and elimination of radioactive carbon tetrachloride by monkeys upon exposure to low vapor concentration. J. Pharmacol. exp. Ther. **102**, 112—124 (1951).
McLEAN, A.E.M., McLEAN, E.K.: The effect of diet and 1,1,1-trichloro-2,2-bis(p-chlorophenyl)ethane (DDT) on microsomal hydroxylating enzymes and on sensitivity of rats to carbon tetrachloride poisoning. Biochem. J. **100**, 564—571 (1966).
— — Diet and toxicity. Brit. med. Bull. **25**, 278—281 (1969).
MILLER, E.P., HAGGARD, H.W.: Intracellular penetration of bromide as a feature in the toxicity of alkyl bromides. J. Ind. Hyg. Toxicol. **25**, 423—433 (1943).
MILNE, G.W.A., GOLDMAN, P., HOLTZMAN, J.L.: The metabolism of 2-fluorobenzoic acid. II. Studies with $^{18}O_2$. J. biol. Chem. **243**, 5374—5376 (1968).
PAUL, B.B., RUBINSTEIN, D.: Metabolism of carbon tetrachloride and chloroform by the rat. J. Pharmacol. exp. Ther. **141**, 141—148 (1963).
PAULING, L.C.: The nature of the chemical bond. Ithaca, N.Y.: Cornell University Press 1960.
RECKNAGEL, R.L.: Carbon tetrachloride hepatotoxicity. Pharmacol. Rev. **19**, 145—208 (1967).
RENSON, J.: Studies on the mechanism of microsomal hydroxylation. Fed. Proc. **23**, 325 (1964).
REYNOLDS, E.S., YEE, A.G.: Liver parenchymal cell injury. VI. Significance of early glucose 6-phosphatase suppression and transient calcium influx following poisoning. Lab. Invest. **19**, 273—281 (1968).
RUBINSTEIN, D., KANICS, L.: The conversion of carbon tetrachloride and chloroform to carbon dioxide by rat liver homogenates. Canad. J. Biochem. **42**, 1577—1585 (1964).
SEAWRIGHT, A.A., McLEAN, A.E.M.: The effect of diet on carbon tetrachloride metabolism. Biochem. J. **105**, 1055—1060 (1967).
SLATER, T.F.: A note on the relative activities of tetrachloromethane and trichloro-fluoromethane on the rat. Biochem. Pharmacol. **14**, 178—181 (1965).
— Stimulatory effect of CCl_4 *in vitro* on lipid peroxidation in rat liver microsomes. Proc. 4th Annual Federation of European Biochemical Society 1967.
— Aspects of cellular injury and recovery. In: The Biological Basis of Medicine. Ed. by E. EDWARD BITTAR, Vol. 1. London and New York: Academic Press 1968.
SMUCKLER, E.A., HULTIN, T.: Effects of SKF 525-A on adrenalectomy and the amino acid incorporation by rat liver microsomes from normal and CCl_4 treated rats. Exp. Molec. Path. **5**, 504—515 (1966).
— Studies on carbon tetrachloride intoxication. IV. Effect of carbon tetrachloride on liver slices and isolated organelles *in vitro*. Lab. Invest. **15**, suppl. January 1966.
SVIRBELY, J.L., HIGHMAN, B., ALFORD, W.C., OETTINGER, W.F., VON: The Toxicity and narcotic action of mono-chloro-mono-bromo-methane with special reference to inorganic and volatile bromide in blood, urine and brain. J. Ind. Hyg. Toxicol. **29**, 382—389 (1947).
VAN DYKE, R.A.: Metabolic pathways and anesthetic detoxification. In: Toxicity of Anesthetics. Ed. by B.R. FINK. Baltimore, Md.: Williams and Wilkins 1968.
WILLIAMS, R.T.: Detoxification Mechanisms, 2nd edition. New York: Wiley and Sons 1959.
WONG, P.T., TERRIERE, L.C.: Epoxidation of aldrin, isodrin and hepatachlor by rat liver microsomes. Biochem. Pharmacol. **14**, 375—377 (1965).

Chapter 45

Glucuronide-Forming Enzymes

G. J. DUTTON

With 1 Figure

Glucuronides, or *β-D*-glucosiduronic acids, are formed when a molecule condenses with the C-1 atom of glucuronic acid; the free carboxyl group at C-6 ensures polarity of the resulting conjugate, which is usually more water-soluble than the free aglycon and therefore more rapidly transported in, or excreted from, the organism. Glucuronide formation is the commonest conjugation in mammals, presumably from the ready availability of glucuronic acid in the tissues and the many chemical groups forming glucuronides. Enzymes catalyzing glucuronide synthesis have been widely, if not deeply, studied and exhaustive references up to 1965 are available (DUTTON, 1966b). Since then several questions, and a few answers, have been clarified; the present review will attempt to cover later significant work, but can only summarise earlier findings and indicate sources of further information.

Glucuronidation of foreign compounds is of obvious pharmacological importance: biologically-active groups may be masked, and excretion of the whole molecule hastened. Many endogenous compounds such as steroids (JAYLE and PASQUALINI, 1966; ROY, 1969), bilirubin (see SCHMID and LESTER, 1966) and the catechol amines (for references see WONG and SOURKES, 1968a), are routinely glucuronidated *in vivo*. Foreign and endogenous molecules both follow the same pathway of glucuronidation, sometimes possibly sharing the same glucuronyltransferase. Administered drugs may therefore profoundly influence the routine conjugations, and this review cannot be restricted to the glucuronidation of drugs but will emphasise pharmacological aspects of glucuronide formation for both foreign and endogenous substrates.

A. Mechanism of Glucuronide Biosynthesis

I. Transference from Uridine Diphosphate Glucuronic Acid

One, possibly the only, major pathway of glucuronide biosynthesis is the transfer of glucuronic acid from UDPglucuronic acid to the aglycon by UDP-glucuronyltransferase (E.C. 2.4.1.17; DUTTON and STOREY, 1954; STOREY and DUTTON, 1955):

$$\text{UDPglucuronic acid} + \text{Aglycon} \rightarrow \text{Aglycon glucuronide} + \text{UDP}$$

Glucuronyl transfer from other nucleotides is not known to be significant.

II. Other Enzymic Pathways of Glucuronide Biosynthesis

Neither free glucuronic acid nor its lactone combine enzymically with the aglycon; glucose and galactose are more direct carbon sources of conjugated glucuronic acid (see DUTTON, 1966b).

Glucuronyl transfer from already-formed glucuronides has been demonstrated by FISHMAN and several Japanese workers (for references see DUTTON, 1966b). Enzymic transference from ether glucuronides to alcohols and amines, and from acyl glucuronides to alcohols and a phenol, occurs in β-glucuronidase preparations, and the responsible 'β-glucuronylase' closely resembles β-glucuronidase (FISHMAN, 1959). There are a number of facts, however, suggesting that this reaction plays an insignificant role *in vivo*. Transfer requires higher concentrations of acceptor than are usually attained *in vivo*. Whenever UDPglucuronyltransferase activity is deficient, a similar deficiency of glucuronidation is demonstrable *in vivo*; no other transfer mechanism appears to fill the gap. β-Glucuronylase, like β-glucuronidase, is inhibited by glucarolactone (FISHMAN, 1959), yet administration of glucarolactone does not diminish glucuronide excretion but raises it. As FISHMAN (1959) acknowledges, speculation on the attractive role of 'β-glucuronylase' in glucuronide formation must await isolation of credible endogenous donor substrates.

Glucuronic acid could theoretically be transferred from aglycon A to aglycon B with intermediate transglucuronylation of UDP, but neither reversibility of UDPglucuronyltransferase nor the presence of a 'high-energy' endogenous glucuronide of A has been demonstrated. It is unlikely that β-glucuronidase catalyzes this kind of transfer because α-UDPglucuronic acid is not a substrate of the enzyme.

III. Non-Enzymic Pathways of Glucuronide Biosynthesis

When certain amines or amino acids are mixed in solution with free glucuronic acid or its lactone, *N*-glucuronides are directly formed (see DUTTON, 1966b). Since such mixing can occur *in vivo*, it has been suggested that the pharmacological action of glucuronate and its derivatives might be exerted by their combination with toxic endogenous amines liberated in disease or fatigue (TAMURA et al., 1966); however, glucuronate injected simultaneously with cyclohexamine did not reduce its toxicity (SMITH and WILLIAMS, 1966).

IV. Study of Glucuronide Biosynthesis

Various methods of studying glucuronide formation are discussed by DUTTON (1966b). Interesting procedures since published (JAAKOMAKI et al., 1967; DOHNÁLEK et al, 1967; MENKEN et al., 1966; FLODGAARD and BRODERSEN, 1967; LAGE and SPRATT, 1968; VAN ROY and HEIRWEGH, 1968; WONG and SOURKES, 1968a) include use of cell cultures (KO, DUTTON and NEMETH, 1967; SKEA and NEMETH, 1969) and suspensions (HENDERSON and DEWAIDE, 1969). Obviously, when intact animals, organs, tissue slices or cells are employed, glucuronide synthesis due to all pathways, known and unknown, is measured, and includes formation of any UDPglucuronic acid; added UDPglucuronic acid will not normally pass the cell membrane (see HENDERSON and DEWAIDE, 1969). Broken-cell preparations require added UDPglucuronic acid for demonstrable synthesis, unless concentrated enough to contain appreciable amounts of the endogenous nucleotide. Addition of UDPglucuronic acid focuses tissue metabolism, and the observer's attention, on the UDPglucuronyltransferase pathway of glucuronide formation; but as this pathway satisfactorily accounts for most glucuronidation phenomena *in vivo* and other pathways are not yet forthcoming, we consider below the factors affecting occurrence, activity — and observation — of UDPglucuronic acid and UDPglucuronyltransferase.

B. UDPGlucuronic Acid

UDPGlucuronic acid in a tissue need not be used there for biosynthesis of a particular, or of any, glucuronide; nor need its concentration indicate its turnover or metabolic importance. The nucleotide has many roles (Fig. 1) and its use by a particular UDPglucuronyltransferase will be controlled by factors of which we know nothing.

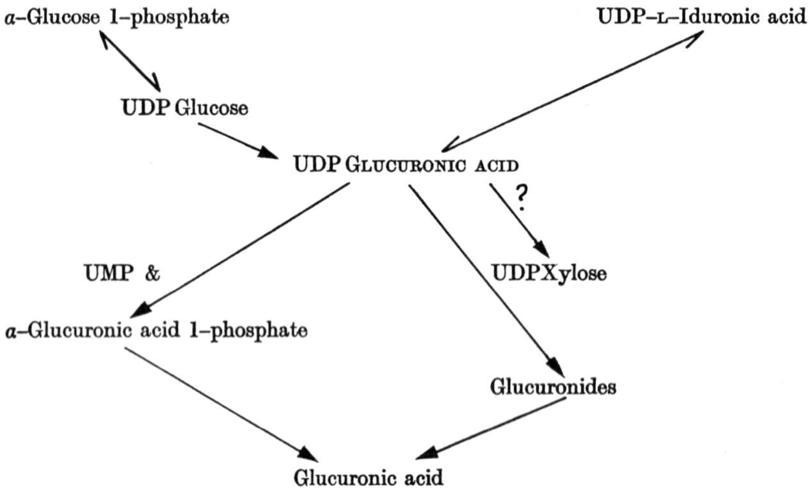

Fig. 1. Principal routes of synthesis and breakdown of UDPglucuronic acid in mammals

UDPGlucuronic acid is formed in animals, plants and bacteria by the NAD-dependent cytoplasmic enzyme UDPglucose dehydrogenase (STROMINGER et al., 1957):

$$\text{UDP-}\alpha\text{-}D\text{-glucose} + \text{NAD} \rightarrow \text{UDP-}\alpha\text{-}D\text{-glucuronic acid} + \text{NAD.H}$$

No intermediate in this reaction has been found (ZALITIS and FEINGOLD, 1968); the products inhibit the reaction.

UDPGlucose derives from *α-D*-glucose 1-phosphate, by UTP and a pyrophosphorylase (MUNCH-PETERSEN et al., 1953), and so ultimately from glucose or glycogen, explaining early observations that glucuronidation required carbohydrate, energy and oxygen (see DUTTON, 1966b).

UDPGlucose dehydrogenase occurs in liver, skin, synovial tissue, kidney, cartilage and alimentary tract, and is reported from mammals, birds, reptiles, amphibians, fish, plants and bacteria; it contains thiol, and possibly carboxyl, groups at the active center; for estimations, see WILSON (1965) and references in DUTTON (1966b).

A 5-epimerase in skin (JACOBSON and DAVIDSON, 1962) interconverts UDP-*L*-iduronic and UDP-*D*-glucuronic acids, but no other source of UDPglucuronic acid formation is known in mammals. Though plants can, and fish may, synthesize the nucleotide from *α*-glucuronic acid 1-phosphate, mammals do not; so administered glucuronic acid or its lactone will not assist glucuronidation by this pathway.

Sources and levels of UDPglucuronic acid are given by DUTTON (1966b) and WONG and SOURKES (1967a, 1968b). It is most abundant in vertebrate liver and kidney, with traces recorded from gastrointestinal tract, cartilage, skin, brain, muscle, testis, spleen, uterus, placenta, milk and various neoplasms (see also REID, 1962); it has not yet been found in insects or mollusks.

Purification, identification and estimation are described in the above references; ultra-violet absorption or chemical methods, such as the carbazole reaction (DISCHE, 1955), may be employed on the chromatographically-pure compound. MARSH (1966) has reviewed chemical syntheses of both α and β forms.

The relative importance *in vivo* of the competing metabolic pathways illustrated in Fig. 1 is unknown, but studies of UDPglucuronyltransferase must allow for breakdown *in vitro* by microsomal UDPglucuronic acid pyrophosphatase; the nucleotide should be added to approximate 'saturation' under the conditions employed, especially when UDPglucuronyltransferase may be 'deficient' or activated (STEVENSON and DUTTON, 1962; STEVENSON, GREENWOOD and McEWEN, 1968; HALAC and SICIGNANO, 1969). The pyrophosphatase is inhibited by its product UMP (OGAWA et al., 1966), and UDPglucuronic acid itself inhibits further breakdown of UMP (ADLARD, 1969); this mechanism may conserve tissue UDPglucuronic acid.

C. UDPGlucuronyltransferase

The term 'UDPglucuronyltransferase' covers an unknown number of closely similar enzymes, possibly with some overlapping specificity; their activity *in vitro* can vary surprisingly, apparently being dependent on sub-microsomal structure, and consequently kinetic, or indeed any quantitative, investigations must be interpreted cautiously.

I. Occurrence of UDPGlucuronyltransferase in Species

All mammals, birds and reptiles investigated possess UDPglucuronyltransferase, though activity towards certain substrates may be low or absent (see DUTTON, 1966b). Cat, for example, exhibits negligible activity towards *o*-aminophenol, menthol, phenolphthalein, 8-hydroxyquinoline, 1-naphthol or *p*-nitrophenol, but glucuronidates metanephrine (AXELROD et al., 1959), bilirubin, thyroxine and iodopanoic acid, and metabolites of some steroids and of *N*-fluorenylacetamide. Cats excrete injected glucuronide, so that conjugation, not excretion, is deficient; UDPglucuronic acid is plentiful in cat liver. Chickens possess transferases for many substrates but not for bilirubin (DUTTON and BURCHELL, 1969). Such differences render extrapolation from one species or substrate to another hazardous, and increase difficulties of drug trials. Hereditary conditions where the usual spectrum of transferase activity for the species is deranged are treated in section D.IV.

Terrestrial adult amphibians possess UDPglucuronyltransferase for the few substrates tested, but not those living wholly in water (see DUTTON, 1966b). Fish are confusing; some species lack UDPglucose dehydrogenase (MAICKEL et al., 1959; BRODIE and MAICKEL, 1962), others possess much (NAGAYAMA et al., 1968); some have no demonstrable, others only weak thermolabile, transferase activity (DUTTON, 1966b; NAGAYAMA et al., 1968). UDPGlucuronic acid occurs in fish, however synthesized (see DUTTON, 1966b), dogfish forms bilirubin glucuronide (ARIAS, 1962), and testosterone glucuronide is reported from salmon (GRAJCER and IDLER, 1963). Even if a fish forms endogenous glucuronides readily, glucuronidation of foreign compounds appears low. As BRODIE (1964) points out, abundant water for dialysis lessens the need for detoxication by conjugation; the need might be greater in salt water (SMITH, 1964) but no induction of transferase is seen during adaptation to salinity (NAGAYAMA et al., 1968).

The insects, crustaceans, mollusks and plants studied exhibited no glucuronidation or transferase activity when foreign phenols were offered, but formed the glucosides (see DUTTON, 1966b). However, plants almost certainly synthesize simple glucuronides of endogenous compounds, utilising a UDPglucuronyltransferase (MARSH, 1960), a metabolic distinction between routine molecules and 'xenobiotics' (see SMITH, 1968), which may persist less obviously in the mammal.

II. Occurrence of UDPGlucuronyltransferase in Tissues

Tissues exposed to the environment usually exhibit UDPglucuronyltransferase activity (see DUTTON, 1966b). Liver, kidney cortex and alimentary tract mucosa possess most; epidermis and urinary tract, but not lung, display some activity. Certain minimum-deviation hepatomas and those induced by diethylnitrosamine contain large amounts of the enzyme (LUEDERS and KUFF, 1967; STEVENSON, 1969). Most investigators employed only a few foreign compounds as aglycons; as implied above, transferases specific to endogenous substrates may exist in certain tissues: placenta, for example, lacks transferases for foreign compounds (see DUTTON, 1966b) but possesses one for estriol (DAHM and BREUER, 1966). For glucuronidation of drugs, liver seems quantitatively the most important tissue, from its weight and level of enzyme; activity resides in the hepatocytes themselves (SKEA and NEMETH, 1969; HENDERSON and DEWAIDE, 1969). In gut, glucuronidation may assist transport of ingested drugs, steroids and amino acids to the blood (for references see DUTTON, 1966b).

III. Location of UDPGlucuronyltransferase in the Cell

UDPglucuronyltransferase is predominantly a microsomal enzyme, its activity intimately associated with the structure of endoplasmic reticulum. However, a 'soluble' (not 'solubilised': but see criticism in section C. IV. below) form, specific for certain steroidal substrates, has been identified in the 150,000 *g* supernatant from human intestinal-mucosa homogenates and, though of weak activity, was not considered to arise from microsomal leakage (DAHM and BREUER, 1966) (see also RAO and BREUER, 1969). In homogenates of alimentary tract mucosa and kidney cortex activity is otherwise always associated with particles sedimenting as 'microsomes', and in liver it occurs in the classical microsomal fraction (see DUTTON, 1966b). Activity towards phenolphthalein appeared equally in both rough and smooth microsomes, but towards *o*-aminophenol and *p*-nitrophenol predominantly in the rough, a distribution unaffected by various treatments (GRAM et al., 1968); WHITE (1967) also noted activity for bilirubin and *p*-nitrophenol in both rough and smooth fractions; it was absent from cytoplasmic membrane. Deranged endoplasmic reticulum can yield microsomes of high transferase activity (SKEA, DUTTON and NEMETH, 1969); disturbance of microsomal membranes may activate or inactivate the enzyme (see section C.VII below).

IV. Purification of UDPGlucuronyltransferase

UDPGlucuronyltransferase can be released from microsomes into the high-speed supernatant fraction by snake venom, digitonin, EDTA, deoxycholate (which is inhibitory: HALAC and REFF, 1967) or sonication (see DUTTON, 1966b; STEVENSON et al., 1968), usually with accompanying activation. Thirty-fold purification of 'solubilised' guinea pig liver enzyme followed ammonium sulphate precipitation and elution from a DEAE column (ISSELBACHER et al., 1962); instability prevented further manipulation. A similar purification has been reported by MOWAT and ARIAS (1969), who found that even after centrifugation of sonication-'solubilised' preparations at 100,000 *g* for 45 min, with subsequent elution from Sephadex, the transferase activity towards *o*-aminophenol and bilirubin remained associated with unsedimentable lipoprotein vesicles 800—2000 Å in size. Transferase-rich vesicles were described by HALAC and REFF (1967) in the high-speed pellet; they inferred that these vesicles were solubilised by increased deoxycholate, but did not examine their supernatant. A truly solubilised transferase preparation has probably not yet been obtained, emphasising dependence of this enzyme's activity on membrane structure (see GRAHAM and WOOD, 1969).

V. Catalytic Center

Because of the insolubility of the UDPglucuronyltransferase complex, kinetic studies designed to silhouette the component enzymes have either not been attempted or have remained unconvincing. References are given by DUTTON (1966b) and further K_m values by TOMLINSON and YAFFE (1966), SCHRIEFERS et al. (1966), HALAC and REFF (1967), VAN ROY and HEIRWEGH (1968), FLODGAARD and BRODERSEN (1967), STEVENSON et al. (1968), WONG and SOURKES (1968a), WINSNES (1969), ADLARD (1969).

Naturally-occurring UDPglucuronic acid has an α-link and all glucuronides formed in this pathway possess the β-link; inversion therefore occurs during transfer, as discussed by Axelrod et al. (1958). Transfer appears irreversible, and approaches 100%.

Ionization (GOLDBERG, 1963) and inhibition (STOREY, 1965b) studies indicate thiol groups at the transferase active center. GOLDBERG (1963) found the K_m value for the nucleotide independent of concentration of acceptor substrate, and suggested two separate combining sites, the nucleotide combining through the NH—CO group of uracil.

VI. Specificity of UDPGlucuronyltransferase

In glucuronide formation, the glucuronyl residue replaces hydrogen from four main chemical groups possible on the aglycon, hydroxyl, carboxyl, sulfhydryl and amino or imino (for subdivisions see SMITH and WILLIAMS, 1966; MARSH, 1966). For the first two groups the linkage is through oxygen and for the others through sulfur and nitrogen respectively. The aglycon may be aromatic, aliphatic or heterocyclic. As *N*,*N*-diethyldithiocarbamate is a substrate (DUTTON and ILLING, 1969), UDPglucuronyltransferase preparations now appear to catalyse glucuronidation of all four main groups and most of their subdivisions (see DUTTON, 1966b).

Evidence for the multiple nature of UDPglucuronyltransferase is discussed fully by DUTTON (1966b) and summarised by ISSELBACHER (1968); though still indirect, it now appears overwhelming. We next must distinguish specificities of the UDPglucuronyltransferases in any one organism. One obvious distinction could concern the chemical linkage. Another could be environmental, between compounds endogenous and foreign to the organism, as noted in plants. So simple a division is unlikely, but illustrates the difficulty. When we administer compounds the species has never encountered in its history, we assail its specifically-evolved transferases with unfamiliar molecules; from the response of these enzymes we are trying to deduce their specificities towards their own natural substrates, most of which remain unknown. A transferase evolved to serve an endogenous substrate may well accept a foreign compound structurally similar to its natural substrate; but two transferases, each specific for their own natural substrates, might in some instances both accept the same foreign substrate; and — a remote possibility — a cellular protein may exist whose catalytic property as a UDPglucuronyltransferase is only manifested when a certain foreign compound is provided as its substrate. 'Foreign' substrates, however valuable pharmacologically, are clumsy tools for investigating the natural specificities — and so the physiological role — of the UDPglucuronyltransferases.

We can only summarise observations on an assortment of foreign and endogenous substrates, refer the investigator to detailed articles, and emphasise the caution required in comparing substrates, species and tissues. Certain species, of course, lack UDPglucuronyltransferase activity towards compounds which are substrates for other species and in this sense there clearly exist several transferases (see Dutton, 1966b), but the present problem concerns identity of separate transferases in the one organism or perhaps specific substrate accessibility to a single enzyme (see C.VII.).

Evidence derives from four main sources: studies on kinetics, activations, developmental rates and on mutants lacking specific transferase activities. The first three especially are difficult to interpret with an insoluble enzyme, and the mutant strains have often been poorly characterized.

One distinguishable UDPglucuronyltransferase activity forms *N*-glucuronides; this is not surprising, for Marsh (1966) points out their chemical peculiarities. Liver slices from Gunn rats cannot synthesize a large number of *O*-glucuronides but form aniline *N*-glucuronide (Arias, 1961), and activity towards *p*-nitrophenol and anthranilate could be solubilised from rabbit liver, but not that towards aniline (Isselbacher et al., 1962). Reports that the Crigler-Najjar child, which has a transferase deficiency similar to the Gunn rat, cannot excrete an *N*-glucuronide (Jansen et al., 1969b), and that activity towards aniline was sonically solubilised with, and behaved exactly as, the activity forming *O*-glucuronides (Leventer et al., 1965), need not invalidate the above conclusion. Walker and Williams (1969) discuss specificity of *N*-glucuronide formation in primates.

Specificity to thiolic aglycons is unknown; thiophenol competitively inhibits transferase activity towards *p*-nitrophenol but not towards *o*-aminophenol (Storey, 1965b).

UDPGlucuronyltransferase activities towards hydroxyl and carboxyl groups are not clearly divisible. Though the acyl glucuronide of bilirubin probably requires a different transferase from those synthesizing phenolic glucuronides, evidence from the Gunn rat, for example, supports no simple division; in some cases the animal is deficient in activity both towards hydroxyl groups (*o*-aminophenol, menthol, 4-methylumbelliferone) and a carboxyl group (bilirubin), but in other cases it possesses normal activity towards these groups (diphenylacetate, Javitt, 1966; tetrahydrocortisone, Drucker, 1968; *p*-nitrophenol, Van Leusden et al., 1962; Temple et al., 1968)—though in some laboratories (White, 1967; Drucker, 1968; Stevenson et al., 1968) it has 'lost' its 'normal' activity for *p*-nitrophenol.

Such confusion is unavoidable at present. The following further divisions are therefore quoted hesitantly; they are from direct substrate comparison in one transferase preparation, with UDPglucuronic acid usually present at high concentration.

(1) Between *p*-nitrophenol, and bilirubin, in various species, from kinetic, ionic and developmental studies, use of mutants, and purification (Isselbacher et al., 1962; Tomlinson and Yaffe, 1966; Halac and Reff, 1967; Cotte et al., 1967; White, 1967; Halac and Sicignano, 1969). (2) Between *p*-nitrophenol and *o*-aminophenol, in various species, from studies on kinetics and with mutants (Storey, 1965b; Temple et al., 1968). (3) Between *p*-nitrophenol and tetrahydrocortisone, with mutants (Drucker, 1968). (4) Between *p*-nitrophenol, phe-

nolphthalein, menthol or bilirubin, and *o*-aminophenol or paracetamol, in rat, from activation studies (STEVENSON et al., 1968). (5) Between *p*-nitrophenol and phenolphthalein in rat, and (6) between *o*-aminophenol and phenolphthalein in mouse, from developmental studies (DUTTON, 1966a).

WINSNES (1969) reports marked differences in activations of various substrates.

Many other suggestive results, not from direct comparison of substrates, appear in the literature quoted here and by DUTTON (1966b). Several reports suggest overlap of specificities.

Probably more meaningful is the study of endogenous substrates, especially steroids. Enzymes forming estrone 3-glucuronide and 17β-estradiol 3-glucuronide in rabbit liver microsomes possess pH optima of 8.1 and 8.7—9.2 respectively (SMITH and BREUER, 1963; BREUER and WESSENDORF, 1966), whereas human gut and rat liver contain a soluble UDPglucuronyltransferase, optimum pH 6.8, for the 17β glucuronides of estriol, 17β-estradiol and testosterone (DAHM and BREUER, 1966); this contrasts with another, microsomal, enzyme there forming 16α glucuronides (DAHM et al., 1967). A further transferase for the 17β group exists in microsomes from human gut (DAHM et al., 1966), its pH optimum at 6.6 resembling that of the soluble '17β' enzyme. Activities of soluble enzymes for the phenolic estrogen and the 16α hydroxyl groups of estriol have also been distinguished by these workers. Others have found differences between glucuronidation of 3α and 17β hydroxyl groups (SCHRIEFERS et al., 1966), and between 3α and 16α hydroxyl groups (SLAUNWHITE et al., 1964). Several minor substrates and non-substrates have been reported from these laboratories (see also DUTTON, 1966b; ROY, 1969; RAO and BREUER, 1969). Specificity towards bilirubin derivatives is discussed by LESTER and KLEIN (1966).

Whether the two glucuronyl residues of a diglucuronide are added simultaneously or consecutively, they might still require a transferase different from the enzyme adding one residue to a free aglycon. After general acceptance that bilirubin 'monoglucuronide' was mixed bilirubin and diglucuronide (see DUTTON, 1966b), VAN ROY and HEIRWEGH's procedure (1968) suggests that although both mono- and diglucuronides occur in bile, only the monoglucuronide is significantly synthesised by liver *in vitro* (but see FLODGAARD and BRODERSEN, 1967); this method has been used clinically (BLACK and BILLING, 1969).

The double conjugate glycyrrhetic acid, a β-*D*-glucuronosyl-β-*D*-glucosiduronic acid (MARSH and LEVVY, 1956) occurs in licorice root; the mammalian double conjugates, estriol-3-sulfate-16-glucuronide and 17α-estradiol-3-glucuronide-17-*N*-acetylglucosaminide, are glucuronidated before the second conjugation (EMERMAN et al., 1967; JIRKU and LAYNE, 1965) so present no specificity problems. Identification of an α-glycosidic link in pregnenediol-3-sulfate-20-α-*N*-acetylglucosaminide (ARCOS and LIEBERMAN, 1967) should be a warning that although no natural α-glucuronides are known, not all 'β-glucuronides' have been checked with purified β-glucuronidase and its specific inhibitor; neither has the uronic acid always been characterized. The extent of glucuronide identification is tabulated by MARSH (1966).

The enzyme(s) catalyzing UDPglucuronyl transfer in polysaccharide biosynthesis appears distinct from the UDPglucuronyltransferases forming simple glucuronides (see SILBERT, 1966; DUTTON, 1966b).

Little is known of transferase specificity towards sugar or nucleotide of the donor substrate; the glucuronyl moiety must be α-, not β-linked (HONJO et al., 1962). Other uronic acid-containing nucleotides exist, and mannuronyl and iduronyl transfer must occur in polysaccharide biosynthesis (LIN and HASSID, 1966; see SILBERT, 1966; DUTTON, 1966b).

VII. Factors Affecting Observed UDPGlucuronyltransferase Activity *in Vitro*

Observed activity of UDPglucuronyltransferase changes strikingly with treatment *in vitro*. Most treatments seem not to affect the enzyme protein directly, but rather the availability of substrates — especially UDPglucuronic acid — in the medium or their accessibility to the insoluble enzyme.

Low concentrations of Mg^{++} increase or decrease activity, depending on preparations and substrates (Tomlinson and Yaffe, 1966; Halac and Reff, 1967; Cotte et al., 1967; Temple et al., 1968; Wong and Sourkes, 1968a; for others see Dutton, 1966b); Ca^{++}, probably antagonistic to Mg^{++}, usually inhibits (Dutton, 1966b; Adlard, 1969). Hydrogen ion concentration, except for those steroid substrates noted earlier, seems not critical, a broad pH optimum existing over 7.3—7.9 (see Dutton, 1966b). Except for one intestinal enzyme (Breuer and Wessendorf, 1966), the transferases are usually inhibited by compounds reacting with thiol groups (see Dutton, 1966b; Halac and Reff, 1967; Flodgaard and Brodersen, 1967). Predictably, thiolic compounds enhance stability (Storey, 1965a).

Stability of UDPglucuronyltransferase varies somewhat with source and purity (see Dutton, 1966b; Halac and Reff, 1967). Liver microsomes lose activity over several weeks at 4°; when solubilized, half is lost in a week (Mowat and Arias, 1969). Freezing or further purification lessens activity.

However, 'ageing' (Lueders and Kuff, 1967; Gram et al., 1968), sonication (Henderson and Dewaide, 1969) or prolonged centrifuging (White, 1967) of homogenate or microsomes activates the enzyme, as do low concentrations of the surface-active agents digitonin, deoxycholate, EDTA and Triton-X (Isselbacher et al., 1962; Huttunen and Miettinen, 1965; Halac and Reff, 1967; Lueders and Kuff, 1967; Halac and Sicignano, 1969; Winsnes, 1969; Adlard, 1969); high concentrations of detergents inhibit activity, and all concentrations inhibit already-'aged' enzyme preparations, suggesting a similar activation mechanism in both procedures. The microsomal structure may 'loosen', allowing easier access of acceptor and donor substrates; or a membrane-bound inhibitor may be removed. Activation with trypsin (Hänninen and Antila, 1969) or venoms (Isselbacher et al., 1962; Temple et al., 1968) may operate similarly. These activations may reach 45-fold, are irreversible, and need not involve release of enzyme into the supernatant fraction or inhibition of UDPglucuronic acid pyrophosphatase (Lueders and Kuff, 1967). Such pyrophosphatase inhibition can occur (Pogell and Leloir, 1961), and Adlard (1969) observed that after solubilisation with deoxycholate a 9-fold activation of transferase towards bilirubin accompanied, and was apparently due to, loss of pyrophosphatase activity. Nucleotides such as UDP-*N*-acetylglucosamine, ATP (Pogell and Leloir, 1961) and UDPglucose (Adlard, 1969) probably 'activate' rat liver microsomal transferase by inhibiting the microsomal pyrophosphatase (Schliselfeld et al., 1965; Ogawa et al., 1966; Adlard, 1969; see Dutton, 1966b); significantly, these nucleotides exert little effect on solubilized rat-liver transferase or the relatively pyrophosphatase-free preparation from guinea pig (Pogell and Leloir, 1961). Yet their activations are additive, and detectable even with excess UDPglucuronic acid. Adlard (1969) suggests ATP may bind inhibitory ions, and Pogell and Leloir (1961) and Winsnes (1969) consider that UDP-*N*-acetylglucosamine also affects accessibility of the active center, as might the other activators, albumin (Pogell and Leloir, 1961; Halac and Reff, 1967) and diethylnitrosamine (Stevenson et al., 1968). Activation by diethylnitrosamine (which strongly inhibits other drug-metabolizing enzymes: STEVENSON and GREENWOOD, 1968) seems so far confined to rat liver and two substrates, and does not affect the pyrophosphatase; it immediately activates certain presumably present but quite inactive transferases in Gunn rat (STEVENSON et al., 1968) and greatly increases activation already produced by detergents (WINSNES, 1969). Increased glucuronidation from inhibition or loss of microsomal β-glucuronidase (see HUTTUNEN and MIETTINEN, 1965, and FISHMAN et al., 1967) has not been observed (HALAC and REFF, 1967; see DUTTON, 1966b); WINSNES (1969) found no change in homogenate β-glucuronidase during transferase activations.

Transferase may be inhibited by drastic interference with microsomal membranes. Their degradation by phospholipases lowers activity towards *p*-nitrophenol, which is restored by added phospholipid micelles (GRAHAM and WOOD, 1969).

SKF 525A may inhibit glucuronidation by acting on cell membranes or on UDPglucuronic acid supply: it inhibits glucuronide formation (COOPER et al., 1954; HENDERSON and DEWAIDE, 1969) or secretion (HARGREAVES, 1967) in slices or cells, but has little effect in homogenates or sonicates (GOLDSTEIN and TAUROG, 1968; HENDERSON and DEWAIDE, 1969).

Certain alcohols also inhibit glucuronidation (see DUTTON, 1966b; HÄNNINEN and ALANEN, 1966), some possibly as competitors for enzyme or, under conditions employed, for nucleotide. Various drugs and steroids inhibiting UDPglucuronyltransferase are, because of the physiological implications, treated in the following section.

D. Factors Affecting Overall Glucuronidation *in Vivo*

Glucuronidation may be controlled at various stages: at uptake of aglycon or its precursor into the cell; at metabolism of precursor into aglycon; at accessibility of enzyme to aglycon; at the level of active enzyme; at availability of UDPglucuronic acid; at secretion of conjugate from the cell; at hydrolysis of conjugate to free aglycon.

Control at any stage will depend on the state of the organism: its age, diet, hormonal or genetic complement, intake of toxins or drugs, its response to external environment and its health.

I. Age

Glucuronidation of many substrates is low or undetectable in diverse preparations of fetal mammalian tissues, from perfusions to microsomes; it increases with age, the rate depending on species, tissue and substrate, until 'adult' capacity is achieved perinatally (see DUTTON, 1966b; TOMLINSON and YAFFE, 1966; FLODGAARD and BRODERSEN, 1967; HALAC and SICIGNANO, 1969).

This phenomenon is of considerable pharmacological importance, explaining both the perinatal toxicity of glucuronidogenic drugs and their icterogenic effect. The human neonate is slow to glucuronidate bilirubin and competition anywhere in this process may precipitate jaundice. Drugs may also decrease glucuronidation of endogenous aglycons not so clinically recognisable as bilirubin.

The causes of any low fetal glucuronidation are complex, but evidence suggests restriction of UDPglucuronic acid, deficient transferase activity and slow excretion of conjugate.

UDPGlucuronic acid must be present in the fetus to synthesise polysaccharides and certain endogenous glucuronides. Its level in fetal liver appeared low (DUTTON, 1959; FLODGAARD and BRODERSEN, 1967), though its greater lability there or the absence of accompanying transferase activators could also explain the results. Restriction of the nucleotide is further suggested by low levels of UDPglucose dehydrogenase (Brown and Zuelzer, 1958), and by transferase activity appearing in UDPglucuronic acid-fortified homogenates before noticeable glucuronidation in slices of the same age (Dutton, 1959); though the last observation could also arise from the defective glucuronide excretion of perinatal liver (Schenker and Schmid, 1964).

Because UDPglucuronyltransferase measurement is so subject to its environment, doubts of a true perinatal deficiency persist. Is active enzyme present in fetal liver homogenates, but unrecordable? Is, for example, added UDPglucuronic acid too rapidly destroyed there for demonstrable transference? Even with high concentrations of the nucleotide, 'deficiency' of the enzyme in early fetal liver remains striking (Stevenson and Dutton, 1962; Halac and Sicignano, 1969); 11-day fetal-rabbit liver homogenate (5mg wet wt.), offered 2.80 mmol UDP-glucuronic acid and 0.29 mmol *o*-aminophenol, formed glucuronide at 1/20 the maternal level over 30 min (Skea and Dutton, 1969). Significantly-higher destruction of UDPglucuronic acid has not been reported in fetal-liver preparations, nor have transferase inhibitors been found there (see Dutton, 1966b). Some species approach adult transferase levels to certain substrates a few days before birth, and at that time high UDPglucuronic acid concentration might raise observed transferase activity up to or above mean adult values, particularly with a limiting factor such as acceptor-substrate concentration.

Because fetal tissues do contain certain glucuronides, presumably some UDPglucuronyltransferases are active there; are other transferases present in less-active form? Halac and Sicignano (1969) activated liver preparations 10-fold, but reported the same developmental pattern; diethylnitrosamine, which unmasks a latent transferase in Gunn rats, has no effect on early-fetal rat liver (Stevenson, 1969) and does not selectively activate newborn rat liver transferase (Winsnes, 1969). There is no evidence that the highly active fetal β-glucuronidase hydrolyses any glucuronides formed; its specific inhibitor, glucaro-1$\rightarrow$4-lactone, does not increase synthesis *in vitro*. Yet formation of this inhibitor is deficient perinatally (Marsh and Carr, 1965), and although β-glucuronidase has low activity at the optimum pH of the transferase, conditions within the microsome (which contains β-glucuronidase) could be decisive.

To produce *in vitro* a fully-active fetal UDPglucuronyltransferase whose catalytic powers are not evident *in vivo* will not of course prove that the fetus can form that particular glucuronide, but should assist understanding of selective glucuronidation.

Such selectivity is illustrated by the formation at adult levels of several glucuronides in fetal tissues. Hirvonen (1966) recorded 'adult' glucuronidation of 4-methylumbelliferone by liver slices from early fetal rats, and many fetal glucuronides are synthesized extrahepatically (see Dutton, 1966b). UDPGlucuronyltransferase for *o*-aminophenol is as low in kidney as in liver of fetal mouse and guinea pig, but is abundant in their alimentary tracts, slices of which glucuronidate above adult levels (Stevenson and Dutton, 1962). Endogenous glucuronides such as those of bilirubin (Bakken and Fog, 1967; Brodersen et al., 1967; Jansen et al., 1969a) or estrogens (see Diczfalusy and Levitz, 1969) may reach human amniotic fluid or fetal perfusates (Bird et al., 1965) from intestinal conjugating sites; steroid glucuronides have, however, been isolated from human fetal liver (Solomon et al., 1967) as well as from intestine (see Diczfalusy and Levitz, 1969), and Engel et al. (1962) reported steroid glucuronidation by human fetal liver slices. Apart from an observation with chick-embryo liver cells (KAPPAS and GRANICK, 1968) there is no direct evidence yet of transferase activity towards steroids in embryonic tissues, but DAHM and BREUER (1966) report it from placenta. If a compound is not placentally conjugated or excreted, then the fetal liver may have to glucuronidate it; LESTER and TROXLER (1969), discussing this, note that fetal primates, able to excrete bilirubin derivatives placentally, have an 'immature' transferase for bilirubin, whereas fetal dogs, with little placental excretion, develop nearly adult levels of the enzyme before birth. Presumably the increasing fetal bilirubin accelerates maturation of its transferase, as strikingly shown by BAKKEN and FOG (see BAKKEN, 1969), who injected pregnant rats with bilirubin and found the offspring (exposed to placentally-passed bilirubin) developed hepatic transferase for bilirubin before control animals.

Impermeability of placenta to conjugated bilirubin (SCHENKER et al., 1964) explains accumulation of bilirubin glucuronide in fetal fluids to levels higher than in neonates (BRODERSEN et al., 1967; BAKKEN and FOG, 1967; JANSEN et al., 1969a), who can more easily excrete it. Another, less likely, hypothesis (JACOBSEN et al., 1967) assumes the transferase reversible for bilirubin, and so the UDPglucuronic acid: UDP ratio, not concentration of UDPglucuronic acid, would determine transferase activity; onset of glycogenesis at birth lowers the ratio and diminishes glucuronidation.

Triggering of transferase activities by accumulation of their natural substrates is an attractive conception; triggering by foreign substrates is obviously much less predictable and, although certain drugs induce fetal transferase activity after crossing the placenta (see section D. V.), more akin to natural maturation are 'spontaneous' inductions such as the precocious appearance of transferase and glucuronidation in cultured chick-embryo liver (KO, DUTTON and NEMETH, 1967; SKEA and NEMETH, 1969). This organ possesses slight transferase activity towards *o*-aminophenol from incubation day 8, which rises rapidly on hatching at 21 days (DUTTON and KO, 1966). In morphologically 'immature' 5-day livers this activity develops from zero up to 5 times adult levels within 8 days' culture in a simple chemically-defined medium containing no obvious inducers; hepatocytes cultured as suspensions or monolayers also showed this induction, which was independent of mitosis. From these and other observations the induction appeared due to removal from a fetal environment. Cultured liver from mammalian fetuses has so far developed transferase only slowly (SKEA, DUTTON and NEMETH, 1969).

UDPGlucuronyltransferase and glucuronidation have not been specially studied in aged animals, but appear lower there.

II. Diet

Although starvation does not markedly affect the transferase, it may affect glucuronide formation. Neonatal development of the liver enzyme and of glucuronide formation is retarded by poor feeding but not accelerated by supplementing an adequate diet (see DUTTON, 1966b). Glucuronidation of several aglycons (though not of bilirubin: ADLARD, 1969) falls on starvation and is restored by administered glucose (see DUTTON, 1966b); as the transferase itself can rise on fasting (MIETTINEN and LESKINEN, 1963), the fall could reflect decreased formation of UDPglucuronic acid and increased breakdown of both nucleotide and conjugate (MIETTINEN and LESKINEN, 1963; WONG and SOURKES, 1967b). Glucose loading increases liver UDPglucuronic acid (WONG and SOURKES, 1967b) and possibly also glucuronidation (see MÜLLER-OERLINGHAUSEN et al., 1967). Vitamin A deficiency does not affect glucuronidation (MAMEESH et al., 1965).

III. Hormones

Sex differences in liver UDPglucuronyltransferase and glucuronide biosynthesis have been observed, and denied, in many species. Except for hamsters, any greater activity appears in males (see DUTTON, 1966b).

Treatment of rats with estradiol eventually decreased male transferase activity, and testosterone brought females up to male level (INSCOE and AXELROD, 1960; KÜNZEL and MÜLLER-OERLINGHAUSEN, 1969). HALAC and SICIGNANO (1969) found that sex difference disappeared after dialysis and suggested removal of an inhibitor. This is unlikely to be estradiol or testosterone itself, for when added *in vitro* either they had no effect (INSCOE and AXELROD, 1960) or testosterone inhibited (KÜNZEL and MÜLLER-OERLINGHAUSEN, 1969; see DUTTON, 1966b); again, the anti-androgen Cyproteron did not reverse induction by testosterone but itself caused stimulation, according to KÜNZEL and MÜLLER-OERLINGHAUSEN (1969), who consider sex differences due to higher UDPglucuronic acid formation by males, a conclusion difficult to reconcile with other work using microsomes and excess nucleotide.

Administration of cortisone, ACTH, thyroxine, insulin or other hormones had little effect on glucuronidation or its enzymes (see DUTTON, 1966b; MARCHI et al., 1964; WONG and SOURKES, 1967b; MÜLLER-OERLINGHAUSEN et al., 1968); adrenaline and hydrocortisone raise liver UDPglucuronic acid (WONG and SOURKES, 1967b). Adrenalectomy (MÜLLER-OERLINGHAUSEN et al., 1969) or male castration (KÜNZEL and MÜLLER-OERLINGHAUSEN, 1969) lowered glucuronide synthesis.

IV. Genetic Factors

A successful species may lack some transferase activities (see section C. I.) but will be well adjusted to its internal and external environments. Within the species slight hereditary variations in transferase activity must occur unnoticed, but grossly defective activity towards endogenous substrates disturbs metabolism and provided such mutants survive till birth they are more easily recognised. Bilirubin, obvious clinically and chemically, is a favourite substrate for genetic studies; other endogenous aglycons, or drugs, are not yet so popular.

The Gunn strain of rats is now of doubtful genetic purity (see discussion to WHITE, 1967) and its transferase deficiencies not wholly reproducible (see section C. VI). Homozygotes all, however, exhibit permanent acholuric jaundice and often kernicterus, due to virtually-absent transferase for bilirubin; bilirubin uptake, conjugate excretion and UDPglucuronic acid availability are normal. Administration of some carcinogens stimulates the defective transferases a little (METGE et al., 1964; see DUTTON, 1966b), but diethylnitrosamine added to microsomal or 'solubilized' liver preparations immediately stimulates activity (for *o*-aminophenol and paracetamol) some 20-fold, to the level in stimulated Wistar rat liver; so, for these substrates at least, the genetic defect lies not in enzyme synthesis but enzyme accessibility (STEVENSON et al., 1968).

Patients with the Crigler-Najjar syndrome also develop soon after birth a severe, usually fatal, unconjugated hyperbilirubinemia, due to lack of transferase activity towards bilirubin; again, glucuronidation of other substrates can be absent (sulfadimethoxine: JANSEN et al., 1969b), low (menthol, *N*-acetyl-*p*-aminophenol: see DUTTON, 1966b) or normal (salicylamide: BILLING et al., 1964; estriol: see HALAC and REFF, 1967). Inheritance is believed autosomal and recessive; the syndrome shades off into a multiplicity of dubiously heritable conditions exhibiting minor elevations of serum bilirubin, including Gilbert's disease, which involves impaired bilirubin uptake and conjugation (BLACK and BILLING, 1969; see SCHMID, 1966).

An inherited disorder in man (Dubin-Johnson syndrome) and sheep (mutant of Corriedale strain) displays defective biliary excretion of several compounds, including glucuronides of bilirubin and, for the sheep, also of metanephrine (see ARIAS, 1966).

V. Administration of Drugs and Steroids

Administration to an organism of compounds not usually encountered in its 'metabolic niche' may alter its glucuronidation pattern. The changes can be studied either for the toxic or therapeutic effect itself, or as an exaggeration of responses controlling normal fluctuation of glucuronide biosynthesis.

UDPGlucuronyltransferase activity and glucuronidation were increased in animals given the carcinogens 3,4-benzpyrene, 3-methylcholanthrene, 1,2,5,6-dibenzanthracene (see DUTTON, 1966b; GOLDSTEIN and TAUROG, 1968) and diethylnitrosamine (STEVENSON et al., 1968), though only diethylnitrosamine activated the enzyme *in vitro*; K_m changes on induction are reported (HOWLAND and BURKHALTER, 1969). Slight increases in liver transferase but not in UDPglucuronic acid appeared with other carcinogens (REID, 1962). Benzpyrene increased liver transferase activity in newborn mice but, on maternal administration, did not induce it in fetuses; chloroquine and chlorcyclizine did so, but could not alleviate human neonatal hyperbilirubinemia (see DUTTON, 1966b).

Barbiturates increase glucuronide excretion (REMMER, 1964; YAFFE et al., 1966) and conjugation (LEVINE et al., 1968; ADLARD et al., 1969); they were given for neonatal and various adult unconjugated hyperbilirubinemias with favourable results (YAFFE et al., 1966; CRIGLER and GOLD, 1966; CATZ and YAFFE, 1962; KREEK and SLEISENGER, 1968; MAURER et al., 1968; TROLLE, 1968; WHELTON et al., 1968; ERTEL and NEWTON, 1969; but see CUNNINGHAM et al., 1969), probably due to stimulation of conjugation, excretion or other metabolic fates of bilirubin. After maternal treatment, offspring had lower serum bilirubin than controls and passed the maximum concentration earlier, consistent with faster development of the transferase. Gunn rats (DELEON et al., 1967) and Crigler-Najjar patients (ARIAS et al., 1964) remained unimproved. Phenobarbitone increases bilirubin uptake by liver cells, but as high levels exist there uptake may not be limiting (ADLARD, 1969); the drug also stimulates formation of a β-glucuronidase inhibitor (HÄNNINEN, 1968). Chloretone and barbital (HOLLMAN and TOUSTER, 1962) rapidly stimulate UDPglucose dehydrogenase, and so increased UDPglucuronic acid formation could partly explain this therapeutic effect, which was also claimed after attempts to increase the nucleotide with precursors unlikely to influence glucuronidating pathways *in vivo* (MATSUDA and SHIRAHATA, 1966). Barbiturates do induce the transferase itself, but so slowly for all substrates tried, including bilirubin (DELEON et al., 1967; ZEIDENBERG et al., 1967; STEVENSON and TURNBULL, 1968; CATZ and YAFFE, 1962), that transferase induction may be a response to products of rapidly induced hydroxylation enzymes; induction appears faster when 'activated' enzyme is measured (HALAC and SICIGNANO, 1969).

Glucuronidation processes are stimulated by other drugs (see DUTTON, 1966b; CAREDDU et al., 1964; HÄNNINEN, 1968), sometimes specifically in certain organs (HÄNNINEN and AITIO, 1968). Tolbutamide may increase liver UDPglucuronic acid (MÜLLER-OERLINGHAUSEN et al., 1968).

No stimulatory drug appears an obvious substrate for the transferase; the probable substrate morphine stimulates UDPglucose dehydrogenase instead (TAKEMORI, 1960). Attempts to induce transferase activity with 'foreign' substrates were unsuccessful (see DUTTON, 1966b); when, with more logic, bilirubin was injected (BAKKEN, 1969) success was achieved.

Much Japanese work suggests that administration of glucuronate or its derivatives assists glucuronidation (see DUTTON, 1966b) or removes toxic endogenous amines (TAMURA et al., 1966). Glucuronate can form *N*-glucuronides (see section A.III.) but not others, and one explanation may be its metabolism to the β-glucuronidase inhibitor glucaro-1→4-lactone (MARSH, 1963; see LEVVY and CONCHIE, 1966).

UDPGlucuronyltransferase itself is inhibited by several drugs such as chloromycetin, streptomycin, phenylbutazone and Ibufenac, some of which are icterogenic (see DUTTON, 1966b). Others inhibit transport rather than conjugation. Novobiocin may inhibit uptake of substrate, and any 'cholephil' (compound concentrated in bile: HARGREAVES and LATHE, 1963) will compete with biliary glucuronides (which are described by SMITH and WILLIAMS, 1966; JAYLE and PASQUALINI, 1966) for excretion; some cholephils also inhibit the transferase itself (HARGREAVES and LATHE, 1963).

Many steroids impair glucuronidation by reducing uptake of aglycon or secretion of glucuronide, by competing for transferase or UDPglucuronic acid, or possibly by non-competitively inhibiting the transferase; as the enzyme is insoluble, 'competition' could occur at microsomal entry or exit as well as at active centers (see DUTTON, 1966b). Interestingly, BEVAN et al. (1965) found that pregnanediol glucuronide inhibited glucuronidation of bilirubin in rat liver slices more strongly than the free steroid. It did not inhibit the transferase but blocked release of bilirubin glucuronide from the slice; other glucuronide inhibitors of glucuronidation probably operate similarly, steroids conjugated at the 5β position seeming the most effective (ADLARD, 1969). This step is also the one blocked by various C-17 alkylated anabolic (see Dutton, 1966b) or oral-contraceptive steroidal drugs (MULLIGAN and SHERLOCK, 1968).

Natural steroids in body fluids can impair glucuronidation, notably when this is already defective, as in neonates; so far all appear to be saturated ring-A metabolites of progesterone or its derivatives, occurring in neonatal or pregnancy serum (LATHE and WALKER, 1958; HOLTON and LATHE, 1963), and some human milk. Serum inhibitors may be glucuronides or free steroids; they inhibited slightly in homogenates (HSIA et al., 1963; JONES and HIPKE, 1964) where they could have competed for insufficient added UDPglucuronic acid, but inhibited strongly with slices (LATHE and WALKER, 1958) and may therefore block cellular transport rather than conjugation. But as UDPglucuronic acid may be limiting in the perinatal liver cell, competition for the nucleotide might well be a factor there. Infants breast-fed by certain mothers develop jaundice, possibly because the milk contains pregnane-3α,20β-diol, an inhibitor of transferase activity towards *o*-aminophenol (ARIAS et al., 1964; ROSENFELD et al., 1967); as this compound does not inhibit bilirubin conjugation (ADLARD, 1969), an associated steroid may be responsible (RAMOS et al., 1966).

Steroid inhibitors may cause the lowered transferase activity reported in pregnancy (RAURAMO et al., 1963; PARKE, 1968; HALAC and SICIGNANO, 1969), though other drug-metabolizing enzymes also seem inhibited (see PARKE, 1968); as liver size and composition change in pregnancy, further data are required.

VI. Environmental Factors

Glucuronidation and total liver UDPglucuronyltransferase fell in rats kept at 3 °C, though microsomal transferase content was constant (INSCOE and AXELROD,

1960). Seasonal changes are mentioned by DUTTON (1966b). X-Irradiation at 400—1200r of isolated intact rodents or their organs decreased tissue glucuronidation and excretion of glucuronide (STEVENS and BERLINER, 1963; see DUTTON, 1966b); yet exposure of isolated chick-embryo liver to 6000r, preventing mitosis, allowed subsequent rapid development of the transferase (SKEA and NEMETH, 1969).

VII. Toxicological and Pathological Factors

Evidence on glucuronide synthesis in damaged tissues is scanty and conflicting, but certain facts should be relevant: liver transferase contains thiol groups, which are susceptible to toxins, but it can survive damage to the endoplasmic reticulum, even showing increased activity; the transferase and UDPglucose dehydrogenase are inducible by drugs and also, presumably, by endogenous molecules; UDPglucuronic acid supply suffers with restricted carbohydrate.

If tissues possess evolved 'priorities' by which less necessary expenditure of enzyme and nucleotide is sacrificed in crises to keep vital processes operative, then gross tissue destruction, or insult by unfamiliar compounds such as chemical poisons or drugs, might well disrupt such control.

Damaged or diseased liver, particularly, may give rise to disturbed glucuronidation. Evidence is contradictory, as expected. Firstly, measurement of glucuronide excretion will include extra-hepatic conjugation. Secondly, in tissue studies the sample taken may be necrotic or cirrhotic, with no transferase; or normal; or possibly, where the endoplasmic reticulum is vesiculated at the periphery of damage, with activated or induced transferase. The extent of injury is also important. Liver has great functional reserve, but eventually toxins administered or produced by tissue damage will compete with routine glucuronidation for diminished nucleotide and enzymes; aglycons then accumulate and hepatic failure becomes evident and rapid.

UDPGlucuronyltransferase does not fall in damage or disease so rapidly as some drug-metabolizing enzymes (see DUTTON, 1969). It may rise after CCl_4 insult (TAKETA, 1962a) but generally falls slowly (ISSELBACHER and MCCARTHY, 1960; CHOJECKI and KERN, 1961; TAKETA, 1962b; METGE et al., 1964); a similar rise (REID, 1962; DOHNÁLEK at al., 1967; BLACK and BILLING, 1969) and fall (MÜTING, 1963; METGE et al., 1964) in glucuronidation accompanies chronic liver disease. Urinary phenolic glucuronides increase in hepatopathias (MÜTING, 1963); they may contribute to the enhanced glucuronic acid output in burns and neoplasia (CORNILLOT, 1962; DOHNÁLEK, 1967).

β-Glucuronidase is liberated in, and from, damaged liver cells (NILIUS and RATH, 1967; WILLIAMS, 1969), reaching high serum levels, and would increase difficulties in glucuronidation: even in healthy tissues some glucuronide hydrolysis must occur (see ACOCELLA et al., 1968). β-Glucuronidase is plentiful in endoplasmic reticulum of regenerating liver (LENTZ and VAN LANCKER, 1968) where the transferase, unlike many drug-metabolizing enzymes, persists at normal levels — at least for an endogenous 'routine' substrate like bilirubin (METGE et al., 1964).

UDPGlucuronic acid supply may be critical in shock or terminal conditions, and deficient also in diabetic liver (SCHRIEFERS et al., 1966, MÜLLER-OERLINGHAUSEN et al., 1967; WONG and SOURKES, 1967b).

Clearly, medication of these conditions should not stress the glucuronidation pathways by inhibiting, competing for, or haphazardly inducing transferases, and so risk impairing the ordered conjugation of both routine and abnormal metabolites. The points of stress should be evident from this review.

Work reported above from the author's laboratory was supported by the Medical Research Council.

References

ACOCELLA, G., TENCONI, L.T., ARMAS-MERINO, R., RAIA, S., BILLING, B.H.: Does deconjugation of bilirubin glucuronide occur in obstructive jaundice? Lancet **1968 I**, 68—69.

ADLARD, B.P.F.: The interaction of steroids and bilirubin glucuronyl transferase in relation to newborn jaundice. Ph. D. Thesis. Leeds (England): University of Leeds 1969.

— LESTER, R.G., LATHE, G.H.: The effect of phenobarbitone treatment of rats and of protein deprivation on the capacity of liver slices to conjugate bilirubin. Biochem. Pharmacol. **18**, 59—63 (1969).

ARCOS, M., LIEBERMAN, S.: 5-Pregnene-3*β*,20*α*-diol-3-sulfate-20-(2′-acetemido-2′-deoxy-*α*-D-glucoside) and 5-pregnene-3*β*,20*α*-diol-3,20-disulfate. Two novel urinary conjugates. Biochemistry **6**, 2032—2039 (1967).

ARIAS, I.M.: Ethereal and *N*-linked glucuronide formation by normal and Gunn rats *in vitro* and *in vivo*. Biochem. biophys. Res. Commun. **6**, 81—84 (1961).

— Studies of bile pigment metabolism in the dogfish (Squalus acanthia) and the goosefish (Lophius piscatorius). Bull. Mt. Desert Island Biol. Lab. **10**, 614 (1962).

— The excretion of conjugated bilirubin by the liver cell. Medicine (Baltimore) **45**, 513—515 (1966).

— GARTNER, L.M., SEIFTER, S., FURMAN, M.: Prolonged neonatal unconjugated hyperbilirubinemia associated with breast feeding and a steroid, pregnane-3*α*, 20*β*-diol, in maternal milk that inhibits glucuronide formation *in vitro*. J. clin. Invest. **43**, 2037—2047 (1964).

AXELROD, J., INSCOE, J., TOMKINS, G.M.: Enzymatic synthesis of *N*-glucosyluronic acid conjugates. J. biol. Chem. **232**, 835—851 (1958).

— WEIL-MALHERBE, H., R. TOMCHICK, R.: The physiological disposition of H^3-epinephrine and its metabolite metanephrine. J. Pharmacol. exp. Ther. **127**, 251—256 (1959).

BAKKEN, A.F.: Effects of unconjugated bilirubin on bilirubin-UDP-glucuronyl transferase activity in liver of newborn rats. Pediat. Res. **3**, 205—209 (1969).

— FOG, J.: Bilirubin conjugates in the newborn. Lancet **1967 I**, 1280.

BEVAN, B.R., HOLTON, J.B., LATHE, G.H.: The effect of pregnanediol and pregnanediol glucuronide on bilirubin conjugation by rat liver slices. Clin. Sci. **29**, 353—361 (1965).

BILLING, B.H., BLACK, M.: Bilirubin metabolism. Gut **10**, 250—254 (1969).

— GRAY, C.H., KULCZYCKA, A., MANFIELD, P., NICHOLSON, D.C.: The metabolism of ^{14}C-bilirubin in congenital nonhemolytic hyperbilirubinemia. Clin. Sci. **27**, 163—170 (1964).

BIRD, C.E., SOLOMON, S., WIQVIST, N., DICZFALUSY, E.: Formation of C-21 steroid sulphates and glucuronides by previable human foetuses perfused with [4-^{14}C] progesterone. Biochim. biophys. Acta (Amst.) **104**, 623—626 (1965).

BLACK, M., BILLING, B.H.: Hepatic bilirubin UDP-glucuronyl transferase activity in liver disease and Gilbert's syndrome. New Engl. J. Med. **280**, 1266—1271 (1969).

BREUER, H., WESSENDORF, D.: Enzymatische Bildung von Östradiol-(17*β*)-glucuroniden in der Mikrosomen-Fraktion der Kaninchenleber. Hoppe-Seylers Z. physiol. Chem. **345**, 1—10 (1966).

BRODERSEN, R., JACOBSEN, J., HERTZ, H., REBBE, H., SORENSEN, B.: Bilirubin conjugation in the human fetus. Scand. J. clin. Lab. Invest. **20**, 41—48 (1967).

BRODIE, B.B.: Physico-chemical factors in drug absorption *and* distribution and fate of drugs; therapeutic implications. In: Absorption and Distribution of drugs. Edinburgh: Livingstone 1964.

— MAICKEL, R.P.: Comparative biochemistry of drug metabolism. In: Proceedings of the 1st. International Pharmacological Meeting, Stockholm, 1961. Vol. 6, Oxford: Pergamon Press 1962.

BROWN, A.K., ZUELZER, W.W.: Studies on the neonatal development of the glucuronide conjugating system. J. clin. Invest. **37**, 332—340 (1958).

CAREDDU, P., PICENI SERENI, L., GUINTA, F., SERENI, F.: Sulle possibilitá di attivare i processi di coniugazione e di escrezione epatica della bilirubina mediante alcuni farmaci. Richerche sperimentale con la dietilamide dell'acido nicotinico (Coramina) e con l'acido fenil-etil-barbiturico (Gardenale). Minerva pediat. **55**, 2559—2565 (1964).

CATZ, C., YAFFE, S.Y.: Pharmacological modification of bilirubin conjugation in the newborn. Amer. J. Dis. Child. **104**, 516—517 (1962).

CHOJECKI, Z., KERN, F.: The effect of dietary cirrhosis and CCl_4 poisoning on glucuronyl transferase activity of rat liver. Gastroenterology **40**, 521—531 (1961).

COOPER, J.R., AXELROD, J., BRODIE, B.B.: Inhibitory effects of *β*-diethylaminoethyl diphenylpropylacetate on a variety of drug metabolic pathways *in vitro*. J. Pharmacol. exp. Ther. **112**, 55—63 (1954).

CORNILLOT, P.: Détermination de l'acide glycuronique dans les urines humaines normales et pathologiques. Clin. chim. Acta 7, 42—50 (1962).

COTTE, J., MATHIEU, M., ANDRÉ, J.P., COLLOMBEL, C., PADIS, L.: Méthode de dosage de l'activité glucuronyl-transferase hépatique applicable en biologie clinique. Enzym. biol. clin. **8**, 387—399 (1967).
CRIGLER, J.F., GOLD, N.: Sodium phenobarbital-induced decrease in serum bilirubin in an infant with congenital nonhemolytic jaundice and kernicterus. J. clin. Invest. **45**, 998—999 (1966).
CUNNINGHAM, M.D., MACE, J.W., PETERS, E.R.: Clinical experience with phenobarbitone in icterus neonatorum. Lancet **1969 II**, 550—551.
DAHM, K., BREUER, H.: Reinigung und Charakterisierung einer löslichen Uridin Diphosphat-Glucuronat:17β-Hydroxysteroid-Glucuronyl Transferase beim Menschen. Biochem. biophys. Acta (Amst.) **128**, 306—316 (1966).
— — LINDLAU, M.: Charakterisierung und Kinetik einer mikrosomalen UDP-Glucuronat:Testosteron-Glucuronyl transferase beim Menschen. Hoppe-Seylers Z. physiol. Chem. **345**, 139—149 (1966).
— LINDLAU, M., BREUER, H.: Biogenese von Östriol-3-monoglucuronid. Acta endocr. (Kbh.) **56**, 403—412 (1967).
DELEON, A., GARTNER, L.M., ARIAS, I.M.: The effect of phenobarbital on hyperbilirubinemia in glucuronyl transferase deficient rats. J. Lab. clin. Med. **70**, 273—278 (1967).
DICZFALUSY, E., LEVITZ, M.: Formation, metabolism and transport of estrogen conjugates. In: Chemical and biological aspects of steroid conjugation. Berlin-Heidelberg-New York: Springer 1970, p. 291.
DISCHE, Z.: New color reactions for determination of sugars in polysaccharides. In: Methods of biochemical analysis. Vol. 2. New York: Interscience 1955.
DOHNÁLEK, J., EYSSELT, M., MARTINEK, K., KADLECOVÁ, D.: Unsere Erfahrungen mit dem OIB-Test (ein Leberfunktionstest durch Verfolgen des *o*-Jodbenzoesäure-^{131}J-Stoffwechsels). Nucl.-Med. **6**, (Stuttg.) 76—86 (1967).
DRUCKER, W.D.: Glucuronic acid conjugation of tetrahydrocortisone and *p*-nitrophenol in the homozygous Gunn rat. Proc. Soc. exp. Biol. (N.Y.) **129**, 308—311 (1968).
DUTTON, G.J.: Glucuronide synthesis in foetal liver and other tissues. Biochem. J. **71**, 141—148 (1959).
— Comparison of glucuronide synthesis in developing mammalian and avian liver. Ann. N.Y. Acad. Sci. **111**, 259—272 (1963).
— Variations in glucuronide formation by perinatal liver. Biochem. Pharmacol. **15**, 947—951 (1966a).
— The biosynthesis of glucuronides. In: Glucuronic acid. New York: Academic Press 1966b.
— Detoxication in normal and damaged liver. In: Alcoholic cirrhosis and other toxic hepatopathias. Skandia International Symposia. Stockholm: Nordiska Bokhandelns Förlag 1970.
— BURCHELL, B.: Unpublished observations, 1969.
— ILLING, H.P.A.: Formation of an *S*-glucuronide by a UDP-glucuronyltransferase and its hydrolysis by β-glucuronidase. Biochem. J. **112**, 16 P. (1969).
— KO, V.: The synthesis of *o*-aminophenyl glucuronide in several tissues of the domestic fowl, *Gallus gallus*, during development. Biochem. J. **99**, 550—556 (1966).
— STOREY, I.D.E.: Uridine compounds in glucuronic acid metabolism. 1. The formation of glucuronides in liver suspensions. Biochem. J. **57**, 275—283 (1954).
EMERMAN, S., TWOMBLY, G.H., LEVITZ, M.: Biliary and urinary metabolites of estriol-15-^{3}H-3-sulfate-^{35}S in women. J. clin. Endocr. **27**, 539—548 (1967).
ENGEL, L.L., BAGGETT, B., HALLA, M.: *In vitro* metabolism of estradiol-17β by human fetal liver: formation of estriol, 16-epistriol, estrone and an estriol glucuronic acid. Endocrinology **70**, 907—914 (1962).
ERTEL, I.J., NEWTON, W.A.: Therapy in congenital hyperbilirubinemia: phenobarbital and diethylnicotinamide. Pediatrics **44**, 43—48 (1969).
FISHMAN, W.H.: Biochemistry of glucuronic acid; lectures in Japan. Tokyo: Faculty of Pharmaceutical Science, University of Tokyo 1959.
— GOLDMAN, S.S., DE LELLIS, R.: Dual localization of β-glucuronidase in endoplasmic reticulum and in lysosomes. Nature (Lond.) **213**, 457—460 (1967).
FLODGAARD, H.J., BRODERSEN, R.: Bilirubin glucuronide formation in developing guinea pig liver. Scand. J. clin. Lab. Invest. **19**, 149—155 (1967).
GOLDBERG, N.D.: The effects of nucleotide substrates containing 5-fluorouracil and 6-azauracil on certain kinetic parameters of UDPG dehydrogenase and UDP-glucuronyltransferase. Ph. D. Thesis. Madison, Wis. (U.S.A.): University of Wisconsin 1963.
GOLDSTEIN, J.A., TAUROG, A.: Enhanced biliary excretion of thyroxine glucuronide in rats pre-treated with benzpyrene. Biochem. Pharmacol. **17**, 1049—1065 (1968).
GRAHAM, A.B., WOOD, G.C.: The phospholipid-dependence of UDP-glucuronyltransferase. Biochem. biophys. Res. Commun. **37**, 567—575 (1969).

Grajcer, D., Idler, D.R.: Conjugated testosterone in the blood and testes of spawned Fraser-river Sockeye salmon (*Oncorhyncus nerka*). Canad. J. Biochem. **41**, 23—30 (1963).
Gram, T.E., Hansen, A.R., Fouts, J.R.: The submicrosomal distribution of hepatic uridine diphosphate glucuronyltransferases in the rabbit. Biochem. J. **106**, 587—591 (1968).
Halac, E., Reff, A.: Studies on bilirubin UDP-glucuronyltransferase, Biochim. biophys. Acta (Amst.) **139**, 328—343 (1967).
— Sicignano, C.: Re-evaluation of the influence of sex, age, pregnancy, and phenobarbital on the activity of UDP-glucuronyltransferase in rat liver. J. Lab. clin. Med. **73**, 677—685 (1969).
Hänninen, O.: On the metabolic regulation in the glucuronic acid pathway in the rat tissues. Ann. Acad. Sci. fenn. A. **II**, No. 142 (1968).
— Aitio, A.: Enhanced glucuronide formation in different tissues following drug administration. Biochem. Pharmacol. **17**, 2307—2311 (1968).
— Alanen, K.: The complete inhibition of *p*-nitrophenyl-*β*-*D*-glucopyranosiduronic acid synthesis by aliphatic alcohols *in vitro*. Biochem. Pharmacol. **15**, 1465—1467 (1966).
— Antila, K.: Personal communication, 1969.
Hargreaves, T.: The effect of diethylaminoethyl diphenylpropylacetic acid (SKF 524A) on uridine 5′-pyrophosphate glucuronyltransferase. Biochem. Pharmacol. **16**, 1481—1488 (1967).
— Lathe, G.H.: Inhibitory aspects of bile secretion. Nature (Lond.) **200**, 1172—1176 (1963).
Heirwegh, K.P.M., Meuwissen, J.A.T.P.: Activation *in vitro* and solubilisation of glucuronyltransferase (assayed with bilirubin as acceptor) with digitonin. Biochem. J. **110**, 31 P (1961).
Henderson, P.Th., Dewaide, J.H.: Metabolism of drugs in isolated hepatocytes. Biochem. Pharmacol. **18**, 2087—2094 (1969).
Hirvonen, T.: Foetal and postnatal development of glucuronide formation in mammalian tissue slices. Ann. Univ. Turkuensis A. **II.**, No. 38 (1966).
Hollman, S., Touster, O.: Alterations in tissue levels of uridine diphosphate glucose dehydrogenase, uridine diphosphate glucuronic acid pyrophosphatase and glucuronyl transferase induced by substances influencing the production of ascorbic acid. Biochim. biophys. Acta (Amst.) **62**, 338—351 (1962).
Holton, J.B., Lathe, G.H.: Inhibitors of bilirubin conjugation in newborn infant serum and male urine. Clin. Sci. **25**, 499—509 (1963).
Honjo, M., Furukawa, Y., Imai, K., Moriyama, H., Tanaka, K.: Synthesis of uridine diphosphate-glucuronic acid. Chem. pharm. Bull. **10**, 225—231 (1962).
Howland, R.D., Burkhalter, A.: Effect of 3-methylcholanthrene on uridine diphosphate glucuronyltransferase. Fed. Proc. **28**, 417 (1969).
Hsia, D. Y.-Y., Riabov, S., Dowben, R. M.: Inhibition of glucuronosyl transferase by steroid hormones. Arch. Biochem. **103**, 181—188 (1963).
Huttunen, J.K., Miettinen, T.A.: Glucuronidation in rats of different ages and strains. Acta physiol. scand. **63**, 133—140 (1965).
Inscoe, J.K., Axelrod, J.: Some factors affecting glucuronide formation *in vitro*. J. Pharmacol. exp. Ther. **129**, 128—131 (1960).
Isselbacher, K.J.: Evidence for the multiplicity of glucuronyl transferases. In: Ikterus. Stuttgart: F.K. Schattauer Verlag 1968.
— Chrabas, M.F., Quinn, R.C.: The solubilisation and partial purification of a glucuronyl transferase from rabbit liver microsomes. J. biol. Chem. **237**, 3033—3036 (1962).
— McCarthy, E.: Effect of carbon tetrachloride on glucuronide formation by guinea pig liver. Proc. Soc. exp. Biol. (N.Y.) **103**, 819—822 (1960).
Jaakomaki, P.I., Yarger, K.A., Horning, E.C.: Gas-liquid chromatographic separation of human urinary steroid glucuronides. Biochim. biophys. Acta (Amst.) **137**, 216—219 (1967).
Jacobson, B., Davidson, E.A.: Biosynthesis of uronic acids by skin enzymes. II. Uridine diphosphate-*D*-glucuronic acid-5-epimerase. J. biol. Chem. **237**, 638—642 (1962).
Jansen, F.H., Heirwegh, K.P.M., Devriendt, A.: Foetal bilirubin conjugation. Lancet **1969**a **I**, 702—704.
— Malvaux, P., Heirwegh, K.P.M., Devriendt, A.: Congenital non-hemolytic jaundice: Crigler-Najjar syndrome. Biol. Neonat. **14**, 53—61 (1969b).
Javitt, N.B.: Ethereal and acyl glucuronide formation in the homozygous Gunn rat. Amer. J. Physiol. **211**, 424—428 (1966).
Jayle, M.F., Pasqualini, J.R.: Implication of conjugation of endogenous compounds — steroids and thyroxine. In: Glucuronic acid. New York: Academic Press 1966.
Jirku, H., Layne, D.S.: The formation of estradiol-3-glucuronoside-17*a*-*N*-acetylglucosaminide by rabbit liver homogenate. Biochemistry **4**, 2126—2131 (1965).
Jones, B., Hipke, M.L.: Glucuronyl transferase inhibition by steroids. J. Pediat. **64**, 815—821 (1964).

KAPPAS, A., GRANICK, S.: Steroid induction of porphyrin synthesis in liver cell culture. II. The effect of heme, uridine diphosphate glucuronic acid, and inhibitors of nucleic acid and protein synthesis on the induction process. J. biol. Chem. **243**, 346—351 (1968).

KO, V., DUTTON, G.J., NEMETH, A.M.: Development of uridine diphosphate-glucuronyltransferase activity in cultures of chick embryo liver. Biochem. J. **104**, 991—998 (1967).

KREEK, M.J., SLEISENGER, M.H.: Reduction of serum-unconjugated bilirubin with phenobarbitone in adult congenital non-haemolytic unconjugated hyperbilirubinemia. Lancet **1968 II**, 73—77.

KÜNZEL, B., MÜLLER-OERLINGHAUSEN, B.: Wirkung von Testosteron and einem Anti-Androgen (Cyproteronacetat) auf die Glucuronbildung in der Rattenleber. Naunyn-Schmiedebergs Arch. exp. Path. Pharmak. **262**, 112—123 (1969).

LAGE, G.L., SPRATT, J.L.: Bilirubin conjugation by hepatic microsomes from adult male guinea pigs. Arch. Biochem. **126**, 175—180 (1968).

LATHE, G.H., WALKER, M.: Inhibition of bilirubin conjugation in rat liver slices by human pregnancy and neonatal serum and steroids. Quart. J. exp. Physiol. **43**, 257—265 (1958).

LENTZ, P.E., VAN LANCKER, J.L.: The transfer or β-glucuronidase from the microsomal to the small mitochondrial fraction in hypoxic livers. Amer. J. Path. **52**, 4a (1968).

LESTER, R., KLEIN, P.D.: Bile pigment excretion: a comparison of the biliary excretion of bilirubin and bilirubin derivatives. J. clin. Invest. **45**, 1839—1846 (1966).

— TROXLER, R.F.: Recent advances in bile pigment metabolism. Gastroenterology **56**, 143—169 (1969).

LEVENTER, L.L., BUCHANAN, J.L., ROSS, J.E., TAPLEY, D.F.: Solubilisation of *N*-glucuronyl transferase. Biochim. biophys. Acta (Amst.) **110**, 428—430 (1965).

LEVINE, W.G., MILLBURN, P., SMITH, R.L., WILLIAMS, R.T.: The effect of phenobarbitone on the biliary excretion of foreign compounds by the rat. Biochem. J. **109**, 35P (1968).

LEVVY, G.A., CONCHIE, J.: β-Glucuronidase and the hydrolysis of glucuronides. In: Glucuronic Acid. New York: Academic Press 1966.

LIN, T-Y., HASSID, W.Z.: Pathway of alginic acid synthesis in the marine brown alga *Fucus gardneri* Silva. J. biol. Chem. **241**, 5284—5297 (1966).

LUEDERS, K.K., KUFF, E.L.: Spontaneous and detergent activation of a glucuronyltransferase *in vitro*. Arch. Biochem. **120**, 198—203 (1967).

MAICKEL, R.P., JONDORF, W.R., BRODIE, B.B.: The conjugation of foreign phenols with glucuronic acid in lower vertebrates. Fed. Proc. **18**, 418 (1959).

MAMEESH, M.S., UTNE, F., BRAEKKAN, O.R.: Studies on glucuronide detoxication mechanisms in vitamin A-deficient rats. Acta pharmacol. (Kbh.) **22**, 235—240 (1965).

MARCHI, S., BERTAZZONI, V., ZAMBOTH, V.: Primi resultati sull' azione dell' idricortisone sull' attivitá UDPG-deidrogenasica del fegato di ratto. Boll. Soc. ital. Biol. sper. **40**, 1493—1495 (1964).

MARSH, C.A.: Reactions of uridine diphosphate sugars catalysed by enzymes of French-bean leaves. Biochim. biophys. Acta (Amst.) **44**, 359—361 (1960).

— Metabolism of *D*-glucuronolactone in mammalian systems. 3. Further studies of *D*-glucuronolactone dehydrogenase of rat liver. Biochem. J. **89**, 108—114 (1963).

— Chemistry of *D*-glucuronic acid and its glycosides. In: Glucuronic acid. New York: Academic Press 1966.

— CARR, A.J.: Changes in enzyme activity, related to *D*-glucaric acid synthesis, with age, pregnancy and malignancy. Clin. Sci. **28**, 209—217 (1965).

— LEVVY, G.A.: Glucuronide metabolism in plants. 3. Triterpene glucuronides. Biochem. J. **63**, 9—14 (1956).

MATSUDA, I., SHIRAHATA, T.: Effects of aspartic acid and orotic acid upon serum bilirubin level in newborn infants. Tohoku J. exp. Med. **90**, 133—136 (1966).

MAURER, H.M., WOLFF, V.A., FINSTER, M., POPPERS, P.J., PANTUCK, E., KUNTZMAN, R., CONNEY, A.H.: Reduction in concentration of total serum-bilirubin in offspring of women treated with phenobarbitone during pregnancy. Lancet **1968 II**, 122—124.

MENKEN, M., BARRETT, P.V.D., BERLIN, N.I.: Assay of hepatic glucuronyl transferase activity using [^{14}C] bilirubin as substrate. Clin. chim. Acta **14**, 777—785 (1966).

METGE, W.R., OWEN, C.A., FOULK, W.T., HOFFMAN, H.N.: Bilirubin glucuronyl transferase activity in liver disease. J. Lab. clin. Med. **64**, 89—98 (1964).

MIETTINEN, T.A., LESKINEN, E.: Enzymic levels of glucuronic acid metabolism in the liver, kidney and intestine of normal and fasted rats. Biochem. Pharmacol. **12**, 565—575 (1963).

MOWAT, A.P., ARIAS, I.M.: 'Solubilization' of UDP-glucuronyl transferase, Pediat. Res. **3**, 352 (1969).

MÜLLER-OERLINGHAUSEN, B., HASSELBLATT, A., JAHNS, R.: Impaired hepatic synthesis of glucuronic acid conjugates in diabetic rats. Life Sci. **6**, 1529—1533 (1967).

MÜLLERE-ORLINGHAUSEN, B., HASSELBLATT, A., JAHNS, R.: Vermehrte Bildung von Bilirubinglucuronid in der Leber der Insulin- und Solfonylharnstoff-Hypoglkämie. Naunyn-Schmiedebergs Arch. exp. Path. Pharmak. **160**, 254—268 (1968).
— JAHNS, R., KÜNZEL, B., HASSELBLATT, A.: Die Wirkung von Tolbutamid auf Blutglucose und Glucuronsäurekonjugation in Lebergewebe normaler und adrenalektomierter Mäuse. Naunyn-Schmiedebergs Arch. exp. Path. Pharmak. **262**, 17—28 (1969).
MÜTING, D.: Detoxication capacity of the diseased liver. Germ. med. Mth. **8**, 198—202 (1963).
MULLIGAN, R., SHERLOCK, S.: The effects of oral contraceptives on hepatic function. Clin. Trials J. **5**, 155—164 (1968).
MUNCH-PETERSEN, A., KALCKAR, H. M., CUTOLO, E., SMITH, E. E. B.: Uridyl transferases and the formation of uridine triphosphate. Nature (Lond.) **172**, 1036—1037 (1953).
NAGAYAMA, F., YAMADA, T., TAUTI, M.: Activities of UDPglucose dehydrogenase, UDPglucuronyl transferase, and some glycosidases of freshwater fish during the adaptation to salt water. Bull. jap. Soc. sci. Fish. **34**, 950—954 (1968).
NILIUS, R., RATH, F. W.: β-Glucuronidase bei akuter Tetrachlorkohlenstoffschädigung der Rattenleber. Z. ges. exp. Med. **144**, 157—172 (1967).
OGAWA, H., SAWADA, M., KAWADA, M.: Purification and properties of a pyrophosphatase from rat liver microsomes capable of catalysing the hydrolysis of UDP-glucuronic acid. J. Biochem. (Tokyo) **59**, 126—134 (1966).
PARKE, D. V.: The biochemistry of foreign compounds. Oxford: Pergamon Press 1968.
POGELL, B. M., LELOIR, L. F.: Nucleotide activation of liver microsomal glucuronidation. J. biol. Chem. **236**, 293—298 (1961).
RAMOS, A., SILVERBERG, M., STERN, L.: Pregnanediols and neonatal hyperbilirubinemia. Amer. J. Dis. Child. **111**, 353—356 (1966).
RAO, G. S., BREUER, H.: Partial purification and kinetic properties of a soluble estrogen glucuronyltransferase from pig intestine. J. biol. Chem. **244**, 5521—5527 (1969).
RAURAMO, L., PULKKINEN, M., HARTIALA, K.: Glucuronide formation in parturients. Ann. Med. exp. Fenn. **41**, 32—37 (1963).
REID, E.: Significant biochemical effects of hepatocarcinogens in the rat. (A review). Cancer Res. **22**, 398—430 (1962).
REMMER, H.: Vermehrte Glucuronidierung von Sulfamethoxin während und nach Phenobarbitalbehandlung bei Ratten. Naunyn-Schmiedebergs Arch. exp. Path. Pharmak. **247**, 461—481 (1964).
ROBERTS, R. J., PLAA, G. L.: Effect of phenobarbital on the excretion of an exogenous bilirubin load. Biochem. Pharmacol. **16**, 827—835 (1967).
ROSENFELD, K. S., ARIAS, I. M., GARTNER, L. M., HELLMAN, L., GALLAGHER, T. F.: Studies of urinary pregnane-3α,20β-diol during pregnancy, post-partum, lactation and progesterone ingestion. J. clin. Endocr. **27**, 1705—1710 (1967).
ROY, A. B.: Enzymological aspects of steroid conjugation. In: Chemical and biological aspects of steroid conjugation. Berlin-Heidelberg-New York: Springer 1970, p. 74.
SCHENKER, S., DAWBER, N. H., SCHMID, R.: Bilirubin metabolism in the fetus. J. clin. Invest. **43**, 32—39 (1964).
— SCHMID, R.: Excretion of C^{14}-bilirubin in newborn guinea pigs. Proc. Soc. exp. Biol. (N.Y.) **115**, 446—448 (1964).
SCHLISELFELD, L. H., VAN EYS, J., TOUSTER, O.: The purification and properties of a nucleotide pyrophosphatase of rat liver nuclei. J. biol. Chem. **240**, 811—818 (1965).
SCHMID, R.: Hyperbilirubinemia. In: The metabolic basis of inherited disease. 2nd ed. New York: Mc Graw-Hill 1966.
— LESTER, R.: Implication of conjugation of endogenous compounds — bilirubin. In: Glucuronic acid. New York: Academic Press 1966.
SCHRIEFERS, H., GHRAF, R., POHL, F.: Biosynthese von Steroidglucuroniden durch Rattenlebermikrosomen. Zur Frage des Verhaltens der UDP-Glucuronyl-Transferase-Activität unter Nahrungsentzug und in Alloxandiabetes. Hoppe-Seylers Z. physiol. Chem. **344**, 25—33 (1966).
SILBERT, J.E.: Metabolism of polysaccharides containing glucuronic acid. In: Glucuronic acid. New York: Academic Press 1966.
SKEA, B. R., DUTTON, G. J.: Unpublished observations, 1969.
— — NEMETH, A. M.: Unpublished observations, 1969.
— NEMETH, A. M.: Factors influencing premature induction of UDP-glucuronyltransferase activity in cultured chick embryo liver cells. Proc. nat. Acad. Sci. (Wash.) **64**, 795—802 (1969).
SLAUNWHITE, W. R., JR., LICHTMAN, M. A., SANDBERG, A. A.: Studies on phenolic steroids in human subjects: VI. Biosynthesis of estriolglucosiduronic acid-16-^{14}C by human liver. J. clin. Endocr. **24**, 638—643 (1964).

SMITH, E.R., BREUER, H.: Enzymic formation of oestriol 3-glucuronide by rabbit liver microsomes. Biochem. J. **88**, 168—172 (1963).
SMITH, J.N.: Comparative biochemistry of detoxification. In: Comparative biochemistry. Vol. 6. New York: Academic Press 1964.
— The comparative metabolism of xenobiotics. Advanc. comp. Physiol. **3**, 173—232 (1968).
SMITH, R.L., WILLIAMS, R.T.: Implication of the conjugation of drugs and other exogenous compounds. In: Glucuronic acid. New York; Academic Press 1966.
SOLOMON, S., BIRD, C.E., LING, W., IWAMIYA, M., YOUNG, P.C.M.: Formation and metabolism of steroids in the fetus and placenta. Recent Progr. Hormone Res. **23**, 297—347 (1967).
STEVENS, W., BERLINER, D.L.: Effect of X-irradiation on the conjugation of steroids by mouse liver and kidney. Radiat. Res. **20**, 510—518 (1963).
STEVENSON, I.H.: Personal communication, 1969.
— DUTTON, G.J.: Glucuronide synthesis in kidney and gastrointestinal tract. Biochem. J. **82**, 330—340 (1962).
— GREENWOOD, D.T.: Inhibition of hexobarbital metabolism by diethylnitrosamine. Biochem. Pharmacol. **17**, 842—845 (1968).
— — MCEWEN, J.: Hepatic UDP-glucuronyltransferase in Wistar and Gunn rats — *in vitro* activation by diethylnitrosamine. Biochem. biophys. Res. Commun. **32**, 866—871 (1968).
— TURNBULL, M.: Hepatic drug-metabolising enzyme activity and duration of hexobarbitone anaesthesia in barbitone-dependent and withdrawn rats. Biochem. Pharmacol. **17**, 2297—2305 (1968).
STOREY, I.D.E.: The inhibition of uridine diphosphate transglucuronylase activity of mouse liver. Biochem. J. **95**, 201—208 (1965a).
— Some differences in the conjugation of *o*-aminophenol and *p*-nitrophenol by the uridine diphosphate transglucuronylase of mouse-liver homogenates. Biochem. J. **95**, 209—214 (1965b).
— DUTTON, G.J.: Uridine compounds in glucuronic acid metabolism. 2. The isolation and structure of 'uridine diphosphate glucuronic acid'. Biochem. J. **59**, 279—288 (1955).
STROMINGER, J.L., MAXWELL, E.S., AXELROD, J., KALCKAR, H.M.: Enzymatic formation of uridine diphosphoglucuronic acid. J. biol. Chem. **224**, 79—90 (1957).
TAKEMORI, A.E.: Enzymic studies on morphine glucuronide synthesis in acutely and chronically morphinized rats. J. Pharmacol. exp. Ther. **130**, 370—374 (1960).
TAKETA, K.: Enzymatic studies of glucuronide formation in impaired liver. III. Effects of carbon tetrachloride and ectromelia virus infection on liver glucuronide formation in mouse. Acta Med. Okayama **16**, 99—111 (1962a).
— Enzymatic studies of glucuronide formation in impaired liver. IV. Liver glucuronyl transferase activity and uridine diphosphate glucuronic acid content in viral hepatitis patients. Acta Med. Okayama **16**, 115—128 (1962b).
TAMURA, S., TOMIZAWA, S., TSUTSUMI, S., SUGORO, M., KIZU, K., ITO, H., NAKAI, K., KITA, S., MASUDA, M.: Metabolism of glucuronic acid in fatigue due to physical exercise. Jap. J. Pharmacol. **16**, 138—156 (1966).
TEMPLE, A.R., CLEMENT, M.S., DONE, A.K.: Studies of glucuronidation. IV. Evidence of different processes for *o*-aminophenol and *p*-nitrophenol. Proc. Soc. exp. Biol. (N.Y.) **128**, 307—314 (1968).
TOMLINSON, G.A., YAFFE, S.J.: The formation of bilirubin and *p*-nitrophenyl glucuronides by rabbit liver. Biochem. J. **99**, 507—512 (1966).
TROLLE, D.: Decrease of total serum-bilirubin concentration in newborn infants after phenobarbitone treatment. Lancet **II**, 705—708 (1968).
VAN LEUSDEN, H.A.J.M., BAKKEREN, J.A.J.M., ZILLIKEN, F., STOLTE, L.A.M.: *p*-Nitrophenylglucuronide formation by homozygous adult Gunn rats. Biochem. biophys. Res. Commun. **7**, 67—69 (1962).
VAN ROY, F.P., HEIRWEGH, K.P.M.: Determination of bilirubin glucuronide and assay of glucuronyltransferase with bilirubin as acceptor. Biochem. J. **107**, 507—518 (1968).
WALKER, S.R., WILLIAMS, R.T.: Metabolites of sulphadimethoxypyrimidine in the urine of various species. Biochem. J. **115**, 61—62 P (1969).
WHELTON, M.J., KUNSTER, L.P., BILLING, B.H.: Reduction in serum bilirubin by phenobarbital in adult unconjugated hyperbilirubinemia. Is enzyme induction responsible? Amer. J. Med. **45**, 160—164 (1968).
WHITE, A.E.: The distribution of glucuronyl transferase in cell membranes. In: Bilirubin metabolism. Oxford: Blackwell 1967.
WILLIAMS, C.H.: *β*-Glucuronidase in serum and liver of rats given pesticides and hepatotoxins. Toxicol. appl. Pharmacol. **14**, 283—292 (1969).
WILSON, D.: Purification of uridine diphosphoglucose dehydrogenase from calf liver. Analyt. Biochem. **10**, 472—478 (1965).

WINSNES, A.: Studies on the activation *in vitro* of glucuronyltransferase. Biochem. biophys. Acta (Amst.) **191**, 279—291 (1969).

WONG, K. P., SOURKES, T. L.: Determination of UDPG and UDPGA in tissues. Analyt. Biochem. **21**, 444—453 (1967a).

— — Measurement of endogenous UDPG in tissues, and some hormonal effects on its concentration in liver. Fed. Proc. **26**, 835 (1967b).

— — Glucuronidation of 3-*O*-methylnoradrenaline, harmalol and some related compounds. Biochem. J. **110**, 99—104 (1968a).

— — Uridine nucleotides in brain. J. Neurochem. **15**, 201—203 (1968b).

YAFFE, S. J., LEVY, G., MATSUZAWA, T., BALIAH, T.: Enhancement of glucuronide-conjugating capacity in a hyperbilirubinemic infant due to apparent enzyme induction. New Engl. J. Med. **275**, 1461—1466 (1966).

ZALITIS, J., FEINGOLD, D. S.: The mechanism of action of UDPG dehydrogenase. Biochem. biophys. Res. Commun. **31**, 693—698 (1968).

ZEIDENBERG, P., ORRENIUS, S., ERNSTER, L.: Increase in levels of glucuronylating enzymes and associated rise of mitochondrial oxidative enzymes upon phenobarbital administration in the rat. J. Cell Biol. **32**, 528—531 (1967).

Chapter 46

Metabolism of Normal Body Constituents by Drug-Metabolizing Enzymes in Liver Microsomes

A.H. CONNEY and R. KUNTZMAN[1]

A. Introduction

The duration and intensity of action of many drugs are determined by the speed at which they are metabolized in the body by enzymes in liver microsomes. The activities of drug-metabolizing enzymes can be altered by dietary and nutritional factors, hormonal changes in the body and by the ingestion of foreign chemicals (CONNEY and BURNS, 1962; GILLETTE, 1963; CONNEY, 1967). Recent studies suggest that steroid hormones, fatty acids, bilirubin and several other normal body constituents are substrates for drug-metabolizing enzymes in liver microsomes. Accordingly, changes in the activities of drug-metabolizing enzymes are reflected by changes in the metabolism of normal body constituents that are metabolized by these enzymes. This review describes some of the normal body constituents that are substrates for drug-metabolizing enzymes in liver microsomes and indicates some of the factors that influence the metabolism of these substances.

B. Steroid Hormones

I. Factors Influencing Steroid Hydroxylation

Evidence indicating that steroid hormones are hydroxylated by NADPH-dependent enzymes in liver microsomes came from the work of MUELLER and RUMNEY (1957). These investigators demonstrated the hydroxylation of estradiol-17β by mouse liver microsomes and indicated that reduced nicotinamide adenine dinucleotide phosphate (NADPH) and oxygen were necessary for enzyme activity. During the past ten years, it has become apparent that numerous estrogens, androgens, progestational steroids and glucocorticoids are hydroxylated by NADPH-dependent enzymes in liver microsomes.

CONNEY and KLUTCH (1963) demonstrated that testosterone and Δ^4-androstene-3,17-dione were hydroxylated in several positions by NADPH-dependent enzymes in rat liver microsomes and they suggested that steroid hormones may be hydroxylated by the same enzymes that hydroxylate drugs. These investigators found that treatment of rats with phenobarbital or other inducers of drug-metabolizing enzymes markedly stimulated the hydroxylation of testosterone and Δ^4-androstene-3,17-dione by enzymes in liver microsomes.

KUNTZMAN et al. (1964) showed that many of the factors that influence the oxidative metabolism of hexobarbital also influence the hydroxylation of estra-

[1] Most of the work on which this chapter is based was carried out in the laboratories of Burroughs Wellcome and Co.

diol-17β and testosterone, and these investigators suggested that estradiol-17β and testosterone were normal body substrates for the enzyme system that oxidizes hexobarbital. Some of the similarities between the enzymatic metabolism of hexobarbital and the hydroxylation of testosterone and estradiol-17β by liver microsomes that were noted in this study include: (1) localization of enzyme activity in liver microsomes and requirement for NADPH and oxygen, (2) higher activity in male rats than in male mice, (3) higher activity in adult male rats than in adult female rats, (4) little or no sex difference in enzyme activity in mice, (5) higher activity in adult male rats than in immature rats, (6) inhibition by the *in vitro* addition of SKF 525-A, (7) increased activity after treatment of rats with phenobarbital or chlordane and (8) little or no increase in activity after treatment of rats with 3-methylcholanthrene. The sex difference for the metabolism of androgens by rat liver was also reported by Leybold and Staudinger (1959), Colas (1962) and Heinrichs et al. (1966). Several of the factors listed above that influence the activity of hexobarbital oxidase in liver microsomes were found to influence the enzymatic oxidation of progesterone by liver microsomes (Kuntzman et al., 1966a). Further support for the concept that steroids are normal body substrates for drug-metabolizing enzymes came from finding that the Michaelis constants for the hydroxylation of testosterone, estradiol-17β and progesterone were lower than those for several representative drug substrates (Kuntzman et al., 1965). More recent studies showed that estradiol-17β, testosterone, androsterone, progesterone and hydrocortisone competitively inhibited the oxidation of ethylmorphine and hexobarbital by rat liver microsomes and that the K_i for this inhibition was similar to the K_m previously reported for the hydroxylation of these steroids (Tephly and Mannering, 1968). These investigators concluded that certain drugs and steroids are alternate substrates for a common microsomal mixed function oxidase system. Thyroidectomy, Walker 256 sarcoma, or treatment with morphine or thyroxin inhibited the metabolism of hexobarbital by liver microsomes of male rats (Kato and Gillette, 1965; Kato et al., 1968a), and these same factors inhibited the oxidation of progesterone by liver microsomes (Kato et al., 1968a).

Treatment of animals with phenobarbital increased the activity of enzymes in liver microsomes that hydroxylate testosterone (Conney and Klutch, 1963), Δ^4-androstene-3,17-dione (Conney and Klutch, 1963), estradiol-17β (Kuntzman et al., 1964; Levin et al., 1968), estrone (Levin et al., 1968), progesterone (Kuntzman et al., 1966a; Conney et al., 1966), deoxycorticosterone (Conney et al., 1966), cortisol, corticosterone and cortisone (Conney and Schneidman, 1964; Conney et al., 1965; Burstein and Bhavnani, 1967). Although treatment of rats with phenobarbital stimulated the activity of liver microsomal enzymes that catalyze reductive processes such as the reduction of the azo linkage of neoprontosil (Hernandez et al., 1967) and the reduction of the nitro group of chloramphenicol (Remmer and Merker, 1963, 1965) and *p*-nitrobenzoic acid (Hart et al., 1962; Cram et al., 1965), phenobarbital administration did not stimulate the A-ring reduction of cortisol (Conney and Schneidman, 1964; Remmer and Merker, 1965). Additional studies indicated that phenobarbital administration did not enhance the A-ring reduction of Δ^4-androstence-3,17-dione in immature male rats (Conney and Klutch, 1963), but did in adult male rats (von Bahr et al., 1969). Since castration of adult male rats increases the A-ring reduction of deoxycorticosterone (Yates et al., 1958) and testosterone (unpublished observations), it is possible that phenobarbital stimulates A-ring reduction in adult male rats by inhibiting the action of endogenous androgens. Drugs other than barbiturates that stimulate the activity of steroid hydroxylases in liver microsomes include diphenylhydantoin, chlorcyclizine, norchlorcyclizine, orphenadrine, phenylbutazone, chlordane, DDT and *o,p'*-DDD (CONNEY and KLUTCH, 1963; CONNEY and SCHNEIDMAN, 1964; CONNEY et al., 1965, 1966; KUNTZMAN et al., 1964; KUPFER and PEETS, 1966; WELCH et al., 1967; LEVIN et al., 1968). The administration of DDT (10 ppm) or dieldrin (2 ppm) for one week to male or female pigeons stimulated the metabolism of testosterone and progesterone by liver microsomes (PEAKALL, 1967). The stimulatory effect of insecticides on steroid metabolism described above and the estrogenic activity of DDT and some of its analogs that was recently reported by LEVIN et al. (1968b), BITMAN et al. (1968) and WELCH et al. (1969) may help explain the decrease in population of certain species of birds which has been reported.

Numerous studies indicate that more than one microsomal system participates in the oxidation of drugs and steroids. Treatment of rats with 3,4-benzpyrene stimulated the hydroxylation of 3,4-benzpyrene, acetanilide, aniline and zoxazolamine, but not the oxidative metabolism of hexobarbital and aminopyrine (CONNEY et al., 1959, 1960). In rats or mice, 3,4-benzpyrene stimulated the 2-hydroxylation of biphenyl, but not its 4-hydroxylation, whereas phenobarbital caused a large increase in the 4-hydroxylation, but only a small increase in the 2-hydroxylation (CREAVEN and PARKE, 1966). Considerable specificity exists in the regulation of testosterone hydroxylation in the 6β-, 7α- and 16α-positions (KUNTZMAN et al., 1968a; CONNEY et al., 1969). Chronic treatment of rats with phenobarbital, phenylbutazone or DDT stimulated the hydroxylation of testosterone in the 16α-position to a greater extent than in the 6β- and 7α-position (CONNEY and SCHNEIDMAN, 1964; WELCH et al., 1967). In contrast, chronic treatment with 3-methylcholanthrene increased the hydroxylation of testosterone in the 7α-position and inhibited hydroxylation at the 16α-position (KUNTZMAN et al., 1968a; CONNEY et al., 1969). In dogs, the administration of phenylbutazone increased the hydroxylation of testosterone in the 6β- and 16α-positions, but no increase was observed in hydroxylation at the 7α-position (CONNEY and SCHNEIDMAN, 1964).

Addition of chlorthion to suspensions of liver microsomes markedly inhibited the 16α-hydroxylation of testosterone, had a smaller effect on the 6β-hydroxylation and had little or no effect on the 7α-hydroxylation reaction (KUNTZMAN et al., 1966a; WELCH et al., 1967). Studies of testosterone hydroxylation as a function of age indicated that the 16α-hydroxylation of this steroid by liver microsomes increased markedly with age in the male rat, whereas a smaller increase was observed for 6β-hydroxylase activity and a decrease with age was observed for 7α-hydroxylase activity (JACOBSON and KUNTZMAN, 1969). The storage of frozen liver microsomal suspensions for 20 days resulted in a large decrease in 16α-hydroxylase activity, a smaller decrease in 6β-hydroxylase activity and no change in 7α-hydroxylase activity (KUNTZMAN et al., 1968a; LEVIN et al., 1969a). The above studies on the effects of age, sex and enzyme induction on the metabolism of drugs and testosterone indicate that the 16α-hydroxylation of testosterone and the oxidative metabolism of hexobarbital, aminopyrine and ethylmorphine are regulated by the same factors and probably proceed via the same enzyme system while the 7α-hydroxylation of testosterone and the oxidation of aniline and zoxazolamine utilize another, but similar enzyme system.

COOPER et al. (1965) provided good evidence that a carbon monoxide-binding pigment (cytochrome P-450) of liver microsomes functions as an oxygen-activating enzyme for several drug oxidations. They found that the liver microsomal oxidation of codeine, 4-monomethylaminoantipyrine and acetanilide was inhibited by CO and that the inhibition was reversed by monochromatic light at 450 mμ to a greater extent than by light at other wavelengths. Recent studies have indicated that cytochrome P-450 also participates in the hydroxylation of testosterone by liver microsomes (CONNEY et al., 1968). Carbon monoxide inhibited the 6β-, 7α- and 16α-hydroxylation of testosterone by rat liver microsomes, but the degree of inhibition of the three hydroxylation reactions differed. The ratios of CO to oxygen required for 50% inhibition of testosterone hydroxylation in the 16α-, 6β- and 7α-positions were 0.93, 1.54 and 2.36, respectively. It was found that low intensity light at 450 mμ antagonized the inhibitory effect of CO on the 7α-hydroxylation reaction to a greater extent than the 6β- and 16α-hydroxylation reactions. These results and the results of other studies described above suggested the possible presence of more than one CO-sensitive cytochrome in liver microsomes that function in the hydroxylation of testosterone in the various positions and that the cytochrome responsible for the 16α-hydroxylation reaction is more sensitive to CO than that which functions for the 6β- and 7α-hydroxylation reactions. The finding that light at 450 mμ was more effective than light at other wavelengths in reversing the CO inhibition of the three hydroxylation reactions suggested the participation in these reactions of cytochrome P-450 and/or other CO-sensitive cytochromes with a similar absorption spectrum for the CO-bound derivative. As in the case of the other mixed function oxygenases studied, the question remains whether the term "cytochrome P-450" actually embraces a group of cytochromes with identical hemes bound to different proteins or whether a single cytochrome P-450 is attended by several specific substrate-binding proteins that put the substrate in the proper position for interaction with the oxygenated cytochrome. The number of cytochromes and other components that participate in each hydroxylation reaction is unknown and must await the solubilization and purification of the microsomal systems.

Evidence was recently obtained for the presence of at least two CO-binding cytochromes in liver microsomes. Whereas treatment of rats with phenobarbital increased the concentration of a CO-binding pigment with a difference spectrum maximum at 450 mμ (REMMER and MERKER, 1965), treatment of rats with 3-methylcholanthrene increased the concentration of a CO-binding pigment with an absorption maximum at 448 mμ (ALVARES et al., 1967; KUNTZMAN et al., 1968a). Since this effect of 3-methylcholanthrene is blocked by inhibitors of protein synthesis (ALVARES et al., 1968), it is believed to represent the formation of a previously unidentified cytochrome. More recently, HILDEBRANDT et al. (1968) showed that treatment of rabbits with 3-methylcholanthrene caused a similar shift in absorption maximum for the CO-binding pigment. Earlier studies, using ethylisocyanide as the ligand, also indicated the induction of different microsomal cytochromes by phenobarbital and 3-methylcholanthrene (SLADEK and MANNERING, 1966).

II. Effect of Enzyme Induction on Steroid Action

The increase in steroid hydroxylation *in vitro* caused by administration of drugs to animals is reflected *in vivo* by an increased metabolism and a decreased physiological action of steroids. The increased hydroxylation of progesterone caused by phenobarbital pretreatment was associated with a decreased anesthetic action of progesterone and with decreased amounts of this steroid and its metabolites in the brain and total body of the rat (KUNTZMAN et al., 1965a; CONNEY et al., 1966). Phenobarbital treatment for four days also decreased the effects of other steroids such as deoxycorticosterone, androsterone, Δ^4-androstene-3,17-dione and testosterone on the central nervous system. Similarly, chronic treatment of rats with chlorcyclizine, phenylbutazone, chlordane or DDT shortened the anesthetic action of progesterone and increased its metabolism by liver microsomal enzymes (KUNTZMAN et al., 1965a; CONNEY et al., 1966).

The administration of physiological amounts of estradiol-17β to immature female rats increased uterine weight, protein synthesis and the activity of phosphofructokinase in the uterus. Treatment of rats with phenobarbital for several days decreased the effect of estradiol-17β in eliciting these responses (LEVIN et al., 1967, 1968; SINGHAL et al., 1967), but a single high dose of phenobarbital administered one hour before the steroid did not inhibit estradiol-17β action (LEVIN et al., 1967). Chronic treatment of rats with phenobarbital also inhibited the uterotropic action of estrone and several synthetic estrogens and progestational steroids used as oral contraceptives (LEVIN et al., 1968, 1968a). The decreased activity of estrogens in phenobarbital-pretreated rats was associated with decreased amounts of estrogen in the uterus and with increased total body metabolism of the steroid (LEVIN et al., 1968 and WELCH et al., 1968). When estrone was administered to control rats, 18% of the dose remained unmetabolized after 40 min; in contrast, following the administration of the steroid to rats previously treated with phenobarbital for 4 days, only 4% of the steroid was unmetabolized after 40 min. The smallest amount of phenobarbital which inhibited estrogen action, decreased the amount of estradiol-17β or estrone in the uterus and increased the hydroxylation of these steroids *in vitro* was 2—5 mg/kg/day for 4 days. Treatment of immature rats with as little as 0.5 mg/kg/day of phenobarbital for 4 days decreased the uterotropic action of mestranol (LEVIN et al., 1968a). The administration of chlorcyclizine, norchlorcyclizine, phenylbutazone, orphenadrine, or chlordane for 4 days stimulated the *in vitro* metabolism of estradiol-17β and estrone, decreased the effect of estrogens on the weight of the uterus and decreased the amount of estradiol-17β found in the uterus following the administration of physiological amounts of tritiated estradiol-17β (LEVIN et al., 1968). Chronic treatment with pentobarbital inhibited the precocious ovulation elicited in immature female rats following estradiol-17β treatment (HAGINO et al., 1966) and it is possible that this effect was caused by enhanced metabolism of estrogens. Similarly, in nursing neonates of phenobarbital-treated rats, uterine responsiveness to exogenous estrogen was reduced (FAHIM and KING, 1968). In contrast to the effect of enzyme inducers on estrogen action, treatment of rats with carbon tetrachloride or other inhibitors of drug hydroxylations inhibited the *in vitro* hydroxylation of estradiol-17β and estrone by liver microsomes and potentiated the effects of these estrogens on the uterus (LEVIN et al., 1970).

Some studies have suggested that barbiturate administration may alter the action of endogenous estrogens. FAHIM et al. (1968a) showed that the administration of phenobarbital (50 mg/kg/day) to adult female mice for 4 days decreased the weight of the uterus when no exogenous estradiol-17β was administered, and this effect did not occur in ovariectomized mice. The authors suggested that the effect of phenobarbital in intact mice was caused by a stimulation of the metabolism of endogenous estrogen. An inhibitory effect of phenobarbital treatment on uterine weight in rats not treated with exogenous estrogen was also observed in our laboratory. During the postnatal development of female rats, the weight of the uterus increases with age; however, when phenobarbital was added to the food of these developing rats (age, 19 days) the rate of increase in uterine size was decreased for several days (WELCH et al., 1970).

Pretreatment of immature male rats with phenobarbital decreased the action of exogenous androgens (LEVIN et al., 1969, 1970a). Treatment with phenobarbital for four days inhibited the growth-promoting effect of testosterone, testosterone propionate 17α-methyltestosterone and fluoxymesterone on the seminal vesicles. It is possible that barbiturate treatment also alters the action of endogenous androgens since the increase in the weight of the seminal vesicles which occurred as rats mature was inhibited in animals treated with phenobarbital (LEVIN et al., 1970a). Treatment of adult male rats with phenobarbital also decreased the weight of the seminal vesicles, without changing testicular weight (LEVIN et al., 1970a). It is not known whether these effects are related to alterations in the metabolism of endogenous androgens.

III. Effect of Enzyme Induction on Steroid Hydroxylation in Man

Some compounds that stimulate the liver microsomal hydroxylation of steroids in animals also alter pathways of steroid metabolism in man. WERK et al. (1964) showed that treatment of humans with diphenylhydantoin increased the urinary excretion of 6β-hydroxycortisol. Other drugs that produce this same effect are phenobarbital (BURSTEIN and KLAIBER, 1965), phenylbutazone (KUNTZMAN et al., 1966), *o,p'*-DDD (BLEDSOE et al., 1964; SOUTHREN et al., 1966) and N-phenylbarbital (KUNTZMAN et al., 1968), and recent studies have shown that people exposed to high levels of DDT in a pesticide factory excreted more 6β-hydroxycortisol in the urine than a control population (POLAND et al., 1970). The effect of DDT was less than that found for the above drugs. The finding that chronic treatment of guinea pigs with several of the above drugs stimulated the activity of an enzyme system in liver microsomes that hydroxylates cortisol in the 6β-position (CONNEY et al., 1965; BURSTEIN and BHAVNANI, 1967; KUNTZMAN et al., 1968) suggested a possible explanation for drug-induced increases in the urinary excretion of 6β-hydroxycortisol in man. The observation that compounds which stimulated drug metabolism also increased the excretion of 6β-hydroxycortisol in human urine has led to the suggestion that the level of urinary 6β-hydroxycortisol may be useful as a measure of microsomal enzyme induction in man. In 8 humans, less than 400 μg of 6β-hydroxycortisol were excreted in the urine per day, but after treatment of these subjects with either N-phenylbarbital or phenylbutazone, the excretion of 6β-hydroxycortisol always exceeded this amount (KUNTZMAN et al., 1968). In addition, treatment of humans with N-phenylbarbital has been shown to decrease the urinary excretion of androsterone and etiocholanolone, the major metabolites of testosterone, and to increase the excretion of unidentified polar metabolites of this steroid (SOUTHREN et al., 1969; KUNTZMAN and SOUTHREN, 1969). It is possible that the measurement of the decrease in excretion of androsterone or etiocholanolone in human urine may be another procedure for the determination of microsomal enzyme induction in man.

Studies by WERK et al. (1966) and SOUTHREN et al. (1966) have suggested that the increased hydroxylation of cortisol observed in man following diphenylhydantoin or *o,p'*-DDD treatment may have therapeutic value in the treatment of Cushing's syndrome. A decrease in the biochemical and clinical signs of this disease was observed following treatment of two subjects with 300—400 mg/day of diphenylhydantoin for three months (WERK et al., 1966). The administration of *o,p'*-DDD also reduced the symptoms of Cushing's syndrome before the drug produced any effect on the rate of cortisol secretion from the adrenal gland (SOUTHREN et al., 1966). However, insufficient work has been done to determine whether enhanced hydroxylation of steroids can decrease the pharmacological action of these substances in man, and additional studies are needed to evaluate the physiological importance of drug-induced increases in steroid hydroxylation.

C. Cholesterol

I. Biosynthesis

Several of the enzymes necessary for the biosynthesis of cholesterol are localized in liver microsomes and require NADPH and oxygen for activity (BLOCH, 1965; MILLER et al., 1967; GAYLOR and MASON, 1968), but the role of cytochrome P-450 in these microsomal reactions is uncertain. A very high concentration of carbon monoxide was needed to inhibit the *in vitro* biosynthesis of cholesterol. The incorporation of C^{14}-acetate, C^{14}-mevalonate and C^{14}-squalene into cholesterol by rat liver homogenate was inhibited 22%, 50% and 75%, respectively, when a 19:1 ratio of carbon monoxide:oxygen was used (WADA et al., 1967, 1969). A 20% inhibition in the incorporation of C^{14}-mevalonate into cholesterol occurred when the ratio of carbon monoxide:oxygen was 4:1 (WADA et al., 1969). It would be of interest to know whether light at 450 mμ prevents the inhibitory effect of carbon monoxide on the incorporation of C^{14}-mevalonate or C^{14}-squalene into cholesterol.

The conversion of lanosterol to cholesterol involves hydroxylation of methyl groups in the 4α-, 4β- and 14α-positions of lanosterol, and this is followed by further metabolism to carbon dioxide (BLOCH, 1965; MILLER et al., 1967; GAYLOR and MASON, 1968). The initial hydroxylation of the methyl groups of lanosterol occurs in liver microsomes in the presence of oxygen and NADPH or NADH, and cytochrome P-450 is not a component of the enzyme system that catalyzes this reaction (MILLER et al., 1967; GAYLOR and MASON, 1968). The demethylation of lanosterol by liver microsomes is insensitive to concentrations of carbon monoxide that inhibit metabolic processes that are dependent on cytochrome P-450, and purification of the sterol demethylase led to a loss of cytochrome P-450 without a proportionate loss of demethylase activity.

Administration of phenobarbital to hamsters or rats increased the activity of hepatic enzymes that incorporate C^{14}-acetate into cholesterol (JONES and ARMSTRONG, 1965; MITOMA et al., 1968; KATO et al., 1968), and recently it was found that phenobarbital administration to rats increased the *in vitro* incorporation of C^{14}-acetate into cholesterol by slices of small intestine (MIDDLETON and ISSELBACHER, 1969). WADA et al. (1967) found that administration of phenobarbital to rats increased the hepatic *in vitro* incorporation of C^{14}-mevalonate into cholesterol to a greater extent than the incorporation of C^{14}-acetate. In contrast to this report, MITOMA et al. (1968) found that treatment of rats with phenobarbital caused a 10-fold increase in the activity of hepatic enzymes that incorporate C^{14}-acetate into cholesterol, but the incorporation of C^{14}-mevalonate into cholesterol was unaffected. The latter investigators found that treatment of rats with 3,4-benzpyrene had no effect on the *in vitro* incorporation of C^{14}-acetate into cholesterol and that the incorporation of C^{14}-mevalonate into cholesterol was inhibited. Treatment of rats with 3,4-benzpyrene increased the serum concentration of cholesterol, whereas treatment of rats with phenobarbital had no effect on the serum concentration of cholesterol (MITOMA et al., 1968; SALVADOR et al., 1969).

WADA et al. (1969a) treated mice for three days with phenobarbital, griseofulvin or allylisopropylacetamide and found enhanced incorporation of C^{14}-acetate into liver cholesterol *in vitro* and *in vivo*. Interestingly, serum cholesterol was decreased 20% by phenobarbital treatment, whereas griseofulvin and allylisopropylacetamide increased the concentration of serum cholesterol by 74 and 67% respectively. A decreased serum cholesterol in mice treated with phenobarbital was also observed by SALVADOR et al. (1969). The above observations suggest a need for more detailed studies on the effects of the various drugs on cholesterol synthesis and metabolism.

II. Metabolism to Bile Acids

The metabolism of cholesterol to bile acids involves hydroxylation at the 7α- and 12α-positions of the sterol nucleus and some of the bile acids are further metabolized by hydroxylation at the 6β-position. These reactions are catalyzed by NADPH-dependent enzymes in liver microsomes (DANIELSSON and EINARSSON, 1966; DANIELSSON and TCHEN, 1968; SHEFER et al., 1968; VOIGT et al., 1968; EINARSSON and JOHANSSON, 1969). The 7α-hydroxylation of cholesterol is an early and possibly rate-determining step in the conversion of cholesterol to bile acids. The 7α-hydroxylase is localized in liver microsomes, requires NADPH and oxygen for activity and the activity of this enzyme is inhibited about 50% by a 1:1 ratio of carbon monoxide:oxygen (WADA et al., 1968; MOSBACH, 1969), suggesting that cytochrome P-450 is a component of the 7α-hydroxylase system. Administration of phenobarbital to rats has been shown to increase the activity of the liver microsomal enzyme that hydroxylates cholesterol and cholestanol in the 7α-position (SHEFER et al., 1968; WADA et al., 1968; MOSBACH, 1969). The stimulatory effect of phenobarbital on the 7α-hydroxylation of cholesterol, however, was not observed by EINARSSON and JOHANSSON (1968) or BOYD et al. (1969). Administration of cholestyramine or breaking the enterohepatic circulation by biliary drainage increased cholesterol-7α-hydroxylase activity (SHEFER et al., 1968; BOYD et al., 1969), but the concentration of cytochrome P-450 in liver microsomes was not affected (BOYD et al., 1969). These observations, coupled with the sensitivity of cholesterol-7α-hydroxylase to carbon monoxide, suggest that although cytochrome P-450 probably participates in the 7α-hydroxylation of cholesterol, this hemoprotein may not be the rate-limiting component of the overall enzyme system.

The 7α-hydroxylation of taurodeoxycholic acid to taurocholic acid by NADPH-dependent enzymes in rat liver microsomes does not appear to require cytochrome P-450, since the 7α-hydroxylase system is refractory to carbon monoxide. Enzyme activity was inhibited only 14% in an atmosphere containing a carbon monoxide: oxygen ratio of 10 (EINARSSON and JOHANSSON, 1969). Liver microsomes from male rats 7α-hydroxylated taurodeoxycholic acid more rapidly than liver microsomes from females, and enzyme activity was increased by treatment of rats with phenobarbital (EINARSSON and JOHANSSON, 1968, 1969) or polycyclic hydrocarbons such as 3-methylcholanthrene and 3,4-benzpyrene (WHITEHOUSE, 1964). The metabolism of cholest-5-ene-3β,7α-diol to 7α-hydroxycholest-4-en-3-one by NAD-fortified microsomes was not affected by phenobarbital administration (EINARSSON and JOHANSSON, 1968).

Studies by SUZUKI et al. (1968) showed that the 12α-hydroxylation of 7α-hydroxycholest-4-en-3-one was not inhibited by a carbon monoxide:oxygen ratio of 9:1, suggesting that cytochrome P-450 does not participate in the 12α-hydroxylation reaction. In contrast to the marked stimulatory effect of phenobarbital on the hydroxylation of many drugs and steroids, treatment of rats with phenobarbital decreased by 50% the 12α-hydroxylation of 7α-hydroxycholest-4-en-3-one by NADPH-fortified liver microsomes (EINARSSON and JOHANSSON, 1968; SUZUKI et al., 1968).

Chenodeoxycholic acid, taurochenodeoxycholic acid and lithocholic acid are hydroxylated in the 6β-position by rat liver microsomes, and NADPH and oxygen are required for this reaction (VOIGT et al., 1968; EINARSSON and JOHANSSON,

1969). Administration of phenobarbital to rats markedly stimulated the activity of liver microsomal enzymes that hydroxylate taurochenodeoxycholic acid and lithocholic acid in the 6β-position (EINARSSON and JOHANSSON, 1969). The 6β-hydroxylation of taurochenodeoxycholate and lithocholate was inhibited by carbon monoxide and the inhibition was partially prevented by white light (VOIGT et al., 1968; EINARSSON and JOHANSSON, 1969). The 6β-hydroxylation of taurochenodeoxycholate was inhibited about 50% by a carbon monoxide:oxygen ratio of 2 (VOIGT et al., 1968a). Studies on the photoreactivation spectrum of the CO-inhibited taurochenodeoxycholate 6β-hydroxylase system revealed that light at 450 mμ was more effective than light at other wavelengths in preventing the inhibitory effect of carbon monoxide (VOIGT et al., 1968a). These observations indicate that cytochrome P-450 participates in the 6β-hydroxylation of taurochenodeoxycholate.

The administration of phenobarbital to rats stimulates bile flow (ROBERTS and PLAA, 1967), but does not change the endogenous serum cholesterol level (MITOMA et al., 1968; SALVADOR et al., 1969). The ability of phenobarbital administration to increase the activity of enzymes involved in the biosynthesis and degradation of cholesterol and to enhance bile flow without changing the endogenous serum cholesterol level in the rat suggests that phenobarbital may enhance the turnover of cholesterol. It was pointed out above that phenobarbital administration in the mouse stimulated cholesterol biosynthesis and lowered serum cholesterol. These results suggest the possibility that phenobarbital administration may have a greater effect on cholesterol metabolism than on cholesterol synthesis in the mouse, but further experiments on this problem are needed. Although treatment of rabbits with phenobarbital did not change the endogenous serum cholesterol level, this treatment did decrease the hypercholesterolemia and the incidence of aortic plaques in rabbits that were fed exogenous cholesterol in the diet (SALVADOR et al., 1967, 1969a).

Chronic exposure to carbon monoxide increased the serum level of cholesterol and enhanced the development of atheromata in cholesterol-fed rabbits (ASTRUP et al., 1967). The authors suggested that carbon monoxide exerted this effect by causing hypoxia and by combining with cytochrome P-450 in liver microsomes. Both effects could result in inhibited oxidation of cholesterol to bile acids. A preliminary report by KJELDSEN (1969) suggested that carbon monoxide may influence serum cholesterol levels in man. These studies indicated that human cigarette smokers had a significantly higher serum cholesterol level than nonsmokers, and there was a significant correlation between carboxyhaemoglobin and serum cholesterol values.

D. Fatty Acids

I. ω-Oxidation

An enzyme system catalyzing the ω-oxidation of fatty acids occurs in liver microsomes and requires NADPH and oxygen for activity (WAKABAYASHI and SHIMAZONO, 1963; PREISS and BLOCH, 1964; ROBBINS, 1968; LU et al., 1969; ICHIHARA et al., 1969). This enzyme system was strongly inhibited by carbon monoxide (LU and COON, 1968, DAS et al., 1968; WADA et al., 1968a; LU et al., 1969), and the inhibition was partially prevented by light (LU et al., 1969), suggesting the participation of cytochrome P-450 in the ω-hydroxylation reaction. The ω-oxidation of lauric acid or stearic acid was inhibited 95% by a carbon monoxide:oxygen ratio of 2 and a ratio of 0.1 caused a 50% inhibition in the ω-oxidation of stearic acid (WADA et al., 1968a). It should be noted that the inhibitory effect of carbon monoxide on the ω-oxidation of stearic acid was considerably greater than the effect of carbon monoxide on the oxidation of several drugs and steroids by enzymes in liver microsomes (Omura et al., 1965; Gillette, 1966; Conney et al., 1968). The ω-oxidation of decanoate by liver microsomes was very sensitive to carbon monoxide, but this reaction was not appreciably inhibited by 1 mM SKF 525-A (Ichihara et al., 1969). The K_m for the ω-hydroxylation of decanoate is 2.6 μM, which is considerably lower than the K_m for the hydroxylation of most drugs. The ω-oxidation of stearic acid was inhibited by rabbit antibody to cytochrome c reductase suggesting that cytochrome c reductase may function as a component of the fatty acid ω-oxidation system (Wada et al., 1968a). Although treatment of rats and rabbits with phenobarbital increased the activity of a liver microsomal enzyme that ω-hydroxylates lauric acid (Lu and Coon, 1968; Das et al., 1968; Lu et al., 1969), treatment of rats with phenobarbital or 3-methylcholanthrene did not stimulate the ω-oxidation of stearic acid (Wada et al., 1968a). These results suggest that the ω-oxidation of laurate and stearate may be catalyzed by different enzymes.

Additional evidence that fatty acids interact with cytochrome P-450 came from the observation that the addition of laurate to liver microsomes gave rise to a "type I" spectral change of the type produced by hexobarbital (Lu et al., 1969; Orrenius and Thor, 1969). The enzyme system catalyzing the ω-hydroxylation of fatty acids was recently solubilized, and chromatography of the soluble preparation on a DEAE cellulose column separated cytochrome P-450, cytochrome P-450 reductase and a heat stable lipid fraction (Lu and Coon, 1968; Lu et al., 1969). All three fractions were necessary for the ω-hydroxylation of laurate. NADPH and oxygen were required for enzyme activity and the system was inhibited by carbon monoxide. This soluble preparation also catalyzed the oxidative metabolism of several drugs such as benzphetamine, aminopyrine, ethylmorphine, hexobarbital, norcodeine and *p*-nitroanisole (Lu et al., 1969a), and cytochrome P-450, NADPH-cytochrome P-450 reductase and the heat stable fraction were necessary for the oxidation of these drugs. Laurate and benzphetamine inhibited each other's metabolism as would be expected if the same hydroxylase system metabolized both substrates.

II. Desaturation

The desaturation of stearyl-CoA to oleate occurs in liver microsomes and requires molecular oxygen and either NADH or NADPH (Bernhard and Wagner, 1959; Stoffel, 1961; Marsh and James, 1962; Holloway et al., 1963; Oshino et al., 1966; Jones et al., 1969). Removal of microsomal lipids by extraction with aqueous acetone inactivated the fatty acid desaturation system, and enzyme activity was restored by the addition of microsomal lipid or a mixture of phospholipids, triglycerides and fatty acids (Jones et al., 1969). Unlike hepatic microsomal enzymes that catalyze the ω-oxidation of fatty acids and the hydroxylation of drugs, the microsomal enzyme that catalyzes the desaturation of fatty acids utilizes NADH, rather than NADPH, as the preferred electron donor (Oshino et al., 1966; Jones et al., 1969). Cytochrome P-450 does not participate in the desaturation of fatty acids, since very high concentrations of carbon monoxide did not inhibit the desaturation of stearyl-CoA by rat liver microsomes. Although pretreatment of rats with phenobarbital increased the concentration of cytochrome P-450 in liver microsomes and increased drug-hydroxylating enzyme activity, NADPH-dependent desaturation activity disappeared (Oshino et al., 1966). It was of considerable interest that fatty acid desaturation was markedly inhibited by cyanide, whereas drug hydroxylation was not (OSHINO et al., 1966). The identity of the cyanide-sensitive component that participates in the desaturation of fatty acids is unknown.

E. Thyroxin

A unique enzyme system which deiodinates thyroxin is present in liver microsomes (STANBURY et al., 1960; WYNN et al., 1962). The enzyme is activated by heat, requires Fe^{+++}, oxygen and a factor which can be replaced by cysteine, reduced glutathione or ascorbic acid. Interestingly, NADPH, NADH, NADP or NAD are not cofactors for this enzyme system. Thyroxin and triiodothyronine deiodination in microsomes followed simple Michaelis-Menton kinetics. The Vmax/mg protein was increased 1.6 to 2.9-fold by treatment of the rats with phenobarbital, and this treatment did not change the Michaelis constant (SCHWARTZ et al., 1969). In contrast to the deiodination of thyroxin, deiodination of monoiodotyrosine by liver microsomes requires NADPH and is not stimulated by phenobarbital administration (SCHWARTZ et al., 1969).

Phenobarbital and chlordane, administered in dosage schedules known to induce liver microsomal enzymes, increased the concentration ratio of I^{125}-thyroxin between liver and plasma in rats that were given an i.v. injection of I^{125}-thyroxin, but the drug pretreatment did not change the ratio of I^{125}-thyroxin between kidney and plasma (BERNSTEIN et al., 1968). Further studies by OPPENHEIMER et al. (1968) indicated that the enhanced hepatocellular binding of thyroxine induced by phenobarbital was reflected by increased deiodination and biliary clearance of this hormone. The enhanced clearance of thyroxin that occurred after phenobarbital treatment appeared to cause increased thyroidal function because the serum protein-bound iodine was unaffected by phenobarbital. In contrast, thyroidectomized animals maintained on a constant replacement dose of thyroxine and treated with phenobarbital exhibited a marked fall in serum protein-bound-iodine (OPPENHEIMER et al., 1968). The above results indicate that administration of phenobarbital to rats increases the deiodinative capacity of hepatic microsomes and this is paralleled by augmented deiodination *in vivo*.

Administration of polycyclic aromatic hydrocarbons to rats also alters the metabolism of I^{131}-thyroxin (NEWMAN and MOON, 1967; GOLDSTEIN and TAUROG, 1968). Rats normally excrete more radioactivity in urine than in feces after a dose of I^{131}-thyroxin. However, after 3-methylcholanthrene administration, more radioactivity was excreted in the feces than in the urine, and protein-bound I^{131} in plasma was decreased (NEWMAN and MOON, 1967). The authors suggested that 3-methylcholanthrene may have enhanced the glucuronidation and biliary excretion of thyroxin. More direct evidence for a stimulatory effect of polycyclic hydrocarbons on the *in vivo* and *in vitro* glucuronidation of thyroxin came from studies by GOLDSTEIN and TAUROG (1968). These investigators found that pretreatment of rats with 3,4-benzpyrene 48 hours before cannulation of the bile duct produced a 3-4-fold increase in the biliary excretion of exogenously administered or endogenously formed thyroxin, while no increase was observed when 3,4-benzpyrene was administered 5—9 hours before cannulation of the bile duct. Almost all of the increase could be accounted for by enhanced excretion of thyroxin glucuronide. The stimulatory effect of 3,4-benzpyrene on the *in vivo* metabolism of thyroxin could be explained by a marked stimulatory effect of 3,4-benzpyrene on thyroxin glucuronyl transferase in the liver (GOLDSTEIN and TAUROG, 1968). These authors found that phenobarbital had only a small stimulatory effect on the excretion of labeled thyroxin (as metabolites) in the bile, and no stimulatory effect of phenobarbital was observed on the activity of thyroxin glucuronyl transferase in the liver.

F. Bilirubin

Drugs, steroids, thyroxin and bilirubin are metabolized to glucuronides by UDPGA-dependent glucuronyl transferases in liver microsomes, and many aspects of this topic have been reviewed elsewhere (DUTTON, 1966). Some of the more recent aspects of the effects of drugs on the metabolism of bilirubin will be described below. INSCOE and AXELROD (1960) were the first to demonstrate enhanced hepatic glucuronyl transferase activity by administration of a foreign chemical. These investigators found that treatment of newborn rats with 3,4-benzpyrene stimulated *o*-aminophenol glucuronyl transferase in liver microsomes, but no such stimulation was observed in newborn rats when their mothers were treated with 3,4-benzpyrene during pregnancy. Treatment of pregnant rats with chloroquine or chlorcyclizine stimulated hepatic bilirubin glucuronide formation in the newborn (ARIAS et al., 1963, 1963a), and treatment of pregnant or newborn animals with barbiturates increased the activity of the bilirubin-conjugating enzyme in the newborn or young animal (CATZ and YAFFE, 1962, 1968). ROBERTS and PLAA (1967) have shown that treatment of mice with phenobarbital enhanced the disappearance of exogenously administered bilirubin from the plasma, and CATZ and YAFFE (1968) showed that pretreatment of adult rabbits with phenobarbital enhanced the excretion of administered bilirubin into bile. The hyperbilirubinemia found after the administration of the antibiotic, novobiocin, could be reduced by prior treatment with phenobarbital (HARBISON and SPRATT, 1967), but this effect may be due to increased metabolism of either bilirubin or novobiocin.

The finding that liver microsomal enzyme inducers increased bilirubin conjugation in animals suggested that these compounds might have a therapeutic effect in diseases of hyperbilirubinemia in man. YAFFE et al. (1966) and CRIGLER and GOLD (1966) found that in two infants with congenital nonhemolytic jaundice, treatment with 15 mg of phenobarbital two to three times a day caused a decrease in the plasma bilirubin levels and a disappearance of the jaundice. When treatment with phenobarbital was stopped, the jaundice returned and the plasma bilirubin levels were elevated. Further treatment with phenobarbital again decreased the hyperbilirubinemia. The decrease in bilirubin levels resulted from a decrease in bilirubin half life without a significant effect on bilirubin turnover (CRIGLER and GOLD, 1969). More recently, WHELTON et al. (1968), KREEK and SLEISENGER (1968) and ERTEL and NEWTON (1969) have confirmed the observation that phenobarbital treatment decreased bilirubin levels in patients with hyperbilirubinemia. SERENI et al. (1967) found that the administration of diethylnicotinamide to newborn infants with nonhemolytic jaundice was effective in decreasing the serum bilirubin levels. THOMPSON et al. (1969a) showed that DDT administration to a subject with nonhemolytic jaundice also decreased bilirubin levels, and after this treatment was stopped, bilirubin levels remained low for several months, possibly because of the prolonged storage of DDT and its metabolites in the fat. The mechanism of this effect appears similar to that postulated for the barbiturates, since THOMPSON and his associates have also shown that in rats, DDT increased hepatic glucuronyl transferase activity. THOMPSON and WILLIAMS (1967) recently treated four subjects with chronic intrahepatic cholestasis with 180 mg of phenobarbital per day for up to 50 days. In all of the subjects, plasma bilirubin decreased markedly and all four subjects reported a striking decrease in itching and an improved feeling of well being. In some humans with hyperbilirubinemia, phenobarbital treatment did not lower serum bilirubin (ARIAS et al., 1969) which is similar to results obtained in the homozygous Gunn rat (DELEON et al., 1967). Bilirubin conjugation is deficient in the Gunn rat and although the metabolism of drugs by liver microsomes can be stimulated by phenobarbital administration, the conjugation of bilirubin is not enhanced. However, in the heterozygous Gunn rat, phenobarbital treatment did stimulate the glucuronidation of bilirubin, and the glucuronide was excreted in the bile (ROBINSON, 1969). Phenobarbital administration not only decreased serum bilirubin in subjects with high bilirubin levels, but THOMPSON et al. (1969) recently showed that phenobarbital, in combination with other anticonvulsants, decreased the serum bilirubin concentration in epileptics with normal serum bilirubin levels.

In the first week of life, there is a transient increase in the level of unconjugated bilirubin in the plasma of human infants. In a retrospective study, TROLLE (1968) found that the hyperbilirubinemia which occurred in the newborn was decreased if the mothers received anticonvulsants containing phenobarbital and primidone throughout pregnancy for the treatment of epilepsy. Recently, MAURER et al. (1968) found that when phenobarbital (30—120 mg/day) was administered orally to pregnant women for 2 weeks or longer prior to delivery, a marked decrease in neonatal serum bilirubin levels was found. Three days after birth, serum bilirubin averaged 5.7 mg% in sixteen control babies, whereas in twelve babies delivered by mothers treated with phenobarbital, the average serum bilirubin level at 3 days after birth was only 2.2 mg%. Two additional studies have substantiated this observation, and it was found that phenobarbital was less effective when it was given to the newborn instead of the mother (TROLLE, 1968a; RAMBOER et al., 1969). BOGGS et al., (1967), found a correlation between the degree of neonatal hyperbilirubinemia and motor and/or mental scores attained at 8 months of age, and these studies suggest that the use of suitable stimulators of bilirubin metabolism to lower serum bilirubin levels in the newborn may prevent the damaging effect of bilirubin on brain function and thereby enhance human intelligence.

G. Miscellaneous

I. Indoles

Tryptamine, N,N-dimethyltryptamine, N,N-diethyltryptamine, N-acetyltryptophan and indolacetic acid are hydroxylated in the 6-position by liver microsomal enzymes that have properties similar to microsomal drug-metabolizing enzymes (JEPSON et al., 1962; JACCARINI and JEPSON, 1968). However, the activities of the enzyme systems that metabolize indoles are not inhibited by the *in vitro* addition of dipyridyl, and the *in vivo* administration of phenobarbital exerts only a weak stimulatory effect on the activity of hepatic enzymes that hydroxylate tryptamine, N,N-diethyltryptamine and N-acetyltryptophan (JACCARINI and JEPSON, 1968). Melatonin, a potent melanocyte-contracting substance that is formed from serotonin by N-acetylation and subsequent O-methylation, is hydroxylated in the 6-position by an NADPH-dependent enzyme system in rat liver microsomes (KOPIN et al., 1961). It is of interest that acute administration of chlorpromazine inhibits the metabolism of melatonin *in vivo* and that chronic administration of phenobarbital stimulates the metabolism of this hormone *in vivo* (WURTMAN et al., 1968).

II. Sympathomimetic Amines

Several normally occurring monophenols are hydroxylated to catecholamines by NADPH-dependent enzymes in liver microsomes (AXELROD, 1963; INSCOE et al., 1965; LEMBERGER et al., 1965). Examples of this metabolic reaction include the conversion of *p*-sympathol to epinephrine and the conversion of tyramine to dopamine. Administration of 3,4-benzpyrene to rats stimulated the activity of liver microsomal enzymes that hydroxylate N-acetylserotonin and N-acetyltyramine, but no effect was observed on the metabolism of tyramine to dopamine (Inscoe et al., 1965). It is of interest that tyramine hydroxylation *in vitro* was markedly inhibited by the adrenergic neuron blocking agents, bethanidine and B.W. 392C60 (N-*o*-chlorobenzyl-N′,N″-dimethylguanidine), which are compounds that do not inhibit the metabolism of hexobarbital (Lemberger et al., 1965). These results indicate that the microsomal enzyme that hydroxylates tyramine differs from the system that oxidizes barbiturates.

III. Heme

Hemoglobin, hematin and myoglobin are converted almost quantitatively to bilirubin *in vivo* and recent studies by Tenhunen et al. (1968, 1969, 1970) have elucidated the enzymatic mechanism of this conversion. An enzyme system, heme oxygenase, that oxidizes heme at the α-methene bridge to form biliverdin is localized in liver and spleen microsomes and requires NADPH and oxygen for activity. The biliverdin is further metabolized to bilirubin by an NADPH-dependent soluble enzyme, biliverdin reductase, which is not rate-limiting in the overall pathway. The activity of heme oxygenase was strongly inhibited by carbon monoxide and the inhibition was reversed by light, suggesting that cytochrome P-450 participates in the oxidation of heme. Studies on the stoichiometry of the metabolism of heme to bilirubin showed that three moles of oxygen were consumed per mole of bilirubin formed. Carbon monoxide and bilirubin were formed in equimolar amounts, and mass spectroscopy studies showed incorporation of atmospheric oxygen into the products, bilirubin and carbon monoxide. Heme oxygenase in spleen microsomes was most active when protohemin IX or methemalbumin was used as a substrate. Less activity in descending order was observed with methemoglobin, the α- and β-chains of hemoglobin, deuterohemin IX, coprohemin I and hemoglobin-haptoglobin complex. Oxyhemoglobin, carboxyhemoglobin, myoglobin and free porphyrins were not metabolized by heme oxygenase. It was of interest that the activity of heme oxygenase per gram tissue protein was several-fold higher in spleen than in liver or brain, and much less activity was present in kidney and lung.

Pretreatment of rats with phenobarbital enhanced the conversion of glycine-2-C^{14} to bilirubin (Schmid et al., 1966), but the mechanism of this effect is not known. A recent report indicated that the administration of phenobarbital to people enhanced their endogenous formation of carbon monoxide which was exhaled in the breath (Coburn, 1967). Phenobarbital may exert this effect by increasing the synthesis of heme or the activity of the microsomal heme oxygenase, which would result in enhanced oxidation of the methene bridge of heme giving rise to carbon monoxide. The stimulatory effect of phenobarbital on the synthesis of microsomal hemoproteins is well known, but the effect of phenobarbital on the activity of microsomal heme oxygenase has not yet been studied.

IV. Kynurenine and Anthranilic Acid

Although L-kynurenine is metabolized to 3-hydroxy-L-kynurenine by liver mitochondria (De Castro et al., 1956; Saito et al., 1957), L-kynurenine is metabolized to 5-hydroxy-L-kynurenine by an NADPH-dependent enzyme system in liver microsomes (Kido et al., 1968). The properties of this microsomal enzyme have not been thoroughly investigated.

Anthranilic acid is metabolized to 5-hydroxyanthranilic acid by rabbit liver microsomes, and no formation of 3-hydroxyanthranilic acid was observed (Kashiwamata et al., 1966). The K_m value for the hydroxylase is 3.8×10^{-4}M.

V. Methylated Purines

Pretreatment of rats with phenobarbital stimulates the demethylation of 6-dimethylaminopurine 6-methylaminopurine, puromycin and puromycin aminonucleoside by NADPH-dependent enzymes in liver microsomes (Mazel et al., 1964, 1966). The effect of phenobarbital on the metabolism of 6-dimethylaminopurine and 6-methylaminopurine is of particular interest, since these methylated purines are constituents of liver ribonucleic acid (Berquist and Matthews, 1959; (Dunn, 1959).

H. Concluding Remarks

The studies described in this review indicate that many normal body constituents are substrates for drug-metabolizing enzymes in liver microsomes and suggest that these enzymes play a role in regulating the physiological actions of the substrates that they metabolize. In agreement with this concept, treatment of rats with phenobarbital enhances the hydroxylation of androgens, estrogens, glucocorticoids and progestational steroids by liver microsomes and this effect is reflected *in vivo* by enhanced metabolism of steroids to polar metabolites and by a decreased action of steroids such as estradiol-17β, estrone, testosterone and progesterone. In contrast to these results, inhibition of microsomal enzymes that hydroxylate estrogens potentiates the action of estradiol-17β and estrone.

Recent studies suggest that inducers of liver microsomal enzymes enhance the hydroxylation of steroids in man. Phenobarbital, diphenylhydantoin and phenylbutazone are examples of drugs that stimulate cortisol hydroxylase activity in guinea pig liver microsomes and enhance the excretion of 6β-hydroxycortisol in human urine. Further research is needed to determine whether the stimulatory effect of drugs on the microsomal metabolism of steroids and other normal body constituents is harmful or beneficial. The answer to this question is particularly important because man is exposed to increasingly large numbers of drugs, pesticides, herbicides, food additives and environmental polycyclic hydrocarbons that stimulate drug metabolism and the metabolism of normal body constituents.

Certain inducers of liver microsomal enzymes have been used therapeutically for the treatment of hyperbilirubinemia in jaundiced children and in adults with chronic intrahepatic cholestasis. The observation that a correlation exists between the degree of neonatal hyperbilirubinemia and motor and/or mental scores attained at 8 months of age also raises the theoretical possibility that the use of suitable stimulators of bilirubin metabolism to lower serum bilirubin levels in the newborn may allow more complete development of potential intelligence. As our knowledge of the functions of microsomal enzymes increases, it seems likely that selective inhibitors and stimulators of these enzymes will be found that are useful for the beneficial regulation of abnormal metabolism peculiar to various human diseases.

References

Alvares, A.P., Schilling, G., Levin, W., Kuntzman, R.: Studies on the induction of CO-binding pigments in liver microsomes by phenobarbital and 3-methylcholanthrene. Biochem. biophys. Res. Commun. **29**, 521—526 (1967).

— — — — Alteration of the microsomal hemoprotein by 3-methylcholanthrene: Effects of ethionine and actinomycin D. J. Pharmacol. exp. Ther. **163**, 417—424 (1968).

Arias, I.M., Gartner, L.M., Cohen, M., Ben Ezzer, J., Levi, A.J.: Chronic nonhemolytic unconjugated hyperbilirubinemia with glucuronyl transferase deficiency: Clinical, biochemical, pharmacologic and genetic evidence for heterogeneity. Amer. J. Med. **47**, 395—409 (1969).

Arias, I.M., Gartner, L.M., Furman, M., Wolfson, S.: Effect of several drugs and chemicals on hepatic glucuronide formation in newborn rats. Proc. Soc. exp. Biol. (N.Y.) **112**, 1037—1040 (1963).

— — — — Studies on the effect of several drugs on hepatic glucuronide formation in newborn rats and humans. Ann. N.Y. Acad. Sci. **111**, 274—280 (1963a).

Astrup, P., Kjeldsen, K., Wanstrup, J.: Enhancing influences of carbon monoxide on the development of atheromatosis in cholesterol-fed rabbits. J. Atheroscler. Res. **7**, 343—354 (1967).

Axelrod, J.: Enzymatic formation of adrenaline and other catechols from monophenols. Science **140**, 499—500 (1963).

Bahr, C., von, Lisboa, B.P., Orrenius, S.: Influence of phenobarbital pretreatment on the *in vitro* ring A reduction of Δ^4-3-oxosteroids in rat liver microsomes. Naunyn-Schmiedeberg's Arch. exp. Path. Pharmak. **264**, 420—426 (1969).

Bernhard, K., von Bulow-Koster, J., Wagner, H.: Die Enzymatische Dehydrierung der Stearinsäure zu Ölsäure. Helv. chim. Acta **42**, 152—155 (1959).

Bernstein, G., Artz, S.A., Hasen, J., Oppenheimer, J.H.: Hepatic accumulation of ^{125}I-thyroxine in the rat: Augmentation by phenobarbital and chlordane. Endocrinology **82**, 406—409 (1968).

Berquist, P.L., Matthews, R.E.F.: Distribution of methylated purines in cell fractions from mouse liver and tumor. Biochim. biophys. Acta (Amst.) **34**, 567—569 (1959).

Bitman, J., Cecil, H.C., Harris, S.J., Fries, G.F.: Estrogenic activity of o,p'-DDT in the mammalian uterus and avian oviduct. Science **162**, 371—372 (1968).

Bledsoe, T., Island, D.P., Ney, R.L., Liddle, G.W.: An effect of o,p'-DDD on the extra-adrenal metabolism of cortisol in man. J. clin. Endocr. **24**, 1303—1311 (1964).

Bloch, K.: The biological synthesis of cholesterol. Science **150**, 19—28 (1965).

Boggs, T.R., Hardy, J.B., Frazier, T.M.: Correlation of neonatal serum total bilirubin concentrations and developmental status at age eight months. A preliminary report from the collaborative project. J. Pediat. **71**, 553—560 (1967).

Boyd, G.S., Scholan, N.A., Mitton, J.R.: Factors influencing cholesterol 7*a*-hydroxylase activity in the rat liver. Plenum Press, New York. Ed. by W.L. Holmes, L.A. Carlson and R. Paoletti. Advanc. exp. Med. Biol. **4**, 443—456 (1969).

Burstein, S., Bhavnani, B.R.: Effect of phenobarbital administration on the *in vitro* hydroxylation of cortisol and on over-all substrate and product metabolism in the guinea pig and rat. Endocrinology **80**, 351—356 (1967).

— Klaiber, E.L.: Phenobarbital-induced increases in 6*β*-hydroxycortisol excretion: Clue to its significance in human urine. J. clin. Endocr. **25**, 293—296 (1965).

Catz, C., Yaffe, S.J.: Pharmacological modification of bilirubin conjugation in the newborn. Amer. J. Dis. Child. **104**, 516—517 (1962).

— — Barbiturate enhancement of bilirubin conjugation and excretion in young and adult animals. Pediat. Res. **2**, 361—370 (1968).

Coburn, R.F.: Effect of phenobarbital on endogenous carbon monoxide production in normal man. J. clin. Invest. **46**, 1046 (1967).

Colas, A.: The 16*a*-hydroxylation of dehydroepiandrosterone (3*β*-hydroxyandrost-5-en-17-one) by rat liver slices. Biochem. J. **82**, 390—394 (1962).

Conney, A.H.: Pharmacological implications of microsomal enzyme induction. Pharmacol. Rev. **19**, 317—366 (1967).

— Burns, J.J.: Factors influencing drug metabolism. Advanc. Pharmacol. **1**, 31—58 (1962).

— Davison, C., Gastel, R., Burns, J.J.: Adaptive increases in drug-metabolizing enzymes induced by phenobarbital and other drugs. J. Pharmacol. exp. Ther. **130**, 1—8 (1960).

— Gillette, J.R., Inscoe, J.K., Trams, E.C., Posner, H.S.: 3,4-Benzpyrene-induced synthesis of liver microsomal enzymes which metabolize foreign compounds. Science **130**, 1478—1479 (1959).

— Jacobson, M., Levin, W., Schneidman, K., Kuntzman, R.: Decreased central depressant effect of progesterone and other steroids in rats pretreated with drugs and insecticides. J. Pharmacol. exp. Ther. **154**, 310—318 (1966).

— — Schneidman, K., Kuntzman, R.: Induction of liver microsomal cortisol 6*β*-hydroxylase by diphenylhydantoin or phenobarbital. An explanation for the increased excretion of 6-hydroxycortisol in humans treated with these drugs. Life Sci. **4**, 1091—1098 (1965).

— Klutch, A.: Increased activity of androgen hydroxylases in liver microsomes of rats pretreated with phenobarbital and other drugs. J. biol. Chem. **238**, 1611—1617 (1963).

— Levin, W., Ikeda, M., Kuntzman, R., Cooper, D.Y., Rosenthal, O.: Inhibitory effect of carbon monoxide on the hydroxylation of testosterone by rat liver microsomes. J. biol. Chem. **243**, 3912—3915 (1968).

CONNEY, A.H., LEVIN, W., JACOBSON, M., KUNTZMAN, R., COOPER, D.Y., ROSENTHAL, O.: Specificity in the regulation of the 6β-, 7α- and 16α-hydroxylation of testosterone by rat liver microsomes, pp. 279—295. "Microsomes and Drug Oxidations" Academic Press (1969).
— SCHNEIDMAN, K.: Enhanced androgen hydroxylase activity in liver microsomes of rats and dogs treated with phenylbutazone. J. Pharmacol. exp. Ther. **146**, 225—235 (1964).
COOPER, D.Y., LEVINE, S., NARASIMHULU, S., ROSENTHAL, O., ESTABROOK, R.W.: Photochemical action spectrum of the terminal oxidase of mixed function oxidase systems. Science **147**, 400—402 (1965).
CRAM, R.L., JUCHAU, M.R., FOUTS, J.R.: Differences in hepatic drug metabolism in various rabbit strains before and after pretreatment with phenobarbital. Proc. Soc. exp. Biol. (N.Y.) **118**, 872—875 (1965).
CREAVEN, P.J., PARKE, D.V.: The stimulation of hydroxylation by carcinogenic and non-carcinogenic compounds. Biochem. Pharmacol. **15**, 7—16 (1966).
CRIGLER, J.F., JR., GOLD, N.I.: Sodium phenobarbital-induced decrease in serum bilirubin in an infant with congenital nonhemolytic jaundice and kernicterus. J. clin. Invest. **45**, 998—999 (1966).
— — Effect of sodium phenobarbital on bilirubin metabolism in an infant with congenital, nonhemolytic unconjugated hyperbilirubinemia and kernicterus. J. clin. Invest. **48**, 42—55 (1969).
DANIELSSON, H., EINARSSON, K.: On the conversion of cholesterol to 7α-, 12α-dihydroxychol-est-4-en-3-one. Bile acids and steroids 168. J. biol. Chem. **241**, 1449—1454 (1966).
DANIELSSON, H., TCHEN, T.T.: Steroid metabolism. In: Metabolic Pathways, pp. 117—168. Ed. by D.M. GREENBERG. New York: Academic Press 1968.
DAS, M.L., ORRENIUS, S., ERNSTER, L.: On the fatty acid and hydrocarbon hydroxylation in rat liver microsomes. Eur. J. Biochem. **4**, 519—523 (1968).
DE CASTRO, R.T., PRICE, J.M., BROWN, R.R.: Reduced triphosphopyridine nucleotide requirement for the enzymatic formation of 3-hydroxykynurenine from L-kynurenine. J. Amer. chem. Soc. **78**, 2904—2905 (1956).
DE LEON, A., GARTER, L.M., ARIAS, I.M.: The effect of phenobarbital on hyperbilirubinemia in glucuronyl transferase deficient rats. J. Lab. clin. Med. **70**, 273—278 (1967).
DUNN, D.B.: Additional components in ribonucleic acid of rat liver fractions. Biochim. biophys. Acta (Amst.) **34**, 286—288 (1959).
DUTTON, D.J.: (ed): Glucuronic acid. New York: Academic Press 1966.
EINARSSON, K., JOHANSSON, G.: Effect of phenobarbital on the conversion of cholesterol to taurocholic acid. Bile acids and steroids 204. Eur. J. Biochem. **6**, 293—298 (1968).
— — Effect of carbon monoxide and phenobarbital on hydroxylation of bile acids by rat liver microsomes. FEBS Letters **4**, 177—180 (1969).
ERTEL, I.J., NEWTON, W.A., JR.: Therapy in congenital hyperbilirubinemia: Phenobarbital and diethylnicotinamide. Pediatrics **44**, 43—48 (1969).
FAHIM, M.S., KING, R.M., HALL, D.G.: Induced alterations in the biologic activity of estrogen. Amer. J. Obstet. Gynec. **100**, 171—175 (1968a).
— KING, T.M.: Effect of phenobarbital on lactation and the nursing neonate. Amer. J. Obstet. Gynec. **101**, 1103—1108 (1968).
GAYLOR, J.L., MASON, H.S.: Investigation of the component fractions of oxidative sterol demethylation. J. biol. Chem. **243**, 4966—4972 (1968).
GILLETTE, J.R.: Metabolism of drugs and other compounds by enzymatic mechanisms. Progr. Drug Res. **6**, 11—73 (1963).
— Biochemistry of drug oxidation and reduction by enzymes in hepatic endoplasmic reticulum. Advanc. Pharmacol. **4**, 219—261 (1966).
GOLDSTEIN, J.A., TAUROG, A.: Enhanced biliary excretion of thyroxine glucuronide in rats pretreated with benzpyrene. Biochem. Pharmacol. **17**, 1049—1065 (1968).
HAGINO, N., RAMALEY, J.A., GORSKI, R.A.: Inhibition of estrogen-induced precocious ovulation by pentobarbital in the rat. Endocrinology **79**, 451—454 (1966).
HARBISON, R.D., SPRATT, J.L.: Novobiocin-induced hyperbilirubinemia and its reduction by phenobarbital pretreatment. Toxicol. appl. Pharmacol. **11**, 257—263 (1967).
HART, L.G., ADAMSON, R.H., DIXON, R.L., FOUTS, J.R.: Stimulation of hepatic microsomal drug metabolism in the newborn and fetal rabbit. J. Pharmacol. exp. Ther. **137**, 103—106 (1962).
HEINRICHS, W.L., FEDER, H.H., COLAS, A.: The steroid 16α-hydroxylase system in mammalian liver. Steroids **7**, 91—98 (1966).
HERNANDEZ, P.H., MAZEL, P., GILLETTE, J.R.: Studies on the mechanism of action of mammalian hepatic azo reductase-II. The effects of phenobarbital and 3-methylcholanthrene on carbon monoxide sensitive and insensitive azo reductase activities. Biochem. Pharmacol. **16**, 1877—1888 (1967).

HILDEBRANDT, A., REMMER, H., ESTABROOK, R.W.: Cytochrome P-450 of liver microsomes — one pigment or many. Biochem. biophys. Res. Commun. **30**, 607—612 (1968).

HOLLOWAY, P.W., PELUFFO, R., WAKIL, S.J.: On the biosynthesis of dienoic fatty acid by animal tissues. Biochem. biophys. Res. Commun. **12**, 300—304 (1963).

ICHIHARA, K., KUSUNOSE, E., KUSUNOSE, M.: Some properties and distribution of the ω-hydroxylation system of medium-chain fatty acids. Biochim. biophys. Acta (Amst.) **176**, 704—712 (1969).

INSCOE, J.K., AXELROD, J.: Some factors affecting glucuronide formation *in vitro*. J. Pharmacol. exp. Ther. **129**, 128—131 (1960).

— DALY, J., AXELROD, J.: Factors affecting the enzymatic formation of o-methylated dihydroxy derivatives. Biochem. Pharmacol. **14**, 1257—1263 (1965).

JACCARINI, A., JEPSON, J.B.: Enzymic 6-hydroxylation of indolealkylamines and related compounds. Biochim. biophys. Acta (Amst.) **156**, 347—363 (1968).

JACOBSON, M., KUNTZMAN, R.: Studies on testosterone hydroxylation and pentobarbital oxidation by rat liver microsomes: Selective effect of age, sex, castration and testosterone propionate treatment. Steroids **13**, 327—341 (1969).

JEPSON, J.B., ZALTZMAN, P., UDENFRIEND, S.: Microsomal hydroxylation of tryptamine indoleacetic acid and related compounds to 6-hydroxy derivatives. Biochim. biophys. Acta (Amst.) **62**, 91—102 (1962).

JONES, A.L., ARMSTRONG, D.T.: Increased cholesterol biosynthesis following phenobarbital induced hypertrophy of agranular endoplasmic reticulum in liver. Proc. Soc. exp. Biol. (N.Y.) **119**, 1136—1139 (1965).

JONES, P.D., HOLLOWAY, P.W., PELUFFO, R.O., WAKIL, S.J.: A requirement for lipids by the microsomal stearyl coenzyme A desaturase. J. biol. Chem. **244**, 744—754 (1969).

KASHIWAMATA, S., NAKASHIMA, K., KOTAKE, Y.: Anthranilic acid hydroxylation by rabbit liver microsomes. Biochim. biophys. Acta (Amst.) **113**, 244—254 (1966).

KATO, R., GILLETTE, J.R.: Sex differences in the effects of abnormal physiological states on the metabolism of drugs by rat liver microsomes. J. Pharmacol. exp. Ther. **150**, 285—291 (1965).

— ONODA, K., OMORI, Y.: Effect of phenobarbital on biosynthesis and elimination of cholesterol in rats. Jap. J. Pharmacol. **18**, 514—515 (1968).

— TAKAHASHI, A., OMORI, Y.: Hydroxylation of steroid hormone by the liver microsomes of rats under pathological states. Life Sci. **7**, 915—920 (1968a).

KIDO, R., NOGUCHI, R., KASEDA, H., KAWAMOTO, M., MATSUMARA, Y.: Formation of 5-hydroxy-L-kynurenine from L-kynurenine by hen liver microsomes. Arch. Biochem. **125**, 1030—1031 (1968).

KJELDSEN, K.: Carboxyhaemoglobin and serum cholesterol levels in smokers correlated to the incidence of occlusive arterial disease. Abstracts of the Second International Symposium on Atherosclerosis (Chicago), 1969, p 30.

KOPIN, I.J., PARE, C.M.B., AXELROD J., WEISSBACH, H.: The fate of melatonin in animals. J. biol. Chem. **236**, 3072—3075 (1961).

KREEK, M.J., SLEISENGER, M.H.: Reduction of serum-unconjugated bilirubin with phenobarbitone in adult congenital nonhemolytic unconjugated hyperbilirubinemia. Lancet **1968 II**, 73—77.

KUNTZMAN, R., JACOBSON, M., CONNEY, A.H.: Effect of phenylbutazone on cortisol metabolism in man. Pharmacologist **8**, 195 (1966).

— — LEVIN, W., CONNEY, A.H.: Stimulatory effect of N-phenylbarbital (phetharbital) on cortisol hydroxylation in man. Biochem. Pharmacol. **17**, 565—571 (1968).

— — SCHNEIDMAN, K., CONNEY, A.H.: Similarities between oxidative drug-metabolizing enzymes and steroid hydroxylases in liver microsomes. J. Pharmacol. exp. Ther. **146**, 280—285 (1964).

— LAWRENCE, D., CONNEY, A.H.: Michaelis constants for the hydroxylation of steroid hormones and drugs by rat liver microsomes. Mol. Pharmacol. **1**, 163—167 (1965).

— LEVIN, W., JACOBSON, M., CONNEY, A.H.: Studies on microsomal hydroxylation and the demonstration of a new CO-binding pigment in liver microsomes. Life Sci. **7**, 215—224 (1968a).

— SANSUR, M., CONNEY, A.H.: Effect of drugs and insecticides on the anesthetic action of steroids. Endocrinology **77**, 952—954 (1965a).

— SOUTHREN, A.L.: The effects of CNS active drugs on the metabolism of steroids in man. Adv. Biochem. Psychopharm. **1**, 206—217 (1969).

— WELCH, R., CONNEY, A.H.: Factors influencing steroid hydroxylases in liver microsomes. In: Adv. Enzyme Reg. **4**, 149—160 (1966a). Ed. by WEBER, G. New York: MacMillan.

KUPFER, D., PEETS, L.: The effect of o,p'-DDD on cortisol and hexobarbital metabolism. Biochem. Pharmacol. **15**, 573—581 (1966).

LEMBERGER, L., KUNTZMAN, R., CONNEY, A.H., BURNS, J.J.: Metabolism of tyramine to dopamine by liver microsomes. J. Pharmacol. exp. Ther. **150**, 292—297 (1965).
LEVIN, W., ALVARES, A.P., JACOBSON, M., KUNTZMAN, R.: Effect of storage of frozen liver microsomal preparations on the hydroxylation of testosterone and pentobarbital and the N-demethylation of ethylmorphine. Biochem. Pharmacol. **18**, 883—889 (1969a).
— WELCH, R.M., CONNEY, A.H.: Effect of chronic phenobarbital treatment On the liver microsomal metabolism and uterotropic action of 17β-estradiol. Endocrinology **80**, 135—140 (1967).
— — — Effect of phenobarbital and other drugs on the metabolism and uterotropic action of estradiol-17β and estrone. J. Pharmacol. exp. Ther. **159**, 362—371 (1968).
— — — Decreased uterotropic potency of oral contraceptives in rats pretreated with phenobarbital. Endocrinology **83**, 149—156 (1968a).
— — — Estrogenic action of DDT and its analogs. Fed. Proc. **27**, 649 (1968b).
— — — Inhibitory effect of phenobarbital or chlordane pretreatment on the androgen-induced increase in seminal vesicle weight in the rat. Steroids **13**, 155—161 (1969).
— — — Effect of carbon tetrachloride and other inhibitors of drug metabolism on the metabolism and action of estradiol-17β and estrone in the rat. J. Pharmacol. exp. Ther. **173**, 247—255 (1970).
— — — Unpublished observations (1970a).
LEYBOLD, K., STAUDINGER, HJ.: Geschlechtsunterschiede im Steroidstoffwechsel von Rattenlebermikrosomen. Biochem. Z. **331**, 389—398 (1959).
LU, A.Y.H., COON, M.J.: Role of hemoprotein P-450 in fatty acid ω-hydroxylation in a soluble enzyme system from liver microsomes. J. biol. Chem. **243**, 1331—1332 (1968).
— JUNK, K.W., COON, M.J.: Resolution of the cytochrome P-450-containing ω-hydroxylation system of liver microsomes into three components. J. biol. Chem. **244**, 3714—3721 (1969).
— STROBEL, H.W., COON, M.J.: Hydroxylation of benzamphetamine and other drugs by a solubilized form of cytochrome P-450 from liver microsomes: Lipid requirement for drug demethylation. Biochem. biophys. Res. Commun. **36**, 545—551 (1969a).
MARSH, J.B., JAMES, A.T.: The conversion of stearic to oleic acid by liver and yeast preparations. Biochim. biophys. Acta (Amst.) **60**, 320—328 (1962).
MAURER, H.M., WOLFF, J.A., FINSTER, M., POPPERS, P., PANTUCK, E., KUNTZMAN, R., CONNEY, A.H.: Reduction in concentration of total serum bilirubin in offspring of women treated with phenobarbitone during pregnancy. Lancet **II**, 122—124 (1968).
MAZEL, P., HENDERSON, J.F., AXELROD, J.: S-Demethylation by microsomal enzymes. J. Pharmacol. exp. Ther. **143**, 1—6 (1964).
— KERZA-KWIATECKI, A., SIMANIS, J.: Studies on the demethylation of puromycin and related compounds by liver microsomal enzymes. Biochim. biophys. Acta (Amst.) **114**, 72—82 (1966).
MIDDLETON, W.R.J., ISSELBACHER, K.J.: The stimulation of intestinal cholesterogenesis in the rat by phenobarbital. Proc. Soc. exp. Biol. (N.Y.) **131**, 1435—1437 (1969).
MILLER, W.L., KALAFER, M.E., GAYLOR, J.L., DELWICH, C.V.: Investigation of the component reactions of oxidative sterol demethylation. Study of the aerobic and anaerobic processes. Biochemistry **6**, 2673—2678 (1967).
MITOMA, C., YASUDA, D., TAGG, J.S., NEUBAUER, S.E., CALDERONI, F.J., TANABE, M.: Effects of various chemical agents on drug metabolism and cholesterol biosynthesis. Biochem. Pharmacol. **17**, 1377—1383 (1968).
MOSBACH, E.H.: Drugs affecting lipid metabolism. In: Effect of drugs on bile acid metabolism, vol. 4, pp. 421—442. Ed. by W.L. HOLMES, L.A. CARLSON and R. PAOLETTI 1969. New York: Plenum Press.
MUELLER, G.C., RUMNEY, G.: Formation of 6β-hydroxy and 6-keto derivatives of estradiol-16-C^{14} by mouse liver microsomes. J. Amer. chem. Soc. **79**, 1004—1005 (1957).
NEWMAN, W.C., MOON, R.C.: Altered thyroxine metabolism resulting from the chemical carcinogen 3-methylcholanthrene. Endocrinology **80**, 896—900 (1967).
OMURA, T., SATO, R., COOPER, D.Y., ROSENTHAL, O., ESTABROOK, R.W.: Function of cytochrome P-450 of microsomes. Fed. Proc. **24**, 1181—1189 (1965).
OPPENHEIMER, J.H., BERNSTEIN, G., SURKS, M.I.: Increased thyroxine turnover and thyroidal function after stimulation of hepatocellular binding of thyroxine by phenobarbital. J. clin. Invest. **47**, 1399—1406 (1968).
ORRENIUS, S., THOR, H.: Fatty acid interaction with the hydroxylating enzyme system of rat liver microsomes. Eur. J. Biochem. **9**, 415—418 (1969).
OSHINO, N., IMAI, Y., SATO, R.: Electron-transfer mechanism associated with fatty acid desaturation catalyzed by liver microsomes. Biochim. biophys. Acta (Amst.) **128**, 13—28 (1966).

PEAKALL, D.B.: Pesticide-induced enzyme breakdown of steroids in birds. Nature (Lond.) **216**, 505—506 (1967).
POLAND, A., KUNTZMAN, R., JACOBSON, M., SMITH, D., CONNEY, A.H.: Clin. Pharmacol. Ther. (in press) (1970).
PREISS, B., BLOCH, K.: Omega-oxidation of long chain fatty acids in rat liver. J. biol. Chem. **239**, 85—88 (1964).
RAMBOER, C., THOMPSON, R.P.H., WILLIAMS, R.: Controlled trials of phenobarbitone therapy in neonatal jaundice. Lancet **I**, 966—968 (1969).
REMMER, H., MERKER, H.J.: Drug-induced changes in the liver endoplasmic reticulum: Association with drug-metabolizing enzymes. Science **142**, 1657—1658 (1963).
— — Effect of drugs on the formation of smooth endoplasmic reticulum and drug-metabolizing enzymes. Ann. N.Y. Acad. Sci. **123**, 79—97 (1965).
ROBBINS, K.C.: *In vitro* enzymic omega oxidation of medium-chain fatty acids in mammalian tissue. Biochem. Biophys. **123**, 531—538 (1968).
ROBERTS, R.J., PLAA, G.L.: Effect of phenobarbital on the excretion of an exogenous bilirubin load. Biochem. Pharmacol. **16**, 827—835 (1967).
ROBINSON, S.H.: Increased bilirubin conjugation in heterozygous Gunn rats treated with phenobarbital. Nature (Lond.) **222**, 990—991 (1969).
SAITO, Y., HAYAISHI, O., ROTHBERG, S.: Studies on oxygenases; Enzymatic formation of 3-hydroxy-L-kynurenine from L-kynurenine. J. biol. Chem. **229**, 921—934 (1957).
SALVADOR, R.A., ATKINS, C., HABER, S., KOZMA, C., CONNEY, A.H.: Changes in the serum concentration of cholesterol, triglycerides and phospholipids in the mouse and rat administered either chlorcyclizine or phenobarbital. Biochem. Pharmacol. **19**, 1463—1469 (1970).
— — — — — Effect of phenobarbital and chlorcyclizine on the development of atheromatosis in the cholesterol-fed rabbit. Biochem. Pharmacol. **19**, 1975—1981 (1970).
— CONNEY, A.H., KOZMA, C.: Inhibitory effect of phenobarbital on cholesterol-induced atherosclerosis in the rabbit. Pharmacologist. **9**, 254 (1967).
SCHMID, R., MARVER, H.S., HAMMAKER, L.: Enhanced formation of rapidly labeled bilirubin by phenobarbital: Hepatic microsomal cytochromes as a possible source. Biochem. biophys. Res. Commun. **24**, 319—328 (1966).
SCHWARTZ, H.L., KOSYREFF, V., SURKS, M.I., OPPENHEIMER, J.H.: Increased deiodination of L-thyroxine and L-triiodothyronine by liver microsomes from rats treated with phenobarbital. Nature (Lond.) **221**, 1262—1263 (1969).
SERENI, F., PERLETTI, L., MARINI, A.: Influence of diethylnicotinamide on the concentration of serum bilirubin of newborn infants. Pediatrics **40**, 446—449 (1967).
SHEFER, S., HAUSER, S., MOSBACH, E.: 7α-Hydroxylation of cholestanol by rat liver microsomes. J. Lipid Res. **9**, 328—333 (1968).
SINGHAL, R.L., VALADARES, J.R.E., LING, G.M.: Influence of chronic phenobarbitone treatment on uterine phosphofructokinase induction. J. Pharm. Pharmacol. **19**, 545—547 (1967).
SLADEK, N.E., MANNERING, G.J.: Evidence for a new P-450 hemoprotein in hepatic microsomes from methylcholanthrene-treated rats. Biochem. biophys. Res. Commun. **24**, 668—674 (1966).
SOUTHREN, A.L., GORDON, G.G., TOCHIMOTO, S., KRIKUN, E., KRIEGER, D.: Effect of N-phenylbarbital (phetharbital) on the metabolism of testosterone and cortisol in man. J. clin. Endocr. **29**, 251—256 (1969).
— TOCHIMOTO, S., STROM, L., RATUSCHNI, A., ROSS, H., GORDON, G.: Remission in Cushing's syndrome with o,p'-DDD. J. clin. Endocr. **26**, 268—278 (1966).
STANBURY, J.B., MORRIS, M.L., CORRIGAN, H.J., LASSITER, W.E.: Thyroxine deiodination by a microsomal preparation requiring Fe^{++}, oxygen and cysteine or glutathione. Endocrinology **67**, 353—362 (1960).
STOFFEL, W.: Biosynthesis of polyenoic fatty acids. Biochem. biophys. Res. Commun. **6**, 270—273 (1961).
SUZUKI, M., MITROPOULOS, K.A., MYANT, N.B.: The electron transport mechanism associated with 12α-hydroxylation of C_{27} steroids. Biochem. biophys. Res. Commun. **30**, 516—521 (1968).
TENHUNEN, R., MARVER, H.S., SCHMID, R.: The enzymatic conversion of heme to bilirubin by microsomal heme oxygenase. Proc. nat. Acad. Sci. (Wash.) **61**, 748—755 (1968).
— — — Microsomal heme oxygenase: Characterization of the enzyme. J. biol. Chem. **244**, 6388—6394 (1969).
— ROSS, M.E., MARVER, H.S., SCHMID, R.: NADPH-Dependent biliverdin reductase: Partial purification and characterization. Biochemistry **9**, 298—303 (1970).
TEPHLY, T.R., MANNERING, G.J.: Inhibition of drug metabolism. V. Inhibition of drug metabolism by steroids. Mol. Pharmacol. **4**, 10—14 (1968).

THOMPSON, R.P.H., EDDLESTON, A.L.W.F., WILLIAMS, R.: Low plasma-bilirubin in epileptics on phenobarbitone. Lancet **I**, 21—22 (1969).
— PILCHER, C.W.T., ROBINSON, J., STATHERS, G.M., MCLEAN, A.E.M., WILLIAMS, R.: Treatment of unconjugated jaundice with dicophane. Lancet **II**, 4—6 (1969a).
— WILLIAMS, R.: Treatment of chronic intrahepatic cholestasis with phenobarbitone. Lancet **II**, 646—648 (1967).
TROLLE, D.: Phenobarbitone and neonatal icterus. Lancet **I**, 251—252 (1968).
— Decrease of total serum bilirubin concentration in newborn infants, after phenobarbitone treatment. Lancet **II**, 705—708 (1968a).
VOIGT, W., HSIA, S.L., COOPER, D.Y., ROSENTHAL, O.: Photoreactivation spectrum of the CO-inhibited taurochenodeoxycholate 6β-hydroxylase system. FEBS Letters **2**, 124—126 (1968a).
— THOMAS, P.J., HSIA, S.L.: Enzymic studies of bile acid metabolism. I. 6β-Hydroxylation of chenodeoxycholic and taurochenodeoxycholic acids by microsomal preparations of rat liver. J. biol. Chem. **243**, 3493—3499 (1968).
WADA, F., HIRATA, K., SAKAMOTO, Y.: Relation of cholesterol synthesis and NADPH oxidation by microsomal electron transport system involving P-450. Biochim. biophys. Acta (Amst.) **143**, 273—275 (1967).
— — — Possible participation of cytochrome P-450 in cholesterol synthesis. J. Biochem. (Tokyo) **65**, 171—175 (1969).
— KAZUYA, H., KASUYASU, N., SAKAMOTO, Y.: Participation of P-450 in 7α-hydroxylation of cholesterol. J. Biochem. (Tokyo) **64**, 415—417 (1968).
— SHIBATA, H., GOTO, M., SAKAMOTO, Y.: Participation of the microsomal electron transport system involving cytochrome P-450 in ω-oxidation of fatty acids. Biochim. biophys. Acta (Amst.) **162**, 518—524 (1968a).
WADA, O., TOYOKAWA, K., URATA, G., YANO, Y., NAKAO, K.: Cholesterol biosynthesis in the liver of experimentally induced porphyric mice. Biochem. Pharmacol. **18**, 1533—1535 (1969a).
WAKABAYASHI, K., SHIMAZONO, N.: Studies on omega-oxidation of fatty acids *in vitro*. I. Overall reaction and intermediate. Biochim. biophys. Acta (Amst.) **70**, 132—142 (1963).
WELCH, R.M., LEVIN, W., CONNEY, A.H.: Insecticide inhibition and stimulation of steroid hydroxylases in rat liver. J. Pharmacol. exp. Ther. **155**, 167—173 (1967).
— — — Stimulatory effect of phenobarbital on the metabolism *in vivo* of estradiol-17β and estrone in the rat. J. Pharmacol. exp. Ther. **160**, 171—178 (1968).
— — — Estrogenic action of DDT and its analogs. Toxicol. appl. Pharmacol. **14**, 358—367 (1969).
— — — Unpublished observations (1970).
WERK, E.E., JR., MACGEE, J., SHOLITON, L.J.: Effect of diphenylhydantoin on cortisol metabolism in man. J. clin. Invest. **43**, 1824—1835 (1964).
— SHOLITON, L.J., OLINGER, C.P.: Amelioration of nontumorous Cushing's syndrome by diphenylhydantoin. International Congress on Hormonal Steroids, 2nd, Milan, (1966) p. 301 (Excerpta Medica Fndn. New York).
WHELTON, M.J., KRUSTEV, L.P., BILLING, B.H.: Reduction of serum bilirubin by phenobarbital in adult unconjugated hyperbilirubinemia. Is enzyme induction responsible ? Amer. J. Med. **45**, 160—164 (1968).
WHITEHOUSE, M.W.: Drugs, hormones and other factors influencing steroid and sterol metabolism. In: Lipid Pharmacology, pp. 185—273. Ed. by R. PAOLETTI. New York: Academic Press 1964.
WURTMAN, R.J., AXELROD, J., ANTON-TAY, F.: Inhibition of the metabolism of H^3-melatonin by phenothiazines. J. Pharmacol. exp. Ther. **161**, 367—372 (1968).
WYNN, J., GIBBS, R., ROYSTER, B.: Thyroxine degradation. I. Study of optimal reaction conditions of a rat liver thyroxine-degrading system. J. biol. Chem. **237**, 1892—1897 (1962).
YAFFE, S.J., LEVY, G., MATSUZAWA, T., BALIAH, T.: Enhancement of glucuronide conjugating capacity in a hyperbilirubinemic infant due to apparent enzyme induction by phenobarbital. New Engl. J. Med. **275**, 1461—1466 (1966).
YATES, F.R., HERBST, A.L., URQUHART, J.: Sex differences in rate of ring A reduction of Δ^4-3-keto-steroids *in vitro* by rat liver. Endocrinology **63**, 887—902 (1958).

Chapter 47

Tissue Distribution Studies of Polycyclic Hydrocarbon Hydroxylase Activity

LEE W. WATTENBERG and J. LIONEL LEONG

I. Introduction

The vast majority of studies of microsomal drug metabolizing systems have been devoted to the liver. There are a number of reasons for this focus of attention. The liver has traditionally been thought of as the principal organ of drug metabolism and, in fact, the microsomal drug metabolizing enzymes have a high activity in this organ. In addition, it is technically advantageous to work with liver because of its size, accessibility, and the large number of methods which have been worked out for enzyme studies in hepatic tissue. However, an accumulating body of knowledge indicates that drug metabolizing systems occur in a wide variety of other tissues (WATTENBERG and LEONG, 1962; WATTENBERG et al., 1962; GELBOIN and BLACKBURN, 1964; JELLINCK and GOUDY, 1967; WATTENBERG, 1969). For demonstrating the full range of tissue distribution of these enzymes, the benzpyrene hydroxylase system has been of considerable importance (CONNEY et al., 1957). Two aspects of this enzyme system are particularly favorable for distribution studies. The first is that a highly sensitive fluorometric technique is available for the quantitative determination of benzpyrene hydroxylase activity (WATTENBERG et al., 1962; WATTENBERG and LEONG, 1965). The second is that there is a morphologic histochemical procedure for demonstrating the localization of this enzyme system in tissue sections (WATTENBERG and LEONG, 1962). Since the histochemical demonstration of the benzpyrene hydroxylase system and other closely related polycyclic hydrocarbon hydroxylases represents a somewhat unique feature not available for other NADPH dependent drug metabolizing systems, studies employing this technique will be discussed initially. This will be followed by a presentation of tissue distribution studies employing the quantitative procedure for determining benzpyrene hydroxylase activity.

II. Histochemical Studies of Polycyclic Hydrocarbon Hydroxylase Systems

While it is evident that tissues are not composed of homogeneous cell populations, the fact that cells of the same general type may show considerable differences in enzyme activity is sometimes not appreciated. In the liver this is true for cells located in different parts of the hepatic lobule. This type of heterogeneity has been demonstrated histochemically for several enzyme systems (CHIQUONE, 1953; SCHUMACHER, 1957), and is also the case for polycyclic hydrocarbon hydroxylases in liver. Histochemical studies of the benzpyrene hydroxylase system in liver of normal rat, mouse, hamster, and monkey show demonstrable activity only in the hepatic cells of the central portion of the hepatic lobule and not in the peripheral portion. While it is quite possible that in the peripheral cells of the liver a weak activity exists which is below the sensitivity of the histochemical procedure, there is unquestionably a marked difference in the activity of the two areas. In addition, WATTENBERG and LEONG (1962) have demonstrated a similar distribution in liver of enzymes which metabolize perylene, 1,2-benzanthracene and 7,12-dimethylbenz(a)anthracene. When the distribution of polycyclic hydrocarbon hydroxylase activity is studied in rats that have received microsomal enzyme inducers such as 1,2-benzanthracene, the activity increases very markedly and is observed in all cells in the hepatic lobule.

Before proceeding further, it might be well to describe briefly the histochemical technique for demonstrating benzpyrene hydroxylase and other polycyclic hydrocarbon hydroxylase systems (WATTENBERG and LEONG, 1962). The basic procedure is quite simple. Small blocks of the tissue to be studied are frozen, and sections cut in a cryostat. The sections are dried, extracted with cold acetone, and coated with a thin layer of benzpyrene or other polycyclic hydrocarbon substrate. The tissue sections thus coated are incubated in a reaction mixture containing NADPH, NADH, and the other constituents conventionally employed for benzpyrene hydroxylase determinations. Following incubation, the tissue sections are studied by fluorescence microscopy. In general, the fluorescence spectra of the hydroxy derivatives is sufficiently close to that of the substrate so as to make interpretation difficult by microscopy when sections are mounted in neutral media. The one exception to this is perylene which will be discussed below. In the earliest work with the histochemical procedure, prolonged incubations were employed in order to allow the conversion of hydroxy derivatives to nonfluorescent quinones. Under these conditions, a loss of fluorescence was used as a method of localizing the enzyme activity. This technique is relatively insensitive, and has been replaced by a procedure in which the tissue sections are mounted in an alkaline medium after incubation. This converts the hydroxy derivatives to phenolates, which have markedly different fluorescence spectra from the unaltered substrates. In general, the most satisfactory substrate from the standpoint of technical considerations is benzo(a)pyrene. As indicated above, perylene has somewhat different properties from the other substrates that have been employed since its fluorescent metabolite(s) have considerably different fluorescence spectra from perylene itself. While the spectral differences between substrate and reaction product(s) are favorable for histochemical work, the relatively weak capacity of perylene to bind to cytoplasmic protein results in a final fluorescence which is less intense than that obtained with benzpyrene. With present procedures, this substrate cannot be used effectively with tissues which have very low hydroxylase activity.

The histochemical procedure is basically quite simple, but the technique for obtaining a uniform coating of the section with the polycyclic hydrocarbon substrate requires some practice. After completion of the incubation, the sections generally are mounted in an alkaline medium in order to obtain the marked shift in fluorescence of the hydroxy metabolites as compared to the unaltered substrates. Under these conditions there is a progressive disappearence of the phenolates from their sites of deposition which makes it necessary to examine the sections and perform any photography within a brief period. Although the histochemical procedure is satisfactory for many purposes, it is inadequate for localizing sites of very weak activity. The quantitative procedure has proved to be more sensitive than the histochemical one.

In addition to liver, the histochemical technique for demonstrating benzpyrene hydroxylase and other polycyclic hydrocarbon hydroxylases has been applied to a number of other tissues in normal animals and in animals which have received enzyme inducers of increased polycyclic hydrocarbon hydroxylase activity such as 1,2 benzanthracene, phenothiazines, and also a number of flavones, in particular, beta-naphthoflavone. The most extensive of these investigations have been carried out in female Sprague Dawley rats of about 7 weeks of age, and unless otherwise indicated, the distribution patterns cited refer to these animals.

Histochemical Studies of Polycyclic Hydrocarbon Hydroxylase Activity in Tissues of Major Portals of Entry. Polycyclic hydrocarbon hydroxylase activity is present in the tissues of all major portals of entry. It is found throughout the entire gastrointestinal tract, but varies quite markedly from one region to another. The greatest activity is found in the proximal portion of the small intestine, where the level of activity is comparable to that of liver. The polycyclic hydrocarbon hydroxylase activity in the small intestine is located in the columnar cells covering the villi both in untreated animals and in animals fed various inducers, but the activity is considerably higher in the latter. The stomach of the rat has two parts, a forestomach lined by squamous epithelium and a glandular portion of the stomach lined by a glandular epithelium. In the forestomach, activity is found in the squamous epithelium of the mucosa. In the glandular stomach, it occurs in the epithelial cells of the surface and in a few cell layers in the adjacent superficial portion of the gastric glands. In the large intestine, activity is most intense in the columnar cells on the surface of the mucosa. A somewhat erratic activity is found in crypt cells.

A second portal of entry in which polycyclic hydrocarbon hydroxylase activity has been demonstrated is the lung. This is of particular interest since the lung represents the most important site of contact of the organism with airborn noxious agents. In lung, activity is demonstrable only in alveolar walls; it has not been detected in tracheal or bronchial mucosa. The precise identification of the specific cell type in the alveolar walls in which the enzyme activity occurs has not been made.

The skin is the third portal of entry in which histochemical studies of polycyclic hydrocarbon hydroxylase activity have been carried out (WATTENBERG, 1969). In normal Ha/ICR animals, the only structure in the skin which shows a positive reaction is the sebaceous glands. When an inducer such as beta-naphthoflavone is painted on the skin, hydroxylase activity increases in these glands and also becomes demonstrable in the surface epithelium and in the superficial portion of the hair follicle beginning at about the level of the entry of the sebaceous gland ducts. In mice in which the inducer has been given intraperitoneally, activity is found in the sebaceous glands and superficial portion of the hair follicles, but not in the surface epithelium.

Histochemical Studies of Polycyclic Hydrocarbon Hydroxylase Activity in Kidney and Adrenal Gland. Benzpyrene hydroxylase activity is found in the distal portion of the proximal convoluted tubules of the kidney in normal rats and in rats which have been given 1,2-benzanthracene. Benzpyrene hydroxylase activity is also demonstrable in the zona fasiculata and zona reticularis of the rat adrenal. No activity is demonstrable in the zona glomerulosa. Unlike other tissues which we have studied, no increase in activity has been found in the adrenal after administration of any of a large number of potent inducers of polycyclic hydrocarbon hydroxylase activity.

Comments on the Results Obtained with the Morphologic Histochemical Procedures for Demonstrating Polycyclic Hydrocarbon Hydroxylase Activity. It is evident from the histochemical studies that there is a marked heterogeneity of the activity in cells of all tissues in which polycyclic hydrocarbon hydroxylase activity has been found. The precise sites of localization would appear to have important functional implications. In some instances these seem evident, but in others they are less clear. Thus, the localization of relatively high levels of activity in the epithelium covering the villi of the small intestine would facilitate contact with potential substrates that are ingested. Similar considerations would hold for localization in surface epithelium of other portions of the gastrointestinal tract. In contrast, the centrilobular localization in normal liver is somewhat puzzling since this would leave the peripheral portion of the hepatic lobule relatively unprotected from the toxic effects of compounds which are detoxified by these systems.

The selective localization of polycyclic hydrocarbon hydroxylase activity in the sebaceous glands of the skin has interesting implications. Physiological or pathological alterations in the state of these glands would presumably change the capacity of the skin to be damaged or otherwise affected by compounds which these enzymes metabolize. Thus, a pathological process which inactivates these enzymes in the sebaceous glands could ultimately result in extensive damage to the entire skin.

A point which is suggested by the histochemical studies is that induction of increased polycyclic hydrocarbon hydroxylase activity may involve two perhaps distinct types of phenomena. The first is the induction of increased activity in cells which have readily demonstrable activity in control animals. The second is induction in cells in which there normally is either a very low activity, i. e. beneath the sensitivity of the histochemical procedure, or possibly even no activity. This second catagory would include cells such as those in the peripheral portion of the hepatic lobule and the surface epithelium of the skin. These sites are negative in control animals, but show an intense reaction following administration of inducers. These cells may simply be responding to inducers in the same way as those in the first category, but it is possible that an additional activation mechanism is involved which converts these non-reactive or weakly reactive cells to a form which responds readily to inducers. If such an activation mechanism does exist, then presumably some inducers could have activation properties as well as inductive ones, others simply the latter capacity (the overall effect on an organ as a whole would then be a weaker induction), and a third category of compound might exist which has an activation capacity but does not induce. With the combined use of morphologic histochemical and quantitative procedures, it is probable that these speculations can be tested experimentally.

III. Quantitative Studies of Polycyclic Hydrocarbon Hydroxylase Systems

Female Sprague Dawley rats of about 7 weeks of age have been used for most of the following studies and unless otherwise specified, the description refers to these animals. Benzpyrene hydroxylase has been the enzyme system studied most thoroughly and has been determined by the technique of WATTENBERG and LEONG (1965) or modification of this technique such as that of GELBOIN and BLACKBURN (1964), and KUNTZMAN et al. (1966).

Polycyclic Hydrocarbon Hydroxylase Activity in Tissues of Major Portals of Entry. Quantitative studies of benzpyrene hydroxylase activity have been carried out in tissues of the gastrointestinal tract, lung and skin. The highest activity in the gastrointestinal tract occurs in the proximal portion of the small intestine. The level of activity at this site is similar to that of liver. There is a gradient of activity in the small intestine in which activity decreases as the ileocecal junction is approached (WATTENBERG et al., 1962). After inducers are fed to the animals, benzpyrene hydroxylase activity increases throughout the entire length of the small intestine, but the activity in the proximal portion is still considerably higher than that in the distal portion. In the large bowel, the activities are lower than in the small intestine. However, as in the small intestine, a gradient of activity is found in which the hydroxylase activity progressively decreases from the proximal portion of the large intestine to the distal portion. Both the forestomach and glandular stomach show a low activity. Following the feeding of inducers, the activity increases in both portions of the stomach. In addition to rat, benzpyrene hydroxylase activity has also been found in the proximal portion of the small intestine of mouse, guinea pig, rabbit, hamster, dog, bull, monkey, baboon, and man (surgical specimens).

Studies of benzpyrene hydroxylase have been carried out in the skin, but up to the present little has been reported (CONNEY, 1967). Benzpyrene hydroxylase activity has been found in the skin of the mouse, rat, and hamster (WATTENBERG, 1969). An increase in this activity can be induced by painting the skin with inducers or by parenteral administration of these compounds. Topical application has proved to be a much more effective means of obtaining induction than parenteral administration.

Benzpyrene hydroxylase activity has been found in lung of the rat, mouse, hamster, rabbit, bull, and man (WATTENBERG et al., 1968a; WATTENBERG and LEONG, 1962; WATTENBERG, 1969). A second drug metabolizing system, aminoazo dye N-demethylase, has also been studied in the lung of the rat (GILMAN and CONNEY, 1963). The relationship between the chemical structure of a number of compounds and their ability to induce benzpyrene hydroxylase has been studied in various tissues including lung (WATTENBERG et al., 1968a; and WATTENBERG et al. 1968b). In a different type of investigation, it has been shown by SUNDERMAN (1967) that nickel carbonyl inhibits the induction of benzpyrene hydroxylase activity by phenothiazine in rat lung. Studies of the effects of a number of inducers on mouse lung have also been carried out as part of an investigation of the capacity of benzpyrene hydroxylase inducers to protect against the carcinogenic effects of polycyclic hydrocarbons (WATTENBERG and LEONG, 1968; WATTENBERG and LEONG, 1970). Benzpyrene hydroxylase activity in the lung has been studied in the hamster. The hamster lung is of particular interest in cancer research because squamous cell carcinomas histologically similar to those occurring in man can be produced in this species (SAFFIOTTI et al., 1968). The benzpyrene hydroxylase activity of the normal hamster lung is extremely low but can be increased by the administration of inducers, especially beta-naphthoflavone and polycyclic hydrocarbons. Investigations with human lung have been carried out only on surgically resected specimens from older individuals. Some specimens showed activity and others did not. Studies of benzpyrene hydroxylase activity have been performed on the tracheal mucosa of the rabbit and the bull; in both, a very weak activity was found (WATTENBERG, 1969).

Lymphoid Tissue. A low benzpyrene hydroxylase activity has been found in thymus, spleen and lymph nodes (axillary and mesenteric) of the rat. An increase in this activity was induced by beta-naphthoflavone (WATTENBERG, 1969).

Kidney and Adrenal. Benzpyrene hydroxylase activity is readily demonstrable in kidney and adrenal. The kidney is highly responsive to a number of inducers. In contrast, a wide variety of inducers have failed to have any effect on the activity of the benzpyrene hydroxylase system of the adrenal.

Placenta. A number of drug metabolizing enzyme systems have been found in the placenta. These include benzpyrene hydroxylase, aminoazo dye N-demethylase, azodye reductase, and zoxazolamine hydroxylase (WELCH et al., 1968; WELCH et al., 1969; VAN PETTEN et al., 1968; DIXON and WILLSON, 1968; and MIRKIN, 1970). The occurrence of polycyclic hydrocarbon hydroxylase activity in placenta is of considerable interest as a possible defense mechanism for protecting the fetus from polycyclic hydrocarbons which have reached the placenta in an unaltered form. Polycyclic hydrocarbon carcinogens which are very widespread environmental pollutants are capable of transplacental passage and thus represent a potential hazard to the conceptus *in utero*. The placenta is the last barrier to the exposure of fetal tissues to these compounds in an unaltered state. Very little is known about factors which might alter drug metabolizing enzyme activity in placenta. However, induction of placental benzpyrene hydroxylase by polycyclic hydrocarbon inducers has been demonstrated. In man, benzpyrene hydroxylase activity is not demonstrable in placentas obtained after childbirth from nonsmokers, but is demonstrable in placentas from women who smoke cigarettes (WELCH et al., 1968). While on initial consideration, this might seem to be a beneficial effect of smoking, the general experience with polycyclic hydrocarbon carcinogens suggests that their carcinogenic hazard outweighs any protective value they might have.

Benzpyrene Hydroxylase Activity in in vitro *Systems.* Polycyclic hydrocarbon hydroxylases have been demonstrated in two types of *in vitro* systems. The most extensively studied are tissue culture systems (ALFRED and GELBOIN, 1967; DIAMOND et al., 1968) which are described by Gelboin elsewhere in this volume. In a second type of system, benzpyrene hydroxylase has been demonstrated in fragments of adult mouse lung maintained in culture (WATTENBERG et al., 1968). In these experiments, it was shown that an increase in benzpyrene hydroxylase activity can be induced in lung tissue *in vitro*. This organ culture system may be useful in studies of enzyme induction in human tissues under conditions where it is not possible to obtain sequential specimens or to administer a particular compound whose inductive effects are under investigation.

IV. Implications of Extra-Hepatic Distribution of Drug Metabolizing Systems

There are profound implications in the widespread distribution of systems metabolizing drugs and other foreign compounds. The presence of these systems in tissues of major portals of entry means that compounds may be metabolized by these enzymes prior to entering the organism. Depending on the dosage and the capacities of the systems, the internal organs of the organism would be partially or totally prevented from coming into contact with the unaltered form of the foreign compound. In those instances where the enzyme system result in detoxification, such as with the polycyclic hydrocarbon hydroxylases, a protective effect would be obtained. Thus, the presence of these systems in the gastrointestinal tract would protect against ingested noxious agents, their location in the lung would protect against inhaled noxious agents, and in the skin they would protect against dermal contact with such agents. The liver represents a second and very potent line of defense. Its function would be aided by the kidney whose microsomal enzyme activity would facilitate excretion.

In addition to these major sites of activity of drug metabolizing systems, there is a possibility that all cells may have at least some activity even though in some instances it might be of a very low order of magnitude. The finding of polycyclic hydrocarbon hydroxylase systems in hamster and mouse embryonic cells as well as other cell lines grown in tissue culture (ALFRED and GELBOIN, 1967 and DIAMOND et al., 1968) indicates that these are not enzymes which are restricted to highly differentiated cells, but, in fact, occur in primitive and undifferentiated cells. Further support for this concept of a possible ubiquitous cell distribution is the fact that with continuing investigation, a progressively increasing list of tissues has been found to have demonstrable polycyclic hydrocarbon hydroxylase activity.

The drug metabolizing systems have come under increasing investigation in the field of oncology (WATTENBERG, 1966). In early studies, it was shown that administration of microsomal enzyme inducers would protect against the carcinogenic effects of aminoazo dyes and 2-acetylaminofluorene (RICHARDSON et al., 1952; MEECHAN et al., 1953; MILLER et al., 1958). More recently, additional studies have shown that protection can be obtained against carcinogenic and other noxious effects of polycyclic hydrocarbons (HUGGINS et al., 1964; WATTENBERG and LEONG, 1965; WATTENBERG and LEONG, 1968; WHEATLEY, 1968; WATTENBERG and LEONG, 1970). Polycyclic hydrocarbon carcinogens occur as atmospheric pollutants resulting from combustion of fuels and other organic materials and they also are present in cigarette smoke. They are the most widely occurring environmental chemical carcinogens known, and thus protective systems against their carcinogenic effects have potential importance. It has been shown that protection can be obtained against pulmonary adenoma formation resulting from oral administration of benzpyrene or 7,12-dimethylbenz(a)anthracene by feeding inducers of increased polycyclic hydrocarbon hydroxylase activity (WATTENBERG and LEONG, 1968; WATTENBERG and LEONG, 1970). The inducers used in experiments of this type were flavones, which occur widely in plants. Those flavones that are fully methylated are moderately potent inducers. These data in addition to other data on naturally occurring inducers support the possibility that dietary factors could be of importance in increasing resistance to at least some environmental carcinogens (SIMS and GROVER, 1967). The feasibility of deliberately attempting to achieve protection against chemical carcinogens in the environment by administering inducers has been discussed in some detail and represents a complex problem because of the possibility of simultaneously inducing an increase in activity of reactions having deleterious effects on the organism (WATTENBERG, 1966).

In addition to consideration of the implications of increased polycyclic hydrocarbon hydroxylase activity on carcinogenesis, the opposite situation, namely the effects of decreased activity is of importance. Various insecticide synergists can inhibit microsomal enzyme activity (CASIDA et al., 1966). Decreases in polycyclic hydrocarbon hydroxylase activity can also be brought about by starvation and other dietary manipulations (WATTENBERG et al., 1962). Accordingly, it is possible that an inadequate diet could enhance the effects of environmental carcinogens. Hopefully, further information on the interplay of drug metabolizing enzyme systems and chemical carcinogens will result in the maximum exploitation of these systems for their protective effects.

References

ALFRED, L. J., GELBOIN, H. V.: Benzpyrene Hydroxylase Induction by Polycyclic Hydrocarbons in Hamster Embryonic Cells Grown *in Vitro*. Science **157**, 75—76 (1967).

CASIDA, J. E., ENGLE, J. L., ESSAC, E. A., KAMIENSKI, F. X., KUWATSUKA: Methylene-C^{14}-Dioxyphenyl Compounds: Metabolism in Relationship to Their Synergistic Action. Science **153**, 1130—1133 (1966).

CHIQUONE, A. D.: Distribution of Glucose-6-phosphatase in the Liver and Kidney of the Mouse. J. Histochem. Cytochem. **1**, 429—435 (1953).

CONNEY, A. H.: Pharmacological Implications of Microsomal Enzyme Induction. Pharmacol. Rev. **19**, 317—366 (1967).

CONNEY, A.H., MILLER, E.C., MILLER, J.A.: Substrate-induced Synthesis and other Properties of Benzpyrene Hydroxylase in Rat Liver. J. biol. Chem. **228**, 753—766 (1957).
COOPER, J.R., BRODIE, B.B.: Enzymatic Oxidation of Pentabarbital and Thiopental. J. Pharmacol. exp. Ther. **120**, 75—83 (1957).
DIAMOND, L., SARDET, C., ROTHBLAT, G.H.: The Metabolism of 7,12-Dimethylbenz(a)anthracene in Cell Cultures. Int. J. Cancer **3**, 838—849 (1968).
DIXON, R.L., WILLSON, V.J.: Metabolism of Hexobarbital and Zoxazolamine by Placentae and Fetal Liver Supernatant Fraction and Response to Phenobarbital and Chlordane Treatment. Arch. int. Pharmacodyn. **172**, 453—466 (1968).
GELBOIN, H.V., BLACKBURN, N.R.: The Stimulatory Effect of 3-Methylcholanthrene on Benzpyrene Hydroxylase Activity in Several Rat Tissues: Inhibition by Actinomycin D. and Puromycin. Cancer Res. **24**, 356—360 (1964).
GILMAN, A.G., CONNEY, A.H.: The Induction of Aminoazo Dye N-Demethylase in Nonhepatic Tissues by 3-Methylcholanthrene. Biochem. Pharmacol. **12**, 591—593 (1963).
HUGGINS, C., LORRAINE, G., FUKUNISHI, R.: Aromatic Influences on the Yields of Mammary Cancers Following Administration of 7,12-Dimethylbenz(a)anthracene. Proc. nat. Acad. Sci. (Wash.) **51**, 737—742 (1964).
JELLINCK, P.H., GOUDY, B.: Effect of Pretreatment with Polycyclic Hydrocarbons on the Metabolism of Dimethylbenzanthracene-12-^{14}C by Rat Liver and Other Tissues. Biochem. Pharmacol. **16**, 131—141 (1967).
KUNTZMAN, R., MARK, L.C., BROND, L., JACOBSON, M., LEVIN, W., CONNEY, A.H.: Metabolism of Drugs and Carcinogens by Human Liver Enzymes. J. Pharmacol. exp. Ther. **152**, 151—156 (1966).
MEECHAN, R.J., MCCAFFERTY, E.D., JONES, R.S.: 3-Methylcholanthrene as an Inhibitor of Hepatic Cancer Induced by 3-Methyl-4-dimethylaminoazo benzene in the Diet of the Rat. Cancer Res. **13**, 802—806 (1953).
MILLER, E.C., MILLER, J.A., BROWN, R.R., MACDONALD, J.C.: On the Protective Action of Certain Polycyclic Aromatic Hydrocarbons Against Carcinogenesis by Aminoazo Dyes and 2-Acetylaminofluorene. Cancer Res. **18**, 469—477 (1958).
MIRKIN, B.L.: Developmental Pharmacology. Ann. Rev. Pharmacol. **10**, (in press) (1970).
RICHARDSON, H.L., STEIN, A.R., BORSON-NACHT-NEBEL, E.: Tumor Inhibition and Adrenal Histologic Responses in Rats in which 3'-Methyl-4-dimethyl Aminoazobenzene and 20-Methylcholanthrene were Simultaneously Administered. Cancer Res. **12**, 356—361 (1952).
SAFFIOTTI, V., CEFIS, F., KOLB, L.H.: A Method of Experimental Induction of Bronchogenic Carcinoma. Cancer Res. **28**, 104—124 (1968).
SCHUMACHER, H.: Histochemical Distribution Pattern of Respiratory Enzymes in the Liver Lobule. Science **125**, 501—503 (1957).
SIMS, P., GROVER, P.L.: Variations Dependent on Aga and Diet in the Metabolism of 7,12-Dimethylbenz(a)anthracene by Rat Liver Homogenates. Nature (Lond.) **216**, 77—78 (1967).
SUNDERMAN, F.W.: Inhibition of Induction of Benzpyrene Hydroxylase by Nickel Carbonyl. Cancer Res. **27**, 950—955 (1967).
VAN PETTEN, G.R., HIRSH, F.H., CHERRINGTON, A.D.: Drug Metabolizing Activity of the Human Placenta. Canad. J. Biochem. **10**, 1057—1061 (1968).
WATTENBERG, L.W.: Chemoprophylaxis of Carcinogenesis: A Review. Cancer Res. **26**, 1520—1526 (1966).
— (unpublished, 1969).
— LEONG, J.L.: Histochemical Demonstration of Reduced Pyridine Nucleotide Dependent Polycyclic Hydrocarbon Metabolising Systems. J. Histochem. Cytochem. **10**, 412—420 (1962).
— — Effects of Phenothiazines on Protective Systems Against Polycyclic Hydrocarbons. Cancer Res. **25**, 365—369 (1965).
— — Inhibition of the Carcinogenic Action of 7,12-Dimethylbenz(a)anthracene by Beta-Naphthoflavone. Proc. Soc. exp. Biol. (N.Y.) **128**, 940—943 (1968).
— — Inhibition of the Carcinogenic Action of Benzo(a)pyrene by Flavones. Proc. of the Tenth Int. Cancer Cong (in press) (1970).
— — GALBRAITH, A.: Induction of Increased Benzpyrene Hydroxylase Activity in Pulmonary Tissue *in Vitro*. Proc. Soc. exp. Biol. (N.Y.) **127**, 467—469 (1968).
— — STRAND, P.J.: Benzpyrene Hydroxylase Activity in the Gastrointestinal Tract. Cancer Res. **22**, 1120—1125 (1962).
— PAGE, MARY ANNE, LEONG, J.L.: Induction of Increased Benzopyrene Hydroxylase Activity by Flavones and Related Compounds. Cancer Res. **28**, 934—937 (1968a).
— — — Induction of Increased Benzpyrene Hydroxylase Activity by 2-Phenylbenzothiazoles and Related Compounds. Cancer Res. **28**, 2539—2544 (1968b).

Welch, R. M., Harrison, Y. E., Conney, A. H., Poppers, P. H., Finster, M.: Cigarette Smoking: Stimulatory Effect of Metabolism of 3,4-Benzpyrene by Enzymes in Human Placenta. Science **160**, 541—542 (1968).

— — Gommi, B. W., Poppers, P. J., Finster, M., Conney, A. H.: Stimulatory Effect of Cigarette Smoking on the Hydroxylation of 3,4-Benzpyrene and the N-Demethylation of 3-Methyl-4-monomethylaminonazobenzene by Enzymes in Human Placenta. Clin. Pharmacol. Ther. **10**, 100—109 (1969).

Wheatley, D. N.: Enhancement and Inhibition of the Induction by 7,12-Dimethylbenz(a)anthracene of Mammary Tumors in Female Sprague-Dawley Rats. Brit. J. Cancer **22**, 787—792 (1968).

Chapter 48

Mechanisms of Induction of Drug Metabolism Enzymes

HARRY V. GELBOIN

With 9 Figures

A. Introduction

A large segment of this review concerns the changes induced by polycyclic hydrocarbons and drugs on the level of certain enzyme activities and the mechanism of these changes. It is, therefore, important to summarize briefly some of the factors which may affect the observed activity of an enzyme system.

Enzyme control mechanisms may be classified into two broad categories. Firstly, there are those factors that affect the enzymatic activity of specific protein molecules, and secondly, those factors that regulate the amount of enzyme protein. In respect to the former, the activity of an enzyme may be affected by the concentration of either substrate or product or the presence of an inhibitor. Isosteric inhibition occurs when an inhibitor that is sterically related to the substrate or cofactor competes with either of them for the catalytic site on the enzyme. This kind of inhibition may occur when the inhibitor is added to the assay system or is present in the enzyme preparation. A stimulation or inhibition of the enzyme can also occur by "allosteric" modification. In this type of interaction the molecule modifying enzyme activity exerts its effect on the enzyme by binding to a site other than the binding site of the substrate. An example of this type of inhibition is feedback inhibition of multi-enzyme systems in which a distal product of a metabolic pathway inhibits an enzyme that catalyzes an early step in the pathway. Another way of altering enzyme activity that is not related to an altered protein amount is illustrated by the activation of the digestive enzymes. Inactive forms of these enzymes are synthesized and subsequently activated by structural modification (NEURATH and DIXON, 1957). Their activation thus mimics enzyme induction, i.e., an increased rate of synthesis of enzyme protein. Activation and inactivation can also occur through an association and dissociation of polypeptide subunits of an enzyme; this type of activation and inactivation has been called "molecular conversion" by MONOD and JACOB (1961).

The amount of enzyme protein may be regulated by factors affecting either the rate of enzyme synthesis or the rate of enzyme degradation. The term "enzyme induction" has been specifically used to describe the process which increases the rate of synthesis of an enzyme relative to its normal rate of synthesis in the uninduced organism. Enzyme repression is the process in which the rate of enzyme synthesis is decreased relative to the normal rate. In many studies in mammalian systems the terms "induction" and "repression" are used to explain a change in enzyme activity even in cases where an increase or decrease in the amount of enzyme protein has not actually been determined. For the purpose of this review the terms "enzyme induction" and "enzyme repression" will be used, although direct evidence for "induction" or "repression", in the strict definition of these terms, is often lacking.

BERLIN and SCHIMKE (1965) have pointed out the importance of both synthesis and degradation in studies on enzyme induction. A stabilization of an enzyme which prevents its degradation mimics enzyme induction. For example, the ten-fold increase in thymidylate kinase activity that occurs after thymidine administration is due to stabilization of thymidine kinase by thymidine and not to enzyme induction (BOJARSKI and HIATT, 1960). Also, tryptophan administration increases the activity of tryptophan pyrrolase by increasing its affinity for a cofactor, hematin (FEIGELSON and GREENGARD, 1962), which stabilizes the enzyme and prevents its degradation (SCHIMKE et al., 1964). Thus, in the absence of tryptophan, the enzyme has a half-life of about 3 hours; in its presence enzyme degradation is not detectable.

B. Effects of Polycyclic Hydrocarbons and Phenobarbital on Protein Synthesis

A single *in vivo* administration of certain polycyclic hydrocarbons and drugs to rats increases a large number of liver microsomal enzyme activities. This phenomenon and types of enzymes involved have been discussed in several broad reviews (GILLETTE, 1963; CONNEY, 1967; GELBOIN, 1967).

ARCOS et al. (1961) showed that many polycyclic hydrocarbons increase liver size, with a proportionate increase in total liver protein. Within 4 days after the administration of 3-methylcholanthrene (MC), naphthacene, or anthanthrene there was a 20—30% increase in liver protein content. Although MC increased total protein content of the liver, it did not change the amount of protein per gram of liver. On the other hand, the administration of phenobarbital and related drugs caused an increase in both the total liver protein and in the amount of protein per gram of wet weight of liver. CONNEY et al. (1960) and CONNEY and GILMAN (1963) found that phenobarbital, chlorcyclizine, orphenadrine, or phenylbutazone caused increases ranging from 22—39% in microsomal protein per gram of wet liver. ORRENIUS et al. (1965) reported an increase in both protein and RNA content of liver microsomes of rats treated with phenobarbital for a 120-hour period. In this case both the agranular and granular endoplasmic reticulum increased, although the phenobarbital effect was considerably greater in the agranular endoplasmic reticulum where a two-fold increase was observed; the granular endoplasmic reticulum increased only 20%. These results are consistent with the reports from several other laboratories that phenobarbital causes a proliferation of the agranular endoplasmic reticulum. Thus, REMMER and MERKER (1963) and FOUTS and ROGERS (1965) have demonstrated by electron microscopy an increase in the agranular endoplasmic reticulum of liver after rats or rabbits were treated with phenobarbital.

C. Enzyme Induction and the Gene-Action System

Although the nature of the genetic code is now almost completely understood, relatively little is known about the processes regulating the transcription of DNA into messenger RNA or those processes regulating the translation of the message into protein. It is known, however, that certain genes may affect the activity of other genes and also that this regulation of one gene by another is sensitive to various molecules in the environment of the cell. These molecules affecting gene activity may be of either endogenous origin, such as certain metabolites, sub-

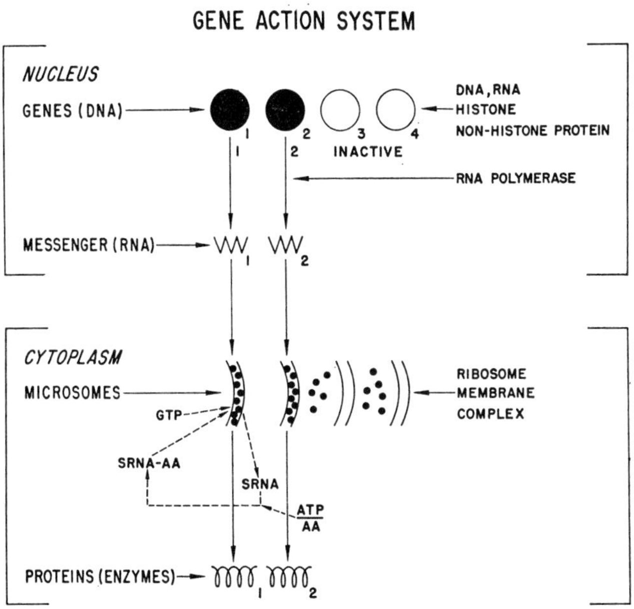

Fig. 1. Model of the gene action system

strates, or hormones; or may be of exogenous origin, for example, certain carcinogens or drugs. In this way genetic activity becomes responsive to the environmental changes to which the cell is exposed.

A simple formulation of the gene-action system is shown in Fig. 1. First is the question of the nature of the mechanism regulating the activity of genes. As shown, certain genes, 1 and 2, are active in the synthesis of messenger RNA's while other genes, 3 and 4, are inactive. Although the mechanisms which regulate gene activity in mammalian cells is not yet known, it is known that when the active DNA is transcribed into messenger RNA the reaction is catalyzed by an enzyme, RNA polymerase. A useful inhibitor which blocks this reaction is actinomycin-D.

After the messenger RNA is made in the nucleus, it is transferred to the cytoplasm and functions on the ribosome-membrane complex. In this ribosome-membrane complex, the messenger RNA directs the assembly of amino acids into specific polypeptide or protein chains. This process requires adapter molecules, amino acyl linked transfer RNAs (SRNA-AAs). These adapter molecules may also have a regulatory function on messenger RNA translation. The amino acyl transfer RNAs are synthesized in the presence of specific amino acids, transfer RNA, ATP and amino acyl transfer RNA synthetases. The process of protein synthesis also requires a variety of other factors including GTP, transferases and initiating factors. Although a fair amount is known about the complex mechanism of protein synthesis, little is known about the mechanisms regulating this process. For example, little is known concerning those factors governing the relative stability of the messenger RNA or the number of times each message is read or the role of SRNA in the translational control. Thus, the factors regulating messenger RNA synthesis in the nucleus are relatively obscure in mammalian systems. This also is the case with our understanding of the factors controlling the rates of messenger RNA translation into proteins. Phenobarbital and a number of polycyclic hydrocarbons and drugs are known to alter the activities of various components of the gene action system. These include activities at the transcriptional level in the nucleus as well as the translational level in the cytoplasm. In studies on the effect of phenobarbital treatment on the *in vivo* incorporation of leucine-C^{14} into the various subcellular fractions of rat liver, KATO et al. (1965) showed that this treatment increased the rate of leucine-C^{14} incorportion into the microsomal fraction by about 25%, but had no effect on amino acid incorporation into the nuclear fraction, the mitochondria, or the soluble fraction of the liver. The increase in leucine-C^{14} incorporation was observed both in the deoxycholate-soluble proteins of the microsomes, that is, in the lipoprotein component, and in the ribosomal component. After pretreating rats with MC, DECKEN and HULTIN (1960) found an increase of 22% in the *in vitro* incorporation of leucine-C^{14} into microsomal protein. Similarly, GELBOIN and SOKOLOFF (1961, 1964) using different types of *in vitro* amino acid incorporating systems, found a 60% and 30% increase in leucine-C^{14} incorporation in microsomes from rats pretreated with MC. By contrast, pretreatment of the rats with phenobarbital caused a 163% increase in the leucine-C^{14} incorporation. GELBOIN and SOKOLOFF (1961) also observed stimulation of amino acid incorporation by MC when SRNA-leucine-C^{14} or SRNA-proline-C^{14} were used in place of free leucine. This result suggests that at least part of the stimulatory effect of MC on amino acid incorporation is independent of soluble factors which may influence the formation of SRNA-bound amino acid. In a subsequent study, GELBOIN and SOKOLOFF (1964) also found evidence for increased levels of GTP in rat liver supernatant of animals treated with MC.

GELBOIN (1964) and KATO et al. (1965, 1966) have examined the mechanism of the MC and phenobarbital stimulation of protein synthesis. They used techniques which enabled them to examine amino acid incorporation directed by endogenous messenger RNA and that directed solely by a synthetic messenger RNA, polyuridylic acid. The microsomal incorporating system can be operationally described as a complex consisting of two parts, the messenger RNA and the microsomal RNA protein complex which serves as the microsomal amino acid incorporation site on which messenger RNA acts to "program" amino acid incorporation. Preincubation of the microsomes in the presence of appropriate cofactors removes endogenous messenger RNA activity by releasing messenger RNA from the microsomal RNA protein complex. Phenylalanine incorporation can be restored by the addition of polyuridylic acid. The latter studies (GELBOIN and SOKOLOFF, 1964; KATO et al., 1965, 1966) showed that with nonpreincubated microsomes, i.e., those containing endogenous RNA, the addition of polyuridylic acid stimulated the incorporation of phenylalanine to the same extent in microsomes from control and MC-treated rats. This suggests that the number of messenger-free binding sites available for poly-U in microsomes is not affected by MC treatment. However, after the removal of endogenous messenger RNA activity, the addition of polyuridylic acid stimulated phenylalanine incorporation to a greater extent in the preparation from MC- and PB-treated rats than in normal preparations. This suggests that after preincubation there are more messenger RNA-free microsomal sites available for the binding of polyuridylic acid in the preparations from MC- and PB-treated rats than there are in the microsomes from normal rats. Also, with no preincubation, the addition of 100 μg of polyuridylic acid was sufficient to saturate the binding sites of microsomes from normal and MC-treated rats. After preincubation, however, 100 μg was sufficient to saturate the active sites of the normal microsomes but was insufficient to saturate the active sites of the microsomes from MC-treated rats. If one assumes that the newly available sites are those that were previously occupied by the

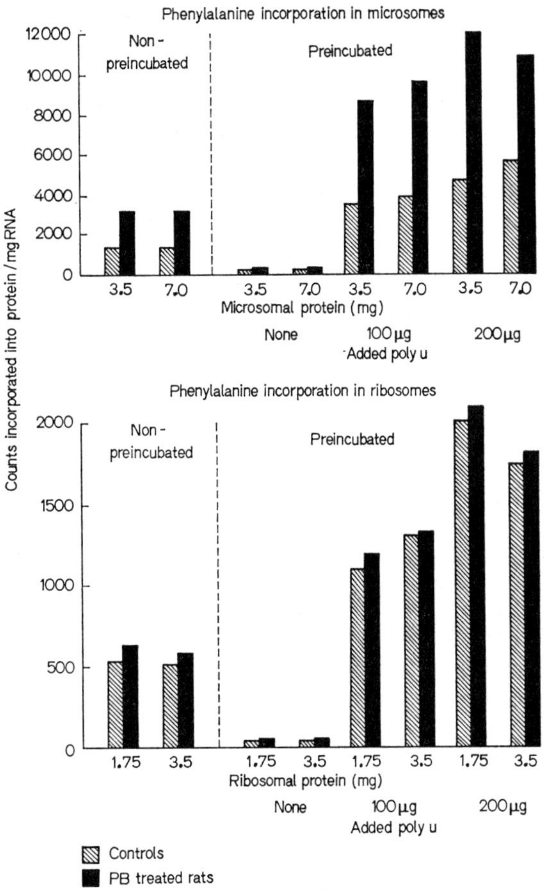

Fig. 2. L-[^{14}C]-phenylalanine incorporation in non-preincubated microsomal and ribosomal preparations from control and phenobarbital-treated rats (KATO et al., 1966)

released messenger RNA, then the results may be interpreted to mean that the MC microsomes contained, prior to preincubation, a greater amount of messenger RNA and, hence, upon preincubation more active sites became available in the MC preparation than in the normal preparation.

KATO et al. (1965, 1966) found that phenobarbital caused similar but quantitatively greater differences than MC in the microsomal protein synthesizing activity. Thus, non-preincubated microsomes from phenobarbital-treated rats are more active than non-preincubated control microsomes in the incorporation of L-phenylalanine-C^{14}. Moreover, preincubated microsomes are much more sensitive than control microsomes to polyuridylic acid-directed L-phenylalanine-C^{14} incorporation. This is probably due to a phenobarbital-induced increase in both the endogenous microsomal messenger RNA content and the total number of microsomal binding sites for messenger RNA. KATO et al. (1965, 1966) found, moreover, that these differences were not observed with ribosomal preparations. Figure 2 from KATO et al. (1966) shows that in non-preincubated microsomes, L-phenylalanine-C^{14} incorporation per mg RNA remains constant when the amount of microsomes is doubled; in each case the microsomes from phenobarbital-treated rats are about twice as active as controls. After preincubation, however, both control and phenobarbital microsomes are inactive until polyuridylic acid is added to the system. On addition of either 100 μg or 200 μg of polyuridylic acid the phenobarbital microsomes are about twice as active as the control preparations. The lower half of the chart shows a similar experiment performed with ribosomes isolated from the same group of rats. Although there are marked differences in microsomal L-phenylalanine-C^{14} incorporation, there are only negligible differences between ribosomes from control and phenobarbital-treated rats. Hence, it seems likely that the factors responsible for the stimulatory activity of phenobarbital are components of the endoplasmic reticulum since they are removed by desoxycholate treatment during the preparation of the ribosomes. Siefert et al. (1968) examined the effect of phenobarbital *in vivo* administration on the *in vitro* phenylalanine incorporating activity of isolated ribosomes at various times. Within 5 hours after phenobarbital treatment, ribosomes showed an increased phenylalanine incorporation; at 17 hours the activity of microsomes and membrane-bound ribosomes diminished. These authors also found that sensitivity to added synthetic messenger RNA was 40% greater in microsomes from phenobarbital-treated rats than in those from controls. They also found that the ribosomal fraction from phenobarbital-treated rats contained a greater number of more rapidly sedimenting polysomal components. They suggest that phenobarbital increases the number of ribosomal binding sites for mRNA attachment. Gelboin (1964) found that actinomycin D, which blocks the synthesis of messenger RNA, not only inhibited the MC induction of benzpyrene hydroxylase but also prevented the MC-induced changes in amino acid incorporation. Thus, the MC-induced changes in microsomal protein synthesis appear dependent on RNA synthesis. Furthermore, the changes in gross protein synthesis parallel the increase in microsomal enzyme activity. These gross changes probably include changes in the rates of synthesis of many proteins, since the microsomal enzymes comprise a relatively small number of the total cell proteins and even marked changes in their rates of synthesis could not account for the overall changes in protein synthesis.

D. Effect of Inducers on the Turnover and Activity of Microsomal Proteins

Jick and Shuster (1966) have investigated the turnover of microsomal reduced NADPH cytochrome *c* reductase and microsomal protein in the livers of mice treated with phenobarbital. Figure 3 shows a phenobarbital-induced increase in the incorporation of L-leucine into microsomal NADPH cytochrome *c* reductase. Figure 4 shows that phenobarbital markedly inhibits the loss of radioactivity from prelabeled NADPH cytochrome *c* reductase. The half-life of *in vivo* loss of radioactivity from enzyme protein averaged 2.8 days in control mice; however, they detected no loss of radioactivity from the purified enzyme in phenobarbital-treated mice. Jick and Shuster concluded from the studies that phenobarbital causes both an increased rate of synthesis and a decreased rate of breakdown of microsomal NADPH cytochrome *c* reductase.

Kuriyama et al. (1969) have also examined the effect of phenobarbital on the synthesis and degradation of total microsomal proteins and two specific proteins of the microsomal endoplasmic reticulum, NADPH-cytochrome *c* reductase and cytochrome b_5. The two proteins were isolated and purified, and the effect of phenobarbital on the synthesis and degradation of the enzymes was determined with both leucine-C^{14} and guanidino-labeled arginine-C^{14}. They reported that a single administration of phenobarbital induced a prompt increase in the rate of

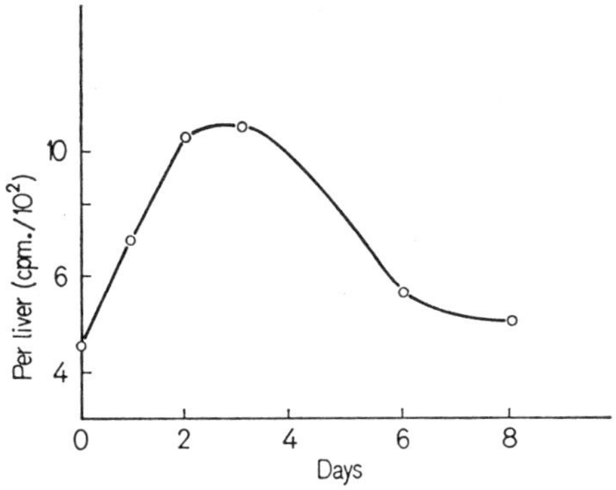

Fig. 3. Effect of phenobarbital treatment on the incorporation of L-leucine into microsomal NADPH-cytochrome *c* reductase. Mice received injections twice daily of sodium phenobarbital, 75 mg per kg, or 0.9% NaCl. At various times after the initiation of phenobarbital treatment one group of four control mice and one group of four phenobarbital-treated mice were injected with 20 μC of L-leucine-^{3}H. The mice were killed 90 min after the injection of labeled leucine. Treatment was stopped after 4 days. Each *point* is the average value based on two separate isolations of enzyme from the pooled steapsin digests obtained from the livers of two mice (JICK and SHUSTER, 1966)

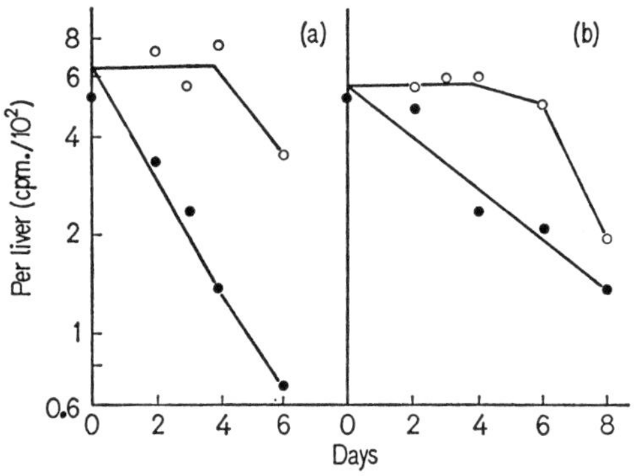

Fig. 4. The loss of radioactivity from prelabeled NADPH-cytochrome *c* reductase in mice treated with phenobarbital. (*a*) phenobarbital treatment was begun 24 hours after the injection of 25 μC of L-leucine-^{3}H. Mice received injections twice daily of sodium phenobarbital, 75 mg per kg, or of 0.25 ml of 0.9% NaCl. Each *point* is the average value based on two separate isolations of enzyme from the pooled steapsin digests obtained from the livers of two or three mice. ●—●, enzyme from control animals; ○—○, enzyme from phenobarbital-treated mice. (*b*) conditions were the same as those in *a* except that treatment was stopped after 4 days. Each *point* is based on two separate isolations of enzyme from the pooled steapsin digests obtained from the livers of two mice (JICK and SHUSTER, 1966)

total microsomal protein and NADPH-cytochrome *c* reductase synthesis but did not effect the rate of cytochrome b_5 synthesis. They also found that the induced reductase was both chromatographically and immunochemically identical to the enzyme normally found in the liver. When repeated phenobarbital doses were given, the increases in NADPH-cytochrome *c* reductase amount became greater and there was a moderate rise in cytochrome b_5 content. Both of these effects seem to be the result of a drastic reduction in the rate of protein degradation in addition to an increased rate of synthesis. In order to minimize the possibility that phenobarbital effects the re-utilization of the C^{14} amino acid, KURIYAMA et al.

also performed their studies with L-arginine-guanidino-C^{14} as the radioactive amino acid. This amino acid is not significantly reutilized because of its rapid degradation through the urea cycle (SWICK and HANDE, 1956; SWICK, 1958; SCHIMKE, 1964; STEPHEN and WATERLOW, 1966). These investigators, however, found that the results with the guanidino-labeled arginine were similar to those with leucine, indicating that the apparent differences in the rates of synthesis and degradation after phenobarbital treatment could not be explained by an altered reutilization of free amino acids (ERNSTER and ORRENIUS, 1965).

KURIYAMA et al. (1969) also found that the phenobarbital induced increase in the rate of incorporation of amino acid into total microsomal membrane protein was an earlier event than the increase in the rate of reductase synthesis. The protein preparation that was labeled at a faster rate contained approximately 50% of the original microsomal protein. The authors suggest that this fraction may reflect a phenobarbital-induced synthesis of a "primary membrane" preceding the synthesis of enzymes that are then deposited on the primary membrane.

Several investigators have suggested the involvement of heme synthesis as a regulating factor in the formation of the microsomal cytochromes (GRANICK, 1966). The biosynthetic pathway of heme involves the condensation of glycine and succinyl CoA in the presence of δ-aminolevulinic acid synthetase and pyridoxal phosphate to form δ-aminolevulinic acid (ALA). The ALA synthetase is a mitochondrial enzyme and is thought to be the rate-limiting step in heme biosynthesis (GRANICK, 1966; GRANICK and URATA, 1963; GRANICK, 1963; TSCHUDY et al., 1965). Since ALA synthetase has a relatively short half-life of 60—70 min (MARVER et al., 1966), its induction and repression may be significant to the changed activities of certain microsomal enzymes. MARVER (1968) has reported a rapid increase of ALA synthetase within several hours after phenobarbital was administered. He suggests that the increase in this activity provides the additional heme required for the drug-induced increases of microsomal cytochromes. MARVER also reports that phenobarbital stimulates Fe^{59} incorporation into microsomes and that the administration of heme largely prevents the increase in cytochrome P-450 induced by phenobarbital. Heme administration also prevents the stimulation of phospholipid synthesis, and the increase in NADPH cytochrome *c* reductase, aminopyrine N-demethylase and hexobarbital oxidase induced by phenobarbital. Since hematin is also a known repressor of heme biosynthesis, the suggestion is that heme biosynthesis plays an important role in the induction of microsomal enzymes. It is possible, however, that the receptor sites for the inducer may be microsomal heme proteins, and that administered hematin may compete with the normal receptor site for the inducer. MARVER's data suggests that heme synthesis is required for the production of increased amounts of microsomal cytochromes. It is not certain, however, whether heme biosynthesis is also necessary for the marked rises in certain enzymes, *e.g.* the aryl hydrocarbon hydroxylases. These increases are observed in tissue culture within 1 hour (NEBERT and GELBOIN, 1968b) and *in vivo* within 4—5 hours after hydrocarbon administration. The work of Marver, however, suggests a role for ALA synthetase regulation and heme biosynthesis in microsomal enzyme induction. Whether the role is initial or concomitant to the general increase in microsomal cytochromes remains to be determined.

LEVIN and KUNTZMAN (1969) have also found that phenobarbital administration stimulates the synthesis of microsomal hemo-proteins as measured by Fe^{59} incorporation, or the incorporation of either glycine or δ-aminolevulinic acid (ALA) into a microsomal fraction containing heme protein. They reported no effect of phenobarbital or MC pretreatment on the incorporation of ALA into

"CO-binding microsomal particles." They did, however, report that the rate of loss of radioactivity from the "particle" was biphasic and that the proportion associated with the second phase was increased by MC treatment. In these studies it would be important to characterize the nature of the radioactivity in the particle.

Several investigators have reported a MC-induced shift in the absorption maxima of CO-binding pigments in liver microsomes from 450 mμ to between 445 and 448. This shift is not observed after phenobarbital administration.

HILDEBRANDT et al. (1968) and SCHENKMAN et al. (1969) have discussed the problem of the possible multiplicity of cytochrome P_{450} and have suggested that the P_{450} exists only in two forms, that of the native enzyme and that of an enzyme substrate complex. In accord with this view, SCHENKMAN and SATO (1968) found that the addition of substrates alters the absolute spectrum of the cytochrome P_{450} and that the spectrum of the P_{450} induced by the polycyclic hydrocarbon appears similar to that of the heme protein in the presence of substrate. On the other hand, KUNTZMAN et al. (1968) have reported that ethionine and actinomycin D prevent the MC-induced shift to 448 from 450, suggesting a role for RNA and protein synthesis in the shift. These authors suggest that these studies provide further evidence that MC stimulates the synthesis of a heme protein which is different from P_{450}.

Studies by SLADEK and MANNERING (1969a, b) have also indicated that the mechanism by which polycyclic hydrocarbons and phenobarbital produce their inductive effects on microsomal N-demethylating systems are different, and that the microsomal N-demethylation stimulated by polycyclic hydrocarbons is also different than that stimulated by phenobarbital. These studies also suggest the possibility of different forms of the enzyme or of two different enzyme systems for N-demethylation.

Studies by GURTOO et al. (1968) and ALVARES et al. (1968) have shown that pretreatment with benzpyrene alters the kinetic behavior of microsomal aryl hydrocarbon hydroxylase. These alterations may be due to allosteric conversion of the control enzyme to a different form or may be due to the induced synthesis of a new and different hydroxylase.

The existence of two forms of the enzyme is also indicated by the different behavior of the control and induced aryl hydrocarbon (benzpyrene) hydroxylase in respect to the inhibitory activity of 7,8-benzoflavone. Thus 7,8-benzoflavone markedly inhibits the induced liver hydroxylase but has no effect on the liver hydroxylase from control rats (DIAMOND and GELBOIN, 1969).

The changes in the spectral properties of microsomal cytochromes and the kinetic behavior of microsomal hydroxylase after pretreatment of the animal with MC and the different sensitivity of the enzyme system to various inhibitors are open to several interpretations. The MC may indeed induce the synthesis of an entirely new enzyme. If the microsomes contained more of this new enzyme they would exhibit different spectral and kinetic behavior. Another possibility is that the enzyme from normal rats is converted to a different form which exhibits different kinetic behavior and shows changed spectral characteristics. Either of the above mechanisms may require RNA and protein synthesis, the first for the direct synthesis of the new enzyme, and the second for the synthesis of a protein needed for the allosteric conversion of the pre-existing enzyme.

Studies from Orrenius' laboratory (ERNSTER and ORRENIUS, 1965; ORRENIUS et al., 1965; ORRENIUS and ERICSSON, 1966) suggested that phenobarbital increases the synthesis of phospholipid in liver endoplasmic reticulum, since they found a 2- to 6-fold greater specific activity of $P^{32}PO_4$ in microsomal phospholipid of treated animals. HOLTZMAN and GILLETTE (1968) have suggested that part of this difference was due to a change in the specific activity of the phosphate pools and to a decrease in the catabolism of microsomal phospholipid. The increased synthesis, however, was not observed in female rats. Thus, it appears that microsomal phospholipid synthesis is stimulated during enzyme induction in male rats and microsomal phospholipid catabolism is reduced by the phenobarbital in both male and female rats. The involvement of phospholipid catabolism in microsomal enzyme induction is an area which is just beginning to be explored and may be highly relevant and central to the induction process. At this time it is difficult to assess the role of the reported alterations in phospholipid metabolism in microsomal enzyme induction.

E. Effects of Inhibitors on the Induction of Enzyme Activities *in Vivo*

I. Enzyme Induction *in Vivo*

Puromycin blocks protein synthesis at the microsomal level by preventing the transfer of soluble RNA-bound amino acid into polypeptide chains (YARMOLINSKY and DE LA HABA, 1959).

GELBOIN and BLACKBURN (1963) examined the effect of puromycin on the MC induction of benzpyrene hydroxylase in liver, kidney, small intestine, and lungs. To avoid the problem of chronic toxicity of the inhibitor these investigators used a short 7-hour period of induction. Puromycin completely inhibited the MC-induced increase in activity in liver, kidney, and small intestine. In lung the stimulatory effect of MC was inhibited by 50%. ORRENIUS et al. (1965) reported that puromycin prevented the phenobarbital-induced increase in N-demethylation, TPNH cytochrome *c* reductase activity, and the CO binding pigment of the microsomes. CONNEY and GILMAN (1963) reported a complete inhibition by puromycin of the increase in aminoazo dye N-demethylase induced by either MC or phenobarbital. Puromycin given simultaneously with either MC or phenobarbital completely prevented the increase in enzyme activity. Puromycin alone had no effect on enzyme activity.

JERVELL et al. (1965) have reported that MC-inducible dimethylaminoazobenzene (DAB) reductase is also increased in rats by starvation. The induction by starvation is prevented by the simultaneous administration of either puromycin or ethionine but not by actinomycin D. This enzyme appears to have a shorter half-life than that suggested by the studies of CONNEY (1965) for aminoazo dye N-demethylase. The administration of puromycin 10 hours after the start of the fast decreased the level of enzyme so that it returned to its normal level within 48 hours. These investigators suggest that carbohydrate represses rat liver DAB reductase formation.

In each case reported, puromycin was found to be an effective inhibitor of polycyclic hydrocarbon or phenobarbital-induced enzyme activity. The question arises as to the dependence of new enzyme synthesis on newly-formed messenger RNA. The induction may require activation of specific genes producing induction of specific RNAs or may involve the activation of stable messenger RNAs at the microsomal or translational level. To examine this aspect of the problem, GELBOIN and BLACKBURN (1963) and CONNEY (1965), have used actinomycin D, an inhibitor of DNA-dependent RNA synthesis (REICH et al., 1961; TAMAOKI and MUELLER, 1962; MERITS, 1963; and KORNER and MUNRO, 1963) on the drug-induced enzyme synthesis. GELBOIN and BLACKBURN (1963) examined the effect of actinomycin D on the MC induction of benzpyrene hydroxylase in liver, lung, kidney, and small intestine. During a 7-hour period of induction and a 9-hour period of exposure to actinomycin, the inhibitor was found to prevent completely the induction of benzpyrene hydroxylase in liver and small intestine and to prevent partially the induction of this enzyme activity in kidney and lungs. It is possible that in liver and small intestine the messenger RNA for this enzyme is rapidly turning over, and a blockage or increase of enzyme synthesis depends on newly synthesized messenger RNA. On the other hand, the failure of actinomycin D to completely block the MC induction in kidney and small intestine may reflect either an inability of the inhibitor to reach its site of action in adequate concentration or alternatively the stability of the messenger RNA for these enzymes may be greater in kidney and lung, and the induction process may take place at least in part at the level of microsomal translation. CONNEY (1965) reported that actinomycin D inhibited the MC-induction of aminoazo dye N-demethylase in the livers of male rats. Actinomycin D also prevented the MC-induced increase in rat liver DAB reductase activity and in the phenobarbital-induced increase in the microsomal content of CO-binding pigment (JERVELL et al., 1965; and ORRENIUS et al., 1965). There have been no reports of failure of actinomycin D to prevent induction of microsomal enzymes by MC or by phenobarbital. JERVELL et al. (1965), however, reported that actinomycin failed to prevent the increase in DAB reductase activity induced by starvation. This suggests that there may be a second mechanism by which microsomal enzymes can be induced which is independent of DNA-dependent RNA synthesis.

II. Enzyme Induction in Isolated Perfused Rat Liver

The stimulatory effect of polycyclic hydrocarbons and drugs on certain liver microsomal enzymes appears not to be mediated through the endocrine system, since the stimulation of at least the aryl hydrocarbon hydroxylase is observed in adrenalectomized and hypophysectomized rats. Moreover, JUCHAU et al. (1965) have shown that microsomal benzpyrene hydroxylase is induced in isolated perfused rat liver when 3,4-benzpyrene is added to the perfusing medium. Maximal enzyme induction was obtained after $6^1/_2$ hours of perfusion and the degree of stimulation at that time was 2- to 3-fold over the control values. These studies demonstrate that the inducer can act directly on the target tissue and its action as an inducer does not require the concomitant functioning of the endocrine system. Hormonal influences, however, are not entirely ruled out in the isolated perfused liver, since endogenous levels of hormones would be expected to be present in the liver. Culturing cells for several weeks would be expected to dilute out any endogenous hormone; in these cells, derived from either the whole embryo or from individual embryonic tissues, the aryl hydrocarbon hydroxylase is still inducible. Thus, the studies of JUCHAU et al. (1965), and NEBERT and GELBOIN (1968b) demonstrate that the inducer acts directly on the target tissue.

F. Enzyme Induction in Cell Culture

The induction of microsomal aryl hydrocarbon hydroxylase in hamster embryo cell culture has been reported and has yielded some new information on the properties of aryl hydrocarbon hydroxylase and its mechanism of induction (ALFRED and GELBOIN, 1967; NEBERT and GELBOIN, 1968a, b). Upon addition of a polycyclic hydrocarbon to the medium, the aryl hydroxylase rises after a lag of about 35 min. The rise continues linearly from 12—16 hours. Upon removal of the inducer from the medium, the enzyme level declines rapidly.

Inducibility	Species (embryo)	Origin of cell	Gestational age (hamster)	Number of subcultures
High	Hamster Mouse	Lung Small intestine, Liver	14 days	2—5
Moderate	Rat	Limb	12 days	6
Low	Chick Guinea pig	Brain	9 days	>6
Absent	—	Established cell lines Transformed cells	—	—

Fig. 5. Characteristics of the aryl hydroxylase induction system (GELBOIN, 1968)

Figure 5 shows some characteristics of the aryl hydrocarbon hydroxylase induction system. This figure should be read only vertically. The enzyme is inducible in cells derived from whole mouse, hamster, or rat embryos. The hydroxylase is also inducible in cells obtained by microdissection from embryonic lung, small intestine, liver, and limb. The inducibility in these tissues is as great as that observed with cells from whole embryos; this suggests that a relatively large proportion of the total cell population is being induced. Optimal induction was observed in cells subcultured 2—6 times. Cells subcultured 11 times were about 50% as inducible as secondary cultures. The enzyme system was not inducible in three established cell lines obtained originally from hamster lung, hamster kidney, and human embryonic lung.

I. Estimation of Half-Life of Induced Aryl Hydroxylase Activity

Figure 6 shows the rate of decay of previously induced aryl hydroxylase activity when inducer is replaced with fresh control medium or when puromycin is added. The half-life of the induced microsomal hydroxylase system was 3.3 ± 1.2 hours; this value does not include the 2- or 3-hour lag period preceding the decline in enzyme activity. In rat liver microsomal membranes, the half-lifes of various protein components *in vivo* ranged from 75—113 hours, with total membrane-lipids having 10—30% shorter half-lifes (OMURA, T. et al., 1967).

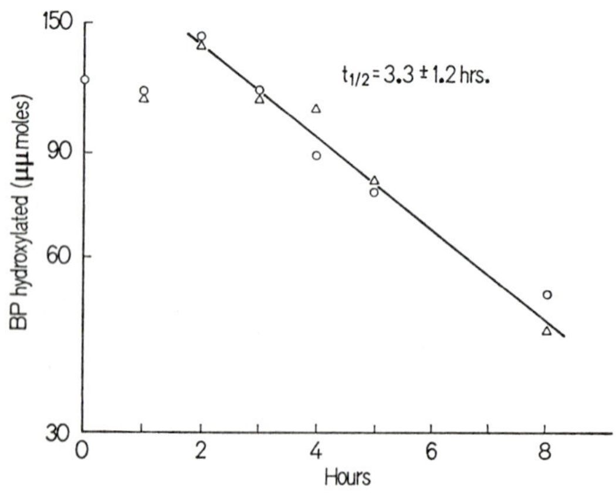

Fig. 6. Semilog plot of the rate of decay of previously induced aryl hydroxylase activity. The effects of 60 μM puromycin (PU) and of fresh control medium alone (CM) were not significantly different (NEBERT and GELBOIN, 1968b)

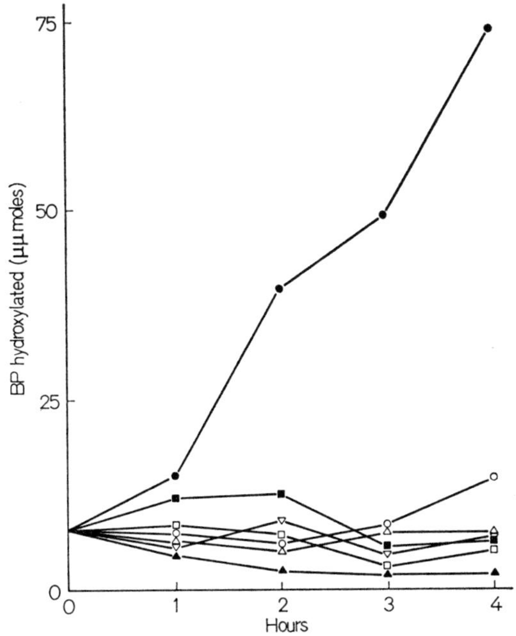

Fig. 7. The effects of 0.4 μM actinomycin D (AD), 60 μM puromycin (PU) and 3.5 μM cycloheximide (CY) on aryl hydroxylase induction by 13 μM 1,2 benzanthracene (BA). The responses to inducer alone (BA) and control medium alone (CM) are also illustrated. The antibiotics and the inducer were added simultaneously. When puromycin or cycloheximide was added alone to cells in control medium, no effect on hydroxylase activity was found. At these concentrations of antibiotics, actinomycin D prevented more than 90% of RNA synthesis, and puromycin and cycloheximide prevented more than 95% of protein synthesis. ●—● BA; ■—■ BA+AD; ▲—▲ BA+AD+PU; ○—○ CM; □—□ AD; △—△ BA+PU; ▽—▽ BA+CY (NEBERT and GELBOIN, 1968b)

II. Effects of Metabolic Inhibitors on Inducible Aryl Hydroxylase

Figure 7 shows the effects of three metabolic inhibitors on aryl hydroxylase induction. The addition of 1,2 benz(a)anthracene (BA) to the medium produced a 9-fold increase in enzymatic activity in 4 hours. The addition of actinomycin D, puromycin, or cycloheximide in combination with the inducer completely prevented the hydroxylase induction. The complete block of induction by actinomycin D indicates a requirement for DNA-dependent RNA synthesis for the induction of microsomal aryl hydroxylase activity. Concomitant analysis of RNA synthesis during this 4-hour experiment showed that actinomycin D inhibited at least 90% of ^{3}H-uridine incorporation into RNA.

That the induction process requires protein synthesis is indicated by the complete prevention of the increase in hydroxylase activity by puromycin and cycloheximide (Fig. 7). Although these data do not show an increase in enzyme protein nor rule out an activation of preexisting enzyme, they do show the requirement of protein synthesis for the increased enzyme activity. Puromycin and cycloheximide inhibited ^{14}C-protein hydrolysate incorporation into cellular protein by at least 95%.

Figure 8 depicts the effects of actinomycin D and puromycin, alone or in combination with the inducer, BA, on aryl hydroxylase activity in cells which

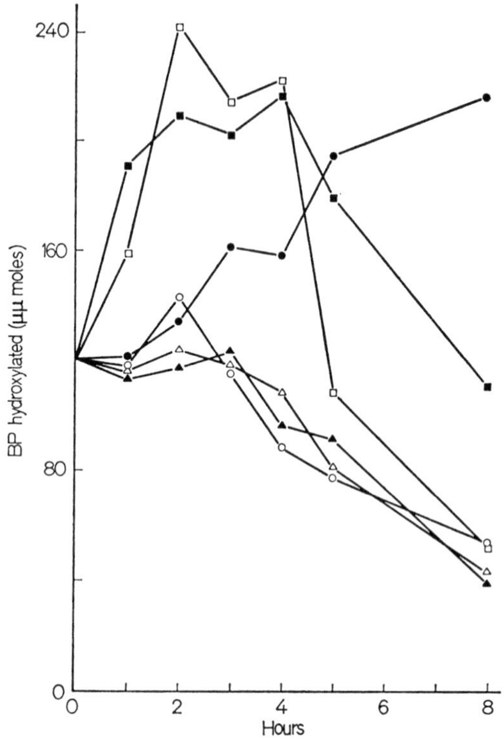

Fig. 8. The effects of 0.4 μM actinomycin D (AD), 60 μM puromycin (PU) and control medium (CM) on hydroxylase activity of previously induced cells. The cultures had been treated with 13 μM 1,2 benzanthracene (BA) for 25 hours, at which time the medium of all dishes was replaced with fresh medium containing the indicated additions. Concomitant experiments to determine the degree of inhibition of RNA and protein synthesis were carried out. Actinomycin D prevented 75% of ^{3}H-uridine incorporation into perchloric acid-precipitable residue in the initial 15 min following its addition; there was 80% inhibition in the second 15-min period, more than 90% inhibition from 30—90 min, and 95—98% during the remaining $6^1/_2$ hours. Puromycin blocked 90% of the ^{14}C-protein hydrolysate incorporation into trichloracetic acid-precipitable protein in the initial 15 min following its addition and 95—99% of incorporation during the remaining $7^3/_4$ hours. ●—● BA; ■—■ BA+AD; □—□ AD; ▲—▲ BA+AD+PU; △—△ PU; ○—○ CM (NEBERT and GELBOIN, 1968b)

had been induced for the preceding 24 hours by BA. Enzyme activity continued to increase at a linear rate in cells exposed to additional inducer. However, the presence of actinomycin D, with or without the hydrocarbon inducer, now produced a greater increase in hydroxylase activity during the initial 4 hours than that observed with BA alone. The addition of puromycin prevented the increased stimulation of hydroxylase activity by actinomycin D, with and without inducer. A similar lack of actinomycin D inhibition has been found during glucocorticoid induction of tyrosine-α-ketoglutarate transaminase in hepatoma tissue culture cells (TOMKINS et al., 1965; THOMPSON et al., 1966; and PETERKOFSKY and TOMKINS, 1967) and has been interpreted as resulting from the inhibition of the synthesis of a labile cytoplasmic translation repressor by relatively high concentrations of actinomycin D. A similar hypothesis has been proposed for the actinomycin D prolongation of the induction of thymidine kinase, which occurs after pox virus infection of HeLa cells (MCAUSLAN, 1963).

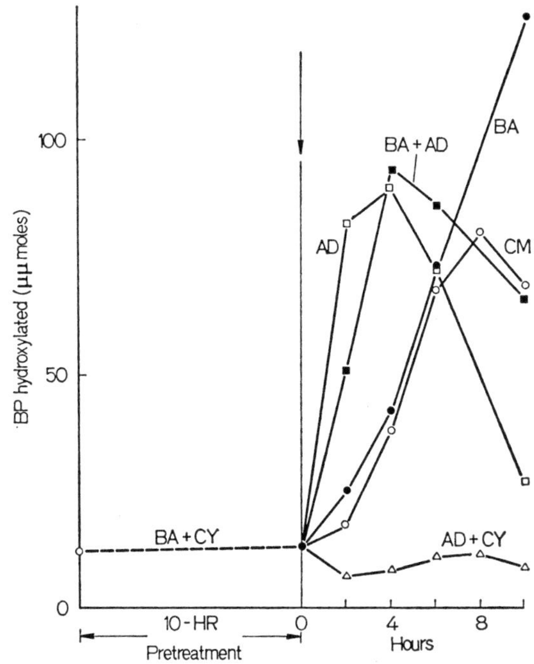

Fig. 9. The effects of 0.40 μM actinomycin D (AD), 13 μM inducer (BA), control medium alone (CM), and 3.5 μM cycloheximide (CY) on aryl hydrocarbon hydroxylase activity in cells previously treated with inducer plus cycloheximide (NEBERT and GELBOIN, 1970)

Following the addition of puromycin, with or without inducer, or the replacement of BA with fresh control medium, aryl hydroxylase activity in the previously induced cells generally remained nearly the same for 3 hours, after which a first order decay rate ensued. The insensitivity to puromycin for several hours may be due to the assembly of already synthesized components of the hydroxylase system. Such a response has been reported for the conversion of subunits to active carbamyl phosphate synthetase in tadpole liver mitochondrial fractions (TATIBANA and COHEN, 1965). The similar delay before the decline of aryl hydroxylase activity, seen when the hydrocarbon inducer was replaced with fresh control medium, suggests that during this period either the induction process is continuing because of the presence of residual amounts of BA or the hydroxylase is being assembled into membrane from previously synthesized precursors.

III. A Translation-independent Phase of Aryl Hydrocarbon Hydroxylase Induction

(NEBERT and GELBOIN, 1970)

The development of insensitivity to actinomycin D inhibition indicates that the early phases of induction involve the synthesis of an induction-specific RNA which accumulates and thereby permits the induction process to become independent of RNA synthesis. One important question is: can this RNA accumulate in the absence of protein synthesis or translation?

The question of whether the induction-specific RNA can be synthesized in the absence of protein synthesis or translation was investigated by the experiments reported in Fig. 9 which show the effect of high levels of actinomycin D on hydroxylase activity in cells previously tratede with BA plus cycloheximide. The addition of high concentrations of actinomycin D, with or without inducer, to cells previously treated with BA plus cycloheximide, stimulated aryl hydrocarbon hydroxylase activity to a greater extent than did BA alone, or control medium alone. The continued presence of cycloheximide prevented the actinomycin D effect. In Figs. 7 and 8 we observed that induction was prevented when actinomycin D was added simultaneously with BA but that induction was not blocked by actinomycin D when the latter was added 16 hours after BA. Very recent findings (Gelboin and Miller, unpublished results) showed that this transition from actinomycin D sensitivity to insensitivity occurred within 2 hours after BA was added, suggesting that the induction of the specific RNA occurs very shortly after addition of the inducer. The results shown in Fig. 9 demonstrate that in the presence of both cycloheximide, which causes an essentially complete block of protein synthesis, and inducer the cells pass from a stage in which actinomycin D inhibits induction to a stage in which it no longer has an inhibitory effect. If this transition represents the synthesis of an induction-specific RNA, one can conclude that this RNA species can be synthesized in the absence of translation. Also, these data suggest that the inducer may be operating at a level independent of translation.

Results of studies in cell culture have suggested the following sequence of events in microsomal enzyme induction. Firstly, upon addition of the inducer to the culture medium, it is rapidly incorporated within several minutes into the cell. This has been found by the use of radioactive inducer and fluorescence microscopy (Miller and Gelboin, unpublished observations). After incorporation, there appears a rapid interaction between inducer and receptor site which is then followed by a period of RNA synthesis. This stage of enzyme induction involving RNA synthesis is sensitive to actinomycin D inhibition. This early RNA synthesis phase occurs within 2 hours after inducer is added and can occur in the absence of translation, since it occurs in the presence of inhibitors of protein synthesis. The next stage is the protein synthesis stage which is sensitive to inhibitors of protein synthesis. This stage can proceed in the absence of RNA synthesis and is therefore not inhibited by actinomycin D. During this stage amino acids are polymerized into polypeptide chains. The next step appears to be an assembly process of the newly-made polypeptide chains. This is independent of protein synthesis and may persist for up to 2 hours. This entire process results in the appearance of increased levels of aryl hydrocarbon hydroxylase. The specific protein, which is made and assembled in the microsomes, may be either the hydroxylase or another protein which may activate an inactive form of the hydroxylase by an allosteric mechanism. All of these events appear before there are gross changes in either protein or RNA synthesis. This suggests that the RNA and protein, which must be synthesized, are very small percentages of total cell RNA and protein and that many of the gross changes of RNA and protein synthesis may be subsequent or parallel to, but not directly responsible for, the appearance of the early increases in enzyme level.

G. The Effect of Inducers on RNA Metabolism

Loeb and Gelboin (1964) and Hishizawa et al. (1964) reported an increased orotic acid incorporation into RNA after MC treatment. Jervell et al. (1965) obtained the same results using liver slices. The latter determined the specific activities of acid-soluble uridine nucleotides in the preparation from MC-treated rats and found them greater than that of the control rats. They pointed out, however, that the higher specific activities of the acid-soluble uridine nucleotides from the MC-treated rats did not account for all of the increase in the specific activity of the RNA. The above investigators suggested that the increased specific activity of the RNA indicates an MC-induced increase in the rate of RNA synthesis. This conclusion must be viewed with caution, since the intracellular and intranuclear pool sizes of precursors of RNA, as well as the rate of degradation of RNA, may markedly affect the specific activity of the RNA. BRESNICK et al. (1966) reported a failure to detect increased orotic acid incorporation after MC pretreatment, but they did not investigate the specific activity of the RNA precursors.

An accumulation of RNA in the nuclei of MC-treated rats may be expected if MC increases the rate of nuclear RNA synthesis and does not concomitantly increase the rate of RNA degradation or the transfer of RNA out of the nucleus. LOEB and GELBOIN (1963, 1964) reported that MC has no effect on the amount of DNA per gram of wet liver; also, 4 hours after MC treatment the RNA content of isolated nuclei was the same as in the controls. However, 16 hours after MC treatment they found a significant increase in the amount of nuclear RNA. In four experiments, there was a 15—50% increase in the RNA content of the isolated nuclei as shown by an increase in the RNA to DNA ratio.

LOEB and GELBOIN (1964) reported that the sedimentation profile of nuclear RNA from control and MC-treated animals was grossly similar. These findings were confirmed by BRESNICK et al. (1966). Normal nuclear RNA showed three peaks of RNA which corresponded to 33S, 19S, and 6S (Svedberg units). The stimulatory effect of MC on orotic acid incorporation was unequal in the various RNA fractions analyzed but was largest in the 9S to 23S region. This area corresponds roughly to some of the RNA fractions reported to have the greater amount of activity in stimulating the incorporation of amino acids into protein in a cell-free *E. coli* system.

LOEB and GELBOIN (1964) tested the nuclear RNA obtained from normal and MC-treated rats for its activity in directing the incorporation of L-phenylalanine-(U)-C^{14} into protein in the cell-free *E.coli* system of MATTHAEI and NIRENBERG (1961). In this system, isolated nuclear RNA had 5—10 times the stimulatory activity of microsomal RNA isolated by a similar procedure. Soluble RNA showed no activity. The nuclear RNA from the MC-treated rats was 29—57% more active than were equivalent amounts of RNA obtained from normal rats.

HOLLAND et al. (1966) have shown that heated ribosomal RNA as well as DNA is able to act as template in the incorporation of amino acids in an *E.coli* system. These results suggest the possibility that the increased template activity may not be due to a greater number of messenger RNA molecules but may be due to an MC-induced alteration in the physical state of the RNA.

GELBOIN et al. (1967) found that 3 hours after MC treatment and 20 hours after phenobarbital treatment, there was a 30—50% increase in RNA polymerase activity of rat liver nuclei.

MADIX and BRESNICK (1967) have reported a stimulation in the template activity of chromatin isolated from the liver of rats pretreated with MC for 16 hours. Thus, in studies with either isolated nuclei or isolated chromatin, MC appears to increase template activity. The increase is not observed when isolated DNA is used as a template and there is no effect of MC on the melting temperature of DNA isolated from rat liver.

BRESNICK et al. (1968) reported changes in cytoplasmic RNA after the administration of MC. These changes were observed by 3 hours after MC was administered and involved an increased incorporation of a nucleic acid precursor to

Table 1. *Summary of Effects of Methylcholanthrene (MC) or Phenobarbital (PB) on Gene-action System*

Microsomes	Nucleus
Increase of:	*Increase of:*
(1) Specific enzymes and protein (MC, PB)	(1) Orotic acid-^{14}C incorporation into RNA (MC)
(2) Amino acid incorporation (MC, PB)	(2) RNA/DNA ratio (MC)
(a) More mRNA (PB)	(3) Messenger RNA content (MC)
(b) More sensitive to added mRNA (PB)	(4) Stimulation of RNA polymerase (MC, PB)
(3) Effects prevented by:	
(a) Puromycin (MC, PB)	
(b) Actinomycin-D (MC, PB)	
(c) Ethionine (MC, PB)	
Inhibition of:	
(1) NADPH cytochrome *c* reductase degradation (PB)	
(2) b_5 degradation (PB)	
Changes in:	
(1) Spectral properties of P_{450} (MC)	
(2) Phospholipid metabolism (MC)	
(3) Kinetic behavior of hydroxylase (MC)	

a 45S cytoplasmic particle in the liver of MC-treated rats. This effect was also observed in adrenalectomized rats. These authors suggest that MC increased the turnover of ribosomal RNA and that ribosomal RNA may have a role in the microsomal enzyme induction. It is possible that this change in ribosomal RNA synthesis is related to the increased amino acid incorporating ability in microsomes from drug-treated rats.

Thus, the various studies on the effect of MC on nuclear RNA metabolism have shown that: 1. MC causes an increase in the uptake of orotic acid into nuclear RNA which suggests increased RNA synthesis; 2. MC increases the amount of RNA in liver cell nuclei; 3. RNA isolated from the liver cell nuclei of MC-treated rats has greater stimulatory activity in an *E. coli* phenylalanine-incorporating system; and 4. the administration of MC *in vivo* stimulates RNA polymerase activity of either isolated liver nuclei or isolated chromatin. These effects of MC suggest an alteration in genetic transcription.

Table 1 is a summary of the various effects of methylcholanthrene (MC) and phenobarbital (PB) on several aspects of nuclear and microsomal metabolism.

References

ALFRED, L. J., GELBOIN, H. V.: Benzpyrene hydroxylase induction by polycyclic hydrocarbons in hamster embryonic cells grown *in vitro*. Science **157**, 75—76 (1967).

ALVARES, A. P., SCHILLING, G. R., KUNTZMAN, R.: Differences in the kinetics of benzpyrene hydroxylation by hepatic drug-metabolizing enzymes from phenobarbital and 3-methylcholanthrene-treated rats. Biochem. biophys. Res. Commun. **30**, 588—593 (1968).

ARCOS, J. S., CONNEY, A. H., BUU-HOI, N. P.: Induction of microsomal enzyme synthesis by polycyclic aromatic hydrocarbons of different molecular sizes. J. biol. Chem. **236**, 1291 to 1296 (1961).

BERLIN, C. M., SCHIMKE, R. T.: Influence of turnover rates on the responses of enzymes to cortisone. Molec. Pharmacol. **1**, 149—156 (1965).

BOJARSKI, T. B., HIATT, H. H.: Stabilization of thymidylate kinase activity by thymidylate and by thymidine. Nature (Lond.) **188**, 1112—1114 (1960).

BRESNICK, E., BRAND, R., KNIGHT, J. A.: Ribonucleic acid biosynthesis in methylcholanthrene-treated rats. Biochim. biophys. Acta (Amst.) **114**, 227—233 (1966).

BRESNICK, E., SYNERHOLM, M.E., TIZARD, G.T.: Changes in liver cytoplasmic RNA after administration of 3-methylcholanthrene. Molec. Pharmacol. **4**, 218—223 (1968).

CONNEY, A.H.: Enzyme induction and drug toxicity. In: Proc. 2nd Intl. Pharmacol. Mtg, Vol. **4**, pp. 277—297, Prague. New York: Pergamon Press 1965.

— Pharmacological implications of microsomal enzyme induction. Pharmacol. Rev. **19**, 317—366 (1967).

— DAVISON, C., GASTEL, R., BURNS, J.J.: Adaptive increases in drug-metabolizing enzymes induced by phenobarbital and other drugs. J. Pharmacol. exp. Ther. **130**, 1—8 (1960).

— GILMAN, A.G.: Puromycin inhibition of enzyme induction by 3-methylcholanthrene and phenobarbital. J. biol. Chem. **238**, 3682—3685 (1963).

DECKEN, A., VON DER HULTIN, T.: Inductive effects of 3-methylcholanthrene on enzyme activities and amino acid incorporation capacity of rat liver microsomes. Arch. Biochem. Biophys. **90**, 201—207 (1960).

DIAMOND, L., GELBOIN, H.V.: Alpha-naphthoflavone: an inhibitor of hydrocarbon cytotoxicity and microsomal hydroxylase. Science **166**, 1023—1025 (1969).

ERNSTER, L., ORRENIUS, S.: Substrate-induced synthesis of the hydroxylating enzyme system of liver microsomes. Fed. Proc. **24**, 1190—1199 (1965).

FEIGELSON, P., GREENGARD, O.: Regulation of liver tryptophan pyrrolase activity. J. biol. Chem. **237**, 1908—1913 (1962).

FOUTS, J.R., ROGERS, L.A.: Morphological changes in the liver accompanying stimulation of microsomal drug metabolizing enzyme activity by phenobarbital, chlordane, benzpyrene or methylcholanthrene in rats. J. Pharmacol. exp. Ther. **147**, 112—119 (1965).

GELBOIN, H.V.: Studies on the mechanism of methylcholanthrene induction of enzyme activities. II. Stimulation of microsomal and ribosomal amino acid incorporation: The effects of polyuridylic acid and actinomycin D. Biochim. biophys. Acta (Amst.) **91**, 130 to 144 (1964).

— Carcinogens, enzyme induction and gene action. Advanc. Cancer Res. **10**, 1—81 (1967).

— Effect of carcinogens on gene action. Monograph of 22nd Annual Symp. on Fundamental Cancer Research, Univ. of Texas, M.D. Anderson Hosp., Houston, Texas (March 1968).

— BLACKBURN, N.: Stimulatory effect of 3-methylcholanthrene on microsomal amino acid incorporation and benzpyrene hydroxylase activity and its inhibition of actinomycin D. Biochim. biophys. Acta (Amst.) **72**, 657—660 (1963).

— SOKOLOFF, L.: The effects of 3-methylcholanthrene and phenobarbital on amino acid incorporation into protein. Science **134**, 611—612 (1961).

— — Studies on the mechanism of methylcholanthrene induction of enzyme activities of rat liver. Biochim. biophys. Acta (Amst.) **91**, 122—129 (1964).

— WORTHAM, J.J., WILSON, R.G.: 3-methylcholanthrene and phenobarbital stimulation of rat liver RNA polymerase. Nature (Lond.) **214**, 281—283 (1967).

GILLETTE, J.R.: Metabolism of drugs and other foreign compounds by enzymatic mechanisms. Progr. Drug. Res. **6**, 11—73 (1963).

GRANICK, S.: Induction of the synthesis of δ-aminolevulinic acid synthetase in liver parenchyma cells in culture by chemicals that induce acute porphyria. J. biol. Chem. **238**, PC 2247—2249 (1963).

— The induction *in vitro* of the synthesis of δ-aminolevulinic acid synthetase in chemical porphyria: A response to certain drugs, sex hormones, and foreign chemicals. J. biol. Chem. **241**, 1359—1375 (1966).

— URATA, G.: Increase in activity of δ-aminolevulinic acid synthetase in liver mitochondria induced by feeding of 3,5-dicarbethoxy-1,4-dihydrocollidine. J. biol. Chem. **238**, 821—827 (1963).

GURTOO, H.L., CAMPBELL, T.C., WEBB, R.E., PLOWMAN, K.M.: Effect of aflatoxin and benzpyrene pretreatment upon the kinetics of benzpyrene hydroxylase. Biochem. biophys. Res. Commun. **31**, 588—595 (1968).

HILDEBRANDT, A., REMMER, H., ESTABROOK, R.W.: Cytochrome P-450 of liver microsomes — one pigment or many. Biochem. biophys. Res. Commun. **30**, 607—612 (1968).

HISHIZAWA, T., OTSUKA, H., TERAYAMA, H.: Metabolic behavior of nucleic acids in subcellular fractions from liver of rats treated with methylcholanthrene. J. Biochem. (Tokyo) **56**, 97—100 (1964).

HOLLAND, J.J., CLAYTON, A.B., MCCARTHY, B.J.: Stimulation of protein synthesis *in vitro* by partially degraded ribosomal ribonucleic acid and transfer ribonucleic acid. Biochem. J. **5**, 358—365 (1966).

HOLTZMAN, J.L., GILLETTE, J.R.: The effect of phenobarbital on the turnover of microsomal phospholipid in male and female rats. J. biol. Chem. **243**, 3020—3028 (1968).

JERVELL, K.F., CHRISTOFFERSEN, T., MORLAND, J.: Studies on the 3-methylcholanthrene induction and carbohydrate repression of rat liver dimethylaminoazobenzene reductase. Arch. Biochem. **111**, 15—22 (1965).

JICK, H., SHUSTER, L.: The turnover of microsomal reduced nicotinamide adenine dinucleotide phosphatecytochrome *c* reductase in the livers of mice treated with phenobarbital. J. biol. Chem. **241**, 5366—5369 (1966).
JUCHAU, M. R., CRAM, R. L., PLAA, G. L., FOUTS, J. R.: The induction of benzpyrene hydroxylase in the isolated perfused rat liver. Biochem. Pharmacol. **14**, 473—482 (1965).
KATO, R., JONDORF, W. R., LOEB, L. A., BEN, T., GELBOIN, H. V.: Studies on the mechanism of drug induced microsomal enzyme activities. V. Phenobarbital stimulation of endogenous messenger RNA and polyuridylic acid-directed L-[^{14}C]-phenylalanine incorporation. Molec. Pharmacol. **2**, 171—186 (1966).
— LOEB, L., GELBOIN, H. V.: Microsome-specific stimulation by phenobarbital of amino acid incorporation *in vivo*. Biochem. Pharmacol. **14**, 1164—1166 (1965).
KORNER, A., MUNRO, A.: Actinomycin inhibition of *in vitro* protein synthesis in rat liver. Biochem. biophys. Res. Commun. **11**, 235—238 (1963).
KUNTZMAN, R., LEVIN, W., JACOBSON, M., CONNEY, A. H.: Studies on microsomal hydroxylation and the demonstration of a new carbon monoxide binding pigment in liver microsomes. Life Sci. **7**, 215—224 (1968).
KURIYAMA, Y., OMURA, T., SIEKEVITZ, P., PALADE, G. E.: Effect of phenobarbital on the synthesis and degradation of the protein components of rat liver microsomal membranes. J. biol. Chem. **244**, 2017—2026 (1969).
LEVIN, W., KUNTZMAN, R.: Studies on the incorporation of δ-aminolevulinic acid into microsomal hemoprotein: Effect of 3-methylcholanthrene and phenobarbital. Life Sci. **8**, 305 to 311 (1969).
LOEB, L. A., GELBOIN, H. V.: Stimulation of aminoacid incorporation by nuclear ribonucleic acid from normal and methylcholanthrene-treated rats. Nature (Lond.) **199**, 809—810 (1963).
— — Methylcholanthreneinduced changes in rat liver nuclear RNA. Proc. nat. Acad. Sci. (Wash.) **52**, 1219—1226 (1964).
MADIX, J. C., BRESNICK, E.: Increased efficacy of liver chromatin as a template for RNA synthesis after administration of 3-methylcholanthrene. Biochem. biophys. Res. Commun. **28**, 445—452 (1967).
MARVER, H. S.: The role of heme in the synthesis and repression of microsomal protein. Proc. Mtg. of Intl. Symposium on Microsomes and Drug Oxidation, Bethesda, Md., Feb. 1968.
— COLLINS, A., TSCHUDY, D. P., RECHCIGL, M., JR.: δ-aminolevulinic acid synthetase. J. biol. Chem. **241**, 4323—4329 (1966).
MATTHAEI, J. H., NIRENBERG, M. W.: Characteristics and stabilization of DNAase-sensitive protein synthesis in *E. coli* extracts. Proc. nat. Acad. Sci. (Wash.) **47**, 1580—1588 (1961).
MCAUSLAN, B. R.: The induction and repression of thymidine kinase in the poxvirus-infected HeLa cell. Virology **21**, 383—389 (1963).
MERITS, I.: Actinomycin inhibition of RNA synthesis in rat liver. Biochem. biophys. Res. Commun. **10**, 254—259 (1963).
MILLER, J., GELBOIN, H. V.: Unpublished observations.
MONOD, J., JACOB, F.: Teleonomic mechanism in cellular metabolism, growth and differentiation. Cold Spr. Harb. Symp. quant. Biol. **28**, 389—401 (1961).
NEBERT, D. W., GELBOIN, H. V.: Substrate-inducible aryl hydroxylase in mammalian cell cultures: I. Assay and properties of induced enzyme. J. biol. Chem. **243**, 6242—6249 (1968a).
— — Substrate-inducible microsomal aryl hydroxylase in mammalian cell culture. II. Cellular responses during enzyme induction. J. biol. Chem. **243**, 6250—6261 (1968b).
— — The role of RNA and protein synthesis in microsomal aryl hydrocarbon hydroxylase induction in cell culture: The independence of transcription and translation. J. biol. Chem. **245**, 160—168 (1970).
NEURATH, H., DIXON, G. H.: Structure and activation of trypsinogen and chymotrypsinogen. Fed. Proc. **16**, 791—801 (1957).
OMURA, T., SIEKEVITZ, P., PALADE, G. E.: Turnover of constituents of the endoplasmic reticulum membranes of rat hepatocytes. J. biol. Chem. **242**, 2389—2396 (1967).
ORRENIUS, S., ERICSSON, J. L. E.: Enzyme-membrane relationship in phenobarbital induction of synthesis of drug-metabolizing enzyme system and proliferation of endoplasmic membranes. J. Cell. Biol. **28**, 181—198 (1966).
— — ERNSTER, L.: Phenobarbital-induced synthesis of the microsomal drug-metabolizing enzyme system and its relationship to the proliferation of endoplasmic membranes. A morphological and biochemical study. J. Cell. Biol. **25**, 627—639 (1965).
PETERKOFSKY, B., TOMKINS, G. M.: Effect of inhibitors of nucleic acid synthesis on steroid-mediated induction of tyrosine aminotransferase in hepatoma cell cultures. J. molec. Biol. **30**, 49—61 (1967).

REICH, E., FRANKLIN, R.M., SHATKIN, A.J., TATUM, E.L.: Effect of actinomycin D on cellular nucleic acid synthesis and virus production. Science **134**, 556—557 (1961).

REMMER, H., MERKER, H.J.: Drug-induced changes in the liver endoplasmic reticulum: Association with drugmetabolizing enzymes. Science **142**, 1657—1658 (1963).

SCHENKMAN, J.B., GRAIN, H., ZANGE, M., REMMER, H.: On the problem of possible other forms of cytochrome P_{450} in liver microsomes. Biochim. biophys. Acta (Amst.) **171**, 23—31 (1969).

— SATO, R.: The relationship between the pH-induced spectral change in ferriprotoheme and the substrate-induced spectral change of the microsomal mixed-function oxidase. Molec. Pharmacol. **4**, 613—620 (1968).

SCHIMKE, R.T.: The importance of both synthesis and degradation in the control of arginase levels in rat liver. J. biol. Chem. **239**, 3808—3817 (1964).

— SWEENEY, E.W., BERLIN, C.M.: An analysis of the kinetics of rat liver tryptophan pyrrolase induction: The significance of both enzyme synthesis and degradation. Biochem. biophys. Res. Commun. **15**, 214—219 (1964).

SIEFERT, J. VON, GREIM, H., CHANDRA, P.: Die Wirkung von Phenobarbital auf die Ribosomenfraktionen der Rattenleber. Hoppe-Seylers Z. physiol. Chem. **349**, 1179—1184 (1968).

SLADEK, N.E., MANNERING, G.J.: Induction of drug metabolism. I. Differences in the mechanisms by which polycyclic hydrocarbons and phenobarbital produce their inductive effects on microsomal N-demethylating systems. Molec. Pharmacol. **5**, 174—185 (1969a).

— — Induction of drug metabolism. II. Qualitative differences in the microsomal N-demethylating systems stimulated by polycyclic hydrocarbons and by phenobarbital. Molec. Pharmacol. **5**, 186—199 (1969b).

STEPHEN, J.M.L., WATERLOW, J.C.: Use of carbon-14-labelled arginine to measure the catabolic rate of serum and liver proteins and the extent of amino-acid recycling. Nature (Lond.) **211**, 978—980 (1966).

SWICK, R.W.: Measurement of protein turnover in rat liver. J. biol. Chem. **231**, 751—764 (1958).

— HANDE, D.T.: The distribution of fixed carbon in amino acids. J. biol. Chem. **218**, 577—585 (1956).

TAMAOKI, T., MUELLER, G.C.: Synthesis of nuclear and cytoplasmic RNA of HeLa cells and the effect of actinomycin D. Biochem. biophys. Res. Commun. **9**, 451—454 (1962).

TATIBANA, M., COHEN, P.P.: Formation and conversion of macromolecular precursor(s) in the biosynthesis of carbamyl phosphate synthetase. Proc. nat. Acad. Sci. (Wash.) **53**, 104—111 (1965).

THOMPSON, E.B., TOMKINS, G.M., CURRAN, J.F.: Induction of tyrosine α-ketoglutarate transaminase by steroid hormones in a newly established tissue culture cell line. Proc. nat. Acad. Sci. (Wash.) **56**, 296—303 (1966).

TOMKINS, G.M., GARREN, L.D., HOWELL, R.R., PETERKOFSKY, B.: The regulation of enzyme synthesis by steroid hormones: The role of translation. J. cell. comp. Physiol. **66**, 137—151 (1965).

TSCHUDY, D.P., PERLROTH, M.G., MARVER, H.S., COLLINS, A., HUNTER, G., JR.: Acute intermittent porphyria: The first "overproduction disease" localized to a specific enzyme. Proc. nat. Acad. Sci. (Wash.) **53**, 841—847 (1965).

YARMOLINSKY, M.B., DE LA HABA, G.L.: Inhibition by puromycin of amino acid incorporation into protein. Proc. nat. Acad. Sci. (Wash.) **45**, 1721—1729 (1959).

Chapter 49

Inhibition of Drug Metabolism

G. J. Mannering

With 1 Figure

Rates of drug metabolism in animals can be reduced in a variety of ways: adrenalectomy (Remmer, 1958a, b), alloxan induced diabetes (Dixon et al., 1961, 1963), administration of inhibitors of protein synthesis, such as ethionine (Conney et al., 1956, 1960; Fujimoto and Plaa, 1961), actinomycin D (Orrenius and Ernster, 1964; Gelboin and Blackburn, 1964), puromycin (Orrenius and Ernster, 1964; Gelboin and Blackburn, 1964) and thioacetamide (Sladek and Mannering, 1969a). Drug metabolism can also be inhibited by X-irradiation (Varagić et al., 1962; Hietbrink and Dubois, 1964; Dubois, 1967) and alkylating agents which mimic the action of X-irradiation (Tardiff and Dubois, 1969), administration of yellow phosphorus (Herken et al., 1958; Neubert and Maibauer, 1959) or radioactive phosphate (Sulser et al., 1966), starvation (Dixon et al., 1960; Kato and Gillette, 1965), and vitamin C deficiency (Axelrod et al., 1954b; Conney et al., 1961). This chapter is not concerned with these indirect means of depressing drug metabolism; it will restrict itself to inhibition as it is more narrowly defined to mean the interference of the metabolism of one agent by another agent at the enzymic site. This automatically excludes such agents as thyroxin (Cochin and Sokoloff, 1960; Conney and Garren, 1961; Mannering et al., 1969), morphine (Axelrod, 1956a; Mannering and Takemori, 1959; Chaplin et al., 1968), CCl_4 (Castro et al., 1968; Dingell and Heimberg, 1968; Sasame et al., 1968), 3-amino-1,2,4-triazole (Kato, 1967; Baron and Tephly, 1969), and *p*-aminosalicylic acid (Rogers et al., 1963a), which are thought to reduce drug metabolism by mechanisms other than direct inhibition at the metabolic site. The chapter will make no attempt to catalog inhibitors of drug metabolism. The probability of any one drug inhibiting the metabolism of another is very high, at least *in vitro*, and the time can be foreseen when the growing list of inhibitors might fill a volume of this size. As a final limitation, the chapter will deal only with the hepatic microsomal enzyme system, known to be responsible for the oxidation and reduction of most drugs. It will not be concerned with the inhibitory action of drugs on enzymes that are primarily involved in the metabolism of natural substrates (e.g., the cholinesterase or monoamine oxidase inhibitors), nor will it be concerned with the inhibition of drug metabolism involving hydrolysis or conjugation reactions.

A. Methods of Determining Inhibition of Drug Metabolism

I. *In Vivo* Methods

The inhibitory effect of an agent on the metabolism of a drug *in vivo* can be determined by three general procedures. After pretreatment of an animal with

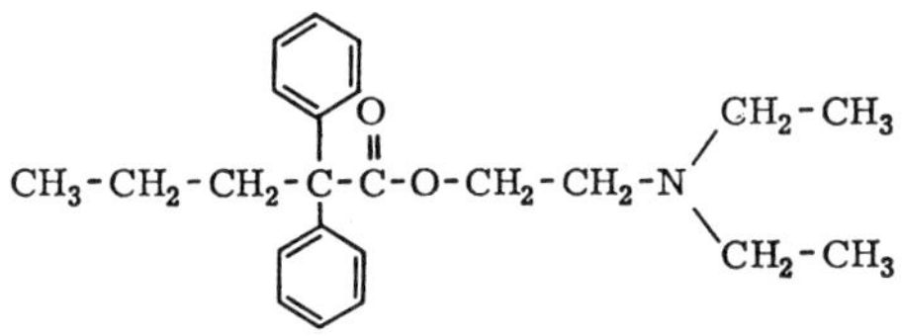

SKF 525-A

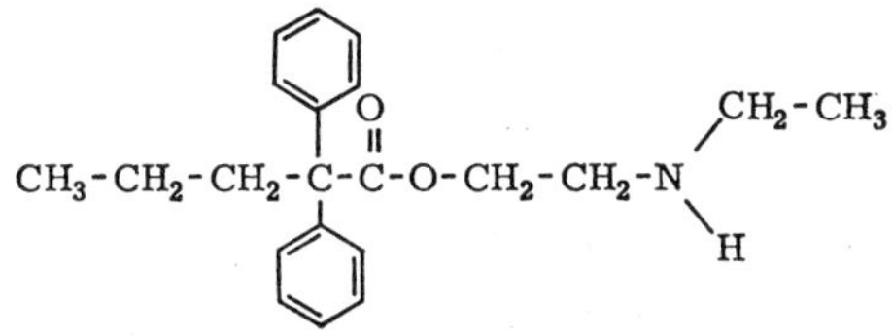

SKF 8742-A

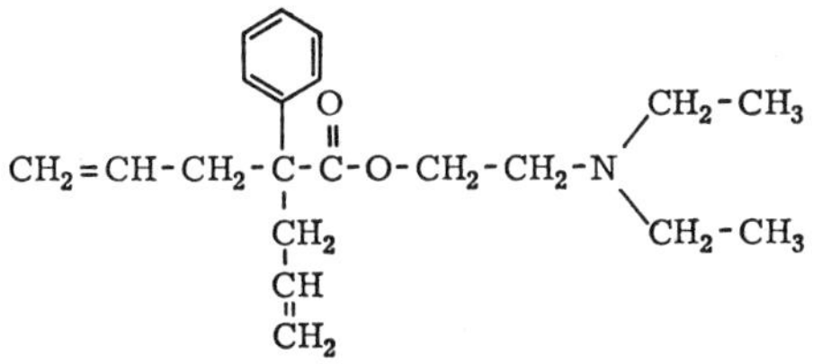

CFT 1201

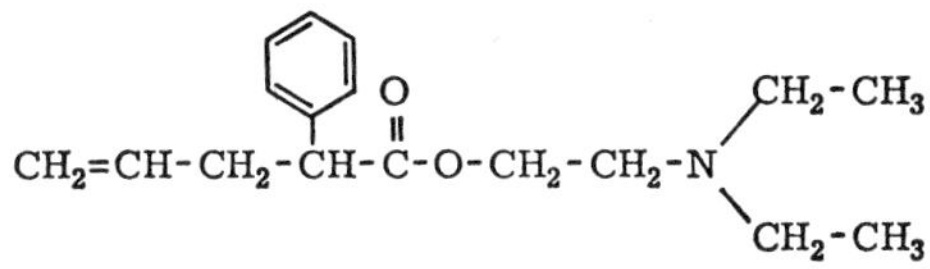

CFT 1208

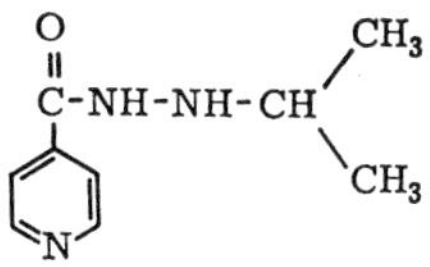

Iproniazid

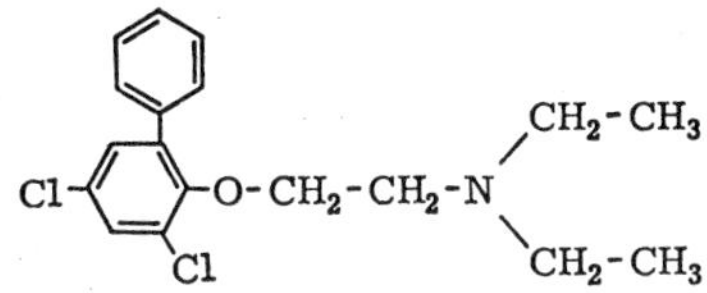

Lilly 18947

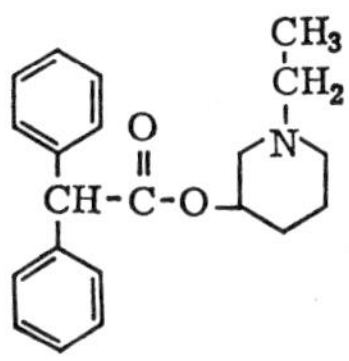

JB 305

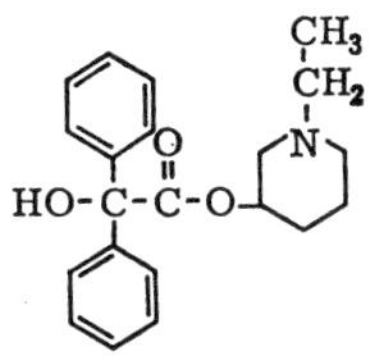

JB 318

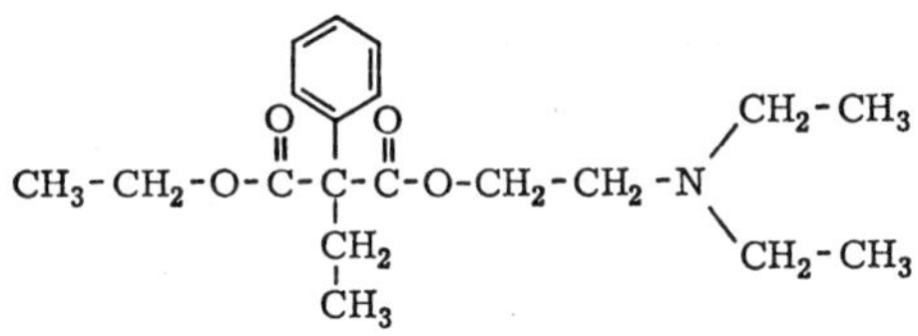

Sch 5705

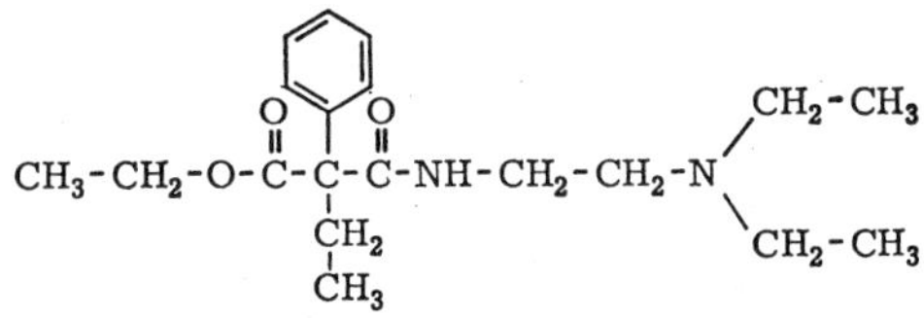

Sch 5706

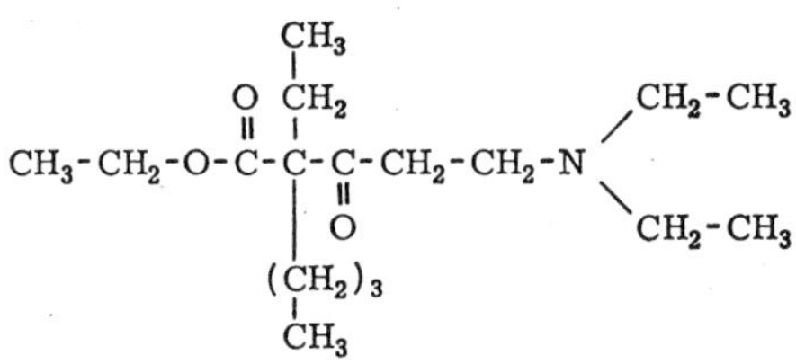

Sch 5712

Fig. 1. Examples of prolonging agents

Table 1. *Inhibitors of drug metabolism*

Code	*Chemical Name*	*Reference*
SKF 525-A	2-Diethylaminoethyl 2,2-diphenylvalerate HCl	COOK et al. (1954b); BRODIE (1956)
SKF 8742-A	2-Ethylaminoethyl 2,2-diphenylvalerate HCl	SCHENKMAN et al. (1967a)
CFT 1201	2-Diethylaminoethyl 2-phenyl-2-(2-propene)-4-penten-1-oate HCl	NEUBERT and HERKEN (1955)
CFT 1208	2-Diethylaminoethyl 2-phenyl-4-penten-l-oate HCl	NEUBERT and HERKEN (1955)
Iproniazid	1-Isopropyl-2-isonicotinyl hydrazine PO_4	FOUTS and BRODIE (1956)
Lilly 18947	2,4-Dichloro-6-phenylphenoxyethyldiethylamine HBr	FOUTS and BRODIE (1955)
JB 305	N-Ethyl-3-piperidyl diphenylacetate HCl	FUJIMOTO et al. (1960)
JB 318	N-Ethyl-3-piperidyl benzilate HCl	FUJIMOTO et al. (1960)
Sch 5705	Ethyl 2-diethylaminoethyl 2-phenyl-2-ethyl-malonate HBr	KRAMER and ARRIGONI-MARTELLI (1959)
Sch 5706	Ethyl N-(2-diethylaminoethyl) 2-phenyl-2-ethylmalonamate HBr	KRAMER and ARRIGONI-MARTELLI (1959
Sch 5712	Ethyl 2-diethylaminoethyl 2-ethyl-2-butyl-malonate HBr	KRAMER and ARRIGONI-MARTELLI (1959)

an inhibitor, the drug is administered, or the two are given simultaneously, and a) plasma or tissue levels of the drug are assayed at intervals after injection of the drug, b) the amounts of drug metabolite excreted over selected time periods are determined, or c) the prolonging effect of the inhibitor on the action of the drug is measured. The plasma level of a drug may not always reflect the rate of drug metabolism accurately because of a highly inequitable distribution of drug between blood and other tissues and the effect the inhibitor may have on this distribution, or because of the roles of biliary and renal excretion in drug disappearance and the effect that the inhibitor may have on these processes. Measuring the rate of drug metabolism by measuring the rate of metabolite formation can also present some problems. The metabolite measured may be only one of several and it may represent the final product of a series of reactions, not all of which are inhibited by the agent in question. Least reliable of the *in vivo* methods is the measurement of the effect of the inhibitor on the duration of action of the drug. The test is limited, *a priori*, to inhibitors which do not in themselves produce actions similar or opposite to that measured. Furthermore, one drug can prolong the action of another in ways other than by inhibiting its biotransformation, even if the effects of the two drugs are not similar or opposite. Diazepam and chlordiazepoxide, drugs without inherent hypnotic effects, increased pentobarbital sleeping time without inhibiting pentobarbital metabolism (JORI et al., 1969). The phenylacetic acid esters, CFT 1201 and CFT 1208 (Fig. 1, Table 1), injected intraperitoneally, potentiated the analgesic action of 0.5 μg of morphine, injected into the posterior portion of the brain of mice 90 min later. This might suggest that the CFT compounds were inhibiting morphine metabolism, especially since they are known to be effective inhibitors of microsomal drug metabolism. However, when very small amounts of the CFT compounds (50 μg) were injected into the brain, they potentiated the analgesic action of morphine injected subcutaneously (10 mg/kg) 80 min later. These small amounts of the CFT compounds could hardly be expected to have inhibited hepatic metabolism of morphine, and it was concluded that they exerted their effects at the level of the central nervous system. SKF 525-A (Fig. 1, Table 1), the potent inhibitor of drug metabolism, is claimed to potentiate the action of curarizing agents by increasing their concentrations at receptors (BETTSCHART et al., 1956; BOVET et al., 1956).

II. *In Vitro* Methods

In systems *in vitro*, inhibitory potency is usually reported as the amount of inhibitor necessary to inhibit a given reaction by 50% (I_{50}) or as its inhibition constant (K_I). The I_{50} is useful for the rapid comparison of large numbers of inhibitors, but these values should not be treated as constants, since they may depend upon the substrate concentration employed in the assay system. The selected substrate concentration should be one that is decidedly on a linear portion of the velocity vs. substrate concentration curve. Inhibitor constants are more meaningful values for purposes of comparison; they also furnish information about the nature of the inhibitory mechanism. The familiar Lineweaver-Burk plot (1/v vs. 1/S) is the most popular method of determining K_I values. For a competitive inhibitor the intercept on the horizontal axis ($1/K'_m$) is represented by the expression, $\frac{1}{K_m(1 + i/K_I)}$, where K_m is the Michaelis constant of the substrate and i is the concentration of the inhibitor (DIXON and WEBB, 1964b). The expression can be rewritten as follows: $K_I = \frac{K_m \cdot i}{K'_m - K_m}$, where K'_m is the apparent K_m of the inhibited reaction. The major, and sometimes very serious, problem presented by the Lineweaver-Burk method is the possibility of drawing plots that are biased. There is a tendency to accord too much weight to velocities obtained at low substrate concentrations. WILKINSON (1961) has pointed out that at substrate concentrations ranging from one-third to three times the K_m, the relative weights of 1/v can vary by factors as high as 80. WILKINSON has minimized this difficulty through the application of weighted and non-linear regression analysis. CLELAND (1963) has written a FORTRAN program for a digital computer to facilitate calculation of the WILKINSON analysis. Using the computer in this manner, we have reexamined a number of published Lineweaver-Burk plots, purported to show either competitive or non-competitive inhibition, and have been unable in certain cases to distinguish one type of inhibition from the other. When plots are not drawn with the aid of statistics, the Hofstee plot (v vs. v/S) appears to have some advantages over the Lineweaver-Burk plot (DOWD and RIGGS, 1965). Even when statistical methods are employed, the Hofstee plot may sometimes be used to advantage; when the plot intersects the y axis very close to the x axis and the standard error is quite large, the computer is not always able to distinguish between a plus and a minus value. Inhibitor constants are frequently determined by the Dixon plot, 1/v vs. i (DIXON, 1953).

Failure to observe certain fundamental principles of enzymology have too often invalidated *in vitro* inhibition studies. The most frequent error is that resulting from unreliable initial velocities, obtained either because the velocity is not linear throughout the incubation period due to deterioration of the enzyme system, or because substrate or enzyme concentrations are such that a high percentage of the substrate is metabolized during the selected incubation period. The latter difficulty can be corrected, in part, by employing an integrated Michaelis equation (DIXON and WEBB, 1964a; ANDERS and MANNERING, 1966a).

III. Combined *in Vivo — in Vitro* Methods

In certain studies, inhibitors are given to animals and at various intervals thereafter livers are removed for *in vitro* studies. Reaction rates are compared with those obtained with liver preparations from untreated animals. Depressed activity usually results from some change produced by the inhibitor in the microsomal enzyme system, e.g., a loss of cytochrome P-450 due to CCl_4 administration (CASTRO et al., 1968, DINGELL and HEIMBERG, 1968; SASAME et al., 1968). *In vitro* activity of liver preparations is often unaffected by pretreatment of the animals with drugs that are inhibitors of liver activity *in vivo*. This is assumed to be due to the loss of the drug during the preparation of the microsomes used in the *in vitro* study. However, administration of compounds like SKF 525-A (ROGERS and FOUTS, 1964; ANDERS et al., 1966; KRATZ and STAUDINGER, 1968), chloramphenicol (DIXON and FOUTS, 1962) and the N,N'-bis (dichloroacetyl) diamines, WIN 13,099 and WIN 18,446 (MEROLA and TURNBULL, 1967), which remain firmly bound to subcellular membrane systems, yields microsomes with depressed drug-metabolizing activities.

B. Implication of a Common Drug Metabolizing System

A wide variety of oxidative and reductive reactions are known to occur in hepatic microsomes: deamination, O-, N- and S-dealkylation, hydroxylation of alkyl and aryl hydrocarbons, epoxidation, formation of alkylol derivatives, N-hydroxylation, N- and S-oxidation, dehalogenation, and azo- and nitro-reduction (reviewed by GILLETTE, 1963, 1966, 1970; GILLETTE and co-editors, 1969; MANNERING, 1968, 1970). All of these varied biotransformations are thought to be catalyzed by a single enzyme complex involving cytochrome P-450, by a limited number of oxidase systems involving one or more CO-sensitive cytochromes, or by enzyme complexes which differ only in the way in which cytochrome P-450 is associated with the microsomal membrane. We reasoned that if the microsomal drug metabolizing system is essentially lacking in substrate specificity, one drug is very likely to competitively inhibit the metabolism of another by acting as an alternative substrate (RUBIN et al., 1964a). This proved to be the case when a variety of structurally unrelated drugs were employed as inhibitors. Hexobarbital, chlorpromazine, zoxazolamine, phenylbutazone and acetanilide were competitive inhibitors of the N-demethylation of ethylmorphine; ethylmorphine, hexobarbital and chlorpromazine inhibited each other's metabolism competitively. When one substrate inhibits the metabolism of another and both substrates compete for the same enzyme, the degree of inhibition will relate to the K_m of the inhibitor; that is, the K_m of the inhibitor should equal the K_I of the reaction inhibited. This proved to be the case when ethylmorphine was employed as an inhibitor of the sulfoxidation of chlorpromazine and when hexobarbital was used to inhibit the N-demethylation of ethylmorphine. The K_m did not equal the K_I when chlorpromazine was the inhibitor of the N-demethylation of ethylmorphine, indicating that in this case inhibition was not a matter of simple substrate competition. Barbital and acetazolamide, drugs that are not metabolized appreciably, did not act as inhibitors.

The competitive inhibition of the metabolism of one agent by another has been demonstrated in several laboratories: the O-demethylation of *p*-nitroanisole by aminopyrine (BOOTH and GILLETTE, cited in GILLETTE, 1966), aldrin epoxidation by dihydroaldrin and γ-hexachlorohexane (BROOKS and HARRISON, 1969), the hydroxylation of dihydroaldrin by dieldrin and γ-hexachlorohexane (BROOKS and HARRISON, 1969), the demethylation of amidopyrine and the O-demethylation of *p*-nitroanisole by disulfiram (HONJO and NETTER, 1969), the O-demethylation of *p*-nitroanisole by diethyldithiocarbamate (HONJO and NETTER, 1969), the metabolism of pentobarbital by quinine and quinidine (BOULOS et al., 1970), and the N-demethylation of aminopyrine by nicotinamide (SCHENKMAN et al., 1967a).

That nicotinamide could inhibit drug metabolism was of particular interest because nicotinamide has been customarily added to incubation mixtures to prevent the loss of NADP due to the action of nucleotidase.[1]

This discussion might end with the conclusion that the kinetic data indicate the involvement of a single microsomal drug metabolizing system if it were not for other studies which showed that inhibition is not always competitive. Inhibition was not competitive in the following interactions: the side chain oxidation of hexobarbital and the hydroxylation of acetanilide by chloramphenicol (DIXON and FOUTS, 1962), the N-demethylation of morphine by nalorphine (LEADBEATER and DAVIES, 1964), the hydroxylation of aniline by nicotinamide (SCHENKMAN et al., 1967a), the O-demethylation of norcodeine by hexobarbital (GEORGE and TEPHLY, 1968), and the hydroxylation of diphenylhydantoin by isonicotinic acid hydrazine and *p*-aminosalicylic acid (KUTT et al., 1968). Since purified enzymes are not available, no definitive explanation of the mixed inhibitor kinetics can be given. The existence of at least two drug metabolizing systems would be one possible explanation. This has already been suggested by observed species and sex differences in the relative rates of drug metabolism; by drug metabolism rate changes due to environmental changes, including the administration of inducing agents; and by two-substrate kinetic studies (ALVARES and MANNERING, 1970). The kinetics of competitive inhibition do not demand that only one enzyme system be involved; the same kinetics will be seen when more than one enzyme is involved in the reaction, if these enzymes share a rate-limiting cofactor. In a multienzyme system, such as that involved in drug metabolism, different components of the same system might be rate-limiting when different drugs are substrates; this situation would yield mixed inhibition kinetics. The most likely explanation for the mixed kinetics will probably be found in the ways different drugs bind to cytochrome P-450. This will be discussed in the section dealing with the role of drug binding to cytochrome P-450.

KATO and associates (1962, 1964) showed that the microsomal metabolism of pentobarbital, hexobarbital, meprobamate, carisoprodol and strychnine was inhibited by 36 drugs. The qualitative nature of these inhibitions was not studied.

The inhibition kinetics of SKF 525-A and other so-called potentiating agents has received a great deal of attention. Because of their somewhat special nature, these agents will be discussed in a separate section.

C. Inhibition of the Metabolism of One Drug by Another Drug *in Vivo*

During the first 30 min following administration to rats, the metabolism of pentobarbital and meprobamate was inhibited by chlorcyclizine, glutethimide, phenaglycodol, imipramine and phenylisopropylhydrazine (KATO et al., 1964). Ethylmorphine and codeine inhibited the metabolism of hexobarbital by rats *in vivo* (RUBIN et al., 1964b). Imipramine and desmethylimipramine inhibited the oxidation of tremorine to oxotremorine in the rat (SJÖQVIST and GILLETTE, 1965; HAMMER and SJÖQVIST, 1966; SJÖQVIST et al., 1968). Desmethylimipramine inhibited oxotremorine metabolism in the rat, but not in the mouse (SJÖQVIST et al., 1968). Imipramine has also been shown to inhibit the metabolism of pento-

1 We were fortunate in our early studies (RUBIN et al., 1964a) not to have used a concentration of nicotinamide in our incubation mixture high enough to produce any significant inhibition of the reactions studied (PARLI and MANNERING, unpublished results). Most investigators no longer include nicotinamide in their reaction mixture.

barbital in rats (KATO et al., 1963a). The enhanced action of amphetamine seen in rats after the administration of desipramine is due to the inhibition of amphetamine metabolism (SULSER et al., 1966; VALZELLI et al., 1966). Phenyramidol inhibited the metabolism of bishydroxycoumarin in the mouse, rabbit and man (SOLOMON and SCHROGIE, 1966). Quinine increased pentobarbital sleeping time in mice and rats, decreased the LD_{50} of pentobarbital in mice, and increased the plasma half-life of pentobarbital in goats (BOULOS et al., 1970). Quinidine also increased the pentobarbital sleeping time of mice (BOULOS et al., 1970). Triparanol and benzmalacene prolonged pentobarbital hypnosis and carisoprodol paralysis in rats (KATO et al., 1963b); the effects were assumed to be due to inhibition of pentobarbital metabolism. Hydroxyzine, chlorpromazine, promazine, orphenodrine, phenobarbital, glutethimide, urethan, trimethadione, 5-ethyl-3-methyl-5-phenylhydantoin, primidone, iproniazid, SKF 525-A, carbutamide, tolbutamide, and azacyclonol increased the hexobarbital sleeping time of mice when tested one hour after administration of each drug, presumably by inhibiting hexobarbital metabolism (RÜMKE and BOUT, 1960).

Interactions of drugs at the metabolic site have been observed in man. In particular the coumarin group of anticoagulants have been implicated as inhibitors of drug biotransformation. Elevated plasma levels and toxic symptoms of diphenylhydantoin (HANSEN et al., 1966) or tolbutamine (KRISTENSEN and HANSEN, 1967) were noted in patients who had also received bishydroxycoumarin. Bishydroxycoumarin was also shown to double the half-life of chlorpropamide in man (KRISTENSEN and HANSEN, 1968). On the other hand, phenyramidol inhibits the metabolism of bishydroxycoumarin and thereby increases the effectiveness and toxicity of the anticoagulant (CARTER, 1965; SOLOMON and SCHROGIE, 1966). Other interactions in man include the inhibition of diphenylhydantoin metabolism by disulfiram (OLESEN, 1966, 1967; KIØRBOE, 1966) isoniazid (MURRAY, 1962; KUTT et al., 1966) and phenyramidol (SOLOMON and SCHROGIE, 1967) and the inhibition of tolbutamide metabolism by sulphaphenazole and phenylbutazone (CHRISTENSEN et al., 1963).

As might be predicted, not all compounds that are effective inhibitors *in vitro* act as inhibitors *in vivo*. Triparanol and chlorpromazine did not affect the metabolism of pentobarbital or meprobamate, and phenobarbital did not inhibit meprobamate metabolism in living rats (KATO et al., 1964). Morphine, norcodeine, dextromethorphan, levomethorphan, meprobamate and acetanilide, compounds known to inhibit the *in vitro* metabolism of hexobarbital, did not delay the disappearance of hexobarbital in living rats (RUBIN et al., 1964b). This is not surprising since many factors govern the overall disposition of drugs. For one drug to inhibit the metabolism of another *in vivo*, it must accumulate at the metabolic site in sufficient quantity to compete with the metabolism of the drug in question. Sufficient accumulation may not be possible because the dose of the inhibitor that can be tolerated by the animal may be too low, the inhibitor may be highly localized in other tissues, the two drugs may be metabolized by different enzymes, or the inhibitor may be eliminated from the animal much more rapidly than the drug by being more rapidly metabolized or excreted. When some of these complexities were circumvented by use of the isolated, perfused rat liver, hexobarbital metabolism was inhibited by drugs which had shown no inhibitory effect *in vivo* (STITZEL et al., 1968). The isolated, perfused liver proved useful in a study with amphetamine, which is hydroxylated by the intact rat and the perfused rat liver, but not by rat microsomes. In both the whole rat and in the perfused liver, amphetamine metabolism was inhibited by desipramine (DINGELL and BASS, 1969).

D. SKF 525-A and other Prolonging Agents

The term *prolonging agent* was proposed by BRODIE (1956) to distinguish between agents which prolong the action of drugs by interfering with their metabolism, and potentiating agents, which produce their effects by altering the responsiveness of animals to drugs. The term is usually applied to compounds which are not used to produce pharmacodynamic effects of their own, or at least not effects similar to those being measured. SKF 525-A is one of the most potent, and certainly the most studied, prolonging agents. A congener of adiphenine, it was synthesized as a possible parasympatholytic agent. It proved not to be useful for this purpose but showed the very interesting property of prolonging the hypnotic action of hexobarbital while lacking any sedative activity of its own (COOK et al., 1954c). Early work by COOK and his associates suggested that SKF 525-A might have some general effect in prolonging the action of many drugs of different pharmacologic activity; they showed that the duration of action of amphetamine, chloral hydrate, many barbiturates and several analgesics was greatly prolonged after its administration (COOK et al., 1954a, b). The answer to the way in which SKF 525-A produced its effects was soon forthcoming from Brodie's laboratory where the prolonging effect was shown to be due to the inhibition of drug metabolism (BRODIE, 1956). Since then, the inclusion of SKF 525-A in the protocols of drug metabolism studies in many laboratories has become almost a reflex action; the list of drugs, the metabolism of which are inhibited by this prolonging agent, both *in vitro* and *in vivo*, is growing steadily.

SKF 525-A does not inhibit the biotransformation of all drugs known to be metabolized by the microsomal system. The inhibitor has little or no effect on: the N-dealkylation by rabbit microsomes of N-methylaniline and several other N-substituted anilines, monoethyl- and monobutyl-4-aminoantipyrine and atabrine (GAUDETTE and BRODIE, 1959); the N-demethylation of 3-methyl-4-methylaminoazobenzene by mouse microsomes (TAKEMORI and MANNERING, 1958); the O-dealkylation of phenacetin by rabbit microsomes (AXELROD, 1956b); the hydroxylation of acetanilide by rabbit microsomes (FOUTS and BRODIE, 1955; MITOMA et al., 1956); the sulfoxidation of chlorpromazine by guinea pig microsomes (GILLETTE and KAMM, 1960); the reduction of chloramphenicol, *p*-nitrobenzoic acid and other aromatic nitro compounds by rabbit microsomes (FOUTS and BRODIE, 1957); and the reduction of aminoazo dyes (KAMM and GILLETTE, 1963) by microsomes from an unidentified species.

The effects of SKF 525-A depend on a number of factors. The compound may inhibit the metabolism of a drug in one species, but not in another. Thus, SKF 525-A inhibits the O-dealkylation of phenacetin by rat microsomes (BURNS, 1966), but not by rabbit microsomes (AXELROD, 1956b). Inducing agents can cause a change in the nature of the microsomal enzymes such that the inhibitory effect of SKF 525-A may be increased or decreased. SKF 525-A inhibits the N-demethylation of 3-methyl-4-methylaminoazobenzene by hepatic microsomes from untreated rats, but has little effect on the metabolism of the aminoazo dye by microsomes from rats induced with 3-methylcholanthrene (SLADEK, 1966; SLADEK and MANNERING, 1966). Conversely, the N-demethylation of N-methylaniline is not inhibited by SKF 525-A when microsomes from untreated rats are employed, but is inhibited when microsomes from phenobarbital treated rats are used (ALVARES and MANNERING, unpublished observations). These differences in the action of SKF 525-A greatly complicate concepts that attempt to explain the mechanism of action of this inhibitor at the molecular level.

Numerous other prolonging agents have appeared since SKF 525-A was synthesized. The structures of some of these are shown in Fig. 1; their code names, chemical names and references to early studies dealing with their inhibitory actions are listed in Table 1.

SKF 525-A was found to inhibit glucuronidation and the hydrolysis of procaine as well as the oxidative biotransformation of drugs. This lack of specificity led to the suggestion that SKF 525-A might interact with the microsomal membrane, thereby decreasing its permeability to drugs (BRODIE, 1956, 1962). However, as GILLETTE (1963) has pointed out, it is difficult to explain the action of SKF 525-A on the basis of altered microsomal membrane permeability when it blocks the metabolism of lipid-soluble substrates, such as nicotine, codeine, hexobarbital and aminopyrine, but does not affect the oxidation of other lipid-soluble compounds, such as monoethyl-4-aminopyrine, methylaniline and acetanilide. The mechanism by which SKF 525-A inhibits procaine esterase has been elucidated by NETTER (1959), who showed that the enzyme is blocked competitively because SKF 525-A is also an ester. Glucuronidation is now known to be inhibited by the action of SKF 525-A on UDP glucuronyltransferase (HARGREAVES, 1967). NETTER (1962) speculated that SKF 525-A might act in a manner analogous to that of an uncoupling agent on oxidative phosphorylation. He proposed that the product of the TPNH oxidase reaction is an "active peroxide" or an "active hydroxyl" and that the drug oxidizing step is coupled to the oxidation of NADPH. SKF 525-A would act in some way to "uncouple" the NADPH oxidative step from the drug oxidizing step. This hypothesis has not been supported experimentally.

Studies by MCMAHON and MILLS (MCMAHON and MILLS, 1961; MCMAHON, 1962) showing that the N-demethylation of butynamine by rat liver microsomes is inhibited competitively by SKF 525-A and a number of other inhibitors, provided good evidence that SKF 525-A was acting directly at the metabolic site. These studies were largely ignored as a clue to the mechanism of action of SKF 525-A. Our attention was drawn to the idea that SKF 525-A might function as a substrate inhibitor by kinetic studies which showed that a variety of structurally unrelated drugs competitively inhibited each other's metabolism by rat liver microsomes (RUBIN et al., 1964a). SKF 525-A offers many possibilities for biotransformation: N-dealkylation, aromatic hydroxylation, penultimate and terminal oxidation of a side chain, and hydrolysis. Not all of these reactions are known to occur, nor are they feasible with all of the prolonging agents shown in Fig. 1; however, all these agents offer the opportunity for N-dealkylation. For this reason, the kinetics of the N-dealkylation reactions of the eleven compounds shown in Fig. 1 were studied with rat liver microsomes in our laboratory (ANDERS and MANNERING, 1966a). All were shown to be competitive inhibitors of the N-demethylation of ethylmorphine. Further support for the concept that SKF 525-A was acting as a substrate inhibitor was derived from a comparison of the K_m's of the N-dealkylations of the inhibitors with corresponding K_I's of their inhibition of the N-demethylation of ethylmorphine. In five of the eleven studies, respective K_m's and K_I's were not statistically different ($P > 0.1$). With four other inhibitors, corresponding K_m's and K_I's differed by about a half order of magnitude, while the difference was about five orders of magnitude for SKF 8742-A and iproniazid. Reasons why the K_m might not always equal the K_I when the inhibitor is acting as a substrate inhibitor were discussed by the authors.

The impression should not be gained from these studies that N-dealkylation of the inhibitor is required for the inhibitory action of prolonging agents. The primary amine of SKF 525-A, SKF 26754-A (2-aminoethyl 2,2-diphenylvalerate), is a potent competitive inhibitor of ethylmorphine N-demethylation by rat liver microsomes (ANDERS et al., 1966). Another primary amine, DPEA (2,4-dichloro-6-phenylphenoxyethylamine HCl) is as potent an inhibitor of drug metabolism as SKF 525-A, and for some substrates, more potent (KATO et al., 1963c; McMAHON et al., 1969). About the only thing that can be said about structure-activity relationships when the configurations of prolonging agents are compared is that none is apparent, except perhaps as they may relate to the lipid solubilities of the compounds. Potencies of thirteen hydrazine prolonging agents correlated well with their lipid solubilities (KATO et al., 1969b).

It remains to be explained why some reactions are inhibited competitively by SKF 525-A and others are not. The O-demethylation of *o*-nitroanisole by rat liver microsomes (NETTER, 1962) and the dealkylation of monomethyl-4-amino-antipyrine by rabbit liver microsomes (LA DU et al., 1954; LA DU, 1962) are inhibited non-competitively by SKF 525-A. Species differences have been observed; SKF 525-A blocks the N-demethylation of aminopyrine competitively when rat liver microsomes are used (KATO et al., 1966), but non-competitively when rabbit or mouse liver microsomes are employed (LA DU et al., 1954; LA DU, 1962; KATO et al., 1966). KATO and associates (1969a) studied species differences in inhibition of microsomal drug metabolism by the four prolonging agents, SKF 525-A, DPEA, chlorcyclizine, and U-16392-A (*o*-chlorisopropylphenyl-hydrazine). Aminopyrine N-demethylation was inhibited competitively by all four agents when rat and mouse microsomes were employed but noncompetitively when microsomes from the rabbit were used; all four agents inhibited the metabolism of hexobarbital competitively when rat microsomes were employed; the hydroxylation of aniline was inhibited noncompetitively by the four agents when either rat or mouse microsomes were used; SKF 525-A inhibited the O-demethylation of *p*-nitroanisole competitively when rat microsomes were the source of enzyme, but the other three agents inhibited the reaction by mixed kinetics. An attempt will be made to explain these species differences when the binding of drugs to cytochrome P-450 is discussed.

SKF 525-A is N-deethylated to its secondary and primary amine derivatives, 2-ethylaminoethyl 2,2-diphenylvalerate (SKF 8742-A) and 2-aminoethyl 2,2-diphenylvalerate (SKF 26754-A) (ANDERS and MANNERING, 1966a; ANDERS et al., 1966). The three compounds are about equally potent as competitive inhibitors of the N-demethylation of ethylmorphine and are equally effective in retarding the disappearance of hexobarbital from the plasma of intact rats (ANDERS and MANNERING, 1966a; ANDERS et al., 1966; STITZEL et al., 1966). The contribution of the metabolites of SKF 525-A to the overall potency of this prolonging agent was demonstrated by comparing the effectiveness of the three amines as inhibitors of hexobarbital metabolism *in vivo* at two time intervals between injections of the amines and hexobarbital (STITZEL et al., 1966). With a 45 min interval, the three compounds were equipotent, but with a 5 h interval, the tertiary amine was more potent than the secondary amine in delaying hexobarbital metabolism, which in turn was more potent than the primary amine. This was interpreted to mean that although SKF 525-A and its dealkylated products were equally effective inhibitors *per se* the longer the route to ultimate inactivation of the amine, the longer the duration of action.

When administered chronically, SKF 525-A and other prolonging agents stimulate rates of drug metabolism (NAVIS et al., 1953; SERRONE and FUJIMOTO, 1962; NEUMANN et al., 1963; ANDERS and MANNERING, 1966b). SKF 525-A and Lilly 18947 were shown to stimulate their own and each other's rate of N-dealkylation (ANDERS and MANNERING, 1966b). At first glance, this would seem to eliminate chronic administration of SKF 525-A as a means of prolonging drug action for extended periods. This proved not to be the case. In rats whose rates of hexobarbital metabolism had been increased by repeated administration of SKF 525-A, hexobarbital metabolism was still inhibited when a final dose of SKF 525-A was given 24 h after the preceding dose (ANDERS and MANNERING, 1966b). In a similar study SKF 525-A and its secondary and primary amine analogs were shown to be effective inhibitors of hexobarbital metabolism in rats whose rates of hexobarbital metabolism had been accelerated by chronic phenobarbital administration. These results were explained on the basis that the inductive process, whether initiated by SKF 525-A or phenobarbital, occurs as a result of the synthesis of new enzymic protein, which is as readily inhibited by SKF 525-A and its N-dealkylated derivatives as that which was present before induction. Even though the rate of metabolism of SKF 525-A is increased as a result of induction, it continues to exert its effects through its N-dealkylated metabolites, which are also excellent inhibitors. Advantage was taken of this ability of SKF 525-A to exert an inhibitory effect, even while producing an inductive effect, in a study where the chronic administration of SKF 525-A was used to protect rat fetuses against the teratogenic effects of chlorcyclizine, presumably by inhibiting the conversion of chlorcyclizine to norchlorcyclizine or to some other highly potent teratogenic metabolite (POSNER et al., 1967). Many commonly used drugs exhibit a biphasic effect on drug metabolism similar to that seen with SKF 525-A; they inhibit drug metabolism immediately after administration, but stimulate the rate of drug metabolism when given repeatedly (KATO et al., 1962, 1964).

SKF 525-A is so thoroughly identified with inhibition that its other pharmacologic properties are frequently overlooked. They are not important therapeutically, but they deserve mention because the question is frequently asked as to why 525-A is not used therapeutically as a prolonging agent. Perhaps the most important deterrant to its use is the finding that its chronic administration (five months) to dogs caused a marked fatty infiltration of the liver, which, however, was rapidly reversible after withdrawal of the compound (DICK et al., 1960). Intravenous injection of SKF 525-A evoked some dramatic responses in cats (GAITONDÉ and BORISON, 1966), including respiratory and gastrointestinal disturbances at doses of 5—10 mg/kg, and clonic convulsions and death at 25 mg/kg. The chief effects of intravenous injection were short-lasting noncholinergic peripheral vasodilation and persistent respiratory depression.

SKF 525-A affects neuromuscular transmission and muscular contraction (NAVIS et al., 1953; HARRIS and MILTON, 1961) and potentiates the blockade caused by a number of compounds (BOVET et al., 1956; DELLA BELLA et al., 1962; DOMER and PINTO-SCOGNAMIGLIO, 1964). The effect is apparently not due to inhibition of the metabolism of the blocking agents, since SKF 525-A did not alter the plasma radioactivity of dogs given ^{14}C-labeled decamethonium or bis (dimethylaminobutoxy) 1,4-benzene diodomethylate (DOMER and PINTO-SCOGNAMIGLIO, 1964). SKF 525-A acted peripherally in rats as a parasympatholytic or sympathomimetic agent or both (CARRANO and MALONE, 1966). It did not inhibit the action of acetylcholinesterase, but was a potent inhibitor of monoamine oxidase (CARRANO and MALONE, 1966; PFEFFER et al., 1968).

Autoregulation of renal blood flow and responsiveness to norepinephrine were found to be inhibited when SKF 525-A was administered via the renal artery (BRODY et al., 1964; MARSHALL and WILLIAMSON, 1964; HOOK and WILLIAMSON, 1964). The brevity of the action makes this inhibitor a useful tool in studies of autoregulation of renal blood flow. Whereas SKF 525-A is diuretic when injected into the renal artery, it is markedly antidiuretic when administered intraperitoneally to rats (ARIMA and KURIAKI, 1959).

SKF 525-A was observed to have an early stimulatory action *in vivo* on liver tryptophan pyrrolase activity in intact or in adrenalectomized, but not in hypophysectomized adult rats (MAGUS and FOUTS, 1967). The effect would therefore seem to involve some form of pituitary activation, but the mechanism remains to be elucidated (MAGUS et al., 1968). SKF 525-A induced tyrosine transaminase activity in intact male rats, but not in adrenalectomized animals, although in the latter, the potentiating effect of administered cortisol on tyrosine transaminase activity was enhanced by SKF 525-A (KUPFER and PEETS, 1967). The administration of SKF 525-A to mice caused a reduction in liver glycogen (WOOLES and McPHILLIPS, 1966). SKF 525-A in high concentration (10^{-3}M) inhibited glycogen synthetase, but had no effect on glycogenolysis *in vitro* (ROGERS et al., 1963b).

SKF 525-A inhibits microsomal enzymes involved in cholesterol biosynthesis and is known to be a hypocholesterolemic agent (GREENBERG et al., 1960; HOLMES and BENTZ, 1960; DICK et al., 1960; HOLMES and DITULLIO, 1962). Cholesterol synthesis was shown to be inhibited *in vitro* at a site lying between lanosterol and zymosterol on the biosynthetic pathway (HOLMES and DITULLIO, 1962). More than one enzyme in the pathway was shown to be inhibited both *in vitro* and *in vivo*.

E. Role of Binding of Inhibitors to Cytochrome P-450

NARASIMHULU and coworkers (1965) observed characteristic spectral changes when 17-hydroxyprogesterone was added to the cytochrome P-450 dependent steroid C-21 hydroxylase system in adrenal cortical microsomes. This prompted studies by REMMER and associates (1966) and IMAI and SATO (1966), published almost simultaneously, which showed that drugs and other foreign compounds combine with hepatic cytochrome P-450 to produce difference spectra of two general types, type I and type II. Compounds giving type I or II difference spectra with hepatic microsomes have come to be known as type I or type II compounds (or drugs). Type I compounds give a difference spectrum with a λ_{max} in the general range of 385—390 mμ and a λ_{min} in the even broader range of 418—427 mμ; the λ_{max} and λ_{min} given by type II compounds are 425—435 and 390—405 mμ, respectively (SCHENKMAN et al., 1967b). Thus, with opposing λ_{max} and λ_{min}, type I and type II spectra are approximate mirror images of each other. Of great interest was the apparent relationship between the kinetics of drug binding to the cytochrome and the kinetics of drug metabolism. The familiar double reciprocal Lineweaver-Burk plot of the magnitude of spectral change vs. concentration of drug can be used to derive the spectral dissociation constant (K_s) in the manner that the Michaelis constant (K_m) is obtained for the metabolism of the same compound. In a number of cases, the K_s and the K_m for a given compound were found to be similar and this encouraged the view that drug binding is an obligatory step in the mechanism of drug hydroxylation.

The question of whether the two types of binding represent complexes of drugs with two different cytochromes or whether they represent complexes with two binding sites on the same cytochrome has not been resolved with certainty, but kinetic studies favor the latter concept. If two cytochrome P-450's exist, one with a type I binding site and the other with a type II binding site, and inhibition is mediated only through the binding sites, then only type I inhibitors would inhibit the metabolism of type I compounds and only type II inhibitors would inhibit the metabolism of type II compounds. Whether or not inhibition was competitive or not would depend on the relevancy of binding spectra to metabolism. If metabolism is a direct function of binding, inhibition should be competitive. The same kinetics would be seen if both binding sites were on the same molecule, and type I and type II compounds reacted only with their respective binding sites, assuming again that metabolism is a function of binding. However, in the case of the single molecule with two binding sites, the possibility must be considered that the binding of a compound to one site might alter the reactivity of the other site. In this event, inhibition might be seen but it would not be competitive. In fact, the result could be stimulation rather than inhibition. IMAI and SATO (1967) believe that binding spectra reflect conformational changes in the protein that occur when drugs combine with cytochrome P-450. Such conformational changes might facilitate rather than retard the flow of electrons through the system. In fact, type I compounds are known to stimulate the activity of NADPH-cytochrome P-450 reductase, the purported rate limiting enzyme in the microsomal drug metabolizing complex (GIGON et al., 1968, 1969; GILLETTE and GRAM, 1969). Type II compounds inhibit the activity of NADPH-cytochrome P-450. In addition to the binding that can be visualized by spectroscopy, it would seem probable that compounds would bind to cytochrome P-450 or to other enzymic components of the complex without producing binding spectra. What would already seem hopelessly complicated, becomes excrutiatingly so when we consider the possibility that a compound may bind and react metabolically with both the type I and the type II binding sites. That any given compound may combine simultaneously with both sites is not idle speculation. When rats are treated with certain polycyclic hydrocarbons for several days, a new cytochrome P-450 (cytochrome P_1-450, cytochrome P-448) replaces the preexisting cytochrome P-450 (SLADEK and MANNERING, 1966, 1969a, 1969b; ALVARES et al., 1967; HILDEBRANDT et al., 1968). Cytochrome P_1-450 is lacking in the type I binding site (SHOEMAN et al., 1969). Hexobarbital, which combines as a type I compound with the cytochrome P-450 from untreated animals, becomes a type II compound when complexed with cytochrome P_1-450. In low concentrations, phenobarbital combines with microsomes from immature rabbits to form a type I spectrum, but in high concentrations, a type II spectrum is produced (JEFCOATE et al., 1969). The alignments of the peaks and troughs of type I and type II compounds are such that the difference spectra tend to cancel each other. However, the alignments are not perfect; if compounds are combining with both sites, this might account for the rather broad ranges of λ_{max} and λ_{min} seen in the spectra obtained with different compounds. Because the two spectra tend to cancel each other, it is not possible to determine the magnitude of the K_s for either the type I or the type II site for a given compound. If the K_s's for both sites are equal, regardless of their magnitude, essentially no difference spectrum would be observed. One criterion of how exclusively a compound binds to either a type I or a type II site may be how closely its K_s approximates its K_m. A compound with a very high K_s for the type I site and a very low K_s for the type II site would yield a type I λ_{max} with a very high molar extinction coefficient; a compound with a very high K_s for the type II site and a very low K_s for the type I site, would give a type II λ_{max} with a high molar extinction coefficient; compounds with K_s's for type I and II binding sites ranging between these two extremes would yield either type I or II λ_{max} with relevant molar extinction coefficients. The picture is complicated further by the probability that absolute as well as relative differences exist among compounds with respect to the degrees of type I and II binding they elicit. Thus, compounds A and B may each combine, say, 75% with the type I site and 25% with the type II site, thereby giving a type I spectrum, but the K_S's of compounds A and B for each of the binding sites may be widely divergent in magnitude. The picture becomes even more complex when we consider that type I compounds stimulate NADPH-cytochrome P-450 reductase whereas type II compounds inhibit it (GIGON et al., 1969). A compound which binds to both sites would stimulate as well as inhibit the reaction; with the right combination of binding to both sites, no metabolism would occur. This might explain why some compounds are poorly metabolized or not metabolized at all. In view of these many complexities, it is not surprising that inhibition was competitive when nicotinamide (type II) inhibited the N-demethylation of aminopyrine (type I) (SCHENKMAN et al., 1967a) and acetanilide (type II) inhibited the N-demethylation of ethylmorphine (type I) (RUBIN et al., 1964a), while the inhibition of the hydroxylation of aniline (type II) by nicotinamide (type II) was not competitive. The summary of a recent study by SASAME and GILLETTE (1970) serves to illustrate the complexity of the inhibition kinetics of microsomal drug metabolism:[2] "Nicotinamide (type II), 2,4-dichloro-6-phenylphenoxyethylamine (DPEA) (type II), and aminoethyldiphenyl propylacetate (SKF 26754A, SKF 525A-PA) (type II) inhibit the hydroxylation of aniline (type II), and the N-demethylation of aminopyrine (type I) and ethylmorphine (type I) by liver microsomes. The mechanism of inhibition, however, depends on the species and the substrate. For example, nicotinamide blocks the aminopyrine demethylating enzyme in rat liver microsomes competitively, and that in mouse liver microsomes by a mixed mechanism. The aniline hydroxylating enzyme in mouse liver microsomes is blocked competitively by nicotinamide, uncompetitively by SKF 525A-PA, and partially uncompetitively by DPEA. The ethylmorphine demethylating enzyme in mouse liver microsomes is inhibited by nicotinamide, SKF 525A-PA and DPEA by dual mechanisms. At low concentrations, the inhibitors block the reaction noncompetitively, but at high concentrations they block it both competitively and non-competitively. Nicotinamide modified the apparent mechanism of inhibition by SKF 525A-PA and DPEA. Thus in the presence of nicotinamide, SKF 525A-PA apparently inhibits the N-demethylation of ethylmorphine by a competitive mechanism."

SKF 525-A binds irreversibly to microsomes (ROGERS and FOUTS, 1964; ANDERS et al., 1966; KRATZ and STAUDINGER, 1968); it is also a type I compound (SCHENKMAN et al., 1967b). The possibility that SKF 525-A might be irreversibly bound to the type I site has been investigated recently in our laboratory (BIDLEMAN, SHOEMAN and MANNERING, unpublished results). Washed microsomes were mixed with a saturating concentration of SKF 525-A (1.2 mM), separated by centrifugation, washed, resedimented and examined for type I and II binding sites, SKF 525-A content, and ability to metabolize ethylmorphine (type I), hexobarbital (type I) and aniline (type II). The type I site was no longer present as was determined by the failure of added SKF 525-A or hexobarbital to evoke a type I difference spectrum. The type II site, as determined by the addition of aniline, was slightly increased (about 10%) over that seen in the microsomes before they were treated with SKF 525-A. The microsomes contained about 56 moles of SKF 525-A per mole of cytochrome P-450. Dialysis reduced this to about 40 moles of SKF 525-A per mole of cytochrome P-450, but did not restore type I binding. The ability of SKF 525-A treated microsomes to metabolize ethylmorphine, hexobarbital and aniline was 63, 31 and 67 percent, respectively, of that observed with untreated microsomes. From these studies it was concluded

2 The liberty has been taken of identifying the type of binding usually associated with the compounds mentioned in the summary.

that a) SKF 525-A binds irreversibly to the type I site, b) SKF 525-A does not bind irreversibly to the type II site, c) SKF 525-A binds firmly to materials in microsomes other than cytochrome P-450 or its binding to cytochrome P-450 is not restricted to the type I site, or both, and d) the metabolism of the type I compounds, ethylmorphine and hexobarbital, is possible without type I binding. While the type I binding site is not obligatory for the metabolism of type I compounds, it would appear to be facilitative. The K_m for ethylmorphine metabolism rose from 0.32 mM when untreated microsomes were used to 4.0 mM when SKF 525-A treated microsomes were employed. These studies recall the warning by DIXON and FOUTS (1962) that kinetic studies of inhibitors that combine irreversibly with enzymes should be interpreted with care because Michaelis-Menten equations assume a reversible combination of enzyme and inhibitor.

F. Some Applications of Inhibitors

Enzyme inhibition can be useful as a generally applicable simple test to determine whether a compound possesses intrinsic pharmacologic activity or whether it owes its action to its metabolic products. The observation that SKF 525-A and other inhibitors of drug metabolism delayed the onset and decreased the intensity of tremors induced by tremorine led to the conclusion that oxytremorine, the metabolite of tremorine, was the pharmacologically active species (WELCH and KOCSIS, 1961; CHO et al., 1962; SJÖQVIST and GILLETTE, 1964). The lethalities of the insecticides, Guthion (MURPHY and DUBOIS, 1958) and Schraden (O'BRIEN, 1962) were decreased by SKF 525-A, which inhibited their metabolism to more toxic products. In contrast, inhibition of drug metabolism with SKF 525-A potentiated the toxicity of Thimet and Tetram, suggesting that these insecticides are metabolized to less toxic substances (O'BRIEN, 1962). The toxicity of DDT is also enhanced by SKF 525-A (MORELLO, 1964). Acetophenetidin is metabolized mainly through the formation of N-acetyl-*p*-aminophenol, which was suggested to be responsible for the analgesic-antipyretic activity of the parent drug (BRODIE and AXELROD, 1949). That this is not the case was shown by the increased antipyretic activity of acetophenetidin in rats that had received SKF 525-A (CONNEY et al., 1966). The hepatotoxicity of CCl_4 (DINGELL and HEIMBERG, 1968; CASTRO et al., 1968; SASAME et al., 1968) and the teratogenic effects of chlorcyclizine (POSNER et al., 1967) are mitigated by SKF 525-A, suggesting that the toxicities of these substances are due to their metabolites. Pressor responses to tyramine and amphetamine were enhanced in cats treated with SKF 525-A, but responses to epinephrine and norepinephrine were unaffected. This and other observations led RAND and TRINKER (1968) to suggest that monoamine oxidase inhibitors potentiate the pressor responses of indirectly acting sympathomimetic amines such as tyramine and amphetamine, not by interfering with the metabolism of endogenous norepinephrine, as was originally supposed, but by inhibiting the metabolism of these amines by the microsomal drug metabolizing system.

The N-dealkylation of tertiary amines has been postulated to proceed through an N-oxide intermediate (FISH et al., 1955), which is formed by a flavoprotein in liver microsomes and rearranged to the demethylated amine (PETTIT and ZIEGLER, 1963; OAE et al., 1963). The demethylation of N,N-dimethylaniline (DMA) is strongly inhibited by SKF 525-A, but the N-oxidation of DMA is not (PETTIT and ZIEGLER, 1963, MACHINIST et al., 1966; ZIEGLER and PETTIT, 1964). Support was given to the concept that the N-oxide pathway to N-demethylation is of importance *in vivo* by the finding that SKF 525-A increased the urinary excretion of the N-oxides of DMA and N,N-dimethyl-n-octylamine (DEHNER et al., 1968).

The hydroxylation by the liver of steroids such as estradiol, testosterone, androsterone, progesterone, and the corticoids are believed to be mediated by the same microsomal system responsible for drug metabolism (reviewed by CONNEY, 1967 and KUNTZMAN, 1969). This conclusion was partly derived from inhibition studies. We showed that estradiol, testosterone, androsterone, progesterone and hydrocortisone competitively inhibited the oxidation of ethylmorphine and hexobarbital by rat liver microsomes (TEPHLY and MANNERING, 1968). Support was gained for the view that steroids were acting as substrate inhibitors by the observation that the K_I's for the inhibition of both drugs by estradiol, testosterone and progesterone were similar to the K_m's of the hydroxylation of these steroids as determined by KUNTZMAN et al., (1965).

The term *synergist* is applied to any compound that increases the toxicity of a pesticide. Synergists usually produce their effects by inhibiting the enzyme system responsible for the biotransformation of pesticides in insects. This enzyme system is located in microsomes, is cytochrome P-450 dependent, and is believed to be similar to the microsomal drug metabolizing system found in mammalian liver. It is found in highest concentration in the mid-gut, but is also found in appreciable concentrations in other organs such as the fat body (CHAKRABORTY et al., 1967). Synergists are particularly useful in controlling insecticide-resistant insects. In general, insecticide-resistant strains of insects arise from the selection of individual variants containing preadaptive genes controlling the level of detoxication enzymes (METCALF and FUKUTO, 1965). The marked synergistic action of the methylenedioxy compounds such as piperonyl butoxide, sesamex, sulfoxide and N-propyl isome for Sevin and other carbamates was first demonstrated by MOOREFIELD (1960), who also showed that piperonyl butoxide suppressed the further development of resistance of houseflies to Sevin. Methylenedioxybenzenes have been shown to inhibit the metabolism of insecticides such as parathion (NAKATSUGAWA and DAHM, 1965, 1967), carbamides (HODGSON and CASIDA, 1961), naphthalene (PHILLEO et al., 1965), and chlorinated hydrocarbons (NAKATSUGAWA et al., 1965; WONG and TERRIERE, 1965; LEWIS et al., 1967). In accordance with the view that insectile and mammalian microsomal systems are very similar, a large number of synergists have been shown to be effective inhibitors of the mammalian drug metabolizing system (FINE and MOLLOY, 1964; EPSTEIN et al., 1967a, 1967b, 1970; ANDERS, 1968; FUJII et al., 1968, 1970; JAFFE et al., 1968, 1969) and SKF 525-A and other prolonging agents have been shown to be effective synergists (MOOREFIELD, 1960; O'BRIEN, 1961; HODGSON and CASIDA, 1961; HEWLETT et al., 1961; MORELLO, 1964; BOND, 1965, BATES et al., 1965; METCALF and FUKUTO, 1965; FORGASH, 1967). Houseflies and other insects contain naturally occurring inhibitors that not only inhibit the activity of insectile microsomes, but that of mammalian microsomes as well (MATTHEWS and HODGSON, 1966; CHAKRABORTY et al., 1967). The inhibitor was removed from housefly microsomes by dialysis and found to be heat stable, water soluble and insoluble in most organic solvents (MATTHEWS and HODGSON, 1966).

SKF 525-A might serve a useful purpose in the routine testing of new drugs. The great variability in the activity of drugs in different species relates largely to the rates at which drugs are metabolized (BRODIE et al., 1965). In a given species the rate of metabolism of a drug can be so rapid that its potential pharmacologic effect might go unrecognized. In many cases, SKF 525-A, used in conjunction with the new drug being investigated, could eliminate or minimize the differences in responses to drugs seen in different species. The number of drugs whose metabolism could be inhibited might be increased by using combinations of inhibitors, e.g. SKF 525-A and DPEA.

G. Therapeutic Implications of Inhibition of Drug Metabolism

The action of most drugs is terminated through biotransformation. Thus anything that will depress the rate of drug metabolism will prolong drug action. If drugs are given repeatedly and drug metabolism is slowed to the degree that the interval between administration is no longer of sufficient duration to allow adequate removal of the drug, accumulation of the drug and toxicity can result. The gradual realization that drugs are metabolized by an enzymic system with very low substrate specificity and the knowledge that one drug can therefore inhibit the metabolism of another is causing the more informed therapist to take another look at the practice of multiple drug therapy, sometimes referred to derogatively as polypharmacy. Adverse reactions due to drug interactions at the metabolic site increase greatly with each increase in the number of drugs given a patient. In a recent survey (SMITH et al., 1966), it was estimated that the average inpatient received six drugs daily. Cases of patients receiving two or three times that number of drugs are not unknown. The problem is complicated further by the fact that some of these drugs must be inducing, as well as inhibiting, drug metabolism. This is certainly one of the reasons many drugs do not perform as well in practice as they do in theory.

An inhibitor with minimal pharmacodynamic activity would fill a need in drug therapy. Many drugs are metabolized more rapidly than we would like, and some individuals metabolize drugs more rapidly than they should. An innocuous inhibitor given with the drug would correct the problem of too rapid drug biotransformation and would avoid the rapid peaking and troughing of tissue or blood drug levels that occur when drugs must be administered with great frequency. Such an inhibitor should not be too hard to locate, for there appears to be little resemblance between the metabolic site and the receptor sites for most drugs.

References

ALVARES, A.P., MANNERING, G.J.: Two substrate kinetics of drug-metabolizing enzyme systems of hepatic microsomes. Molec. Pharmacol. **6**, 206—212 (1970).

— SCHILLING, G., LEVIN, W., KUNTZMAN, R.: Studies on the induction of CO-binding pigments in liver microsomes by phenobarbital and 3-methylcholanthrene. Biochem. biophys. Res. Commun. **29**, 521—526 (1967).

ANDERS, M.W.: Inhibition of microsomal drug metabolism by methylenedioxybenzenes. Biochem. Pharmacol. **17**, 2367—2370 (1968).

— ALVARES, A.P., MANNERING, G.J.: Inhibition of drug metabolism. II. Metabolism of 2-diethylaminoethyl 2,2-diphenylvalerate HCl (SKF 525-A). Molec. Pharmacol. **2**, 328 to 334 (1966).

— MANNERING, G.J.: Inhibition of drug metabolism. I. Kinetics of the inhibition of the N-demethylation of ethylmorphine by 2-diethylaminoethyl 2,2-diphenylvalerate HCl (SKF 525-A) and related compounds. Molec. Pharmacol. **2**, 319—327 (1966a).

— — Inhibition of drug metabolism. IV. Induction of drug metabolism by 2-diethylaminoethyl 2,2-diphenylvalerate HCl (SKF 525-A) and 2,4-dichloro-6-phenylphenoxyethyldiethylamine HBr (Lilly 18947) and the effect of induction on the inhibitory properties of SKF 525-A type compounds. Molec. Pharmacol. **2**, 341—346 (1966b).

ARIMA, K., KURIAKI, K.: Some pharmacological studies on the renal carbonic anhydrase activity and electrolytes excretion in the rat. Jap. J. Pharmacol. **8**, 165—169 (1959).

AXELROD, J.: Possible mechanism of tolerance to narcotic drugs. Science **124**, 263—264 (1956a).

— The enzymic cleavage of aromatic ethers. Biochem. J. **63**, 634—639 (1956b).

AXELROD, J., REICHENTHAL, J., BRODIE, B.B.: Mechanism of the potentiating action of β-diethylaminoethyl diphenylpropylacetate. J. Pharmacol. exp. Ther. **112**, 49—54 (1954a).
— UDENFRIEND, S., BRODIE, B.B.: Ascorbic acid in aromatic hydroxylation. II. Effect of ascorbic acid on hydroxylation of acetanilide, aniline and antipyrine *in vivo*. J. Pharmacol. exp. Ther. **111**, 176—181 (1954b).
BARON, J., TEPHLY, T.R.: Effect of 3-amino-1,2,4-triazole on the stimulation of hepatic microsomal heme synthesis and induction of hepatic microsomal oxidases produced by phenobarbital. Molec. Pharmacol. **5**, 10—20 (1969).
BATES, A.N., HEWLETT, P.S., LLOYD, C.J.: Synergistic effects of some compounds related to 2-diethylaminoethyl 2,2-diphenyl-n-pentanoate (SKF 525-A) on the insecticidal activity of pyrethrins. J. Sci. Food Agric. **16**, 289—292 (1965).
BETTSCHART, A., DELLA BELLA, D., BOVET, D.: Potenzierung der curareähnlichen Eigenschaften von 1815 I. S. durch SKF 525-A. Helv. physiol. pharmacol. Acta **14**, C 58 (1956).
BOND, E.J.: Comparative effects of oxygen and of pyrethrum synergists on the action of certain insecticides. J. econ. Ent. **58**, 642—645 (1965).
BOOTH, J., GILLETTE, J.R.: (1966) unpublished observations cited by J.R. GILLETTE (1966).
BOULOS, B.M., SHORT, C.R., DAVIS, L.E.: Quinine and quinidine inhibition of pentobarbital metabolism. Biochem. Pharmacol. **19**, 723—732 (1970).
BOVET, D., BOVET-NITTI, F., BETTSCHART, A., PINTO-SCOGNAMIGLIO, W.: Mécanisme de la potentialization par le chlorhydrate de diéthylamino-éthyl-diphényl-propylacétate deseffets de quelques agents curarisants. Helv. physiol. pharmacol. Acta **14**, 430—440 (1956).
BRODIE, B.B.: Pathways of drug metabolism. J. Pharm. Pharmacol. **8**, 1—17 (1956).
— Drug metabolism-subcellular mechanism. *Ciba Foundation Symposium on Enzymes and Drug Action*, pp. 317—343. Eds. J.E. MONGAR and A.V.S. DE REUCK. Boston: Little Brown 1962.
— AXELROD, J.: The fate of acetophenetidin (Phenacetin) in man and method for the estimation of acetophenetidin and its metabolites in biological material. J. Pharmacol. exp. Ther. **97**, 58—67 (1949).
— COSMIDES, G.J., RALL, D.P.: Toxicology and the biomedical sciences. Science **148**, 1547 to 1554 (1965).
BRODY, M.J., LUKENSMEYER, W.A., WILLIAMSON, H.E.: Inhibition of autoregulation of renal blood flow by SKF 525-A and fluoracetate. Proc. Soc. exp. Biol. (N.Y.) **117**, 79—83 (1964).
BROOKS, G.T., HARRISON, A.: The oxidative metabolism of aldrin and dihydroaldrin by houseflies, housefly microsomes and pig liver microsomes and the effect of inhibitors. Biochem. Pharmacol. **18**, 557—568 (1969).
BURNS, J.J. (1966). Personal communication cited by J.R. GILLETTE (1966).
CARRANO, R.A., MALONE, M.H.: New pharmacologic aspects of β-diethylaminoethyl 2,2-diphenylpentanoate. J. pharm. Sci. **55**, 563—567 (1966).
CARTER, S.A.: Potentiation of the effect of orally administered anticoagulants by phenyramidol hydrochloride. New Engl. J. Med. **273**, 423—426 (1965).
CASTRO, J.A., SASAME, H.A., SUSSMAN, H., GILLETTE, J.R.: Diverse effects of SKF 525-A and antioxidants on carbon tetrachloride-induced changes in liver microsomal P-450 content and ethylmorphine metabolism. Life Sci. **7**, 129—136 (1968).
CHAKRABORTY, J., SISSONS, C.H., SMITH, J.N.: Inhibitors of microsomal oxidations in insect homogenates. Biochem. J. **102**, 492—497 (1967).
CHAPLIN, M.D., SLADEK, N.E., MANNERING, G.J.: Effects of age and sex on the depression of drug metabolism produced by repeated administration of morphine (M). Fed. Proc. **27**, 349 (1968).
CHO, A.K., HASLETT, W.L., JENDEN, D.J.: The peripheral actions of oxotremorine, a metabolite of tremorine. J. Pharmacol. exp. Ther. **138**, 249—257 (1962).
CHRISTENSEN, L.K., HANSEN, J.M., KRISTENSEN, M.: Sulphaphenazole-induced hypoglycemic attack in tolbutamide-treated diabetics. Lancet **1963** II, 1298—1301.
CLELAND, W.W.: Computer programmes for processing enzyme kinetic data. Nature (Lond.) **198**, 463—465 (1963).
COCHIN, J., SOKOLOFF, L.: Effects of administration of L-thyroxin on liver N-demethylating activity in normal and morphine-treated rats. Proc. Soc. exp. Biol. (N.Y.) **104**, 504—506 (1960).
CONNEY, A.H.: Pharmacological implications of microsomal enzyme induction. Pharmacol. Rev. **19**, 317—366 (1967).
— BRAY, G.A., EVANS, C., BURNS, J.J.: Metabolic interaction between L-ascorbic acid and drugs. Ann. N.Y. Acad. Sci. **92**, 115—127 (1961).
— DAVISON, C., GASTEL, R., BURNS, J.J.: Adaptive increases in drug-metabolizing enzymes induced by phenobarbital and other drugs. J. Pharmacol. exp. Ther. **130**, 1—8 (1960).

CONNEY, A.H., GARREN, L.: Contrasting effects of thyroxin on zoxazolamine and hexobarbital metabolism. Biochem. Pharmacol. **6**, 257—262 (1961).
— MILLER, E.C., MILLER, J.A.: The metabolism of methylated aminoazo dyes. V. Evidence for induction of enzyme synthesis in the rat by 3-methylcholanthrene. Cancer Res. **16**, 450—459 (1956).
— SANSUR, M., SOROKO, F., KOSTER, R., BURNS, J.J.: Enzyme induction and inhibition in studies on the pharmacological actions of acetophenetidin. J. Pharmacol. exp. Ther. **151**, 133—138 (1966).
COOK, L., MACKO, E., FELLOWS, E.J.: The effect of β-diethylaminoethyl-diphenylpropyl-acetate hydrochloride on the action of a series of barbiturate and CNS depressants. J. Pharmacol. exp. Ther. **112**, 382—386 (1954a).
— NAVIS, G., FELLOWS, E.J.: Enhancement of the action of certain analgetic drugs by β-diethylaminoethyldiphenylpropylacetate hydrochloride. J. Pharmacol. exp. Ther. **112**, 473—479 (1954b).
— TONER, J.J., FELLOWS, E.J.: The effect of diethylaminoethyldiphenylpropylacetate hydrochloride (SKF 525-A) on hexobarbital. J. Pharmacol. exp. Ther. **111**, 131—141 (1954c).
DEHNER, E.W., MACHINIST, J.M., ZIEGLER, D.M.: Effect of SKF 525-A on the excretion of amine oxides by the rat. Life Sci. **7**, 1135—1146 (1968).
DELLA BELLA, D., RAGONI, F., TEOTINO, U.: Effect of β-diethylaminoethyl 3,3-diphenyl-propylacetate on the action of suxamethonium and other neuromuscular blocking drugs. Brit. J. Pharmacol. **18**, 563—571 (1962).
DICK, E.C., GREENBERG, S.M., HERNDON, J.F., JONES, M., VAN LOON, E.J.: Hypochol-esteremic effect of β-diethylaminoethyldiphenylpropylacetate hydrochloride (SKF 525-A) in the dog. Proc. Soc. exp. Biol. (N.Y.) **104**, 523—526 (1960).
DINGELL, J.V., BASS, A.D.: Inhibition of the hepatic metabolism of amphetamine by desi-pramine. Biochem. Pharmacol. **18**, 1535—1538 (1969).
— HEIMBERG, M.: The effects of aliphatic halogenated hydrocarbons on hepatic drug metab-olism. Biochem. Pharmacol. **17**, 1269—1278 (1968).
DIXON, M.: The determination of enzyme inhibition constants. Biochem. J. **55**, 170—171 (1953).
— WEBB, E.C.: *Enzymes*, 2nd ed. p. 114. New York: Academic Press 1964a.
— — *Enzymes*, 2nd ed. p. 319. New York: Academic Press 1964b.
DIXON, R.L., FOUTS, J.R.: Inhibition of microsomal drug metabolic pathways by chlor-amphenicol. Biochem. Pharmacol. **11**, 715—720 (1962).
— HART, L.G., FOUTS, J.R.: The metabolism of drugs by liver microsomes from alloxan-diabetic rats. J. Pharmacol. exp. Ther. **133**, 7—11 (1961).
— — ROGERS, L.A., FOUTS, J.R.: The metabolism of drugs by liver microsomes from alloxan-diabetic rats: long term diabetes. J. Pharmacol. exp. Ther. **142**, 312—317 (1963).
— SHULTICE, R.W., FOUTS, J.R.: Factors affecting drug metabolism by liver microsomes. IV. Starvation. Proc. Soc. exp. Biol. (N.Y.) **103**, 333—335 (1960).
DOMER, F.R., PINTO-SCOGNAMIGLIO, W.: Effect of β-diethylaminoethyl diphenyl-n-propyl acetate (SKF 525-A) on the plasma concentration of C^{14}-labeled neuromuscular blockers. J. pharm. Sci. **53**, 225—226 (1964).
DOWD, J.E., RIGGS, D.S.: A comparison of estimates of Michaelis-Menten constants for various linear transformations. J. biol. Chem. **240**, 863—869 (1965).
DUBOIS, K.P.: Inhibition by radiation of the development of drug-detoxification enzymes. Radiat. Res. **30**, 342—350 (1967).
EPSTEIN, S.S., ANDREA, J., CLAPP, P., MACKINTOSH, D.: Enhancement by piperonyl butoxide of acute toxicity due to freons, benzo [a]pyrene, and greseofulvin in infant mice. Toxicol. appl. Pharmacol. **11**, 442—448 (1967a).
— CSILLAG, R.G., GUERIN, H., FRIEDMAN, M.A.: Biochem. Pharmacol. (1970). In press.
— JOSHI, S., ANDREA, J., CLAPP, P., FALK, H., MANTEL, N.: Synergistic toxicity and car-cinogenecity of "freons" and piperonyl butoxide. Nature (Lond.) **214**, 526—528 (1967b).
FINE, B.C., MOLLOY, J.O.: Effects of insecticide synergists on duration of sleep induced in mice by barbiturates. Nature (Lond.) **204**, 789—790 (1964).
FISH, M.S., JOHNSON, N.M., LAWRENCE, E.R., HORNING, E.C.: Oxidative N-dealkylation. Biochim. biophys. Acta (Amst.) **18**, 564—565 (1955).
FORGASH, A.J.: Joint action of SKF 525-A and sesamex with insecticides in susceptible and resistant house flies. J. econ. Ent. **60**, 1596—1600 (1967).
FOUTS, J.R., BRODIE, B.B.: Inhibition of drug metabolic pathways by the potentiating agent, 2,4-dichloro-6-phenylphenoxyethyl diethylamine. J. Pharmacol. exp. Ther. **115**, 68—73 (1955).
— — On the mechanism of drug potentiation by iproniazid (2-isopropyl-1-isonicotinyl hydrazine). J. Pharmacol. exp. Ther. **116**, 480—485 (1956).

FOUTS, J.R., BRODIE, B.B.: The enzymatic reduction of chloramphenicol, p-nitrobenzoic acid and other aromatic nitro compounds in mammals. J. Pharmacol. exp. Ther. **119**, 197—207 (1957).
FUJII, K., JAFFE, H., BISHOP, Y., ARNOLD, E., MACKINTOSH, D., EPSTEIN, S.S.: Structure-activity relations for methylenedioxyphenyl and related compounds on hepatic microsomal enzyme function, as measured by prolongation of hexobarbital narcosis and zoxazolamine paralysis in mice. Toxicol. appl. Pharmacol. **16**, 482—494 (1970).
— — EPSTEIN, S.S.: Factors influencing the hexobarbital sleeping time and zoxazolamine paralysis time in mice. Toxicol. appl. Pharmacol. **13**, 431—438 (1968).
FUJIMOTO, J.M., PEARCE, K.B., PLAA, G.L.: Barbiturate metabolism as affected by certain agents acting on the liver. J. Pharmacol. exp. Ther. **129**, 139—143 (1960).
— PLAA, G.L.: Effect of ethionine and carbon tetrachloride on urethan and phenobarbital induced changes in hexobarbital action. J. Pharmacol. exp. Ther. **131**, 282—286 (1961).
GAITONDÉ, B.B., BORISON, H.L.: Toxicity of β-diethylaminoethyl diphenylpropylacetate (SKF 525-A) in cats. Toxicol. appl. Pharmacol. **8**, 118—125 (1966).
GAUDETTE, L.E., BRODIE, B.B.: Relationship between the lipid solubility of drugs and their oxidation by liver microsomes. Biochem. Pharmacol. **2**, 89—96 (1959).
GELBOIN, H.V., BLACKBURN, N.R.: The stimulatory effect of 3-methylcholanthrene on benzpyrene hydroxylase activity in several rat tissues: Inhibition by actinomycin D and puromycin. Cancer Res. **24**, 356—360 (1964).
GEORGE, W.J., TEPHLY, T.R.: Studies on hepatic microsomal N- and O-dealkylation of morphine analogues. Molec. Pharmacol. **4**, 502—509 (1968).
GIGON, P.L., GRAM, T.E., GILLETTE, J.R.: Effect of drug substrates on the reduction of hepatic microsomal cytochrome P-450 by NADPH. Biochem. biophys. Res. Commun. **31**, 558—562 (1968).
— — — Studies on the rate of reduction of hepatic microsomal cytochrome P-450 by reduced nicotinamide adenine dinucleotide phosphate: effect of drug substrates. Molec. Pharmacol. **5**, 109—122 (1969).
GILLETTE, J.R.: Metabolism of drugs and other foreign compounds by enzymatic mechanisms. Fortschr. Arzneimittelforsch. **6**, 13—73 (1963).
— Biochemistry of drug oxidation and reduction by enzymes in hepatic endoplasmic reticulum. Advanc. Pharmacol. **4**, 219—261 (1966).
— Mechanisms of oxidation by enzymes in the endoplasmic reticulum. In: *Biochemical Aspects of Antimetabolites and Drug Hydroxylation*, No. 16 in the Federation of European Biochemical Society Symposia Series. Ed. by D. SHUGAR, pp. 109—124. New York: Academic Press 1969.
— CONNEY, A.H., COSMIDES, G.J., ESTABROOK, R.W., FOUTS, J.R., MANNERING, G.J., (eds.): *Microsomes and Drug Oxidations*, New York: Academic Press 1969.
— GRAM, T.E.: Cytochrome P-450 reduction in liver microsomes and its relationship to drug metabolism; in *Microsomes and Drug Oxidations*, pp. 133—149. Eds. J.R. GILLETTE, A.H. CONNEY, G.J. COSMIDES, R.W. ESTABROOK, J.R. FOUTS and G.J. MANNERING New York: Academic Press 1969.
— KAMM, J.J.: The enzymatic formation of sulfoxides: the oxidation of chlorpromazine and 4,4-diaminodiphenyl sulfide by guinea pig liver microsomes. J. Pharmacol. exp. Ther. **130**, 262—267 (1960).
GREENBERG, S.M., HERNDON, J.F., DICK, E.C., LIN, T.H.: Antihypercholesteremic properties of a new compound, tris-(2-dimethylaminoethyl) phosphate trihydrochloride (SK&F No. 7732-A_3). Circulation **22**, 680 (1960).
HAMMER, W., SJÖQVIST, F.: Inhibition of the metabolism of tremorine and oxotremorine in rats by antidepressants of the imipramine type. In: *Ist Symposium Antidepressant Drugs, Milan*, Excerpta Med. Int. Congr., series 122, pp. 279—289, 1966.
HANSEN, J.M., KRISTENSEN, M., SKOVSTED, L., CHRISTENSEN, L.K.: Dicoumarol induced diphenylhydantoin intoxication. Lancet 1966II, 265—266.
HARGREAVES, T.: The effect of diethylaminoethyl diphenylpropylacetic acid (SKF 525-A) on uridine 5′-pyrophosphate glucuronyltransferase. Biochem. Pharmacol. **16**, 1481—1488 (1967).
HARRIS, E.D., MILTON, A.S.: Inhibitory actions of β-diethylaminoethyl diphenyl-n-propyl acetate (SKF 525-A) on muscle contraction. Proc. Soc. exp. Biol. (N.Y.) **107**, 157—160 (1961).
HERKEN, H., MAIBAUER, D., NEUBERT, D.: Der Einfluß von Athionin und anderen Lebergiften auf Fermentosysteme der Lebermikrosonen. Naunyn-Schmiedeberg's Arch. exp. Path. Pharmak. **233**, 139—150 (1958).
HEWLETT, P.S., LLOYD, C.J., BATES, A.N.: Effects of 2-diethylaminoethyl 2,2-diphenylpentanoate (SKF 525-A) on insecticidal potency. Nature (Lond.) **192**, 1273—1275 (1961).

Hietbrink, B.E., Dubois, K.P.: Influence of X-radiation on development of enzymes responsible for desulfuration of an organic phosphorothioate and reduction of p-nitrobenzoic acid in the livers of male rats. Radiat. Res. **22**, 598—605 (1964).
Hildebrandt, A., Remmer, H., Estabrook, R.W.: Cytochrome P-450 of liver microsomes — one pigment or many. Biochem. biophys. Res. Commun. **30**, 607—612 (1968).
Hodgson, E., Casida, J.E.: Metabolism of N:N-dialkyl carbamates and related compounds by rat liver. Biochem. Pharmacol. **8**, 179—191 (1961).
Holmes, W.L., Bentz, J.D.: Effect of SK&F 7732 and SK&F 7997 on cholesterol biosynthesis *in vitro*. Circulation **22**, 663—664 (1960).
— Di Tullio, N.W.: Inhibitors of cholesterol biosynthesis which act at or beyond the mevalonic acid stage. Amer. J. clin. Nutr. **10**, 310—322 (1962).
Honjo, T., Netter, K.J.: Inhibition of drug demethylation of disulfiram *in vivo* and *in vitro*. Biochem. Pharmacol. **18**, 2681—2683 (1969).
Hook, J.B., Williamson, H.E.: Addition of the natruretic action of SKF 525-A to the action of certain other natruretic agents. J. Pharmacol. exp. Ther. **146**, 265—269 (1964).
Imai, Y., Sato, R.: Substrate interaction with hydroxylase system in liver microsomes. Biochem. biophys. Res. Commun. **22**, 620—626 (1966).
— — Studies on the substrate interactions with P-450 in drug hydroxylation by liver microsomes. J. Biochem. (Tokyo) **62**, 239—249 (1967).
Jaffe, H., Fujii, K., Guerin, H., Sengupta, M., Epstein, S.S.: Bi-modal effect of piperonyl butoxide on the o- and p-hydroxylations of biphenyl by mouse liver microsomes. Biochem. Pharmacol. **18**, 1045—1051 (1969).
— — Sengupta, M., Guerin, H., Epstein, S.S.: *In vivo* inhibition of mouse liver microsomal hydroxylating systems by methylenedioxyphenyl insecticidal synergists and related compounds. Life Sci., Part I, **7**, 1051—1062 (1968).
Jefcoate, C.R.E., Gaylor, J.L., Calabrese, R.L.: Ligand interactions with cytochrome P-450. I. Binding of primary amines. Biochemistry **8**, 3455—3463 (1969).
Jori, A., Prestini, P.E., Pugliatti, C.: Effect of diazepam and chlordiazepoxide on the metabolism of other drugs. J. Pharm. Pharmacol. **21**, 387—390 (1969).
Kamm, J.J., Gillette, J.R.: Unpublished observations cited by J.R. Gillette (1963).
Kato, R.: Effect of administration of 3-aminotriazole on the activity of microsomal drug-metabolizing enzyme systems of rat liver. Jap. J. Pharmacol. **17**, 56—63 (1967).
— Chiesara, E., Vassanelli, P.: The *in vitro* inhibition of pentobarbital metabolism by chlorpromazine. Experientia (Basel) **18**, 269—270 (1962).
— — — Mechanism of potentiation of barbiturates and meprobamate actions by imipramine. Biochem. Pharmacol. **12**, 357—364 (1963a).
— — — Further studies on the inhibition and stimulation of microsomal drug-metabolizing enzymes of rat liver by various compounds. Biochem. Pharmacol. **13**, 69—83 (1964).
— Gillette, J.R.: Effect of starvation on NADPH-dependent enzymes in liver microsomes of male and female rats. J. Pharmacol. exp. Ther. **150**, 279—284 (1965).
— Onoda, K., Takayanagi, M.: Species difference in the inhibition of drug metabolism by liver microsomes by different inhibitors. Jap. J. Pharmacol. **19**, 438—450 (1969a).
— Sasame, H.A., Gillette, J.R.: Unpublished results cited by J.R. Gillette (1966).
— Takanaka, A., Shoji, H.: Inhibition of drug-metabolizing enzymes of liver microsomes by hydrazine derivatives in relation to their lipid solubility. Jap. J. Pharmacol. **19**, 315—322 (1969b).
— Vassanelli, P., Chiesara, E.: Inhibition of some microsomal drug-metabolizing enzymes by inhibitors of cholesterol biosynthesis. Biochem. Pharmacol. **12**, 349—351 (1963b).
— — — A new potent inhibitor of microsomal drug-metabolizing enzymes 2:4-dichloro-6-phenylphenoxyethylamine hydrochloride (DPEA) (Lilly 32391). Biochem. Pharmacol. **12**, 353—356 (1963c).
Kiørboe, E.: Phenytoin intoxication during treatment with antabuse (disulfiram). Epilepsia **7**, 246—249 (1966).
Kramer, M., Arrigoni-Martelli, E.: Die Verstärkung des narkotischen Effekts und die Abbauhemmung von Hexobarbital durch Malonsäurederivate. Naunyn-Schmiedeberg's Arch. exp. Path. Pharmak. **237**, 264—275 (1959).
Kratz, F., Staudinger, H.: Spektrale Änderungen von Kaninchenlebermikrosomen durch Cumarin. Hoppe-Seylers Z. physiol. Chem. **349**, 455—458 (1968).
Kristensen, M.D., Hansen, J.M.: Potentiation of the tolbutamide effect by dicoumarol. Diabetes **16**, 211—214 (1967).
— — Accumulation of chlorpropamide caused by dicoumarol. Acta med. scand. **183**, 83—86 (1968).
Kuntzman, R.: Drugs and enzyme induction. Ann. Rev. Pharmacol. **9**, 21—36 (1969).
— Lawrence, D., Conney, A.H.: Michaelis constants for the hydroxylation of steroid hormones and drugs by rat liver microsomes. Molec. Pharmacol. **1**, 163—167 (1965).

KUPFER, D., PEETS, L.: Potentiation of cortisol induction of hepatic tyrosine transaminase by β-diethylaminoethyl diphenylpropylacetate. Nature (Lond.) **215**, 637—638 (1967).

KUTT, H., VEREBELY, K., McDOWELL, F.: Inhibition of diphenylhydantoin metabolism in rats and in rat liver microsomes by antitubercular drugs. Neurology (Minneap.) **18**, 706 to 710 (1968).

— WINTERS, W., McDOWELL, F.: Depression of parahydroxylation of diphenylhydantoin by antituberculosis chemotherapy. Neurology (Minneap.) **16**, 594—602 (1966).

LA DU, B.N.: Metabolic factors controlling duration of drug action. *Proceedings of the First International Pharmacological Meeting*, vol. 6, pp. 229—233. Eds. B.B. BRODIE and E.G. ERDOS. New York: The Macmillan Co. 1962.

— HORNING, E.C., WOOD, H.B., TRUSOF, N., BRODIE, B.B.: Inhibition of enzymatic dealkylation by compounds related to β-diethylamino-diphenyl-propylacetate (SKF 525-A). Fed. Proc. **13**, 377 (1954).

LEADBEATER, L., DAVIES, D.R.: The inhibition of the liver microsomal N-demethylation of morphine by N-allyl normorphine and its pharmacological implications. Biochem. Pharmacol. **13**, 1569—1576 (1964).

LEWIS, S.E., WILKINSON, C.F., RAY, J.W.: The relationship between microsomal epoxidation and lipid peroxidation in houseflies and pig liver and the inhibitory effect of derivatives of 1,3-benzodioxole (methylenedioxybenzene). Biochem. Pharmacol. **16**, 1195—1210 (1967).

MACHINIST, J.M., ORME-JOHNSON, W.H., ZIEGLER, D.M.: Microsomal oxidases. II. Properties of a pork liver microsomal N-oxidase-dealkylase. Biochemistry **5**, 2939—2943 (1966).

MAGUS, R.D., FOUTS, J.R.: Multiple action of 2′-diethylaminoethyl 2,2-diphenylpentanoate HCl (SKF 525-A) on rat liver tryptophan pyrrolase *in vivo*. Biochem. Pharmacol. **16**, 1323—1337 (1967).

— RICKERT, D.E., FOUTS, J.R.: Activation of hydrocortisone-induced tryptophan pyrrolase of rat liver by SKF 525-A. The possible involvement of antidiuretic hormone. Biochem. Pharmacol. **17**, 2071—2080 (1968).

MANNERING, G.J.: Significance of stimulation and inhibition of drug metabolism in pharmacological testing; in *Selected Pharmacological Testing Methods*, pp. 51—119. Ed. by A. BURGER. New York: Marcel Dekker 1968.

— Microsomal enzyme systems which catalyze drug metabolism; in *Fundamentals of Drug Metabolism and Disposition*, eds. B.N. LA DU, H.G. MANDEL and E.L. WAY, Baltimore/Maryland: Williams and Wilkins 1970 (in press).

— SLADEK, N.E., PARLI, C.J., SHOEMAN, D.W.: Formation of a new P-450 hemoprotein after treatment of rats with polycyclic hydrocarbons. In: *Microsomes and Drug Oxidations*, pp. 303—330. Eds. J.R. GILLETTE, A.H. CONNEY, G.J. COSMIDES, R.W. ESTABROOK, J.R. FOUTS and G.J. MANNERING. New York: Academic Press 1969.

— TAKEMORI, A.E.: The effect of repeated administration of levorphan, dextrophan and morphine on the capacity of rat liver preparations to demethylate morphine- and morphinan-type analgesics. J. Pharmacol. exp. Ther. **127**, 187—190 (1959).

MARSHALL, F.N., WILLIAMSON, H.E.: Natruretic response during infusion of β-diethylaminoethyldiphenylpropylacetate hydrochloride. J. Pharmacol. exp. Ther. **143**, 395—400 (1964).

MATTHEWS, H.B., HODGSON, E.: Naturally occurring inhibitor(s) of microsomal oxidations from the house fly. J. econ. Ent. **59**, 1286—1288 (1966).

McMAHON, R.E.: The competitive inhibition of N-demethylation of butynamine by 2,4-dichloro-6-phenylphenoxyethylamine (DPEA). J. Pharmacol. exp. Ther. **138**, 382—386 (1962).

— MILLS, J.: Demethylation studies. II. The competitive inhibition of microsomal N-demethylating enzyme by a primary amine, 2,4-dichloro-6-phenylphenoxyethylamine. J. med. pharm. Chem. **4**, 211—213 (1961).

— — CULP, H.W., GIBSON, W.R., MILLER, W.M, MARSHALL, F.J.: Demethylation studies. VI. The inhibition of hepatic microsomal oxygenation by 2,4-dichloro(6-phenylphenoxy) ethylamine and related compounds. J. med. Chem. **12**, 207—211 (1969).

MEROLA, A.J., TURNBULL, J.D.: The inhibition of drug metabolism by antispermatogenic N,N′-bis(dichloroacetyl) diamines. Biochem. Pharmacol. **16**, 211—215 (1967).

METCALF, R.L., FUKUTO, T.R.: Carbamate insecticides. Effects of chemical structure on intoxication and detoxication of phenyl N-methylcarbamates in insects. J. agr. Fd. Chem. **13**, 220—231 (1965).

MITOMA, C., POSNER, H.S., REITZ, H.C., UDENFRIEND, S.: Enzymatic hydroxylation of aromatic compounds. Arch. Biochem. **61**, 431—441 (1956).

MOOREFIELD, H.H.: Insecticide resistance to the carbamate insecticides; in Symposium on research progress in insecticide resistance. Misc. Pubs. ent. Soc. Am. **2**, 145—152 (1960).

MORELLO, A.: Role of DDR-hydroxylation in resistance. Nature (Lond.) **203**, 785—786 (1964).

MURPHY, S. D., DUBOIS, K. P.: The influence of various factors on enzymatic conversion of organic thiophosphates to anticholinesterase agents. J. Pharmacol. exp. Ther. **124**, 194 to 202 (1958).
MURRAY, F. J.: Outbreak of unexpected reactions among epileptics taking isoniazid. Amer. Rev. resp. Dis. **86**, 729—732 (1962).
NAKATSUGAWA, T., DAHM, P. A.: Parathion activation enzymes in the fat body microsomes of the American cockroach. J. econ. Ent. **58**, 500—509 (1965).
— — Microsomal metabolism of parathion. Biochem. Pharmacol. **16**, 25—38 (1967).
— ISHIDA, M., DAHM, P. A.: Microsomal epoxidation of cyclodiene insecticides. Biochem. Pharmacol. **14**, 1853—1865 (1965).
NARASIMHULU, S., COOPER, D. Y., ROSENTHAL, O.: Spectrophotometric properties of a triton-clarified steroid 21-hydroxylase system of adrenocortical microsomes. Life Sci. **4**, 2101—2107 (1965).
NAVIS, G. J., TONER, J. J., COOK, L.: Effect of β-diethylaminoethyl-diphenylpropylacetate hydrochloride (SKF 525-A) on the activity of d-tubocurarine chloride. Fed. Proc. **12**, 354 (1953).
NETTER, K. J.: Die Hemmung der Procainhydrolyze durch die Diäthyläminoäthanolester der Diephenylpropylessigsäure (SKF 525-A) und der Diphenylessigsäure („Trasentin"). Naunyn-Schmiedeberg's Arch. exp. Path. Pharmak. **235**, 498—512 (1959).
— Drugs as inhibitors of drug metabolism; in *Metabolic Factors Controlling Drug Action, Proceedings of the First International Pharmacological Meeting*, vol. 6, pp. 213—233. Eds. B. B. BRODIE and E. G. ERDOS. New York: The Macmillan Co. 1962.
NEUBERT, D., HERKEN, H.: Wirkungssteigerung von Schlafmitteln durch den Phenyldiallylessigsäureester des Diäthylaminoäthanols. Naunyn-Schmiedeberg's Arch. exp. Path. Pharmak. **225**, 453—462 (1955).
— MAIBAUER, D.: Vergleichende Untersuchungen der oxydativen Leistungen von mitochondrien und Microsomen bei experimenteller Leberschädigung. Naunyn-Schmiedeberg's Arch. exp. Path. Pharmak. **235**, 291—300 (1959).
NEUMANN, N. R., MIYA, T. S., BOUSQUET, W. F.: Mechanism of development of tolerance to β-diethylaminoethyl diphenylpropylacetate (SKF 525-A) in the rat. Proc. Soc. exp. Biol. (N.Y.) **114**, 141—145 (1963).
OAE, S., KITAO, T., KAWAMURA, S.: Model pathways for enzymic oxidative demethylation. II. Polonovskii reaction of N,N-dimethylaniline N-oxide, Pummerer reactions of dimethyl, butyl methyl, and methionine sulfoxide with acetylating agents and their implications in enzymic demethylation. Tetrahedron **19**, 1783—1788 (1963).
O'BRIEN, R. D.: The effect of SKF 525-A (2-diethylaminoethyl 2:2-diphenylvalerate hydrochloride) on organophosphate metabolism in insects and mammals. Biochem. J. **79**, 229—235 (1961).
— Desulfuration; in Proceedings of the First International Pharmacological Meeting, Stockholm. Vol. 6, pp. 111—119. Eds. B. B. BRODIE and E. G. ERDOS. New York: Pergamon Press 1962.
OLESEN, O.: Disulfiram (antabuse) as inhibitor of phenytoin metabolism. Acta pharmacol. (Kbh.) **24**, 317—322 (1966).
— The influence of disulfiram and calcium carbimide on the serum diphenylhydantoin. Arch. Neurol. (Chic.) **16**, 642—644 (1967).
ORRENIUS, S., ERNSTER, L.: Phenobarbital-induced synthesis of the oxidative demethylating enzyme of rat liver microsomes. Biochem. biophys. Res. Commun. **16**, 60—65 (1964).
PETTIT, F. H., ZIEGLER, D. M.: The catalytic demethylation of N,N-dimethylaniline-N-oxide by liver microsomes. Biochem. biophys. Res. Commun. **13**, 193—197 (1963).
PFEFFER, M., SEMMEL, M., SCHOR, J. M.: Rat brain monoamine oxidase inhibition by β-diethylaminoethyl diphenylpropylacetate (SKF 525-A). Enzymologia **34**, 299—303 (1968).
PHILLEO, W. W., SCHONBROD, R. D., TERRIERE, L. C.: Methylenedioxyphenyl compounds as inhibitors of the hydroxylation of naphthalene in houseflies. J. agr. Fd. Chem. **13**, 113—115 (1965).
POSNER, H. S., GRAVES, A., KING, C. T. G., WILK, A.: Experimental alteration of the metabolism of chlorcyclizine and the incidence of cleft palate in rats. J. Pharmacol. exp. Ther. **155**, 494—505 (1967).
RAND, M. J., TRINKER, F. R.: The mechanism of the augmentation of responses to indirectly acting sympathomimetic amines by monoamine oxidase inhibitors. Brit. J. Pharmacol. **33**, 287—303 (1968).
REMMER, H.: Die Beschleunigung des Evipanabbaues unter der Wirkung von Barbituraten. Naturwissenschaften **45**, 189 (1958a).
— Die Verstärkung der Abbaugeschwindigkeit von Evipan durch Glykocorticoide. Naunyn-Schmiedeberg's Arch. exp. Path. Pharmak. **233**, 184—191 (1958b).

REMMER, H., SCHENKMAN, J., ESTABROOK, R.W., SASAME, H., GILLETTE, J., NARASIMHULU, S., COOPER, D.Y., ROSENTHAL, O.: Drug interaction with hepatic microsomal cytochrome. Molec. Pharmacol. **2**, 187—190 (1966).

ROGERS, L.A., ALCANTARA, G.A., FOUTS, J.R.: p-Aminosalicylic acid induced prolongation of hexobarbital sleeping time. J. Pharmacol. exp. Ther. **142**, 242—247 (1963a).

— DIXON, R.L., FOUTS, J.R.: The effects of SKF 525-A on hepatic glycogen and rate of hepatic drug metabolism. Biochem. Pharmacol. **12**, 341—348 (1963b).

— FOUTS, J.R.: Some of the interactions of SKF 525-A with hepatic microsomes. J. Pharmacol. exp. Ther. **146**, 286—293 (1964).

RUBIN, A., TEPHLY, T.R., MANNERING, G.J.: Kinetics of drug metabolism by hepatic microsomes. Biochem. Pharmacol. **13**, 1007—1016 (1964a).

— — — Inhibition of hexobarbital metabolism by ethylmorphine and codeine in the intact rat. Biochem. Pharmacol. **13**, 1053—1057 (1964b).

RÜMKE, C.L., BOUT, J.: Die Beeinflussung der Hexobarbitalnarkose durch vorher verabfolgte Pharmaka. Naunyn-Schmiedeberg's Arch. exp. Path. Pharmak. **240**, 218—223 (1960).

SASAME, H.A., CASTRO, J.A., GILLETTE, J.R.: Studies on the destruction of liver microsomal cytochrome P-450 by carbon tetrachloride administration. Biochem. Pharmacol. **17**, 1759—1768 (1968).

— GILLETTE, J.R.: Studies on the inhibitory effects of various substances on drug metabolism by liver microsomes: the effect of nicotinamide in altering the apparent mechanism of inhibition. Biochem. Pharmacol. **19**, 1025—1041 (1970).

SCHENKMAN, J.B., BALL, J.A., ESTABROOK, R.W.: On the use of nicotinamide in assays for microsomal mixed-function oxidase activity. Biochem. Pharmacol. **16**, 1071—1081 (1967a).

— REMMER, H., ESTABROOK, R.W.: Spectral studies of drug interaction with hepatic microsomal cytochrome. Molec. Pharmacol. **3**, 113—123 (1967b).

SERRONE, D.M., FUJIMOTO, J.M.: The effect of certain inhibitors in producing shortening of hexobarbital action. Biochem. Pharmacol. **11**, 609—615 (1962).

SHOEMAN, D.W., CHAPLIN, M.D., MANNERING, G.J.: Induction of drug metabolism. III. Further evidence for the formation of a new P-450 hemoprotein after treatment of rats with 3-methylcholanthrene. Molec. Pharmacol. **5**, 412—419 (1969).

SJÖQVIST, F., GILLETTE, J.R.: Potentiation of oxotremorine by "anti-tremorine" drugs. Pharmacologist **6**, 245 (1964).

— — Prolongation and potentiation of oxotremorine effects by desmethylimipramine, an "anti-tremorine" drug. Life Sci. **4**, 1031—1036 (1965).

— HAMMER, W., SCHUMACHER, H., GILLETTE, J.R.: The effect of desmethylimipramine and other "anti-tremorine" drugs on the metabolism of tremorine and oxotremorine in rats and mice. Biochem. Pharmacol. **17**, 915—934 (1968).

SLADEK, N.E.: Studies on the stimulation of drug metabolism by phenobarbital and polycyclic hydrocarbons, Ph. D. thesis, Univ. of Minnesota (1966).

— MANNERING, G.J.: Evidence for a new P-450 hemoprotein in hepatic microsomes from methylcholanthrene treated rats. Biochem. biophys. Res. Commun. **24**, 668—674 (1966).

— — Induction of drug metablism. I. Differences in the mechanism by which polycyclic hydrocarbons and phenobarbital produce their inductive effects on microsomal N-demethylating systems. Molec. Pharmacol. **5**, 174—185 (1969a).

— — Induction of drug metabolism. II. Qualitative differences in the microsomal N-demethylating systems stimulated by polycyclic hydrocarbons and by phenobarbital. Molec. Pharmacol. **5**, 186—199 (1969b).

SMITH, J.W., SEIDL, L.G., CLUFF, L.E.: Studies on the epidemiology of adverse drug reactions. Ann. intern. Med. **65**, 629—640 (1966).

SOLOMON, H.M., SCHROGIE, J.J.: The effect of phenyramidol on the metabolism of bishydroxycoumarin. J. Pharmacol. exp. Ther. **154**, 660—666 (1966).

— — The effect of phenyramidol on the metabolism of diphenylhydantoin. Clin. Pharmacol. Ther. **8**, 554—556 (1967).

STITZEL, R.E., ANDERS, M.W., MANNERING, G.J.: Inhibition of drug metabolism. III. Inhibition of hexobarbital metabolism in the intact rat and in the isolated perfused liver by 2-diethylaminoethyl 2,2-diphenylvalerate HCl (SKF 525-A) and its N-deethylated derivatives. Molec. Pharmacol. **2**, 335—340 (1966).

— TEPHLY, T.R., MANNERING, G.J.: Inhibition of drug metabolism. VI. Inhibition of hexobarbital metabolism in the isolated perfused liver of the rat. Molec. Pharmacol. **4**, 15—19 (1968).

SULSER, F., OWENS, M.L., DINGELL, J.V.: On the mechanism of amphetamine potentiation by desipramine (DMI). Life Sci. **5**, 2005—2010 (1966).

TAKEMORI, A.E., MANNERING, G. J.: Metabolic N- and O-demethylation of morphine- and morphinan-type analgesics. J. Pharmacol. exp. Ther. **123**, 171—179 (1958).

TARDIFF, R.G., DUBOIS, K.P.: Inhibition of hepatic microsomal enzymes by alkylating agents. Arch. int. Pharmacodyn. **177**, 445—456 (1969).
TEPHLY, T.R., MANNERING, G.J.: Inhibition of drug metabolism. V. Inhibition of drug metabolism by steroids. Molec. Pharmacol. **4**, 10—14 (1968).
VALZELLI, L., CONSOLO, S., MORPURGO, C.: Influence of imipramine-like drugs on the metabolism of amphetamine; in Symposium on Antidepressant Drugs, pp. 61—69. Excerpta Medica Foundation, series 122, 1966.
VARAGIĆ, V., STEPANOVIĆ, S., HAJDUKOVIĆ, S.: The effect of X-irradiation and cysteamine on the barbiturate sleeping time in rats. Arch. int. Pharmacodyn. **138**, 113—119 (1962).
WELCH, R.M., KOCSIS, J.J.: Activation of tremorine by liver. Proc. Soc. exp. Biol. (N.Y.) **107**, 731—739 (1961).
WILKINSON, G.N.: Statistical estimation in enzyme kinetics. Biochem. J. **80**, 324—332 (1961).
WONG, D.T., TERRIERE, L.C.: Epoxidation of aldrin, isodrin and heptachlor by rat liver microsomes. Biochem. Pharmacol. **14**, 375—377 (1965).
WOOLES, W.R., McPHILLIPS, J.J.: Hepatic glycogen concentration and hexobarbital-sleeping time in mice. Proc. Soc. exp. Biol. (N.Y.) **121**, 399—401 (1966).
ZIEGLER, D.M., PETTIT, F.H.: Formation of an intermediate N-oxide in the oxidative demethylation of N,N-dimethylaniline catalyzed by liver microsomes. Biochem. biophys. Res. Commun. **15**, 188—193 (1964).

Subsection B: Nonmicrosomal Enzymes

Chapter 50

Esterases of Human Tissues

BERT N. LA DU and HARRY SNADY

With 2 Figures

A. Introduction

This chapter is a brief survey of the esterases which have been identified in human tissues. The literature on esterases is voluminous; a comprehensive review of even the relatively limited number of esterases that are known to be present in the blood and other tissues of man would be an enormous task. We have arbitrarily selected only certain references from the available source material to emphasize those aspects which we feel will be of greatest usefulness and interest to biochemical pharmacologists.

There are special problems concerning the classification and the identification of esterases which should be noted. In general, esterases have been characterized by their pattern of substrate specificity and their sensitivity to a variety of inhibitors. Most esterases, however, are not unique in these features; different esterases are likely to show common properties in their substrate requirements as well as in their inhibitor sensitivity. Identification is based upon a series of quantitative responses rather than the result of highly specific tests for each esterase. The problem of identification is even more difficult when the tests have been made on a mixture of esterases, such as plasma or tissue extracts. The development of the zymogram technique, using starch gel electrophoresis as described by SMITHIES (1955) followed by histochemical tests for esterase activity in the gel, as introduced by HUNTER and MARKERT (1957), has provided a valuable method both to obtain physical separation of the individual esterases as discrete bands and to determine the characteristics of the separated esterases in regard to substrate requirements and susceptibility to many inhibitors applied directly to the gel strips.

B. Properties of Different Types of Esterases

The characteristics of seven major types of esterases which have been found in one or more human tissues are summarized in Tables 1 and 2. Of the seven types of esterases only three have been extensively investigated: acetylcholinesterase, serum cholinesterase (pseudocholinesterase) and carbonic anhydrase, the esterase activity of the last enzyme having been recognized in recent years.

Acetylcholinesterase (true cholinesterase) is well known. It is believed to play an important role in the hydrolysis of acetylcholine in nervous tissue. The esterase is widely distributed and has been found to be present in all nervous tissues and erythrocytes of all species examined (Table 1). It appears to be intimately involved in the neurohumoral functions of acetylcholine in nerve transmission and in

Table 1. *Distribution and substrate specificity of esterases of human tissues*[a]

	Acetylcholinesterase (True cholinesterase)	Serum Cholin-esterase (Pseudocholin-esterase)	Aliesterase (B-esterase)	Acetyl esterase	Arylesterase (Aromatic esterase)	Carbonic Anhydrase	C-esterase
Tissue distribution	Central nervous system (grey matter) Sympathetic ganglia Motor end plates Erythrocytes	Plasma Intestinal nucosa Liver Central nervous system (White matter)	Liver Erythrocytes Muscle Kidney	Liver Kidney Erythrocytes Muscle	Plasma Erythrocytes	Erythrocytes Renal Cortex Gastric mucosa	Erythro-cytes
Choline esters	ACh > PrCh > BuCh acetyl-β-methyl-choline +; benzoyl-choline —	BuCh > PrCh > ACh acetyl-β-methyl-choline —; benzoyl-choline +	—	ACh	—	?	—
Acetate esters	Preferentially hydrolyzed	Hydrolyzed; not best substrates	Most are hydrolyzed	Characteristic substrates	Only of aromatic type	?	Many are hydrolyzed
Aliphatic esters	+, not triglycerides	+, including triglycerides	Characteristic substrates	+ of acetic acid	—[c]	?	Many are hydrolyzed
Long Chain fatty acid esters	—	+	—[b]	—	—	?	—
Aromatic esters	∅Ac > ∅Pr > ∅Bu	∅Bu > ∅Pr > ∅Ac	∅Bu > ∅Ac	∅Ac	∅Ac > ∅Pr	p-NO_2∅Ac	∅Ac
α-naphthyl-acetate	+	+	+	+	+	+	+

[a] +, compound hydrolyzed; —, compound not hydrolyzed.
[b] These substrates are hydrolyzed by lipases.
[c] Aliphatic substrates with a double bond α to the ethereal oxygen (e.g. vinylacetate) are hydrolyzed.

Table 2. *Inhibitors of esterases of human tissues*

Inhibitors	Acetylcholin-esterase (True Colin-esterase)	Serum Cholin-esterase (Pseudocholin-esterase)	Aliesterase (B-esterase)	Acetylesterase	Arylesterase (Aromatic esterase)	Carbonic Anhydrase	C-esterase
Eserine	Inhibition at 10^{-5}	Inhibition at 10^{-5}	Inhibition at 10^{-3} to 10^{-4}	Inhibition at 10^{-4} to 10^{-5}	No inhib.	?	No inhib.
DFP	Inhibition at 10^{-6}	Inhibition at 10^{-6}	Inhibition at 10^{-4} to 10^{-5}	Inhibition at 10^{-4} to 10^{-5}	No inhib.[b]	?	No inhib.
Paraxon	Inhibition at 10^{-6}	Inhibition at 10^{-6}	Inhibition at 10^{-5}	Inhibition at 10^{-3} to 10^{-4}	No inhib.[b]	?	No inhib.
p-HMB and p-CMB	No inhib.	No inhib.	No inhib.	?	Inhibition at 10^{-2} to 10^{-4}[c]	?	Activation at 10^{-3}
NaF	?	Inhibition at 10^{-2}[a]	No inhib.	No inhib.	No inhib.[c]	No inhib.	?
Acetazolamide .	No inhib.	No inhib.	No inhib.	No inhib.	No inhib.	at 10^{-5}	No inhib.
La^{+++}	No inhib.	No inhib.	No inhib.	?	Inhibition at 10^{-4} to 10^{-6}[c]	?	?
EDTA	No inhib.	No inhib.	No inhib.	No inhib.	Inhibition at 10^{-2} or Act.[c]	No inhib.[d]	?

[a] = Inhibition may be incomplete; [b] = Compounds may be substrates; [c] = Arylesterases differ in their sensitivity to inhibitor; [d] = Inhibition on prolonged incubation.

nerve conduction (Nachmansohn and Wilson, 1951; Wilson, 1961; Koelle, 1963). Wilson (1961) has studied the molecular properties, substrate binding, catalytic mechanism of ester hydrolysis, and interaction with inhibitors; and Nachmansohn (1969) has described the cellular localization of the enzyme and the properties of purified acetylcholinesterase.

Of all the esters studied, acetylcholinesterase catalyzes the hydrolysis of acetylcholine most rapidly, followed by propionylcholine and butyrylcholine. It has some hydrolytic activity with acetyl-β-methylcholine but none with benzoylcholine or methylbutyrate. Hydrolysis of some other aliphatic and aromatic esters occurs, especially acetyl derivatives, but the rates are considerably less than that of acetylcholine hydrolysis.

Inhibition studies with acetylcholinesterase have shown that excess acetylcholine inhibits the rate of its own hydrolysis, a feature that is not generally seen with other esterases. Inhibition by excess substrate is believed to be due to the formation of an enzyme-disubstrate complex, with the quaternary ammonium group of one molecule of substrate bound at the anionic site and the ester group of the second molecule bound at the esteratic site. This causes either molecular strain or an impedence of the reaction with water in the hydrolysis of the acyl-enzyme complex.

Acetylcholinesterase is "irreversibly" inhibited by organophosphate compounds, such as DFP, TEPP and paraoxon, which interact with the enzyme at the esteratic site (Wilson, 1961). It is well known that the inhibited dialkylphosphoryl-enzyme is reactivated by certain nucleophilic agents, such as hydroxamic acids and oximes (including PAM)[1], and that the reactivation is inhibited by quaternary ammonium ions. This implies that the anionic site is still available in the dialkylphosphoryl-enzyme. The esterase is also inhibited by eserine at relatively low concentrations of the inhibitor (10^{-5}M).

Until quite recently the only known catalytic function of carbonic anhydrase was the rapid hydration of carbon dioxide with water to yield carbonic acid. The enzyme is found primarily in the erythrocytes, and seems to aid the diffusion or transport of carbon dioxide, hydrogen ion, bicarbonate and sodium ions. A few years ago Tashian and his collaborators (Shaw et al., 1962; Tashian et al., 1963) reported the esterase activity of carbonic anhydrase. Although the range of esterase activity of carbonic anhydrase has not been fully studied, it is clear that the enzyme will catalyze the hydrolysis of the acetates and butyrate esters of α- and β-naphthol in the following order: β-naphthylacetate > α-naphthylacetate > β-naphthylbutyrate > α-naphthylbutyrate.

There have been several studies and reviews on the molecular properties of carbonic anhydrase (Davis, 1961; Nyman and Lindskog, 1964; Rickli et al., 1964). Human erythrocytes have at least three carbonic anhydrases, designated carbonic anhydrases A, B and C by Rickli et al. (1964) and Nyman and Lindskog (1964). Carbonic anhydrase A is present in small amounts and has low specific activity; it has not been investigated in detail. Carbonic anhydrases B and C have been highly purified and characterized (Rickli et al., 1964: Nyman and Lindskog, 1964; Tashian, 1965). Both enzymes have molecular weights of approximately 30,000 and contain one atom of zinc per molecule. They differ in their amino acid composition, isoelectric points and other physical properties. The specific activities of the carbonic anhydrase activity of the two enzymes also differ; carbonic anhydrase C has about thirty times greater a specific activity than carbonic

1 The following abbreviations are used: PAM, pyridine-2-aldoxime methiodide; DFP, diisopropylfluorophosphate; TEPP, tetraethylpyrophosphate; EDTA, ethylenediamine tetracetate; *p*HMB, *p*-hydroxymercuribenzoate; *p*CMB, *p*-chloromercuribenzoate.

anhydrase B. Since there is about five times more carbonic anhydrase B than C present in the erythrocytes, both enzymes are believed to contribute significantly in the total carbonic anhydrase activity of the red cells. The esterase activity of the major carbonic anhydrases seems to be an intrinsic property of these proteins, and it is of interest that the esterase activity is also inhibited by the carbonic anhydrases inhibitor, acetazolamide at 10^{-5}M (SHAW et al., 1962). Several genetic variant forms with different electrophoretic migration patterns have been identified. These will be described in the following section on erythrocyte esterases.

Serum cholinesterase (pseudocholinesterase) catalyzes the hydrolysis of many of the same choline esters as acetylcholinesterase, but the relative rate of hydrolysis of the series of esters is quite different. For example, butyrylcholine is hydrolyzed much faster than acetylcholine. In addition, cholinesterase catalyzes the hydrolysis of benzoylcholine, procaine, acetylsalicylate and succinylcholine but not acetyl-β-methylcholine. Succinylcholine is an especially important drug substrate; studies of unusual individual differences in its metabolism led to the discovery of variant forms of cholinesterase in human serum. (This will be discussed in a later section).

Divalent metal ions, such as Ca^{++} and Mg^{++} activate serum cholinesterase, but are not absolutely required for activity. Other activators are narcotic agents, amino acids and alcohols (AUGUSTINSSON, 1961a). The molecular weight of the enzyme is rather high, about 300,000, and serine seems to be present in the esteratic site (AUGUSTINSSON, 1961a). In human serum, cholinesterase exists in at least four molecular forms that can be identified by the zymogram technique. The slowest migrating band, C_4, has over 80% of the total serum cholinesterase activity; the minor components, C_3, C_2 and C_1, each migrate progressively faster and are of lower molecular weight. Component C_1 is about one-fourth (80,000) the size of C_4 (LA MOTTA et al., 1970; DEWALD and LA DU, 1970). Interconversion of the cholinesterase components has been reported by LAMOTTA et al. (1968), and the conversion of C_4 to a product resembling C_1 can be accomplished using urea and mercaptoethanol (DEWALD and LA DU, 1970). The derived C_1 and native C_1 have essentially the same molecular weights and show similar properties as far as gel migration, substrate affinity characteristics and kinetic properties.

Cholinesterase is much less sensitive to inhibition by excess substrate than acetylcholinesterase (MYERS, 1953), but it is inhibited by organophosphates, carbamates, quaternary ammonium salts and eserine (AUGUSTINSSON, 1961a). Inhibition by the organophosphates and carbamates most likely involves strong binding to the serine hydroxyl group of the esteratic site; the cationic inhibitors combine with the anionic site. A book on cholinesterases has recently been published (GOEDDE et al., 1967).

Aliesterases (B-esterases) are characterized by the fact that they catalyze the hydrolysis of both aliphatic and aromatic esters, but not choline esters. The active site of these enzymes contains an imidazole group and a serine hydroxyl group but no complementary anionic site is present (AUGUSTINSSON, 1961a). They are distinguished from lipases by their selective action on water soluble substrates rather than on water insoluble substrates, such as esters of glycerol and long chain fatty acids. Lipases are, however, frequently included in the group of aliesterases, which have been shown to catalyze the hydrolysis of some triglycerides, such as triacetin and tributyrin (MOUNTER and WHITTAKER, 1953), and some long chain fatty acid esters (ECOBICHON and KALOW, 1962).

AUGUSTINSSON (1961b) compared the forms of esterases in the plasma of many vertebrate species and noted that aliesterases are the main esterases in the plasma of the lower vertebrates. Since aliesterases are absent from human, monkey, dog and pig plasmas it was suggested that during phylogenetic development and biochemical evolution the aliesterases have been replaced by cholinesterases.

It is noteworthy that some aliesterases readily catalyze the hydrolysis of aromatic esters, but their behavior towards certain inhibitors should prevent their misclassification as arylesterases. The aliesterases are inhibited by organophosphates at a concentration of 10^{-5}M, but are not appreciably inhibited by eserine at 10^{-5}M, though they may be inhibited at higher concentrations. In contrast cholinesterases are usually inhibited by eserine at 10^{-6}M.

Arylesterases (aromatic esterases) preferentially catalyze the hydrolysis of aromatic esters but not choline esters. Among the aromatic esters, there is a further preference for esters of acetic acid. Phenylacetate seems to be the best substrate for these enzymes. The substrate requirement and specificity of the arylesterases suggests that the hydrolytic mechanism involves the formation of a thiol-ester intermediate, through the combination of a sulfhydryl group of enzyme with a double bond of the substrate to form an activated complex. The hydrolysis of aromatic substrates was not well understood until it was recently shown that the double bond of the alcohol moiety must be in a position alpha to the ester linkage (as phenol in phenyl acetate). Thus, aliphatic esters such as vinylacetate, with a double bond in the correct position, are also hydrolyzed by arylesterase (Augustinsson, 1964; Augustinsson and Ekedahl, 1962). Evidence that a cysteine sulfhydryl group is part of the active site is furnished by the results of inhibition studies. For example, the sulfhydryl agents, *p*-hydroxymercuribenzoate and *p*-chloromercuribenzoate, are strong inhibitors of arylesterases and cysteine reverses the inhibition (Augustinsson, 1961b; Blanco and Zinkham, 1966). Furthermore, the esterases are inhibited by the heavy metals, Hg^{++}, Ag^{+} and Cu^{++} (Augustinsson, 1961b). It is presumed that the sulfhydryl group of the active site acts in conjunction with an imidazole group (Augustinsson, 1964).

Arylesterases are not inhibited by organophosphates. In fact, these compounds sometimes act as substrates for the arylesterases. The lack of inhibition has been attributed to the relatively great susceptibility to hydrolysis of P-S bonds than P-O bonds (Augustinsson, 1964). Another important characteristic of the arylesterases is that they are not inhibited by 10^{-3}M eserine. The activity of many arylesterases depends upon calcium ions, since calcium stimulates and EDTA impairs activity. However, recent studies have shown that certain arylesterases are not only unaffected by calcium, but are actually activated by 0.01 M EDTA (Björklund et al., 1962). Various arylesterases have been characterized by the rates at which they hydrolyze *p*-nitrophenylacetate, and by the minimum concentration of *p*-chloromercuribenzoate or urea required to inactivate the esterase (Tashian, 1965).

Relatively little is known about C-esterases. They were first found by Bergmann et al. (1957) in hog kidney, and catalyze the hydrolysis of aliphatic and aromatic acetates preferentially (Bergmann et al., 1957; Tashian, 1965). Substituents which increase the electrophilic character of the ethereal oxygen atom of the ester group increase the rate of hydrolysis (Bergmann and Rimon, 1958). Whether they catalyze the hydrolysis of choline esters and fatty acid esters has not been determined.

Copper and mercury salts inhibit C-esterase activity, but it is not known whether the inhibition is due to the binding of essential sulfhydryl groups (Bergmann et al., 1957). Studies on the effect of pH on C-esterase activity, however, suggests that there is an imidazole group at the active site (Bergmann and Rimon, 1958).

C-esterases are activated by organic mercurials at low concentrations, 10^{-5}M, which inhibit the arylesterases. As the concentration of the mercurials is increased to 10^{-3}M the activation diminishes and at concentrations between 10^{-3}M and 10^{-2}M inhibition occurs. This inhibition seems to be due to a loss by denaturation rather than to combination with the active site of the esterase (BERGMANN et al., 1957). Studies of the pH dependence of the inhibition by organic mercurials has provided further evidence for the presence of an imidazole group at the active site (BERGMANN and RIMON, 1958). C-esterases are not inhibited by organophosphates, such as DFP or TEPP, nor do they catalyze the hydrolysis of these substances (BERGMANN et al., 1957; BERGMANN and RIMON, 1958).

The last major category of esterases, acetylesterases, is the most general in its characteristics. In fact, several of the other esterases, such as the arylesterases and C-esterases, are often considered to be subtypes of acetylesterases because of the similarity in the substrate specificities of these esterases. The acetylesterases preferentially catalyze the hydrolysis of acetyl esters. Certain acetylesterases are active with other esters, but the order is acetate > propionate > butyrate. The acetylesterases vary in their behavior towards most organophosphates, but they are relatively resistant to these inhibitors. For example, DFP inhibits only at concentrations of approximately 10^{-4}M and no inhibition occurs at 10^{-6}M (ECOBICHON and KALOW, 1962). Acetylesterases are not inhibited by low concentrations of eserine, but are inhibited at 10^{-4}M.

The above discussion has emphasized the properties of the general types of esterases and the characteristics which have been used in their classification. Some esterases have been identified which do not fit neatly into any of the established classes. In some cases, this can be attributed to the difficulty in separating and isolating individual esterases, and the confusion is due to the presence of more than one esterase. In other instances, the properties of the isolated esterase must be accepted as distinctive features of that enzyme, and the limitations of our present classification methods become evident.

The value of the zymogram technique for the identification and characterization of esterases must be mentioned again, since it has been of such importance in recent years in the studies of esterases. This technique has been used by several investigators to determine the pattern of the esterase activities of various human tissues, such as blood, liver, kidney, muscle, heart, brain and other organs. These patterns show some similarities, but there are also interesting differences from tissue to tissue. Our knowledge of the esterases of particular human tissues is still very incomplete, but the following sections will describe some of the esterases in specific tissues of man.

C. Blood Esterases

1. Serum Esterases

The main esterases of human serum are listed in Table 3. AUGUSTINSSON (1959) made a comparative study of the esterases of plasma from a variety of mammalian species, including man, and measured the rates of hydrolysis of a series of substrates (Table 4). Of considerable pharmacological interest is the lack of uniformity in the plasma esterase activities in various mammalian species. Succinylcholine was the only drug included in the series of substrates tested, but it can be predicted that other drugs containing ester groups would also show similar wide variation from species to species.

AUGUSTINSSON (1959) employed the technique of preparative electrophoresis on cellulose columns followed by elution to fractionate the plasma proteins of many mammalian species for detecting the presence of esterases. Again, there were significant species differences in the types and relative concentrations of the

Table 3. *Esterases of human serum*

Name	Forms	Remarks
Cholinesterase (Pseudocholinesterase)	Usual (normal) Dibucaine resistant Fluoride resistant Silent (little or no act.)	Particular esterase determined at E_1 genetic locus; homozygous individuals with dibucaine resistant esterase (atypical), fluoride resistant or silent genes are *sensitive* to succinylcholine.
	C_5	Determined by a gene at another locus, E_2. C_5^+ adds about 25 % cholinesterase activity over that of C_5^-.
	Cynthiana	Genetic locus not established. Individuals with this gene have about three times the normal serum cholinesterase activity; they are *resistant* to succinylcholine.
Arylesterase (Aromatic esterase)	Arylesterase I	Major aromatic esterase; requires calcium, inhibited by EDTA; more labile to heat; inhibited by 5×10^{-5}M La^{+++}; may hydrolyze organophosphates.
	Arylesterase II	Minor aromatic esterase activated by EDTA, no calcium required; inhibited only 50% by 10^{-4}M La^{+++}.
Serum albumin	—	Weak esterase activity with phenylacetate and β-naphthylacetate. May contribute in hydrolysis of compounds such as paraoxon.

Table 4. *Relative rates of hydrolysis of some esters by different mammalian plasma*

Species	Acetyl-choline	Butyryl-choline	Benzoyl-choline	Succinyl-choline	Tributyrin	Phenyl-acetate
Man	135	360	50	3	55	3,330
Monkey (Macaque)	22	71	9	1	10	655
Monkey (Mangabey)	180	540	70	8	90	225
Horse	130	365	40	1	100	2,200
Cow	3	2	0	0	4	4,700
Sheep	7	2	< 1	< 1	2	5,500
Swine	16	23	3	2	3	450[a]
Cat	50	150	12	1	80	5,700
Dog	70	180	30	0	12	2,800
Guinea Pig	50	170	20	0	530	1,700
Rabbit	16	10	2	0	50	7,500[a]
Rat	20	15	10	1	90	3,000

From Augustinsson (1959).

Activity determined manometrically at 25° in a bicarbonate-CO_2 buffer at pH 7.4; substrate concentrations were 0.01 *M*; total liquid volume of incubation mixture, 2.0 ml per flask. Results are expressed in µl of CO_2 evolved during 30 min incubation period per 0.1 ml of plasma, based upon initial rate of reaction, corrected for nonenzymatic hydrolysis.

[a] Marked individual variation in values noted.

esterases in the series of mammalian plasmas. He found human plasma to have two major regions with high esterase activity: one produced rapid hydrolysis of phenylacetate and was presumed to be a peak of arylesterase activity; the other region was rich in cholinesterase activity. Benzoylcholine, succinylcholine and the butyrates of phenol and aliphatic alcohols were hydrolyzed by this fraction. In addition, he found this zone to hydrolyze procaine, atropine and Tween 20, but not cocaine or heroin.

Better resolution of the esterases of human serum was obtained with the zymogram technique. Starch gel electrophoresis methods developed by SMITHIES (1955, 1959) and histochemical procedures (HUNTER and MARKERT, 1957; ECOBICHON and KALOW, 1962) with α-naphthylacetate and Fast Blue RR (diazotized 4-benzoyl-2,5-dimethoxyaniline) gave a dye complex which precipitated at the zones in the gel where α-naphthol had been released by hydrolysis of the ester. Recently, even more sensitive zymogram methods have been published that are particularly well suited for the detection of serum cholinesterases. For example, separation of the proteins by polyacrylamide-agarose gel electrophoresis (URIEL, 1966) followed by the butyrylthiocholine-copper stain described by JUUL (1968).

By the zymogram techniques it is possible to detect one major band (C_4) and three or four minor bands of cholinesterase activity in normal human serum (Fig. 1). One also finds some esterase activity in the albumin region with α-naphthylacetate. This was previously thought to be an artifact and to represent

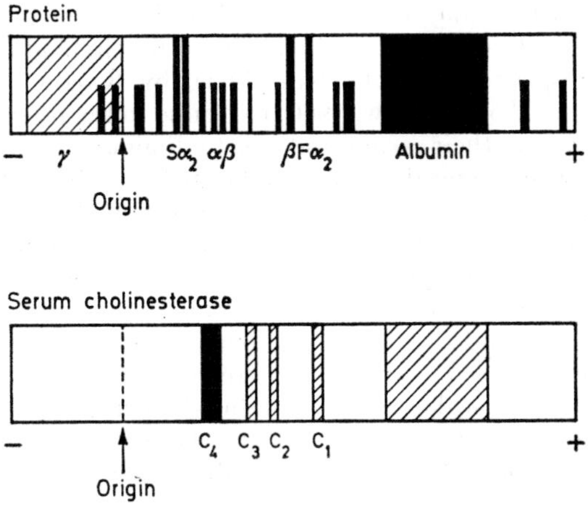

Fig. 1. Comparison of serum proteins separated by starch gel electrophoresis stained for proteins (above) and cholinesterase (below). The weak esterase activity found in the albumin region is indicated as well as the major (C_4) and minor (C_3, C_2 and C_1) bands of cholinesterase

protein binding of the naphthol-dye complex by albumin rather than the presence of esterase activity of albumin. ERDÖS and BOGGS (1961) have shown that albumin is able to catalyze the hydrolysis of naphthylacetate, and ZELLER (1956) found hydrolysis of phenylacetate in the albumin region. It is still not absolutely clear whether the esterase activity observed is due to esterases contaminating the albumin or to an esterase activity of albumin itself. SIMPSON (1968), using phenylacetate and Fast Black as the dye-coupling agent, observed a faster moving band of esterase activity, which migrated with the albumin fraction, in 4% of Cree Indians. The esterase was not sensitive to eserine or to EDTA. Apparently this esterase variant is identical to the albumin variant described by MELARTIN and BLUMBERG (1966) in Naskapi Indians. This would seem to be further evidence that human serum albumin does have some intrinsic esterase activity. Further studies are needed to evaluate the importance of this property, particularly whether it is able to catalyze the hydrolysis of any drugs which contain ester linkages.

The α-naphthylacetate-Fast Blue RR system is not suitable for the detection of arylesterases of human plasma, but a simple method based on the hydrolysis of phenylacetate in a weakly buffered solution of phenol red (La Du, 1970) can be used. The zymogram shows yellow bands, where acid has been produced, against a pink colored background. In human plasma the arylesterase bands are found behind albumin, but well in front of the cholinesterase C_4 band. Thus, drug substrates used in place of phenylacetate would produce a yellow color with phenol red if they are hydrolyzed at an appreciable rate in the appropriate zones. Succinylcholine, as expected, is hydrolyzed in the cholinesterase C_4 region; acetylsalicylic acid is also hydrolyzed in the C_4 band and not where phenylacetate is hydrolyzed.

The above methods, with further refinements, will serve not only to indicate which plasma esterases will hydrolyze specific drugs, but also to allow investigators to detect whether altered proteins, such as genetic variant forms of the esterases, possess the ability to catalyze these hydrolyses.

Soon after the muscle relaxant drug, succinylcholine, was introduced clinical experience led to the realization that serum cholinesterase was of critical importance in determining how much of the drug reaches its sites of action at the myoneural junction and how long the drug remained in the body. The exaggerated response to the usual dose of succinylcholine by certain individuals with prolonged paralysis of the respiratory muscles was shown by Kalow and his coworkers (Kalow and Davies, 1958; Kalow, 1960) to be due to the presence of an atypical type of cholinesterase in their serum and not to diminished amounts of the usual type of enzyme. The atypical esterase inherited by these individuals differs qualitatively from normal esterase in having a lower affinity for choline ester substrates, and thus is a much less efficient catalyst in hydrolyzing succinylcholine at concentrations present in the blood. The atypical esterase also is less susceptible to inhibition by dibucaine and several other inhibitors than is normal cholinesterase. Kalow and Genest (1957) developed a useful diagnostic test for the atypical esterase, based upon the difference in dibucaine inhibition under standard conditions. Atypical esterase is inhibited about 20% and normal esterase about 80%. The test also permitted the detection of carriers of the trait, since their serum showed about 60% inhibition by dibucaine in the test. The incidence of heterozygous carriers in the Canadian population studied by Kalow was 3.8%. About 1:2,500 individuals have atypical esterase and would be sensitive to succinylcholine if given the drug. Heterozygous carriers have a mixture of normal and atypical esterase in their serum, but do not show sensitivity to the drug under ordinary circumstances.

The atypical (dibucaine resistant) esterase variant form of serum cholinesterase accounts for the largest fraction of exaggerated responses to succinylcholine, at least for the cases that can be explained on a genetic basis and directly attributed to functional alterations in the esterase. A number of additional variant forms of serum cholinesterase have been recognized in recent years that are also associated with unusual clinical responses to succinylcholine. One variant, called the "fluoride resistant" type of cholinesterase, was discovered by Harris and Whittaker (1961). It also has a reduced affinity for choline esters and is detected by its greater resistance to fluoride inhibition than normal cholinesterase. Occasionally, people have been found with essentially no detectable cholinesterase activity in their serum. This deficiency is inherited and the individuals are homozygous for the "silent" gene (see GOEDDE et al., 1967). Family studies and pedigree analyses indicate that one genetic locus, E_1, determines the type of serum cholinesterase each person inherits. At that locus, four allelic genes, *normal*, *dibucaine resistant*, *fluoride resistant* and *silent*, permit many genotypic combinations and types of serum esterase. Practically, succinylcholine sensitivity is observed only in those individuals with no normal esterase, since heterozygous individuals carrying half of the usual amount of normal enzyme are protected adequately.

The above variants in cholinesterase are associated with decreased activity, but there is an interesting family in which several members have unusually high serum cholinesterase activity (NEITLICH, 1966). In zymograms of their serum an additional or double band of esterase is found in the C_4 region, and their serum has nearly three times as much esterase activity as normal. YOSHIDA and MOTULSKY (1969), who named this variant "Cynthiana", believe that the specific activity of the esterase is normal and that the high activity is due to an unusually large amount of enzyme.

Although the E_1 locus mentioned above is of greatest importance in determining the characteristics of serum cholinesterase, another locus, E_2 also affects serum cholinesterase activity. The presence of an extra band of cholinesterase in about 10% of the people is determined by the E_2 locus. The esterase called C_5, was discovered by HARRIS et al. (1962) using electrophoresis in two dimensions, but it is not easily detected by the usual zymogram techniques. Since it contributes to the total cholinesterase activity of serum, C^+_5 individuals have about 25% more esterase activity than C^-_5 people.

The range of cholinesterase activity is extremely broad when we consider not only the variation in activity of individuals with normal esterase, but the exterme limits represented by the genetic variants which extend from essentially no activity (individuals homozygous for the silent gene) to the triple-normal value (individuals with the Cynthiana variant). Since people lacking cholinesterase have no metabolic disorder it seems that this enzyme serves no vital role in normal metabolism. In the hydrolysis of succinylcholine, however, it is evident that the problems encountered clinically with this drug arise because of the wide individual variations in rate of hydrolysis of the drug. Even though a highly charged compound, such as succinylcholine, would ordinarily not require metabolic transformation for it to be eliminated from the body in a reasonably short time, the enzyme in normal individuals markedly shortens the drug's biological half-life and high doses are needed to elicit the therapeutic effect. Thus, the usual dose is in great excess of that required by individuals with reduced cholinesterase activity.

The importance of cholinesterase in the metabolism of drugs other than succinylcholine is still uncertain. Procaine and acetylsalicylic acid are both hydrolyzed by cholinesterase, but there is no evidence that the rate of hydrolysis in serum is critical in determining their pharmacological effectiveness or their toxicity. However, the variety of cholinesterases and levels of activity in man which have been found as a result of the experience with succinylcholine should enable investigators to evaluate some of these possibilities with appropriate subjects.

Two forms of arylesterase in human serum have been separated by continuous flow curtain electrophoresis by BJÖRKLUND et al. (1962). Arylesterase I, which migrates faster than arylesterase II in curtain electrophoresis, is more labile to heat, the activity being lost after heating to 56°C for 30 min. It is inhibited by 0.01 *M* EDTA and by 5×10^{-5}M La^{+++}. Arylesterase II withstands heating to 68°C for 30 min and is activated by 0.01 *M* EDTA. It is more resistant to inhibition by La^{+++}; it is inhibited only 50% by La^{+++} at $10^{-4} M$. Human plasma contains about five times as much arylesterase I activity as arylesterase II. The low activity of plasma of newborn infants may be due to a lack of one of these two forms of the enzyme, which apparently cannot pass from the maternal circulation to the infant *in utero* (Augustinsson and Brody, 1962). The level of arylesterase activity is low in newborn infants, but increases during the first six months after birth and reaches adult levels in two year old children. No sex differences were found in the rate of increase or in adult levels of activity (Augustinsson and Barr, 1963; Augustinsson, 1964).

Although there is evidence that the level of serum arylesterase in pigs is genetically determined (Augustinsson and Olsson, 1960), this has not been proved for man. Augustinsson (1964) suggests this possibility, and he found that serum esterase levels in monozygotic and dizygotic twins gave correlation values which supported this view. The site of synthesis of the serum arylesterase is not known, but Augustinsson and Brody (1962) have proposed that it may be mainly in the kidney rather than the liver. However, the finding of reduced levels of the esterase in patients with liver disease and cachexia (Marton and Kalow, 1959) suggests that the liver is also a source of serum arylesterase. On the basis of the rate of decline of arylesterase contained in blood given to infants needing transfusions, Augustinsson and Barr (1963) estimated the half-life of the serum enzyme to be about 16 h.

2. Erythrocyte Esterases

Several types of esterases have been identified in human red blood cells. These include acetylcholinesterase, carbonic anhydrase, aliesterase, arylesterase and C-esterase. The acetylcholinesterase of erythrocytes has been shown to catalyze the hydrolysis of phenylacetate and acetylcholine at equally rapid rates. A series of para-substituted phenylacetates was also studied, and all but *p*-nitrophenyl derivatives were hydrolyzed to some extent (Mounter and Whittaker, 1953). Inhibition studies indicated that the red cell acetylcholinesterase had the same sensitivity to inhibitors as acetylcholinesterase of the nervous tissue (Table 2).

The physiological significance of the low but significant esterase activity shown by the different molecular forms of carbonic anhydrase is not known. It has been calculated that one molecule of carbonic anhydrase C can catalyze the hydration of 36×10^6 molecules of CO_2/min at pH 7 and 25° C, and the hydrolysis of about 2,200 molecules of *p*-nitrophenylacetate under similar experimental conditions (Edsall, 1968). A third distinct chemical reaction that carbonic anhydrase can also catalyze is the hydration of aldehydes (Pocker and Meany, 1965).

Several variant forms of carbonic anhydrase B have been described and all of these may be different products of allelic genes at the locus which determines the structure of this protein (Tashian et al., 1963). These are summarized in Table 5. The variant forms have been discovered by their unusual mobilities during electrophoresis. Carbonic anhydrase variants have been reported in many other species as well as man (Tashian et al., 1968). The different forms of carbonic anhydrase have varying amounts of esterase activity, but no forms have been observed which have unusually high esterase activity. Nevertheless, these esterases might contribute to the hydrolysis of drugs and other esters foreign to the body. This possibility must still be explored, and the known genetic variants should be useful in these investigations.

The aliphatic esterase found in human erythrocytes (Mounter and Whittaker, 1953) was shown to be sensitive to DFP but not eserine. The esterase catalyzed the hydrolysis of tributyrin faster than most of the aromatic esters

Table 5. *Forms of carbonic anhydrase with esterase activity detected in human erythrocytes*

Carbonic anhydrases[a]	Other designations				Usual and variant forms of enzyme		
	NYMAN (1961	RICKLI and EDSALL (1962)	LAURENT (1962)	TASHIAN, (1965) TASHIAN et al. (1966)	Variant	Incidence	Distinguishing characteristics
Carbonic anhydrase A	II		X_2	Ia (+1)	—	all populations	Minor normal component
					CA-Ia	Found in all populations tested	Normal form; prefers β-over α-naphthylacetate as esterase substrate.
					CA-Ib	First observed in hemolysates from a patient with mongolism (Trisomy-21 Karyotype) (SHAW et al., 1962)	Alternate form of enzyme appears to be under the contro of a single autosomal gene. Only heterozygous individuals have been detected. Altered enzyme not associated with mongolism.
Carbonic anhydrase B	III	I	X_1	I	CA-Ic Guam	First observed in 4 of 500 Micronesians (TASHIAN et al., 1963)	Modified form of enzyme appears to be under control of a single autosomal gene. Esterase activity of enzyme like that of normal form. Only heterozygous individuals have been detected. Structural modification appears to be a replacement of glycine for argenine in the mutant enzyme (TASHIAN, 1966).
					CA-Id	Found in 2 of 600 American negroes (TASHIAN, 1965)	Only heterozygous individuals have been detected. Variant form of enzyme may be product of a gene alletic with above (TASHIAN, 1965).
Carbonic anhydrase C	V	II	Y	II	—	All populations	Normal major component. No variants detected in man; a few have been found in other species (TASHIAN et al., 1968).

[a] Named according to RICKLI et al. (1964).

tested, but both types of esters were hydrolyzed. It should be noted that in this study the enzyme had not been highly purified, and was not separated from an arylesterase that was also present. Recently, Tashian (1965) has been able to find in human erythrocytes three distinct types of arylesterases called A_1, A_2, and A_3. On electrophoresis, they migrated to different positions and could be differentiated by their distinctive sensitivities to iodoacetate, *p*-CMB and urea.

Genetic studies by Tashian (1965) revealed some variant forms of A esterases with altered electrophoretic mobility of all three components. This would suggest that they share a common polypeptide subunit and are isoenzymes.

A C-esterase, activated by $10^{-3}\,M$ *p*-CMB and not inhibited by $10^{-4}\,M$ DFP, was found to be a normal constituent of the red blood cells of humans and many other primate species (Tashian, 1965). The profile of esterases of the red blood cells of 23 primate species is carefully documented in Tashian's paper.

D. Tissue Esterases

The analysis of the esterases of other human tissues is even more complicated than it is in red blood cells, and the classification and description of the individual esterases of other tissues is far from complete. Aside from the difficulties in separating complex mixtures of proteins with esterase activity, there is the added complication that some of the esterases exist in multiple molecular forms. A series of investigations by Ecobichon and Kalow (1962, 1963, 1964, 1965; Ecobichon, 1965) deal with the types and properties of the soluble esterase of a number of human tissues. Bernsohn et al. (1959), Barron et al. (1963) and Blanco and Zinkham (1966) also have contributed to this area of investigation.

1. Liver

Ecobichon and Kalow (1962) found three zones of esterase activity in liver extracts which, due to their method of preparation, should represent only soluble esterases or those very loosely bound to the particulate fractions of liver. They (Ecobichon and Kalow, 1962, 1963) prepared extracts of human liver obtained at autopsy by homogenizing the tissue in distilled water, freezing and thawing the homogenate, and then centrifuging at $11{,}000 \times g$. The clear supernatant fraction was concentrated and analyzed by starch gel electrophoresis followed by histochemical tests for esterases with β-naphthylacetate and other substrates. They compared the zymograms of liver extracts with those of human serum to see if there were any bands common to both tissues (Fig. 2). Serum showed two major zones of esterase activity; the band moving fastest toward the anode (S-1) had arylesterase activity (aromatic esterase), and the slower moving zone (S-2) had cholinesterase activity; the latter was the C_4 band of serum pseudocholinesterase.

Liver extracts contained many esterase bands which were difficult to resolve, but they could be grouped into three general zones by their migration and enzymatic characteristics:

L-1, the zone that migrates most rapidly toward the anode, has a mobility similar to that of albumin. More than one type of esterase was present, but characteristics of an *aliesterase* were detected by substrate and inhibitor studies. Fatty acid esters were hydrolyzed, but choline esters were not. The enzymes were inhibited by organophosphates and eserine when tested at concentrations greater than $10^{-5}\,M$. The presence of a *lipase* in this zone was indicated by the activating effect of sodium cholate with long chain fatty acid esters. Other substrates hydrolyzed in this area were: 6-bromo-2-naphthyl-gluco- and galacto-pryanosides and L-leucyl-β-naphthyl-amide. L-2, a broad zone moving more slowly toward the anode, was also a mixture of esterases. Acid phosphatase and a lipase were present. Weak cholinesterase activity in this region was attributed to serum trapped in the liver. Acetylthiocholine was not hydrolyzed in the L-2 zone, but β-carbonaphthoxycholine was a substrate. The esterase

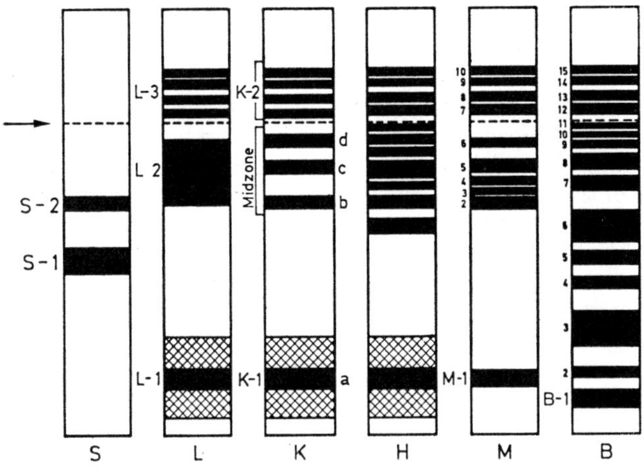

Fig. 2. Schematic drawing of the esterase of several human tissue extracts separated by starch gel electrophoresis at pH 7.4. The arrow indicates the origin, and S (serum), L (liver), K (kidney), H (heart), M (skeletal muscle) and B (brain) indicate the tissues. The bottom of the figure is the anode. Figure modified from ECOBICHON (1966)

activity was inhibited by $10^{-4} M$ DFP and by malathion but not by eserine. Partial inhibition of the L-2 zone by NaF and by TEPP was noted, suggesting that several types of esterases were present in the L-2 zone.

L-3, a zone of 3 or 4 bands, moved toward the cathode and appeared to be one or more acetylesterases. Aliphatic and aromatic esters of acetic acid were hydrolyzed, but fatty acid esters were not. Low concentrations of DFP or eserine did not cause inhibition, but higher concentrations of these agents ($10^{-4} M$) and TEPP were inhibitory.

It is evident that all three zones contained multiple bands of esterases which were difficult to resolve, and conclusions as to the identity of the individual esterases within each zone were necessarily tentative until more complete separation and further analyses could be made. ECOBICHON (1965) presented evidence that in some cases the multiple bands of the three zones of liver extracts probably represented multiple forms of the same enzyme. For example, the enzymes in the L-3 zone, consisting of 4 bands of acetylesterase, were remarkably similar in their substrate specificity and sensitivity to several inhibitors. The enzymes in these bands were also very much alike in their molecular size and shape, but differed in their net charge. The L-2 zone was found to contain 5 bands of esterase activity, and the zone L-1 had 8 distinct bands. Of the latter, 7 seemed to represent multiple forms of an aliesterase. The eighth band was clearly another esterase. It catalyzed the hydrolysis of α-naphthylbutyrate and valerate more rapidly than α-naphthylacetate, whereas the reverse order was found for the other 7 bands.

Much less is known about the esterases associated with liver microsomes of human liver. KRISCH (1963a) isolated a hydrolytic enzyme from hog liver microsomes by glycerol extraction. He proposed the name "microsomal liver esterase" for the enzyme and found that it catalyzed the hydrolysis of acetanilide, procaine, xylocaine, L-tyrosine ethyl ester and simple aliphatic esters. Thus, the enzyme has the properties of an amidase, a procaine esterase, and an amino acid esterase.

Glycerol extraction of human liver microsomes (HAMMER and LA DU, 1968) followed by fractionation on a column of Sephadex G-200 gave at least three peaks with high esterase activity in the eluted fractions. p-Nitrophenylacetate was the substrate used to detect esterase activity. Esterases of the peak zones were further characterized by starch gel electrophoresis and histochemical tests, and by evaluating the activity with a number of substrates and esterase inhibitors. The first peak of esterase activity eluted from the column had high activity with both *p*-nitrophenylacetate and benzoylcholine. It contained a major esterase component which migrated on starch gel electrophoresis like serum cholinesterase (C_4) and had similar properties as far as its inhibition by dibucaine and by fluoride. Since the microsomes had been carefully washed before glycerol extraction, the cholinesterase of the liver microsomes is probably not a contaminant from plasma. It may represent the liver precursor form of serum cholinesterase but the evidence is not conclusive. The esterases of the other two peaks have not been studied in detail, but it is clear that they have little or no benzoylcholine hydrolyzing activity.

2. Kidney

Ecobichon and Kalow (1964) investigated the soluble esterases of human kidney by essentially the same techniques described above for liver extracts. They found 5 areas of esterase activity:

K-1, a zone of *aliesterase* activity migrating toward the anode in the region of serum albumin. Several aliphatic and aromatic esters were hydrolyzed, but, unlike L-1, no long chain fatty acid esters were hydrolyzed.

K-2, a zone of *acetylesterase* activity consisting of 4 bands that migrate toward the cathode. Aromatic and aliphatic acetic acid esters were hydrolyzed. The activities and location of this esterase were essentially the same as the acetylesterase of zone L-3 from liver extracts.

In addition, 4 bands (*a*, *b*, *c* and *d*) were detected in the K-1 and the middle zones using α-naphthylbutyrate as the histochemical substrate. These bands did not appear when the routine naphthylacetate esters were used. Band *b* was thought to be serum cholinesterase, arising from serum present in the tissue. The other three bands were not inhibited by eserine at $10^{-4} M$ or *p*-HMB at $10^{-3} M$; they were inhibited by DFP at $10^{-5} M$, but not at $10^{-7} M$. Bands *c* and *d* were inhibited at lower concentrations of organophosphates than was band *a*. The *c* and *d* bands showed identical behavior in their sensitivities to all inhibitors tested, and they may be isozymes.

None of the esterases of human kidney extracts were sensitive to acetazolamide, so no carbonic anhydrase activity could be detected by the zymogram technique in kidney extracts. There was no evidence for an aromatic esterase (arylesterase) in kidney, since none of the enzymes was stimulated by calcium and migrated like the arylesterase of serum (S-1). A search for a C-esterase with properties like those of the C-esterase of hog kidney (Bergmann et al., 1957) was unsuccessful. *p*-Hydroxymercuribenzoate produced inhibition rather than activation in crude kidney extracts. Human kidney apparently does not contain a C-esterase like that of hog kidney.

Although several of the esterase bands in human kidney extracts have not been identified beyond their migration patterns and general substrate and inhibition characteristics, the major zones (K-1 and K-2) are very much like the L-1 and L-3 zones of liver. The K-2 and L-3 zones are probably 4 isozymic forms of an acetylesterase common to both tissues.

3. Skeletal and Smooth Muscle

Using samples of pectoral and gastrocnemius muscle obtained at autopsy as the source of skeletal muscle and the pyloric sphincter and strips of duodenum as sources of smooth muscle, Ecobichon and Kalow (1965) studied the soluble esterases of these human tissues.

Ten bands of esterase activity were found in skeletal muscle extracts, and 9 of these bands (all but band 1) were present in smooth muscle.

Bands 1—5 catalyzed the hydrolysis of α-naphthylbutyrate rapidly, whereas bands 7—10 showed relatively higher activity with α-naphthylacetate. Band 2 was presumed to be serum cholinesterase (S-2) as it disappeared when the muscle preparations were thoroughly washed before homogenization. Bands 7—10, migrating toward the cathode, resemble closely the equivalent 4 bands of liver and kidney, and bands 2, 5 and 6 appear to be the same as the midzone three bands in kidney extracts (Fig. 2).

On the basis of substrate specificity and sensitivity to inhibitors, band 1 was classified as a butyrate hydrolyzing *aliesterase,* bands 3—6 were called *non-specific aliesterases,* and bands 7—10 as *acetylesterase.*

No band of acetylcholinesterase was found, but this is not unexpected in view of the method used to prepare the soluble esterases. Acetylcholinesterase is localized in specific cellular structures; it is not loosely bound or in a free form in the tissues (Nachmansohn, 1969).

4. Brain

The esterase profile observed in extracts of human brain is more complex than that of any of the other tissues examined. A wide variety of esterases are present in the soluble fraction of brain. Since the individual esterases have not been fully studied, little is known about their classification and enzymatic properties.

Ecobichon (1966) was able to identify 15 distinct bands of esterase activity in human brain extracts with the zymogram technique. Two of the bands (bands 5 and 6) had the properties of an arylesterase. They catalyzed the hydrolysis of aromatic esters, were inhibited by *p*-HMB and were resistant to inhibition by organophosphates and eserine. They were not inhibited by 10^{-3} *M* EDTA and did not require calcium for activity. These characteristics correspond to those of arylesterase II of serum (Björklund et al., 1962). Bernsohn et al. (1959) noted earlier that brain arylesterase does not require calcium for optimal activity, and this observation is in agreement with Ecobichon's findings.

Although an esterase band with the properties of a C-esterase (because of activation by *p*-HMB) was detected in human brain extracts by Barron et al. (1963), a careful search for the esterase by Ecobichon (1966) was unsuccessful.

Cholinesterase activity was not found by Ecobichon (1966) in any of the 15 bands of the aqueous extracts of human brain, but two additional bands active with acetylthiocholine and butyrylthiocholine were obtained by extracting brain homogenates with solutions of desoxycholate or cholate. Ecobichon suggested that the enzymes responsible for the hydrolysis of these substrates were associated with membranes and were not easily extracted by water. In accord with this view, cholinesterase and acetylcholinesterase have been found in the nuclear, mitochondrial and microsomal fractions of brain (Parmar et al., 1961; Aldridge and Johnson, 1959). The two bands of acetylcholinesterase activity obtained by cholate extraction may be isozymic forms of the enzyme, since Bernsohn et al. (1963) presented substantial evidence that brain acetylcholinesterases have essentially the same optimal pH and Km values, substrate specificities and pI_{50} values with various inhibitors. Evidently acetylcholinesterase and cholinesterase of brain are present in several molecular forms. Their relationship to the multiple forms of cholinesterase in serum (mentioned in an earlier section) is not clear.

Four bands of acetylesterase in brain extracts migrating toward the cathode (B 12—15) are probably the same series of isoenzymes found in many tissues (Fig. 2). They catalyzed the hydrolysis of esters in which the acid group was not longer than two carbons (no fatty acid esters were hydrolyzed), and they were inhibited by low concentrations of organophosphate compounds.

Some of the other bands of brain extracts showed substrate specificities characteristic of aliesterases. Esters with acid groups containing up to five carbon atoms long were hydrolyzed, and these bonds were sensitive to organophosphate inhibitors.

5. Esterases of Other Human Tissues

Blanco and Zinkham (1966) studied the esterases of several other human tissues (stomach, diaphragm, heart, testis and adrenal gland). The individual enzymes were not characterized and only α-naphthyl esters were used as substrates. However, the paper is of particular interest because it compares liver esterases from fetal, premature, neonatal-term and older human subjects.

Paul and Fottrell (1961) examined the esterases of many human and mouse tissues, and extracts of cultured cell strains of mouse and human origin. The esterases were separated by starch gel electrophoresis and detected by the usual histochemical tests. Characteristic patterns of esterases were found for the two species; additional esterase profiles were characteristic for particular tissues. Cultured cells maintained their individual esterase patterns after many years of subculturing; there is little doubt that these enzymatic markers are genetically determined. Culture cells derived from tumors (cervical carcinoma), amnionic cells and other cell lines were studied by Komma (1963), who found amniotic cells to have a variety of esterases including C-esterase, arylesterase, aliesterase and cholinesterase.

A useful, general reference for further details on the numerous histochemical techniques utilized in the studies cited in this section and the earlier sections is the book by Pearse (Pearse, 1960).

E. Hydrolysis of Drugs Containing Ester Groups in Man

Several years ago Kalow (1962b) noted that there are many drugs and pharmacologically active agents with ester linkages, and many esterases in mammalian tissues but that it was impossible to give a comprehensive description of the role of esterases in drug metabolism and drug action. Unfortunately, this is still true today.

A few comments follow about the metabolism of some specific drugs with ester groups to illustrate some of the ways we believe esterases participate in the metabolic transformation of these agents.

Succinylcholine. Succinylcholine is hydrolyzed by serum cholinesterase (Kalow, 1962a). The duration and effects of the drug are closely related to the efficiency of its hydrolytic inactivation. The concentration of serum cholinesterase and the qualitative properties of the enzyme, as controlled by genetic factors, determine how rapidly the drug will be metabolized. If the enzyme is either deficient or inhibited by anticholinesterase agents, the rate of hydrolysis of succinylcholine will be affected.

Procaine. The local anesthetic, procaine, and a number of other structural analogues are also hydrolyzed by serum cholinesterase (Kalow, 1952). There seems to be no additional "procaine esterase" in human blood. The contribution of esterases in tissues, such as liver, in the hydrolysis of procaine *in vivo* is not clear. It has been suggested that a major portion of the procaine absorbed is hydrolyzed by serum cholinesterase during its circulation (Brodie et al., 1948).

Modification of the ester by substituting an amide linkage to give procainamide reduces the susceptibility to hydrolysis. Procainamide is hydrolyzed very slowly by plasma cholinesterase (Mark et al., 1951).

Aspirin. The hydrolysis of aspirin to salicylate takes place very rapidly in man, but there is evidence that the ester is hydrolyzed after its absorption into the blood (MANDEL et al., 1954). Hydrolysis of aspirin by serum *in vitro* is due to serum cholinesterase, but the relative importance of hydrolysis in blood and other tissues has not been clarified.

Atropine. Certain strains of rabbits carry a gene which determines the presence of a serum enzyme called "atropine esterase" (see KALOW, 1962a). Human serum does not hydrolyze atropine; hence the breakdown of atropine to tropic acid is a minor route of metabolism in man.

Tromexan. The anticoagulant, Tromexan (ethylbiscoumacetate), is metabolized in man primarily by hydroxylation of one of the benzene rings and relatively little is hydrolyzed to Tromexan acid. It is of interest that the rate of disappearance of Tromexan from the blood is about the same in man and rabbit, about 20% per hour, but the major route of metabolism in rabbits is by hydrolysis rather than ring hydroxylation (BURNS et al., 1953). Dogs metabolize the drug very slowly, about 3% per hour, and thus are deficient in both of these metabolic systems.

Meperidine. In man, meperidine is metabolized by two major pathways: hydrolysis to meperidine acid, and demethylation to normeperidine (BURNS et al., 1955). Hydrolysis of meperidine to meperidine acid does not take place in the blood, but occurs mainly in liver microsomes (WAY et al., 1947; KRISCH, 1963b). Human and rabbit plasma contain an activator of "demerol esterase" (AMMON and TAKEO, 1966), but the significance of this activator in the metabolism of the drug in man has not been determined.

Paraoxon and DFP. The active form of parathion is paraoxon and the latter is hydrolyzed to some extent by human serum. Serum arylesterase accounts for most of the hydrolysis, but the esterase activity of albumin contributed to some degree (ERDÖS and BOGGS, 1961). Hydrolysis of DFP is reportedly catalyzed by human serum arylesterases (AUGUSTINSSON and CASIDA, 1959).

Acetylated Derivatives of Morphine. Heroin undergoes deacetylation by rabbit serum; removal of the acetyl groups in positions 3 and 6 however, is catalyzed by two different enzymes. Human serum contains neither of these enzymes, but human liver has both activities (see BERNHEIM, 1952). The deacetylation of acetyl groups in both ester and amide linkages may be catalyzed by the same enzyme if it has a sufficiently nonspecific substrate requirement The microsomal esterase of hog liver, described by KRISCH (1963b), is an example of such an enzyme. A more complete discussion of the deacetylation enzymes is given in Chapter 54 by W. WEBER.

Chloromycetin palmatate, Cortisol succinate, Prednisolone succinate. Chloromycetin was not suitable for oral administration because of its bitter taste. GLAZKO et al. (1952) showed that chloromycetin palmitate is a tasteless ester that is hydrolyzed in the small intestine to release the active drug. Some corticosteroids are also given in an ester form, especially when high concentrations are needed, and the 1600-fold increase in water solubility of cortisol-21-succinate over free cortisol (MELBY and SILBER, 1961) is of considerable advantage. The steroid esters are believed to be hydrolyzed in the gut, plasma and tissues, but the enzymes involved in the hydrolysis of these agents have not been carefully identified.

Clofibrate. The cholesterol lowering agent, ethyl *a-p*-chlorophenoxyisobutyrate, is absorbed as the ester and rapidly hydrolyzed by tissue and serum esterases (THORP, 1962). Which esterases in the serum catalyze the hydrolysis is not known, and the relative importance of esterases in other tissues is uncertain.

Summary

The classification and types of esterases present in human tissues have been reviewed. Unfortunately, there are relatively few studies on the esterases of human tissues in which a variety of drug substrates containing ester groups have been used. It is clear, however, that the esterases vary considerably from tissue to tissue in the same species, and from one species to another. The extrapolation of data on the metabolism of ester drugs from animals to man is of limited value and may be incorrect for these reasons.

Acknowledgement: The preparation of this chapter was supported by grant GM-17184 from the National Institutes of Health.

References

ALDRIDGE, W.N., JOHNSON, M.K.: Cholinesterase, succinic dehydrogenase, nucleic acids, esterase and glutathione reductase in sub-cellular fractions from rat brain. Biochem. J. **73**, 270—276 (1959).

AMMON, R., TAKEO, K.: Die Dolantin-Esterase. Enzymologia **30**, 69—79 (1966).

AUGUSTINSSON, K.B.: Electrophoresis studies on blood plasma esterases. I. Mammalian plasmata. Acta chem. scand. **13**, 571—592 (1959).

— Acetylcholine Esterase and Cholinesterase. *In:* BOYER, PAUL D., LARDY, HENRY, and MYRBACK, KARL: The Enzymes, 2nd ed., Vol. **4**. New York, N.Y. and London: Academic Press 1961a.

— Multiple forms of esterase in vertebrate blood plasma. Ann. N.Y. Acad. Sci. **94**, 844—860 (1961b).

— Arylesterases. J. Histochem. Cytochem. **12**, 744—747 (1964).

— BARR, M.: Age variation in plasma arylesterase activity in children. Clin. chim. Acta **8**, 568—573 (1963).

— BRODY, S.: Plasma arylesterase activity in adults and newborn infants. Clin. chim. Acta **7**, 560—565 (1962).

— CASIDA, J.E.: Enzymic hydrolysis of N:N-dimethylcarbamoyl fluoride. Biochem. Pharmacol. **3**, 60—67 (1959—1960).

— EKEDAHL, G.: On the specificity of arylesterases. Acta chem. scand. **16**, 240—241 (1962).

— OLSSON, B.: A genetically determined enzyme in the pig. Nature (Lond.) **187**, 924—925 (1960).

BARRON, K.D., BERNSOHN, J., HESS, A.R.: Separation and properties of human brain esterases. J. Histochem. Cytochem. **11**, 139—156 (1963).

BERNHEIM, F.: Enzymes in detoxication. *In:* The Enzymes, SUMNER, J.B. and MYRBACK, KARL, 1st ed., Vol. II, Pt. 2, pp. 850—854. New York: Academic Press 1952.

BERGMANN, F., RIMON, S.: The effect of pH variations on the activities of C-esterase. Biochem. J. **70**, 339—344 (1958).

— SEGAL, R., RIMON, S.: A new type of esterase in hog-kidney extract. Biochem. J. **67**, 481—486 (1957).

BERNSOHN, J., BARRON, K.D., HEDRICK, M.T.: Some properties of acetylcholinesterase. Biochem. Pharmacol. **12**, 761—763 (1963).

— POSSLEY, L., LIEBERT, E.: Study of esterase activity in human brain and serum. J. Neurochem. **4**, 191—201 (1959).

BJÖRKLUND, B., PAULSSON, J.E., EKBERG, S.: Curtain electrophoretic separation of phenyl acetate hydrolysing esterases of human serum. Demonstration of an EDTA-dependent enzyme. Proc. Soc. exp. Biol. (N.Y.) **110**, 458—463 (1962).

BLANCO, A., ZINKHAM, W.H.: Soluble esterases in human tissues: characterization and ontogeny. Bull. Johns Hopk. Hosp. **118**, 27—39 (1966).

BRODIE, B.B., LIEF, P.A., POET, R.: The fate of procaine in man following its intravenous administration and methods for the estimation of procaine and diethylaminoethanol. J. Pharmacol. exp. Ther. **94**, 359—366 (1948).

BURNS, J.J., BERGER, B.L., LIEF, P.A., WOLLACK, A., PAPPER, E.M., BRODIE, B.B.: The physiological diposition and fate of meperidine (demerol) in man and a method for its estimation in plasma. J. Pharmacol. exp. Ther. **114**, 289—298 (1955).

— WEINER, M., SIMSON, G., BRODIE, B.B.: The biotransformation of ethyl biscoumacetate (Tromexan) in man, rabbit and dog. J. Pharmacol. exp. Ther. **108**, 33—41 (1953).

DAVIS, R.P.: Carbonic Anhydrase. *In:* BOYER, PAUL D., LARDY, HENRY, and MYRBACK, KARL: The Enzymes, 2nd ed., Vol. 5. New York, N.Y. and London: Academic Press 1961.

DEWALD, B., LA DU, B.N.: Properties and interrelationship of multiple molecular forms of human serum cholinesterase. Fed. Proc. **29**, 803 (1970).
ECOBICHON, D.J.: Multiple forms of human liver esterases. Canad. J. Biochem. **43**, 595—602 (1965).
— Properties and classification of the soluble esterases of human brain. Canad. J. Physiol. Pharmacol. **44**, 225—232 (1966).
— KALOW, W.: Properties and classification of the soluble esterases of human liver. Biochem. Pharmacol. **11**, 573—583 (1962).
— — Action of organophosphorus compounds upon esterases of human liver. Canad. J. Biochem. **41**, 1537—1546 (1963).
— — Properties and classification of the soluble esterases of human kidney. Canad. J. Biochem. **42**, 277—286 (1964).
— — Properties and classification of the soluble esterases of human skeletal and smooth muscle. Canad. J. Biochem. **43**, 73—79 (1965).
EDSALL, J.T.: Multiple molecular forms of carbonic anhydrase in erythrocytes. Ann. N.Y. Acad. Sci. **151**, 41—63 (1968).
ERDÖS, E.G., BOGGS, L.E.: Hydrolysis of paraoxon in mammalian blood. Nature (Lond.) **190**, 716—717 (1961).
GLAZKO, A.J., EDGERTON, W.H., DILL, W.A., LENZ, W.R.: Chloromycetin palmitate-a-synthetic ester of chloromycetin. Antibiot. and Chemother. **2**, 234—242 (1952).
GOEDDE, H.W., DOENICKE, A., ALTLAND, K.: Pseudocholinesterasen. Berlin-Heidelberg-New York: Springer 1967.
GREENWAY, R.M., QUASTEL, J.H.: Hydrolysis of succinylmonocholine by a liver esterase. Proc. Soc. exp. Biol. (N.Y.) **90**, 72—74 (1955).
HAMMER, G.S., LA DU, B.N.: Evidence for the liver being the source of human serum cholinesterase. Pharmacologist **10**, 202 (1968).
HARRIS, H., HOPKINSON, D.A., ROBSON, E.B.: Two dimensional electrophoresis of pseudocholinesterase components in normal human serum. Nature (Lond.) **196**, 1296—1298 (1962).
— WHITTAKER, M.: Differential inhibition of human serum cholinesterase with fluoride. Recognition of two new phenotypes. Nature (Lond.) **191**, 496—498 (1961).
HUNTER, R.L., MARKERT, C.L.: Histochemical demonstration of enzymes separated by zone electrophoresis in starch gels. Science **125**, 1294—1295 (1957).
JUUL, P.: Human plasma cholinesterase isozymes. Clin. chim. Acta **19**, 205—213 (1968).
KALOW, W.: Hydrolysis of local anesthetics by human serum cholinesterase. J. Pharmacol. exp. Ther. **104**, 122—134 (1952).
— Cholinesterase types. Ciba Foundation Symposium, Biochemistry of Human Genetics, pp. 39—56. Boston: Little, Brown & Co. 1960.
— Pharmacogenetics. Heredity and the Response to Drugs. Philadelphia: W.B. Saunders Co. 1962a.
— Esterase action. *In:* Proc. 1st. intnatl. pharm. mtg., Metabolic factors controlling duration of drug action, B.B. BRODIE and E.G. ERDÖS (eds.), Vol. 6. New York: MacMillian Co. 1962b.
— DAVIES, R.O.: The activity of various esterase inhibitors towards atypical human serum cholinesterase. Biochem. Pharmacol. **1**, 183—192 (1958).
— GENEST, K.: A method for the detection of atypical forms of human serum cholinesterase. Determination of dibucaine numbers. Canad. J. Biochem. **35**, 339—346 (1957).
KOELLE, G.B. (Ed.): Cholinesterases and anticholinesterase agents. Handb. exp. Pharmak., Suppl. 15. Berlin-Göttingen-Heidelberg: Springer 1963.
KOMMA, D.: Characteristics of the esterases of human cells grown in vitro. J. Histochem. Cytochem. **11**, 619—623 (1963).
KRISCH, K.: Isolierung einer Esterase aus Schweinelebermikrosomen. Biochem. Z. **337**, 531—545 (1963a).
— Eigenschaften und Substratspezifitat einer Esterase aus Schweinelebermikrosomen. Biochem. Z. **337**, 546—573 (1963b).
LA DU, B.: Plasma esterase activity and the metabolism of drugs with ester groups. Ann. N.Y. Acad. Sci. (in press) (1970).
LAMOTTA, R.V., MCCOMB, R.B., NOLL, C.R., JR., WETSTONE, H.J., REINFRANK, R.F.: Multiple forms of serum cholinesterase. Arch. Biochem. **124**, 299—305 (1968).
— WORONICK, C.L., REINFRANK, R.F.: Multiple forms of serum cholinesterase: Molecular weights of the isoenzymes. Arch. Biochem. **136**, 448—451 (1970).
LAURENT, G., MARRIQ, C., NAHON, D., CHARREL, M., DERRIEN, Y.: Isolement des proteines «lentes» Y, X_1, et X_2 accompagnant l'hemoglobine humaine dans ses preparations. C. R. Soc. Biol. (Paris) **156**, 1456—1461 (1962).

Mandel, H.G., Cambosos, N.M., Smith, P.K.: The presence of aspirin in human plasma after oral administration. J. Pharmacol. exp. Ther. **112**, 495—500 (1954).
Mark, L.C., Kayden, H.J., Steele, J.M., Cooper, J.R., Berlin, I., Rovenstine, E.A., Brodie, B.B.: The physiological disposition and cardiac effects of procaine amide. J. Pharmacol. exp. Ther. **102**, 5—15 (1951).
Marton, A., Kalow, W.: Studies on aromatic esterase and cholinesterase of human serum. Canad. J. Biochem. **37**, 1367—1373 (1959).
Melartin, L., Blumberg, B.S.: Albumin Naskapi: A new variant of serum albumin. Science **153**, 1664—1666 (1966).
Melby, J.C., Silber, R.H.: Clinical pharmacology of water-soluble corticosteroid esters. Amer. Practit. **12**, 156—161 (1961).
Mounter, L.A., Whittaker, V.P.: The hydrolysis of esters of phenol by cholinesterases and other esterases. Biochem. J. **54**, 551—559 (1953).
Myers, D.K.: Studies on cholinesterase. 9. Species variation in the specificity pattern of the pseudocholinesterases. Biochem. J. **55**, 67—79 (1953).
— Studies on ali-esterases. 4. Differentiation of esterases in pancreas and brain by the use of organophosphorus inhibitors. Biochem. J. **64**, 740—747 (1956).
Nachmansohn, D.: Proteins of excitable membranes. In: Membrane Proteins. Proceedings of a symposium sponsored by the New York Heart Association. Boston: Little, Brown & Co. 1969.
— Wilson, I.B.: The enzymatic hydrolysis and synthesis of acetylcholine. Advanc. Enzymol. **12**, 259—339 (1951).
Neitlich, H.W.: Increased plasma cholinesterase activity and succinylcholine resistance: A genetic variant. J. clin. Invest. **45**, 380—387 (1966).
Nyman, P.O.: Purification and properties of carbonic anhydrase from human erythrocytes. Biochim. biophys. Acta (Amst.) **52**, 1—12 (1961).
— Lindskog, S.: Amino acid composition of various forms of bovine and human erythrocyte carbonic anhydrase. Biochim. biophys. Acta (Amst.) **85**, 141—151 (1964).
Parmar, S.S., Sutter, M.C., Nickerson, M.: Localization and characterization of cholinesterase in subcellular fractions of rat brain and beef pituitary. Canad. J. Biochem. **39**, 1335—1345 (1961).
Paul, J., Fottrell, P.: Tissue-specific and species-specific esterases. Biochem. J. **78**, 418—424 (1961).
Pearse, A.G.E.: Histochemistry-Theoretical and Applied, 2nd ed., chapter XVI, pp. 456 to 490. Boston, Mass.: Little, Brown & Co. 1960.
Pocker, Y., Meany, J.E.: The catalytic versatility of erythrocyte carbonic anhydrase. I. Kinetic studies of the enzyme-catalyzed hydration of acetaldehyde. Biochemistry **4**, 2535—2541 (1965).
Rickli, E.E., Edsall, J.T.: Zinc binding and the sulfhydryl group of human carbonic anhydrase. J. biol. Chem. **237** PC 258—260 (1962).
— Ghazanfar, S.A.S., Gibbons, B.H., Edsall, J.T.: Carbonic anhydrases from human erythrocytes. Preparation and properties of two enzymes. J. biol. Chem. **239**, 1065—1078 (1964).
Shaw, C.R., Syner, F.N., Tashian, R.E.: New genetically determined molecular form of erythrocyte esterase in man. Science **138**, 31—32 (1962).
Simpson, N.: Genetics of esterases in man. Ann. N.Y. Acad. Sci. **151**, 699—709 (1968).
Smithies, O.: Zone electrophoresis in starch gels: group variations in the serum proteins of normal human adults. Biochem. J. **61**, 629—641 (1955).
— An improved procedure for starch-gel electrophoresis: Further variations in the serum proteins of normal individuals. Biochem. J. **71**, 585—587 (1959).
Tashian, R.E.: Multiple forms of esterases from human erythrocytes. Proc. Soc. exp. Biol. (N.Y.) **108**, 364—366 (1961).
— Genetic variation and evolution of the carboxylic esterases and carbonic anhydrases of primate erythrocytes. Amer. J. hum. Genet. **17**, 257—272 (1965).
— Douglas, D.P., Yu, Y.S.L.: Esterase and hydrase activity of carbonic anhydrase-I from primate erythrocytes. Biochem. biophys. Res. Commun. **14**, 256—261 (1964).
— Plato, C.C., Shows, T.B., Jr.: Inherited variant of erythrocyte carbonic anhydrase in Micronesians from Guam and Saipan. Science **140**, 53—54 (1963).
— Riggs, S.K., Yu, Y.S.L.: Characterization of a mutant human erythrocyte carbonic anhydrase: carbonic anhydrase Ic Guam. Arch. Biochem. **117**, 320—327 (1966).
— Shaw, M.W.: Inheritance of an erythrocyte acetylesterase variant in man. Amer. J. hum. Genet. **14**, 295—300 (1962).
— Shreffler, D.C., Shows, T.B.: Genetic and phylogenetic variation in the different molecular forms of mammalian erythrocyte carbonic anhydrases. Ann. N.Y. Acad. Sci. **151**, 64—77 (1968).

THORP, J.M.: Experimental evaluation of an orally active combination of androsterone with ethyl chlorophenoxyisobutyrate. Lancet **1**, 1323—1326 (1962).
URIEL, J.: Methode d'electrophorese dans des gels d'acrylamide-agarose. Bull. Soc. Chim. biol. (Paris) **48**, 969—982 (1966).
WAY, E.L., SWANSON, R., GIMBLE, A.I.: Studies *in vitro* and *in vivo* on the influence of the liver on isonipecaine (demerol) activity. J. Pharmacol. exp. Ther. **91**, 178—184 (1947).
WILSON, I.B.: Acetylcholinesterase. *In:* BOYER, P.D., LARDY, H. and MYRBACK, K.: The Enzymes, 2nd ed., Vol. 4. New York, N.Y. and London: Academic Press 1961.
YOSHIDA, A., MOTULSKY, A.G.: A pseudocholinesterase variant (E Cynthiana) associated with elevated plasma enzyme activity. Amer. J. hum. Genet. **21**, 486—498 (1969).
ZELLER, E.A.: Enzymology of the refractory media of the eye. IV. Direct photometric determination of cholinesterase and aliesterase of corpus vitreum. Arch. Biochem. **61**, 231—240 (1956).

Chapter 51

Enzymatic Oxidation and Reduction of Alcohols, Aldehydes and Ketones

R. E. McMahon

The TPNH dependent monooxygenases, which are localized in the endoplasmic reticulum of the liver cell, have been implicated in the majority of drug oxidations. In addition to these enzymes, however, there are a number of other classes of enzymes which are involved in the oxidation and reduction of foreign chemicals in the body. These include among others the oxido-reductases as well as those enzymes responsible for the oxidation of aldehydes to carboxylic acids. The oxido-reductases are a class of dehydrogenases that catalyze the conversion of alcohols to aldehydes or ketones or alternatively the reduction of carbonyl compounds to alcohols.

A number of years ago, Gillette (1959) studied the *in vivo* stepwise oxidation of p-nitrotoluene to p-nitrobenzoic acid. p-Nitrotoluene first undergoes microsomal hydroxylation to p-nitrobenzyl alcohol which is in turn oxidized to p-nitrobenzaldehyde by an alcohol dehydrogenase. Finally this aldehyde is enzymatically oxidized to p-nitrobenzoic acid.

The metabolism of p-nitrotoluene represents a prototype of a reaction sequence frequently encountered in studies of the biotransformation of drugs. For example, the antidiabetic drug tolbutamide is oxidized in the body by the same three-step process yielding carboxytolbutamide as the main metabolite (Tagg et al., 1967; Thomas and Ikeda, 1966; McDaniel et al., 1969). When the alcohol is a secondary alcohol rather than primary, oxidation stops at the carbonyl stage instead and ketones rather than carboxylic acids are end products. The metabolism of hexobarbital (Toki and Tsukamoto, 1964), pentobarbital (Kuntzman et al., 1967), and the hydrocarbon indane (Billings et al., 1970) illustrate this point.

Oxido-reductases, acting as reductases, can convert ketones and aldehydes to carbinols. Drugs metabolized in this fashion include acetohexamide (McMahon et al., 1965) and tetrabenazine (Schwartz et al., 1966).

The best known example of the involvement of these enzymes in drug metabolism is the *in vivo* oxidation of ethyl alcohol. The first step of the reaction is dehydrogenation to acetaldehyde. This reaction is mediated by liver alcohol dehydrogenase (LADH), the most thoroughly characterized of the oxido-reductases involved in the metabolism of carbinols. The second step, the oxidation of acetaldehyde to acetate, is catalyzed by DPN^+-dependent aldehyde dehydrogenase.

Aldehyde dehydrogenase is one of at least three enzymes which have been implicated in the oxidation of foreign aldehydes. The others are aldehyde oxidase and xanthine oxidase. The oxidation of aldehydes to carboxylic acids is a vital step in the metabolism of foreign compounds. Aldehydes are in general relatively toxic compounds and due to their lipid solubility not readily excreted. Carboxylic acids on the other hand, are substantially less toxic and in addition are usually readily excreted. Aldehydes are formed metabolically by a number of routes, the two most important being dehydrogenation of primary alcohols and the oxidation of amines by amine oxidases, principally monoamine oxidase.

Both the oxido-reductases and the aldehyde oxidizing enzymes are considered in this chapter. Emphasis, of necessity, will be on those enzymes which have a sufficiently broad substrate specificity to implicate them in the metabolism of foreign compounds. In addition, although these enzymes are commonly found in almost all living organisms only those of mammalian origin will be described.

A. Oxido-Reductases

I. Liver Alcohol Dehydrogenase

1. General Properties

Liver alcohol dehydrogenase (LADH) is undoubtedly the most important of the oxido-reductases involved in the metabolism of foreign alcohols and carbonyl compounds. The alcohol dehydrogenases are widely distributed in nature. In mammals it is found as a soluble enzyme in liver. ADH from horse liver was crystallized in Stockholm in 1948 (Bonnichsen and Wassen, 1948). Alcohol dehydrogenase has been purified from human liver (von Wartburg et al., 1964) and has been crystallized (Mourad and Woronick, 1967). Its properties are very similar to those of the horse liver enzyme (Li and Theorell, 1969).

Alcohol dehydrogenase has become one of the most widely studied of enzymes. This is due in part to the ready availability of crystalline horse liver ADH and in part due to the recognition of the important role played by LADH in ethanol oxidation. The literature of the structure and function of LADH has been critically reviewed (Theorell, 1967; Sund and Theorell, 1963).

Horse LADH has a molecular weight of about 80,000. Electrophoretic studies suggest that as many as nine isoenzymes may be present in the crystalline material (Pietruszko et al., 1969). The number of subunits present is still an unsettled question (Pietruszko et al., 1969; Green and McKay, 1969). Each molecule contains four zinc atoms (cf. Drum et al., 1969), two binding sites for coenzyme, and two binding sites for substrate. The two active sites may have different affinities for ethanol and for sterols (Theorell et al., 1966).

LADH can catalyze both the oxidation of carbinols to ketones and aldehydes and the reduction of these carbonyl compounds to carbinols. The coenzyme for these transformations are DPN^+ and DPNH. TPN^+ and TPNH can also serve as cosubstrates but at greatly reduced rates (Dalziel and Dickinson, 1965). The overall stoichiometry of the reversible reaction is:

$$DPN^+ + \text{alcohol} \rightleftarrows DPNH + \text{ketone} + H^+$$

Since a proton is involved in the reaction, pH would be expected to greatly influence the position of equilibrium. Thus ketone formation is optimal near pH 10 while alcohol formation occurs most readily near pH 7 (Sund and Theorell, 1963). In the intact animal, the reaction usually proceeds in the direction of oxidation, because the aldehyde is further oxidized to acids and DPNH is reoxidized to DPN^+ by other enzymes in liver.

2. Substrate Selectivity of LADH

Despite the fact that LADH is one of the most extensively studied enzymes, its main physiological role remains a mystery. Since ethanol does not occur naturally in mammals, ethanol oxidation cannot be the normal role of LADH.

LADH possesses a relatively low degree of substrate specificity and can accept a variety of primary alcohols and aldehydes and secondary alcohols and ketones as substrates (Sund and Theorell, 1963). This fact suggests that LADH may play an important part in the metabolism of foreign alcohols. It should be pointed out that the demonstration that a given alcohol is oxidized by LADH does not prove that the same oxidation occurring *in vivo* is indeed mediated by LADH in the intact cell. Considerably more research will be needed to define the sole of LADH in drug metabolism. The current status of substrate activity studies with LADH is summarized in the following paragraphs.

In early studies of substrate selectivity, Theorell and Bonnichsen (1951) found that primary alcohols ($-\overset{|}{\underset{|}{C}}-CH_2OH$) in general serve as substrates for LADH. Later work by several authors including Winer (1958), Merritt and Tomkins (1959) and Tsai (1968) indicates that maximum activity among the straight chain aliphatic alcohols is seen with butanol-1. Many branched chain primary alcohols such as isobutanol are also oxidized. The reverse reaction, the reduction of aldehydes to primary alcohols, has also been studied. Winer (1958) has found that again the C-4 analog, butyraldehyde is the most active substrate. It is reduced about 15 times more rapidly than is acetaldehyde.

An interesting group of aliphatic primary alcohols are the prenols which Christophe and Popják (1961) have reported to be substrates for LADH. Of these the most interesting one is trans-trans-farnesol because of its possible role in cholesterol biosynthesis in liver. Indeed, Waller (1965) has shown that trans-trans-farnesol is sufficiently active as a LADH substrate to support the suggestion that this may be a normal physiological function of LADH in the intact animal.

Secondary alcohols are also oxidized by LADH but at greatly reduced rates. Thus butanol-2 is oxidized about one-third as rapidly as butanol-1. At least one group (Dickinson and Dalziel, 1967) has observed activity with propanol-2. Others (Winer, 1958; Merritt and Tomkins, 1959) found no activity. Interestingly enough, neither acetone nor methyl ethyl ketone appear to be reduced by LADH (Winer, 1958). In contrast, it has been reported that methyl ethyl ketone and higher analogs undergo reduction in the intact animals (Smith et al., 1954). This suggests that an enzyme other than LADH may be involved in aliphatic ketone reduction.

Among the halogenated compounds, chloral hydrate has been found to be readily reduced to trichloroethanol by LADH (Friedman and Cooper, 1960). Contrariwise, the oxidation of 2-fluoroethanol has been reported to be mediated by an oxido-reductase not identical with LADH (Treble, 1962).

LADH differs from yeast alcohol dehydrogenase in that LADH readily mediates the interconversion of cyclohexanol and cyclohexanone (Winer, 1958; Merritt and Tomkins, 1959). The alicyclic carbinols and ketones are for that matter the most widely studied group of LADH substrates.

Prelog and his coworkers have carried out extensive studies on the stereospecificity of microbiological reductions of alicyclic ketones. In an extension of this work the reduction of a number of substituted cyclohexanones and decalones by LADH was studied. From these studies (Prelog, 1964) it was concluded that LADH should be classed as an e-enzyme since it is the equatorial hydrogen that is transferred.

Graves et al. (1965) have reported both kinetic studies and product determination on the reduction of alkyl cyclohexanones and the isomeric 10-methyl-2-decalones. Among the methyl cyclohexanones they found (±)3-methyl cyclohexanone to be reduced more rapidly than either (±)2-methyl or 4-methyl cyclohexanone. In the decalone series, cis-2-decalone was a more efficient substrate than trans-2-decalone. In both cases the 10-methyl derivatives were less active than the unsubstituted ketone. Among the optical isomers *d*-10-methyl-cis-2-decalone was 25 times more active than the *l*-isomer while *l*-10-methyl-trans-2-decalone was 100 times as active as its antipod. Product determinations showed the reaction to be only partially stereospecific in that both axial and equatorial carbinols were formed in most but not all cases.

ELLIOTT and coworkers (ELLIOTT et al., 1965, 1966; CHEO et al., 1967) have carried out extensive studies on the fate of oxygenated alicyclics in the intact rabbit. With the isomeric methyl cyclohexanones as well as with isomeric decalones, they found that reduction to the thermodynamically more stable carbinol was the preferred pathway. The administration of each of the cis and trans isomers of the methyl cyclohexanols resulted in the excretion (as conjugates) of those that represented the thermodynamically more stable isomer of a given pair. The unstable isomers, on the other hand, underwent conversion to the stable isomer before excretion. ELLIOTT et al. (1969) proposed that this transformation occurs by a two-step process in which the unstable isomer is first dehydrogenated to the ketone. The ketone then undergoes reduction to the more stable isomer. Both of these reactions are catalyzed by LADH in *in vitro* studies. On the basis of their studies with crystalline horse LADH these authors (ELLIOTT et al., 1969) make the reasonable suggestion that the *in vivo* interconversions between the alicyclic alcohols and ketones are very likely catalyzed by LADH.

It should be pointed out that none of the substituted cyclohexanones or the decalones are as active substrates as is the parent compound itself, i. e. cyclohexanone. The same is true for the carbinols in that cyclohexanol is the most active substrate among the alicyclic carbinols. Of all of the substituted alicyclic compounds studied (—)3-methyl cyclohexanone and (+)-cis-3-methyl cyclohexanol were the most active with rates of about 2/3 those of cyclohexanone and cyclohexanol (ELLIOTT et al., 1969). Adamantanone was essentially without activity (RINGOLD et al., 1967). Despite the apparent similarity of cyclopentanone and cyclopentanol to cyclohexanone and cyclohexanol, the 5-ring analogs are without substrate activity (GRAVES et al., 1965).

Part of the interest in the alicyclic substrates has arisen because they represent partial structures of the sterol molecules. It is not surprising then that certain sterol derivatives can serve as substrates. Substrate structural requirements are, however, fairly rigid. WALLER et al. (1965) found that bile acids containing a 3-β-hydroxy or a 3-keto group were substrates for horse LADH. Hydroxy groups at 5, 7 or 12 were not oxidized. Bile acids with a 3-α-hydroxy group were also inactive. WALLER et al. (1965) found that certain sterols containing a primary alcohol group were also oxidized by LADH. In this connection, MOIR et al. (1968) have studied the enzyme system responsible for demethylation of 4,4-dimethyl sterols and reported that the dehydrogenase step may be catalyzed by an enzyme identical with LADH. These studies suggest that one of the physiological roles of LADH may be as a sterol dehydrogenase. Further research is needed, however, to establish this role.

A variety of aromatic aldehydes including benzaldehyde are excellent substrates for LADH (WINER, 1958; WRATTEN and CLELAND, 1965). In fact the K_m for benzaldehyde has been reported to be two orders of magnitude less than for cyclohexanone (GRAVES et al., 1965). BLOMQUIST (1966) has studied the effect of ring substitution on the reduction of benzaldehydes. He found that the rate of reduction is increased by the presence of electron-withdrawing groups in the para-position.

The reverse reaction, the oxidation of benzyl alcohols to benzaldehydes, also proceeds well, benzyl alcohol being about one-half as active a substrate as is ethanol (Wratten and Cleland, 1965). The oxidation of a substituted benzyl alcohol to an aldehyde is an important step in the conversion of aromatic methyl groups to carboxyl groups, a pathway often encountered in *in vivo* drug metabolism (cf. McDaniel et al., 1969; Smith et al., 1965; Gillette, 1959). It seems likely that LADH is the relevant enzyme in these *in vivo* dehydrogenations. As a matter of fact, it is probable that, for this group of substrates at least, LADH serves mainly as a dehydrogenase *in vivo* since there is at present no evidence that aromatic aldehydes undergo *in vivo* reduction to carbinols (Williams, 1959).

Thus, LADH demonstrates a very broad substrate specificity. It appears to show a preference for primary carbinols. Indeed there have been very few reports of inactive primary alcohols. Even methanol, once thought to be inactive, has been shown to be oxidized by LADH when the methanol concentration is sufficiently high (Kini and Cooper, 1961). Secondary alcohols are not as efficient substrates as the primary alcohols. Even the alicyclic carbinols are substantially less active than the simpler primary alcohols. Among the inactive substrates already mentioned are propanol-2, cyclopentanol and cholic acids not having the 3-β-OH group. Other inactive substrates include secondary aromatic alcohols such as methylphenylcarbinol, indanol-1 and tetralol-1 (Billings, unpublished observations, this laboratory).

3. Stereochemistry and Mechanism

It is not the purpose of this review to present a critical discussion of the mechanistic aspects of oxidation and reduction by oxido-reductases. However, a brief commentary on the salient features of stereochemistry and mechanism should be helpful in understanding substrate specificity and the possible physiological roles of LADH[1].

The two hydrogen atoms at carbon-4 of DPNH (or TPNH) are stereochemically distinct, i.e. carbon atom-4 is potentially an assymetric center and is referred to as a "prochiral" carbon (cf. Arigoni and Eliel, 1969). Thus the replacement of one of the two hydrogen atoms at a "prochiral" center with isotopic hydrogen produces a chiral or assymetric center. By the use of isotopic labeling it has been shown (Westheimer et al., 1951; Fisher et al., 1953) that only one of the two hydrogens is transferred when acetaldehyde is reduced by yeast ADH. This hydrogen has been designated H_A. In the reverse reaction, the dehydrogenation of ethanol, the hydrogen atom is returned to the A-side. Enzymes which transfer a hydrogen atom to or from the A-side of DPN^+ or DPNH (or TPN^+ or TPNH) are referred to as Class A or A-side specific enzymes. Class B or B-side specific enzymes utilize the opposite side of DPNH. LADH was shown to be A-side specific by Levy and Vennesland (1957) when ethanol and acetaldehyde were substrates. LADH has also been shown to be A-side specific when 2-butanol (Dickinson and Dalziel, 1967) and when various substituted cyclohexanones and cyclohexanols (Elliott et al., 1969) are substrates. Not surprisingly, LADH is also A-side specific in the reduction of p-chlorobenzaldehyde with TPNH as cosubstrate (Culp and McMahon, 1968).

The question of the absolute configuration of the reduced pyridine nucleotides has been resolved by Cornforth et al. (1962). By the degradation of enzymatically

1 For further discussion of the mechanism of pyridine nucleotide dependent oxido-reductases see Sund (1968) and Sund et al. (1964).

prepared deuterium labeled DPNH to structures of known configuration they have established the following absolute configuration for DPNH (I).

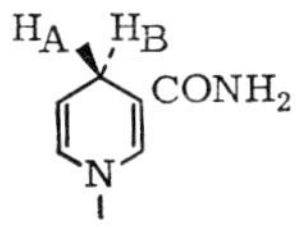

I

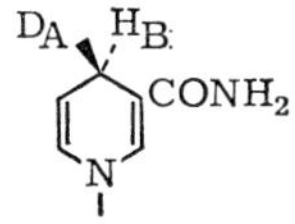

II

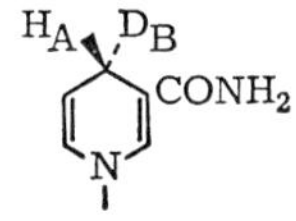

III

Thus, 4-d-DPNH obtained by the reduction of DPN^+ with *a,a*-dideuteroethanol has the 4R-configuration (II) while 4-d-DPNH prepared by LADH mediated reduction of 4-d-DPN^+ with unlabeled ethanol has the 4S-configuration (III) (R and S terms are defined in CAHN et al., 1966). Since TPNH and DPNH have been interrelated (NAKAMOTO and VENNESLAND, 1960) the absolute configuration of TPNH is also known.

The next question to be considered is the stereospecificity with respect to substrate. The interconversion of aldehydes and primary alcohols will first be considered. The crucial studies are those of VENNESLAND, WESTHEIMER and coworkers beginning about 1951. For example, LOEWUS et al. (1953) found that reduction of acetaldehyde-1-d with DPNH and yeast ADH gave ethanol-1-d which upon enzymatic oxidation reformed acetaldehyde-1-d without loss of deuterium. Alternatively reduction of unlabeled acetaldehyde with 4RS-4-d-DPNH produced ethanol-1-d which upon reoxidation regenerated acetaldehyde containing no deuterium. Work in several laboratories (LEMIEUX and HOWARD, 1963; WEBER et al., 1966; STREITWIESER and GRANGER, 1967) has clearly established that the ethanol-1-d formed by reduction of acetaldehyde-1-d is S(—)-ethanol-1-d (IV) while that formed by reduction of acetaldehyde with RS-4-d-DPNH is R(+)-ethanol-1-d (V).

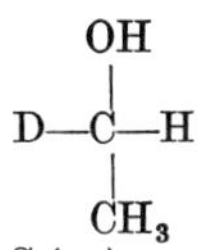

S (—)

IV

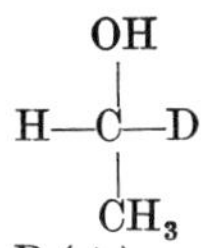

R (+)

V

Surprisingly, similar studies were not carried out with LADH until 1969. UMANI-RONCHI, WEBER and ARIGONI (unpublished, cf. ARIGONI and ELIEL, 1969) have now established that the stereospecificity of the interconversion of ethanol and acetaldehyde by LADH has the same stereospecificity as the yeast enzyme studied earlier.

An interesting report is that of ZAGALAK et al. (1966). They report that the LADH mediated reduction of R- and S-lactaldehyde with 4RS-4-d-DPNH yields R- and S- propandiols of identical configuration at C-1. Thus the stereochemical course of reduction by LADH is not influenced by the configuration of the carbon atom adjacent to the center being reduced.

The stereospecificity of LADH catalyzed interconversions of secondary alcohols and ketones has not yet been clearly defined. The studies of PRELOG and associates are of particular interest. They have been especially interested in the reduction of cyclic ketones by oxido-reductases from fungi and by LADH. On the basis of studies with a very large number of substrates they have formulated the following simplified scheme to describe the stereochemical nature of the reaction (PRELOG, 1964; ACKLIN et al., 1965):

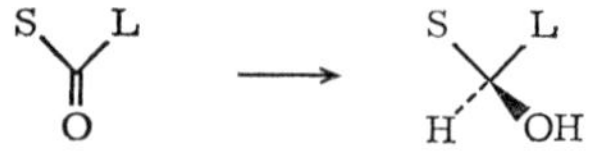

In this projection, the S represents the smaller of the alkyl groups and L the larger. Thus the carbinol formed has the S configuration in the Cahn-Ingold-Prelog terminology (Cahn et al., 1966). In general the experimental evidence confirms this generalization. Thus in the reduction of 25 bicyclic and tricyclic ketones by a reductase from *Curvularia falcata*, Acklin et al. (1965) obtained the S carbinol in 24 instances. In general the limited number of studies with LADH indicate the S-carbinols are preferentially formed as well as preferentially oxidized. The indications are, however, that although LADH is stereoselective for S-carbinol formation and oxidation, it is not stereospecific in this respect in all cases (cf. Elliott et al., 1969; Graves et al., 1965). A significant report is that of Dickinson and Dalziel (1967) who found S and R-2-butanol were oxidized by LADH at almost the same rate. The dehydrogenation of cholanic acids by LADH on the other hand is completely stereospecific for the 3β-hydroxy isomers (Waller et al., 1965). Finally, it should be noted that the stereospecific reduction of acetaldehyde-1-d to S(—)-ethanol-1-d is in accord with the Prelog scheme.

A substantial amount of work is needed before a complete understanding of the stereochemistry of LADH action is at hand.

Space does not permit a detailed discussion of the extensive kinetic studies which have been carried out on crystalline horse LADH. Early studies (Theorell and Bonnichsen, 1951; Theorell and Chance, 1951) led to the formulation of the Theorell-Chance mechanism. In simple terms, this mechanism proposes that the enzyme reacts in an obligatory sequence first with coenzyme then with substrate. This simple mechanism has been subjected to remarkably penetrating kinetic analyses in several laboratories (cf. Theorell and McKinley-McKee, 1961; Dickinson and Dalziel, 1967a; Dalziel and Dickinson, 1966; Wratten and Cleland, 1965). The mechanism does indeed appear to be valid in reactions involving primary alcohols but does not appear to describe the reaction with secondary alcohols.

The nature of the orientation of substrate and cosubstrate to each other in the transition state has been the subject of numerous speculatory reports (Ringold et al., 1966; Graves et al., 1965; Prelog, 1964; Elliott et al., 1969). Prelog has proposed that the substrate binding site can be characterized by a specific volume of a diamond lattice. Ringold et al. (1967), on the other hand, suggest that LADH does not have a fixed template type substrate recognition pocket but instead it is of the induced fit type which depends on the particular substrate.

II. Other Alcohol Dehydrogenases

In addition to LADH, numerous other oxido-reductases have been described from mammalian sources. These enzymes play a crucial role in the metabolism of steroids, lipids, carbohydrates and other vital body constituents. However, the substrate specificities of many of these oxido-reductases are relatively narrow and it is not likely that they participate to an important extent in the metabolism of foreign compounds[2]. A few, however, may be of some interest in drug metabolism and are discussed below.

One such group of enzymes which may be of significance are the brain alcohol dehydrogenases. A soluble enzyme from brain has been described by Raskin and

2 For a survey of oxido-reductases involved in steroid metabolism, the reader is referred to Talalay (1963) and to Clayton (1969).

SOKOLOFF (1968). They report that its properties are very similar to those of the liver enzyme and suggest that it may play a role in the metabolism of ethanol in the brain. Another possible function of brain oxido-reductases is suggested by work on the metabolism of catecholamines and of serotonin. AXELROD et al. (1959) reported the discovery of 3-methoxy-4-hydroxy phenylglycol among the metabolites of epinephrine. Later, KVEDER et al. (1962) described the formation of 5-hydroxytryptophol as a metabolite of 5-hydroxytryptamine in rats. *In vivo* experiments by FELDSTEIN and WONG (1965) showed that 5-hydroxytryptamine could be converted to 5-hydroxytryptophol in rat liver. It is also reported to be a major metabolite of 5-hydroxytryptamine in isolated platelets (BARTHOLINI et al., 1964). Later, a careful study by ECCLESTON et al. (1966) revealed that human and rat brain homogenates could convert serotonin to 5-hydroxytryptophol. The conversion occurred by way of the intermediate formation of 5-hydroxyindole acetaldehyde, a step mediated by monoamine oxidase. The intermediate 5-hydroxyindole acetaldehyde then underwent either oxidation to hydroxyindole acetic acid or alternatively was reduced by an alcohol dehydrogenase to 5-hydroxytryptophol. They report that this alcohol dehydrogenase differs from LADH in that TPNH is the preferred cofactor for the reduction. The nature and function of oxido-reductases in the central nervous system have not as yet been adequately investigated.

An important part of the chemical cycle of vision involves the interconversion of $retinol_1$ and $retinal_1$ and of $retinol_2$ and $retinal_2$ (WALD, 1968). For many years it was thought that these reactions were catalyzed by an enzyme very similar to or identical with LADH. It is now known, however, that there is an oxido-reductase present in the eyes which is distinctly different from LADH and is absent from liver (KOEN and SHAW, 1966).

Recent studies on the microsomal hydroxylation of indane to 1-indanol led to the discovery of a microsomal oxido-reductase which readily dehydrogenated 1-indanol to 1-indanone (BILLINGS et al., 1970). Both DPN^+ and TPN^+ served as cosubstrates for the reaction. In the case of TPN^+ the TPNH formed is reoxidized to TPN^+ by oxygen and microsomal TPNH oxidase, thus regenerating TPN^+. In this cyclic process, which occurs with oxygen present, several moles of indanone are formed for each mole of TPN^+ present. Other aromatic alcohols oxidized by liver microsomes include methylphenylcarbinol, acenaphthenol and 1-tetralol. None of these carbinols are substrates for LADH (BILLINGS et al., unpublished data). In a related study, HOPKINS (1968) and DRUMMOND and HOPKINS (1969) have reported that rat liver microsomes can catalyze the dehydrogenation of cis- and trans-acenaphthene-1, 2-diols.

Although oxido-reductases are characteristically soluble enzymes, a number of other examples of microsomal bound activities have been recorded. For example, BERSÉUS et al. (1967) report that liver microsomal fraction fortified with either DPN^+ or TPN^+ readily converts cholest-5-ene-3β,7α,12α-triol to 7α,12α-dihydroxycholest-4-ene-3-one. Similarly, liver microsomes plus DPN^+ convert 7α-hydroxycholesterol to cholest-4-ene-3-one-7α-ol (HUTTON and BOYD, 1966). HURLOCK and TALALAY (1959) have described a rat liver microsomal 11β-hydroxy steroid dehydrogenase which can utilize either DPN^+ or TPN^+ as a cosubstrate. It is relatively nonspecific in the sense that a variety of 11β-hydroxy steroids serve as substrate (KOERNER, 1969). INANO et al. (1969) have described a Δ5-3β-hydroxy steroid dehydrogenase from the microsomal fraction of adrenals which may be involved in corticogenesis. What role these and other microsomal oxido-reductases play in the metabolism of foreign lipid soluble compounds remains to be determined.

In 1957 Gillette et al. described the oxidation of methanol to formaldehyde by liver microsomes in the presence of TPNH and oxygen. The reaction was catalyzed by catalase and utilized hydrogen peroxide generated by the TPNH oxidase system. Ethyl alcohol is oxidized by the same system (cf. Roach et al., 1969). Other reports (Orme-Johnson and Ziegler, 1965 and Lieber and Decarli, 1970) suggest that ethanol may be oxidized directly by the mixed function oxidases of hepatic microsomes. However, in a recent study Isselbacher and Carter (1970) demonstrated the presence of ADP in the liver microsome fraction and presented evidence that it may be the major factor responsible for the microsomal oxidation of ethyl alcohol.

Studies on the enzymatic dehydrogenation of indanol have been extended (Billings, Sullivan and McMahon, unpublished) and a soluble enzyme partially purified from the 100,000 g supernate of liver homogenates which readily dehydrogenates 1-indanol, 1-tetralol and cyclohexenol-3. It does not however dehydrogenate aliphatic cyclic alcohols or open chain aromatic carbinols such as methylphenylcarbinol. This enzyme which is clearly distinct from LADH, may be related to or identical with 3-hydroxymethylhexabarbital dehydrogenase which has been partially purified by Toki and Tsukamoto (1964). These authors report that the enzyme they have isolated readily dehydrogenates 3-hydroxymethylhexabarbital and cyclohexenol-3 but not ethanol, cyclohexanol or benzyl alcohol.

Arene dihydrodiols such as 1,2-dihydro-1,2-dihydroxybenzene (VI) undergo *in vivo* dehydrogenation to an enol (VII) which

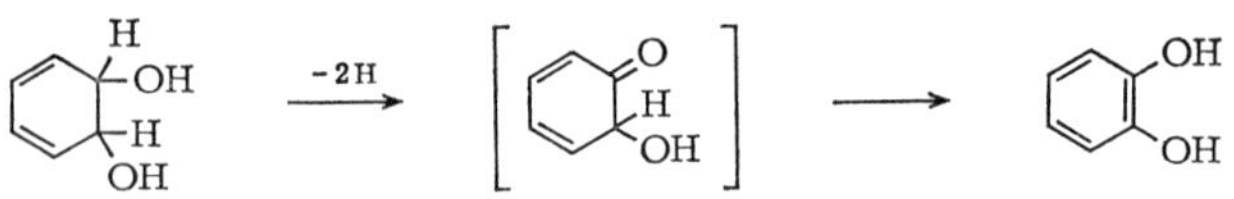

VI VII VIII

spontaneously rearranges to catechol (VIII). The dehydrogenase responsible for this reaction is present in liver (Ayengar et al., 1959). Recently Jerina et al. (1970) have investigated the stereoselectivity of this soluble liver enzyme. They found, for example, that (+)-trans-1,2-dihydro-1,2-dihydroxybenzene underwent dehydrogenation several times more rapidly than the (—) isomer. The (+) isomer has the 1S,2S configuration so that this stereoselectivity is consistent with the Prelog generalization discussed above. Since the (+) isomer is a minor product of the enzymatic hydrolysis of arene oxides it is not surprising that catechols are not important metabolites of aromatic compounds. More work is needed to adequately characterize this dihydrodiol dehydrogenase and to differentiate it from other oxido-reductases. Whether dihydrodiols are intermediates in the formation of catechols as drug metabolites is unknown. Such a metabolite has, however, been reported by Tatsumi et al. (1967) for phenacetylurea in rabbits.

III. Reductases

The oxido-reductases that have been discussed so far appear to function in the body mainly as dehydrogenases rather than as reductases. There are, however, a number of other oxido-reductases which have been reported from mammalian sources which appear to function as true reductases. For many of these, the preferred coenzyme is TPNH rather than DPNH. This is not surprising since TPNH has been shown to exist almost exclusively in the reduced form in extramitochondrial space in the liver cell (Jacobson and Kaplan, 1957). A number of these reductases which may be of interest in drug metabolism, are described in the following paragraphs.

1. 4-Ketoproline Reductase

SMITH and MITOMA (1962) have described the partial purification of a soluble enzyme from rat kidney which mediates the reduction of ketoproline to hydroxyproline. This enzyme for which DPNH is the preferred cosubstrate also reduces pyruvate and α-ketobutyrate although it clearly is not lactate dehydrogenase. The normal function of this enzyme, which does not catalyze the reverse reaction, i. e. hydroxyproline to ketoproline, is unknown.

2. Aromatic Aldehyde-Ketone Reductase

Another kidney reductase has recently been described by CULP and McMAHON (1968). Aromatic aldehyde-ketone reductase was purified from rabbit kidney cortex homogenate about 200-fold and its properties studied. The enzyme had an absolute requirement for TPNH as cosubstrate and readily reduced many aromatic aldehydes and ketones. The reverse reaction, the oxidation of aromatic carbinols to ketones and aldehydes, was not catalyzed. The reduction was stereoselective since methylphenylcarbinol formed by the reduction of acetophenone was a mixture of 75% S-carbinol and 25% R-carbinol. The enzyme was also shown to utilize the tritium of 4S-4-t-TPNH and not that of 4R-4-t-TPNH. Thus, aromatic aldehyde-ketone reductase is B-side specific (opposite that of LADH which is A-side specific). Both substituted benzaldehydes and acetophenones were reduced. Ring substitution of electron withdrawing groups such as para-nitro and para-chloro greatly enhanced the rate while electron donating groups such as para-methoxy slowed the rate of reduction. HERMANN et al. (1969) have studied the structure-activity relationships among the substituted acetophenones. They have obtained significant correlations using simple linear models for regression analysis which employ substituent constants based on several different molecular parameters. All of the structure-activity work on substrates so far is consistent with a mechanism involving the transfer of the elements of hydride ion from TPNH to the carbonyl compound (cf. SUND, 1968). Aromatic aldehyde-ketone reductase reduced straight chain aliphatic ketones and aldehydes only very slowly, if at all. However, certain alicyclic ketones were readily reduced. Both cyclohexanone and 2-decalone were excellent substrates. Even the highly hindered ketone, adamantanone, was efficiently reduced. CULP and McMAHON (1966) have also partially purified this enzyme from the soluble fraction of rabbit liver homogenate. The liver enzyme was reported to be very similar to the kidney enzyme with respect to substrate specificity, inhibitor activity, pH optimum and K_m for TPNH.

3. Pig Liver Reductase

Workers in PRELOG's laboratory (PRELOG, 1964; WALDVOGEL, 1965) have described a ketone reductase from pig liver. The activity was purified about 120-fold from the soluble fraction of pig liver homogenate. One unusual property of this protein is its high molecular weight which is about 525,000. Like aromatic aldehyde-ketone reductase, the pig liver reductase was found to utilize TPNH and to be B-side specific. Substrate activity studies showed that a wide variety of cyclohexanones, decalones and other alicyclic ketones were reduced. Cyclopentanone, however, was not an active substrate. It will be of interest to find out whether or not benzaldehydes and acetophenones serve as substrates for the pig liver reductase, since it is altogether possible that this enzyme is identical to the liver enzyme described by CULP and McMAHON (1966).

Some of the substrates reduced by pig liver reductase are the same substrates which have been shown to be reduced by liver alcohol dehydrogenase. This is of special interest since LADH is an A-side specific enzyme while pig liver reductase is a B-side specific. If it is assumed that S-carbinols are formed in each case, it can be concluded that either the relative positioning of substrate and coenzyme in the transition state is quite different for the two enzymes or alternatively that the the 3-carboxamide group is not important in product stereospecificity control (cf. Karabatsos, 1966, for further discussion of this point). Although the function of this enzyme in the intact animal remains obscure, it is possible that the *in vivo* reduction of cyclohexanones and decanones (*vida supra*) is mediated by this enzyme rather than by LADH as suggested by Elliott et al. (1969).

4. α-β-Unsaturated Ketone Reductase

Another TPNH-dependent ketone reductase is *α,β*-unsaturated ketone reductase which has been studied by Fraser et al. (1967). This enzyme was isolated and purified from both dog erythrocytes and from human liver. It mediates the reduction of a number of unsaturated ketones but not of saturated ketones or unsaturated compounds without the keto group. The enzyme activity was shown to be distinct from aromatic aldehyde-ketone reductase, aromatic *α*-keto acid reductase, LADH and lactic dehydrogenase. Like aromatic aldehyde-ketone reductase, the reverse reaction was not catalyzed. When 4-phenyl-3-butene-2-one was used as substrate, the products were 4-phenylbutane-2-one and 4-phenylbutane-2-ol (Fraser et al., 1968).

5. Kidney Lactaldehyde Reductase

Gupta and Robinson (1960) have purified from pig kidney an enzyme which catalyzes the reduction of *l*-lactaldehyde to propanediol. The enzyme has an absolute requirement for TPNH and catalyzes the reverse reaction only with great difficulty. Unlike LADH, which catalyzes the reduction of both the *l* and *d* isomers of lactaldehyde, kidney lactaldehyde reductase utilizes only the *l*-isomer as substrate. Other compounds reduced included glucuronic acid, methylglyoxal, glyceraldehyde, ribose and xylose.

6. Retinal Reductase from Rat Intestine

During intestinal absorption of *β*-carotene, the carotene undergoes cleavage to 2 moles of retinal. The retinal, in turn, is reduced by a soluble enzyme from intestinal mucosa to retinol. Fidge and Goodman (1968) have partially purified this reductase and found it to have a molecular weight in the range of 60,000 to 80,000. Either DPNH or TPNH served as cofactor. Although the enzyme is A-side specific, it was shown to differ from LADH. The enzyme was relatively nonspecific and reduced straight-chain aliphatic aldehydes of short and medium chain. Benzaldehyde was also reduced. This interesting enzyme appears to be primarily a reductase.

7. Aromatic α-Keto Acid Reductase

Zannoni and Weber (1966) have isolated an enzyme from beef and dog heart which catalyzes the reduction of aromatic *α*-keto acids to phenyllactic acids. This enzyme requires DPNH and is distinct from lactic dehydroganese. It is widely distributed in mammalian tissues and is the main enzyme responsible for the reduction of aromatic *α*-keto acids in mammals (Weber and Zannoni, 1966). A variety of substituted phenylpyruvic acids were shown to be active substrates. The phenyllactic acids formed had the L configuration.

8. Other Reductases

Many reductases other than those listed above have been reported. An interesting example is beef liver microsomal *d*-3-oxo-sphinganine oxido-reductase (Stoffel et al., 1968). This enzyme catalyzes the reduction of D-3-oxodihydrosphingosine to D-erythrodihydrosphingosine. It is TPNH-dependent and is B-side specific. Wakil and Bressler (1962) have purified a soluble enzyme, acetoacetyl-CoA reductase from pigeon liver. This TPNH-dependent enzyme reduces acetoacetyl coenzyme A to D(—)-β-hydroxybutyryl-CoA. Their results indicate that this enzyme may not be involved in fatty acid synthesis but may have some other function on the body. Yet another reductase is mavaldate reductase, an important enzyme in cholesterol biosynthesis. It utilizes either DPNH or TPNH and is A-side specific (Donninger and Popják, 1965).

B. Aldehyde Oxidation

The oxidation of aldehydes to carboxylic acids at the enzyme level is not well understood. Aldehydes are produced in the body principally through the action of monoamine oxidase on amines and by the oxidation of primary alcohols by oxido-reductases as discussed above. Aldehydes also may rise by more obscure pathways. For example, one of the primary metabolites of cephalothin, when given orally, is thienylacetamidoacetylaldehyde (Sullivan and McMahon, 1967). Aldehydes are rarely, if ever, excreted as such. For the most part they are rapidly and completely oxidized to the corresponding carboxylic acid before excretion. In a few rare cases such as the metabolism of catecholamines, serotonin or orally administered cephalothin, some of the aldehyde is reduced to the primary alcohol. Three enzymes or groups of enzymes have been implicated in the *in vivo* oxidation of aldehydes. These are the aldehyde dehydrogenases, aldehyde oxidases and xanthine oxidase. Each of these are discussed below with respect to properties and substrate specificity. In addition to these enzymes, it has also been shown that formaldehyde undergoes a dismutation to formic acid and methanol in the presence of liver LADH and DPN^+ (Abeles and Lee, 1960). Pyruvaldehyde, acetaldehyde and acrolein also show this reaction.

I. Aldehyde Dehydrogenases

The first aldehyde dehydrogenase to be isolated and distinguished from LADH was beef liver aldehyde dehydrogenase (Racker, 1949). It was shown to oxidize formaldehyde, acetaldehyde, glycolaldehyde, propionaldehyde, butyraldehyde and isovalerylaldehyde. Deitrich et al. (1962) have shown that liver aldehyde dehydrogenase will also dehydrogenate aromatic aldehydes. A study of the effect of substitution in the benzaldehyde ring produced a biphasic Hammett plot in which benzaldehyde itself gave the maximum rate. Erwin and Deitrich (1966) have also prepared aldehyde dehydrogenase from bovine brain. A study of the oxidation of aliphatic aldehydes by this soluble brain enzyme produced a linear Taft plot which showed that the rate increased as the carbonyl carbon became more electropositive. No steric effect was observed. A number of other aldehyde dehydrogenases have been described in the literature (Jacoby, 1963). However, to date, none has been obtained in sufficient purity to allow a complete characterization of the protein responsible for aldehyde dehydrogenation. It is known however that in the reaction the aldehyde hydrogen is transferred directly to DPN^+ and that this transfer is to the A-side of DPN^+ (Levy and Vennesland, 1957).

Although more work is needed it seems likely that the aldehyde dehydrogenases do play an important role in the oxidation of aldehydes to carboxylic acids *in vivo*.

II. Aldehyde Oxidase

In addition to aldehyde dehydrogenase, liver contains a second enzyme, aldehyde oxidase, capable of oxidizing aldehydes. This enzyme has been studied by Mahler et al. (1954) and more recently by Rajagopalan et al. (1962) and Rajagopalan and Handler (1964) 1964a). Aldehyde oxidase is a very complex enzyme having a molecular weight of 300,000. It is a metalloflavoprotein with a molar ratio content of Mo:FAD:Fe of 2:2:8. Hepatic aldehyde oxidase has a dual substrate specificity since both aldehydes and N-heterocyclic substrates are oxidized. Although this substrate specificity is similar to that of xanthine oxidase there are important differences. For example, aldehyde oxidase oxidizes purine to 8-hydroxy purine whereas xanthine oxidase converts it in three steps to uric acid. In the oxidative reactions catalyzed by aldehyde oxidase, several compounds can serve as electronic acceptors. Oxygen, however, is an excellent electron acceptor and may be the physiological acceptor (cf. Rajagopalan and Handler, 1968).

III. Xanthine Oxidase

Xanthine oxidase is a complex metalloflavoprotein whose physical properties are very similar to those of aldehyde oxidase with respect to molecular weight and to the molar ratio of molybdenum, FAD and iron. The enzyme has a wide distribution in nature, cow's milk or calf's liver being particularly good sources of enzyme. The xanthine oxidase literature has been reviewed by Bray (1963) and by Rajagopalan and Handler (1968). As with aldehyde oxidase the precise physiological function of xanthine oxidase is unknown. However, the oxidation of xanthine and hypoxanthine in the presence of oxygen is particularly rapid and may be a clue to its natural function. In addition to these substrates, many other nitrogen heterocyclics as well as aldehydes are oxidized by this enzyme. Although almost all aldehydes are oxidized, the K_m's are significantly greater than for the heterocyclics indicating that aldehyde oxidation may be of less importance. Oxygen is a good electron acceptor for xanthine oxidase and indeed may be the physiological acceptor. Presently it appears that the aldehyde dehydrogenases are the most important enzymes with respect to aldehyde oxidation. However, a possible role of aldehyde oxidase and xanthine oxidase cannot be ruled out.

C. Summary

It is clear that there is a very large number of enzymes which have been shown to have the capability of oxidizing alcohols and aldehydes and of reducing aldehydes and ketones. The unanswered question is which of these are of importance in the *in vivo* metabolism of foreign alcohols, aldehydes and ketones. Because of the mass of the liver and its uniquely efficient blood circulation system, it is probable that those enzymes present in the liver are of greatest importance in drug metabolism. Enzymes present in other tissues, however, may be involved. Further experimental investigation of this question would be of value. In particular, the oxido-reductases present in erythrocytes and platelets may be important.

The oxidation of foreign compounds is frequently a multistep process. For example, in the intact rat S(—) methylphenylcarbinol is efficiently converted to S(—) mandelic acid (McMahon and Sullivan, 1968): S-$PhCHOHCH_3$ → $PhCOCH_3$ → $PhCOCH_2OH$ → S-$PhCHOHCH_2OH$ → S-PhCHOHCHO → S-PhCHOHCOOH. In the five step reaction sequence, three of the steps are catalyzed by oxido-reductases, one by a microsomal hydroxylase and one by aldehyde dehydrogenase. The question is whether in the intact cell these enzymes exist in close proximity in some sort of a multienzyme system that can efficiently carry out a multistep oxidation of a foreign substance. The alternative is a random process in which the substrate at each step distributes randomly until it becomes bound to the appropriate enzyme. This is yet another question that requires experimental investigation.

References

ABELES, R.H., LEE, JR., H.E.: The dismutation of formaldehyde by liver alcohol dehydrogenase. J. biol. Chem. **235**, 1499—1503 (1960).

ACKLIN, W., PRELOG, V., SCHENKER, F., SERDAREVIC, B., WALTER, P.: Reduktion von stereoisomeren Dekalonen-(1) und einigen verwandten bicyclischen und tricyclischen Ketonen durch *Curvularia falcata*. Helv. chim. Acta **48**, 1725—1746 (1965).

ARIGONI, D., ELIEL, E.: Chirality due to the presence of hydrogen isotopes at noncyclic positions. In: Topics in Stereochemistry, Vol. 4, N. ALLINGER, ed. New York: Interscience-Wiley 1969.

AXELROD, J., KOPIN, I.J., MANN, J.D.: 3-Methoxy-4-hydroxyphenylglycol sulfate, a new metabolite of epinephrine and norepinephrine. Biochim. biophys. Acta (Amst.) **36**, 576—577 (1959).

AYENGAR, P.K., HAYAISHI, O., NAKAJIMA, M., TOMIDA, I.: Enzymic aromatization of 3,5-cyclohexadiene-1,2-diol. Biochim. biophys. Acta (Amst.) **33**, 111—119 (1959).

BARTHOLINI, G., PLETSCHER, A., BRUDERER, H.: Formation of 5-hydroxytryptophol from endogenous 5-hydroxytryptamine by isolated blood platelets. Nature (Lond.) **203**, 1281 to 1283 (1964).

BERSÉUS, O., DANIELSSON, H., EINARSSON, K.: Synthesis and metabolism of cholest-5-ene: $3\beta,7\alpha,12\alpha$-triol. J. biol. Chem. **242**, 1211—1219 (1967).

BILLINGS, R.E., SULLIVAN, H.R., MCMAHON, R.E.: The oxidation of indane to indanol and indanone by the hepatic microsomal system. Biochem. J. **9**, 1256—1260 (1970).

BLOMQUIST, C.H.: Electronic effects in horse liver alcohol dehydrogenase catalysis. Acta chem. scand. **20**, 1747—1757 (1966).

BONNICHSEN, R.K., WASSEN, A.M.: Crystalline alcohol dehydrogenase from horse liver. Arch. Biochem. **18**, 361—363 (1948).

BRAY, R.C.: Xanthine oxidase. In: The Enzymes, 2nd ed., Vol. 7, P.D. BOYER, H. LARDY and K. MÝRBACK, Eds. New York: Academic Press 1963.

CAHN, R.S., INGOLD, C., PRELOG, V.: Specification of molecular chirality. Angew. Chem. Intern. Ed. Engl. **5**, 385—415 (1966).

CHEO, K.L., ELLIOTT, T.H., TAO, R.C.C.: The metabolism of the isomeric *tert.*-butylcyclohexanones. Biochem. J. **104**, 198—204 (1967).

CHRISTOPHE, J., POPJÁK, G.: Studies on the biosynthesis of cholesterol. XIV. The origin of prenoic acids from allyl pyrophosphates in liver enzyme systems. J. Lipid Res. **2**, 244—257 (1961).

CLAYTON, R.B., ed.: Steroids and Terpenoids. In: Methods in Enzymology, Vol. 15, S.P. COLOWICK and N.O. KAPLAN, Editors in Chief. New York: Academic Press 1969.

CORNFORTH, J.W., RYBACK, G., POPJÁK, G., CONNINGER, C., SCHROEPFER, JR., G.: Stereochemistry of enzymic hydrogen transfer to pyridine nucleotides. Biochem. biophys. Res. Commun. **9**, 371—375 (1962).

CULP, H.W., MCMAHON, R.E.: A TPNH dependent benzaldehyde reductase from kidney and liver. Abstracts, Amer. Chem. Soc. 152nd Meeting, Div. of Biol. Chem., Abstract No. 190 (1966).

— — Reductase for aromatic aldehydes and ketones, the partial purification and properties of a reduced triphosphopyridine nucleotide-dependent reductase from rabbit kidney cortex. J. biol. Chem. **243**, 848—852 (1968).

DALZIEL, K., DICKINSON, F.M.: The activity of liver alcohol dehydrogenase with nicotinamide-adenine dinucleotide phosphate as coenzyme. Biochem. J. **95**, 311—230 (1965).

— — Substrate activation and inhibition in coenzyme-substrate reactions. Cyclohexanol oxidation catalyzed by liver alcohol dehydrogenase. Biochem. J. **100**, 491—500 (1966).

DEITRICH, R.A., HELLERMAN, L., WEIN, J.: Diphosphopyridine nucleotide-linked aldehyde dehydrogenase I. Specificity and *sigma-rho* function. J. biol. Chem. **237**, 560—564 (1962).

DICKINSON, F.M., DALZIEL, K.: Substrate specificity and stereospecificity of alcohol dehydrogenases. Nature (Lond.) **214**, 31—33 (1967).

— — The specificities and configurations of ternary complexes of yeast and liver alcohol dehydrogenases. Biochem. J. **104**, 165—172 (1967a).

Donninger, C., Popják, G.: Studies on the biosynthesis of cholesterol, XVIII. The stereospecificity of mevaldate reductase and the biosynthesis of asymmetrically labelled farnesyl pyrophosphate. Proc. roy. Soc. B **163**, 465—491 (1965).

Drum, D.E., Li, T.-K., Vallee, B.L.: Considerations in evaluating the zinc content of horse liver alcohol dehydrogenase preparations. Biochem. J. **8**, 3783—3791 (1969).

Drummond, E.C., Hopkins, R.P.: Microsomal dehydrogenation of *cis*- and *trans*-acenaphthene-1,2-diol to acenaphthenequinone. Biochem. J. **113**, 13p (1969).

Eccleston, D., Moir, A.T.B., Reading, H.W., Ritchie, I.M.: The formation of 5-hydroxytryptophol in brain *in vitro*. Brit. J. Pharmacol. **28**, 367—377 (1966).

Elliott, T.H., Jacob, E., Tao, R.C.C.: The *in vitro* and *in vivo* metabolism of optically active methylcyclohexanols and methylcyclohexanones. J. Pharm. Pharmacol. **21**, 561—572 (1969).

— Robertson, J.S., Williams, R.T.: The metabolism of the isomeric decalones. Biochem. J. **100**, 393—402 (1966).

— Tao, R.C.C., Williams, R.T.: Stereochemical aspects of the metabolism of the isomeric methylcyclohexanols and methylcyclohexanones. Biochem. J. **95**, 59—69 (1965).

Erwin, V.G., Deitrich, R.A.: Brain aldehyde dehydrogenase localization, purification and properties. J. biol. Chem. **241**, 3533—3539 (1966).

Feldstein, A., Wong, K.K.: Enzymatic conversion of serotonin to 5-hydroxytryptophol. Life Sci, **4**, 183—191 (1965).

Fidge, N.H., Goodman, D.S.: The enzymatic reduction of retinal to retinol in rat intestine. J. biol. Chem. **243**, 4372—4379 (1968).

Fisher, H.F., Conn, E.E., Vennesland, B., Westheimer, F.H.: The enzymatic transfer of hydrogen I. The reaction catalyzed by alcohol dehydrogenase. J. biol. Chem. **202**, 687—697 (1953).

Fraser, I.M., Fancher, D.A., Strother, A.: Products and sites of reduction of 4-phenyl-3-buten-2-one and 4-phenylbutan-2-one in the rat and dog. Pharmacologist **10**, 203 (1968) (Abstract).

— Peters, M.A., Hardinge, M.G.: Purification and some characteristics of an α,β-unsaturated ketone reductase from dog erythrocytes and human liver. Molec. Pharmacol. **3**, 233—247 (1967).

Friedman, P.J., Cooper, J.R.: The role of alcohol dehydrogenase in the metabolism of chloral hydrate. Pharm. J. **129**, 373—376 (1960).

Gillette, J.R.: Side chain oxidation of alkyl substituted ring compounds I. Enzymatic oxidation of *p*-nitrotoluene. J. biol. Chem. **234**, 139—143 (1959).

— Brodie, B.B., La Du, B.N.: The oxidation of drugs by liver microsomes: on the role of TPNH and oxygen. J. Pharm. exp. Ther. **119**, 532—539 (1957).

Graves, J.M.H., Clark, A., Ringold, H.J.: Stereochemical aspects of the substrate specificity of horse liver alcohol dehydrogenase. Biochem. J. **4**, 2655—2671 (1965).

Green, R.W., McKay, R.H.: The behavior of horse liver alcohol dehydrogenase in guanidine hydrochloride solutions. J. biol. Chem. **244**, 5034—5043 (1969).

Gupta, N.K., Robinson, W.G.: The enzymatic conversion of lactaldehyde to propanediol. J. biol. Chem. **235**, 1609—1612 (1960).

Hermann, R.B., Culp, H.W., McMahon, R.E., Marsh, M.M.: Structure-activity relationhips among substrates for a rabbit kidney reductase. Quantum chemical calculation of substituent parameters. J. med. pharm. Chem. **12**, 749—754 (1969).

Hopkins, R.P.: Microsomal ring-fission of *cis*- and *trans*-acenapthene-1,2-diol. Biochem. J. **108**, 577—582 (1968).

Hurlock, B., Talalay, P.: Microsomal 3α- and 11β-hydroxysteroid dehydrogenase. Arch. Biochem. **80**, 468—470 (1959).

Hutton, H.R.B., Boyd, G.S.: The metabolism of cholest-5-en-$3\beta,7\alpha$-diol by rat liver cell fractions. Biochim. biophys. Acta (Amst.) **116**, 336—361 (1966).

Inano, H., Machino, A., Tamaoki, B.: Localization of the $\Delta 5$-3β-hydroxysteroid dehydrogenase and 21-hydroxylase activities in smooth-surfaced microsomes of adrenals Steroids **13**, 357—363 (1969).

Isselbacher, K.J., Carter, E.A.: Ethanol oxidation by liver microsomes: Evidence against a separate and distinct enzyme system. Biochem. biophys. Res. Commun. **39**, 530—537 (1970).

Jacobson, K.B., Kaplan, N.O.: Pyridine coenzymes of subcellular tissue fractions. J. biol. Chem. **226**, 603—613 (1957).

Jacoby, W.B.: Aldehyde dehydrogenases. In: The Enzymes, 2nd ed., Vol. 7, P.D. Boyer, H. Lardy and K. Myrback, Eds., New York: Academic Press 1963.

Jerina, D.M., Ziffer, H., Daly, J.W.: The role of the arene oxide-oxepin system in the metabolism of aromatic substrates. IV. Stereochemical considerations of dihydrodiol formation and dehydrogenation. J. Amer. chem. Soc. **92**, 1056—1061 (1970).

KARABATSOS, G.J., FLEMING, J.S., HSI, N., ABELES, R.H.: Comments on the factors controlling product stereospecificity in the reduction of carbonyl compounds with alcohol dehydrogenase and diphosphopyridine nucleotide. J. Amer. chem. Soc. **88**, 849—850 (1966).
KINI, M.M., COOPER, J.R.: Biochemistry of methanol poisoning III. The enzymic pathway for the conversion of methanol to formaldehyde. Biochem. Pharmacol. **8**, 207—215 (1961).
KOEN, A.L., SHAW, C.R.: Retinol and alcohol dehydrogenases in retina and liver. Biochim. biophys. Acta (Amst.) **128**, 48—54 (1966).
KOERNER, D.R.: Assay and substrate specificity of liver 11β-hydroxysteroid dehydrogenase. Biochim. biophys. Acta (Amst.) **176**, 377—382 (1969).
KUNTZMAN, R., IKEDA, M., JACOBSON, M., CONNEY, A.H.: A sensitive method for the determination and isolation of pentobarbital-C^{14} metabolites and its application to *in vitro* studies of drug metabolism. J. Pharmacol. exp. Ther. **157**, 220—226 (1967).
KVEDER, S., ISKRIC, S., KEGLEVIC, D.: 5-Hydroxytryptophol: a metabolite of 5-hydroxytryptamine in rats. Biochem. J. **85**, 447—449 (1962).
LEMIEUX, R.U., HOWARD, J.: The absolute configuration of *dextro*-1-deuterioethanol. Canad. J. Chem. **41**, 308—316 (1963).
LEVY, H.R., VENNESLAND, B.: The stereospecificity of enzymatic hydrogen transfer from diphosphopyridine nucleotide. J. biol. Chem. **228**, 85—96 (1957).
LI, T., THEORELL, H.: Human liver alcohol dehydrogenase: inhibition by pyrazole and pyrazole analogs. Acta chem. Scand. **23**, 892—902 (1969).
LIEBER, C.S., DECARLI, L.M.: Hepatic microsomal ethanol-oxidizing system. *In vitro* characteristics and adaptive properties *in vivo*. J. biol. Chem. **245**, 2505—2512 (1970).
LOEWUS, F.A., WESTHEIMER, F.H., VENNESLAND, B.: Enzymatic synthesis of the enantiomorphs of ethanol-1-d. J. Amer. Genat. Soc. **75**, 5018—5023 (1953).
MAHLER, H.R., MACKLER, B., GREEN, D.E., BOKK, R.M.: Studies on metalloflavoproteins III. Aldehyde oxidase: a molybdoflavoprotein. J. biol. Chem. **210**, 465 (1954).
MCDANIEL, H.G., PODGAINY, H., BRESSLER, R.: The metabolism of tolbutamide in rat liver. J. Pharmacol. exp. Ther. **167**, 91—97 (1969).
MCMAHON, R.E., MARHSALL, F.J., CULP, H.W.: The nature of the metabolites of acetohexamide in the rat and in the human. J. Pharmacol. exp. Ther. **149**, 272—279 (1965).
— SULLIVAN, H.R.: The nature of the *in vivo* conversion of L(—)methylphenylcarbinol to D(—)mandelic acid in the rat. Pharmacologist **10**, 203 (1963) (Abstract).
MERRITT, A.D., TOMKINS, G.M.: Reversible oxidation of cyclic secondary alcohols by liver alcohol dehydrogenase. J. biol. Chem. **234**, 2778—2782 (1959).
MOIR, N.J., MILLER, W.L., GAYLOR, J.L.: Investigation of the component reactions of oxidative sterol demethylation. Alcohol dehydrogenase. Biochem. biophys. Res. Commun. **33**, 916—921 (1968).
MOURAD, N., WORONICK, C.L.: Crystallization of human liver alcohol dehydrogenase. Arch. Biochem. **121**, 431—439 (1967).
NAKAMOTO, T., VENNESLAND, B.: The enzymatic transfer of hydrogen VII. The reactions catalyzed by glutamic and isocitric dehydrogenases. J. biol. Chem. **235**, 202—204 (1960).
ORME-JOHNSON, W.H., ZIEGLER, D.M.: Alcohol mixed function oxidase activity of mammalian liver microsomes. Biochem. biophys. Res. Commun. **21**, 78—82 (1965).
PIETRUSZKO, R.H., RINGOLD, H.J., LI, T.-K., VALLEE, B.L., AKESON, A., THEORELL, H.: Structure and function relationships in isoenzymes of horse liver alcohol dehydrogenase. Nature (Lond.) **221**, 440—443 (1969).
PRELOG, V.: Specification of the stereospecificity of some oxido-reductases by diamond lattice sections. Pure appl. Chem. **9**, 119—130 (1964).
RACKER, E.: Aldehyde dehydrogenase, a diphosphopyridine nucleotide-linked enzyme. J. biol. Chem. **177**, 883—892 (1949).
RAJAGOPALAN, K.V., FRIDOVICH, I., HANDLER, P.: Hepatic aldehyde oxidase I. Purification and properties. J. biol. Chem. **237**, 922—928 (1962).
— HANDLER, P.: Hepatic aldehyde oxidase II. Differential inhibition of electron transfer to various electron acceptors. J. biol. Chem. **239**, 2022—2026 (1964).
— — Hepatic aldehyde oxidase III. The substrate-binding site. J. biol. Chem. **239**, 2027 to 2035 (1964a).
— — Metalloflavoproteins. In: Biological Oxidation, T.P. SINGER, ed., New York, London and Sydney: Interscience 1968.
RASKIN, N.H., SOKOLOFF, L.: Brain alcohol dehydrogenase. Science **162**, 131—132 (1968).
RINGOLD, H.J., BELLAS, T., CLARK, A.: Adamantanone as a probe for the dimensions and characteristics of the substrate binding pocket of certain alcohol dehydrogenases. Biochem. biophys. Res. Commun. **27**, 361—367 (1967).
— GRAVES, J.M.H., CLARK, A., BELLAS, T.: Experimental strategy for delineation of the enzyme region involved in substrate recognition. Proc. nat. Acad. Sci. (Wash.) **56**, 255 to 261 (1966).

Roach, M.K., Reese, W.N., jr., Creaven, P.J.: Ethanol oxidation in the microsomal fraction of rat liver. Biochem. biophys. Res. Commun. **36**, 596—602 (1969).
Schwartz, D.E., Bruderer, H., Rieder, J., Brossi, A.: Metabolic studies of tetrabenazine, a psychotropic drug in animals and man. Biochem. Pharmacol. **15**, 645—655 (1966).
Smith, D., Forist, A.A., Dulin, W.E.: 5-Methylpyrazole-3-carboxylic acid. The potent hypoglycemic metabolite of 3,5-dimethylpyrazole in the rat. J. med. pharm. Chem. **8**, 350—353 (1965).
Smith, J.N., Smithies, R.H., Williams, R.T.: Studies in detoxication. 59. The metabolism of alkylbenzenes. The biological reduction of ketones derived from alkylbenzenes. Biochem. J. **57**, 74—76 (1954).
Smith, T.E., Mitoma, C.: Partial purification and some properties of 4-ketoproline reductase. J. biol. Chem. **237**, 1177—1180 (1962).
Stoffel, W., LeKim, D., Sticht, G.: Stereospecificity of the NADPH-dependent reduction reaction of 3-oxodihydrosphingosine (2-amino-1-hydroxyoctadecane-3-one). Hoppe-Seylers Z. physiol. Chem. **349**, 1637—1644 (1968).
Streitwieser, A., jr., Granger, M.R.: Stereochemistry of the primary carbon. XV. Preparation of optically active ethanol-1-*d* by asymmetric induction and its absolute configuration. J. Org. Chem. **32**, 1528—1529 (1967).
Sullivan, H.R., McMahon, R.E.: Metabolism of oral cephalothin and related cephalosporins in the rat. Biochem. J. **102**, 976—982 (1967).
Sund, H.: The pyridine nucleotide coenzymes and the pyridine nucleotide-dependent dehydrogenases. In: Biological Oxidations, T.P. Singer, ed., New York, London and Sydney: Interscience 1968.
— Diekmann, H., Wallenfels, K.: Die Wasserstoffübertragung mit Pyridinnucleotiden. Advanc. Enzymol. **26**, 115—145 (1964).
— Theorell, H.: Alcohol dehydrogenases. In: The Enzymes, 2nd ed., Vol. **7**, P.D. Boyer, H. Lardy and K. Myrback, Eds., New York: Academic Press 1963.
Tagg, J., Yasuda, D.M., Tanabe, M., Mitoma, C.: Metabolic studies of tolbutamide in the rat. Biochem. Pharmacol. **16**, 143—153 (1967).
Talalay, P.: Steroid dehydrogenases. In: The Enzymes, 2nd ed., Vol. **7**, P.D. Boyer, H. Lardy and K. Myrback, Eds., New York: Academic Press 1963.
Tatsumi, K., Yoshimura, H., Tsukamoto, H.: Metabolism of drugs LVI. The metabolic fate of phenacetylurea. Biochem. Pharmacol. **16**, 1941—1951 (1967).
Theorell, H.: Function and structure of liver alcohol dehydrogenase. In: Harvey Lectures, Series 61. New York and London: Academic Press 1967.
— Bonnichsen, R.: Studies on liver alcohol dehydrogenase I. Equilibria and initial reaction velocities. Acta chem. scand. **5**, 1105—1126 (1951).
— Chance, B.: Studies on liver alcohol dehydrogenase II. The kinetics of the compound of horse liver alcohol dehydrogenase and reduced diphosphopyridine nucleotide. Acta Chem. scand. **5**, 1127—1144 (1951).
— McKinley-McKee, J.S.: Liver alcohol dehydrogenase I. Kinetics and equilibria without inhibitors. Acta chem. scand. **15**, 1797—1810 (1961).
— Taniguchi, S., Akeson, A., Skursky, L.: Crystallization of a separate steroid-active liver alcohol dehydrogenase. Biochem. biophys. Res. Commun. **24**, 603—609 (1966).
Thomas, R.C., Ikeda, G.J.: The metabolic fate of tolbutamide in man and in the rat. J. med. pharm. Chem. **9**, 507—510 (1966).
Toki, K., Tsukamoto, H.: Metabolism of drugs XL. Enzymatic oxidation of methylhexabital. 3. Purification and properties of 3-hydroxy-methylhexabital dehydrogenase. J. Biochem. (Tokyo) **55**, 142—147 (1964).
Treble, D.H.: The metabolism of 2-fluoroethanol. Biochem. J. **82**, 129—134 (1962).
Tsai, C.S.: Relative reactivities of primary alcohols as substrates of liver alcohol dehydrogenase. Canad. J. Biochem. **46**, 381—385 (1968).
Wakil, S.J., Bressler, R.: Studies on the mechanism of fatty acid synthesis X. Reduced triphosphopyridine nucleotide-acetoacetyl coenzyme a reductase. J. biol. Chem. **237**, 687—693 (1962).
Wald, G.: Molecular basis of visual excitation. Science **162**, 230—239 (1968).
Waldvogel, G.: Über eine E-Oxydoreduktase aus Schweineleber. Ph. D. Dissertation No. 3681. Eidgenössische Technische Hochschule, Zürich 1965.
Waller, G.R.: Dehydrogenation of trans-trans farnesol by horse liver alcohol dehydrogenase. Nature (Lond.) **207**, 1389—1390 (1965).
— Theorell, H., Sjövall, J.: Liver alcohol dehydrogenase as a 3β-hydroxy-5β-cholanic acid dehydrogenase. Arch. Biochem. **111**, 671—684 (1965).
Wartburg, von, J.-P., Bethune, J.L., Vallee, B.L.: Human liver-alcohol dehydrogenase. Kinetic and physiochemical properties. Biochem. J. **3**, 1775—1782 (1964).

WEBER, H., SEIBL, J., ARIGONI, D.: Die absolute Konfiguration von 1-$^{2}H_{1}$-Äthanol. Helv. chim. Acta **49**, 741—748 (1966).

WEBER, W.W., ZANNONI, V.G.: Reduction of phenylpyruvic acids to phenyllactic acids in mammalian tissues. J. biol. Chem. **241** 1345—1349 (1966).

WESTHEIMER, F.H., FISHER, H.F., CONN, E.E., VENNESLAND, B.: The enzymatic transfer of hydrogen from alcohol to DPN. J. Amer. chem. Soc. **73**, 2403 (1951).

WILLIAMS, R.T.: Detoxication Mechanisms, 2nd Ed. p. 333. New York: Wiley 1959.

WINER, A.D.: A note on the substrate specificity of horse liver alcohol dehydrogenase. Acta chem. scand. **12**, 1695—1696 (1958).

WRATTEN, C.C., CLELAND, W.W.: Kinetic studies with liver alcohol dehydrogenase. Biochem. J. **4**, 2442—2451 (1965).

ZAGALAK, B., FREY, P.A., KARABATSOS, G.L., ABELES, R.H.: The stereochemistry of the conversion of D and L 1,2-propanediols to propionaldehyde. J. biol. Chem. **241**, 3028—3035 (1966).

ZANNONI, V.G., WEBER, W.W.: Isolation and properties of aromatic α-keto acid reductase. J. biol. Chem. **241**, 1340—1344 (1966).

Chapter 52

Amine Oxidases

E. A. Zeller

Oxidative deamination of biogenic amines occurs throughout the living kingdom, from bacteria to mammals. The enzymes catalyzing this reaction belong to flavoproteins, to pyridoxal phosphate enzymes, to enzymes using pyridine nucleotides as hydrogen acceptors, and to the cobamide enzymes. In this section, only members of the first two groups are considered, in particular mammalian amine oxidases which use oxygen as an electron acceptor.

Flavoproteins: Included are the pyridoxamine phosphate oxidase (pyridoxaminephosphate:O_2 oxidoreductase [deaminating] 1.4.3.5) (Pogell, 1958) and the monoamine oxidases (MAO, monoamine:O_2 oxidoreductase [deaminating] 1.4.3.4).

Pyridoxal phosphate enzymes: They comprise the semicarbazide sensitive diamine oxidases (DAO, diamine:O_2 oxidoreductase [deaminating] 1.4.3.6), spermine (or plasma amine) oxidases (spermine:O_2 oxidoreductase [donor cleaving] 1.5.3.3) and the enzymes which attack ethanolamine phosphate, converting it to acetaldehyde, ammonia, and inorganic phosphate (Fleshood and Pitot, 1969).

I limit my discussion to the so-called monoamine oxidases, and to a few remarks about plasma amine oxidases, and the diamine oxidases.

Monoamine Oxidases

Ewins and Laidlaw (1910—1911) added tyramine to the perfusion fluid of surviving rabbit liver and isolated p-hydroxyphenylacetic acid from the fluid. In analogous experiments with intact animals, Guggenheim and Löffler (1916) demonstrated a nearly quantitative transformation of phenylethylamine to phenylacetic acid. These results found their explanation by the truely pioneering work of Mary Hare-Bernheim (1928, 1931) who discovered "tyramine oxidase" in mammalian livers which attacked these two amines. Later, two other enzymes, called amine oxidase (Pugh and Quastel, 1937a) and adrenaline oxidase (Blaschko et al., 1937a) were found to catalyze the oxidative deamination of aliphatic amines and epinephrine respectively. Within the same year Kohn (1937), Blaschko et al. (1937b), and Pugh and Quastel (1937b) concluded that the three enzymes were identical. These classical papers and several other important early publications on amine oxidases appeared in a single volume of the Biochemical Journal!

After this creative pulse, the enzyme stayed in relative obscurity until 1952, when the Prince Charming iproniazid, the first *in vivo* inhibitor of MAO, appeared on the scene (Zeller et al., 1952). Then, the interest in this group of enzymes grew rapidly, and successful investigations were carried out all over the world. Unfortunately, only a small fraction of the results can be reported here. Several reviews that appeared during the Sixties are available for further information

(BLASCHKO, 1963; GORKIN, 1966; LÉVY, 1968; PLETSCHER et al., 1960, 1965; ZELLER and FOUTS, 1963).

In contrast to the diamine oxidases, the MAO's form a tightly knit group of similar enzymes with widely overlapping substrate and inhibitor patterns. To differentiate these enzymes from diamine oxidases, ZELLER et al. (1939) proposed the name "monoamine oxidase." This way, the term "amine oxidases" could serve as the very necessary general term for all amine oxidases defined as enzymes catalyzing oxidative deamination of biogenic amines and using molecular oxygen as an electron acceptor. It was a very unfortunate event when YAMADA and YASUNOBU (1962) applied the same term to the spermine oxidase when they had accomplished the isolation of amine oxidase. A terrible confusion reigns ever since throughout the field of amine oxidases, because two enzymes of entirely different nature, one containing pyridoxal phosphate and copper, the other FAD, carry the same name. This hydra of disorder is as hard to slay as was its namesake of antiquity.

1. Isolation of MAO

For many years, unsuccessful attempts have been made in several laboratories to purify MAO. The main obstacle consisted of transferring the tightly bound enzyme from the structured part of cell organelles into aqueous solution and eliminating the accompanying lipids and other structural elements. The first partially successful solubilization was reported as late as 1953 (BARSKY et al.). With sonic oscillations and deoxycholic acid an active material was obtained which remained non-sedimentable after one hour's centrifugation at $105{,}000 \times g$. In the past years, several other detergents and various oscillators were successfully employed in solubilizing mitochondrial MAO (GUHA and KRISHNA MURTI, 1965; GABAY and VALCOURT, 1968) After solubilization, most often a fractionation with ammonium sulfate is carried out, followed by a variety of chromatographic procedures. When the first MAO preparations were obtained which were pure enough to permit some insight into their molecular properties, it was surprising to find that a 68-fold (beef liver, NARA et al., 1966) or even a 34-fold purification (beef kidney, ERWIN and HELLERMAN, 1967) was needed to reach this level. In other instances, a 1000-fold purification was accomplished (pig brain, TIPTON, 1968). Today, we have reports pertaining to the purification of MAO from 5 species and from 4 different organs. The methods range from a 3-step procedure (SEN et al., 1968) to a rather elaborate sequence of GOMES et al. (1969).

2. Molecular Properties of MAO

In view of the short time elapsed since purified MAO preparations became available, it is not surprising that our knowledge of the molecular properties of this enzyme is still rather limited. Calculations based on gel filtration and ultracentrifugation led to molecular weights from 150,000 to 2,800,000 (YOUDIM and SOURKES, 1966; GOMES et al., 1969). With flavine as a yardstick, molecular weights from 100,000 (GOMES et al., 1969) to 150,000 (YASUNOBU et al., 1968; SOURKES, 1968) were proposed. Apparently, this multiplicity is due to the isolation of the enzyme in different molecular forms.

On the basis of incomplete circumstantial evidence, it was suggested that MAO is a flavoenzyme. This assumption has been confirmed by the successful work of two research groups, one at the University of Hawaii (NARA et al., 1966) and the other at Johns Hopkins University (ERWIN and HELLERMAN, 1967). The flavoprotein spectra are somewhat anomalous and need more detailed analysis, as also is true for the excitation and emission fluorescence spectra. Some of the difficulties encountered in this area stem from the fact that the flavine moiety is not easily removable from the holoenzyme. Apparently, the pigment is attached to the enzyme covalently. Flavopeptides were isolated after pronase digestion (Gomes et al., 1969). The enzyme purified from pig brain by Tipton (1968), however, can be converted into its apo-enzyme and the latter is re-activated by FAD, but not by the flavine mononucleotide.

Since the observations of Singer and Barron (1945) regarding the inactivation of MAO by p-chloromercuribenzoate (PCMB), it became apparent that at least one sulfhydryl residue is present. According to Hellerman and Erwin (1968), 7 to 8 SH-groups per 100,000 g of protein can be titrated. The same authors were also able to demonstrate that beef kidney MAO is *not* a copper protein, despite a lot of evidence which was brought forth in favor of this concept (Barbato and Abood, 1963; Nara et al., 1966). Recently, Symes et al. (1969) suggested that iron is an integral part of MAO. They came to their conclusion on the basis of feeding rats with an iron-free diet and of inhibiting the enzyme with three iron-chelating agents.

3. Methods of Measurement of MAO Activities

Only a very short survey of the many proposed methods can be given here. Either we follow the rate of disappearance of substrate, or oxygen, or the rate of the appearance of aldehyde, ammonium, or hydrogen peroxide (equation I).

a) In Vitro Procedures

We may separate the methods into two groups: one which can be carried out — in principle — with every substrate, and another reserved for specific substrates. To the former belong measurements of oxygen by manometric or polarographic procedures, assessment of ammonium (or alkylamines) and hydrogen peroxide by a variety of methods. In addition, the application of isotopically labelled substrates belong to this group. The deaminated products are so much more soluble in typical organic solvents than the substrates that a separation of the product from the remaining substrate is fairly easily accomplished (Otsuka and Kobayashi, 1964).

To the second group belong spectrophotometric procedures based on the high optical density of benzaldehyde and its derivatives at approximately 250 mμ and the much smaller density of the benzylamines. Tabor et al. (1954) introduced this principle for the evaluation of plasma amine oxidase. When an amino group is placed in the ortho-position to the alkylamine side chain, the aldehyde formed under the influence of MAO will rapidly react with the aromatic amino residue and form a cyclic compound of vastly different chemical and spectroscopic properties as compared to the substrate. Kynuramine (Weissbach et al., 1960), 5-hydroxykynuramine (which is converted into a fluorescent product, Takahashi and Takahara, 1968), and 2-(2′-aminophenyl)ethylamine are suitable substrates for this type of reaction. The last one yields indole, which can be determined photometrically in microgram quantities and less (Zeller et al., 1969); since indole is absent from tissues, the "enzyme blanks" are extremely low.

For purely enzymological kinetic studies, we like to have methods which permit continuous reading or automatic recording. The methods based on oxygen consumption and spectrophotometric procedures measuring benzaldehydes obviously fulfill this requirement. 3-Nitro-4-hydroxy-benzylamine (Gorkin et al., 1964), m-iodobenzylamine (Zeller et al., 1965), dimethylamino benzylamine (Deitrich and Erwin, 1969) served as satisfactory sources for highly absorbing aldehydes.

b) Determination of MAO Activity in Materials Obtained from Living Persons

In disregarding pharmacological or metabolic procedures used for indirect *in vivo* evaluation of MAO inhibitors, only biopsy materials were available for the assessment of MAO activity in specimens obtained from living persons. Liver (TAKAHASHI, 1955) and intestinal mucosa (LEVINE and SJOERDSMA, 1962) have been used so far. Obviously, these approaches are rarely open to investigators. When the occurrence of MAO in human platelets was discovered (PAASONEN et al., 1964) a better chance for *in vivo* determinations arose. Isotopically labelled tyramine (ROBINSON et al., 1968) and 2-(2′-aminophenyl)ethylamine were found to be suitable substrates for the measurement of platelet MAO. With the latter compound, a method was developed which requires 10 ml or less of human blood (ZELLER et al., 1969). Thus, we now have a method permitting us to test MAO activity in the course of the treatment of patients with inhibitors.

4. Substrate Specificity and Multiple Forms of MAO

Instead of presenting here the very long list of substrates, I prefer to describe a few properties a compound must have to be accepted by MAO as a substrate. The basic structure is found in methylamine, viz. a non-protonated methylene amino group (see section 5), attached to a hydrophobic moiety, represented in a minuscule form by a hydrogen atom: $H\text{-}CH_2\text{-}NH_2$. Occasionally, methylamine itself is attacked by MAO (ALLES and HEEGAARD, 1943). When, however, we substitute one, and only one, of the hydrogen atoms of the methylene by alkyl, aralkyl, or aryl residues, we often obtain excellent substrates. Among the aromatic rings we find not only carbocyclic, but also heterocyclic systems. The enzyme imposes some restrictions on the hydrophobic backbone with respect to size and shape. Within homologous series, optima in chain length for alkylamines (ALLES and HEEGAARD, 1943) and arylalkylamines (ZELLER, 1961; SARKAR, 1962) are discernible. When we shift a substituent of relatively small van der Waals' radius from the meta- to the ortho-position of benzylamine, an excellent substrate is dramatically converted into a competitive inhibitor (ZELLER, 1963a, b).

Electron withdrawing residues appear to improve the substrate character, as seen by the positive slopes of Hammett plots.

In contrast to the behavior of DAO, MAO does accept mono- and dimethylated amino residues (ALLES and HEEGAARD, 1943). The second methyl group usually reduces reaction rates considerably unless, as in the case of N-dimethyl-o-bromo-phenyl-ethylamine, the substrate molecule is locked into a favorable (eutopic) position by ortho-substitution (HOLTZ et al., 1967).

The term monoamine oxidase covers more than one entity. In considering the outcome of countless experiments pertaining to the substrate and inhibitor pattern, we have to face the possibility of finding a different MAO wherever this enzyme occurs, in every animal species and in every tissue of each species. We do not know, however, the chemical basis for the existence of this suspected enormous number of multiple forms. Since not a single MAO has been sufficiently purified to permit its chemical and physical analysis, we are at present unable to decide whether various monoamine oxidases are polymers of one or several unit proteins (see section 2), whether there are variations in primary, secondary, and tertiary structure or of the architecture of the active and allosteric sites, whether the localization of MAO in different cell organelles influences the enzyme response, or whether the functional state of mitochondria or the presence of cell components unrelated to MAO affects the outcome of an inhibition test. Most likely more than one factor is responsible for the diversity of monoamine oxidases.

Each MAO preparation, whether obtained from different species, organs, tissues, organelles, or from a set of "isozymes," displays a similar substrate pattern. However, a few cases of restrictive specificities are known, e.g. the inability of the thyroid MAO to attack m-iodobenzylamine (Fischer et al., 1968), and the failure of human placental MAO to initiate the degradation of 2-(2′-aminophenyl)ethylamine (Danforth and Zeller, 1969). These differences may not be absolute and may simply reflect the sensitivity of our methods.

5. Kinetic Studies

When we look at the previous reviews, we become painfully aware how much the kinetics of MAO reaction have been neglected in the past. Two recent studies, however, have begun to fill up a few of these glaring gaps; McEwen et al. (1968, 1969a, b), on the basis of a careful kinetic analysis, have demonstrated that substrates and related competitive inhibitors react as non-protonated amines with the active site of MAO and that the Michaelis constant K_m is very close to the equilibrium constant K_s. These important results make it possible to calculate changes in free energies occurring during enzyme-substrate complex formation.

During the past years, extensive kinetic measurements were made in order to analyze the effect of electron density, hydrophobic bonding, and steric factors on the interaction between MAO and some of its substrates. Recently, the degradation rates of a large number of ring-substituted benzylamines were followed polarographically in the presence of a partially purified beef liver MAO (Miller and Zeller, 1968). When the results were organized on the basis of the Hammett relationship, which included Taft's steric factors, E_s, a linear relationship for the $\ln(V/V_o)$ was obtained by regression analysis with correlation coefficients > 0.94!

6. MAO Inhibitors

The number of inhibitors described for MAO is probably larger than that for any other enzyme. To organize this multitude of chemically different compounds, a new classification is attempted here.. It is based on the diminishing degree of structural similarity existing between substrate and inhibitor. This order should ease the difficult task of bringing to light the mechanism of inhibitor action. Previous lists (Pletscher et al., 1960, 1965; Zeller, 1968) were more chemically and less functionally designed than the present one. The two reviews written by Pletscher's group contain a welter of reliable and pertinent data and are, therefore, a major source of information in this field.

a) List of Inhibitors

1. Substrates and substrate analogues
  - 1.1. Compounds containing amino nitrogen
    - 1.1.1. Alkyl and aralkylamines
      - 1.1.1.1. Substrates and potential substrates
        - 1.1.1.1.1. Substrates
        - 1.1.1.1.2. Potential substrates
        - 1.1.1.1.3. Propargylamines
      - 1.1.1.2. α-alkylated alkyl and aralkylamines
      - 1.1.1.3. Cyclopropylamines
      - 1.1.1.4. N-substituted alkyl and aralkylamines
    - 1.1.2. Hydrazine derivatives
      - 1.1.2.1. Alkyl and aralkyl hydrazine derivatives
      - 1.1.2.2. Aromatic hydrazines
      - 1.1.2.3. Acyl hydrazides
      - 1.1.2.4. Furazolidines

1.1.3. Amides, amidines, and guanidines
 1.1.3.1. S-n-alkylisoureas
 1.1.3.2. Alkyl, aryl, and aralkylamidines
 1.1.3.3. Alkyl and aralkylguanidines
1.1.4. Aromatic amines
1.1.5. N-Heterocyclic compounds without alkylamine side chain
2. Sulfhydryl reagents
3. Agents of unknown mechanism
 3.1. Organic nitrates
 3.2. Carbon disulfide

b) Substrates as Inhibitors and Inhibitors as Substrates

When we consider the co-existence of more than one biogenic amine in certain cells, it becomes conceivable that they mutually influence their respective degradation rates and thus affect their relative intracellular concentrations (ZELLER, 1962). Therefore, studies of competitive substrate inhibition not only provide us with important kinetic data, but may also contribute to our understanding of the biofunction of MAO. Valuable pertinent data were recently presented by McEwen's group (see section 5), who demonstrated that for a number of substrates K_m, the Michaelis constant, and K_i, the dissociation constant of the enzyme-inhibitor complex, are practically identical.

A second group of competitive inhibitors display all the expected structural features of a substrate without being one. As typical competitors, they do react with the binding site, apparently in a non-productive (dystopic) way, and form a complex with the enzyme which is not capable of breaking down to the usual reaction products. To this group of inhibitors belong o-iodobenzylamine (ZELLER, 1963a, b) and mescaline (MCEWEN et al., 1969a).

Thus, normal and dystopically bound substrates act as inhibitors. On the other hand, one very powerful inhibitor, phenylethylhydrazine (CHESSIN et al., 1959; ZELLER et al., 1959), has been demonstrated to be a substrate of MAO. Using isotopically labelled phenylethylhydrazine, CLINESCHMIDT and HORITA (1969) were able to demonstrate elegantly its conversion into phenylacetic acid. Whether this enzyme-substrate interaction is a part of the inhibitory mechanism is not clear as yet.

c) Propargylamine Derivatives

Pargyline, N-benzyl-N-methylpropynylamine, is one of the strongest MAO inhibitors, and causing a marked inhibition at 10^{-7} and 10^{-8}M concentrations (SWETT et al., 1963; ZELLER, 1963b). In the past few years, several other effective inhibitory propargylamine derivatives were synthesized and tested (phenyl-isopropyl-methyl-propynylamine, KNOLL et al., 1965; N-methyl-N-2-propynyl-1-indanamine, MAÎTRE and WYSS, 1967). As has been shown for many MAO inhibitors, there is a strong difference of action in the absence and presence of substrates. According to MCEWEN et al. (1969b), simultaneous addition of pargyline and substrate to MAO preparations leads to competitive inhibition. In the absence of the substrate, this inhibition is a function of time and follows second order kinetics.

HELLERMAN and ERWIN (1968) found pargyline irreversibly bound to purified bovine kidney MAO. This inhibitor appears to be capable of reducing the flavine moiety of the enzyme and thus serves as a substrate. Again the question arises whether this interaction with the enzyme is an integral part of the inhibitory action. The fact that another pargyline derivative, clorgyline, N-methyl-N propargyl-3(2,4-dichlorophenoxy)propylamine (HALL and LOGAN, 1969), acts without a lag phase with MAO would, in this instance, argue against the obligatory oxidation of the inhibitor molecule prior to its action as an inhibitor.

d) α-Alkylamines

The similarity of this group of compounds to the classical substrates is quite apparent. They never serve as substrates, but display a fair affinity for MAO, acting presumably as competitive inhibitors. Whether a substantial *in vivo* inhibition can be produced with all the members of this group of substances is uncertain. With α-ethyltryptamine, however, the high affinity of the indole nucleus for the binding site confers a strong MAO blocking power to this compound, as some pharmacological tests seem to indicate (GREIG et al., 1959, 1961).

e) Cyclopropylamine Derivatives

Cyclopropylamine moieties are found in several powerful MAO inhibitors. Chemically, these compounds are closely related to α-alkylamines. In fact, the first one presented, tranylcypromide (*d,1*-trans-2-phenylcyclopropylamine, TEDESCHI et al., 1959), was patterned after amphetamine (BURGER and YOST, 1948). Other derivatives are N-(2-chlorophenoxy)-cyclopropylamine, Lilly 51641 (FULLER, 1968), trans-3-phenylcyclopropylhydrazine (GORKIN et al., 1967), and 5-oxo-(D-trans-2-phenylcyclopropyl)-L-2-pyrrolidonecarboxamide (EX 4883) (McMONIGLE and HORITA, 1969). With tranylcypromine, substantial inhibitions were observed at 10^{-7} to 10^{-8}M concentrations (SARKAR et al., 1960; ZELLER and SARKAR, 1962; FULLER, 1968). For Lilly 51641, a marked reduction of activity was seen at 10^{-9}M concentration (FULLER, 1968). Tranylcypromine is an instantaneous competitive inhibitor as well as a time-dependent non-competitive inhibitor (SARKAR et al., 1960). The optical configuration of the α-carbon affects the process of inactivation. The constant for the second order reaction between enzyme and inhibitor is 60 times higher for the *d*(+)-trans phenylcyclopropylamine than for the *l*(—)enantiomer (McEWEN et al., 1969b). In contrast to many other inhibitor reactions, the inactivation of MAO is reversible (ZELLER and SARKAR, 1962; HELLERMAN and ERWIN, 1968). Although tranylcypromine is structurally very closely related to the phenylethylamines, they are like other α-substituted amines in that they are not transformed by MAO. The compound mentioned by McMONIGLE and HORITA is hydrolyzed *in vivo* to phenylcyclopropylamine prior to its action.

f) Hydrazine Derivatives

The analysis of the action of iproniazid indicated that the alkylamine moiety is mainly responsible for its inhibitory action (ZELLER, 1956). Methyl-, benzyl-, and isopropyl-hydrazine were shown to be much stronger inhibitors than iproniazid itself (ZELLER, 1956; DAVISON, 1957). The similarity of the alkyl- and aralkylhydrazines to some typical MAO substrates is apparent when we consider the NH-group as an isosteric replacement of the α-methylene residue (ZELLER, 1956). When homologous series of substrates and inhibitors are compared, the same optimal geometric patterns for both groups of compounds appear (BARSKY et al., 1959; ZELLER et al., 1959; ZELLER, 1961).

In the absence of substrate, all hydrazine derivatives so far tested produce a time-dependent decrease of MAO activity (DAVISON, 1957; GREEN, 1962; McEWEN et al., 1969b). This inactivation seems to be irreversible; only a few exceptions are known, e.g. the reversal of inhibition by α-naphthylmethylhydrazine by dialysis (GREEN, 1962).

A number of drugs belong to this group of hydrazine derivatives, e.g. phenylisopropyl hydrazine (pheniprazine, BIEL et al., 1959), phenelzine (see section 6b), and α-methylbenzylhydrazine (mebamazine).

Since these compounds are carbonyl reagents which are able to react with pyridoxalphosphate enzymes, their pharmacological action may involve components that are not related to MAO.

g) Acylhydrazides

For iproniazid no obvious counterpart appears to exist in the substrate pattern of MAO. Actually, iproniazid is not much of an inhibitor either. When added simultaneously with tyramine to an MAO preparation, a modest 50% inhibition is achieved with a 0.01 M concentration! Only after pre-incubation of the enzyme in the absence of substrates does iproniazid reach its full inhibitory potential (ZELLER et al., 1955). It is now fairly certain that iproniazid is first converted to isopropylhydrazine, which appears to be the active substance. With the help of isotopically labelled iproniazid and isocarboxazid (N_1-(5-methyl-3-isoxazolylcarbonyl)-N_2-benzylhydrazine), isonicotinic acid and benzylhydrazine respectively were isolated (PLETSCHER et al., 1960, 1965). SEIDEN and WESTLEY (1963) isolated the MAO molecule responsible for the hydrolysis of iproniazid. More studies, however, are needed to settle the question pertaining to the agent effecting the hydrolysis of acyl hydrazides. Certain peptidases are capable of catalyzing the hydrolysis of acyl hydrazides, as shown by chymotrypsin, which is known to act on nicotinyl tyrosylhydrazide (DIXON and WEBB, 1964). In any event, the acyl hydrazides generate aralkyl hydrazines and thus fit well into the general picture of structural requirements for MAO inhibitors.

h) Furazolidines

A number of bacteriostatic nitrofurans, e.g. the condensation product between 5-nitrofuran and 3-amino-2-oxazolidinone were found to be effective *in vivo* inhibitors of MAO. These compounds are even farther removed from the structural inhibitor requirements for MAO inhibitors than the acylhydrazides. They seem, however, to be metabolically transformed into hydrazine derivatives with a free amino residue, and possibly into 2-hydroxyethylhydrazine (STERN et al., 1967; QUIRING and PALM, 1970).

i) Aromatic Amines and N-Heterocyclic Compounds

Aromatic amines, e.g. methylene blue (PLETSCHER et al., 1960, 1965), and multiple ring systems with and without alkylamine side chains are to be mentioned here. To the latter belong the β-carbolines, pyridine, and quinoline derivatives, to the former, chlorpromazine and atabrine. Harmaline and other β-carbolines are strong and reversible MAO inhibitors (UDENFRIEND et al., 1958; BOUCHAUD et al., 1967; PLETSCHER et al., 1960, 1965), depressing MAO activity at levels as low as 10^{-9}M (FULLER, 1968)! While for β-carbolines, the relationship to tryptamine, an MAO substrate, was obvious, such structural correlations between substrate and inhibitors were overlooked for the so-called chelating agents, e.g. 1,10-phenanthroline (BARBATO and ABOOD, 1963) and 9-hydroxyquinoline (SEVERINA and GORKIN, 1964). These chelating agents share with many substrates of the fundamental property of possessing a nucleophilic nitrogen at a distance > Å from an aromatic — hydrophobic — system. Thus, many investigators were mislead and assumed that these inhibitors acted as chelating agents with copper, which was suspected to be in the MAO molecule, an assumption that is no longer tenable (section 2). In our laboratory, we became alerted to an alternative explanation of the inhibitor potency when it turned out that 1,9-phenanthroline, which unlike the 1,10-isomer is not a chelating agent, is a better inhibitor than the latter substance. Hellerman and Erwin (1968) carefully compared copper-chelating and inhibitory action of a number of substances and found no correlation between the two properties.

j) *Alcohols, Phenol, and Ethers*

When we replace isosterically the amino group of an MAO substrate by a hydroxyl residue, we then obtain competitive inhibitors. As measured by the K_i-values, there is a difference of approximately 2 kcal/mole between the two in free energy of binding. For the rest of the molecule, qualitatively and quantitatively the same conditions for binding of the amines or the alcohols to the active site prevail. Thus, for both types of compounds, the contribution of each methylene residue to the change in standard free energy of binding is constant and amounts to 1.3 kcal/mole (McEwen et al., 1968). In times gone by, octanol was used to differentiate MAOs from the diamine oxidases (Zeller et al., 1958), because the latter were entirely unaffected by this alcohol, while MAO, at least in part, was inhibited by it.

Some phenols, e.g. β-naphthol ($K_i = 13$ [uM]), are competitive inhibitors of MAO (McEwen et al., 1969a). β-Naphthol fulfills the structural requirements as outlined in the preceding section, since it possesses a nucleophilic group located approximately 3 Å from the center of the (unsubstituted) benzene ring.

p-Tolylcholine ether was one of the more potent inhibitors available prior to the arrival of iproniazid (Pletscher et al., 1960, 1965). Since we have no indication that the ammonium residue is involved in the critical binding of the molecule to the active site of MAO, it seems more likely that the compound acts with its nucleophilic ether-oxygen.

k) *Effect of the Substrate on Modality and Efficiency of MAO Inhibition*

In 1963, a new inhibitor phenomenon was discovered when cis- and trans-2-phenylcyclopropylamines were tested. The outcome of the experiments depended a great deal on the kind of substrate added to the enzyme system. With phenylbutylamine, an excellent MAO substrate, a 20 to 800-fold greater concentration was required to produce 50% inhibition than with tyramine (Zeller and Sarkar, 1962). Since then, similar phenomena were observed by various authors with other inhibitors. While proflavine, harmine, α-methyltryptamine, and the cyclopropylamine derivative Lilly 51641 were much more effective in the presence of serotonin than of tyramine, the reverse was true for the propargylamines, pargyline and SU-11,730. In some instances, differences of 1000-fold and greater were noted (Fuller, 1968; Gorkin and Romanova, 1968; Maître and Wyss, 1967). The results of analogous *in vivo* experiments were in agreement with these *in vitro* studies (for a review of the studies of Gorkin and his group, see Gorkin and Romanova, 1968). Although comprehensive kinetic data are unavailable, the results with phenylcyclopropylamines suggest that this "substrate effect" is linked with two other phenomena: (a) with the reversibility of the inactivation (which leaves out most hydrazine derivatives) and (b) with the time-dependency observed with many MAO-inhibitor interactions (sections 6c and 6e). GORKIN and OREKHOVICH (1967) considered the multiplicity of MAO as one of the reasons for the selectivity of the inhibitory effects. Whatever the ultimate explanation will be, we hope some day to have sufficient information for developing or recognizing agents which are capable of *selectively* blocking the metabolism of one biogenic amine without substantially affecting the degradation of others (HUSZTI and BORSY, 1968). Thus, we can anticipate a more sophisticated and effective use of MAO in pharmacology and therapy than the present shotgun procedures.

7. Mechanism of Interaction Between MAO and its Substrates

As during a foggy day in the Alps, we see through a few holes in the clouds some sections of our way to the peak, without being able to connect them to an uninterrupted line of ascent, so knowledge concerning the mechanism of MAO action is still quite limited. Some general ideas of the modalities of the reaction can be gleaned from the stochiometric equation which summarizes the overall reaction. Equation I was first established by MARY BERNHEIM-HARE (1931). Obviously, the reaction represented by equation I is so complex that it will take several steps to reach its goal.

$$RCH_2NR'R'' + H_2O + O_2 = RCHO + NHR'R'' + H_2O_2 \qquad \text{(I)}$$
$$R' \text{ and } R'' \text{ are H or } CH_3$$

The only function of the following reaction sequence is to serve as a means of organizing present and future information and thus of paving the way for a real understanding of the mechanism involved.

Step I: The nucleophilic attack of a thioester by the non-protonated amino residue of the substrate, followed by the formation of an amide bond.

Step II: The deprotonation of an α-carbon atom.

Step III: The two-electron transfer to molecular oxygen by way of FAD.

Step IV: Re-establishment of the thioester and formation of an "aldimine."

Step V: The breakdown of the aldimine and release of the end products.

In essence, the enzyme oscillates between a thioester and an amide. When the amide bond (a covalent bond) is established, the rest of the substrate molecule is bound to the active site by the secondary forces, and the α-carbon is brought into such a functional and geometrical situation, that a proton and two electrons can then be removed. After this electron loss, the terminal area of the residue which represents the original substrate is less able to hold the carbonyl and the sulfur gains the upper hand and thus reforms the thioester bond. The dehydrogenated substrate (aldimine) breaks down and the products, aldehyde and ammonium ion, are released.

More than 10 years ago, we suggested that a peptide or ester bond may be the receptor for the amino group (BARSKY et al., 1959; ZELLER, 1959). The peptide concept is to be dismissed, because the liberated peptide amino residue would be protonated and thus become unavailable for the return reaction. Two events have strengthened the ester hypothesis: the discovery that copper is *not* a part of the active site of MAO (section 2) and the demonstration that the non-protonated amino group of the substrate reacts with the enzyme (section 5). A thioester is preferable to an ordinary oxygen ester because the former reacts with nucleophils such as amines under conditions in which ordinary oxygen esters do not react (CONNORS and BENDER, 1961). As mentioned in section 2, there is at least one SH-residue essential for MAO action which, as indicated by the protective effect of the substrate toward inactivation by p-chloromercuribenzoate, appears to be close to or a part of the binding site (MCEWEN et al., 1969b).

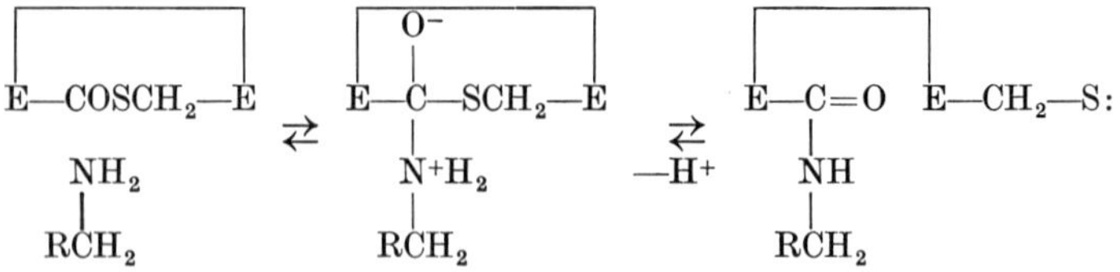

(II)

The aminolysis of thioesters has been studied intensively in non-enzymic systems, particularly the intramolecular aminolysis of acetyl mercaptoethanol (JENCKS, 1969). The reaction consists of two or more steps and is subject to general acid and general base catalysis. Obviously, it is too early for attempting analogous detailed interpretations of the MAO-substrate interaction.

Reaction II is proposed on the basis of positive slopes of Hammett plots (section 5) and if the interpretation of the isotope effects are correct, this reaction represents a rate limiting step. When the hydrogens attached to the α-carbon atoms are stereospecifically replaced by deuterium, in tyramine (BELLEAU et al., 1960; BELLEAU and MORAN, 1963) or in m-methoxybenzylamine or p-methoxyphenylethyl amine (KAUFMAN et al., 1963), different reaction rates are observed for the R-α-d and the S-α-d configurations.

Since we have very few experimental facts concerning the electron transport system, a discussion of this process is omitted.

In order to constrain the substrate molecule to the active site of MAO, or to any enzyme for that matter, van der Waals' and hydrophobic attractions must produce free-energy changes to compensate for the translational entropy lost in forming the complex (WESTHEIMER, 1962). The entropy gain of the release of the products favors the last phase of the reaction. The loss of (approximately 2 kcal) free energy of binding by the removal of the amino residue from the rest of the substrate molecule, makes the dissociation of the enzyme-product complex that much easier.

8. Interaction between Inhibitors and MAO

In considering the wide range of chemical structures capable of inactivating MAO, one may assume that many different inhibitor mechanisms will be found. If we disregard sulfhydryl reagents and a few compounds which leave us completely in the dark, an amazingly large number of inhibitors mimic substrate structures to a larger or smaller degree (section 6). It is, therefore, possible to bring order into a heterogeneous material and to characterize the inhibitors of group I (section 6a) with respect to the number of steps they have in common within the sequence of enzyme-substrate interaction.

This concept is not generally accepted, as demonstrated by a recent statement made by MCEWEN et al. (1969b). These authors think "it is still possible that time-dependent inhibition by hydrazine derivatives is caused by other enzyme interactions which are not analogous to the formation of enzyme-substrate complexes."

Most of the compounds belonging to the "pseudosubstrates" appear to be capable of interacting with a thioester group. Alcohols may reversibly form oxygen esters and aliphatic amines and the nitrogen of heteroaromatic rings may reversibly react as nucleophiles with the thioester carbonyl. Hydrazines can irreversibly lead to hydrazides. The majority of the members of this set of compounds do not undergo oxidative degradation, as they are either α-substituted, or because they are dystopically attached to the active site, or since they do not carry an amino group. One propargylamine derivative (section 6c) and phenylethylhydrazine (section 6b) seem to be dehydrogenated while bound to MAO.

9. On the Biological Function of MAO

If we think of MAO only in terms of an agent responsible for the elimination of unwanted amines, as most biologists do, we are likely to miss some of its important biofunctions.

a) Occurrence of MAO in the Mammalian Organism

Some pertinent information may be gained by studying the distribution of this enzyme in the animal organism. MAO occurs widely in normal as well as in neoplastic mammalian cells. The presence of MAO was asserted in the cells of all three germinal layers. It would not be surprising if some day it were found in all cells equipped with mitochondria. Within the cell, most of the activity is present in the mitochondria. In this organelle, the major part of the activity was found in the outer membrane (SCHNAITMAN and GREENAWALT, 1968), or in the inner membrane (ALLMANN et al., 1968), or between the two membranes (TIPTON, 1967)! Today, MAO activity frequently serves as a *leitfossil* for the identification of the outer membrane during the fractionation of mitochondria. If our computations give the correct order of magnitude, as much as 5% of the protein of the outer membrane in the liver may consist of MAO molecules!

Within a given organ, however, the distribution is usually quite uneven. This is particularly true for the human brain (BIRKHÄUSER, 1941) and the kidney (EDER, 1957).

b) Ontogenetic Changes in MAO Activity

For a real understanding of the biological role of MAO, it is important to remember that this enzyme's activity does not remain the same throughout the lifetime of the cell and that within a few days marked changes can and do occur. A long time ago, BIRKHÄUSER (1941) and ZELLER et al. (1940) showed that the MAO activity in brain and kidney of newborn children is much lower than in adult organs. In the male rat heart, the MAO activity never stops increasing (NOVICK, 1961; GEY et al., 1964). Probably related to this phenomenon is HORITA's observation (1968) that the initial rate of recovery of cardiac MAO after *in vivo* inhibition by pargyline is greater in older than in younger rats. A major contribution to the significance of ontogenetic changes came from BRODIE's laboratory (KARKI et al., 1962). These authors showed that brain levels of norepinephrine, serotonin, and MAO were low in the brains of newborn rats. The low levels are associated with the low functional ability of these animals, who are relatively helpless in the newborn state. Several weeks later, when functional ability had developed, the levels reached those of adults. The levels of the amines and MAO in the brains of guinea pigs (which showed good locomotor and other forms of functional ability shortly after birth) were almost as high in the newborn as in the adult animals.

c) Effect of Hormones on MAO

There are several known ways of regulating MAO activity. Two groups of hormones, the thyroid and sex hormones, produce marked changes in MAO activity. In both instances, the MAO present in various organs responds differently to hormone treatment. In 1951, SCHWEPPE et al. found a marked sex difference in the activity of rat liver MAO. In recent years, CHORDIKIAN et al. (1970) studied the role of sex hormones on the MAO levels in various organs of mice. The efficiency in reducing liver MAO activity drops from androgens to estrogens to progesterone. Furthermore, MAO activities were reduced to zero by inhibitors and the rate of recovery was followed in the presence and absence of puromycin and of the sex hormones. The results suggest that the sex hormones affect MAO activity by reducing the rate of synthesis.

In two laboratories, detailed investigations were carried out which showed that the MAO activity of the rat hypothalamic region strongly responded to the changing hormone levels during estrus (T. KOBAYASHI et al., 1965; KAMBERI and Y. KOBAYASHI, 1970). The mechanism of these remarkable changes is not as yet known.

Recently, the sex differences were found to be reflected in the MAO activities of human platelet MAO. The values in women were 67% higher than in men (ZELLER and STANICH, 1969).

d) Protective Function of MAO

There was a time when clinicians were sure that the biogenic amines originating from the intestinal flora would contribute heavily to the intestinal autointoxication (BECHER, 1931). The animal organism, however, is well protected against such an invasion, because active mono and diamine oxidases are strategically located in the intestinal mucosa. This almost forgotten role of MAO became dramatically apparent a few years ago, when patients treated with MAO inhibitors suffered acutely from severe circulatory ills. Cheese and a few other foods were found to be the culprits. Some, but not all, forms of cheese contain large amounts of tyramine which enters the human body unimpeded when MAO is inactivated by inhibitor treatment. The danger can easily be avoided by omitting these foods from the patient's diet (AIRAKSINEN et al., 1966; HORWITZ et al., 1964; KAYAALP et al., 1968; TEDESCHI and FELLOWS, 1964).

e) Specific Functions of MAO

The chemistry and reaction mechanism of MAO presumably is much the same in various organs and tissues and yet it seems that the biological *consequences* of MAO action vary from organ to organ.

For one, MAO is involved in the determination of the serotonin/catecholamine ratio in the brain system which in turn appears to influence the sleep pattern, aggressiveness and depression, EEG patterns, body temperature, etc. With the help of MAO inhibitors, this ratio can be changed and with that the functions just mentioned above (VALZELLI and GARATTINI, 1968; BUENO et al., 1968).

There is a growing awareness that not only the biogenic amines themselves, but also products of the amine oxidases may be capable of exerting substantial biological functions. BARONDES (1962) and SABELLI et al. (1969) presented experimental evidence that in some instances indoleacetaldehydes, rather than the parent serotonin and tryptamine, produce the effects ascribed to tryptamine and serotonin. In this case, MAO would be instrumental in producing an active hormone rather than in destroying it.

In the thyroid, a high MAO activity was first observed by LANGEMANN (1942). Upon addition of tyramine to a thyroid microsomal fraction, the tyramine/MAO system replaces the requirement for an exogenous hydrogen peroxide generating system for both iodination and iodothyronin biosynthesis (FISCHER et al., 1966). In turn, the thyroid hormones depress MAO activity in some organs.

The role of amines and their control by MAO is also apparent in the dynamics of the aqueous humor of the rabbit eye. MAO inhibitors, alone or in combination with amine releasing agents (reserpine, benzoquinolizine Ro 4-1284), produce a marked and highly significant depression of the aqueous humor formation, as indicated by tonographic measurements (ZELLER et al., 1967; HSU et al., 1970).

References

AIRAKSINEN, M.M., MUSTALA, O., TORSTI, P.: Effects of some biogenic amines on the blood pressure of pargyline-treated rabbits. Ann. Med. exp. Fenn. **44**, 376—381 (1966).

ALLES, G.A., HEEGAARD, E.V.: Substrate specificity of amine oxidase. J. biol. Chem. **147**, 487—503 (1943).

ALLMANN, D.W., BACHMANN, E., ORME-JOHNSON, N., TAN, W.C., GREEN, D.E.: Membrane systems of mitochondria. VI. Membranes of liver mitochondria. Arch. Biochem. **125**, 981—1012 (1968).

BARBATO, L.M., ABOOD, L.G.: Purification and properties of monoamine oxidase. Biochim. biophys. Acta (Amst.) **67**, 531—541 (1963).

BARONDES, S.H.: The influence of neuroamines on the oxidation of glucose by the anterior pituitary. J. biol. Chem. **237**, 204—207 (1962).

BARSKY, J., BERMAN, E.R., ZELLER, E.A.: On the solubilization and iproniazid inhibition of monoamine oxidase. XIX Internat. Physiol. Congress, Montreal, 1953; Abstr. of Communicat., pp. 191—192.

— PACHA, W.L., SARKAR, S., ZELLER, E.A.: Amine oxidases. XVII. Mode of action of 1-isonicotinyl-2-isopropylhydrazine. J. biol. Chem. **234**, 389—391 (1959).

BECHER, E.: Zur Frage der intestinalen Autointoxication. Klin. Wschr. **10**, 1009—1013, 1057—1060 (1931).

BELLEAU, B., FANG, M., BURBA, J., MORAN, J.: The absolute optical specificity of monoamine oxidase. J. Amer. chem. Soc. **82**, 5752—5754 (1960).

— MORAN, J.: Deuterium isotope effects in relation to the chemical mechanism of monoamine oxidase. Ann. N.Y. Acad. Sci. **107**, 822—839 (1963).

BERNHEIM, M.L.C.: Tyramine oxidase. II. The course of the oxidation. J. biol. Chem. **93**, 299—309 (1931).

BIEL, J.H., DRUKKER, A.E., MITCHELL, T.F., SPRENGELER, E.P., NUHFER, P.A., CONWAY, A.C., HORITA, A.: Central stimulants. Chemistry and structure-activity relationships of arakyl hydrazines. J. Amer. chem. Soc. **81**, 2805—2813 (1959).

— NUHFER, P.A., CONWAY, A.C.: Structure and activity relationships of monoamine oxidase inhibitors. Ann. N.Y. Acad. Sci. **80**, 568—582 (1959).

BIRKHÄUSER, H.: Fermente im Gehirn geistig normaler Menschen (Cholinesterase, Mono- und Diamin-oxydase, Cholin-oxydase). Helv. chim. Acta **23**, 1071—1086 (1941).

BLASCHKO, H.: Amine oxidase. In: The Enzymes, vol. 8, pp. 337—351, ed. P.D. BOYER, H. LARDY and K. MYRBÄCK. New York and London: Academic Press 1963.

— RICHTER, D., SCHLOSSMANN, H.: The inactivation of adrenaline. J. Physiol. (Lond.) **90**, 1—17 (1937a).

— — — The oxidation of adrenaline and other amines. Biochem. J. **31**, 2187—2196 (1937b).

BOUCAUD, J., BOUCHAUD, C., COUPEAUX, R.: Histochemical study of the *in vitro* action of serotonin, tryptophane and their derivatives on rat brain monoamine oxidases. C.R. Acad. Sci. (Paris) **264**, Ser. D 775—778 (1967).

BUENO, J.R., PSCHEIDT, G.R., HIMWICH, H.E.: Interactions of monoamine oxidase inhibitors and reserpine: an EEG (electro-encephalograph), gross behavioral, and biochemical analysis. Psychopharmacologia (Berl.) **12**, 400—413 (1968).

BURGER, A., YOST, W.L.: Arylcycloalkylamines. I. 2-Phenylcyclopropylamine. J. Amer. chem. Soc. **70**, 2198—2201 (1948).

CHESSIN, M., DUBNICK, B., LEESON, G., SCOTT, C.C.: Biochemical and Pharmacological studies of β-phenylethylhydrazine and selected related compounds. Ann. N.Y. Acad. Sci. **80**, 597—608 (1959).

CHORDIKIAN, F.K., OTIENO, S., SCHWEPPE, J.S., ZELLER, E.A.: Sex hormone-enzyme interrelationships. VII. Action of sexual hormones monoamine oxidase levels in mouse organs. Agents and Actions (Basel) 1970.

CLINESCHMIDT, B.V., HORITA, A.: Monoamine oxidase catalyzed degradation of phenelzine-1-^{14}C, an irreversible inhibitor of monoamine oxidase — I. Studies *in vitro*. Biochem. Pharmacol. **18**, 1011—1120 (1969).

CONNORS, K.A., BENDER, M.L.: Kinetics of alkaline hydrolysis and butylaminolysis of ethyl p-nitrobenzoate and ethyl p-nitrothiolbenzoate. J. Org. Chem. **26**, 2498—2504 (1961).

DANFORTH, D., ZELLER, E.A.: Unpublished data (1969).

DAVISON, A.N.: The mechanism of the irreversible inhibition of rat liver monoamine oxidase by iproniazid. Biochem. J. **67**, 316—322 (1957).

DEITRICH, R.A., ERWIN, V.G.: Spectrophotometric assay for monoamine oxidase. Analyt. Biochem. **30**, 395—402 (1969).

DIXON, M., WEBB, E.C.: Enzymes, p. 230. New York: Academic Press 1964.

EDER, M.: Der histochemische Nachweis des Ferments Monoaminoxydase. Entwicklung einer Nachweismethode und deren Anwendung. Beitr. path. Anat. **117**, 343—396 (1957).

ERWIN, V.G., HELLERMAN, L.: Mitochondrial monoamine oxidase. I. Purification and characterization of the bovine kidney enzyme. J. biol. Chem. **242**, 4230—4238 (1967).
FISCHER, A.G., SCHULZ, A.R., OLINER, L.: The possible role of thyroid monoamine oxidase in iodothryonine synthesis. Life Sci. **5**, 995—1002 (1966).
— — — Thyroidal biosynthesis of iodothyronines. II. General characteristics and purification of mitochondrial monoamine oxidase. Biochim. biophys. Acta (Amst.) **159**, 460—471 (1968).
FLESHOOD, H.L., PITOT, H.C.: O-Phosphorylethanolamine ammonia lyase, a new pyridoxal phosphate-dependent enzyme. Biochem. biophys. Res. Commun. **36**, 110—118 (1969).
FULLER, R.W.: Influence of substrate in the inhibition of rat liver and brain monoamine oxidase. Arch. int. Pharmacodyn. **174**, 32—36 (1968).
GABAY, S., VALCOURT, A.J.: Monoamine oxidases. I. Purification and properties of the rabbit liver mitochondrial enzyme. Biochim. biophys. Acta (Amst.) **159**, 440—450 (1968).
GEY, K.F., BURKARD, W.P., PLETSCHER, A.: Age-dependent changes in catecholamine metabolism in the rat heart. Helv. physiol. pharmacol. Acta **22**, C17—C20 (1964).
GOMES, B., IGAUE, I., KLOEPFER, H.G., YASUNOBU, K.T.: Amine oxidase. XIV. Isolation and characterization of the multiple beef liver amine oxidase components. Arch. Biochem. **132**, 16—27 (1969).
GORKIN, V.Z.: Monoamine oxidases. Pharmacol. Rev. **18**, Part I, 115—120 (1966).
— et al.: Effect of some hydrazine and nonhydrazine inhibitors on the activity of mitochondrial monoamine oxidase. Vop. med. Khim. **13**, 413—417 (1967); Chem. Abstr. **67**, No. 79170 (1967).
— KITROSSKY, N.A., KLYASHTORIN, L.B., KOMISAROVA, N.V., LEONTYEVA, G.A., POUCHKOV, V.A.: On the substrate specificity of amine oxidases. Biokhimiya **29**, 88—96 (1964).
— OREKHOVICH, V.N.: Monoamine oxidases: new data on their nature, possible biological role, and specific inhibition by pharmaceutical preparations. Biochim. appl. (Parma) **14**, 343—358 (1967).
— ROMANOVA, L.A.: Selective inhibition by some monoamine oxidase inhibitors of deamination of biogenic monoamines *in vivo*. Biochem. Pharmacol. **17**, 855—860 (1968).
GREEN, A.L.: The inhibition of monoamine oxidase by arylalkylhydrazines. Biochem. J. **84**, 217—223 (1962).
GREIG, M.E., SEAY, P.H., FREYBURGER, W.A.: Pharmacology of etryptamine. J. Neuropsychiat. **2**, S131—S135 (1961).
— WALK, R.A., GIBBONS, A.J.: Effect of three tryptamine derivatives on serotonin metabolism *in vitro* and *in vivo*. J. Pharmacol. exp. Ther. **127**, 110—115 (1959).
GUHA, S.R., KRISHNA MURTI, C.R.: Purification and solubilization of monoamine oxidase of rat liver mitochondria. Biochem. biophys. Res. Commun. **18**, 350—354 (1965).
HALL, D.W.R., LOGAN, B.W.: Inhibition of monoamine oxidase by M and B 9302 (clorgyline). II. Comparison of M and B 9302 inhibition with that of iproniazid. Biochem. Pharmacol. **18**, 1955—1959 (1969).
HARE, M.L.C.: Tyramine oxidase. I. A new enzyme system in liver. Biochem. J. **22**, 968—979 (1928).
HELLERMAN, L., ERWIN, V.G.: Mitrochondrial monoamine oxidase II. Action of various inhibitors for the bovine kidney enzyme. Catalytic mechanisms. J. biol. Chem. **243**, 5234—5243 (1968).
HOLTZ, P., MENKENS, K., PALM, D.: Pharmacology of quarternary β-phenylethylamine derivatives. Arch. Pharm. exp. Path. **25**, 193—220 (1967).
HORITA, A.: Influence of age in the recovery of cardiac monoamine oxidase after irreversible inhibition. Biochem. Pharmacol. **17**, 2091—2096 (1968).
HORWITZ, D., LOVENBERG, W., ENGELMAN, K., SJOERDSMA, A.: Monoamine oxidase inhibitors, tyramine, and cheese. J. Amer. med. Ass. **188**, 1108—1110 (1964).
HSU, M., KNEPPER, P.A., SHOCH, D., ZELLER, E.A.: On the effect of reserpine and the benzoquinolizine RO 4-1284 on the tonographic parameters of the rabbit eye. Invest. Ophthal. **9**, 551—552 (1970).
HUSZTI, Z., BORSY, J.: Comparative studies on the oxidation of 5-hydroxytryptamine and 3,4-dimethoxyphenylethylamine in rat, dog, and human brain. J. Neurochem. **15**, 1407 to 1413 (1968).
JENCKS, W.P.: Catalysis in chemistry and enzymology. New York: McGraw-Hill Book Co. 1969.
KAMBERI, I.A., KOBAYASHI, Y.: Monoamine Oxidase activity in the hypothalamus and various other brain areas and in some endocrine glands of the rat during the estrus cycle. J. Neurochem. **17**, 261—268 (1970).
KARKI, N., KUNTZMAN, R., BRODIE, B.B.: Storage, synthesis, and metabolism of monoamine in the developing brain. J. Neurochem. **9**, 53—58 (1962).

KAUFMAN, K.D., MAYERS, D.F., ZELLER, E.A.: A study of the active site of monoamine oxydase by the use of deuterium labeled amines. (Dissertation, 1963) unpublished.
KAYAALP, S.O., KAYMAKCALAN, S., OZER, A.: Interaction between some cheeses and monoamine oxidase inhibitors. Arzneimittel-Forsch. **18**, 1195—1198 (1968).
KNOLL, J., ECSERI, Z., KELEMEN, K., NIEVEL, J., KNOLL, B.: Phenyl isopropylmethylpropynylamine (E-250). A new psychic energizer. Arch. int. Pharmacodyn. **155**, 154—164 (1965).
KOBAYASHI, T., TOBAYASHI, T., KATO, J., NINAGUCHI, H.: Fluctuation in monoamine oxidase activity in the hypothalamus of rat during the estrous cycle and after castrations. Endocr. jap. **11**, 283—290 (1965).
KOHN, H.I.: Tyramine oxidase. Biochem. J. **31**, 1693—1704 (1937).
LANGEMANN, H.: Cholin-esterase in menschlichen Organen mit innerer Sekretion. Helv. chim. Acta **25**, 464—472 (1942).
LEVINE, R.J., SJOERDSMA, A.: Monoamine oxidase activity in human tissues and intestinal biopsy specimens (27160). Proc. Soc. exp. Biol. (N.Y.) **109**, 225—227 (1962).
LÉVY, J.: Amine-oxidases. Therapie **23**, 1003—1036 (1968).
MAÎTRE, L., WYSS, E.: Monoamine oxidase inhibiting properties of SU 11739 in the rat. Comparison with pargyline, tranylcypromine, and iproniazid. J. Pharmacol. exp. Ther. **157**, 81—88 (1967).
MCEWEN, C.M., JR., SASAKI, G., JONES, D.C.: Human liver mitochondrial monoamine oxidase. II. Determinants of substrate and inhibitor specificities. Biochemistry **8**, 3952—3962 (1969a).
— — — Human liver mitochondrial monoamine oxidase. III. Kinetic studies concerning time-dependent inhibitions. Biochemistry **8**, 3963—3972 (1969b).
— — LENZ, W.R., JR.: Human liver mitochondrial monoamine oxidase. I. Kinetic studies of model interactions. J. biol. Chem. **243**, 5217—5225 (1968).
MCMONIGLE, J.J., HORITA, A.: Bioactivation of 5-Oxo-(D-trans-2-phenylcyclopropyl)-L-2-pyrrolidonecarboxamide (EX 4883) into a monoamine oxidase inhibitor by a soluble fraction enzyme system. Arch. int. Pharmacodyn. **178**, 53—61 (1969).
MILLER, J.C., ZELLER, E.A.: Unpublished data (1968).
NARA, S., GOMES, B., YASUNOBU, K.T.: Amine oxidase. VII. Beef liver mitochondrial monoamine oxidase, a copper-containing protein. J. biol. Chem. **241**, 2774—2780 (1966).
NOVICK, W.J., JR.: The effect of age and thyroid hormones on the monoamine oxidase of rat heart. Endocrinology **69**, 55—59 (1961).
OGAWA, K., GUDBJARNASON, S.: A correlation between the inhibition of monoamine oxidase activity and the relief of angina pain by organic nitrates. Arch. int. Pharmacodyn. **172**, 172—182 (1968).
OTSUKA, S., KOBAYASHI, Y.: A radioisotopic assay for monoamine oxidase determinations in human plasma. Biochem. Pharmacol. **13**, 995—1006 (1964).
PAASONEN, M.K., SOLATUNTURI, E., KIVALO, E.: Monoamine oxidase activity of blood platelets and their ability to store 5-hydroxytryptamine in some mental deficiencies. Psychopharmacologia (Berl.) **6**, 120—124 (1964).
PLETSCHER, A., GEY, K.F., BURKARD, W.P.: Inhibitors of monoamine oxidase and decarboxylase of aromatic amino acids. Handb. Exp. Pharmacol. **19**, 593—735 (1965).
— — ZELLER, P.: Monoaminoxydase-Hemmer. Biochemie — Chemie — Pharmakologie — Klinik. In: Progress in drug research, vol. **2**, p. 417, ed. E. JUCKER. Basel: Birkhäuser 1960.
POGELL, B.M.: Enzymatic oxidation of pyridoxal phosphate in rabbit liver. J. biol. Chem. **232**, 761—776 (1958).
PUGH, C.E.M., QUASTEL, J.H.: Oxidation of aliphatic amines by brain and other tissues. Biochem. J. **31**, 286—291 (1937a).
— — Oxidation of amines by animal tissues. Biochem. J. **31**, 2306—2321 (1937b).
QUIRING, K., PALM, D.: Inhibition of amine oxidases by nitrofuran derivatives: possible structure-activity relations and criteria of irreversibility. Naunyn-Schmiedeberg's Arch. exp. Path. Pharmak. **265**, 397—410 (1970).
ROBINSON, D.S., LOVENBERG, W., KEISER, H., SJOERDSMA, A.: Effects of drugs on human blood platelet and plasma amine oxidase activity *in vitro* and *in vivo*. Biochem. Pharmacol. **17**, 109—119 (1968).
SABELLI, H.C., GIARDINA, W.J., ALIVISATOS, S.G.A., SETH, P.K., UNGAR, F.: Indoleacetaldehydes: serotonin-like effects on the central nervous system. Nature (Lond.) **223**, 73—74 (1969).
SARKAR, S.: Characterization of the active center of monoamine oxidases with substrates and inhibitors. Dissertation Abstr. **22**, 2973 (1962).
— BANERJEE, R., ISE, M.S., ZELLER, E.A.: Über die Wirkung von 2-Phenylcyclopropylaminen auf die Monoamin-oxydase und andere Enzymsysteme. 18. Mitteilung über Amin-oxydasen. Helv. chim. Acta **43**, 439—447 (1960).

Schnaitman, C., Greenawalt, J.W.: Enzymic properties of the inner and outer membranes of rat liver mitochondria. J. Cell. Biol. **38**, 158—175 (1968).
Schweppe, J.S., Zeller, E.A., Higgins, G.M.: Interrelationships between enzymes and hormones. VI. Influence of age, sex, adrenalectomy, and cortisone acetate upon the concentration of monoamine oxidase in the livers of white rats. Proc. Mayo Clin. **26**, 371—375 (1951).
Seiden, L.S., Westley, J.: Mechanism of iproniazid inhibition of brain monoamine oxidase. Arch. int. Pharmacodyn. **146**, 145—162 (1963).
Sen, R., Parmar, S.S., Guha, S.R.: Monoamine oxidase of rat heart mitochondiia. I. Purification and properties. Acta biol. med. germ. **21**, 1—11 (1968).
Severina, I.S., Gorkin, V.Z.: Selective inhibition by various hydroxyquinolines of the activity of monoamine oxidases of the rat liver in mitochondria. Biokhimiya **29**, 1093 to 1102 (1964).
Singer, T.P., Barron, E.S.G.: Studies on biological oxidations. XX. Sulphydryl enzymes in fat and protein metabolism. J. biol. Chem. **157**, 241—253 (1945).
Sourkes, T.L.: Properties of the monoamine oxidase of rat liver mitochondria. Advanc. Pharmacol. **6** (Pt.A), 61—69 (1968).
Stern, I.J., Hollifield, R.D., Wilk, S., Buzard, J.A.: The antimonoamine oxidase effects of furazolidone. J. Pharmacol. exp. Ther. **156**, 492—499 (1967).
Swett, L.R., Martin, W.B., Taylor, J.D., Everett, G.M., Wykes, A.A., Gladish, Y.C.: Structure-activity relations in the pargyline series. Ann. N.Y. Acad. Sci. **107**, 891—898 (1963).
Symes, A.L., Sourkes, T.L., Youdim, M.B.H., Gregoriadis, G., Birnbaum, H.: Decreased monoamine oxidase activity in liver of iron-deficient rats. Canad. J. Biochem. **47**, 999 to 1002 (1969).
Tabor, C.W., Tabor, H., Rosenthal, S.M.: Purification of amine oxidase from beef plasma. J. biol. Chem. **208**, 645—661 (1954).
Takahashi, H., Takahara, S.: A sensitive fluorimetric assay for monoamine oxidase based on the formation of 4,6-quinolinediol from 5-hydroxykynurenamine. J. Biochem. (Tokyo) **64**, 7—11 (1968).
Takahashi, Y.: Amine oxidase activity of liver tissues obtained by needle biopsy together with other liver function tests on schizophrenic patients. A preliminary report. Folia psychiat. neurol. jap. **10**, 263—278 (1955).
Tedeschi, D.H., Fellows, E.J.: Monoamine oxidase inhibitors: augmentation of pressor effects of peroral tyramine. Science **144**, 1225—1226 (1964).
Tedeschi, R.E., Tedeschi, D.H., Ames, P.L., Cook, L., Mattis, P.A., Fellows, E.J.: Some pharmacological observations on tranylcypromine (SKF trans-385), a potent inhibitor of monoamine oxidase. Proc. Soc. exp. Biol. (N.Y.) **102**, 380—381 (1959).
Tipton, K.F.: The submitochondrial localization of monoamine oxidase in rat liver and brain. Biochim. biophys. Acta (Amst.) **135**, 910—920 (1967).
— The purification of pig brain mitochondrial monoamine oxidase. Europ. J. Biochem. **4**, 103—107 (1968).
Udenfriend, S., Witkop, B., Redfield, B.G., Weissbach, H.: Studies with reversible inhibitors of monoamine oxidase: Harmaline and related compounds. Biochem. Pharmacol. **1**, 160—165 (1958).
Valzelli, L., Garattini, S.: Biogenic amines in discrete brain areas after treatment with monoamine oxidase inhibitors. J. Neurochem. **15**, 259—261 (1968).
Weissbach, H., Smith, T.E., Faly, J.W., Witkop, B., Udenfriend, S.: A rapid spectrophotometric assay of monoamine oxidase based on the rate of disappearance of kynuramine. J. biol. Chem. **235**, 1160—1163 (1960).
Westheimer, F.H.: Mechanism related to enzyme catalysis. Advances in Enzymology, vol. **24**, pp. 441—482. New York: Interscience Publ. Inc. 1962.
Yamada, H., Yasunobu, K.T.: Monoamine oxidase. I. Purification, crystallization, and properties of plasma monoamine oxidase. J. biol. Chem. **237**, 1511—1516 (1962).
Yasunobu, K.T., Igaue, I., Gomes, B.: Purification and properties of beef liver mitochondrial monoamine oxidase. Advanc. Pharmacol. **6** (Pt.A), 43—59 (1968).
Youdim, M.B.H., Sourkes, T.L.: Properties of purified, soluble monoamine oxidase. Canad. J. Biochem. **44**, 1397—1400 (1966).
Zeller, E.A.: On the nature of the reactive surface of amine oxidases. In: Cornell University, Symposium papers on biochemistry and nutrition. 1955, pp. 25—33; Ithaca, N.Y. 1956.
— The role of amine oxidase in the destruction of catecholamines. Pharmacol. Rev. Vol. **II**, 387—393 (1959).
— Some remarks about monoamine oxidase and monoamine oxidase inhibitors. J. Neuropsychiat. **2**, S125—S130 (1961).

ZELLER, E. A.: Monoamine oxidase. In: Monoamines et systeme nerveux central, p. 51, ed. J. DE AJURIA-GUERRA, Geneva et Paris: Georg et Co. S. A. 1962.
— Über eutope und dystope Substratkomplexe der Monoaminoxydase. 20. Mitteilung über Amin-oxydasen. Biochem. Z. **339**, 13—22 (1963a).
— A new approach to the analysis of the interaction between monoamine oxidase and its substrates and inhibitors. Ann. N.Y. Acad. Sci. **107**, 811—820 (1963b).
— Structure-activity relationship of monoamine oxidase inhibitors. In: Proceed. 3rd Internat. Pharmacological Meeting, Sao Paulo, 1966, Vol. **10**, pp. 3—13. J. Cheymol and J.R. BOISSIER, editors. Oxford: Pergamon Press 1968.
— BABU, B.H., STANICH, G., CAVANAUGH, M.: *In vivo* inhibition of human platelet monoamine oxidase by pargyline. Pharmacol. Res. Commun. **1**, 20—24 (1969).
— BARSKY, J., BERMAN, E.: Amine oxidases. XI. Inhibition of monoamine oxidase by 1-isonicotinyl-2-isopropylhydrazine. J. biol. Chem. **214**, 267—274 (1955).
— — FOUTS, J.R., KIRCHHEIMER, W.F., VAN ORDEN, L.S.: Influence of isonicotinic acid hydrazide (INH) and 1-isonicotinyl-2-isopropyl hydrazide (IIH) on bacterial and mammalian enzymes. Experientia (Basel) **8**, 349 (1952).
— BIRKHÄUSER, H., MISLIN, H., WENK, M.: Über das Vorkommen der Diamin-oxydase bei Mensch, Säugetier und Vogel. Mit einem Anhang über das Vorkommen der Cholin-esterase beim Vogel. 5. Mitteilung über den enzymatischen Abbau von Polyaminen. Helv. chim. Acta **22**, 1381—1395 (1939).
— BLANKSMA, L.A., BURKARD, W.P., PACHA, W.L., LAZANAS, J.C.: *In vitro* and *in vivo* inhibition of amine oxidases. Ann. N.Y. Acad. Sci. **80**, 583—588 (1959).
— FOUTS, J.R.: Enzymes as primary targets of drugs. Ann. Rev. Pharmacol. **3**, 9—32 (1963).
— SARKAR, S.: Amine oxidases. XIX. Inhibition of monoamine oxidase by phenylcyclopropylamine and iproniazid. J. biol. Chem. **237**, 2333—2336 (1962).
— SHOCH, D., COOPERMAN, S.C., SCHNIPPER, R.I.: On the role of monoamine oxidase (EC 1.4.3.4) in the regulation of aqueous humor dynamics of the rabbit eye. Invest. Ophthal. **6**, 215 (1967).
— STANICH, G.J.: Unpublished data (1969).
— STERN, R., WENK, M.: Über die Diamin-Diamin-oxydase-Reaktion. 6. Mitteilung über den enzymatischen Abbau von Poly-aminen. Helv. chim. Acta **23**, 3—17 (1940).
ZELLER, V., RAMACHANDER, G., ZELLER, E.A.: Amine oxidases. XXI. A rapid method for the determination of the activity of monoamine oxidase and monoamine oxidase inhibitors. J. med. Chem. **8**, 440—443 (1965).
— — — CHERKAS, M.S., FOUTS, J.R.: Degradation of mescaline by amine oxidases. J. Pharmacol. exp. Ther. **124**, 282—289 (1958).

Chapter 53

Sulphate Conjugation Enzymes

A.B. Roy

With 3 Figures

A. General Introduction

In biochemistry the term 'sulphate ester' means an ion having the structure $RO.SO_3^-$. These compounds are therefore half-esters of sulphuric acid (not to be confused with the fully covalent diesters, $R.OSO_2O.R'$, e.g. dimethyl sulphate) and are usually isolated or prepared as the corresponding potassium salts although other cations may confer useful properties. In the following discussion the compound called, for example, phenyl sulphate should therefore strictly be named potassium phenyl sulphate, trimethylammonium phenyl sulphate, etc. as appropriate. In metabolic experiments the nature of the cation is unimportant, except in so far as it itself may have biological effects, because the sulphate esters are salts of strong acids and so are fully ionised at any pH likely to be encountered in biological systems. The corresponding free acids, for example phenyl hydrogen sulphate, $C_6H_5O.SO_3H$, are unstable and cannot normally be isolated. The preparation and some properties of various types of sulphate ester have recently been summarised by Roy and Trudinger (1970).

The formation of such sulphate esters in the animal body has been known since the last century when phenyl sulphate was found in the urine of patients who had been exposed to phenol. This early observation has been greatly extended during the past ninety years, as is obvious from the work described by Williams (1959), and it is now clear that sulphation is a major pathway in the metabolism of substances which either contain phenolic hydroxyl groups or can be converted *in vivo* to those containing such groups. Compounds containing alcoholic hydroxyl groups or primary amino groups can also form sulphate esters *in vivo* but the quantitative importance of these conversions is apparently less.

The physiological significance of these sulphations, by reactions very expensive in energy, is not obvious but the chemical and physical properties of the esters differ considerably from those of the parent compounds. In particular, sulphation converts an unionised or poorly ionised group into a fully ionised group and so generally increases the solubility in aqueous solvents. This may aid the urinary excretion of the parent compounds. On the other hand, many sulphate esters, both of steroids (Wang and Bulbrook, 1967) and of simple phenols (Hearse et al., 1969), are firmly bound to proteins. Although this is probably a non-specific phenomenon, similar to the binding of other simple or complex anions to proteins (Steinhardt and Beychok, 1964), it could nevertheless be important in controlling the movements of compounds between blood and tissue fluids or between blood and urine. For example, Wang and Bulbrook (1967) have shown that the different rates of clearance of steroid sulphates from human and rabbit blood can be correlated with the greater binding of steroid sulphates to the plasma proteins in the former. This in turn may be related to the quite different types of metabolism undergone by, for example, androstenolone and androstenolone sulphate in man (BAULIEU et al., 1965). Again, many sulphate esters can, with cations having large hydrophobic residues (such as methylene blue, cationic detergents or some phospholipids), form complexes which are soluble in non-polar solvents (BURSTEIN, 1962). Such complexes could be important in the transfer of materials through membranes, as has been suggested by the model experiments of KELLER and BLENNEMANN (1961). At present these examples must suffice to point to some of the ways in which sulphation could greatly alter the behaviour of a drug.

Finally in this connection it should perhaps be pointed out that the general acceptance of sulphation as a detoxication reaction may be wrong, or at least an oversimplification. Both holuthurin A, a neurotoxin in the sea cucumber *Actinopyga agassizi* (FRIESS et al., 1967), and phyllokinin, a hypotensive peptide in the skin of the reptile *Phyllomedusa rohdei* (ANASTASI et al., 1966), are sulphate esters. The former has the sulphate group esterified with the carbohydrate part of a complex steroid glycoside and the latter contains tyrosyl *O*-sulphate residues: in both cases the toxicity is greatly decreased by desulphation. A brief but useful review of some aspects of this work has recently appeared (GORDON and HUNTER, 1969).

A more direct demonstration of toxicity being increased by sulphation comes from the suggestion (DEBAUN et al., 1970) that the carcinogenicity of *N*-hydroxy-2-acetamidofluorene is due to the formation *in vivo* of its sulphate ester which, unlike the parent compound, rapidly reacts with nucleophilic components of proteins and nucleic acids. DEBAUN et al. (1970) describe the ester as an *N*-sulphate, an unfortunate name because this term is usually, although incorrectly, applied to compounds such as heparin which contain sulphamate groups ($—NH.SO_3^-$). The sulphate ester of *N*-hydroxy-2-acetamidofluorene contains the quite different group $—N(OC.CH_3).OSO_3^-$, similar to the $>N.OSO_3^-$ group in the mustard oil glycosides (ETTLINGER and LUNDEEN, 1956) and in the oxime *O*-sulphonates (SMITH, 1948). An enzyme capable of forming the sulphate ester of *N*-hydroxy-2-acetamidofluorene occurs in rat liver but the relation of this to the sulphotransferases to be discussed below is unknown.

The ability to form sulphate esters of one type or another is widespread in nature and is found not only in most, if not all, animals but also in plants and microorganisms. Only the situation in animals will be considered in this discussion.

The synthesis of sulphate esters can conveniently be regarded as being made up of two parts: first, the activation of sulphate, itself a two stage process, and secondly the transfer of the sulphate group to the appropriate acceptor through the action of a sulphotransferase. The importance of the activation of sulphate in other metabolic processes, particularly in microorganisms, must not be forgotten but information on this topic must be sought elsewhere (ROY and TRUDINGER, 1970).

B. The Activation of Sulphate

I. The Sulphate-Activating System

This enzyme system catalyses the over-all conversion of sulphate ions to 'active sulphate', 3′-phosphoadenylyl sulphate (3′-phosphoadenosine 5′-phosphosulphate, 3′-phosphoadenosine 5′-sulphatophosphate, PAPS) with adenylyl sulphate (adenosine 5′-sulphatophosphate, APS) as an intermediate. The structures of these compounds are shown below (I and II). Their characteristic feature is the sulphatophosphate group which identifies them as derivatives of a mixed anhydride of phosphoric and sulphuric acids. As such, they are very acid-labile substances, the half-life of the sulphatophosphate group in PAPS being only 6 min in 0.1 N HCl at 37°. They are, on the other hand, quite stable to alkali.

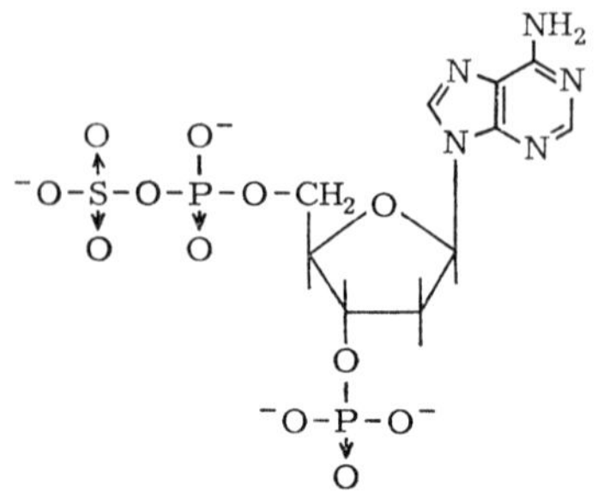

I
PAPS

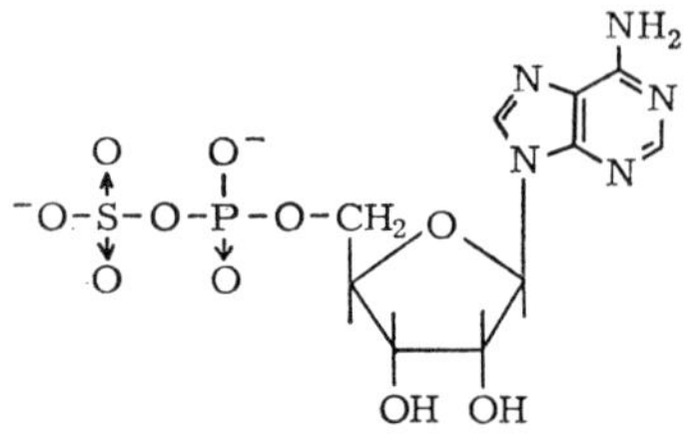

II
APS

The reaction catalysed by the sulphate-activating system is shown in equation (1): it has an absolute requirement for Mg^{2+} ions as cofactor, its pH optimum is

$$2\,ATP + SO_4^{2-} \rightarrow PAPS + ADP + PP_i \quad (1)$$

very flat between pH 7 and pH 9, and its optimum substrate concentration is about 1—2 mM SO_4^{2-} with an apparent K_m of 0.15 mM SO_4^{2-}. The occurrence of the system has been directly demonstrated in only a few tissues but it must be presumed in all those which can form sulphate esters because the only known pathway for this involves PAPS. If this evidence be accepted, then the sulphate-activating system must occur in all mammals, lower vertebrates and many, if not all, invertebrates. In the higher mammals, at least, it is present in most tissues including the adrenal, brain, cartilage, intestinal mucosa, kidney, liver, mast cells, muscle, ovary and testis to mention only a few. This widespread distribution is not unexpected in view of the apparently fundamental importance of the sulphate-containing mucopolysaccharides such as chondroitin sulphate whose synthesis is dependent upon the formation of PAPS.

The intracellular distribution of the system has not been studied in detail but at least in liver it is present in the soluble fraction obtained by the usual cell fractionation techniques.

Little is known of physiological changes in the level of the sulphate activating system in the higher mammals and nothing in other species. The activity is low in the livers of foetal and new-born rats, the latter showing only about 10% of the adult activity (Wengle, 1963), but the same is not necessarily true in other species or in other tissues. There is some evidence to suggest that the level of the sulphate-activating system is high in rapidly growing tissues, both in the rat (Balasubramanian and Bachhawat, 1961; Gerlach, 1963) and in the human (Sasaki, 1967).

Likewise there is little information on the level of the system in pathological conditions but it has been reported (Koizumi et al., 1969) that in liver it rises during chronic poisoning with CCl_4.

Much effort was devoted to an investigation of the relationship between vitamin A and sulphate activation following the observation by Varandani et al. (1960) that in rats deficient in vitamin A the ability to form PAPS was depressed. One striking feature of this work has been the variable results obtained by different workers (see Roels, 1967; Roy and Trudinger, 1970) and it has only recently become apparent that vitamin A has no *direct* action on the formation of PAPS although it undoubtedly does have an indirect one through the sensitivity of one of the enzymes of the system, ATP-sulphurylase, to the nutritional status of the animal. This will be discussed below. In hypovitaminosis A, however, rats do show a decreased ability to form PAPS and this can be reflected in a decreased ability to form sulphate esters, either mucopolysaccharides (DZIEWIATKOWSKI, 1954) or the sulphate esters excreted in the urine (SUBBA RAO et al., 1963). It is therefore not impossible that in the human, or other mammal, a deficiency of vitamin A might be reflected in a lowered ability to form sulphate esters.

MUKHERJI and BACHHAWAT (1966) have claimed that in the converse situation of hypervitaminosis A the ability to synthesise PAPS is also decreased in cartilage, although not in colon or brain. On the other hand, KOIZUMI et al. (1969) have stated that hypervitaminosis A increases the ability of healthy liver to form PAPS but decreases it in liver damaged by CCl_4. It was suggested that the latter effect was caused by an increased activity of enzymes capable of destroying PAPS (see below).

Another group of compounds which have an indirect effect on the formation of PAPS is that of the anti-inflammatory drugs, either salicylates, steroids such as cortisone or anti-inflammatory agents such as phenylbutazone (BOSTRÖM, BERNTSEN and WHITEHOUSE, 1964). These act through their influence on the formation of ATP, either by uncoupling oxidative phosphorylation or by directly affecting the oxidative reactions in the mitochondria. Any defect in the synthesis of ATP is likely to be reflected in the synthesis of PAPS as has been shown with preparations from a mastocytoma *in vitro*. SPOLTER et al. (1967) showed that the addition of NAD^+ to this system caused greatly increased amounts of PAPS to be produced: in the absence of NAD^+ the ratio PAPS/APS was 3 but in the presence of NAD^+ it was 15. This effect was almost certainly due to the stimulation of glycolysis by NAD^+ with the consequent increase in ATP production. It is therefore possible that treatment with anti-inflammatory agents could modify the metabolism of other drugs through inhibiting their conversion to sulphate esters: certainly BOSTRÖM, BERNTSEN and WHITEHOUSE (1964) showed that such treatment decreased the excretion of ester sulphates in the urine. This is the rationale behind the suggestion (COTTY and HARRIS, 1966) that metachromatic leucodystrophy which is associated with, if not caused by, an accumulation of cerebroside sulphates in the tissues, might be treated by massive doses of salicylates. To judge by the work of MEHL and JATZKEWITZ (1965) such treatment would be unlikely to be successful.

II. ATP-Sulphurylase

This enzyme (ATP: sulphate adenylyltransferase, 2.7.7.4), which was originally obtained from yeast by ROBBINS and LIPMANN (1958a, b), catalyses the first stage in the formation of PAPS, the reaction between ATP and SO_4^{2-} to give APS

$$ATP + SO_4^{2-} \rightleftharpoons APS + PP_i \qquad (2)$$

(equation 2). The equilibrium of (2) lies far in favour of ATP, the equilibrium constant being about 10^{-8} so that the standard free energy change for the reaction is about +11,000 cal.

The unfavourable equilibrium has made the direct assay of ATP-sulphurylase difficult. In the forward direction it is only possible if the equilibrium is displaced by the inclusion of pyrophosphatase in the system but even so the assay is not satisfactory because of product inhibition by APS. The best method is undoubtedly that of LEVI and WOLF (1969) which uses the reverse reaction, the formation of ATP from APS and pyrophosphate, This can be made extremely sensitive by adopting the luciferase method for the determination of ATP. In the past such assays were limited by the difficulty of obtaining APS but reliable methods are now available for the preparation of this in substrate amounts (Cherniak and Davidson, 1964). Another assay which has been much used depends upon the fact that ATP-sulphurylase is not absolutely specific for sulphate but can use analogous group VI anions such as selenate, chromate, molybdate or tungstate. With these ions the mixed anhydride produced by the reaction with ATP is unstable and immediately hydrolyses to AMP and the anion: if pyrophosphatase is present in the system then ATP-sulphurylase can be assayed by determining the amount of orthophosphate produced, as is represented in equation (3) (Wilson and Bandurski, 1958).

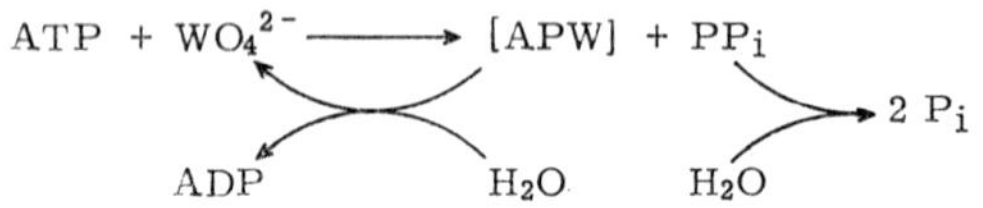

(3)

Although this method is apparently simple, in practice there are difficulties in obtaining adequate control determinations: for example, Wheldrake and Pasternak (1965) have shown that molybdate can displace phosphate bound to proteins in bacterial extracts.

The ATP-sulphurylase from rat liver has only recently been obtained in a highly purified state (Levi and Wolf, 1969) although no evidence has yet been presented as to the homogeneity of the final preparation. Despite previous claims to the contrary, this enzyme is quite stable and many of the difficulties encountered in earlier studies have undoubtedly been caused by it being quite rapidly inactivated in Tris buffers, although it is stable in phosphate buffers of the same pH. Again, despite claims to the contrary, it is not stabilised by SO_4^{2-} ions. The enzyme has the high molecular weight of about 900,000, as judged by gel filtration.

Detailed studies of the kinetics of the reaction have not been made. The pH optimum is about 8 and Mg^{2+} ions are required as cofactor. It is probably an SH enzyme because it is inhibited by p-chloromercuribenzoate and by Cu^{2+} or Co^{2+} ions. The inhibition by the former is reversed by glutathione. The available values of K_m for the various substrates (Levi and Wolf, 1969) are summarised in Table 1.

Table 1. *The apparent values of K_m for the ATP-sulphurylases of rat and sheep liver*

Substrate	K_m (mM) rat liver	sheep liver
ATP	1.6	—
SO_4^{2-}	0.1	—
Adenylyl sulphate	0.25	2.0
Pyrophosphate	0.037	1.7

These values may have little absolute significance because they were determined under arbitrary conditions and were not shown to be independent. In fact, if the enzyme does have the mechanism proposed by Levi and Wolf (1969) then the K_m values for the different substrates cannot be independent. The mechanism suggested was a ping-pong reaction, as represented below:

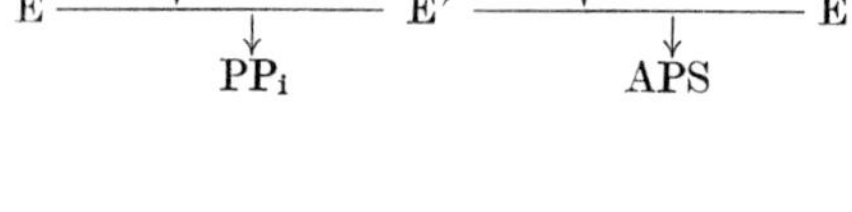

The only other ATP-sulphurylase from animal tissues that has been studied is that from sheep liver (PANIKKAR and BACHHAWAT, 1968). This sulphurylase also has a molecular weight in excess of 200,000 and a pH optimum of 8.5. The available information on K_m, subject to the same reservations as above, is summarised in Table 1.

It has in the past been suggested that the ATP-sulphurylase of animal tissues was activated by some metabolite of vitamin A or perhaps required this metabolite as a cofactor (SUNDARESAN, 1966). The evidence for this was scanty and contradictory, being based essentially on the different levels of ATP-sulphurylase activity in the tissues of normal animals and of those deficient in vitamin A. It is now clear that the effect is an indirect one due to the sensitivity of the level of ATP-sulphurylase to the nutritional state of the animal, starvation of rats for even 2 days causing a considerable drop in the activity of the system (LEVI et al., 1968; GEISON et al., 1968). Further evidence for the lack of any direct relationship between vitamin A and ATP-sulphurylase has been provided by LEVI and WOLF (1969). They isolated and purified ATP-sulphurylase from the livers of rat which had been treated with [6.7—$^{14}C_2$] vitamin A after having been rendered deficient in the vitamin. Although initially the enzyme was associated with radioactivity, the final purified material was devoid of ^{14}C and so could contain neither the vitamin nor any metabolite which still retained carbon atoms 6 and 7 of the vitamin. This would seem to show conclusively that vitamin A plays no direct role in the ATP-sulphurylase reaction.

III. APS-Kinase

This enzyme (ATP: adenylyl sulphate 3′-phosphotransferase, 2.7.1.25) has been much less studied than ATP-sulphurylase. It catalyses the essentially irreversible conversion of APS to PAPS with ATP as the phosphate donor, as shown in equation (4). APS-kinase was first identified in yeast by ROBBINS and LIPMANN

$$\text{APS} + \text{ATP} \rightarrow \text{PAPS} + \text{ADP} \tag{4}$$

(1958a) and this is still the only such enzyme for which any reliable information is available although it must be present in all tissues which can form PAPS.

The assay of APS-kinase is not easy. One method determines the amount of PAPS formed by means of the sulphotransferase reaction (see below; GREGORY, 1962; ROBBINS, 1962) and another uses [^{35}S]APS as substrate, separates the [^{35}S]PAPS by paper electrophoresis and determines this by some suitable method (WHELDRAKE and PASTERNAK, 1965).

The yeast enzyme requires Mg^{2+} ions as cofactor, has a pH optimum of between 8.5 and 9.0 and is completely saturated at 5 μM APS, a property which makes it admirably suited for trapping the small amounts of APS produced by the energetically unfavourable sulphurylase reaction.

There is no information on the enzyme in animal tissues.

C. The Hydrolysis of Adenylyl Sulphates

It was early noted (e.g. SUZUKI and STROMINGER, 1960) that animal tissues could degrade APS and PAPS to a mixture of products and several pathways seemed to be involved. One was the attack of phosphatases and nucleotidases, and another the attack of sulphatases of a hitherto unknown type. The latter were investigated by BALASUBRAMANIAN and BACHHAWAT (1962) who used sheep brain as a source of the enzymes. It appears that such degradative enzymes are of widespread occurrence, having been found in virtually all tissues capable of synthesising or utilising the adenylyl sulphates. Although their significance *in vivo* is obscure, they can be very troublesome in crude tissue preparations *in vitro* where they effectively compete with, for instance, the sulphotransferases.

Bailey-Wood et al. (1969) have considerably purified from the soluble fraction of rat liver an enzyme which hydrolyses APS to AMP and SO_4^{2-} at an optimum pH of 5.2 and with a K_m of 0.5 mM APS. This preparation could not hydrolyse PAPS although crude extracts of rat liver did so. ATP was not hydrolysed by the enzyme but was an inhibitor of the hydrolysis of APS (70% inhibition at 0.1 mM ATP), as were also all other nucleotides studied. Unfortunately the closest analogue of APS, ADP, was apparently not tested as a possible substrate.

Koizumi et al. (1969) have shown that the lysosomes of rat liver contain an enzyme hydrolysing PAPS: this could well be the same enzyme as found by Bailey-Wood et al. (1969) in their unpurified preparations of APS-hydrolase. The enzyme was released from the lysosomes by chronic poisoning with CCl_4 or by hypervitaminosis A, a further factor which must be taken into account when assessing the action of vitamin A on sulphate activation *in vivo*.

D. Sulphotransferases

I. General Considerations

The final step in the biosynthesis of sulphate esters is the transfer of the sulphate group from PAPS to the appropriate acceptor, as shown in equation (5), in which R.OH may be an alcohol or a phenol. The reaction is, except in special

$$R.OH + PAPS \rightarrow PAP + R.OSO_3^- \qquad (5)$$

circumstances, irreversible. Certain amines, $R.NH_2$, can replace R.OH in equation (5) and so give rise to sulphamates. The latter reaction is definitely enzymic in contrast to the formation of *N*-glucuronides which may be non-enzymic, either *in vivo* or *in vitro* (Dutton, 1966 and Chapter 45, this volume).

Thiols might be expected to react similarly to form thiosulphate esters but no such reaction has been observed *in vitro* although Williams (1959) mentions the possibility of phenyl thiosulphate ($C_6H_5.SSO_3^-$) being a metabolite of thiophenol. The only thiosulphate esters known to occur naturally in higher animals are *S*-sulphocysteine and *S*-sulphoglutathione and although the sulpho groups of these compounds can arise from PAPS, it seems that they are derived from sulphite produced by the reduction of the nucleotide rather than directly from the latter itself. Robinson (1965) suggested that the biosynthesis of these esters proceeds via equations (6) and (7), of which only (6) is enzymatic. Although this sequence was postulated to explain only the formation of the *S*-sulpho derivatives of cysteine

$$PAPS + NADPH_2 \rightarrow PAP + NAD^+ + H_2O + SO_3^{2-} \qquad (6)$$

$$SO_3^{2-} + R.S.S.R \rightleftarrows R.SH + R.SSO_3^- \qquad (7)$$

or glutathione, it could occur with any suitable disulphide (Milligan and Swan, 1962) and so account for the excretion of ester sulphate (Parke, 1952) in the urine of rabbits dosed with thiophenol, which is readily oxidised to diphenyl disulphide.

No sulphotransferase has been obtained in a pure state and these enzymes have been studied mostly in crude tissue preparations. It is therefore by no means certain how many separate enzymes must be considered but in connection with drug metabolism the *activities* of phenol sulphotransferase, of alcohol sulphotransferase, of steroid sulphotransferases and of arylamine sulphotransferase must be taken into account. Other sulphotransferases are known — for example, cerebroside sulphotransferase, mucopolysaccharide sulphotransferase and choline sulphotransferase to name only three — but at present there is no reason to associate these with drug metabolism in mammals. Although choline sulphotransferase might be a likely candidate for such a role, as far as is known it is not present in animal tissues but only in certain higher fungi.

The assay of the sulphotransferases is, in principle, simple. Some of the methods which have been used are not, however, satisfactory. For example, assays which depend upon the presence of the PAPS generating system are suspect because the steady-state concentration of PAPS is not known and could well be vanishingly small. Assays which use a sulphate-activating system to produce PAPS before the addition of the sulphotransferase are better but again the concentration of the nucleotide is unknown. Both types of assay suffer from the fact that other nucleotides such as ADP or PAP are likely to be produced during the formation of PAPS and these are powerful general inhibitors of the sulphotransferases. The only reliable assays use known concentrations of PAPS as the sulphate donor. Since either unlabeled or ^{35}S labeled PAPS may be prepared chemically (Baddiley and Sanderson, 1963; Cherniak and Davidson, 1964) or enzymically (Banerjee and Roy, 1966; Balasubramanian et al., 1967; Hodson and Schiff, 1969) such assays of sulphotransferases should always be used. Details of the assay vary with the particular sulphotransferase under consideration and the only general techniques, suitable for use with most acceptors, depend upon the separation of [^{35}S]PAPS from [^{35}S]sulphate esters either by chromatography (Vestermark and Boström, 1959a; Spencer, 1960) or by precipitation with Ba^{2+} (Wengle, 1964). Another fairly general method is that of Banerjee and Roy (1966) which makes use of the solubility in chloroform of the methylene blue complexes of certain sulphate esters. This technique can be used with many phenols, steroids and arylamines but it cannot be used with very water-soluble acceptors such as the simple alcohols or carbohydrates. Specific methods are available for determining the sulphation of p-nitrophenol (Gregory and Lipmann, 1957), m-aminophenol (Bernstein and McGilvery, 1952) or serotonin (Hidaka et al., 1967). The use of amino phenols as sulphate acceptors should perhaps be discouraged in view of the likelihood of sulphamation also occurring (see section D.V.).

Two general points regarding the assay of the sulphotransferases must be kept in mind. The first is the apparently ubiquitous occurrence of enzymes capable of destroying PAPS. The second is the fact, already mentioned, that sulphate esters may bind very firmly to proteins so that careful recovery experiments are necessary. It may be essential to denature the protein before attempting to determine the ester (Banerjee and Roy, 1967).

There is little information on the sulphotransferase activities in different species because different workers have used very different conditions in the assay of these enzymes. Table 2 summarises some of these data but the values must be considered only as indications of the relative activities because they represent the combined activity of the sulphate-activating system and the sulphotransferases. At high levels of synthesis the former system could be rate-limiting. Some values showing the change in activity of the sulphotransferases of the liver during growth are shown in Table 3: in general the level seems to be low in the foetus and to increase slowly to the adult value. For more detailed consideration of this topic the very thorough investigations of Boström and his coworkers must be consulted (Wengle, 1963, 1966; Boström and Wengle, 1967).

It may be difficult to relate the values given in Tables 2 and 3 to the situation *in vivo*. This is exemplified by the observations of Boyland et al. (1957) on the excretion of 2-naphthyl sulphamate, a metabolite of 2-naphthylamine which can easily be detected in the urine of rats dosed with the amine although not in the

Table 2. *The rates of synthesis of some sulphate esters in the livers of some mammals. The assays were carried out under constant conditions, not necessarily the optimum, and depended upon the endogenous sulphate-activating systems to form PAPS*

Species and Sex	Rate of formation (nMoles/g liver/h) of sulphate ester of p-Nitrophenol	Androstenolone	Oestrone	2-Naphthylamine
Rat, male	—	53[a]	—	—
Rat, female	—	150[a]	—	—
Rat, male	1500	120	78	140
Rat, female	1200	390	47	320
Rat, female[b]	—	—	—	170
Mouse, male	—	7[a]	—	—
Mouse, female	—	34[a]	—	—
Guinea pig[c]	—	75[a]	—	—
Guinea pig[c]	370	260	72	1200
Guinea pig[b]	—	—	—	1600
Rabbit[c]	—	17[a]	—	—
Ox	—	19[a]	—	—
Brush tailed possum (*Trichosurus vulpecula*)				
male	17	—	—	—
female	49	—	—	—

[a] These results are known to be low because low concentrations of uncrystallised ATP were used in the assays.
[b] Different strain of animal.
[c] No sex differences were noted in these species.

Table 3. *The rates of synthesis of some sulphate esters at different stages of development. The assays were carried out under standard conditions with preformed PAPS as the sulphate donor. The results are not directly comparable to those given in Table 2* (From Wengle, 1963, 1966; Boström and Wengle, 1967)

Species and Sex	Rate of formation (nMoles/g liver/h) of sulphate ester of Phenol	Androstenolone	Oestrone	Testosterone
Rat, foetus[a]	0	0	—	—
Rat, new born, male	170	130	—	—
Rat, new born, female	70	80	—	—
Rat, adult, male	3200	410	—	—
Rat, adult, female	1490	2080	—	—
Human, foetus[b]	653	120	147	15
Human, adult[b]	2513	498	214	99

[a] These assays were carried out using ATP and SO_4^{2-} as a source of PAPS and so may reflect a lowered sulphate-activating system as well as lowered sulphotransferases.
[b] No sex difference was noted here.

urine of guinea pigs similarly treated. Nevertheless, according to Table 2, guinea pig liver contains considerably more arylamine sulphotransferase than does rat liver. This point is considered further below (section D. V.). On the other hand, the very low sulphotransferase activity of possum liver is matched by the negligible excretion of ester sulphates by this species (Roy, 1963).

There is little information on any factors influencing the activity of the sulphotransferases *in vivo*. The only study of possible pathological changes is that of Boström and Wengle (1967) and this, unfortunately, provided nothing of interest. There have been reports that in rats deficient in vitamin A there is a decreased sulphotransferase activity in liver (Subba Rao et al., 1963; Subba Rao and Ganguly, 1964) but there is nothing to show that this is due to a direct action on the sulphotransferases (CARROLL, 1969). CARROLL and SPENCER (1965) suggested that the low activity of sulphotransferases in foetal rat liver was due to a physiological hypovitaminosis A but no evidence for this was given except that the addition of retinol or retinoic acid (1 μg/ml) *in vitro* caused an increased sulphotransferase activity. Ascorbic acid is involved in the synthesis of mucopolysaccharide sulphates (KODICEK and LOEWI, 1955) but this effect need not be mediated through the sulphotransferases and ROY (1958) found no difference from normal in the ability of the livers of scorbutic guinea pigs to form androstenolone sulphate. Another factor influencing the formation of mucopolysaccharide sulphates is the serum sulphation factor (SALMON and DAUGHADAY, 1957; DAUGHADAY and PARKER, 1965) but this probably affects protein synthesis so there is again no need to invoke an action on the sulphotransferases.

In general terms, the sulphotransferases appear to be localised in the soluble fraction of the cell, to have molecular weights of about 65,000 (as judged by gel filtration), and to tend to form interacting systems. Their pH optima lie in the region of pH 5.5—8, some require exogenous Mg^{2+} ions as activators while others do not, and probably all are activated by SH compounds although there is no real evidence that there are SH groups present in the active centres of the enzymes. They are all inhibited by PAP, ADP and related nucleotides. Detailed studies of their kinetics have been made with only one phenol sulphotransferase (see below) but the available results would be consistent with their generally catalysing rapid equilibrium random bi bi reactions.

II. Phenol Sulphotransferase

This type of sulphotransferase activity seems to be quite ubiquitous in animals, if it be accepted that all species which form aryl sulphates must contain phenol sulphotransferases, but in only a few cases has the enzyme been isolated. All mammals so far investigated can form sulphate esters, as can at least some birds, reptiles, amphibia, insects, arachnids, crustaceans, molluscs and echinoderms (SMITH, 1968). There seems to be no report of a phenol sulphotransferase being present in fish but this may reflect insufficient investigation rather than a fundamental difference from other groups. Again in mammals, the enzyme must be present in most tissues, to judge by the situation in the ox (HOLCENBERG and ROSEN, 1965) and the human (BOSTRÖM and WENGLE, 1967), but liver, kidney, intestinal mucosa and placenta are probably among the richer sources. As has been shown in Table 3, the activity in rat and human foetal tissues seems to be lower than that in adult tissues.

No phenol sulphotransferase has been obtained as a single protein. The most highly purified enzyme of this type is that from guinea pig liver (BANERJEE and ROY, 1966, 1968) which had no detectable steroid, alcohol or arylamine sulphotransferase activity. It had a molecular weight of about 65,000, did not require Mg^{2+} ions as cofactor and was stabilised, or reactivated, by mercaptoethanol. Its pH optimum (with p-nitrophenol as acceptor) was 5.6 and the dissociation constants of the various enzyme-substrate complexes are given in Table 4. The mech-

Table 4. *The dissociation constants, K_s, of the enzyme-substrate complexes of the phenol sulphotransferase of guinea pig liver*

	K_s (mM)
p-Nitrophenol	0.070
3′-Phosphoadenylyl sulphate	0.036
p-Nitrophenyl sulphate	0.068
Adenosine 3′,5′-diphosphate	0.024

anism of the reaction catalysed by this enzyme has been investigated in some detail (Banerjee and Roy, 1968) and shown to be a rapid-equilibrium random bi bi reaction with one dead-end complex, as represented in the scheme below, where E is the phenol sulphotransferase and NP is p-nitrophenol.

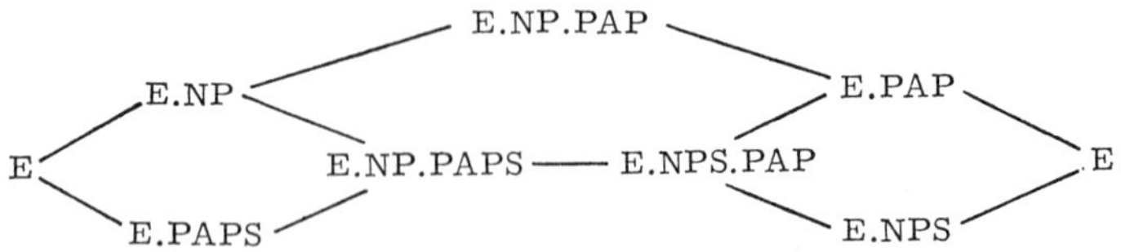

With acceptors such as p-nitrophenol or 3,5-dinitrophenol the sulphotransferase reaction is reversible because the sulphate esters of these phenols have a 'sulphate group potential' comparable to that of PAPS (Gregory and Lipmann, 1957) thereby allowing equilibrium to be readily attained. The 'sulphate group potential' is a function of the pK of the phenolic group; the more acidic the phenol, the more easily hydrolysed is the sulphate ester (see Fendler and Fendler,

Table 5. *Some relations between the structure and the excretion of phenols as sulphate esters. The column 'Excretion' gives the percentage of a dose of the phenol excreted as the sulphate ester by the rabbit; K′ is the apparent equilibrium constant for the phenol sulphotransferase reaction with the appropriate phenol as substrate, and k′ is the apparent first order rate constant for the acid hydrolysis of the appropriate sulphate ester*

	pK	Excretion[a]	K′	k′ (× 10^5)
Phenol	9.8	19	∞	3.2[d]
p-Nitrophenol	7.1	—	26[b], 3[c]	43.5[e]
2,4-Dinitrophenol	4.0	—	—	135[e]
2,5-Dinitrophenol	5.1	—	—	45[e]
3,5-Dinitrophenol	6.7	—	4[b]	—
2,4-Dichlorophenol	7.7	16	—	—
2,6-Dichlorophenol	6.8	—	—	—
Pentachlorophenol	5.3	—	—	—

[a] From Dodgson et al. (1950).
[b] At room temperature and pH 7.8. Gregory and Lipmann (1957).
[c] At 37° and pH 5.6. Banerjee and Roy (1968).
[d] At 40° in 1 M HCl. Kice and Anderson (1966).
[e] At 45° in 1 M HCl. Fendler and Fendler (1968).

1968). Table 5 summarises some pertinent data. With simple phenols, such as phenol itself, it must be stressed that the sulphotransferase reaction is quite irreversible.

The reversibility with p-nitrophenol means that under suitable conditions phenol sulphotransferase(s) can catalyse a transfer of sulphate from p-nitrophenyl sulphate to, say, phenol, with PAP acting as a cofactor. This reaction, represented below, was first studied in a crude preparation from rabbit liver (Gregory and Lipman, 1957). It is not known if only one sulphotransferase is involved in this

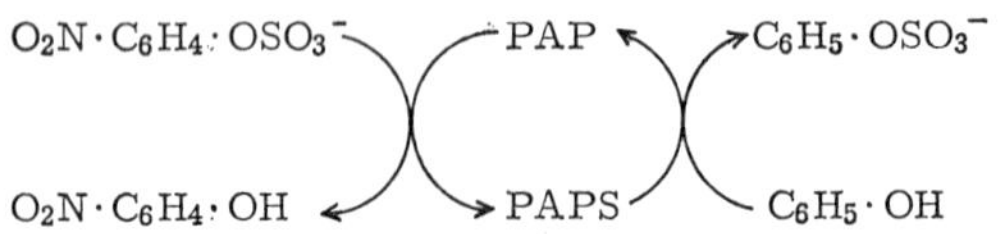

sequence of reactions and it is perhaps pertinent that the purified phenol sulphotransferase from guinea pig liver could not catalyse such a transfer (Banerjee and Roy, 1968). Gregory and Lipmann (1957) stated that acceptors other than phenols, for example steroids, could not be used in this reaction but Wortman (1961) showed that extracts from ox cornea could transfer sulphate from p-nitrophenyl sulphate to mucopolysaccharides with PAP as a cofactor.

The specificity of phenol sulphotransferase is not completely understood because no homogeneous enzyme is available but studies *in vivo* (see Williams, 1959) suggest that almost any phenol can be converted to a sulphate ester. Therefore, either there must be many rather specific phenol sulphotransferases or only a few, perhaps one, less specific enzymes. Some preliminary studies of the specificity of the phenol sulphotransferase of guinea pig liver are summarised in Table 6: this

Table 6. *The values of K_m and relative maximum velocities, V, for different substrates for the phenol sulphotransferase of guinea pig liver. The roman numerals refer to formulae in the text*

	K_m (mM)	V
Phenol	2.50	0.30
Thiophenol	—	0.00
p-Nitrophenol	0.070	1.00
1-Naphthol	0.025	1.02
4-Nitro-1-naphthol	0.018	0.39
2-Naphthol (III)	0.025	0.95
5,6,7,8-Tetrahydro-2-naphthol	0.056	0.63
2-Phenanthrol (IV)	0.017	0.51
15,16-Dihydro-3-hydroxy-17-oxocyclopentena-[a]phenanthrene (V)	0.015	0.13
Equilenin (VI)	0.015	0.10
Equilin (VII)	0.020	0.21
Oestrone (VIII)	—	0.00

seems to suggest that the specificity for phenols is not high although the reason why oestrone, a typical phenol, is not a substrate remains obscure. The structures of some of these acceptors are given in formulae III to VIII. It seems likely that

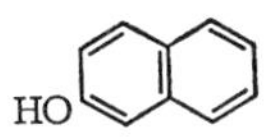

III
2-Naphthol

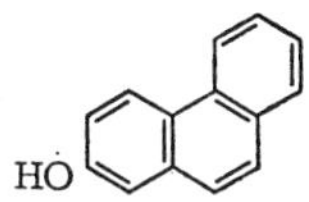

IV
2-Phenanthrol

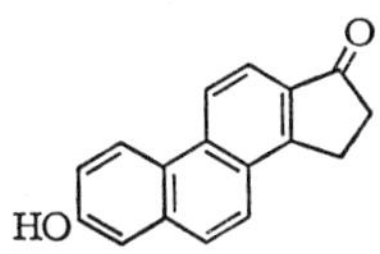

V
15, 16-Dihydro-3-hydroxy-17-oxocyclopentena-[a]phenanthrene

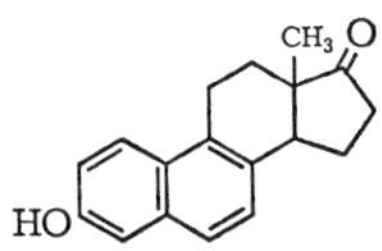

VI
Equilenin

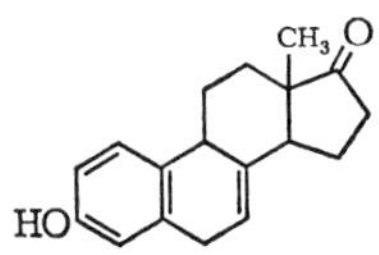

VII
Equilin

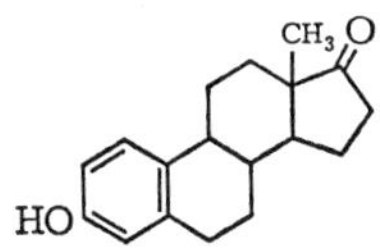

VIII
Oestrone

general phenol sulphotransferases will prove to be involved in the synthesis of adrenalin sulphate (Boström and Wengle, 1964), serotonin sulphate (Hidaka et al., 1969), and triiodothyronine sulphate (Cohn, 1965) in mammals; of bufothionin in the toad (Wieland and Vocke, 1930) and of ommatin D in insects (Butenandt et al., 1960) but the participation of more specific enzymes cannot yet be excluded. Finally, it must be mentioned that polyphenols can form disulphates (Vestermark and Boström, 1960a) and that at least one mixed conjugate, a sulphate-glucuronide, of a diphenol is known, that of 4-nitrocatechol (Flynn et al., 1967).

A sulphotransferase of potential interest in pharmacology is that involved in the formation of the tyrosyl *O*-sulphate residues found in fibrinogen and in the pharmacologically active peptides gastrin II (Gregory et al., 1964), phyllokinin (Anastasi et al., 1966) and caerulein (Anastasi et al., 1967). Whether this sulphation is catalysed by a general phenol sulphotransferase or by a specific enzyme is not known. Kinetic studies (Mattock and Jones, 1970; Mattock et al., 1970) certainly suggest that simple derivatives of tyrosine are sulphated by an enzyme distinct from phenol sulphotransferase but this cannot be taken as proven and, further, the relation between this reaction and the sulphation of tyrosine-containing peptides is still obscure.

Finally it must be pointed out that a given tissue may contain more than one phenol sulphotransferase: for instance, guinea pig liver contains not only the specific phenol sulphotransferase considered above but also two others associated with oestrone sulphotransferase and with androstenolone sulphotransferase, respectively. The relation between these activities has not yet been clarified (Banerjee and Roy, 1966).

Although much remains to be discovered about the phenol sulphotransferases, it seems a safe generalisation that most phenols and related heterocyclic compounds such as 3-hydroxypyridine will be converted to sulphate esters *in vivo*. Exceptions may arise if the hydroxyl group is heavily hindered (although thyroxin can probably be sulphated) or if the pK of the phenol is less than 7. Anderton et al. (1948) suggested that for a phenol to be capable of forming a sulphate ester *in vivo* it must have a pK of between 7 and 10, a view supported by Dodgson et al. (1950) who showed that of a series of chlorinated phenols only those with pK values greater than 7 (all being less than 10) were excreted by the rabbit as sulphate esters. It must be borne in mind that this may reflect not the specificity of the sulphotransferase so much as the effect of the pK of the phenol on the stability of its sulphate ester; with very acidic phenols the esters might not accumulate either because of their inherent instability or because of the unfavourable equilibrium of the sulphotransferase reaction.

III. Alcohol Sulphotransferase

This enzyme has been little studied, even in crude preparations, but it presumably occurs in extracts of rat and human liver which can form the sulphate esters of simple alcohols (Vestermark and Boström, 1959b; Boström and Wengle, 1964). Embryonic chick liver can also form alkyl sulphates (Spencer and Raftery, 1966), an interesting observation because the only alkyl sulphate known to occur naturally in animals, isopropyl sulphate, has been isolated from hen eggs (Yagi, 1964, 1966).

The specificity of this presumed alcohol sulphotransferase is quite unknown but enzyme preparations from rat liver can form sulphate esters not only of the primary alcohols from methanol to pentanol (Vestermark and Boström, 1959b), but also of the more complex polyols (Vestermark and Boström, 1960b). The latter type of reaction is important because of the use of propylene glycol as a solvent for poorly water-soluble substrates, such as steroids, in many studies of sulphotransferases (Banerjee and Roy, 1967) and indeed in metabolic experiments in general (see Cooke and Taylor, 1961).

Although such sulphations could be of obvious pharmacological interest, alkyl sulphates do not appear to have been recognised as products of drug metabolism apart from the observation by LAW et al. (1963) that dimetridazole (IX) is excreted by turkeys as the alkyl sulphate (X). BOSTRÖM and VESTERMARK (1960)

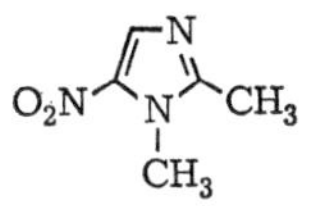

IX
Dimetridazole

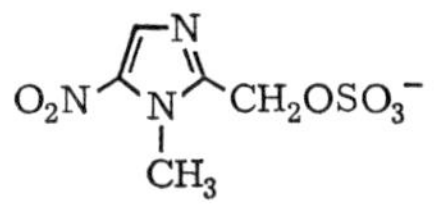

X
Hydroxydimetridazole sulphate

have discussed the possible significance of the formation of alkyl sulphates and have suggested that, under certain conditions, the excessive consumption of alcohol might disturb the conversion of other foreign compounds into their sulphate esters by competing for the available PAPS.

Further consideration of this activity must await proof that it is due to a specific sulphotransferase and is not simply a facet of the activity of some other enzyme, for example, desoxycorticosterone sulphotransferase, which also sulphates primary hydroxyl groups.

IV. Steroid Sulphotransferases

1. Introduction

This group of sulphotransferases certainly contains several distinct enzymes; exactly how many is still not certain but the following *activities* can be recognised: oestrone sulphotransferase, androstenolone sulphotransferase, aetiocholanolone sulphotransferase, testosterone sulphotransferase and desoxycorticosterone sulphotransferase. The formulae of the typical substrates of these enzymes are given below (VIII and XI—XIV) and some aspects of steroid nomenclature which are per-

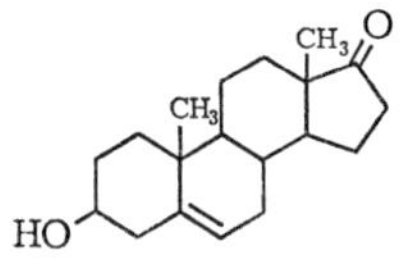

XI
Androstenolone

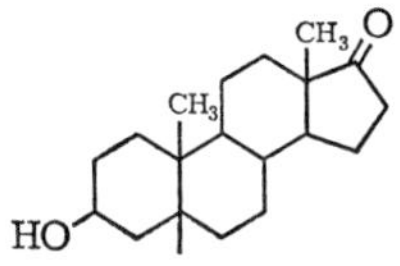

XII
Aetiocholanolone

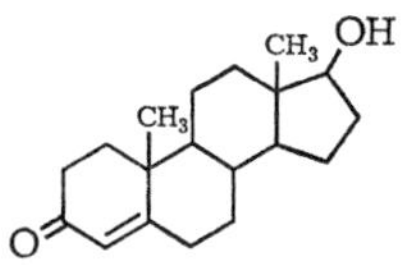

XIII
Testosterone

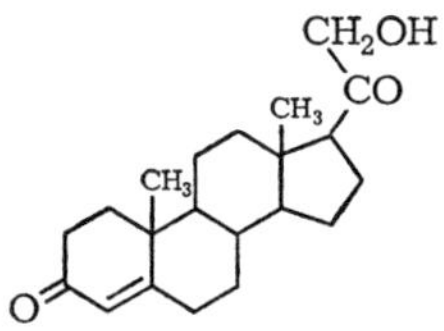

XIV
Desoxycorticosterone

tinent to the subsequent discussion are shown in Fig. 1. In Fig. 2 are shown the conformations of some important classes of steroid. Regardless of how many separate *enzymes* are involved it is clear that mammals at least are capable of sulphating many different types of steroid. Between them the above activities allow the sulphation of the phenolic hydroxyl group of oestrogens, the 3α- and 3β-secondary hydroxyl groups of the 5α and Δ^5 series of steroids, the 3α- and 3β-

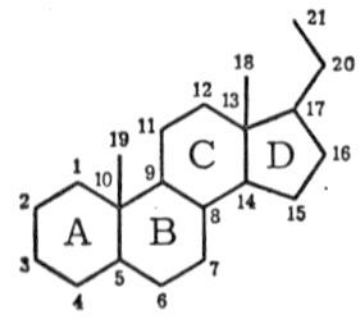

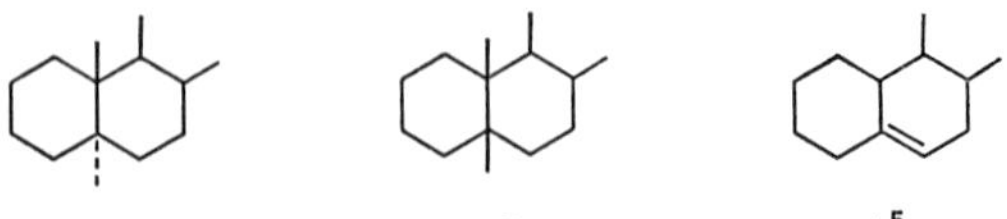

5α 5β Δ5

Fig. 1. The numbering of the steroid nucleus and the general structures of the 5α, 5β and Δ^5 series of steroids (for the conformation of these steroids see Fig. 2). The nomenclature of substituents at other positions in the molecule is similar to that shown for those at position 5. In all steroids of animal origin the C/D ring junction is trans so that these compounds are 14α steroids

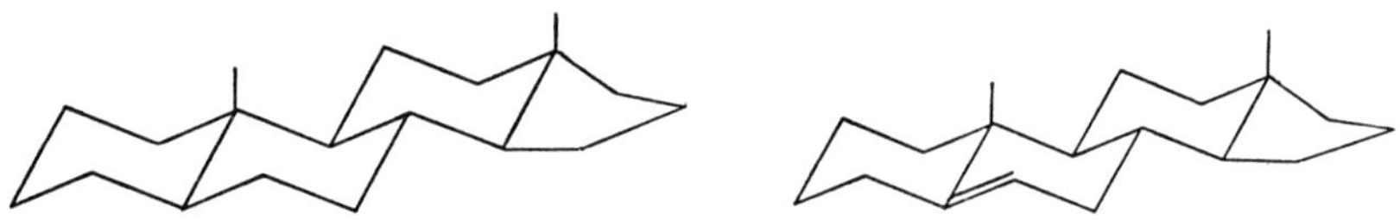

5α Δ5

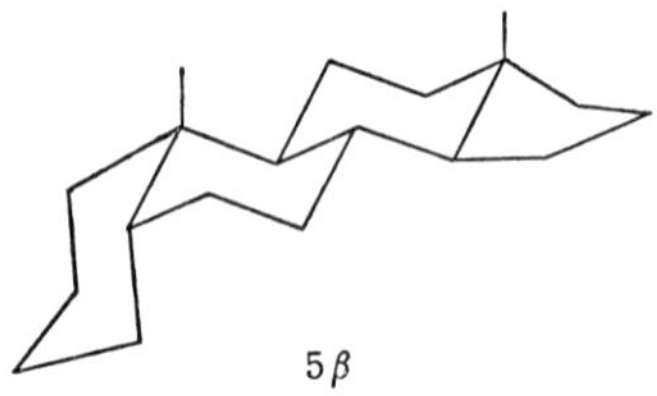

5β

Fig. 2. The conformations of the 5α, 5β and Δ^5 series of steroids

secondary hydroxyl groups of the 5β series of steroids, the 17α- and 17β- secondary hydroxyl groups of C_{18} and C_{19} steroids, and the primary hydroxyl group at position 21 of certain pregnane derivatives. As pointed out by Wengle and Boström (1963), steroid disulphates can also be formed, especially of the 3β, 17β- and 3β, 20β- dihydroxy steroids, and many of the observations made by these authors can be correlated with the behaviour of such steroids *in vivo*. It must be assumed, therefore, that sulphation is a likely fate of any steroid in the animal body and this can lead to its further metabolism diverging greatly from that of the original free steroid (Baulieu et al., 1965). Such sulphation may occur not only with the usual steroids of animal origin and their analogues but also with steroids having, for animals, quite unusual structures: for example Herrmann and Repke (1964) have shown that a number of cardioactive genins, of both the 5α and 5β series, are sulphated by preparations from the livers of several mammalian species. These genins differ from steroids of animal origin in that the C/D ring junction is *cis*. The formulae of a typical 'animal' steroid, cholesterol, and a cardioactive genin, digitoxigenin, are given below (XV, XVI). It should be noted that the change from the 14α configuration of cholesterol to the 14β configuration of digitoxigenin alters

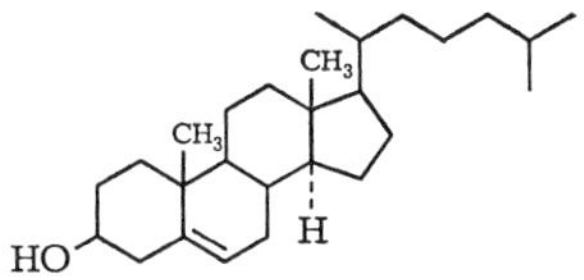

XV
Cholesterol

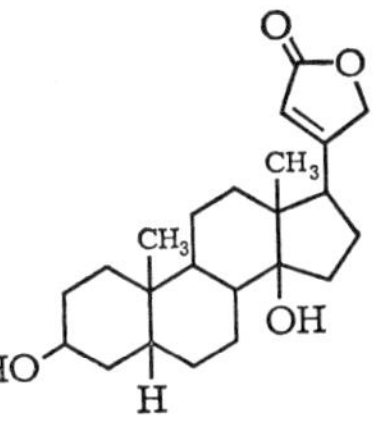

XVI
Digitoxigenin

the conformation at the C/D ring junction in a way quite analogous to that shown in Fig. 2 for the change of a 5α to a 5β steroid.

Finally, the occurrence of double conjugates must be noted: for example, oestradiol 3-sulphate 16-glucuronide (LEVITZ et al., 1966), pregnenediol 3-sulphate 20-glucuronide (ARCOS and LIEBERMAN, 1967), taurolithocholic acid 3-sulphate and glycolithocholic acid 3-sulphate (PALMER, 1967) have been found *in vivo*. Although these compounds are of obvious interest in connection with the specificities of the various conjugating systems, they cannot be considered here.

The steroid sulphotransferases are less widely distributed than the phenol sulphotransferases but at least some representatives of the group have been found in all the higher mammals studied; their distribution in some human tissues is shown in Table 7. Whether they occur in marsupials and in the lower vertebrates

Table 7. *The rates of synthesis of certain steroid sulphates in adult and foetal human tissues. The values are comparable with those in Table 3* (From BOSTRÖM and WENGLE, 1967)

	Rates of formation (nMoles/g tissue/h) of sulphate ester of				
	Oestrone	Andro-stenolone	Aetiochol anolone	Testo-sterone	Desoxycorti-costerone
Liver, adult	214	498	483	99	155
Liver, foetal	147	120	108	15	34
Adrenal, adult	83	295	326	56	63
Adrenal, foetal	661	3741	3521	553	932
Jejunum, adult	85	52	60	a	a
Jejunum, foetal	141	99	112	18	43
Kidney, adult	a	a	a	a	a
Kidney, foetal	127	120	108	15	34

a No significant activity detected.

is not clear. At least some amphibia and fish must contain the apparently quite different sulphotransferases which are involved in the formation of the bile alcohol sulphates (BRIDGWATER and RYAN, 1957; HASLEWOOD, 1967).

2. Oestrone Sulphotransferase

In the tissue of the adult mammal this enzyme is of restricted occurrence and in the ox and human only the liver, adrenal and jejunal mucosa are quantitatively significant sources (HOLCENBERG and ROSEN, 1965; BOSTRÖM and WENGLE, 1967). On the other hand, in the human foetus oestrone sulphotransferase is present in significant amounts in almost all tissues (WENGLE, 1966). It also occurs in chick embryo (ADAMS, 1963; SPENCER and RAFTERY, 1966), in the adult hen (MATHUR et al., 1969) and in the gut of the sea urchin *Strongylocentrotus franciscanus*

(Creange and Szego, 1967). The enzyme may be particularly important in the hen, which, apparently alone among the animals investigated, excretes oestrogens almost entirely as sulphate esters.

Banerjee and Roy (1966) partially purified the oestrone sulphotransferase of guinea pig liver but were unable to separate it from phenol sulphotransferase and arylamine sulphotransferase activities. All three types of activity could have been associated with a single protein. Adams and Poulos (1967), on the other hand, obtained from ox adrenal gland an oestrone sulphotransferase which had no arylamine sulphotransferase activity and only a very restricted phenol sulphotransferase activity. It could utilise the synthetic oestrogens stilboestrol and hexoestrol, but not phenol nor the naphthols, as acceptors. The rates of sulphation of the synthetic oestrogens were much less than those of the steroid oestrogens and it was not established that a single enzyme was involved. Some kinetic parameters of these enzymes are given in Table 8. The oestrone sulphotransferase of ox adrenal

Table 8. *The properties of some partly purified steroid sulphotransferases*

	Oestrone sulphotransferase Guinea pig liver	Ox adrenal	Androstenolone Guinea pig liver	sulphotransferase Human adrenal
Optimum pH	6	8	7.5	7.7
K_m (mM) PAPS	>0.1[a]	0.07	.05	[b]
K_m (mM) Oestrone	0.025	0.014	—	—
K_m (mM) Oestradiol	—	0.014	—	—
K_m (mM) Androstenolone		—	.02	[b]
K_m (mM) Cholesterol	—	—	.02	—
Requirement for Mg^{2+}	+	+	+	+
Activation by SH	—	+	—	+

[a] Probably high because of the presence of PAPS-degrading enzymes.
[b] The kinetic behavior was extremely complex and no meaningful values of K_m were obtained.

gland can exist either as a monomer, of molecular weight about 67,000, or as a trimer (or tetramer) of this (Adams and Chulavatnatol, 1967): the kinetics of the reaction catalysed by the polymeric form are complex and the values in Table 8 refer to the monomer.

Detailed specificity studies have not been carried out but the adrenal enzyme can apparently sulphate only the phenolic hydroxyl groups (at position 3) of oestrogens. The rates of sulphation, under empirical conditions, of oestriol, 17β-oestradiol, 16-oxo-17β-oestradiol, oestrone and equilenin did not vary by more than a factor of 2.5 (Adams and Poulos, 1967) and the values of K_m by little more (Adams, 1967). With the liver enzyme the variation was greater but the results were not unambiguous because other steroid sulphotransferases were present (Roy and Banerjee, 1967). It is not known if oestrone sulphotransferases can sulphate the hydroxyl group at position 2 of 2-hydroxyoestrone (XVII). The two

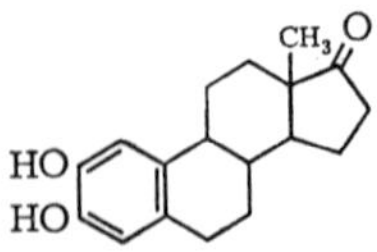

XVII
2-Hydroxyoestrone

hydroxyl groups are chemically similar and it might have been expected that either could be sulphated *in vivo*. That this is indeed the case has been shown by Yoshi-

ZAWA and FISHMAN (1969) and some implications of this finding have been considered by these authors and by MIYAZAKI et al. (1969).

It must be pointed out that although BANERJEE and ROY (1968) could find no evidence for oestrone being a substrate for the phenol sulphotransferase of guinea pig liver, the related oestrogens equilin and equilenin were substrates (Table 6). The possibility remains, therefore, that some phenol sulphotransferases may be able to function as oestrone sulphotransferases. The converse, that some oestrone sulphotransferases may be general phenol sulphotransferases, also remains a possibility.

3. Androstenolone Sulphotransferase

The distribution of this enzyme is similar to that of oestrone sulphotransferase in the ox and in the human so that only the liver, adrenal and jejunal mucosa are quantitatively important sources in the adult (Table 7). Nevertheless other tissues, such as the testis, must contain the enzyme. In the human foetus the kidney also shows activity but by far the greatest concentration of androstenolone sulphotransferase occurs in the foetal adrenal gland, as can be seen from the data in Table 7 (WENGLE, 1966). The enzyme also occurs in chick embryo (SPENCER and RAFTERY, 1966) and in at least some insects because HUTCHINS and KAPLANIS (1969) have shown that the meconium from the tobacco hookworm *Manduca sexta*, contains cholesteryl, campesteryl and β-sitosteryl sulphates. The parent steroids occurred in the diet of the larvae and it was suggested that sulphation was a preliminary to their excretion.

The typical substrate for the enzyme is, as the name implies, androstenolone (XI) dehydro*epi*androsterone), but as far as is known the same enzyme is responsible for the synthesis of the 3α- or 3β- sulphates of related steroids with relatively planar molecules, that is, of the 5α and Δ^5 steroids (Fig. 2). This could be an over-simplification and a number of more specific enzymes may yet be separated (c.f. NOSE and LIPMANN, 1958).

BANERJEE and ROY (1966) also partly purified an androstenolone sulphotransferase from guinea pig liver; again the steroid sulphotransferase was associated with phenol and arylamine sulphotransferase activities from which it could not be separated.

ADAMS and EDWARDS (1968) have examined an androstenolone sulphotransferase in crude extracts of human adrenal gland. The enzyme apparently existed as a number of slowly interconvertible polymers, the equilibrium between them being influenced by the substrates, PAPS causing dissociation to the monomer and androstenolone favouring association. Such behaviour might make androstenolone sulphotransferase an ideal site for the operation of a control mechanism but further observations on a purer enzyme are required before too much significance can be attached to the results.

Some properties of these enzymes are also shown in Table 8. The pH optima quoted therein are much higher than that of about 6 given by BOSTRÖM and WENGLE (1967) for the androstenolone sulphotransferases they obtained from human adrenal and liver. The reason for this discrepancy is not obvious but the latter authors used an assay in which the concentration of PAPS was unknown and inhibitors were likely to have been present: these could well have introduced complicating effects. In the case of the enzyme from guinea pig liver, the rate of formation of cholesteryl sulphate was about 40% that of androstenolone sulphate and this reaction was competitively inhibited by androstenolone methyl ether (K_i 0.09 mM). Some implications of this have been considered by BANERJEE and ROY (1967) (see also section D.V.).

4. Aetiocholanolone Sulphotransferase

The existence of this enzyme is suggested by the fact that the ratios of sulphotransferase activities with androstenolone (XI) and with aetiocholanolone (XII) as substrates vary considerably in different tissues. In preparations from rat liver (Roy, 1956) and rabbit liver (Nose and Lipmann, 1958) the two 3-hydroxy-5β-androstan-7-ones (aetiocholanolones) are sulphated much more slowly than androstenolone, but in preparations from human liver (Boström and Wengle, 1964) or adrenal (Adams, 1964; Boström, Franksson and Wengle, 1964) the aetiocholanolones and androstenolone are sulphated at quite similar rates. Obviously one interpretation of this could be that there is a separate aetiocholanolone sulphotransferase, a conclusion which seems justified by the very different conformations of the 5α (or Δ^5) and 5β series of steroids (Fig. 2).

5. Testosterone Sulphotransferase

The ability of crude preparations from rat (Roy, 1956; Schneider and Lewbart, 1956) and guinea pig (Roy, 1960a) liver to sulphate testosterone (XIII) and epitestosterone has been known for some time but the relation of this activity to other steroid sulphotransferases remains obscure. Roy and Banerjee (1967) showed that in guinea pig liver the testosterone sulphotransferase activity was distinct, but not separable, from androstenolone and oestrone sulphotransferases. Again, therefore, it is not possible to give any information on the specificity of the enzyme. Presumably, however, it could utilise the 17-hydroxy group of an oestrogen as an acceptor but this has not been demonstrated.

6. Desoxycorticosterone Sulphotransferase

This also is distinct but inseparable from the androstenolone and oestrone sulphotransferases in guinea pig liver but its activity closely parallels that of testosterone sulphotransferase (Roy and Banerjee, 1967). The relation between these sulphotransferases must remain in doubt but the very different chemistry of the 17β-hydroxy group of testosterone (XIII) and 21-hydroxy group of desoxycorticosterone (XIV) makes it unlikely that a single sulphotransferase could react with both types of steroid.

Again nothing can be said of the specificity of the enzyme except that the presence of a 17α-hydroxyl group in the molecule, as in cortisone or cortisol, seems to inhibit sulphation at position 21 (Wengle and Boström, 1963). Such a specificity would be in keeping with the metabolism of corticosteroids *in vivo*.

V. Arylamine Sulphotransferase

Although Boyland et al. (1957) showed that 2-naphthyl sulphamate (XVIII)

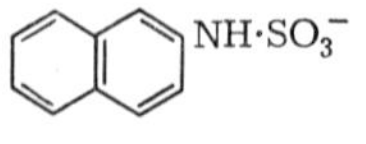

XVIII
2-Naphthyl sulphamate

was a metabolic product of 2-naphthylamine in rats and rabbits and Roy (1960a) showed that the sulphamation took place in preparations from rat or guinea pig liver, there is still no certain indication that a specific arylamine sulphotransferase exists. As already mentioned, Banerjee and Roy (1966) found arylamine and phenol sulphotransferase activities to be closely and inseparably associated with both oestrone and androstenolone sulphotransferases in guinea pig liver.

An interesting property of the presumed arylamine sulphotransferase is its sensitivity to many 17-oxosteroids which activate the enzyme from rat liver but inhibit that from guinea pig liver (Roy, 1960a, 1961). Previous interpretations of these effects (Roy, 1962, 1964) are open to criticism now that guinea pig liver has been shown to contain two separable arylamine sulphotransferases. Both of these, however, are inhibited by 17-oxosteroids (Banerjee and Roy, 1966) so that the observations are still of interest because they show how the metabolism of one compound, an arylamine, could be greatly altered by the presence of another quite unrelated compound, a 17-oxosteroid. *In vitro* the effects were obvious at concentrations of 17-oxosteroid as low as 1 μM so it is possible that they could occur *in vivo* and perhaps be responsible for the fact, already mentioned, that guinea pigs do not excrete 2-naphthyl sulphamate whereas rats do, although the livers of the latter contain much lower amounts of arylamine sulphotransferase (see Table 2).

The specificity of this presumed arylamine sulphotransferase has not been examined but preparations from rat or guinea pig liver can use aniline and 1- or 2-naphthylamine, but not benzylamine, as substrates. Likewise the distribution of the activity has been little studied and apart from the livers of various mammals the only known sources are sheep colonic mucosa (Kent and Pasternak, 1958), chick embryo (Spencer and Raftery, 1966) and certain spiders (Hitchcock and Smith, 1964).

Although such sulphamations have been noted only with simple arylamines, this type of conjugation could be important in the metabolism of more complex molecules containing arylamine residues. That such sulphamates have not been detected in the past could due to their lability to acid. Aryl sulphamates will hydrolyse more or less completely under the conditions of diazotisation normally used in the determination of arylamines so that such methods would not, in general, distinguish aryl sulphamates from the parent arylamine (Boyland et al., 1957; Roy, 1960a). Peters (1969) has recently considered the possibility of the sulphamate, N^1-sulphato-N^2-isonicotinylhydrazine, being a metabolite of isonicotinylhydrazine in man and animals but was unable to find evidence for the formation of such a conjugate (which is not an aryl sulphamate) *in vivo*.

E. The Synthesis of Sulphate Esters *in Vivo*

There can be no doubt that the enzymes described above are those responsible for the synthesis of sulphate esters *in vivo*. The only alternative pathway to have received much consideration is the reaction of cysteine and a phenol to give an aryl sulphate without the intermediate formation of inorganic sulphate. This thesis, which is reminiscent of the suggestion (Shiple et al., 1924) that sulphate esters are formed by the oxidation of mercapturic acids, has recently been forcefully propounded by Wellers (1960), mainly as a result of most thorough sulphur-balance studies on rats (Wellers and Chevan, 1959; Wellers and Boelle, 1960). These have clearly shown that cysteine is a more efficient precursor of urinary aryl sulphates than is dietary inorganic sulphate: almost certainly, however, this reflects only the poor absorption of sulphate from the gastrointestinal tract and does not imply a direct reaction between cysteine and the phenol. In the rabbit also the sulphur amino acids are better precursors of sulphate esters than is sulphate, although no more efficient than sulphite (Bray et al., 1952).

The recent discovery (Mead and Finamor, 1969) of ascorbic acid 3-sulphate in the undeveloped cysts of the brine shrimp, *Artemia salina*, does, however, open up the possibility of the existence of a further pathway leading to sulphate esters.

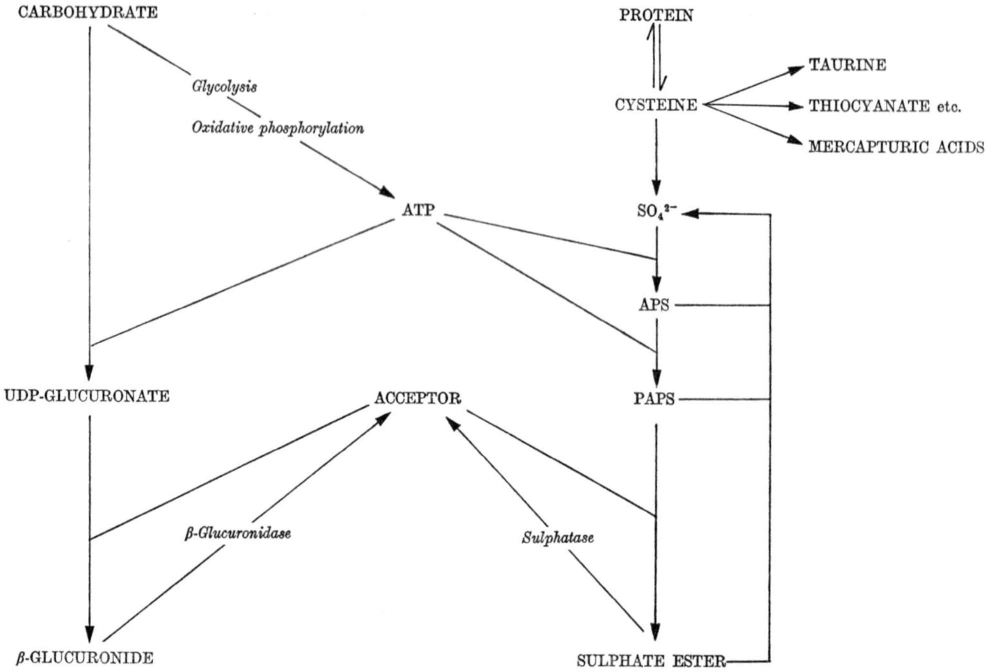

Fig. 3. The relationship of sulphate metabolism to some other metabolic pathways

Ascorbic acid 3-sulphate (or its isopropylidene derivative) can certainly act as a sulphate donor *in vitro* and under mildly oxidising conditions the sulphate group is transferred to suitable acceptors such as octanol (Mumma, 1968) or steroids (Chu and Slaunwhite, 1968). There seems no reason why similar reactions could not occur *in vivo* so that ascorbic acid 3-sulphate, a rather stable compound, might well act as a store of 'active sulphate'. It is to be hoped that information on the distribution of this interesting ester in other species will soon be forthcoming.

That the synthesis of sulphate esters is closely related to other metabolic pathways is shown in Fig. 3 and it should be obvious that disturbances to any of these pathways could greatly alter the ability to form sulphate esters *in vivo*.

A key reaction is obviously the production of sulphate from cysteine and any decrease in this could well result in a deficiency of sulphate because, quite apart from its poor absorption from the gut, this ion is not present to any extent in most normal diets. In protein deficiency the ability to synthesise sulphate esters is therefore likely to be depressed through a deficiency of sulphate, as well as through diminished levels of ATP-sulphurylase (see section B II). Any specific lack of cysteine could similarly diminish the ability to form sulphate esters; such a lack could occur in chronic poisoning with halogenated aromatic hydrocarbons, where cysteine in the form of glutathione is required for the synthesis of mercapturic acids (see Williams, 1959), or in the chronic degenerative neuropathy recently described by Osuntokun (1968) where cysteine is apparently utilised for the detoxication of cyanide coming from cyanogenic glycosides in the diet.

The oxidation of cysteine to sulphate is a complex sequence of reactions (see Roy and Trudinger, 1970) but the only known defect in the pathway is at the terminal stage, the oxidation of sulphite to sulphate. A child showing an inability to carry out this step was found to have a congenital deficiency of sulphite oxidase

(IRREVERRE et al., 1967). Although detailed investigations have not been reported, there was no obvious change from normal in the ability to form sulphate esters (PERCY et al., 1968) but the disease was so severe in its effects that alterations in the metabolism of foreign compounds were unlikely to have been of much practical importance.

The other essential requirement for the synthesis of sulphate esters is ATP. This presumably arises through glycolysis or oxidative phosphorylation. Any disturbance of these processes would almost certainly disrupt the formation of PAPS and so of sulphate esters. That this can happen *in vivo* seems to have been clearly established by BOSTRÖM, BERNTSEN and WHITEHOUSE (1964) in their study of the effects of anti-inflammatory drugs on sulphate metabolism. As already discussed (section B. I), these seem to act by limiting the production of ATP and so preventing the activation of sulphate.

Finally, the effects of protein deficiency and of vitamin A deficiency in causing a lowered level of ATP-sulphurylase activity must again be mentioned (see section B. II). This must be reflected in a decreased ability to form sulphate esters.

Acting in opposition to the formation of the adenylyl sulphates and sulphate esters are several hydrolytic reactions. The hydrolysis of APS and of PAPS has already been considered above and, as pointed out, the appropriate enzymes occur both in the lysosomes and the soluble fraction of the cell. The sulphatases, which hydrolyse sulphate esters (ROY, 1960b), occur principally in the lysosomes although some occur in the microsomes. It might be expected, therefore, that in any condition in which the lysosomes were more labile than normal the net production of sulphate would be decreased, either because of the destruction of PAPS or because the esters which had been formed were subsequently hydrolysed by sulphatases. Among the factors which seem to cause an increased lability of the lysosomes are hypervitaminosis A (DINGLE, 1961; DINGLE, 1963); hypovitaminosis E (ZALKIN et al., 1962; TAPPEL et al., 1963); poisoning with CCl_4 (DIANZANI, 1963) and radiation (ROTH and HILTON, 1963). It is not suggested that the labilisation of the lysosomes is the dominant action of these agents but there is no doubt that it is a major facet of it. Furthermore, it must be stressed that there are complex and ill-understood interactions between these agents, for example, between vitamins A and E (GUHA and ROELS, 1965; ROELS et al., 1965) or vitamin E and CCl_4 (GALLAGHER, 1961), and still other interactions which involve selenite (BIERI, 1964). These problems cannot be considered here but it seems likely that they could cause widespread disruption of the ability to synthesis sulphate esters *in vivo* through their actions on the lysosomes.

In metachromatic leucodystrophy there is the converse situation of an almost complete lack of sulphatase A, which may or may not be associated with a lack of sulphatases B and C (AUSTIN et al., 1965) but no defect in the formation of ester sulphates was noted in this condition.

Finally it should be stressed that there is essentially a competition between the formation of sulphate esters and of β-glucuronides. All the types of compounds which have been considered above as being precursors of sulphate esters can form β-glucuronides *in vivo*, and, at least in the case of phenols, the glucuronide pathway appears to be the dominant one in the rabbit, if not in other species (WILLIAMS, 1959). Probably all that need be said here is that the formation of glucuronides is perhaps less likely to be influenced by factors such as protein deficiency than is the formation of sulphate esters so that the balance between the two processes could easily be altered *in vivo*. Certainly a deficiency of glucuronide precursors is much less likely to occur than a deficiency of sulphate, the former being essentially unlimited so long as glucose (and ATP) is available. On the other hand, the availability of sulphate may easily become limiting: the normal daily urinary excretion of sulphate ions in man is about 30 mmole and this presumably corresponds to the maximum amount of sulphate ester which can be produced without disturbing the normal metabolic pattern of the body. At least in the rat, the availability of sulphate may become limiting at quite low levels of xenobiotic: for example, following the administration of harmine, at a dose of 5 mg/kg, the ratio of harmol sulphate to harmol glucuronide in the urine steadily falls unless sulphite is simultaneously administered to the animals (Slotkin et al., 1970).

References

Adams, J.B.: Sulfate metabolism in avian and mammalian cartilage extracts. Arch. Biochem. Biophys. **101**, 478—488 (1963).
— Enzymic synthesis of steroid sulphates. I. Sulphation of steroids by human adrenal extracts. Biochim. biophys. Acta (Amst.) **82**, 572—580 (1964).
— Enzymic synthesis of steroid sulphates. V. On the binding of estrogens to estrogen sulphotransferase. Biochim. biophys. Acta (Amst.) **146**, 522—528 (1967).
— Chulavatnatol, M.: Enzymic synthesis of steroid sulphates. IV. The nature of the two forms of estrogen sulphotransferase of bovine adrenals. Biochim. biophys. Acta (Amst. **146**, 509—521 (1967).
— Edwards, A.M.: Enzymic synthesis of steroid sulphates. VII. Association-dissociation equilibria in the steroid alcohol sulphotransferase of human adrenal gland extracts. Biochim. biophys. Acta (Amst.) **167**, 122—140 (1968).
— Poulos, A.: Enzymic synthesis of steroid sulphates. III. Isolation and properties of estrogen sulphotransferase of bovine adrenal glands. Biochim. biophys. Acta (Amst.) **146**, 493—508 (1967).
Anastasi, A., Bertaccini, G., Erspamer, V.: Pharmacological data on phyllokinin (bradykinyl-isoleucyl-tyrosine O-sulphate) and bradykinyl-isoleucyl-tyrosine. Brit. J. Pharmacol. **27**, 479—485 (1966).
— Erspamer, V., Endean, R.: Isolation and structure of caerulein, an active decapeptide from the skin of *Hyla caerulea*. Experientia (Basel) **23**, 699—700 (1967).
Anderton, J.I., Smith, J.N., Williams, R.T.: Observations on the type of hydroxyl group undergoing the ethereal sulphate synthesis in rabbits. Biochem. J. **43**, XXXV (1948).
Arcos, M., Lieberman, S.: 5-Pregnene-3β, 20α-diol-3-sulfate-20-(2′-acetamido-2′-deoxy-α-D-glucoside) and 5-Pregnene-3β, 20α-diol-3,20-disulfate. Two novel urinary conjugates. Biochemistry **6**, 2032—2039 (1967).
Austin, J., Armstrong, D., Shearer, L.: Metachromatic form of diffuse cerebral sclerosis. V. The nature and significance of low sulfatase activity. A controlled study of brain, liver and kidney in four patients with metachromatic leucodystrophy. Arch. Neurol. (Chic.) **13**, 593—614 (1965).
Baddiley, J., Sanderson, A.R.: Adenosine 3′-phosphate 5′-sulfatophosphate, "Active sulfate". Biochem. Prep. **10**, 3—5 (1963).
Bailey-Wood, R., Dodgson, K.S., Rose, F.A.: A rat liver sulphohydrolase enzyme acting on adenylyl sulphate. Biochem. J. **112**, 257—258 (1969).
Balasubramanian, A.S., Bachhawat, B.K.: Formation of active sulphate in rat brain. J. Sci. Ind. Res. **20**c, 202—204 (1961).
— — Enzymic degradation of active sulphate. Biochim. biophys. Acta (Amst.) **59**, 389—397 (1962).
— Spolter, L., Rice, L.I., Sharon, J.B., Marx, W.: Preparation of 3′-phosphoadenylyl sulfate in substrate quantities using mastocytoma enzymes. Analyt. Biochem. **21**, 22—33 (1967).
Banerjee, R.K., Roy, A.B.: The sulfotransferases of guinea pig liver. Mol. Pharmacol. **2**, 56—66 (1966).
— — The formation of cholesteryl sulphate by androstenolone sulphotransferase. Biochim. biophys. Acta (Amst.) **137**, 211—213 (1967).
— — Kinetic studies of the phenol sulphotransferase reaction. Biochim. biophys. Acta (Amst.) **151**, 573—586 (1968).
Baulieu, E.E., Corpéchot, C., Dray, F., Emiliozzi, R., Lebeau, M.C., Mauvais-Jarvis, P., Robel, P.: An adrenal secreted 'androgen': dehydroisoandrosterone sulfate. Its metabolism and a tentative generalisation on the metabolism of other steroid conjugates in man. Recent Progr. Hormone Res. **21**, 411—500 (1965).
Bernstein, S., McGilvery, R.W.: The enzymatic conjugation of *m*-aminophenol. J. biol. Chem. **198**, 195—203 (1952).

BIERI, J.G.: Synergistic effects between antioxidants and selenium or vitamin E. Biochem. Pharmacol. **13**, 1465—1470 (1964).

BOSTRÖM, H., BERNTSEN, K., WHITEHOUSE, M.W.: Biochemical properties of anti-inflammatory drugs. II. Some effects on sulphate-^{35}S metabolism *in vivo*. Biochem. Pharmacol. **13**, 413—420 (1964).

— FRANKSSON, C., WENGLE, B.: Studies on ester sulphates. 22. Sulphate conjugation in adult human adrenal extracts. Acta endocr. (Kbh.) **47**, 633—644 (1964).

— VESTERMARK, A.: Studies on ester sulphates. 7. On the excretion of sulphate conjugates of primary aliphatic alcohols in the urine of rats. Acta physiol. scand. **48**, 88—94 (1960).

— WENGLE, B.: Studies on ester sulphates. 19. On sulphate conjugation in adult human liver extracts. Acta Soc. Med. upsalien. **69**, 41—63 (1964).

— — Studies on ester sulphates. 23. Distribution of phenol and steroid sulphokinase in adult human tissues. Acta endocr. (Kbh.) **56**, 691—704 (1967).

BOYLAND, E., MANSON, D., ORR, S.F.D.: The biochemistry of aromatic amines. 2. The conversion of arylamines into arylsulphamic acids and arylamine-*N*-glucosiduronic acids. Biochem. J. **65**, 417—423 (1957).

BRAY, M.G., HUMPHRIS, B.G., THORPE, W.V., WHITE, K., WOOD, P.B.: Kinetic studies of the metabolism of foreign organic compounds. 4. The conjugation of phenols with sulphuric acid. Biochem. J. **52**, 419—423 (1952).

BRIDGWATER, R.J., RYAN, D.A.: Sulphate conjugation with ranol and other steroid alcohols in liver homogenates from *Rana temporaria*. Biochem. J. **65**, 24p (1957).

BURSTEIN, S.: Interaction of [7*a*-^{3}H]- androstenolone sulphate with cationic detergents and phosphatides. Biochim. biophys. Acta (Amst.) **62**, 576—578 (1962).

BUTENANDT, A., BIEKERT, E., KOGA, N., TRAUB, P.: Über Ommochrome. XXI. Konstitution und Synthese des Ommatins D. Hoppe-Seylers Z. physiol. Chem. 2. **321**, 258—275 (1960).

CARROLL, J.: Phenolsulphotransferase in the developing rat. Amer. J. clin. Nutr. **22**, 978—985 (1969).

— SPENCER, B.: Vitamin A and sulphotransferases in foetal rat liver. Biochem. J. **96**, 79P (1965).

CHERNIAK, R., DAVIDSON, E.A.: Synthesis of adenylyl sulfate and adenylyl sulfate 3′-phosphate. J. biol. Chem. **239**, 2986—2990 (1964).

CHU, T.M., SLAUNWHITE, W.R.: The nonenzymic sulfation of androsterone with L-ascorbic acid 3-sulfate. Steroids **12**, 309—321 (1968).

COHN, G.L.: Biosynthesis of triodothyronine sulfate by beef thyroid *in vitro*. Nature (Lond.) **208**, 80 (1965).

COOKE, B.A., TAYLOR, W.: Inhibition of 'conjugate' formation by ethanol and propylene glycol during metabolism of [4-^{14}C] progesterone by female-rat liver *in vitro*. Biochem. J. **81**, 12P (1961).

COTTY, V.F., HARRIS, A.F.: Salicylates for leucodystrophy? Lancet **1966**, 1421.

CREANGE, J.E., SZEGO, C.M.: Sulphation as a metabolic pathway for oestradiol in the sea urchin *Strongylocentrotus franciscanus*. Biochem. J. **102**, 898—903 (1967).

DAUGHADAY, W.H., PARKER, M.L.: Human pituitary growth hormone. Ann. Rev. Med. **16**, 47—66 (1965).

DEBAUN, J.R., SMITH, J.Y.R., MILLER, E.C., MILLER, J.A.: Reactivity *in vivo* of the carcinogen *N*-hydroxy-2-acetyl-aminofluorene. Increase by sulfate ion. Science **167**, 184—186 (1970).

DIANZANI, M.U.: Lysosome changes in liver injury. In: Lysosomes. London: Churchill 1963.

DINGLE, J.T.: Studies on the mode of action of excess vitamin A. 6. Release of a bound protease by the action of vitamin A. Biochem. J. **79**, 509—512 (1961).

— Action of vitamin A on the stability of lysosomes *in vivo* and *in vitro*. In: Lysosomes. London: Churchill 1963.

DODGSON, K.S., SMITH, J.N., WILLIAMS, R.T.: Studies in detoxication. 29. The orientation of glucuronic acid conjugation in chloroquinols. Biochem. J. **46**, 124—128 (1950).

DUTTON, J.G.: The biosynthesis of glucuronides. In: Glucuronic Acid. New York: Academic Press 1966.

DZIEWIATKOWSKI, D.D.: Vitamin A and endochrondral ossification in the rat as indicated by the use of sulfur-35 and phosphorus-32. J. exp. Med. **100**, 11—24 (1954).

ETTLINGER, M.G., LUNDEEN, A.J.: The structure of sinigrin and sinalbin. An enzymatic rearrangement. J. Amer. chem. Soc. **78**, 4172—4173 (1956).

FENDLER, E.J., FENDLER, J.H.: Hydrolysis of nitrophenyl and dinitrophenyl sulfate esters. J. org. Chem. **33**, 3852—3859 (1968).

FLYNN, T.G., DODGSON, K.S., POWELL, G.M., ROSE, F.A.: The metabolism of dipotassium 2-hydroxy-5-nitrophenyl [^{35}S] sulphate, a substrate for lysosomal arylsulphatases A and B. Biochem. J. **105**, 1003 (1967).

Friess, S.L., Durant, R.C., Chanley, J.D., Fash, F.J.: Role of the sulphate charge center in irreversible interactions of holuthurin A with chemoreceptors. Biochem. Pharmacol. **16**, 1617—1625 (1967).
Gallagher, C.H.: Protection by antioxidants against lethal doses of carbon tetrachloride. Nature (Lond.) **192**, 881—882 (1961).
Geison, R.L., Rogers, W.E., Johnson, B.C.: Comparative effects of vitamin A deficiency and controlled food consumption on adenosine 5′-triphosphate sulfate adenylyltransferase. Biochim. biophys. Acta (Amst.) **165**, 448—458 (1968).
Gerlach, U.: Über die Altersabhängigkeit der Aktivität sulfataktivierender Enzyme im Herzen. Klin. Wschr. **41**, 873—876 (1963).
Gordon, M., Hunter, A.S.: Organic sulphate esters of potential biological interest. J. heterocyclic Chem. **6**, 739—744 (1969).
Gregory, H., Hardy, P.M., Jones, D.S., Kenner, G.W., Sheppard, R.C.: The antral hormone gastrin. Nature (Lond.) **204**, 931—933 (1964).
Gregory, J.D.: Sulfate-transferring enzymes. Meth. Enzymol. **5**, 977 (1962).
— Lipmann, F.: The transfer of sulfate among phenolic compounds with 3′,5′-diphosphoadenosine as coenzyme. J. biol. Chem. **229**, 1081—1090 (1957).
Guha, A., Roels, O.A.: The influence of α-tocophenol on arylsulphatases A and B in the livers of vitamin A deficient rats. Biochim. biophys. Acta (Amst.) **111**, 364—374 (1965).
Haslewood, G.A.D.: Bile Salts. London: Methuen 1967.
Hearse, D.J., Powell, G.M., Olavesen, A.H., Dodgson, K.S.: The influence of some physico-chemical factors on the biliary excretion of a series of structurally related aryl sulphate esters. Biochem. Pharmacol. **18**, 181—195 (1969).
Herrmann, I., Repke, K.: Konjugation von Cardenolidgeninen mit Schwefelsäure oder Glucuronsäure. Naunyn-Schmiedebergs Arch. exp. Path. Pharmak. **248**, 370—386 (1964).
Hidaka, H., Nagatsu, T., Yagi, K.: A rapid and simple assay of serotonin sulfokinase activity. Analyt. Biochem. **17**, 388—392 (1967).
— — — Formation of serotonin *O*-sulphate by sulphotransferase of rabbit liver. Biochim. biophys. Acta (Amst.) **177**, 354—357 (1969).
Hitchcock, M., Smith, J.N.: Comparative detoxication. 13. Detoxication of aromatic acids in Arachnids: arginine, glutamic acid and glutamine conjugations. Biochem. J. **93**, 392—400 (1964).
Hodson, R.C., Schiff, J.A.: Preparation of adenosine 3′-phosphate 5′-phosphosulfate (PAPS). An improved enzymatic method using *Chlorella pyrenoidosa*. Arch. Biochem. Biophys. **132**, 151—156 (1969).
Holcenberg, J.S., Rosen, S.W.: Enzymatic sulfation of steroids by bovine tissues. Arch. Biochem. Biophys. **110**, 551—557 (1965).
Hutchins, R.F.N., Kaplanis, J.N.: Sterol sulfates in an insect. Steroids **13**, 605—614 (1969).
Irreverre, F., Mudd, S.H., Heizer, W.D., Laster, L.: Sulfite oxidase deficiency. Studies of a patient with mental retardation, dislocated ocular lenses, and abnormal urinary excretion of *S*-sulfo-L-cysteine, sulfite and thiosulfate. Biochem. Med. **1**, 187—217 (1967).
Keller, H., Blennemann, H.: Modell aktiver Transportleistung mit enzymatischer Steuerung der Energietransformation aus ATP. Hoppe-Seylers Z. physiol. Chem. **324**, 134—146 (1961).
Kent, P.W., Pasternak, C.A.: Sulphate activation by intestinal mucosa enzymes. Proc. IV Int. Cong. Biochem. 4—74 (1958).
Kice, J.L., Anderson, J.M.: The mechanism of the acid hydrolysis of sodium aryl sulfates. J. Amer. chem. Soc. 88, 5242—5245 (1966).
Kodicek, E., Loewi, G.: The uptake of [^{35}S] sulphate by mucopolysaccharides of granulation tissue. Proc. roy. Soc. B **144**, 100—115 (1955).
Koizumi, T., Suematsu, T., Kawasaki, A., Hiramatsu, K., Iwabori, N.: Synthesis and degradation of active sulfate in liver. Biochim. biophys. Acta (Amst.) **184**, 106—113 (1969).
Law, G.L., Mansfield, G.P., Muggleton, D.F., Parnell, E.W.: Dimetridazole: absorption, excretion and metabolism in turkeys. Nature (Lond.) **197**, 1024—1025 (1963).
Levi, A.S., Geller, S., Root, D.M., Wolf, G.: The effect of vitamin A and other dietary constituents on the activity of adenosine triphosphate sulphurylase. Biochem. J. **109**, 69—74 (1968).
— Wolf, G.: Purification and properties of the enzyme ATP-sulfurylase and its relation to vitamin A. Biochim. biophys. Acta (Amst.) **178**, 262—282 (1969).
Levitz, M., Katz, J., Twombly, G.H.: The biosynthesis of labeled estriol-3-sulfate-16-glucosiduronate. Steroids **6**, 553—559 (1966).
Mathur, R.S., Common, R.H., Collins, D.C., Layne, D.S.: Steroid estrogen conjugates of hen's urine. Formation *in vivo* of steroid estrogen monosulphates and disulphates from injected estradiol-17β. Biochim. biophys. Acta (Amst.) **176**, 394—402 (1969).

MATTOCK, P., BARFORD, D.J., BASFORD, J.M., JONES, J.G.: The effect of substrate concentration and pH on the enzymic sulphation of *L*-tyrosyl derivatives. Biochem. J. **116**, 805—810 (1970).
— JONES, J.G.: Partial purification and properties of an enzyme from rat liver that catalyses the sulphation of *L*-tyrosyl derivatives. Biochem. J. **116**, 797—803 (1970).
MEAD, C.G., FINAMORE, F.J.: The occurrence of ascorbic acid sulfate in the brine shrimp, *Artemia salina*. Biochemistry **8**, 2652—2655 (1969).
MEHL, E., JATZKEWITZ, H.: Evidence for the genetic block in metachromatic leucodystrophy. Biochem. biophys. Res. Commun. **19**, 407—411 (1965).
MILLIGAN, B., SWAN, J.M.: Bunte salts. Rev. Pure appl. Chem. **12**, 72—94 (1962).
MIYAZAKI, M., YOSHIZAWA, I., FISHMAN, J.: Directive *O*-methylation of oestrogen catechol sulfates. Biochemistry **8**, 1669—1672 (1969).
MUKHERJI, B., BACHHAWAT, B.K.: Role of vitamin A in sulphate metabolism. Part II and III. Indian J. Biochem. **3**, 1—4 and 4—6 (1966).
MUMMA, R.O.: Ascorbic acid sulfate as a sulfating agent. Biochim. biophys. Acta (Amst.) **165**, 571—573 (1968).
NOSE, Y., LIPMANN, F.: Separation of steroid sulfokinases. J. biol. Chem. **233**, 1348—1351 (1958).
OSUNTOKUN, B.: An ataxic neuropathy in Nigeria. Brain **91**, 215—248 (1968).
PALMER, R.H.: The formation of bile and sulfates. A new pathway of bile acid metabolism in humans. Proc. nat. Acad. Sci. (Wash.) **58**, 1047—1050 (1967).
PANIKKAR, K.R., BACHHAWAT, B.K.: Purification and properties of ATP-sulphate adenylyltransferase from liver. Biochim. biophys. Acta (Amst.) **151**, 725—727 (1968).
PARKE, D.V. (1952). Quoted by WILLIAMS (1959).
PERCY, A.K., MUDD, S.H., IRREVERRE, F., LASTER, L.: Sulfite oxidase deficiency. Sulfate esters in tissues and urine. Biochem. Med. **2**, 198—208 (1968).
PETERS, H.: N^1-sulfato-N^2-isonicotinyl hydrazine. A potential metabolite of Isoniazid. J. med. pharm. Chem. **12**, 702—703 (1969).
ROBBINS, P.W.: Sulfate-activating enzymes. Meth. Enzymol. **5**, 964—977 (1962).
— Enzymatic synthesis of adenosine-5′-phosphosulfate. J. biol. Chem. **233**, 686—690 (1958b).
— LIPMANN, F.: Separation of the two enzymatic phases in active sulfate synthesis. J. biol. Chem. **233**, 681—685 (1958a).
ROBINSON, H.C.: The reduction of inorganic sulphate to inorganic sulphite in the small intestine of the rat. Biochem. J. **94**, 687—691 (1965).
ROELS, O.A.: In: The Vitamins, 2nd Vol. 1. New York: Academic Press 1967.
— TROUT, M., GUHA, A.: The effect of vitamin A deficiency and dietary α-tocopherol on the stability of rat liver lysosomes. Biochem. J. **97**, 353—359 (1965).
ROTH, J.S., HILTON, S.: The effect of whole-body X-irradiation on the distribution of acid deoxyribonuclease and β-glactosidase in subcellular fractions of rat spleen. Radiat. Res. **19**, 42—49 (1963).
ROY, A.B.: The enzymic synthesis of steroid sulphates. Biochem. J. **63**, 294—300 (1956).
— Comparative studies on the liver sulphatases. Biochem. J. **68**, 519—528 (1958).
— The enzymic synthesis of aryl sulphamates. Biochem. J. **74**, 49—56 (1960a).
— The synthesis and hydrolysis of sulfate esters. Advanc. Enzymol. **22**, 205—235 (1960b).
— The enzymic synthesis of aryl sulphamates. 2. The effect of 3β-methoxyandrost-5-en-17-one on arylamine sulphokinase. Biochem. J. **79**, 253—261 (1961).
— The enzymic synthesis of aryl sulphamates. 3. The specificity and mechanism of the activation of rat-liver arylamine sulphokinase by 17-oxosteroids. Biochem. J. **82**, 66—71 (1962).
— The arylsulphatases and some related enzymes in the livers of some lower vertebrates. Aust. J. exp. Biol. med. Sci. **41**, 331—342 (1963).
— Possible allosteric effects with arylamine sulphokinase. J. molec. Biol. **10**, 176—179 (1964).
— BANERJEE, R.K.: The steroid sulphotransferases. Proc. 2nd Int. Cong. Hormonal Steroids, Excerpta Medica International Congress Series no. **132**, 397—403 (1967).
— TRUDINGER, P.A.: The biochemistry of inorganic compounds of sulphur. Cambridge: University Press 1970.
SALMON, W.D., DAUGHADAY, W.H.: A hormonally controlled serum factor which stimulates sulfate incorporation by cartilage *in vitro*. J. Lab. clin. Med. **49**, 825—836 (1957).
SASAKI, S.: The PAPS synthetic enzyme system in granulation tissue. Clin. chim. Acta **17**, 215—217 (1967).
SCHNEIDER, J.J., LEWBART, M.L.: Enzymatic synthesis of steroid sulfates. J. biol. Chem. **222**, 787—794 (1956).
SHIPLE, G.J., MULDOON, J.A., SHERWIN, C.P.: The formation of ethereal sulfates. J. biol. Chem. **60**, 59—67 (1924).

Slotkin, T. A., Distefano, V., Au, W. Y. W.: Blood levels and urinary excretion of harmine and its metabolites in man and rats. J. pharm. exp. Therap. **173**, 26—30 (1970).
Smith, J. N.: The comparative metabolism of xenobiotics. Advanc. comp. Physiol. Biochem. **3**, 173—232 (1968).
Smith, P. A. S.: Ketoxime-*O*-sulfonic acids. J. Amer. chem. Soc. **70**, 323—326 (1948).
Spencer, B.: Endogenous sulphate acceptors in rat liver. Biochem. J. **77**, 294—304 (1960).
— Raftery, J.: Sulphate activation and sulphotransferase in foetal guinea-pigs and in developing hen's eggs. Biochem. J. **99**, 35P (1966).
Spolter, L., Rice, L. I., Yamada, R., Marx, W.: Stimulation of sulfate activation by nicotinamide-adenine dinucleotide in presence of mastocytoma fractions free of mitochondria. Biochem. Pharmacol. **16**, 229—232 (1967).
Steinhardt, J., Beychock, S.: Interaction of proteins with hydrogen ions and other small ions and molecules. In: The Proteins, vol. 2, 2nd ed., pp. 139—304. New York: Academic Press 1964.
Subba Rao, K., Ganguly, J.: Studies on metabolism of vitamin A. 6. The effect of vitamin A deficiency on the activation of sulphate and its transfer to p-nitrophenol in rat liver. Biochem. J. **90**, 104—109 (1964).
— Sastry, P. S., Ganguly, J.: Studies on metabolism of vitamin A. 2. Enzymic synthesis and hydrolysis of phenolic sulphates in vitamin-A-deficient rats. Biochem. J. **87**, 312—317 (1963).
Sundaresan, P. R.: Vitamin A and the sulfate-activating enzymes. Biochim. biophys. Acta (Amst.) **113**, 95—109 (1966).
Suzuki, S., Strominger, J.: Enzymatic sulfation of mucopolysaccharides in hen oviduct. J. biol. Chem. **235**, 257—276 (1960).
Tappel, A. L., Sawant, P. L., Shibko, S.: In: Lysosomes. Distribution in animals, hydrolytic capacity and other properties. London: Churchill 1963.
Varandani, P. T., Wolf, G., Johnson, B. C.: Function of vitamin A in the synthesis of 3'-phosphoadenosine-5'-phosphosulphate. Biochem. biophys. Res. Commun. **3**, 97—100 (1960).
Vestermark, A., Boström, H.: Studies on ester sulfates. 1. Application of two-dimensional paper chromatography in studies on the biosynthesis of ester sulfates. Acta chem. scand. **13**, 827—830 (1959a).
— — Studies on ester sulfates. V. On the enzymatic formation of ester sulfates of primary aliphatic alcohols. Exp. Cell Res. **18**, 174—177 (1959b).
— — On the sulphurylation of mono-, di- and trihydric phenols. Experientia (Basel) **16**, 408 (1960a).
— — On the enzymatic formation of ester sulphates of aliphatic polyols. Acta chem. scand. **13**, 2133 (1960b).
Wang, D. Y., Bulbrook, R. D.: Binding of the sulphate esters of dehydroepiandrosterone, testosterone, 17-acetoxypregnenolone and pregnenolone in the plasma of man, rabbit and rat. J. Endocr. **39**, 405—413 (1967).
Wellers, G.: La sulfoconjugaison des phenols *in vivo* et son mecanisme. Prod. pharm. **15**, 307—316 (1960).
— Boelle, G.: Recherches sur la sulfoconjugaison de l'indol. VI. L'utilisation du soufre de la methionine et de la cysteine et la non-utilisation du soufre des sulfates mineraux *in vivo* par le rat adulte. Arch. int. Physiol. Biochim. **68**, 299—313 (1960).
— Chevan, J.: Recherches sur la metabolisme du soufre. J. Physiol. (Paris) **51**, 723—748 (1959).
Wengle, B.: Studies on ester sulphates. 17. Sulphate-conjugation in extracts of foetal and juvenile rat liver. Acta Soc. Med. upsalien **68**, 154—166 (1963).
— Studies on ester sulphates. 16. Use of ^{35}S-labelled inorganic sulphate for quantitative studies of sulphate conjugation in liver extracts. Acta chem. scand. **18**, 65—76 (1964).
— Distribution of some steroid sulphokinases in foetal human tissues. Acta endocr. (Kbh.) **52**, 607—618 (1966).
— Boström, H.: Studies in ester sulphates. 14. The *in vitro* formation of steroid disulphates in rat liver extracts. Acta chem. scand. **17**, 1203—1217 (1963).
Wheldrake, J. F., Pasternak, C. A.: The control of sulphate activation in bacteria. Biochem. J. **96**, 276—280 (1965).
Wieland, H., Vocke, F.: Über die Giftstoffe der japanischen Kröte. Justus Liebigs Ann. Chem. **481**, 215—232 (1930).
Williams, R. T.: Detoxication Mechanisms. London: Chapman Hall 1959.
Wilson, L. G., Bandurski, R. S.: Enzymatic reactions involving sulfate, sulfite, selenate and molybdate. J. biol. Chem. **233**, 975—981 (1958).

WORTMAN, B.: Enzymic sulfation of corneal mucopolysaccharides by beef cornea epithelial extract. J. biol. Chem. **236**, 974—978 (1961).
YAGI, T.: Isopropylsulfuric acid in chick embryos. Biochim. biophys. Acta (Amst.) **82**, 170—172 (1964).
— Sulfate esters in developing eggs. J. Biochem. (Tokyo) **59**, 495—500 (1966).
YOSHIZAWA, I., FISHMAN, J.: Conjugation of 2-hydroxyoestrone in man. J. clin. Endocr. **29**, 1123—1125 (1969).
ZALKIN, H., TAPPEL, A.L., CALDWELL, K.A., SHIBKO, S., DESAI, I.D., HOLLIDAY, T.A.: Increased lysosomal enzymes in muscular dystrophy of vitamin E-deficient rabbits. J. biol. Chem. **237**, 2678—2682 (1962).

Chapter 54

Acetylating, Deacetylating and Amino Acid Conjugating Enzymes

WENDELL W. WEBER[1]

With 3 Figures

Foreign compounds, including many different amines and carboxylic acids, undergo acylation in mammalian species and, in the process, are converted to amide conjugates prior to excretion. Acylation reactions are catalyzed by enzymes (acyltransferases) which are specific for the foreign compound and involve coenzyme A (CoA-SH) derivatives. These reactions are of two general types. In the first type, foreign amines are acylated by acetyl-S-CoA to form acetylated derivatives:

$$CH_3CO{-}S{-}CoA + R{-}NH_2 \xrightarrow{\text{N-acetyltransferase}} CoA{-}SH + R{-}NH{-}COCH_3$$

In the second type, foreign carboxylic acids are converted in the presence of ATP and CoA to acyl-S-CoA derivatives which acylate glycine or another endogenous amino acid:

$$CoA{-}SH + R{-}COOH \xrightarrow[\text{ATP}]{\text{Activating enzyme}} R{-}CO{-}S{-}CoA + H_2O$$

$$R{-}CO{-}S{-}CoA + H_2NCH_2COOH \xrightarrow{\text{Acyltransferase}} CoA{-}SH + R{-}CO{-}HNCH_2COOH$$

The properties of the acyltransferases which catalyze these reactions in mammalian tissues and the factors which modify their activity will be discussed in this chapter. Enzymes which catalyze the acetylation of drugs and other foreign compounds will be considered first, and discussion of deacetylating enzymes will be included with them.

A. Acetylation and Deacetylation Enzymes

Acetylation of NH_2, OH and SH groups can occur *in vivo*, but only a few examples of acetylation of OH (e.g. choline) and SH (e.g. coenzyme A) normally occur in mammalian species. No examples of acetylation of these groups in foreign compounds appear to be known (WILLIAMS, 1967). Acetylation of the NH_2 group of foreign compounds, however, occurs frequently and the enzymes which catalyze the acetylation of aryl amines, hydrazines and certain aliphatic amines have been the subject of numerous investigations.

Following the discovery by MARSHALL et al. (1937) and FULLER (1937) that man and rabbit were capable of acetylating the aryl NH_2 group of sulfanilamide (N^4-acetylation), KLEIN and HARRIS (1938) showed by an *in vitro* technique with

1 Career Scientist of the Health Research Council of the City of New York, Contract I-441.

rabbit liver slices that the liver was a major site of this reaction. The properties of the acetylating enzyme, however, were first investigated in cell free preparations by LIPMANN (1945) in his pioneering studies on the acetylation mechanism in pigeon and rabbit liver homogenates. The requirement for a coenzyme A derivative, ultimately shown to be acetyl coenzyme A, as an essential cofactor of the enzyme was established. Partially purified preparations of the pigeon liver enzyme were noted to have a broad specificity for acetyl acceptor substrates, including sulfonamides (other than sulfanilamide), *p*-aminobenzoic acid, numerous other aryl amines, and histamine (LIPMANN, 1945; TABOR et al., 1953). The enzyme, found in the soluble portion of the cell, was shown to have a broad pH range of activity and to contain essential sulfhydryl groups. This acyltransferase is called acetyl coenzyme A: arylamine N-acetyltransferase (E.C. 2.3.1.5).

Early studies of arylamine acetylation in human volunteers and in animals showed that large differences in the capacity to excrete acetylated derivatives of foreign amines existed between the species (WILLIAMS, 1967). The rabbit, for example, has a relatively high capacity to excrete sulfanilamide in the form of N^4-acetylsulfanilamide, while man has a moderate capacity to carry out this process compared to other mammalian species. At the lower end of the spectrum are the dog and fox, which have little or no capacity to acetylate sulfanilamide in the N^4 position. These two species, however, acetylate the sulfamoyl group of sulfanilamide and excrete N^1-acetylsulfanilamide. From findings of this sort, the existence of different N-acetyltransferases has been suggested to account for such differences in the excretion patterns of the acetylated metabolites of sulfanilamide in different species (WILLIAMS, 1967). Study of N^1-acetylation has proven to be more difficult than N^4-acetylation, and consequently the properties of N^1-acetyltransferases have not been investigated by *in vitro* techniques.

Attempts to determine the site and distribution of arylamine acetylation in tissues indicated at first that acetylating activity was perhaps confined to liver (KLEIN and HARRIS, 1938). Later, with acetyl coenzyme A generating systems and still later with purified preparations of this cofactor, it was possible to demonstrate acetylation in many different tissues from man and other animals that excrete acetylated amines. These studies show, as will be described more fully later, that the level of acetylating activity in different tissues from an individual varies greatly, and that different patterns of activity are found with different substrates, such as sulfamethazine and *p*-aminobenzoic acid, when a series of such tissues is examined (HEARSE and WEBER, 1970). To account for these findings various investigators have proposed the existence of more than one N-acetyltransferase in tissues from a single species (MOTULSKY, 1964; EVANS and WHITE, 1964; HEARSE and WEBER, 1970). Attempts to determine the cellular sites responsible for acetylation have also yielded some interesting findings; studies with relatively homogenous cell populations isolated from rabbit liver indicate that acetylation of sulfanilamide and *p*-aminobenzoic acid is a property of reticuloendothelial cells and not of hepatic parenchymal cells (GOVIER, 1965). It has also been noted in other studies that gastrointestinal tract tissue acetylates sulfamethazine in rabbits (HEARSE and WEBER, 1970), and isoniazid (INH) in humans (JENNE, 1965); these activities appear to be associated with mucosal (epithelial) elements and not with supporting connective and muscle tissue. Although it remains to be shown conclusively, one might anticipate from these findings that several types of cells will be found to contain arylamine N-acetyltransferase activity and that different types of cells may contain different N-acetyltransferases.

Recent studies in man and in certain other species of mammals have shown that genetic and developmental factors are important modifiers of the rate and pattern of drug acetylation. Isoniazid (INH), various sulfonamides, and several other structurally related drugs, including hydralazine and *p*-diaminodiphenylsulfone, undergo acetylation prior to excretion. The rate of acetylation of these drugs is low in the early stages of rabbit development (COHEN and WEBER, 1968) and in human adults is subject to wide variation between individuals; this variation has been shown to be correlated in man and rabbit with the variation in activity of liver N-acetyltransferase (EVANS and WHITE, 1964; FRYMOYER and JACOX, 1963b). In mature individuals, the level of liver N-acetyltransferase activity has been shown to be genetically determined in both man (KALOW, 1962) and rabbit (FRYMOYER and JACOX, 1963a), and it is well known that individuals of both species can be classified as either "rapid" or "slow" acetylators (inactivators) of INH. EVANS et al. (1960) have shown for man that this inherited trait is transmitted by two autosomal alleles and that the slow acetylator is homozygous for the recessive slow allele. The same conclusions have been reached for the mode of inheritance of this trait in rabbit (FRYMOYER and JACOX, 1963a). In humans, slow acetylators have been noted to be much more susceptible to INH toxicity than rapid acetylators (HUGHES et al., 1954; DEVADATTA et al., 1960); it has also been shown that slow acetylators are likely to be especially susceptible to adverse effects from other drugs which are inactivated by acetylation, such as phenelzine (EVANS et al., 1965), hydralazine (PERRY et al., 1967), and *p*-diaminodiphenylsulfone (PETERS et al., 1970). Slow acetylators also appear to be predisposed in certain unexpected ways to adverse drug-drug interactions; for example, some develop diphenylhydantoin intoxication while receiving this drug in combination with INH (KUTT et al., 1966; BRENNAN et al., 1968). The importance of the acetylation polymorphism, as this trait is now usually termed, to an understanding of adverse drug reactions and drug-drug interactions in man is clearly brought out by these examples.

Within the past few years attempts to understand how species differences and various other genetic and environmental factors result in differences in the acetylating capacity of individuals have greatly stimulated the biochemical study of mammalian arylamine drug acetylating enzymes. Most of the previous studies were concerned with the pigeon liver enzyme, but much of the recent information about acetylating enzymes has been acquired through the study of the acetylation of INH and other compounds by human and rabbit liver N-acetyltransferase. This information will be emphasized in the discussion which follows. It should be pointed out that several other enzymes that catalyze the transfer of the acetyl group to aromatic amines have been described in addition to the acetyl coenzyme A: arylamine N-acetyltransferase described here. FRANZ and KRISCH (1968) have isolated and characterized, from pig liver, pig kidney, and bovine liver, three carboxyl esterases (E.C. 3.1.1.) which enzymatically acetylate aromatic amines such as aniline and *p*-phenetidin. BOOTH (1966) has characterized an N-acetyltransferase in rat tissues that transfers the acetyl group from N-hydroxyacetamidoaryl compounds (hydroxamic acids) to arylamines. The evidence indicates that none of these enzymes is identical with the N-acetyltransferase under consideration here and no further reference to them will be made.

1. Acetylator Phenotyping

Knowledge of the acetylator phenotype of an individual is sometimes useful and phenotyping methods are available for both man and animals. Humans can be classified as rapid or slow acetylators with either INH or sulfamethazine according to techniques developed by EVANS (EVANS et al., 1965; EVANS, 1969). The INH technique uses the concentration of free INH remaining in the blood 6 hours after ingestion of a test dose of the drug to determine the acetylator phenotype of an individual; the sulfamethazine method uses the ratio of free to acetylated sulfamethazine excreted in the urine over an 8 hour period as the basis for such classification. SCOTT has shown that the half-life of INH in the blood may also be used to discriminate the two phenotypes (SCOTT et al., 1969). Rabbits may be classified as rapid or slow acetylators on the basis of the half-life of free sulfadiazine in the blood determined according to the method of FRYMOYER and JACOX (1963b).

2. Assay Methods for N-Acetyltransferase in Mammalian Tissues

Activity levels of the enzyme can be measured *in vitro* by colorimetric, spectrophotometric and isotopic procedures. For precise determination of N-acetyltransferase activity, purified acetyl coenzyme A is required rather than an acetyl coenzyme A generating system, since the initial rate of the acetylation reaction depends upon the initial concentration of this cofactor (WEBER, 1970). A method has also been developed which uses N,S-diacetylcysteamine instead of acetyl coenzyme A as the acetyl donor (GOEDDE et al., 1967). A number of arylamines and other compounds have been used as acetyl acceptor substrates. Drugs used for this purpose include INH, several sulfonamides (sulfamethazine, sulfadiazine, and sulfanilamide), *p*-aminosalicylic acid, and hydralazine; various other compounds which have been used include *p*-aminobenzoic acid, aniline, and aminophenol (WEBER et al., 1968).

Colorimetric assay methods that have been used for quantitative study of N-acetyltransferase activity are based upon the well known Bratton-Marshall diazotization procedure (BRATTON and MARSHALL, 1939). This technique for color development can be used with a variety of primary arylamines. Methods based upon this technique have the advantage of rapidity and good sensitivity. They are suitable for studying the enzyme in crude tissue homogenates, as well as in more highly purified preparations of the enzyme. The technique can also be readily adapted to microassay methods. Specific tests, based upon the Bratton-Marshall procedure for measuring N-acetyltransferase activity in tissue preparations, have used either sulfamethazine or sulfadiazine as the drug substrate (WEBER, 1970). Either of these compounds can be replaced by other sulfonamides or by *p*-aminobenzoic acid; with slight modifications the procedure may be used with other primary aryl amines, such as *p*-aminosalicylic acid (MARSHALL, 1948) and aniline (BRODIE and AXELROD, 1948). Colorimetric procedures for INH (MAHER et al., 1957) and hydralazine (SHULERT, 1961), which have been used for acetylation studies have also been described. A disadvantage of all these colorimetric methods is their nonspecificity. Since the acetylated drug is not diazotized in these procedures, it is determined indirectly as the disappearance of free drug after the reaction. Thus, other methods that are specific for the isolation and identification of the acetylated product must be used for this purpose.

Several spectrophotometric methods are available which are suitable for following the acetylation reaction continuously. One of these methods uses INH as the acetyl acceptor substrate and depends on the change in absorbance at 303 mμ to measure the formation of the reaction product, acetyl-INH (2-acetyl-1-isonicotinyl hydrazide) (JENNE and BOYER, 1962). This method has been used with partially purified N-acetyltransferase preparations obtained from liver of pigeon (JENNE and BOYER, 1962); a modification of the original method has been used to assay N-acetyltransferase from a number of mammalian species including man, monkey, rabbit and rat (WEBER et al., 1968). Another spectrophotometric procedure, which employs *p*-aminobenzoic acid as the substrate, has been used to determine N-acetyltransferase activity in studies of the pigeon liver enzyme

(TABOR et al., 1953). This method can also be used with other compounds (e.g., aniline) for study of purified preparations of mammalian enzyme. Still another spectrophotometric procedure uses DTNB (5,5′-dithio-(2-nitrobenzoic acid)) to detect the appearance of thiol groups in coenzyme A, a product of the acetylation reaction (WEBER and COHEN, 1968). This reagent reacts rapidly and stoichiometrically at pH 8.0 with the thiol group according to the following equations:

$$\text{AcCoA} + \text{Drug} \longrightarrow \text{CoASH} + \text{Acetylated drug}$$
$$\text{CoASH} + \text{DTNB} \longrightarrow \text{CoA—S—S—MTNB} + \text{MTNB}$$

The monothio-nitrobenzoic acid, MTNB, which is an anion at pH 8.0, absorbs strongly at 412 mμ and has a molar extinction coefficient of 13,600 (ELLMAN, 1959). Another reagent, DTDP (4,4′dithio-dipyridine), which reacts with thiol groups in the same manner as DTNB, yields an anion with a molar extinction coefficient of 19,900 at 324 mμ (GRASSETTI and MURRAY, 1967). Thiol groups can be determined over a wider pH range with the latter reagent than with DTNB. Since both DTNB and DTDP also react with sulfhydryl groups in protein, use of these reagents is limited to study of N-acetyltransferase activity in extensively purified preparations of the enzyme.

Isotopic methods which use 1-^{14}C-AcCoA or labeled substrates with other markers (e.g. ^{3}H-aniline) have also been developed and used in the author's laboratory (STEINBERG et al., 1969; STEINBERG, 1970). These methods involve incubation of the enzyme in the presence of the isotopic substrate, followed by isolation and quantitative determination of the labeled acetylated product. Isolation of the acetylated product from other labeled components in the assay can usually be done efficiently by chromatography on regular or ion-exchange paper. High specificity and the small quantity of enzyme required are the main advantages of this technique.

3. Properties of Mammalian Liver N-Acetyltransferase

N-Acetyltransferase obtained from livers of mature individuals of various species of mammals including man, monkey (cynomolgous), rabbit, and rat has been purified 300—500 fold from the 100,000 g supernatant fraction (WEBER and COHEN, 1967; WEBER et al., 1968); it has also been purified from monkey (rhesus) liver by a somewhat different procedure (GOEDDE et al., 1967). The most highly purified preparations of the enzyme retain about 80% of their activity for 4-5 days when stored at pH 7.2 in the presence of 0.001 M EDTA at 4°. Sucrose-gradient studies indicate the enzyme has a sedimentation coefficient of 2.84, which corresponds to a molecular weight of approximately 37,000 (BAUMGARTNER et al., private communication). The enzyme is relatively unstable below pH 6.5. The pH for optimum activity and the shape of the pH-activity curve both vary with the acetyl acceptor substrate; e.g. with sulfamethazine there is a broad optimal pH range between 5.7 and 7.4 but the activity with INH and with sulfanilamide, on the other hand, varies little between pH 5 and 9. With sulfadiazine the optimal pH is 5.7 and activity drops rapidly to either side of this pH. From the pH dependency of N-acetyltransferase activity with these compounds *in vitro* (WEBER and COHEN, 1967) and *in vivo* (SMITH and WILLIAMS, 1948), it appears that the enzyme interacts preferentially with the uncharged form of the substrate.

N-Acetyltransferase from all species studied has a broad substrate specificity. It catalyzes the acetylation of drugs and foreign compounds which contain an NH_2 group attached either directly or via a carbonyl group to unsaturated rings. Human liver has been shown to catalyze the acetylation of 4-aminoantipyrine, aniline, *p*-aminobenzoic acid, *p*-aminosalicylic acid, furfurylamine, *p*-phenetidin, sulfamerazine, sulfamethazine, sulfanilamide, INH, and hydralazine. Several investigators have noted that N-acetyltransferase preparations from various mammalian species can catalyze the acetylation of non-arylamines such as 5-hydroxytryptamine and histamine (WEISSBACH et al., 1960; STEINBERG et al., 1969; SCHLOOT et al., 1969; WHITE et al., 1969). In the rabbit the acetylation of 5-hydroxytryptamine and INH both appear to be catalyzed by the same acetylating enzyme, since it was not possible to separate the two acetylating activities through extensive purification; moreover, the relative rates of acetylation of 5-hydroxytryptamine and INH were substantially the same in enzyme preparations obtained from rabbits which were rapid and slow acetylators (STEINBERG et al., 1969). In contrast to these findings for rabbit, EVANS and his associates (WHITE et al., 1969) have found for man that the rate of acetylation of 5-hydroxytryptamine does not correlate with the rate of acetylation of INH or sulfamethazine in partially purified human liver enzyme preparations. Although this species difference between rabbit and man is not understood, the findings suggest that the human enzyme preparation may contain an N-acetyltransferase activity other than that which is responsible for acetylating INH and sulfamethazine (see below: Evidence for Multiple N-Acetyltransferases). Mammalian liver N-Acetyltransferase does not acetylate *p*-nitroaniline (GOEDDE et al., 1967; WEBER, 1970) and thus appears to differ in at least one respect from the pigeon liver enzyme (TABOR et al., 1953). Furthermore, it does not acetylate cyclohexamine, glucosamine, pyridoxamine, phenylalanine, anthranilic acid, or glutamine (STEINBERG, 1970). Inhibition of N-acetyltransferase activity by *p*-chloromercuribenzoate or by N-ethylmaleimide coupled with inhibition by various metals (Cu^+, Zn^{++}, Mn^{++}, and Ni^{++}) indicate that sulfhydryl groups are essential for catalytic function of the enzyme. Electrophoretic studies on starch and on polyacrylamide/agarose gels indicate that N-acetyltransferase activity is distributed between two major bands of protein (SZABADI and WEBER, unpublished observations).

4. Mechanism of Acetylation

The mechanism of acetylation catalyzed by INH N-acetyltransferase has been shown to be a two-step process involving the formation and breakdown of an

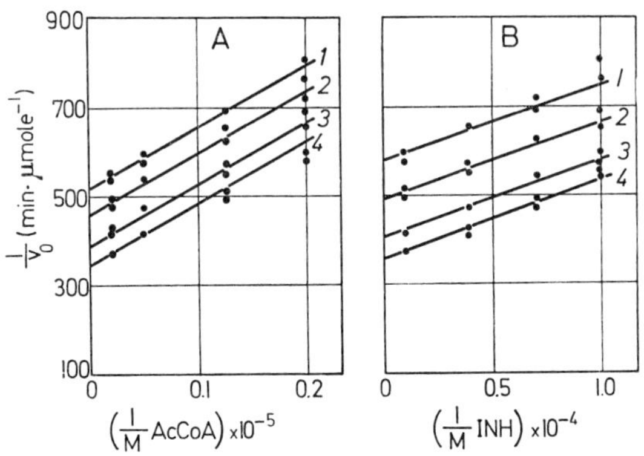

Fig. 1. Initial velocity patterns with human liver N-acetyltransferase from a rapid inactivator. *A*. AcCoA as the variable substrate. INH concentration: Line 1, 0.1×10^{-3}M; line 2, 0.14×10^{-3}M; line 3, 0.25×10^{-3}M and line 4, 1.0×10^{-3}M. *B*. INH as the variable substrate. AcCoA concentration: Line 1, 0.05×10^{-3}M; line 2, 0.08×10^{-3}M; line 3, 0.20×10^{-3}M and line 4, 0.50×10^{-3}M. The enzyme preparation used was the DEAE-cellulose fraction (0.34 mg protein/ml). Reaction velocities were determined by assay with 5,5′-dithio (*p*-nitrobenzoic acid) at pH 8.0 (WEBER and COHEN, 1968). The initial velocity was calculated as μmoles AcINH formed/min/ml DEAE-cellulose fraction. From STEINBERG (1970)

acetylated enzyme intermediate. This concept was proposed initially by BESSMAN and LIPMANN from their work on acetylation with the pigeon liver enzyme (BESSMAN and LIPMANN, 1953), and was later put forward by others (JENNE and BOYER, 1962). Relatively recently, however, an approach to the analysis of complex enzymatic processes based on initial velocity, product inhibition and isotope exchange techniques has been developed (CLELAND, 1968). Application of these techniques to the study of acetylation of aryl amines and hydrazine compounds by mammalian liver enzyme led to the proposal that acetylation proceeds according to a "ping-pong Bi-Bi" mechanism (WEBER and COHEN, 1967; WEBER and COHEN, 1968; STEINBERG, 1970). Initial velocity and product inhibition patterns from a typical study of this type on the acetylation of INH by human liver INH N-acetyltransferase are shown in Figs. 1 and 2. Results of exchange reactions between AcCoA and ^{3}H-CoA in the absence of an amine substrate and between ^{3}H-aniline and acetanilide in the absence of AcCoA are shown in Fig. 3. It can be seen that the initial velocity studies yielded families of parallel lines (Fig. 1). The patterns of inhibition by each of the products of the reaction, CoA and AcINH, were as follows (Fig. 2):

Product inhibitor	*Variable substrate*	*Inhibition pattern found*
CoA	AcCoA	Non-competitive
CoA	INH	Competitive
AcINH	AcCoA	Competitive

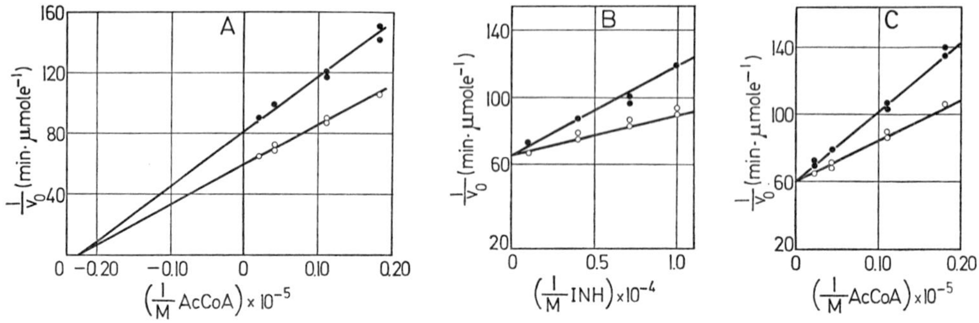

Fig. 2. Product inhibition studies with human liver N-acetyltransferase from a rapid inactivator. Assays were made up in a total volume of 0.20 ml in 0.1 M potassium phosphate buffer, pH 7.0, 10^{-3}M EDTA. The INH and acetyl-INH (AcINH) were dissolved in this buffer. The AcCoA used was prepared by diluting 1-^{14}C-AcCoA (45.0 mC/mmole) with unlabeled AcCoA so that one-fifth of the total AcCoA was labeled. When INH and AcCoA were used as the fixed substrate, their concentrations in the assay were 10^{-3}M and 2×10^{-4}M respectively. The enzyme preparation was the DEAE-cellulose fraction (75 μg protein/assay) and each reaction mixture was incubated at 27°. *A*. AcCoA as the variable substrate (○); in the presence of CoA (10^{-3}M) as inhibitor (●); *B*. INH as the variable substrate (○); in the presence of CoA (2×10^{-3}M) as inhibitor (●); *C*. AcCoA as the variable substrate (○); in the presence of AcINH (5×10^{-4}M) as inhibitor (●). From STEINBERG (1970)

Also, the liver N-acetyltransferase was capable of reversibly catalyzing each exchange reaction in the absence of the other substrate-product pair. It should be noted that although each of these reactions is reversible, the overall reaction appears to proceed only toward the formation of acetylated drug. These findings fulfill the

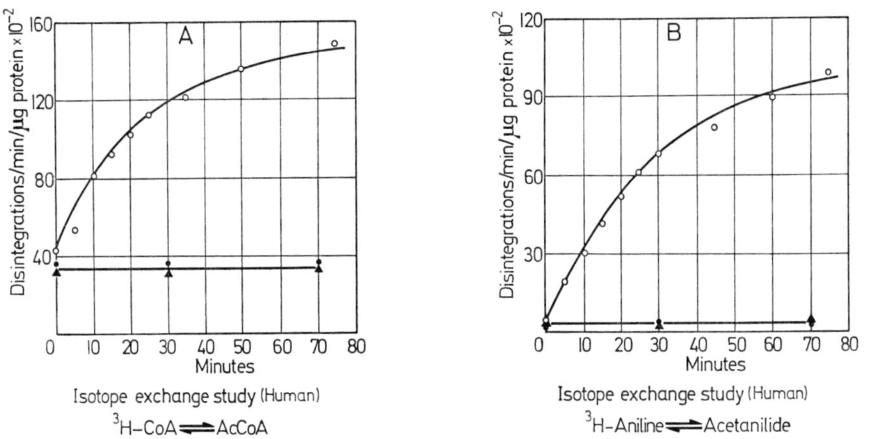

Fig. 3. Exchange reactions. A. Between AcCoA and ^{3}H-CoA. The reaction mixture contained 0.01 ml of ^{3}H-CoA solution (0.027 μmoles), 0.07 ml of 4×10^{-2}M AcCoA (2.8 μmoles) prepared in water, 0.10 ml of DEAE-cellulose enzyme fraction (30 μg protein) from a rapid inactivator human and 0.8 M potassium borate buffer, pH 8.0 in a total volume of 0.27 ml at 27°. Aliquots of 0.02 ml were removed and immediately mixed with 0.05 ml of 3×10^{-3}M DTNB dissolved in 0.05 M sodium acetate buffer, pH 5.0 (0.15 μmoles) at 4° to stop the reaction. Aliquots of 0.01 ml were then removed from this mixture, and the Ac-^{3}H-CoA was separated from the ^{3}H-CoA on DEAE-cellulose ion-exchange paper. The Ac-^{3}H-CoA area was cut out, placed in a counting vial, eluted with 0.02 ml of 0.6 N HCl and counted. Complete reaction mixture (○); mixture without AcCoA (●); mixture with enzyme previously inactivated by heating at 55° for 15 min (▲). B. Between ^{3}H-aniline and acetanilide. INH and AcINH could not be used to demonstrate this reaction since isotopically labeled INH of adequate purity was not available. The reaction mixture contained 0.005 ml of ^{3}H-aniline dissolved in water (115 mC/mmole, 0.0019 μmoles), 0.20 ml of 3×10^{-2}M acetanilide dissolved in 0.1 M sodium pyrophosphate buffer, pH 8.0 (6.0 μmoles), 0.10 ml of DEAE-cellulose enzyme fraction from a rapid inactivator human (30 μg protein) and 0.10 M sodium pyrophosphate buffer, pH 8.0, in a total volume of 0.305 ml at 27°. Aliquots of 0.01 ml were removed, placed on CM-cellulose strips, and treated with 0.005 ml of acetone-absolute ethanol (1:1) to stop the reaction. The ^{3}H-acetanilide was separated from the ^{3}H-aniline by eluting the strips with glycine buffer at pH 2.8. The ^{3}H-acetanilide area was cut out, placed in a counting vial, eluted with 0.20 ml of 0.6 N HCl and counted. Complete reaction mixture (○); mixture without acetanilide (●); mixture with enzyme previously inactivated by heating at 55° for 15 min (▲). From STEINBERG (1970)

minimal criteria expected for a ping-pong Bi-Bi reaction mechanism. Acetylation of INH by this mechanism may be written as follows:

$$\begin{array}{ccccccc} & \text{AcCoA} & \text{CoA} & & \text{INH} & \text{AcINH} & \\ & \downarrow & \uparrow & & \downarrow & \uparrow & \\ \hline \text{NAT} & & & \text{AcNAT} & & & \text{NAT} \end{array}$$

or as two partial reactions:

$$\text{NAT} + \text{AcCoA} \rightleftarrows \text{AcNAT} + \text{CoA—SH}$$

$$\text{AcNAT} + \text{INH} \rightleftarrows \text{AcINH} + \text{NAT}$$

where NAT is N-acetyltransferase and AcNAT represents the acetylated enzyme intermediate formed in the first reaction and utilized in the second with regeneration of the enzyme. The existence of an acetylated enzyme intermediate capable of transferring acetyl groups to INH has also been demonstrated (STEINBERG, 1970). In addition, the enzyme has also been shown to be capable of catalyzing transacetylation, i.e. acetyl group transfer between such compounds as aniline and AcINH.

The equation which describes the initial velocity (v_o) of INH acetylation can be written in double reciprocal form as follows:

$$\frac{1}{v_o} = \frac{1}{V} + \frac{K_m, AcCoA}{V} \frac{1}{(AcCoA)} + \frac{K_m, INH}{V} \frac{1}{(INH)}$$

where V is the maximum velocity of the reaction when AcCoA and INH are both at infinite concentration, and K_m is the limiting apparent Michaelis constant for each substrate, i.e. the concentration of one substrate which half saturates the enzyme in the presence of an infinite concentration of the other substrate. Limiting values of the apparent Michaelis constants for AcCoA and INH are given in Table 1 for man, monkey, rabbit and rat. The values for each of these substances do not differ significantly from each other between the species.

Table 1. *Limiting values of the apparent K_m,AcCoA and K_m,INH determined with liver N-acetyltransferase from 4 mammalian species*

	K_m,AcCoA (M) × 10^5	K_m,INH (M) × 10^5
Human	3.9	5.8
Monkey	2.7	10.4
Rabbit	2.0	18.2
Rat	2.2	6.0

For the same four species values of the ratio of the apparent K_m for other acetyl acceptor substrates to the K_m for INH are given in Table 2. The values for hydralazine and aniline do not differ greatly between these species, but those for *p*-aminosalicylic acid, sulfamethazine, and *p*-phenetidin are much greater for the human and monkey enzyme than for the rabbit and rat enzyme. The fact that this functional difference occurs only with substrates which have substituents on the aromatic ring para to the group which is acetylated may be an expression of an underlying molecular difference between the primate and rodent enzymes, but this remains to be proven.

Table 2. $\frac{K_m,\text{Substrate}}{K_m,\text{INH}}$ *determined with liver N-acetyltransferase from four mammalian species*

Substrate	Human	Monkey	Rabbit	Rat
INH	1.0	1.0	1.0	1.0
p-Aminosalicylic acid	6.3	4.3	0.042	0.039
Sulfamethazine	1.5	0.59	0.048	0.12
Hydralazine	0.50	0.34	0.41	0.11
p-Phenetidin	0.15	0.18	0.001	0.0008
Aniline	0.04	0.02	0.03	0.11

5. Comparison of Liver N-Acetyltransferases from Rapid and Slow INH Acetylators

Comparative studies of the properties of partially purified liver N-acetyltransferase from rapid and slow acetylators of both man (JENNE, 1965; WEBER et al., 1968; STEINBERG, 1970) and rabbit (WEBER et al., 1968) have been carried out using the techniques described above. The total N-acetyltransferase activity contained in the liver of a rapid acetylator is estimated to be at least an order of magnitude greater than in the liver of a slow acetylator. Despite such a large difference, no definite evidence has been obtained which would point to a qualitative difference between enzymes from the two acetylator phenotypes in either species. These enzymes can be purified by the same procedure and their pH characteristics, heat stability, kinetic properties, and specificity for a variety of drug substrates and other compounds are indistinguishable (JENNE, 1965; WEBER et al., 1968; STEINBERG, 1970); moreover, initial velocity patterns and product inhibition studies suggest that acetylation is carried out by the same mechanism by the enzyme from both phenotypes (WEBER et al., 1968; STEINBERG, 1970). In addition, the possibility that an inhibitor of N-acetyltransferase is present in liver preparations of slow acetylators appears unlikely (JENNE, 1965). Thus, the difference in levels of N-acetyltransferase activity in liver of the two INH acetylator phenotypes is not yet accounted for and further investigation is needed. Although the presence of a subtle functional or structural difference between these enzymes has not been excluded, it seems more likely from the evidence accumulated so far that the difference between the acetylator phenotypes may be due to a difference in liver N-acetyltransferase content, resulting from a difference in either the rate of formation or degradation of the same enzyme.

6. Comparison of Liver N-Acetyltransferases from Adult and Developing Rabbits

The enzyme has also been partially purified from livers of developing rabbits by means of the purification procedure already mentioned (WEBER, 1970). The level of activity per gram of liver is only about 3—5% of the adult level in 6 day old rabbits, 20% in 14 day old rabbits, 16% in 20 day old rabbits and reaches adult levels at about 1 month of age. Comparative studies of the properties of the enzyme from immature and adult rabbits indicate, in contrast to the findings described in the previous paragraph, that the developmental variation in acetylating capacity may be associated with a "fetal" form of N-acetyltransferase (COHEN and WEBER, 1968). This form of the enzyme has been found to be more heat labile than the adult enzyme and to have a limiting value for the K_m for INH which is approximately one-third that obtained for the adult enzyme (BAUMGARTNER, STEINBERG and COHEN, private communication). A transition from the "fetal" form to the adult form appears to occur during the third week after birth, when the N-acetyltransferase activity is relatively constant.

7. Evidence for Multiple N-Acetyltransferases

From *in vitro* studies of the acetylating capacity of mammalian tissues, several investigators have obtained evidence suggesting that these tissues contain more than one N-acetyltransferase. The capacity of homogenates prepared from human liver to acetylate INH, sulfamethazine, and hydralazine are quite similar to each other, but bear no relation to their capacity to acetylate *p*-aminobenzoic acid, sulfanilamide and *p*-aminosalicylic acid (EVANS and WHITE, 1964; JENNE, 1965). Also, the data on acetylation of *p*-aminosalicylic acid in red cell homogenates indicates that the red cell activity is not concordant with the INH acetylator phenotype (MOTULSKY and STEINMAN 1962; MOTULSKY, 1964). Observations made on the excretion patterns of INH, sulfamethazine and sulfanilamide (PETERS et al., 1965) and of *p*-aminosalicylic acid (JENNE, 1965) in human volunteers appear to substantiate these *in vitro* findings (PETERS et al., 1965).

Additional evidence has been obtained recently for N-acetyltransferase multiplicity from systemic *in vivo* studies of N-acetylation in rapid and slow acetylator rabbits and from *in vitro* studies with various tissues from these animals (HEARSE and WEBER, 1970; HEARSE et al., 1970). It has been shown in a rabbit population that while sulfamethazine acetylating capacity is bimodally distributed, *p*-aminobenzoic acid acetylating activity is unimodal. Analogous findings in the rabbit have been noted previously by FRYMOYER and JACOX (1963b) for sulfadiazine and *p*-aminosalicylic acid. *In vitro* tissue distribution studies in the rabbit further revealed a wide distribution of *p*-aminobenzoic acid and sulfamethazine acetylating activities throughout the body. Moreover, the sulfamethazine acetylating activity of partially purified N-acetyltransferase preparations from different rabbits was found to vary by several thousand fold, while that for *p*-aminobenzoic acid remained high and relatively constant. A large tissue-to-tissue variation in the ratio of sulfamethazine/*p*-aminobenzoic acid acetylating activity was also found. These findings strongly suggest the presence of two or more acetylating enzymes in differing proportions in certain rabbit tissues. One of these enzymes, INH N-acetyltransferase which is responsible for sulfamethazine acetylation, is dependent upon the INH acetylator phenotype and has a level of activity which fluctuates widely between individuals; another which is primarily responsible for the acetylation of *p*-aminobenzoic acid is independent of the INH acetylator phenotype and appears to be subject to relatively little variation between individuals. The properties of the two activities are very similar but appear to differ in pH and stability characteristics; a partial separation has been achieved (HEARSE et al., 1970).

8. Deacetylation Enzymes

Enzymes which split N-acetyl arylacetamido compounds to the unconjugated form according to the following reaction:

$$R\text{—}NH\text{—}COCH_3 + H_2O \longrightarrow RNH_2 + CH_3COOH$$

belong to the general class of arylacylamide amidohydrolases (E.C. 3.5.1.13). They are sometimes referred to more briefly as arylacylamidases. The discussion which follows will deal with specific amidases of this class which are capable of hydrolyzing arylacetamido compounds, such as acetanilide, N^4-acetylsulfonamides, and *p*-acetamidobenzoic acid, into their arylamines.

Several investigators have obtained evidence that deacetylation of aryl acetamido compounds occurs in the intact animal (WILLIAMS, 1959). A summary of information on such compounds is given in Table 3. KREBS et al. (1947) showed that N^4-acetylsulfamethazine was deacetylated to a considerable extent by the pigeon, dog, and cat, but that man and rabbit were unable to hydrolyze this acetyl compound in significant quantities. Similar results have been obtained by others for man and for rabbit as the table indicates. Although some arylacetamido compounds appear to undergo slight hydrolysis ($< 5\%$ of the dose) in the rabbit, this conversion seems to be accounted for by spontaneous hydrolysis (KREBS et al., 1947). Recently, a series of systematic studies on acetylation and deacetylation have been carried out by PETERS and his associates (GORDON et al., 1969; GORDON et al., 1970; PETERS et al., 1970; PETERS, private communication) on animals and man as indicated in Table 3. These studies have brought out some rather striking species differences in the deacetylation of N^4-acetylsulfamethazine between Old World (rhesus) and New World (squirrel) monkeys. After receiving an injection of N^4-acetylsulfamethazine, the squirrel monkey deacetylated this compound, as shown by both plasma and urine assays. In contrast, rhesus monkey was found to

Table 3. *In vivo deacetylation of arylacetamido compounds in various species*

Species	Arylacetamido Compound	*In vivo* Deacetylation Observed	Reference
Pigeon . .	N^4-acetylsulfamethazine	+	KREBS et al. (1947)
Chicken . .	N^1-acetylsulfanilamide	+	BRIDGES and WILLIAMS (1963)
	N^4-acetylsulfanilamide	+	BRIDGES and WILLIAMS (1963)
Dog	N^4-acetylsulfamethazine	+	KREBS et al. (1947)
Cat	N^4-acetylsulfamethazine	+	KREBS et al. (1947)
Rat	Acetanilide, Phenacetin	+	ELSON et al. (1946)
Mouse . . .	Monoacetyldiaminodiphenylsulfone	+	GORDON et al. (1970)
Rabbit . .	N^1-acetylsulfanilamide	—	BRIDGES and WILLIAMS (1963)
	N^4-acetylsulfanilamide	—	SMITH and WILLIAMS (1948)
	N^4-acetylsulfadiazine	—	SMITH and WILLIAMS (1948)
	N^4-acetylsulfamerazine	—	SMITH and WILLIAMS (1948)
	N^4-acetylsulfamethazine	—	SMITH and WILLIAMS (1948)
	N^4-acetylsulfapyrazine	—	SMITH and WILLIAMS (1948)
	N^4-acetylsulfathiazole	—	SMITH and WILLIAMS (1948)
	Acetanilide	—	SMITH and WILLIAMS (1948)
	Phenacetin	—	SMITH and WILLIAMS (1948)
	p-Acetamidobenzoic acid	—	SMITH and WILLIAMS (1948)
	p-Acetamidophenol	—	SMITH and WILLIAMS (1948)
	p-Acetamidophenylacetic acid	—	SMITH and WILLIAMS (1948)
	Monoacetyldiaminodiphenylsulfone	—	GORDON et al. (1970)
Rhesus monkey	N^4-acetylsulfamethazine	—	GORDON et al. (1969)
	Monoacetyldiaminodiphenylsulfone	—	GORDON et al. (1970)
Squirrel monkey	N^4-acetylsulfamethazine	+	GORDON et al. (1969)
	Monoacetyldiaminodiphenylsulfone	+	GORDON et al. (1970)
Man	N^4-acetylsulfamethazine	—	SYKES (1944); KREBS et al. (1947); PETERS (1970)
	Monoacetyldiaminodiphenylsulfone	+	GORDON et al. (1970)

resemble man and rabbit since it did not deacetylate N^4-acetylsulfamethazine. Studies with diaminodiphenylsulfone and its monoacetyl derivative, monoacetaminodiphenylsulfone, have also been carried out by these investigators on various animal species and man. Their findings on primates show that the rhesus monkey does not deacetylate monoacetyldiaminodiphenylsulfone but that both squirrel monkey and man do deacetylate it. Thus, the occurrence of deacetylation even within a species, as these findings show for man, may or may not be evident depending upon the acetylated compound which is used for the test.

Deacetylation of arylacetamido compounds has also been observed *in vitro*. MICHEL et al. (1937) were first to note that hydrolysis of acetanilide occurred in the presence of homogenates of several rat tissues but especially in those of kidney and liver; the presence of deacetylase activity was also found in liver of dog, cat, rabbit and ox. KOHL and FLYNN (1940) observed deacetylation by extracts of rat liver of N-acetylsulfanilamide and various other N-acylsulfanilamides, including 4:4′-acetylaminodiphenylsulfone and acetanilide. BIETER et al. (1941) noted the occurrence of deacetylation of acetylsulfonamides in their studies on chicken kidney and other tissues. KREBS et al. (1947) demonstrated that pigeon liver and sheep kidney cortex, liver, and intestinal mucosa contained an active deacetylase for various acetamidosulfonamides at pH 7.3. BRAY et al. (1949, 1950) studied the action of liver and kidney deacetylase extracts from a variety of mammalian species on acetanilide, acetyl-glycine and various other N-acylated compounds. They concluded on the basis of different responses of the activity in these preparations toward acetanilide and acetylglycine during treatment with various organic solvents and with heat, that the deacetylase for acetanilide was different from that for acetyl-glycine. SHAFFER and BIETER (1950) found that chicken kidney contained a heat labile enzyme which was capable of converting N^4-acetylsulfonamides to their deacetylated forms, and in further studies with this tissue, NIMMO-SMITH (1960) reported that chick kidney rapidly deacylated acetanilide and a number of acylanilides, and that the activity for these substrates was associated with mitochondrial fractions. Further studies of the activity in mitochondrial suspensions showed that deacylation was most rapid at pH 7.3 at 44° and was inhibited by heavy metals and by *p*-chloromercuribenzoate. Inhibition with the latter compound was partially reversible with the sulfhydryl protecting agents, glutathione and cysteine. The optimum N-acyl group substitution was found to be either an acetyl or propionyl group; substitution in the para position of acetanilide resulted in an increase in the relative rate of deacetylation and a decrease in the apparent K_m. These mitochondrial suspensions also deacetylated *p*-acetamidobenzoic acid, N^4-acetylsulfanilamide, and phenacetin. Although this enzyme appeared to be absent from mitochondria of kidney and liver of a number of mammalian species, N-acetanilide deacetylase activity has been noted quite recently by other investigators in different subcellular fractions isolated from mammalian kidney (FRANKLIN et al., 1969). Acetanilide deacetylase activity was noted to be present mainly in the microsomes of this tissue, although its characteristics were not further described. Some acetanilide deacetylase activity was also found in the soluble fraction from rat kidney. Of greater interest, however, is the finding that this fraction also deacetylated *p*-acetamidobenzoic acid to a greater extent than acetanilide, but did not deacetylate N^4-acetylsulfanilamide. These observations suggest that more than one arylacetamido deacetylase may exist in rat kidney, perhaps in different subcellular compartments, and that partial separation of different deacetylases may have been achieved. Additional studies with the *p*-acetamidobenzoic acid deacetylase activity in the soluble fraction revealed the presence of two types of activity, one dependent on the Mn^{+2} concentration and the other independent of this metal ion. These observations were interpreted as evidence that soluble rat kidney deacetylase may possess two active sites.

Thus there is ample evidence that arylacetamido deacetylating activity occurs in intact animals of various species and is associated with several different tissues. In all species studied, it seems to be primarily localized in the kidney and in liver. It is evident that wide differences in the levels of deacetylating activity may exist not only between species (KREBS et al., 1947; BRIDGES and WILLIAMS, 1963) and within different strains of the same species (GORDON et al., 1969), but also occurs within the same species for different acetyl derivatives. Moreover, variation between individuals of the same species must also occur, but not enough data are available for any one species to establish this. It also appears that tissues from various species of birds, such as chicken and pigeon, possess higher levels of arylacetamido deacetylase activity than do tissues of mammals, although the data from which this conclusion is drawn is rather sparse. Only a few *in vitro* studies of the biochemical properties of deacetylating enzymes have been carried out, and these have been done with either crude tissue homogenates and extracts prepared from various species, or with subcellular preparations which have not been fractionated further. Among these studies, several have provided suggestive evidence for the existence of different deacetylases. The data of FRANKLIN et al. (1969), referred to in the previous paragraph, provide the most recent evidence for this possibility as well as interesting new information about the properties of deacetylases. Procedures for separating individual deacetylating enzymes, however, have not been reported in detail. Moreover, their biochemical properties and the factors which alter their activity have not been elucidated.

9. Comments on Evaluating the Relative Importance of Acetylating and Deacetylating Enzymes in Different Species

It is apparent from the foregoing discussion on N-acetylating and N-deacetylating enzyme systems in various species that these are independent systems which act in opposition to each other. Whenever they occur in the same individual, the problem arises of evaluating their relative importance in determining the extent to which foreign arylamines are excreted as acetyl conjugates.

Species diversity for both of these enzyme systems is evidently so broad that either one or the other may be absent, or if present may be inoperative in the intact individual. The dog, for example, has been shown to possess an active deacetylase system; as already mentioned in another connection, this species has little or no capacity to excrete foreign amines as acetylated derivatives and has been found to be deficient in an active liver N-acetyltransferase (LEIBMAN and ANACLERIO, 1962). The reverse situation appears to exist in the rabbit, particularly the rapid acetylator, which has a very active acetylating enzyme system in its tissues and a correspondingly high capacity to excrete foreign amines as acetylated derivatives, but lacks an operative deacetylating system. This condition in rabbit also appears to exist in man for N^4-acetylsulfamethazine. Thus, whenever only one of the two opposing enzyme systems is functional, the problem of predicting the extent of acetylation of a particular arylamine is somewhat simplified. It should be pointed out that this prediction may still be rather difficult; acetylation of an arylamine may vary with the structure and other properties of the compound and is subject to modification by genetic, developmental and various other environmental factors. A great deal of information, however, is now known about the effects of these factors on acetylation, which frequently permits such predictions to be made with a fair degree of confidence.

The investigations of KREBS et al. (1947) appear to be the only systematic study on record that has attempted to evaluate the relative importance of acetylation and deacetylation in animal species having functional systems of both kinds in their tissues. Carrying out correlative studies on intact animals and *in vitro* studies on tissues obtained from animals of the same species, they concluded that the degree of acetylation of various sulfonamides depended on both acetylating and deacetylating systems. Although their quantitative data with tissues were not in good agreement with this concept, their *in vitro* studies were conducted with crude, rather unstable enzyme preparations. They also observed that the activity in their deacetylating systems was dependent upon factors, such as the presence of an inhibitor in sheep kidney suspensions, which they did not study in detail. It is possible that the problems they encountered in the *in vitro* studies may at least partially account for discrepancies between their *in vivo* and *in vitro* data. Since then, various studies have been conducted in intact animals to obtain information about the extent of acetylation of different arylamines, but these studies provide very little insight into the action of individual acetylation and deacetylation systems which operate in tissues of the body. Also, much remains to be learned about the biochemical properties of deacetylation enzymes, although some advances toward understanding their complex nature have been made recently. Another important but little known area concerns the effects of genetic and environmental factors which may modify deacetylating activity in individuals, such as those discussed in relation to the acetylation enzymes. As further information in each of these areas becomes available about both of these enzyme systems, and particularly about deacetylating systems, it should be possible to evaluate their action and their relative importance in various species.

B. Amino Acid Conjugating Enzymes

Acylation reactions also include conjugation of aromatic carboxylic acids with the α-amino group of certain amino acids including glycine, glutamine, cysteine and ornithine. Glycine and glutamine conjugating enzyme systems are surveyed in the following discussion and cysteine conjugation is discussed elsewhere in this volume (Chapter 55). Ornithine conjugation, which so far has been found only in birds and reptiles, is of less direct interest and will not be discussed in detail (WILLIAMS, 1959).

Following Lipmann's fundamental work on coenzyme A, rapid progress was made in the identification of glycine acylating activity in tissues and in the determination of its distribution and other properties. With a view toward studying peptide bond synthesis in model systems, COHEN and MCGILVERY (1946) observed the condensation of *p*-aminobenzoic acid and glycine to form *p*-aminobenzoylglycine (*p*-aminohippurate) by rat liver slices, but KIELLEY and SCHNEIDER (1950) first showed, with a cell-free preparation from mouse liver, that this condensation activity was associated with the mitochondria. From studies of the enzyme in rat liver extracts, CHANTRENNE (1950) suggested the possibility that an active coenzyme A derivative was involved in the enzymatic synthesis of hippurate. Evidence for this possibility was obtained by SCHACHTER and TAGGART (1953) who showed, in a partially purified system derived from pig kidney cortex, that benzoyl coenzyme A was utilized directly in the enzymatic synthesis of hippurate, and thus concluded that benzoic acid, and not glycine, was the activated member in the condensation of these two substances. These studies were extended to include further purification and characterization of the enzyme from beef liver mitochondria (SCHACHTER and TAGGART, 1954a, b). The series of studies by MOLDAVE and MEISTER (1957a, b, c) on the synthesis of phenylacetylglutamine by human tissues provided further understanding of the acylation of aromatic carboxylic acids and led to our present concept of this reaction. These investigators demonstrated both that coenzyme A and ATP were required for the formation of phenylacetylglutamine from phenylacetate and glutamine; they also obtained evidence which strongly indicated that phenylacetyl AMP and phenylacetyl CoA were intermediates in this process. They proposed that the enzymatic synthesis of phenylacetylglutamine consisted of three steps as follows:

(1) Phenylacetate + ATP ⟶ Phenylacetyl AMP + Pyrophosphate
(2) Phenylacetyl AMP + CoA—SH ⟶ Phenylacetyl—S—CoA + AMP
(3) Phenylacetyl—S—CoA + L-glutamine ⟶ Phenylacetylglutamine + CoA—SH.

Accordingly, they concluded that activation involved a process similar to that proposed for activation of fatty acids (JENCKS and LIPMANN, 1957), with the participation of an acyl-AMP intermediate as had been originally suggested for the acetate-activating enzyme system by BERG (1955). From the earlier evidence of SCHACHTER and TAGGART (1953) and from their own studies, MOLDAVE and MEISTER also suggested that benzoylglycine and phenylacetylglutamine were formed by similar mechanisms. Isolation and partial purification of the acetylating enzyme (acyltransferase) which catalyzes only the third reaction has been achieved (MOLDAVE and MEISTER, 1957c), but whether separate enzymes are responsible for the first two reactions has not been established.

1. Properties of the Acyl Activating Enzyme System

The properties of the activating enzyme system (reactions 1 and 2) have been studied in preparations of beef (SCHACHTER and TAGGART, 1954a) and in human and rat liver mitochondria (Moldave and Meister, 1957b, c) and are presumed to be identical with the fatty acid-activating enzyme described by Mahler et al. (1953). It should be noted that these purified preparations still possessed considerable acylating (reaction 3) activity (Moldave and Meister, 1957c). Studies with the human liver preparations showed that the acetylating enzyme catalyzed the formation of phenylacetylglutamine and phenylacetylglycine in the presence of phenylacetate, CoA-SH, ATP and either glutamine or glycine; it also catalyzed the formation of benzoylglycine from benzoate, glycine, ATP and CoA-SH. The beef and rat liver preparations catalyzed phenylacetylglutamine formation from phenylacetate CoA-SH and ATP in the presence, but not in the absence, of human acylating enzyme. Moldave and Meister suggested, therefore, that the activation of phenylacetate and benzoate might be catalyzed by enzymes from several species, but that a marked species specificity existed for the transfer of the acyl group from the acyl CoA compound to glutamine.

2. Properties of the Acyltransferases

The enzymes which catalyze reaction 3 have been found in both particulate (mitochondrial) and soluble sub-cellular fractions. Schachter and Taggart (1954a) described the 53-fold purification of a stable glycine N-acylase (E.C. 2.3.1.13) from beef liver mitochondria. This enzyme catalyzes the transfer of various aliphatic (C_2—C_{10}) and aromatic acyl CoA derivatives, including benzoate and phenylacetate, to glycine. The purified preparation showed a single peak in the analytical ultracentrifuge from which the molecular weight of the enzyme was estimated to be approximately 190,000. An electrophoretic study of the enzyme, however, showed that it consisted of two major components, one of which accounted for 70—90% of the total activity, depending upon the pH, and had the same specific activity as the original sample. Tests of the specificity of the enzyme for various acyl acceptors showed that it was specific for glycine. When the influence of pH on hippurate synthesis from benzoyl CoA was examined, a broad range for optimal activity (pH 7.3—9.7) was found.

The activity of the acylating component of this acylation system from the rat has been shown to vary with age in a pattern similar to that observed during development (Brandt, 1964). Studies using benzoyl CoA as the acyl donor substrate showed that very little glycine acyltransferase activity was present in liver of fetal and neonate animals (Brandt, 1966). By the age of weaning (20 days), activity had increased appreciably. It reached a maximum by about 30 days after birth and then decreased slightly. In the course of these studies, the glycine acyltransferase from adult rat liver was purified 780-fold from acetone powder extracts and some of its characteristics were determined (Brandt et al., 1968). Evidence obtained during purification revealed the presence of inhibiting factors in the starting material and the presence of more than one enzyme with glycine acyltransferase activity. The pH characteristics of the purified rat liver enzyme were noted to differ from those of the beef liver enzyme.

Acylating enzyme activity in human autopsy tissue has been purified about 90-fold from the soluble fraction of liver and about 50-fold from that of kidney (Moldave and Meister, 1957c). Both of these purified human acyltransferase (E.C. 2.3.1.14 phenylacetyl-CoA: L-glutamine α-N-phenylacetyltransferase) preparations catalyzed the formation of phenylacetylglutamine from phenylacetyl CoA and glutamine (reaction 3 above). These preparations also catalyzed benzoylglycine formation from benzoyl CoA and glycine and, at a relatively slow rate, the formation of phenylacetylglycine from phenylacetyl CoA and glycine, but did not catalyze the condensation of glycine with indolylacetyl CoA or with various aliphatic acyl CoA derivatives. Since the formation of phenylacetylglutamine did not occur with preparations from beef and rat liver, it was suggested that the reaction between phenylacetyl CoA and glutamine may be catalyzed specifically by human tissues and possibly also by the chimpanzee (POWER, 1936).

C. Concluding Remarks

Recent studies on the effects of inherited and developmental factors on acetylation reactions in man and animals have generated a great deal of new interest in this area of drug metabolism. As a result, considerable progress has been made toward the development of improved isolation procedures for the enzymes (N-acetyltransferases) which are responsible for these reactions and toward a description of their properties in biochemical terms. Evidence is accumulating that N-acetyltransferase activity from a single individual comprises several distinct proteins with closely related enzyme activities, a phenomenon now recognized to be very general among enzymes and other proteins, and of great importance to an understanding of their biological action (VESELL, 1968). Many problems remain in the identification and separation of these proteins with N-acetyltransferase activity, but there is also considerable promise of advancement in our understanding of acetylation processes from such investigations. The available information on deacetylation and other acylation processes is much more limited in scope. Although the importance of these processes is apparent for certain drugs and other foreign compounds, very little is known about the diversity of these enzymes in mammalian tissues, their properties, and the extent to which their actions may be influenced by genetic and environmental factors in the individual.

References

BAUMGARTNER, R., STEINBERG, M.S., COHEN, S.N.: Private communication 1970.

BERG, P.: Participation of adenyl-acetate in the acetate-activating system. J. Amer. chem. Soc. **77**, 3163—3164 (1955).

BESSMAN, S.P., LIPMANN, F.: The enzymatic transacetylation between aromatic amines. Arch. Biochem. Biophys. **46**, 252—254 (1953).

BIETER, R.N., BAKER, A.B., BEATON, J.G., SHAFFER, J.M., SEERY, T.M., ORR, B.A.: Nervous injury produced by sulfanilamide. J. Amer. med. Ass. **116**, 2231—2236 (1941).

BOOTH, J.: Acetyltransfer in arylamine metabolism. Biochem. J. **100**, 745—753 (1966).

BRANDT, I.K.: The development of the hippuric acid-synthesizing system in the rat. Develop. Biol. **10**, 202—215 (1964).

— Glycine acyltransferase activity in developing rat liver. Biochem. Pharmacol. **15**, 994—995 (1966).

— SIMMONS, P., GUTFINGER, T.: Rat liver glycine acyltransferase: Partial purification and some properties. Biochim. biophys. Acta (Amst.) **167**, 196—198 (1968).

BRATTON, A.C., MARSHALL, E.K., JR.: A new coupling component for sulfanilamide determination. J. biol. Chem. **128**, 537—550 (1939).

BRAY, H.G., JAMES, S.P., RAFFAN, I.M., RYMAN, B.E., THORPE, W.V.: The fate of certain organic acids and amides in the rabbit. 7. An amidase of rabbit liver. Biochem. J. **44**, 618—625 (1949).

— — THORPE, W.V., WASDELL, M.R.: Deacetylation of acetamido compounds by tissue extracts. Biochem. J. **47**, 483—488 (1950).

BRENNAN, R.W., DEHEJIA, H., KUTT, H., MCDOWELL, F.: Diphenylhydantoin intoxication attendant to slow inactivation of INH. Neurology **18**, 283 (1968).

BRIDGES, J.W., WILLIAMS, R.T.: Species differences in the acetylation of sulphanilamide. Biochem. J. 19P (1963).

BRODIE, B.B., AXELROD, J.: The estimation of acetanilide and its metabolic products, aniline, N-acetyl p-aminophenol and p-aminophenol (free and total conjugated) in biological fluids and tissues. J. Pharmacol. exp. Ther. **94**, 22—28 (1948).

CHANTRENNE, H.: The requirement for coenzyme A in the enzymatic synthesis of hippuric acid synthesis. J. biol. Chem. **189**, 227—233 (1950).
CLELAND, W.W.: Enzyme kinetics. Ann. Rev. Biochem. **36**, 77—112 (1968).
COHEN, P.P., McGILVERY, R.W.: Peptide bond synthesis. I. The formation of p-aminohippuric acid by rat liver slices. J. biol. Chem. **166**, 261—272 (1946).
COHEN, S.N., WEBER, W.W.: Drug conjugating enzymes in the newborn: Evidence for a "fetal" form of N-acetyltransferase in infant rabbit liver. Pharmacologist **10**, 191 (1968).
DEVADATTA, S., GANGADHARAM, P.R.J., ANDREWS, R.H., FOX, W., RAMAKRISHNAN, C.V., SELKON, J.B., VELU, S.: Peripheral neuritis due to isoniazid. Bull. Wld Hlth Org. **23**, 587—598 (1960).
ELLMAN, G.L.: Tissue sulfhydryl groups. Arch. Biochem. Biophys. **82**, 70—77 (1959).
ELSON, L.A., GOULDEN, F., WARREN, F.L.: The metabolism of aromatic amines. Biochem. J. **40**, XXIX (1946).
EVANS, D.A.P.: An improved and simplified method of detecting the acetylator phenotype. J. Med. Gen. **6**, 405—407 (1969).
— DAVISON, K., PRATT, R.T.C.: The influence of acetylator phenotype on the effects of treating depression with phenelzine. Clin. Pharmacol. Ther. **6**, 430—435 (1965).
— MANLEY, K., McKUSICK, V.A.: Genetic control of isoniazid metabolism in man. Brit. med. J. **II**, 485—491 (1960).
— WHITE, T.A.: Human acetylation polymorphism. J. Lab. clin. Med. **63**, 394—403 (1964).
FRANKLIN, M.R., BRIDGES, J.W., WILLIAMS, R.T.: The enzymic deacetylation of p-acetamido benzoic acid. Biochem. J. **114**, 6P (1969).
FRANZ, W., KRISCH, K.: Acylgruppenübertragung auf aromatische Amine durch Carboxylesterasen. Hoppe-Seylers Z. physiol. Chem. **349**, 1413—1422 (1968).
FRYMOYER, J.W., JACOX, R.F.: Investigation of the genetic control of sulfadiazine and isoniazid metabolism in the rabbit. J. Lab. clin. Med. **62**, 891—904 (1963a).
— — Studies of genetically controlled sulfadiazine acetylation in rabbit livers: Possible identification of the heterozygous trait. J. Lab. clin. Med. **62**, 905—909 (1963b).
FULLER, A.T.: Is p-aminobenzene sulphonamide the active agent in prontosil therapy? Lancet **I**, 194—198, (1937).
GOEDDE, W., SCHLOOT, W., VALESKY, A.: Individual different response to drugs: Characterisation of an INH-acetylating system in rhesus monkeys. Biochem. Pharmacol. **16**, 1793—1799 (1967).
GORDON, G.R., PETERS, J.H., GELBER, R., LEVY, L.: Metabolic disposition of dapsone (4,4'-diaminodiphenyl sulfone) in animals and man. Proc. Western Pharmacol. Soc. (in press) (1970).
— SHAFIZADEH, A.G., PETERS, J.H.: Demethylation and acetylation of drugs by rhesus and squirrel monkeys. Fed. Proc. **28**, 545 (1969).
GOVIER, W.C.: Reticuloendothelial cells as the site of sulfanilamide acetylation in the rabbit. J. Pharmacol. exp. Ther. **150**, 305—308 (1965).
GRASSETTI, D.R., MURRAY, J.F.: Determination of sulfhydryl groups with 2,2'- or 4,4'-dithiopyridine. Arch. Biochem. Biophys. **119**, 41—49 (1967).
HEARSE, D.J., SZABADI, R., WEBER, W.W.: Enzyme multiplicity in the N-acetylation of drugs. Pharmacologist (in press) (1970).
— WEBER, W.W.: Evidence for genetic and enzymic heterogeneity in the "slow" INH acetylator. Fed. Proc. **29**, 803 (1970).
HUGHES, H.B., BIEHL, J., JONES, A.P., SCHMIDT, L.H.: Metabolism of isoniazid in man as related to the occurrence of peripheral neuritis. Amer. Rev. Tuberc. **70**, 266—273 (1954).
JENCKS, W.P., LIPMANN, F.: Studies on the initial step of fatty acid activation. J. biol. Chem. **225**, 207—223 (1957).
JENNE, J.W.: Partial purification and properties of the isoniazid transacetylase in human liver. Its relationship to the acetylation of p-aminosalicylic acid. J. clin. Invest. **44**, 1992—2002 (1965).
— BOYER, P.D.: Kinetic characteristics of the acetylation of isoniazid and p-aminosalicylic acid by a liver enzyme preparation. Biochim. biophys. Acta (Amst.) **65**, 121—127 (1962).
KALOW, W.: Pharmacogenetics. Heredity and response to drugs. Philadelphia and London: W.B. Saunders Co. 1962.
KIELLEY, R.K., SCHNEIDER, W.C.: Synthesis of p-aminohippuric acid by mitrochondria of mouse liver homogenates. J. biol. Chem. **185**, 869—880 (1950).
KLEIN, J.R., HARRIS, J.S.: The acetylation of sulfanilamide *in vitro*. J. biol. Chem. **124**, 613—626 (1938).
KOHL, M.F.F., FLYNN, L.M.: Deacetylation of N^4-n-acylsulfanilamides and N^4-n-acylsulfanilylhydroxamides *in vitro*. Proc. Soc. exp. Biol. (N.Y.) **44**, 455—457 (1940).

KREBS, H.A., SYKES, W.O., BARTLEY, W.C.: Acetylation and deacetylation of the p-amino group of sulphonamide drugs in animal tissues. Biochem. J. **41**, 622—630 (1947).
KUTT, H., VEREBELY, K., McDOWELL, F.: Depression of parahydroxylation of diphenylhydantoin by anti-tuberculous therapy. Neurology **16**, 594 —602 (1966).
LEIBMAN, K.C., ANACLERIO, A.M.: Comparative studies on sulfanilamide acetylation; an inhibitor in dog liver. In: Proc. 1st Int. Pharm. Meeting, Metabolic Factors Controlling Duration of Drug Action. B.B. BRODIE and E.G. ERDOS (eds.), Vol. 6. New York: MacMillan Co. 1962.
LIPMANN, F.: Acetylation of sulfanilamide by liver homogenates and extracts. J. biol. Chem. **160**, 173—190 (1945).
MAHER, J.R., WHITNEY, J.M., CHAMBERS, J.S., STANONIS, D.J.: The quantitative determination of isoniazid and para-aminosalicylic acid in body fluids. Amer. Rev. Tuberc. **76**, 852—861 (1957).
MAHLER, H.R., WAKIL, S.J., BOCK, R.M.: Studies on fatty acid oxidation. I. Enzymatic activation of fatty acids. J. biol. Chem. **204**, 453—467 (1953).
MARSHALL, E.K., JR.: Determination of para-aminosalicylic acid in blood. Proc. Soc. exp. Biol. (N.Y.) **68**, 471—472 (1948).
— CUTTING, W.C., EMERSON, K.: Acetylation of para-aminobenzene sulfonamide in the animal organism. Science **85**, 202—203 (1937).
MICHEL, H.O., BERNHEIM, F., BERNHEIM, M.L.C.: The hydrolysis of acetanilide by various tissues. J. Pharmacol. **61**, 321—327 (1937).
MOLDAVE, K., MEISTER, A.: Enzymatic acylation of glutamine by phenylacetic acid. Biochim. biophys. Acta (Amst.) **24**, 654—655 (1957a).
— — Participation of phenylacetyladenylate in the enzymic synthesis of phenylacetylglutamine. Biochim. biophys. Acta (Amst.) **25**, 434—435 (1957b).
— — Synthesis of phenylacetylglutamine by human tissue. J. biol. Chem. **229**, 463—476 (1957c).
MOTULSKY, A.: Pharmacogenetics. Chapter 2 in Progress in Medical Genetics. III. A.G. STEINBERG and A. BEARN (eds.). New York, N.Y.: Grune & Stratton 1964.
— STEINMAN, L.: Aryl amine acetylation in human red cells. J. clin. Invest. **41**, 1387 (1962).
NIMMO-SMITH, R.H.: Aromatic deacylation by chick-kidney mitochondria. Biochem. J. **75**, 284—293 (1960).
PERRY, H.M., JR., SAKAMOTO, A., TAN, E.M.: Relationship of acetylating enzyme to hydralazine toxicity. J. Lab. clin. Med. **70**, 1020 (1967).
PETERS, J.H.: Private communication (1970).
— GORDON, G.R., GELBER, R., LEVY, L., GLAZKO, A.J.: Polymorphic acetylation of dapsone (4,4′-diaminodiphenyl sulfone, DDS) in man. Fed. Proc. **29**, 803 (1970).
— MILLER, K.S., BROWN, P.: Studies on the metabolic basis for the genetically determined capacities for isoniazid inactivation in man. J. Pharmacol. exp. Ther. **150**, 298—304 (1965).
POWER, F.W.: Detoxication of phenylacetic acid by the chimpanzee. Proc. Soc. exp. Biol. (N.Y.) **33**, 598—600 (1936).
SCHACHTER, D., TAGGART, J.V.: Benzoyl coenzyme A and hippurate synthesis. J. biol. Chem. **203**, 925—934 (1953).
— — Glycine N-acylase: Purification and properties. J. biol. Chem. **208**, 263—275 (1954a).
— — Product inhibition in the glycine N-acylase reaction. J. biol. Chem. **211**, 271—278 (1954b).
SCHLOOT, W., TIGGES, F.J., BLAESNER, H., GOEDDE, H.W.: N-acetyltransferase and serotonin metabolism in man and other species. I. Hoppe-Seylers Z. Physiol. Chem. **350**, 1353—1361 (1969).
SCOTT, E.M., WRIGHT, R.C., WEAVER, D.D.: The discrimination of phenotypes for rate of disappearance of isonicotinyl hydrazide from serum. J. clin. Invest. **48**, 1173—1176 (1969).
SHAFFER, J.M., BIETER, R.N.: Conversion of acetylsulfonamides to the unconjugated form by the chick kidney. J. Pharmacol. **100**, 192—200 (1950).
SHULERT, A.R.: Physiological disposition of hydralazine (1-hydrazinophthalazine) and a method for its determination in biological fluids. Arch. int. Pharmacodyn. **CXXXII**, 1—15 (1961).
SMITH, J.N., WILLIAMS, R.T.: The metabolism of sulphonamides. 5. A study of the oxidation and acetylation of sulphonamide drugs and related compounds in the rabbit. Biochem. J. **42**, 351—356 (1948).
STEINBERG, M.S.: Purification and properties of human liver N-acetyltransferase from rapid and slow isoniazid inactivators. Ph.D. Thesis, New York University 1970.
— COHEN, S.N., WEBER, W.W.: Acetylation of 5-hydroxytryptamine by isoniazid N-acetyltransferase. Biochim. biophys. Acta (Amst.) **184**, 210—212 (1969).
SYKES, W.O.: Observations on the metabolism of sulphamethazine in the intact body and in isolated tissues. Biochem. J. **38**, XIX (1944).

SZABADI, R., WEBER, W.W.: Unpublished observations.
TABOR, H., MEHLER, A.H., STADTMAN, E.R.: The enzymatic acetylation of amines. J. biol. Chem. **204**, 127—138 (1953).
VESELL, E. (ed.): Multiple molecular forms of enzymes. Ann. N.Y. Acad. Sci. **151**, 1—689 (1968).
WEBER, W.W.: N-acetyltransferase (mammalian liver). In: Metabolism of amino acids and amines in Methods in Enzymology, Vol. 17B. Ed. by H. TABOR and C.W. TABOR. New York: Academic Press 1970 (in press).
— COHEN, S.N.: N-acetylation of drugs: Isolation and properties of an N-acetyltransferase from rabbit liver. Mol. Pharmacol. **3**, 266—273 (1967).
— — The mechanism of isoniazid acetylation by human N-acetyltransferase. Biochim. biophys. Acta (Amst.) **151**, 276—278 (1968).
— — STEINBERG, M.S.: Purification and properties of N-acetyltransferase from mammalian liver. Ann. N.Y. Acad. Sci. **151**, 734—741 (1968).
WEISSBACH, H., REDFIELD, B.G., AXELROD, J.: Biosynthesis of melatonin. Enzymic conversion of serotonin to N-acetyl serotonin. Biochim. biophys. Acta (Amst.) **43**, 352—353 (1960).
WHITE, T.A., JENNE, J.W., EVANS, D.A.P.: Acetylation of serotonin *in vitro* by a human N-acetyltransferase. Biochem. J. **113**, 721—725 (1969).
WILLIAMS, R.T.: Detoxication Mechanisms, 2nd edition. New York, N.Y.: John Wiley and Sons 1959.
— Comparative patterns of drug metabolism. Fed. Proc. **26**, 1029—1039 (1967).

Chapter 55

Mercapturic Acid Conjugation

E. Boyland

With 1 Figure

Baumann and Preusse (1879) and Jaffé (1879) investigated the metabolism of bromobenzene and chlorobenzene and showed that they were excreted as unstable complexes of S-(*p*-bromophenyl) acetylcysteine (1, X = Br) and S-(*p*-chlorophenyl) acetylcysteine (1, X = Cl) respectively. The structures of the complexes were not realised at the time, but the derivatives isolated after treatment with acid and other excretion products containing acetylcysteine residues are called mercapturic acids. Iodobenzene (Mills and Wood, 1953), 1:2-dichlorobenzene and 1:3; dichlorobenzene (A3003, Parke and Williams, 1955) are also excreted as the corresponding phenyl mercapturic acid derivatives (1, X = I; 2 and 3) which still contain the halogen atoms. The isomeric 1:4-dichlorbenzene does not appear to

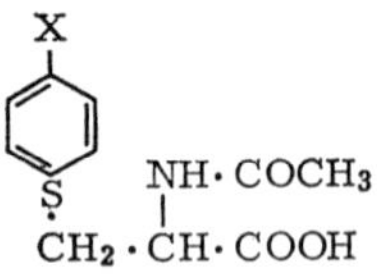

(1)

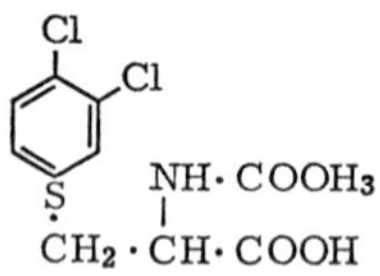

(2)

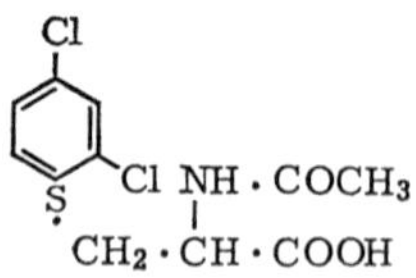

(3)

be metabolised to a mercapturic acid. In these benzene derivatives, in which the halogen residues of the original compounds are not reactive, the metabolic route is probably analogous to that of naphthalene described below; the active chemical group which reacts with the sulphydryl derivative (which eventually yields the mercapturic acid) must be introduced by some preliminary metabolic step.

Aromatic hydrocarbons are also metabolised to mercapturic acids. 1-Naphthyl mercapturic acid (4) was isolated from the acidified urine of rabbits treated with naphthalene (Bourne and Young, 1934). 1-Anthryl mercapturic acid (5) was similarly isolated by Boyland and Levi (1936), phenylmercapturic acid (6) by Zbarsky and Young (1943) and *p*-diphenylmercapturic acid (7) by West et al. (1956). Some of the compounds metabolised to mercapturic acids are listed in Table 1.

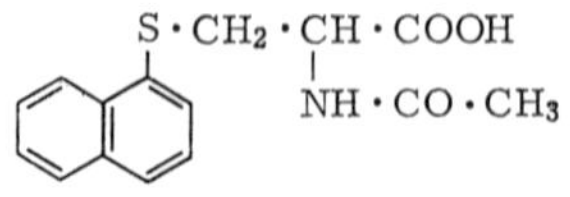

(4)

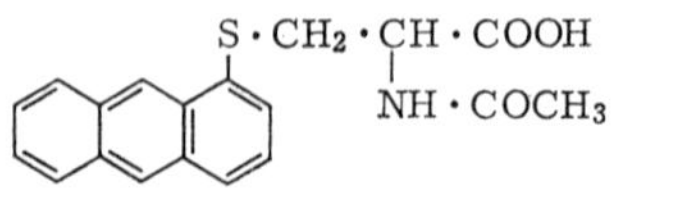

(5)

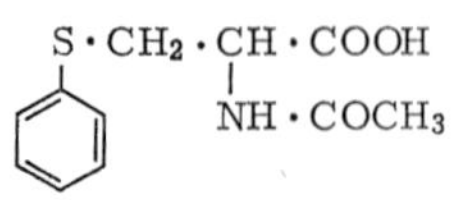

(6)

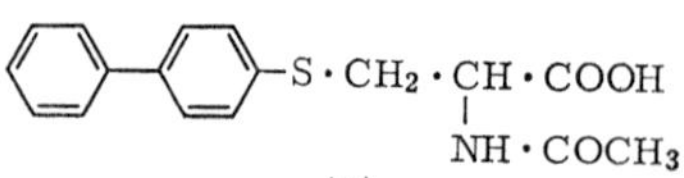

(7)

Table 1. *Mercapturic acid precursors*

Precursor	Group reacting with thiol	Reference to mercapturic acid excretion
Aromatic hydrocarbon[a]		
Benzene		ZBARSKY and YOUNG (1943b)
Naphthalene		BOURNE and YOUNG (1934)
Anthracene	Epoxide	BOYLAND and LEVI (1936)
Phenanthrene	intermediate	BOYLAND and SIMS (1962)
Benz[a]anthracene		BOYLAND and SIMS (1964a)
Styrene		JAMES and WHITE (1967)
Arylamine		
Aniline	Hydroxylamine	BOYLAND, et al., (1963)
2-Naphthylamine	intermediate	BOYLAND et al. (1963)
Acetophenetidine[b]		JAGENBURG and TOCZKO (1964)
Arylhalide[a]		
Bromobenzene		BAUMANN and PREUSSE (1879)
Chlorobenzene	Epoxide	JAFFÉ (1879)
Iodobenzene	intermediate	MILLS and WOOD (1953)
1,2-Dichlorobenzene		PARKE and WILLIAMS (1955)
1-Chloronaphthalene		CORNISH and BLOCK (1958)
Halogenonitrobenzene		
1,2-Dichloro-4-nitrobenzene	Cl	BRAY, et al., (1957a)
1-Bromo-3-chloro-6-nitrobenzene	Br	BRAY et al. (1957a)
Pentachloronitrobenzene	NO_2	BETTS, JAMES and THORPE (1955)
Aralkyl halide		
Benzyl chloride	Cl	STEKOL (1938)
Phenethyl bromide	Br	JAMES and WHITE (1967)
1-Menaphthyl chloride	Cl	HYDE and YOUNG (1965)
Aralkyl ester		
Benzyl acetate	$O\cdot CO\cdot CH_3$	CLAPP (1967)
1-Menaphthyl acetate		HYDE and YOUNG (1968)
Alkyl phenol		
3,5-Di-*tert.*-butyl-4-hydroxytoluene	H of ring-methyl	DANIEL, GAGE and JONES (1968)
Alkyl halide		
Iodomethane	I	BARNSLEY and YOUNG (1965)
Bromoethane	Br	THOMSON, MAW and YOUNG (1958)
Allyl chloride	Cl	CLAPP (1967)
Nitroalkane		
1-Nitropropane	NO_2	BRAY and JAMES (1958)
Cycloalkene[a]		
Cyclopentene	Epoxide intermediate	JAMES, WARING and WHITE (1967)
Halogenocycloalkane		
Bromocyclohexane	Br	JAMES and JEFFERY (1964)
Carboxylic acid[b]		
Maleic acid (or fumaric acid)	$\alpha\beta$-Double bond	KUWAKI and MIZUHARA (1966)
Isovaleric acid	H on α-carbon	OHMORI and MIZUHARA (1962)
Ester		
Ethyl methanesulphonate	$HO_3S\cdot CH_3$	ROBERTS and WARWICK (1958a)
Urethane	$O\cdot CO\cdot NH_2$	BOYLAND and NERY (1965)
Sulphonamide		
Benzothiazole-2-sulphonamide	$SO_2.NH_2$	COLUCCI and BUYSKE (1965)
Sulphur mustard		
Bis-β-chloroethyl sulphide[c]	Cl	DAVISON, ROZMAN and SMITH (1961)

Table 1. (Continued)

Precursor	Group reacting with thiol	Reference to mercapturic acid excretion
aβ-Unsaturated compound		
Ethacrynic acid[b]	*aβ*-Double bond	BEYER, BAER, MICHAELSON and RUSSO (1965)
Arecoline	*aβ*-Double bond	BOYLAND and NERY (1969)
Allyl acetate	*aβ*-Double bond	CLAPP, KAYE and YOUNG (1969)

[a] These compounds are first converted to an intermediate epoxide.
[b] Excreted as a cysteine conjugate.
[c] Excreted as glutathione and cysteine conjugates.

I. Sources of the Cysteine Group that have been Proposed

The cysteine for mercapturic acid formation might come from dietary protein, cysteine residues of tissue proteins, and glutathione which is present in most mammalian tissues (BOYLAND, 1938).

STEKOL (1937a—e, 1939a) showed that addition of glutathione or sulfur-containing amino acids to the diets of animals did not increase mercapturic acid formation from bromobenzene or naphthalene. BARNES and JAMES (1957) also showed that administration of cysteine, cystine, or methionine to rabbits with chlorobenzene, 1,2,3,5-tetrachloro-6-nitrobenzene, 1,2,3-trichloro-5-nitrobenzene, or benzyl chloride did not increase mercapturic acid excretion. GUTMAN and WOOD (1950) and MARSDEN and YOUNG (1958) administered [^{35}S]-cystine to rats with bromobenzene and naphthalene, and found that only a small proportion of labeled material was excreted as a mercapturic acid. BINKLEY (1949) demonstrated that the administration of bromobenzene to cystinuric dogs did not reduce excretion of cystine.

STEKOL (1939b) and MILLS and WOOD (1956) considered that the initial stage in mercapturic acid formation involved conjugation of the foreign compound with the cysteine of tissue proteins. Following oral administration of [^{131}I]-iodobenzene to the rat, labeled tissue proteins were isolated (MILLS and WOOD, 1956), but the radioactivity could have been due to adsorbed molecules not removed by washing (MILLS and WOOD, 1956). Assessment of the relative rates of liver protein synthesis and of mercapturic acid formation led BARNES et al. (1959) to conclude that tissue proteins could not provide sufficient cysteine for mercapturic acid production.

The suggestion of SHERWIN (1922) that bromobenzene was hydroxylated to *p*-bromophenol and the hydroxyl group was replaced with cysteine seems unlikely as halogenophenols are not metabolized to mercapturic acids (SPENCER and WILLIAMS, 1950). RHODE (1922) suggested that an intermediate dihydrobenzene was formed *in vivo* from bromobenzene, containing both hydroxyl and cysteine groups.

II. Glutathione as the Source of Cysteine

All three amino acids of the tripeptide glutathione (*L*-glutamyl-*L*-cysteinylglycine) are used in the metabolism of foreign compounds; phenylacetic acid is excreted as the glutamine conjugate, benzoic acid as the glycine conjugate (hippuric acid), and bromobenzene as *p*-bromophenylmercapturic acid (WAELSCH, 1930) and (BRAND and HARRIS, 1933).

NAKASHIMA (1934) showed that administration of naphthalene, which causes cataract, to rabbits depleted the glutathione content of the lens and liver. Mercapturic acid precursors decrease liver glutathione but not glutathione levels of blood, kidney or intestine (BINET and WELLERS, 1951; JOHNSON, 1965; SUGA et al., 1966b; BARNES et al., 1959); the turnover rate of glutathione in liver is sufficient to account for mercapturic acid biosynthesis.

STEKOL (1940, 1941) showed that glutathione derivatives of benzyl chloride and *p*-bromobenzyl bromide were excreted as the corresponding mercapturic acids by rats. S-ethylglutathione is excreted as ethylmercapturic acid by rats (ROBERTS and WARWICK, 1958a). FOXWELL and YOUNG (1964) isolated alkylmercapturic acids from the urine of rats dosed with different S-alkylglutathiones. Glutathione conjugates have been detected in liver after the administration of *p*-chlorobenzyl chloride (BRAY et al., 1959a) and methyl iodide (JOHNSON, 1966b). These findings indicate that conjugation of glutathione with the foreign compound is a step in mercapturic acid formation.

BOOTH et al. (1961) showed that an enzyme present in the supernatant fraction of rat liver homogenates catalyzed the conjugation of glutathione with several compounds, including some that are metabolized to mercapturic acids. This enzyme, which was first named glutathione kinase and later glutathione S-aryltransferase (GROVER and SIMS, 1964) was specific for glutathione but active towards many second substrates. COMBES and STAKELUM (1961) independently described an enzyme that catalyzed the conjugation of glutathione with sulfobromophthalein, a dye used as a test for hepatic function (ROSENTHAL and WHITE, 1924). This enzyme is possibly glutathione S-aryltransferase. A biliary metabolite considered to be the glutathione conjugate has been found in rats (COMBES, 1959) and in man (GRODSKY et al., 1959) after the administration of sulfobromophthalein.

Bile collected from rats dosed with naphthalene contained dihydroxynaphthalene conjugates of glutathione, cysteinylglycine, cysteine and *N*-acetylcysteine. Similarly, bile of rats treated with 1,2-dihydronaphthalene and 1,2-epoxy-1,2,3,4-tetrahydronaphthalene contained analogous conjugates which can be considered as derivatives of 1,2,3,4-tetrahydronaphthalene (BOYLAND et al., 1961). The γ-glutamyl-S-cysteine derivatives were not detected. These findings led BOYLAND (1962) to propose that the sequence of events in mercapturic acid biosynthesis proceeds in the following order: R-glutathione → R-cysteinylglycine → R-cysteine → R-*N*-acetylcysteine.

III. Conversion of Glutathione Conjugates into Mercapturic Acids

BRAY and FRANKLIN (1957) demonstrated that liver homogenates of rats, rabbits and guinea pigs liberated S-*p*-chlorobenzyl-L-cysteine from S-*p*-chlorobenzylglutathione, and the rate of cysteine derivative liberation was parallel to the glutathionase (γ-glutamyltransferase) activity of the preparations. BOOTH et al. (1960) have shown that the glutathione conjugate of dihydrohydroxynaphthalene was converted into the cysteine derivative by rat kidney homogenates. This probably proceeds by a transpeptidation reaction, by γ-glutamyltransferase, to give the cysteinylglycine derivative which is converted to the cysteine derivative. In rats, only the kidney and pancreas are able to transfer glutamyl residues (REVEL and BALL, 1959), but in the rabbit, all the stages of mercapturic acid formation occur in the liver. Cysteinylglycine derivatives are hydrolyzed by peptidases (i.e., cysteinylglycinase), present in rat kidney, liver and pancreas, to cysteine derivatives (BRAY et al., 1959a; BOOTH et al., 1960; SUGA et al., 1966a).

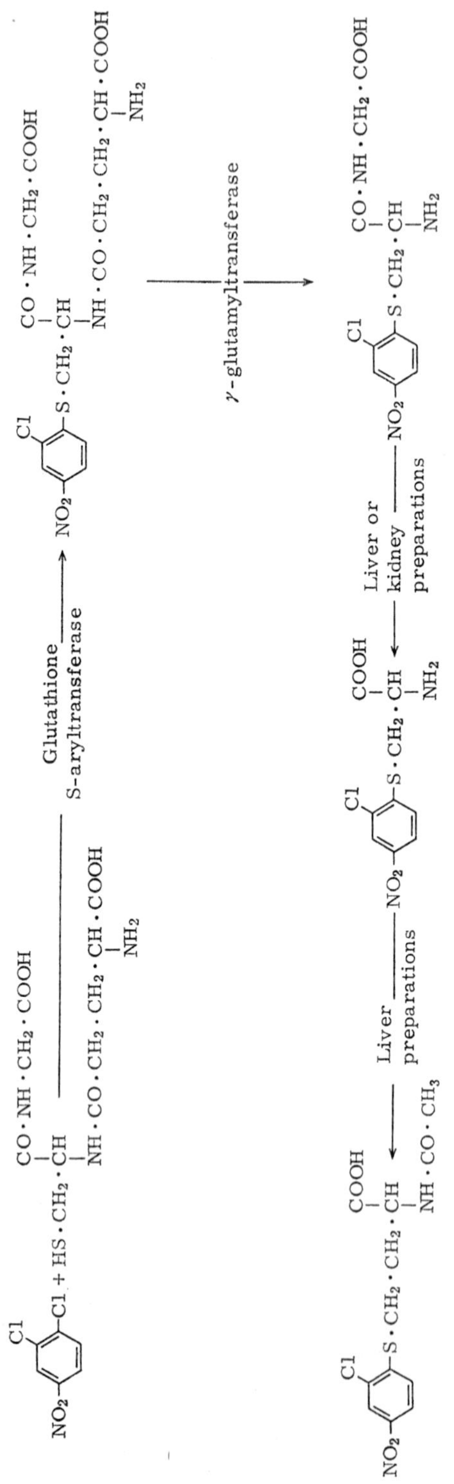

STEKOL (1938) isolated N-acetyl-S-benzylcysteine (benzylmercapturic acid) from the urine of dogs, rats and rabbits dosed with S-benzylcysteine and ZBARSKY and YOUNG (1943) isolated phenylmercapturic acid from the urine of rats following administration of S-phenylcysteine. WEST and MATHURA (1954) showed that many arylcysteines were acetylated by rats. Acetylation of the cysteine derivative which is the final stage in mercapturic acid biosynthesis has been demonstrated *in vivo* and *in vitro* with liver homogenates and with slices (GUTMAN and WOOD, 1951; WEST et al., 1951; BRAY et al., 1959b; BOOTH et al., 1960; THOMSON et al., 1963; BARNSLEY et al., 1966).

The reactions involved in the formation of a mercapturic acid from 1,2-dichloro-4-nitrobenzene are shown in Fig. 1.

IV. Glutathione S-Transferases

The initial step in mercapturic acid formation is conjugation of the foreign compound with glutathione, a reaction usually catalyzed by glutathione S-transferases. Since glutathione S-aryltransferase was described (BOOTH et al., 1961), several other glutathione S-transferases have been found: glutathione S-epoxidetransferase, catalyzing the reaction of glutathione with epoxides (BOYLAND and WILLIAMS, 1965); glutathione S-alkyltransferase, catalyzing the S-alkylation of alkyl halides (JOHNSON, 1966a); and several glutathione S-alkenetransferases catalyzing the reaction of glutathione with $\alpha\beta$-unsaturated compounds (BOYLAND and CHASSEAUD, 1967, 1968).

The reaction of glutathione with some compounds is negligible at neutral pH and 37° C in the presence or absence of an enzyme. Other com-

Fig. 1. Mercapturic acid formation from 1,2-dichloro-4-nitrobenzene

pounds react nonenzymatically with glutathione, although the rate is increased by the addition of enzyme (BOOTH et al., 1961; JOHNSON, 1966a; BOYLAND and CHASSEAUD, 1968). In some cases the reaction of mercapturic acid precursors with glutathione is unaffected by rat liver supernatant, and conjugate formation apparently takes place nonenzymically; arecoline, an alkaloid present in betel nuts is an example of such a substance (BOYLAND and NERY, 1969).

V. Glutathione S-Aryltransferase

Glutathione S-aryltransferase was first described by BOOTH et al. (1961) who showed that it catalyzed the reaction of 1,2-dichloro-4-nitrobenzene with glutathione. This enzyme present in the supernatant fraction of rat liver homogenates had a broad pH optimum about pH 8.0. Glutathione S-aryltransferase occurs in the livers of many vertebrates (GROVER and SIMS, 1964; WIT and LEEUWANGH, 1969); as shown with rats, however, only small amounts of the enzyme are present in other organs.

1,2-Dichloro-4-nitrobenzene (cf. Fig. 1) is particularly suitable for the estimation of glutathione S-aryltransferase because on conjugation with glutathione the peak in the absorption spectrum of the nitrobenzene derivative changes to a longer wavelength (280—350 mμ) (BOOTH et al., 1961). Measurement of absorption at 350 mμ gives a direct reading of the enzymic reaction. Other glutathione S-transferases are generally estimated by measuring loss of glutathione (BOYLAND and WILLIAMS, 1965; JOHNSON, 1966a; BOYLAND and CHASSEAUD, 1967), release of labile groups (AL-KASSAB et al., 1963; BOYLAND and WILLIAMS, 1965; JOHNSON, 1966a), or by chromatography (SUGA et al., 1967).

Glutathione S-aryltransferase appears to catalyze reactions of glutathione with aromatic and other cyclic compounds containing labile halogen or nitro groups. Compounds of this type, which are metabolized to mercapturic acids in rabbits include mono-, di-, and trihalogenonitrobenzenes (BRAY et al., 1955a, b, 1956, 1957a, 1958a) and certain tetrahalogenonitrobenzenes that are metabolized (BRAY et al., 1953; BETTS et al., 1955) by replacement of nitro groups (AL-KASSAB et al., 1963). The nitro group is also replaced in certain trihalogenonitrobenzenes and in pentahalogenonitrobenzene (BETTS et al., 1955; BETTS et al., 1957). No mercapturic acid is formed from 1,3-dichloro-2-nitrobenzene (BRAY et al., 1957b). The reactivity of groups in the aromatic ring is governed by electronic and steric effects exerted by neighbouring groups. Lability of the halogen or nitro groups during alkaline hydrolysis *in vitro* is related to mercapturic acid formation *in vivo* (BETTS et al.,

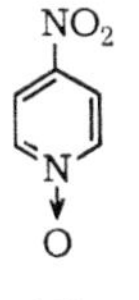

(8)

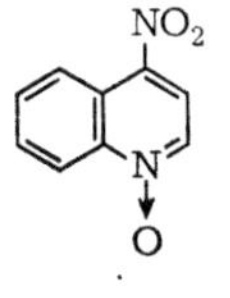

(9)

1955; BRAY et al., 1957a). Pentachloronitrobenzene and tetrachloronitrobenzenes induce tumours when applied to mouse skin (SEARLE, 1966) and the compound with a stable nitro group, 1,2,3,4-tetrachloro-6-nitrobenzene, was the most active.

The reactions of glutathione with 4-nitropyridine N-oxide (8) and the carcinogenic 4-nitroquinoline N-oxide (9) are probably catalyzed by glutathione S-aryltransferase (AL-KASSAB et al., 1963) although the latter reacts rapidly with thiols even in the absence of the enzyme (NAKAHARA and FUKUOKA, 1959).

Conjugation of sulfobromophthalein (BSP) with glutathione (COMBES and STAKELUM, 1961) is catalyzed by glutathione S-aryltransferase and the conjugate is transported to bile more rapidly than the free dye (COMBES, 1965), but results of BOYLAND and GROVER (1967) indicate that conjugation was not always the rate-limiting step in dye clearance. In a study of species variation in metabolism of the dye, KLAASSEN and PLAA (1967) showed that biliary excretion was probably the limiting factor in the elimination of BSP from the plasma.

Glutathione S-aryltransferase is present in several insect species (COHEN and SMITH, 1964; COHEN et al., 1964). CLARK et al. (1967) found differences in the glutathione-binding sites of glutathione S-aryltransferase from sheep liver and grass grub. House fly supernatant preparations can carry out the mercapturic acid biosynthesis (SIMS and GROVER, 1965).

VI. Glutathione S-Epoxidetransferase

Mono-, di- and trihalogenobenzenes are metabolized to arylmercapturic acids (SMITH et al., 1950; AZOUZ et al., 1955; JONDORF et al., 1955; PARKE and WILLIAMS, 1955), the proportion of which decreases with increased halogen substitution in the ring. A free *para* position is required (AZOUZ et al., 1955) since the hydrogen atom *para* to the halogen is generally replaced by the acetylcysteine residue. Arylmercapturic acids have been isolated from the acidified urine of animals dosed with aromatic hydrocarbons, e.g., 1-anthrylmercapturic acid (5) (BOYLAND and LEVI, 1936) and *p*-biphenylmercapturic acid (7) (WEST et al., 1956) from anthracene and biphenyl.

The early workers on monohalogenobenzene metabolism (BAUMANN and PREUSSE, 1879; JAFFÉ, 1879) recognized that the isolated mercapturic acids were excreted as acid-labile precursors. These precursors have been called "premercapturic acids" and are excreted from animals after administration of benzene, naphthalene, anthracene and monohalogenobenzenes (KNIGHT and YOUNG, 1958), but

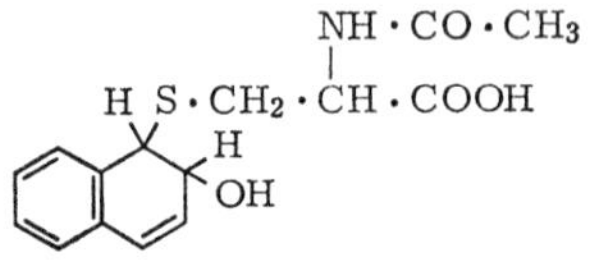

(10)

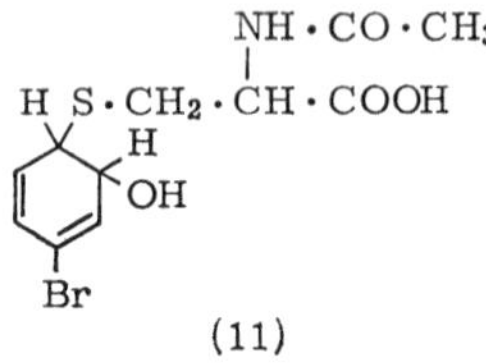

(11)

they are mercapturic acids and the term "premercapturic acid" seems unnecessary. The ammonium salt of the acid-labile mercapturic acid formed from naphthalene by rabbits has been isolated and shown to be N-acetyl-S(1,2-dihydro-2-hydroxy-1-naphthyl)-L-cysteine (10) (BOYLAND and SIMS, 1958). Treatment of this compound (10) with cold mineral acid yielded 1-naphthylmercapturic acid (4) together with naphthalene, 1-naphthol and 2-naphthol. The acid-labile mercapturic acid (11) produced by rats and rabbits dosed with bromobenzene has been isolated as the dicyclohexylamine salt (GILLHAM and YOUNG, 1967). Acid-labile mercapturic acids are probably formed through an intermediate epoxide (BOYLAND and SIMS, 1958, 1960) that is conjugated with glutathione. Further evidence for the existence of the epoxide intermediate suggested by BOYLAND (1950) and BOYLAND and SIMS (1958, 1960) was obtained when BOOTH et al. (1961) showed that *in vitro* conjugations of glutathione with iodobenzene, naphthalene and phenanthrene would only occur in the presence of rat liver microsomes, NADPH and oxygen. Although the intermediates were not isolated, the microsomal enzyme system presumably caused the formation of the epoxide derivatives, since the conjugation of glutathione with 1,2-epoxy-1,2,3,4-tetrahydronaphthalene was catalyzed by rat liver supernatant alone.

Boyland and Williams (1965) showed that the enzyme in rat liver supernatant catalyzing conjugations of glutathione with epoxides was different from glutathione S-aryltransferase. 2,3-Epoxypropyl phenyl ether was employed as the second substrate in studies with this enzyme because it reacted only slowly with glutathione in the absence of the enzyme. This enzyme, glutathione S-epoxidetransferase, has a pH optimum at pH 6.5 (Boyland and Williams, 1965; Wit and Snel, 1968). It is probably responsible for *in vivo* conjugations of glutathione with epoxy derivatives of halogenobenzenes, aromatic hydrocarbons and other compounds. Some epoxides react with glutathione in the absence of enzyme, some only if the enzyme is present and others do not react even with the enzyme (Table 2).

Table 2. *Reaction of epoxides with glutathione at pH 6.5 and 25°*

Epoxides which do not react either chemically or enzymically	Epoxides which react chemically and at an increased rate enzymically	Epoxides which react enzymically but not chemically
1,2-Epoxyethane-1,2-dicarboboxylic acid	1,2-Epoxypropane	2,3-Epoxypropyl phenyl ether
9,10-Epoxystearic acid	DL-1,2:3,4-Diepoxy butane	2,3-Epoxypropyl butyrate
1,4-2,3-Diepoxyl,2,3,4-tetrahydronaphthalene	1,2:5,6-Diepoxyhexane	Styrene oxide
Scopolamine	Triethylene glycol bis-2,3-epoxypropyl ether (Epidyl)	1,2-Epoxy-1,2,3,4-tetrahydronaphthalene
Dieldrin	2,3-Epoxypropyl methacrylate	Resorcinol bis-2,3-epoxypropyl ether

The intermediate epoxide from naphthalene has been synthesised (Vogel and Klärner, 1968) and shown to be formed in naphthalene metabolism by Jerina et al. (1968). The existence of this compound as an intermediate was indicated by studies on the metabolism of 1,2-dihydronaphthalene and 1,2-epoxy-1,2,3,4-tetrahydronaphthalene (13) (Boyland and Sims, 1960).

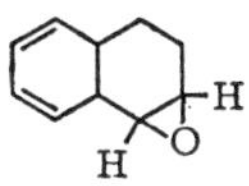

(13)

Acid-labile mercapturic acid derivatives have also been obtained as metabolites of the polycyclic hydrocarbons, phenanthrene (Boyland and Sims, 1962) and benz[a]anthracene (Boyland and Sims, 1964a). Formation of acid-labile mercapturic acids from these hydrocarbons proceeds through intermediate epoxides that may also be synthesized chemically (Boyland and Sims, 1965a). In these molecules there are five reactive double bonds which can undergo epoxidation, but the nature and amounts of the detected metabolites indicated that mercapturic acid formation occurred mainly on the double bond in the K region, which is the position in the molecule of the greatest electron density: a measure of this property is given by the bond order of the bond concerned. The amounts of the metabolites of phenanthrene and benz[a]anthracene produced is related to bond order (Boyland, 1964), and it was shown that the relative amounts of metabolites derived from a particular bond increased with increasing bond order in these non-carcinogenic compounds.

Most known carcinogenic polycyclic hydrocarbons have a region of high electron density, that is, a K region, but the role that this bond plays in carcinogenesis remains unknown. The importance of the K region is illustrated by the fact that the metabolism of these compounds preferentially yields mercapturic acids in which the K region is involved. However, the biochemical changes which phenanthrene and benz[a]anthracene undergo are different from the addition reactions which they undergo in the absence of enzymes. The biological oxidation of these compounds gives products in which not only the K region but also other double bonds with less chemical reactivity are involved. On the other hand the reactions of phenanthrene and benz[a] anthracene with ozone, osmium tetroxide, diazoacetic acid, or perbenzoic acid are almost entirely with the double bond with the highest chemical reactivity, i.e. the K region. Biological oxidations are thus in closer agreement with theoretical predictions of bond order than are the non-enzymic chemical reactions.

Oxidation of the same hydrocarbons with rat liver microsomes and reduced pyridine nucleotides gave products analogous to those found in urine and bile of animals (BOYLAND et al., 1964). The bile of rats treated with phenanthrene, benz[a]anthracene, and pyrene contained the acid-labile mercapturic acid, cysteine, cysteinylglycine and glutathione derivatives of the corresponding hydrocarbon epoxides (BOYLAND and SIMS, 1962, 1964a, b), thus providing further evidence as to the nature of the intermediates involved in mercapturic acid biosynthesis.

The polycyclic hydrocarbons, benz[a]anthracene, dibenz[a,h]anthracene (BOYLAND and SIMS, 1965b), 3-methylcholanthrene (SIMS, 1966), and 7- and 12-methylbenz[a]anthracene (SIMS, 1967) formed glutathione conjugates in the presence of rat liver homogenates and are probably partly metabolized as mercapturic acids *in vivo*. The carcinogenic hydrocarbons 7,12-benzanthracene and 3,4-benzopyrene are not metabolised in the K region (SIMS, 1969).

The mercapturic acids detected *in vivo* after administration of lower chlorinated naphthalenes (CORNISH and BLOCK, 1958) and the herbicide, 2,6-dichlorobenzonitrile (WIT and VAN GENDEREN, 1966), to animals were probably formed through intermediate epoxides. Styrene was probably metabolized as hydroxyphenylethylmercapturic acid (14) *in vivo* by rabbits and rats (JAMES and WHITE, 1967) through the intermediate styrene epoxide (15), as the reaction of this epoxide with glutathione is catalyzed by rat liver supernatant (BOYLAND and WILLIAMS, 1965). BRAY and CARPANINI (1968) showed that about 40% of thiophene (16) was excreted as thiophenyl 2- and 3-mercapturic acids by rabbits: these metabolites were

$Ph \cdot CH(OH) \cdot CH_2 \cdot S \cdot CH_2 \cdot CH(NH \cdot CO \cdot CH_3) \cdot COOH$

(14)

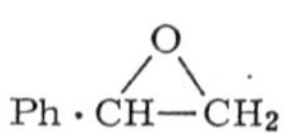

(15)

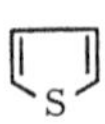

(16)

possibly formed through the intermediate 2,3-epoxy-2,3-dihydrothiophene, which conjugates with glutathione.

VII. Glutathione S-Alkyltransferase

BOOTH et al. (1961) showed that conjugation of 1-bromopropane (17) with glutathione was catalyzed by rat liver supernatant. JOHNSON (1963) described an enzyme that catalyzed the S-alkylation of glutathione *in vitro* by iodomethane, other alkyl halides, and the carcinogenic β-propiolactone (18).

$$CH_3 \cdot CH_2 \cdot CH_2 \cdot Br \qquad \begin{array}{l} CH_2 - C{=}O \\ \;| \qquad\quad | \\ CH_2 - O \end{array}$$

(17) (18)

This enzyme, glutathione S-alkyltransferase, differed from glutathione S-epoxidetransferase (BOYLAND and WILLIAMS, 1965) and from glutathione S-aryltransferase (JOHNSON, 1966a). With iodomethane as the second substrate, the enzyme had a pH optimum at about pH 8.5 and occurred in rat liver and rat kidney in similar amounts.

JAMES (1961) and BRAY et al. (1964) found that in addition to the alkylmercapturic acids (19), a divalent-sulfur-containing metabolite identical with those formed from the corresponding 1,2-alkenes was excreted (JAMES and JEFFERY, 1964). BARNSLEY (1964a, b) showed that the second metabolite produced from 1-bromopropane was N-acetyl-S-(2-hydroxy-1-propyl)-L-cysteine (20), which is a hydroxyalkylmercapturic acid. This compound (20) has also been detected in the urine of rats dosed with 1-chloropropane, 1-iodopropane, 1,2-epoxypropane and 1-chloropropan-2-ol (BARNSLEY, 1966). Hydroxyalkylmercapturic acids were also formed as metabolites of the corresponding bromocycloalkanes, 1,2-epoxycycloalkanes and 1,2-cycloalkenes by rabbits (JAMES et al., 1967).

$$\text{Alkyl}\cdot S\cdot CH_2\cdot \underset{NH\cdot CO\cdot CH_3}{\underset{|}{CH}}\cdot COOH \qquad CH_3\cdot CH(OH)\cdot CH_2\cdot S\cdot CH_2\cdot \underset{NH\cdot CO\cdot CH_3}{\underset{|}{CH}}\cdot COOH$$

(19) (20)

SIMS and GROVER (1965) reported that the chlorocyclohexenes, α-3,4,5,6-tetrachlorocyclohex-1-ene and γ-2,3,4,5,6-pentachlorocyclohex-1-ene, are conjugated with glutathione by a rat liver enzyme that is probably glutathione S-aryltransferase.

JAMES and JEFFERY (1964) have suggested that mercapturic acids are formed from alkyl halides by two mechanisms: the first by replacement of the halogen atom by glutathione catalyzed by glutathione S-alkyltransferase (eq. A), and the second by an intermediate stage involving dehydrodebromination, epoxidation, and conjugation of the epoxide with glutathione catalyzed by glutathione S-epoxidetransferase (eq. B). The epoxide may also arise by hydroxylation of the alkyl halide and elimination of HBr (eq. C). Hydroxyalkylmercapturic acids could also be formed by hydroxylation of the corresponding alkylmercapturic acid or precursor before excretion, as rat liver slices convert S-butylcysteine and butylmercapturic acid to hydroxyalkylmercapturic acids (JAMES et al., 1968).

$$R\cdot CH_2\cdot CH_2\cdot Br + \text{glutathione} \rightarrow R\cdot CH_2\cdot CH_2\cdot SG + H^+ + Br^- \qquad (A)$$

$$R\cdot CH_2\cdot CH_2\cdot Br \xrightarrow{-HBr} \text{Alkyl}\cdot CH{=}CH_2 \xrightarrow{+\text{“O”}} \text{Alkyl}\cdot \overset{O}{\overbrace{CH - CH_2}} \qquad (B)$$

$$\xrightarrow{+\text{ glutathione}} \text{Alkyl}\cdot CH(OH)\cdot CH_2\cdot SG$$

$$R\cdot CH_2\cdot CH_2\cdot Br \xrightarrow{+\text{“O”}} \text{Alkyl}\cdot CH(OH)\cdot CH_2\cdot Br \xrightarrow{-HBr} \text{Alkyl}\cdot \overset{O}{\overbrace{CH - CH_2}} \qquad (C)$$

Hydroxyalkylmercapturic acid formation is restricted to alkyl halides containing more than two carbon atoms since hydroxyalkylmercapturic acids are not metabolites of iodomethane (BARNSLEY and YOUNG, 1965) or bromoethane

(THOMSON et al., 1963). Bromoethane and 1-bromopropane are also partly metabolized to the alkylmercapturic acid sulfoxides (BARNSLEY et al., 1964; BARNSLEY et al., 1966). Some S-alkyl-L-cysteine sulfoxides occur naturally in plants, e.g. alliin (21) in garlic (VIRTANEN, 1962).

$$CH_2{=}\,CH{\cdot}CH_2{\cdot}\overset{\overset{\displaystyle O}{\|}}{S}{\cdot}CH_2{\cdot}CH(NH_2){\cdot}COOH$$

(21)

Rabbits and rats dosed with 1-bromobutane excrete butylmercapturic acid, (2-hydroxybutyl)mercapturic acid, (3-hydroxybutyl)-mercapturic acid, and 3-(butylthio)lactic acid. The latter was also formed from S-butylcysteine by rabbit liver slices and may arise by reduction of 3-(butylthio)pyruvic acid produced from S-butylcysteine (JAMES et al., 1968).

The glutathione alkyl transferase, described by HUTSON et al. (1968) appears to utilize glutathione as an acceptor of alkyl groups for the detoxication of phosphoric acid triesters, such as 2-chloro-1-(2,4,5-trichlorphenyl)vinyldimethyl phosphate (22) and related alkyl homologues by O-dealkylation (HUTSON et al., 1967). Products formed on incubation of a rat liver supernatant containing glutathione

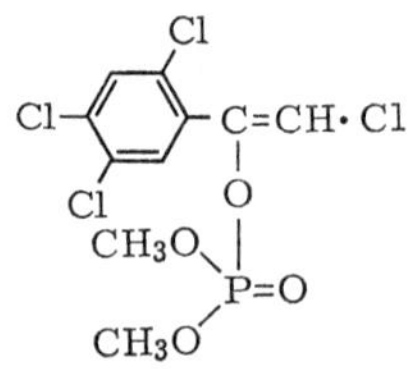

(22)

and (22) included S-methylglutathione and the O-demethylated phosphate diester (HUTSON et al., 1968).

FUKAMI and SHISHIDO (1966) showed that the enzyme system that hydrolyzes methyl parathion to desmethyl parathion in rat tissues and insect larvae was glutathione-dependent. The metabolism of *cis* and *trans* isomers of dimethyl 1-carbomethoxy-1-propen-2-yl phosphate (Phosdrin) by mouse liver preparations is different: the *cis* form is O-demethylated by a glutathione-dependent enzyme to S-methylglutathione and *cis*-mono-methyl 1-carbomethoxy-1-propen-2-yl phosphate and the *trans* form is cleaved by a glutathione-independent system to dimethyl phosphate and a ketoester (MORELLO et al., 1967). Traces of S-ethylcysteine which have been detected after hydrolysis of urine from rats dosed with a triethyl phosphate (ROBERTS and WARWICK, 1958b) may have arisen by a mechanism similar to that acting on the *cis* form. The enzymes concerned with these processes may be glutathione S-alkyltransferase or separate enzymes.

VIII. Glutathione S-Aralkyltransferase

STEKOL (1938) isolated benzylmercapturic acid (23) from the urine of dogs

$$Ph{\cdot}CH_2{\cdot}S{\cdot}CH_2{\cdot}\underset{\underset{\displaystyle NH{\cdot}CO{\cdot}CH_3}{|}}{CH}{\cdot}COOH$$

(23)

dosed with benzyl chloride. Mercapturic acids have been isolated after administration of other aralkyl halides to animals (STEKOL, 1941; BRAY et al., 1958b; HYDE and YOUNG, 1965, 1968; JAMES and WHITE, 1967). BRAY et al. (1958b) found that the proportion of aralkylmercapturic acid excreted decreased with increasing alkyl chain length of the aralkyl halide precursor from 49% for benzyl chloride to 4% for 4-bromobutylbenzene. HYDE and YOUNG (1968) have isolated 1-menaphthylmercapturic acid (24) and the corresponding glutathione and cysteine conjugates from the urine of rats dosed with 1-menaphthyl chloride, bromide, alcohol, acetate, or benzoate. CLAPP (1967) detected mercapturic acids in the urine of rats dosed

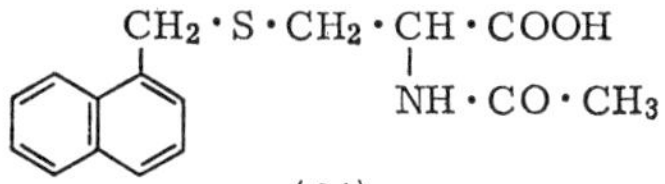

(24)

with 1-menaphthyl sulfate, phenanthrene 9-carbinol, phenanthrene 9-methylchloride and acetate, anthracene 9-carbinol and anthracene 9-methylchloride and acetate. Benzylmercapturic acid (23) was isolated from the urine of rats dosed with benzyl acetate; and 1-menaphthyl alcohol and esters were excreted by rats as 1-menaphthylmercapturic acid (CLAPP, 1967).

The enzyme catalyzing the conjugation of benzyl chloride with glutathione has a pH optimum at pH 6.8, and the ratio of activities in rat liver and rat kidney is 10:7 compared with 100:8 for glutathione S-aryltransferase (SUGA et al., 1967). SUGA suggested that glutathione S-aralkyltransferase was different from glutathione S-aryltransferase. This would agree with the findings of BOOTH et al. (1961) that benzyl chloride was a noncompetitive inhibitor of glutathione S-aryltransferase. Glutathione S-aralkyltransferase has been partially separated from glutathione S-alkyltransferase and S-aryltransferase (E. BOYLAND and L.F. CHASSEAUD, 1969). CLAPP (1967) has shown that rat liver supernatant catalyzes reactions between 1-menaphthyl esters and glutathione. Rat liver supernatant catalyzes the reaction of glutathione with benzyl formate, but the reaction is slow (BOYLAND and CHASSEAUD, 1969).

Phenethylbromide (25) is metabolized to hydroxyaralkylmercapturic acid (26) as well as phenethylmercapturic acid (JAMES and WHITE, 1967), and similar

$Ph{\cdot}CH_2{\cdot}CH_2{\cdot}Br$ (25)

$Ph{\cdot}CHOH{\cdot}CH_2{\cdot}S{\cdot}CH_2{\cdot}CH(NH{\cdot}CO{\cdot}CH_3){\cdot}COOH$ (26)

hydroxyaralkylmercapturic acids are produced from other related aralkyl precursors. S-Phenethylcysteine and phenethylmercapturic acid are also converted *in vivo* and *in vitro* to the hydroxyaralkylmercapturic acid (26), so that hydroxylation of the mercapturic acid can occur after conjugation with glutathione and subsequent degradation to the cysteine derivative.

The urine of rats dosed with allyl chloride contained allylmercapturic acid (27) and 2- or 3-hydroxypropylmercapturic acid, and a metabolite similar to the latter was produced by rats dosed with allyl acetate (CLAPP et al., 1969).

$CH_2{=}CH{\cdot}CH_2{\cdot}S{\cdot}CH_2{\cdot}CH(NH{\cdot}CO{\cdot}CH_3){\cdot}COOH$

(27)

IX. Glutathione S-Alkenetransferases

Reactions of glutathione with $\alpha\beta$-unsaturated compounds RR′C=CR″A, including acetals, aldehydes, esters, ketones, lactones, nitriles, nitrocompounds and sulfones, are catalyzed by preparations from various animal species (BOYLAND

Table 3. *αβ-Unsaturated carbonyl compounds that are substrates for glutathione S-alkenetransferases* (from BOYLAND and CHASSEAUD, 1969)

Enzyme	Type of αβ-unsaturated compound catalyzed	Example
1	*cis*-Ester	Diethyl maleate, Ethyl acrylate
2	*trans*-Ester	Diethyl fumarate
3	Cyclic ketone and possibly some lactones	Cyclohex-2-en-1-one, Parasorbic acid
4	Vinyl ketone	2,3-Dimethyl-4-(2-methylenebutyryl) phenoxyacetic acid
5	Open-chain *trans* ketone (substituted vinyl ketone)	*trans*-Benzylidene-acetone
6	*trans* Aldehyde and possibly acetals	*trans*-Cinnamaldehyde, *trans*-Hex-2-en-1-al, Cinnamaldehyde dimethylacetal

Table 4. *Reactions catalyzed by glutathione transferases.*

Enzyme	Reaction catalysed	References
GSH S-aryltransferase	Replacement of labile aryl halogen and nitro groups by GSH	BOOTH, BOYLAND and SIMS (1961); COMBES and STAKELUM (1961); AL-KASSAB, BOYLAND and WILLIAMS (1963)
GSH S-epoxide-transferase	Conjugation of some alkyl and aryl epoxides with GSH	BOYLAND and WILLIAMS (1965)
GSH S-alkyl-transferase	Replacement of some alkyl halogen and possibly nitro groups by GSH	JOHNSON (1966a)
GSH S-aralkyl-transferase	Replacement of labile aralkyl halogen and possibly ester groups by GSH	SUGA, OHATA, KUMAOKA and AKAGI (1967)
GSH S-alkene-transferases (see Table 3)	Conjugation of αβ-unsaturated compounds with GSH	BOYLAND and CHASSEAUD (1967), BOYLAND and CHASSEAUD (1968), CHASSEAUD (1967)
Phosphoric acid triester: glutathione alkyl transferase	O-Dealkylation of phosphate triesters in the presence of GSH	FUKAMI and SHISHIDO (1966), HUTSON, PICKERING and DONNINGER (1968)
Nitroglycerine reductase	Denitration of glyceryl trinitrate in the presence of GSH	HEPPEL and HILMOE (1950), NEEDLEMAN and HUNTER (1965)

and CHASSEAUD, 1966, 1967, 1968; CHASSEAUD, 1967). At least six different enzymes appear to catalyze reactions of glutathione with various αβ-unsaturated carbonyl compounds (Table 3) (BOYLAND and CHASSEAUD, 1968, 1969). Evidence for this was obtained from heat inactivation experiments, ammonium sulfate fractionation studies, enzyme-inhibition studies with S-(αβ-dicarbethoxyethyl)glutathione, and the distribution of activities in rat liver and rat kidney in the livers of other animals. These enzymes, glutathione S-alkenetransferases, differ from glutathione S-alkyltransferase, S-aryltransferase, and S-epoxidetransferase and occur in the supernatant fraction of rat liver homogenates (BOYLAND and CHASSEAUD, 1968).

The glutathione S-alkenetransferase catalyzing the reaction of diethyl maleate with glutathione has a pH optimum at pH 7.6 (BOYLAND and CHASSEAUD, 1967), is inhibited by the reaction product (CHASSEAUD, 1967; BOYLAND and CHASSEAUD, 1968) and occurs in the livers of several animal species (BOYLAND and CHASSEAUD, 1967; WIT and SNEL, 1968). Within 2 hours of the administration of a dose (0.7

g/kg) of diethyl maleate to the rat, liver glutathione content fell by 90% (Chasseaud, 1967).

Other substrates for glutathione S-alkenetransferases (Boyland and Chasseaud, 1967; Chasseaud, 1967) include ethyl acrylate, vinyl acetate, and acrylonitrile used in the plastics industry, a series of alk-2-en-1-als which are present as autoxidation products in fats (Wishner and Keeney, 1965; Day, 1966), β-nitrostyrenes and αβ-unsaturated ketones possessing antifungal and antibacterial properties (Geiger and Conn, 1945; McGowan et al., 1948; Schales and Graefe, 1952). Substrates that occur naturally include cinnamaldehyde, parasorbic acid (Hauschka et al., 1945) and hex-2-en-1-al (Watanabe, 1958; Forss et al., 1962; Nursten and Williams, 1967).

Because of their widespread use and occurrence, the toxicities and properties of several of these compounds have been determined (see Fassett and Irish, 1963). The existence of glutathione S-alkenetransferases suggests that these compounds are partly metabolized to mercapturic acids and the probable pathway is outlined in Fig. 1. The initial reaction with glutathione probably takes place by addition of the nucleophile (GS^-) to the β-carbon atom of the αβ double bond strongly polarized by conjugation with electron-withdrawing groups; thiols are known to react with αβ-unsaturated compounds in this manner (Mayo and Walling, 1940; Hurd and Gershbein, 1947; Knuth et al., 1954; Patai and Rappoport, 1964; Friedman et al., 1965).

Ethacrynic acid, a diuretic (Baer and Beyer, 1966), is metabolized in animals to the cysteine conjugate (Porter, 1966).

Glutathione and cysteine conjugates of maleic acid have been found in extracts of calf lens (Calam and Waley, 1963) and the cysteine derivative (28) is also present in human urine and animal kidney (Kuwaki and Mizuhara, 1966). Boyland

$$HOOC\cdot CH(NH_2)\cdot CH_2S\cdot CH(COOH)\cdot CH_2\cdot COOH$$

(28)

and Chasseaud (1967) found that the reaction of glutathione with maleic acid is catalyzed by an enzyme present in rat liver and rat kidney in comparable amounts (Chasseaud, 1967), but a mercapturic acid has not been reported as a metabolite of maleic acid (e.g., Taggart et al., 1962). Angielski and Rogulski (1961) suggested that increased losses of glutathione in the presence of kidney homogenates were due to its conversion into cysteine which then reacted nonenzymically with maleic acid.

Parasorbic acid is one of several lactones that are carcinogenic on subcutaneous injection into rats (Dickens, 1964). However, no carcinogenic effect was observed when this compound was administered orally (Dickens et al., 1966).

Arecoline (29), an alkaloid present in the seeds of the betel nut palm, is metabolized to a mercapturic acid in the rat (E. Boyland and Nery, 1969). Nonenzymic reaction of glutathione with this alkaloid occurs readily at pH 7.4.

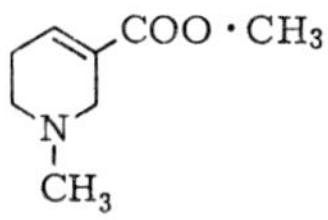

(29)

Reactions of glutathione with deca-2,4-dien-1-al (30) and the acetylenic compound, dimethylacetylenedicarboxylate (31) are catalyzed by rat liver preparations (Chasseaud, 1967).

$CH_3 \cdot (CH_2)_4 \cdot CH{=}CH \cdot CH{=}CH \cdot CHO$ (30)

$H_3C \cdot OOC \cdot C{\equiv}C \cdot COO \cdot CH_3$ (31)

Although some quinones react with glutathione (NICKERSON et al., 1963) and the reaction of glutathione with menadione (32) is catalyzed by rat liver prepara-

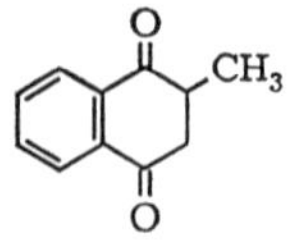

(32)

tions (CHASSEAUD, 1967), BRAY and GARRETT (1961) found no mercapturic acids excreted after administration of this and other quinones to animals.

X. Other Mercapturic Precursors

It is not clear whether glutathione S-transferases are involved in the metabolism of several compounds that are excreted as mercapturic acids by animals.

1. Arylamines

Two mercapturic acids have been identified in the urine of animals dosed with 2-naphthylamine, a compound that causes bladder cancer (BOYLAND et al., 1963; BOYLAND and MANSON, 1966). One is N-acetyl-S-(2-acetamido-5,6-dihydro-6-hydroxy-5-naphthyl)-L-cysteine (33) and is probably formed through an intermediate epoxide.

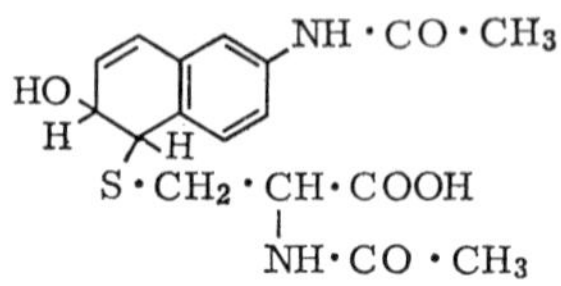

(33)

The second mercapturic acid probably arises through the formation of 2-naphthylhydroxylamine (34) which yields mercapturic acid (35) (BOYLAND et al., 1963).

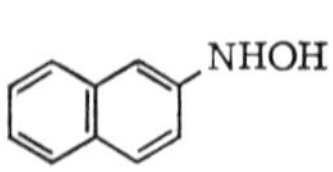

(34)

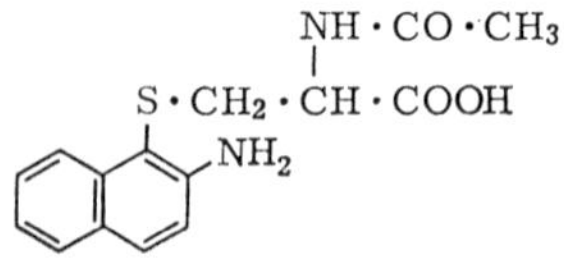

(35)

Ortho and *p*-Aminophenyl- and *p*-acetamidophenylmercapturic acids have been detected in the urine of rats and rabbits dosed with aniline and were probably formed through an intermediate hydroxylamine derivative since phenylhydroxylamine, administered to rats, was converted into *p*-aminophenylmercapturic acid (E. BOYLAND, D. MANSON and R. NERY, unpublished work).

After administration of the analgesic acetophenetidine, 2% was metabolized in man to the cysteine derivative (36) (JAGENBURG and TOCZKO, 1964). This conjugate could have been formed by N-hydroxylation and reaction of this derivative with glutathione.

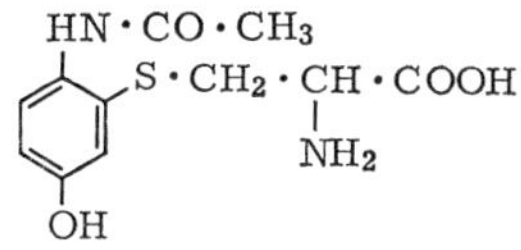

(36)

2. Urethane

In rats, urethane is metabolized and largely excreted in the expired air as carbon dioxide (BOYLAND and RHODEN, 1949). Metabolites detected in the urine of animals dosed with urethane include ethylmercapturic acid, N-acetyl-S-carbethoxycysteine (37), and ethylmercapturic acid sulfoxide (BOYLAND and NERY, 1965) and are probably formed through an intermediate N-hydroxyurethane which reacts *in vitro* with cysteine producing small amounts of S-ethyl and S-carbethoxy derivatives.

$$HOOC{\cdot}\underset{\displaystyle NH.CO.CH_3}{CH}{\cdot}CH_2{\cdot}S{\cdot}CO{\cdot}O{\cdot}CH_2{\cdot}CH_3$$

(37)

3. Benzothiazole-2-Sulfonamide

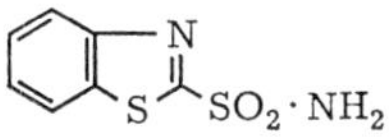

(38)

Metabolites of benzothiazole-2-sulfonamide (38) in rats, rabbits and dogs include benzothiazole-2-mercapturic acid, benzothiazole-2-mercaptan, and benzothiazole-2-thioglucuronic acid (COLUCCI and BUYSKE, 1965). The reaction between benzothiazole-2-sulfonamide (38) and glutathione is not increased on addition of rat liver supernatant (COLUCCI and BUYSKE, 1965).

4. Alkyl Methanesulfonates

Alkylmercapturic acids have been detected as metabolites of alkyl methanesulfonates administered to animals (ROBERTS and WARWICK, 1958a; PILLINGER et al., 1964; BARNSLEY, 1968). Reaction of ethyl methanesulfonate ("half myleran") with glutathione is catalyzed by rat liver supernatant (BOOTH et al., 1961), by replacement of the methanesulfonate ($SO_3.CH_3$) moiety by glutathione (ROBERTS and WARWICK, 1958a).

The major urinary metabolite of the antileukemia agent, myleran, in rats was monohydroxytetrahydrothiophene-1,1-dioxide, probably formed by condensation of myleran with glutathione (eq. D) (ROBERTS and WARWICK, 1959).

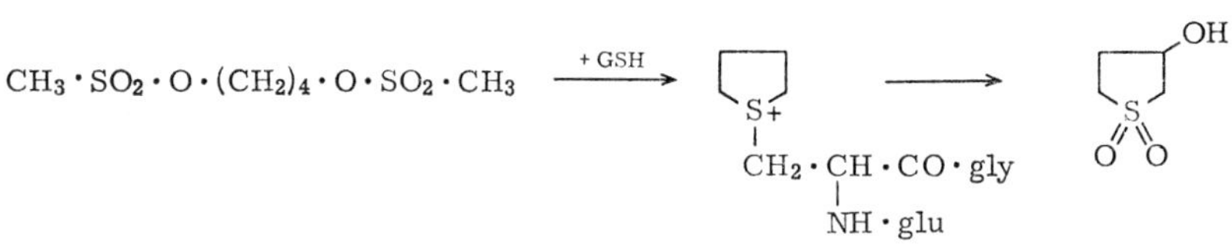

(D)

S-methylglutathione has been detected in the bile of rats dosed with methyl methanesulfonate, but the principal urinary metabolites are S-methylcysteine sulfoxide, methylmercapturic acid, and methylmercapturic acid sulfoxide (PILLINGER et al., 1964). BARNSLEY (1968) has also shown that other metabolites include 2-hydroxy-3-methylsulfinylpropionic acid, methylsulfinylacetic acid, and N-(methylthioacetyl)glycine. Similar metabolites have also been identified in the urine of rats dosed with iodomethane (BARNSLEY and YOUNG, 1965), S-methyl-glutathione (FOXWELL and YOUNG, 1964), and S-methylcysteine (BARNSLEY, 1964b). SKLAN and BARNSLEY (1968) isolated 2-hydroxy-3-methylsulfinylpropionic acid and methylsulfinylacetic acid as dicyclohexylamine salts from the urine of rats dosed with S-methyl-L-cysteine.

5. 3,5-Di-tert-butyl-4-hydroxytoluene

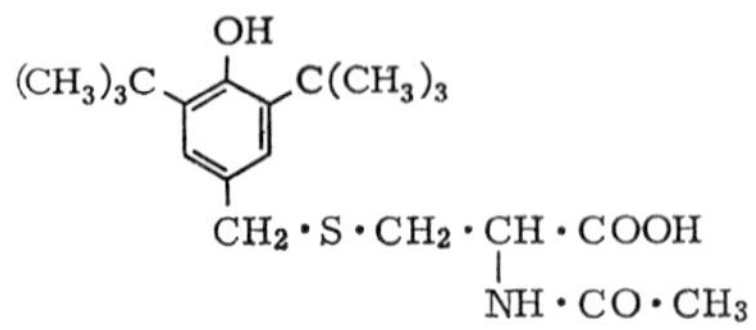

(39)

DANIEL et al. (1968) showed that a major metabolite of the food antioxidant 3,5-di-*tert*-butyl-4-hydroxytoluene (BHT) in the rat was the mercapturic acid (39). Only a trace of this metabolite was present in human urine. Although benzyl alcohol is not excreted as a mercapturic acid (STEKOL, 1939b), benzyl chloride is (STEKOL, 1938), and it is possible that the mercapturic acid (39) is formed from BHT through the intermediate radical or carbonium ion reacting with glutathione.

6. Isovalthine

The amino acid, isovalthine (S-(1-carboxyisobutyl)cysteine) (40) occurs in the urine of hypercholesterolemic patients and of cats (OHMORI and MIZUHARA, 1962).

$$(CH_3)_2\cdot CH\cdot CH(COOH)\cdot S\cdot CH_2\cdot CH(NH_2)\cdot COOH$$

(40)

The biosynthesis of this compound may need the presence of ATP (KUWAKI et al., 1963). The glutathione-isovaleric acid conjugate is probably converted to iso-valthine by the enzymes that catabolize the glutathione conjugates of other mer-capturic acid precursors (KUWAKI, 1965).

Other cysteine derivatives isolated or detected include S-(β-carboxy-*n*-propyl)-L-cysteine (also known as β-isobuteine) and S-(β-carboxy-ethyl)-L-cysteine in normal children's urine (OHMORI et al., 1965), and S-(carboxymethyl)cysteine in some animal tissues and in the urine of hypertensive and diabetic patients (UBUKA et al., 1967).

7. Bis-β-chloroethyl Sulfide

Glutathione conjugates of sulfur mustard (41) (bis-β-chloroethyl sulfide) and of bis-β-chloroethyl sulfone are the major urinary metabolites of mustard gas in rodents: some thiodiglycol and other hydrolysis and oxidation products are also formed (DAVISON et al., 1961).

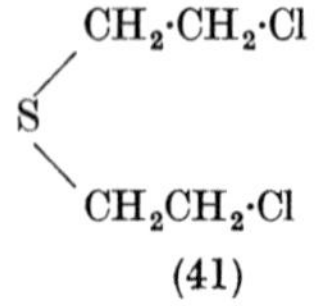

(41)

8. Nitrofurans

Rat liver supernatant catalyzes reactions of glutathione with nitrofurans containing labile nitro groups, e.g., 2-cyano-5-nitrofuran (42) (E. Boyland, B.E. Speyer and K. Williams, unpublished work). The enzyme catalyzing these reactions may be glutathione S-aryltransferase. Known carcinogenic nitrofurans (Morris, 1967) such as (43) hardly react with glutathione (E. Boyland, B.E. Speyer and K. Williams, unpublished work).

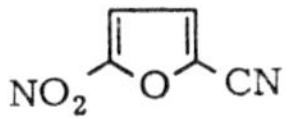

(42)

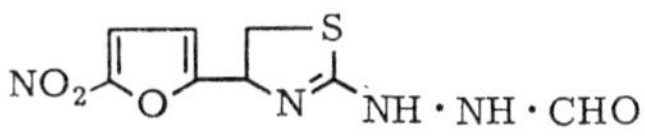

(43)

Conclusion

Mercapturic acid biosynthesis is an important pathway for the elimination of foreign compounds. The initial stage is usually the conjugation of glutathione with the foreign compound or a more reactive form of it (e.g., an epoxide). These conjugations are generally catalyzed by glutathione S-transferases, although in some cases, nonenzymic reactions predominate. At least ten different glutathione S-transferases are known (cf. Tables 3 and 4) although one enzyme would theoretically be sufficient to activate glutathione which could then react with foreign compounds. It is therefore probable that both glutathione and the foreign compound are bound to enzymic active sites and that the function of glutathione S-transferases in the cell is to bring glutathione and the foreign compound together.

The glutathione conjugates are probably catabolized to cysteine derivatives along the same pathway that operates for glutathione. Acetylation of the cysteine derivative to form a mercapturic acid generally occurs before excretion from the body. Further catabolism of the mercapturic acid, such as oxidation to the sulfoxide and products may occur (Barnsley, 1964b; Sklan and Barnsley, 1968). West and Miller (1962) found that administration of *p*-chlorophenylmercapturic acid and [^{35}S]-L-methionine simultaneously to animals resulted in the excretion of [^{35}S]-*p*-chlorophenylmercapturic acid (75% of the dose), suggesting that there was exchange between the sulphur containing amino acids.

Whereas other conjugative detoxication processes such as glucuronide or sulfate conjugation require the initial formation of a "high energy" or "active" intermediate involving ATP, the reaction of foreign compounds with glutathione does not appear to require this except for the reaction of glutathione and isovaleric acid (Kuwaki et al., 1963).

The importance of the mercapturic acid biosynthesis in man is difficult to assess. Conjugation with glutathione occurs, but enzyme activities are low compared with other species (Grover and Sims, 1964; Boyland and Chasseaud, 1967, 1968). Glutathione-conjugating ability is present in the foetus (Grover and Sims, 1964; Boyland and Chasseaud, 1967, 1968) and in the newborn (Vest and Rossier, 1963). Stekol (1946) has shown that acetylation of arylcysteines to mercapturic acids occurs in man. Although it is unlikely that the pathway for the catabolism of glutathione conjugates is absent (cf. Revel and Ball, 1959), Wainer and Lorincz (1963) were unable to isolate the mercapturic acid after administration of bromobenzene to human subjects. Some animal species may form little or no mercapturic acid due to deficiency in some stage of the mercapturic acid biosynthesis (Bray et al., 1959b).

There are probably many other foreign compounds, at present undescribed, that are substrates for glutathione S-transferases. These would be expected to include some compounds capable of providing a sufficiently electrophilic centre for reaction with the nucleophilic glutathione.

Glutathione S-transferases do not appear to catalyze reactions of glutathione with endogenous substances. The thyroid hormone, thyroxine, and related compounds are not substrates for glutathione S-transferases (Grover, 1965). Endogenous compounds that may be substrates include *αβ*-unsaturated compounds formed by autoxidation of polyenoic acids, alkyl and acyl groups released as carbonium ions in dealkylation or deacylation reactions, or epoxides formed as intermediates in oxidative metabolic reactions. However, the original function of glutathione S-transferases is unknown. Boyland (1962) has suggested that nature adapted the existing compound glutathione for a new purpose, that of detoxication.

This investigation has been supported by grants to the Chester Beatty Research Institute (Institute of Cancer Research: Royal Cancer Hospital) from the Medical Research Council and the British Empire Cancer Campaign for Research.

References

Al-Kassab, S., Boyland, E., Williams, K.: An enzyme from rat liver catalysing conjugations with glutathione. Replacement of nitro groups. Biochem. J. **87**, 4—9 (1963).

Angielski, S., Rogulski, J.: The influence of kidney homogenate upon the reaction between glutathione and maleic acid. Acta biochim. pol. **8**, 89—110 (1961).

Azouz, W.M., Parke, D.V., Williams, R.T.: Studies in detoxication. 62. The metabolism of halogenobenzenes. *ortho*- and *para-dichlorobenzenes*. Biochem. J. **59**, 410—415 (1955).

Baer, J.E., Beyer, K.H.: Renal pharmacology. Ann. Rev. Pharmacol. **6**, 261 (1966).

Barnes, M.M., James, S.P.: Glutathione and formation of mercapturic acid *in vivo*. Biochem. J. **66**, 3P (1957).

— — Wood, P.B.: The formation of mercapturic acids. 1. Formation of mercapturic acid and the levels of glutathione in tissues. Biochem. J. **71**, 680—690 (1959).

Barnsley, E.A.: The formation of N-acetyl-S-(2-hydroxypropyl)-L-cysteine from 1-bromopropane in the rat. Biochem. J. **93**, 15P (1964a).

— The metabolism of S-methyl-L-cysteine in the rat. Biochim. biophys. Acta (Amst.) **90**, 24—36 (1964b).

— The formation of 2-hydroxypropylmercapturic acid from 1-halogenopropanes in the rat. Biochem. J. **100**, 362—372 (1966).

— The metabolism of methyl methanesulphonate in the rat. Biochem. J. **106**, 18P—19P (1968).

— Grenby, T.H., Young, L.: Biochemical study of toxic agents. The metabolism of 1- and 2-bromopropane in rats. Biochem. J. **100**, 282—288 (1966).

— Thomson, A.E.R., Young, L.: Biochemical studies of toxic agents. 15. The biosynthesis of ethylmercapturic acid sulphate. Biochem. J. **90**, 588—596 (1964).

— Young, L.: Biochemical studies of toxic agents. The metabolism of iodomethane. Biochem. J. 77—81 (1965).

Baumann, E., Preusse, C.: Über Bromphenylmercaptursäure. Ber. dtsch. Ges. **12**, 806—810 (1879).

Betts, J.J., Bray, H.G., James, S.P., Thorpe, W.V.: The metabolism of the trichloronitrobenzenes in the rabbit. Biochem. J. **66**, 610—621 (1957).

— James, S.P., Thorpe, W.V.: The metabolism of pentachloronitrobenzene and 2:3:4:6-tetrachloronitrobenzene and the formation of mercapturic acids in the rabbit. Biochem. J. **61**, 611—617 (1955).

Beyer, K.H., Baer, J.E., Michaelson, J.K., Russo, H.E.: Renotropic characteristics of ethacrynic acid: A phenoxyacetic saluretic-diuretic agent. J. Pharmacol. exp. Ther. **147**, 1—22 (1965).

Binet, L., Wellers, G.: Role du glutathion lors de l'intoxication du rat par le monobromobenzène. Bull. Soc. Chim. biol. (Paris) **33**, 279—285 (1951).

Binkley, F.: Formation of mercapturic acids by cystinuric and normal dogs. J. biol. Chem. **178**, 811—820 (1949).

Booth, J., Boyland, E., Sato, T., Sims, P.: The reaction of 1:2-dihydronaphthalene and 1:2-epoxy-1:2:3:4-tetrahydronaphthalene with glutathione catalysed by tissue preparations. Biochem. J. **77**, 182—186 (1960).

BOOTH, J., BOYLAND, E., SIMS, P.: The conversion of naphthalene into a derivative of glutathione by rat liver slices. Biochem. J. **74**, 117—122 (1960).

— — — An enzyme from rat liver catalysing conjugations with glutathione. Biochem. J. **79**, 516—524 (1961).

BOURNE, M.C., YOUNG, L.: The metabolism of naphthalene in rabbits. Biochem. J. **28**, 803—808 (1934).

BOYLAND, E.: Some chemical constituents and biochemical reactions of tumours. Acta Un. int. Cancr. **3**, 3—12 (1938).

— Biological significance of metabolism of hydrocarbons. Biochem. Soc. Symp. **5**, 40—54 (1950).

— Mercapturic Acid Conjugation. In: Proc. 1st International Pharmacological Meeting "Mode of action of drugs", Vol. 6, pp. 65—74. Oxford: Pergamon Press 1962.

— Polycyclic hydrocarbons. Brit. med. Bull. **20**, 121—126 (1964).

— CHASSEAUD, L.F.: An enzyme catalysing the reaction of glutathione with unsaturated compounds. Biochem. J. **99**, 13P (1966).

— — Enzyme-catalysed conjugations of glutathione with unsaturated compounds. Biochem. J. **104**, 95—102 (1967).

— — Enzymes catalysing conjugations of glutathione with *αβ*-unsaturated carbonyl compounds. Biochem. J. **109**, 651—661 (1968).

— — Glutathione S-aralkyltransferase. Biochem. J. **115**, 985—991 (1969).

— GROVER, P.L.: The relationship between hepatic glutathione conjugation and BSP excretion and the effect of therapeutic agents. Clin. chim. Acta **16**, 205—213 (1967).

— KIMURA, M., SIMS, P.: The hydroxylation of some aromatic hydrocarbons by the ascorbic acid model hydroxylating system and by rat-liver microsomes. Biochem. J. **92**, 631—638 (1964).

— LEVI, A.A.: Anthrylmercapturic acid. Biochem. J. **30**, 1225—1227 (1936).

— MANSON, D.: The biochemistry of aromatic amines. The metabolism of 2-naphthylamine and 2-naphthylhydroxylamine derivatives. Biochem. J. **101**, 84—102 (1966).

— — NERY, R.: The biochemistry of aromatic amines. 9. Mercapturic acids as metabolites of aniline and 2-naphthylamine. Biochem. J. **86**, 263—271 (1963).

— NERY, R.: The metabolism of urethane and related compounds. Biochem. J. **94**, 198—208 (1965).

— — Mercapturic acid formation during the metabolism of arecoline and arecaidine in the rat. Biochem. J. **113**, 123—130 (1969).

— RAMSAY, G.S., SIMS, P.: The secretion of metabolites of naphthalene, 1,2-dihydronaphthalene and 1,2-epoxy-1,2,3,4-tetrahydronaphthalene in rat bile. Biochem. J. **78**, 376—384 (1961).

— RHODEN, E.: The distribution of urethane in animal tissues, as determined by a microdiffusion method, and the effect of urethane treatment on enzymes. Biochem. J. **44**, 528—531 (1949).

— SIMS, P.: An acid-labile precursor of 1-naphthylmercapturic acid and naphthol: an N-acetyl-S-(1:2-dihydroxynaphthyl)-L-cysteine. Biochem. J. **68**, 440—447 (1958).

— — The metabolism of 1:2-dihydronaphthalene and 1:2-epoxy-1:2:3:4-tetrahydronaphthalene. Biochem. J. **77**, 175—181 (1960).

— — The metabolism of phenanthrene in rabbits and rats: mercapturic acids and related compounds. Biochem. J. **84**, 564—570 (1962).

— — The metabolism of benz[a]anthracene. Biochem. J. **91**, 493—506 (1964a).

— — The metabolism of pyrene in rats and rabbits. Biochem. J. **90**, 391—398 (1964b).

— — The metabolism of 9,10-epoxy-9,10-dihydrophenanthrene in rats. Biochem. J. **95**, 788—792 (1965a).

— — The metabolism of benz[a]anthracene and dibenz[a,h]anthracene and their 5,6-epoxy-5,6-dihydro derivatives by rat-liver homogenates. Biochem. J. **97**, 7—16 (1965b).

— WILLIAMS, K.: A new enzyme, catalysing the conjugations of epoxides. Biochem. J. **94**, 190—197 (1965).

BRAND, E., HARRIS, M.M.: Some aspects of intermediary protein metabolism. Science **77**, 589—590 (1933).

BRAY, H.G., CARPANINI, F.M.B.: The metabolism of thiophen and benzo[b]thiophen. Biochem. J. **109**, 11P (1968).

— CAYGILL, J.C., JAMES, S.P., WOOD, P.B.: Formation of mercapturic acids. 5. Metabolism of some halogenoparaffins and nitroparaffins. Biochem. J. **90**, 127—132 (1964).

— FRANKLIN, T.J.: Glutathione and formation of mercapturic acid *in vitro*. Biochem. J. **66**, 3P (1957).

— — JAMES, S.P.: The formation of mercapturic acids. 2. The possible role of glutathione, Biochem. J. **71**, 690—696 (1959a).

— — — The formation of mercapturic acids. 3. N-acetylation of S-substituted cysteines in the rabbit, rat and guinea pig. Biochem. J. **73**, 465—473 (1959b).

Bray, H.G., Garrett, A.J.: The metabolism of 1:4-quinones and their reactivity with sulphydryl groups. Biochem. J. **80**, 6P (1961).
— Hybs, Z., James, S.P., Thorpe, W.V.: The metabolism of 2:3:5:6- and 2:3:4:5-tetrachloronitrobenzenes in the rabbit and the reduction of aromatic nitro compounds in the intestine. Biochem. J. **53**, 266—273 (1953).
— James, S.P., Thorpe, W.V.: The metabolism of 3:4-dichloronitrobenzene in the rabbit with special reference to the formation of mercapturic acids. Biochem. J. **60**, 23P—24P (1955a).
— — The formation of mercapturic acids from aliphatic compounds *in vivo*. Biochem. J. **69**, 24P (1958).
— — — The metabolism of the trichloronitrobenzenes in the rabbit. Biochem. J. **61**, 5P—6P (1955b).
— — — The metabolism of the monochloronitrobenzenes in the rabbit. Biochem. J. **64**, 38—44 (1956).
— — — The metabolism of 2:4-dichloronitrobenzene in the rabbit. Biochem. J. **65**, 483—490 (1957a).
— — — The metabolism of 2:3-, 2:6- and 3:5-dichloronitrobenzene and the formation of a mercapturic acid from 2:3:4:5-tetrachloronitrobenzene in the rabbit. Biochem. J. **67**, 607—616 (1957b).
— — — Metabolism of *o*-, *m*- and *p*-fluoro-, bromo- and iodo-nitrobenzenes in the rabbit. Biochem. J. **68**, 561—568 (1958a).
— — — Metabolism of some ω-halogenoalkylbenzenes and related alcohols in the rabbit. Biochem. J. **70**, 570—579 (1958b).
Calam, D.H., Waley, S.G.: Acidic peptides of the lens. 8. S-($\alpha\beta$-dicarboxyethyl)glutathione. Biochem. J. **86**, 226—231 (1963).
Chasseaud, L.F.: Enzyme-catalysed conjugations of glutathione with unsaturated compounds. Ph.D. Thesis, University of London, 1967.
Clapp, J.J.: Biochemical studies on arylalkyl mercapturic acids. Ph.D. Thesis, University of London, 1967.
— Kaye, C.M., Young, L.: Observations on the metabolism of allyl compounds in the rat. Biochem. J. **114**, 6P—7P (1969).
Clark, A.G., Darby, F.J., Smith, J.N.: Species differences in the inhibition of glutathione S-aryltransferase by phthaleins and dicarboxylic acids. Biochem. J. **103**, 49—54 (1967).
Cohen, A.J., Smith, J.N.: Comparative detoxication. 9. The metabolism of some halogenated compounds by conjugation with glutathione in the locust. Biochem. J. **90**, 449—456 (1964).
— — Turbert, H.: Comparative detoxication. 10. The enzymic conjugation of chloro compounds with glutathione in locusts and other insects. Biochem. J. **90**, 457—464 (1964).
Colucci, D.F., Buyske, D.A.: The biotransformation of a sulfonamide to a mercaptan and to mercapturic acid and glucuronide conjugates. Biochem. Pharmacol. **14**, 457—466 (1965).
Combes, B.: The biliary excretion of sulfobromophthalein sodium (BSP) in the rat as a conjugate of glycine and glutamic acid. J. clin. Invest. **38**, 1426—1433 (1959).
— The importance of conjugation with glutathione for sulfobromophthalein sodium (CBSP) transfer from blood to bile. J. clin. Invest. **44**, 1214—1224 (1965).
— Stakelum, G.S.: A liver enzyme that conjugates sulfobromophthalein sodium with glutathione. J. clin. Invest. **40**, 981—988 (1961).
Cornish, H.H., Block, W.D.: Metabolism of chlorinated naphthalenes. J. biol. Chem. **231**, 583—588 (1958).
Daniel, J.W., Gage, J.C., Jones, D.I.: The metabolism of 3,5-di-*tert*.-butyl-4-hydroxytoluene in the rat and in man. Biochem. J. **106**, 783—790 (1968).
Davison, C., Rozman, R.S., Smith, P.K.: Metabolism of bis-β-chloroethyl sulfide (sulfur mustard gas). Biochem. Pharmacol. **7**, 65—74 (1961).
Day, E.A.: Role of milk lipids in Flavours of dairy products. Advanc. Amer. Chem. Ser. **56**, 94—120 (1966).
Dickens, F.: Carcinogenic lactones and related substances. Brit. med. Bull. **20**, 96—101 (1964).
— Jones, H.E.H., Waynforth, H.B.: Oral subcutaneous and intratracheal administration of carcinogenic lactones and related substances: the intratracheal administration of cigarette tar in the rat. Brit. J. Cancer **20**, 134—144 (1966).
Fassett, D.W., Irish, D.D.: Industrial hygiene and toxicology. 2nd rev. ed., Vol. 2. New York: Interscience 1963.
Forss, D.A., Dunstone, E.A., Ramshaw, E.H., Stark, W.: The flavor of cucumbers. J. Food Sci. **27**, 90—93 (1962).
Foxwell, C.J., Young, L.: The metabolism of S-alkylglutathiones. Biochem. J. **92**, 50P (1964).
Friedman, M., Cavins, J.F., Wall, J.S.: Relative nucleophilic reactivities of amino groups and mercaptide ions in addition reactions with $\alpha\beta$-unsaturated compounds. J. Amer. chem. Soc. **87**, 3672—3682 (1965).

FUKAMI, J., SHISHIDO, T.: Nature of a soluble glutathione dependent enzyme system active in cleavage of methylparathion to demethyl parathion. J. Econ. Entomol. **59**, 1338—1346 (1966).
GEIGER, W.B., CONN, J.E.: The mechanism of antibiotic action of clavacin and penicillic acid. J. Amer. chem. Soc. **67**, 112—116 (1945).
GILLHAM, B., YOUNG, L.: Isolation of biosynthetic p-bromophenylmercapturic acid. Biochem. J. **103**, 24P—25P (1967).
GRODSKY, G.M., CARBONE, J.V., FANSKA, R.: Identification of metabolites of sulfobromophthalein. J. clin. Invest. **38**, 1981—1988 (1959).
GROVER, P.L.: Conjugations with glutathione. Ph.D. Thesis, University of London, 1965.
— SIMS, P.: Conjugations with glutathione. I. Distribution of glutathione S-aryltransferase in vertebrate species. Biochem. J. **90**, 603—606 (1964).
GUTMANN, H.R., WOOD, J.L.: The effect of bromobenzene and 3,4-benzpyrene on the metabolism of radioactive L-cystine. Cancer Res. **10**, 8—12 (1950).
— — A note on the acetylation of sulfur amino acids by liver and kidney. J. biol. Chem. **189**, 473—477 (1951).
HAUSCHKA, T., TOENNIES, G., SWAIN, A.P.: The mechanism of growth inhibition by hexenolactone. Science **101**, 383—385 (1945).
HEPPEL, L.A., HILMOE, R.J.: Metabolism of inorganic nitrite and nitrate esters. Il The enzymatic reduction of nitro-glycerin and erythritol tetranitrate by glutathione. J. biol. Chem. **183**, 129—138 (1950)
HURD, C.D., GERSHBEIN, L.L.: Reactions of mercaptans with acrylic and methacrylic derivatives. J. Amer. chem. Soc. **69**, 2328—2335 (1947).
HUTSON, D.H., AKINTONWA, D.A.A., HATHWAY, D.E.: The metabolism of 2-chloro-1-(2′,4′-dichlorophenylvinyl diethyl phosphate (Chlorfenvinphos) in the dog and rat. Biochem. J. **102**, 133—142 (1967).
— PICKERING, B.A., DONNINGER, C.: Phosphoric acid triester: glutathione alkyltransferase. Biochem. J. **106**, 20P (1968).
HYDE, C.W., YOUNG, L.: Biosynthesis of 1- and 2-menaphthylmercapturic acid. Biochem. J. **94**, 34P (1965).
— — Biochemical studies of toxic agents. The metabolic formation of 1- and 2-menaphthylmercapturic acid. Biochem. J. **107**, 519—522 (1968).
JAFFÉ, M.: Über die nach Einführung von Bromobenzol und Chlorbenzol in Organismus entstehenden schwefelhaltigen Säuren. Ber. dtsch. chem. Ges. **12**, 1092—1098 (1879).
JAGENBURG, O.R., TOCZKO, K.: The metabolism of acetophenetidine. Isolation and characterization of S-(1-acetamido-4-hydroxyphenyl)-cysteine, a metabolite of acetophenetidine. Biochem. J. **92**, 639—643 (1964).
JAMES, S.P.; The metabolism of some bromo paraffins. Biochem. J. **80**, 4P (1961)
— JEFFERY, D.J.: The biosynthesis of N-acetyl-S-hydroxyalkylcysteines. Biochem. J. **93**, 16P (1964).
— — WARING, R.H., WOOD, P.B.: Some metabolites of 1-bromobutane in the rabbit and the rat. Biochem. J. **109**, 727—736 (1968).
— WARING, R.H., WHITE, D.A.: Some metabolites of bromocyclopentane, bromocyclohexane and bromocycloheptane. Biochem. J. **103**, 25P (1967).
— WHITE, D.A.: The metabolism of phenethyl bromide, styrene and styrene oxide in the rabbit and rat. Biochem. J. **104**, 914—921 (1967).
JERINA, D.M., DALY, J.W., WITKOP, B., ZALTZMAN-NIRENBERG, P., UDENFRIEND, S.: The role of arene oxide-oxepin systems in the metabolism of aromatic substrates. III. Formation of 1,2-naphthalene oxide from naphthalene by liver microsomes. J. Amer. chem. Soc. **90**, 6525—6527 (1968).
JOHNSON, M.K.: A distinct enzyme of rat liver and kidney coupling glutathione with some aliphatic halogen compounds. Biochem. J. **87**, 9P—10P (1963).
— The influence of some aliphatic compounds on rat liver glutathione levels. Biochem. Pharmacol. **14**, 1383—1385 (1965).
— Metabolism of iodomethane in the rat. Biochem. J. **98**, 38—43 (1966a).
— Studies on glutathione S-alkyltransferase of the rat. Biochem. J. **98**, 44—56 (1966b).
JONDORF, W.R., PARKE, D.V., WILLIAMS, R.T.: Studies in detoxication. 66. The metabolism of halogenobenzenes. 1:2:3-, 1:2:4- and 1:3:5-trichlorobenzenes. Biochem. J. **61**, 512—521 (1955).
KLAASSEN, C.D., PLAA, G.L.: Species variation in metabolism storage and excretion of sulfobromophthalein. Amer. J. Physiol. **213**, 1322—1326 (1967).
KNIGHT, R.H., YOUNG, L.: Biochemical studies of toxic agents. 11. The occurrence of premercapturic acids. Biochem. J. **70**, 111—119 (1958).
KNUTH, C., BAVLEY, A., LAZIER, W.A.: Reaction of thiols with unsaturated compounds. J. Org. Chem. **19**, 845—850 (1954).

Kuwaki, T.: Enzymatic cleavage of S-(isopropylcarboxymethyl) glutathione into isovalthine. J. Biochem. (Tokyo) **57**, 125—130 (1965).
— Mizuhara, S.: S-(1-2-dicarboxyethyl)cysteine in urine and kidney. Biochim. biophys. Acta (Amst.) **115**, 491—493 (1966).
— Ohmori, S., Mizuhara, S.: Biosynthesis of isovalthine precursor in liver homogenates. Biochim. biophys. Acta (Amst.) **78**, 553—555 (1963).
Marsden, C.M., Young, L.: Biochemical studies of toxic agents. 10. Observations of the metabolism of ^{35}S-labelled mercapturic acids. Biochem. J. **69**, 257—265 (1958).
Mayo, F.R., Walling, C.: The peroxide effect in the addition of reagents on saturated compounds and in rearrangement reactions. Chem. Rev. **27**, 351—412 (1940).
McGowan, J.C., Brian, P.W., Hemming, H.G.: Fungistatic activity of ethylenic and acetylenic compounds. Effect of the affinity of the substituents for electrons upon the biological activity of ethylenic compounds. Ann. appl. Biol. **35**, 25—36 (1948).
Mills, G.C., Wood, J.L.: Metabolism of iodobenzene. J. biol. Chem. **204**, 547—552 (1953).
— — Mercapturic acid precursors. J. biol. Chem. **219**, 1—8 (1956).
Morello, A., Vardanis, A., Spencer, E.Y.: Differential glutathione-dependent detoxication of two geometrical vinyl organophosphorus (mevinphos) isomers. Biochem. biophys. Res. Commun. **29**, 241—245 (1967).
Morris, J.E.: The carcinogenic activity in the rat of some derivatives of 5-nitrofuran. Dissertation Abstr. **28**, 1594—1595 (1967).
Nakahara, W., Fukuoka, F.: Study of carcinogenic mechanisms based on experiments with 4-nitroquinoline N-oxide. Gann **50**, 1—15 (1959).
Nakashima, T.: Chemical studies on the origin of naphthalene cataracts. J. Biochem. (Tokyo) **19**, 281—314 (1934).
Needleman, P. Hunter, F.E.: The transformation of glyceryl trinitrate and other nitrates by glutathioneorganic nitrate reductase. Molec. Pharmacol. **1**, 77—86 (1965).
Nickerson, W.J., Falcone, G., Strauss, G.: Studies on quinone-thioethers. I. Mechanism of formation and properties of thiodione. Biochemistry **2**, 537—543 (1963).
Nursten, H.E., Williams, A.A.: Fruit aromas: a survey of components identified. Chem. Ind. (Lond.) 486—497 (1967).
Ohmori, S., Mizuhara, S.: Structure of a new sulfur-containing amino acid. Arch. Biochem. Biophys. **96**, 179—185 (1962).
— Shimomura, T., Azumi, T., Mizuhara, S.: S-(β-carboxy-n-propyl)-L-cysteine and S-(β-carboxyethyl)-L-cysteine in urine. Biochem. Z. **343**, 9—15 (1965).
Parke, D.V., Williams, R.T.: Studies in detoxication. 63. The metabolism of halogenobenzenes. (a) *Meta*-dichlorobenzene. (b) Further observations on the metabolism of chlorobenzene. Biochem. J. **59**, 415—422 (1955).
Patai, S., Rappoport, Z.: Nucleophilic attacks on carbon-carbon double bonds. In: The chemistry of alkenes, pp. 469—584. S. Patai, ed. New York and London: Interscience 1964.
Pillinger, D.J., Craig, A.W., Jackson, H.: Tracer studies of the metabolism of methyl methanesulphonate. Biochem. J. **90**, 43P (1964).
Porter, C.C.: Cited in Baer, J.E., and Beyer, K.H.: Renal Pharmacology. Ann. Rev. Pharmacol. **6**, 261—292 (1966).
Revel, J.P., Ball, E.G.: The reaction of glutathione with amino acids and related compounds as catalyzed by γ-glutamyl transpeptidase. J. biol. Chem. **234**, 577—582 (1959).
Rhode, H.: The excretion of ethereal sulfates by rabbits after feeding phenol, bromophenol and bromobenzene. Hoppe-Seylers Z. physiol. Chem. **124**, 15—36 (1922).
Roberts, J.J., Warwick, G.P.: Studies on the mode of action of tumour-growth-inhibiting alkylating agents. I. The fate of ethyl methanesulphonate ("half Myleran") in the rat. Biochem. Pharmacol. **1**, 60—75 (1958a).
— — The metabolism of alkyl alkanesulphonates and related compounds. A.R. Brit. Emp. Cancer Campgn. **36**, 53—54 (1958b).
— — Metabolic and chemical studies of 'Myleran': formation of 3-hydroxy-tetrahydrothiophene-1,1-dioxide *in vivo* and reactions with thiols *in vitro*. Nature (Lond.) **184**, 1288—1289 (1959).
Rosenthal, S.M., White, E.C.: Hepatic function. VI. The pharmacological behavior of certain phthalein dyes. The value of selected phthalein compounds in the estimation of hepatic function. J. Pharmacol. **24**, 265—288 (1924).
Schales, O., Graefe, H.A.: Arylnitroalkenes. A new group of antibacterial agents. J. Amer. chem. Soc. **74**, 4486—4490 (1952).
Searle, C.E.: Tumour initiatory activity of chloromononitrobenzenes. Cancer Res. **26**, 12—17 (1966).
Sherwin, C.P.: The fate of foreign organic compounds in the animal body. Physiol. Rev. **2**, 238—276 (1922).

SIMS, P.: The metabolism of 3-methylcholanthrene and some related compounds by rat-liver homogenates. Biochem. J. **98**, 215—228 (1966).
— The metabolism of 7- and 12-methylbenz[a]anthracene and their derivatives. Biochem. J. **105**, 591—598 (1967).
— The metabolism of some aromatic hydrocarbons by mouse embryo cell cultures. Biochem. Pharmacol. (in press) (1969).
— GROVER, P.L.: Conjugations with glutathione. The enzymic conjugation of some chlorocyclohexenes. Biochem. J. **95**, 156—160 (1965).
SKLAN, N.M., BARNSLEY, E.A.: The metabolism of S-methyl-L-cysteine. Biochem. J. **107**, 217—223 (1968).
SMITH, J.N., SPENCER, B., WILLIAMS, R.T.: Studies in detoxication. 34. The metabolism of chlorobenzene in the rabbit. Isolation of dihydrodihydroxychlorobenzene, p-chlorophenylglucuronide, 4-chlorocatechol glucuronide and p-chlorophenylmercapturic acid. Biochem. J. **47**, 284—293 (1950).
SPENCER, B., WILLIAMS, R.T.: Studies in detoxication. 33. The metabolism of halogenobenzenes. A comparison of the glucuronic acid, ethereal sulphate and mercapturic acid conjugations of chloro-, bromo- and iodo-benzenes and of the o-, m- and p-chlorophenols. Biosynthesis of o-, m- and p-chlorophenylglucuronides. Biochem. J. **47**, 279—284 (1950).
STEKOL, J.A.: Studies on the mercapturic acid synthesis in animals. I. The extent of the synthesis of p-bromophenylmercapturic acid in dogs as affected by diets of varying sulfur content. J. biol. Chem. **117**, 147—159 (1937a).
— Studies on the mercapturic acid synthesis in animals. III. The extent of the synthesis of p-bromophenylmercapturic acid in dogs as related to the time of administration of food and bromobenzene. J. biol. Chem. **118**, 155—160 (1937b).
— Studies on the mercapturic acid synthesis in animals. VI. The dependence of the extent of the synthesis of p-bromophenylmercapturic acid in dogs on the body weight. J. biol. Chem. **121**, 93—98 (1937c).
— Studies on the mercapturic acid synthesis in animals. V. The effect of naphthalene on the growth of rats as related to diets of varying sulfur content. J. biol. Chem. **121**, 87—91 (1937d).
— Studies on the mercapturic acid synthesis in animals. VIII. l-cystine dl-methionine, glutathione and taurine in relation to the synthesis of mercapturic acids in the rat. J. biol. Chem. **122**, 333—342 (1937e).
— Studies on the mercapturic acid synthesis in animals. IX. The conversion of benzyl chloride and S-benzylcysteine into benzylmercapturic acid in the organism of the dog, rabbit and rat. J. biol. Chem. **124**, 129—132 (1938).
— Studies on the mercapturic acid synthesis in animals. X. Glutathione in relation to growth of rats on a low casein diet which contained bromobenzene and naphthalene. J. biol. Chem. **127** 131—136 (1939a).
— Studies on the mercapturic acid synthesis in animals. XI. The detoxication of benzyl chloride, benzyl alcohol, benzaldehyde and S-benzylhomocysteine in the rabbit and rat. J. biol. Chem. **128**, 199—205 (1939b).
— Conversion of S-benzylglutathione to benzylmercapturic acid. Proc. Soc. exp. Biol. (N.Y.) **43**, 108—110 (1940).
— Studies on the mercapturic acid synthesis in animals. XII. The synthesis of N-acetyl-S-p-bromobenzyl-l-cysteine in the rat from p-bromobenzyl bromide, S-p-bromobenzyl-l-cysteine, and S-p-bromobenzylglutathione. J. biol. Chem. **138**, 225—229 (1941).
— Studies on the mercapturic acid synthesis in animals. XIV. On the synthesis of mercapturic acids in man. J. biol. Chem. **164**, 651—656 (1946).
SUGA, T., KUMAOKA, H., AKAGI, M.: Studies on mercapturic acids. Participation of glutathionase in the conversion of glutathione derivatives to cysteine derivatives. J. Biochem. (Tokyo) **60**, 133—139 (1966a).
— OHATA, I., AKAGI, M.: Studies on mercapturic acids. Effect of some aromatic compounds on the level of glutathione and the activity of glutathionase in the rat. J. Biochem. (Tokyo) **59**, 209, 215 (1966b).
— — KUMAOKA, H., AKAGI, M.: Studies on mercapturic acids. Investigation of glutathione-conjugating enzyme by the method of thin-layer chromatography. Chem. Pharmacol. Bull. **15**, 1059—1064 (1967).
TAGGART, J.V., ANGIELSKI, S., MORELL, H.: Complete oxidation of maleic acid via D(+) malate in the kidney. Biochim. biophys. Acta (Amst.) **58**, 141—144 (1962).
THOMSON, A.E.R., BARNSLEY, E.A., YOUNG, L.: Biochemical studies of toxic agents. 14. The biosynthesis of ethylmercapturic acid. Biochem. J. **86**, 145—152 (1963).
— MAW, G.A., YOUNG, L.: Ethylmercapturic acid and its formation *in vivo*. Biochem. J. **69**, 23P (1958).

UBUKA, T., KODAMA, H., MIZUHARA, S.: Isolation of S-(carboxymethyl)-cysteine from urine. Biochim. biophys. Acta (Amst.) **141**, 266—269 (1967).
VEST, M.F., ROSSIER, R.: Detoxification in the newborn: the ability of the newborn infant to form conjugates with glucuronic acid, glycine, acetate and glutathione. Ann. N.Y. Acad. Sci. **111**, 183—198 (1963—1964).
VIRTANEN, A.I.: Some organic sulfur compounds in vegetables and fodder plants and their significance in human nutrition. Angew. Chem. Internat. Ed. **1**, 299—306 (1962).
VOGEL, E., KLÄRNER, F.G.: 1,2-Naphthalene oxide. Angew. Chem. Internat. Ed. **7**, 374—375 (1968).
WAELSCH, H.: Detoxication in the animal organism. Arch. exp. Pathol. Pharmakol. **156**, 356—369 (1930).
WAINER, A., LORINCZ, A.E.: Studies on mercapturic acid synthesis by humans. Life Sci. **7**, 504—508 (1963).
WATANABE, T.: Substances in mulberry leaves which attract silkworm larvae (*Bombyx mori*). Nature (Lond.) **182**, 325—326 (1958).
WEST, H.D., LAWSON, J.R., MILLER, I.H., MATHURA, G.R.: The fate of diphenyl in the rat. Arch. Biochem. Biophys. **60**, 14—20 (1956).
— MATHURA, G.R.: Synthesis of some aryl-substituted L-cysteines and their fate in the animal body. J. biol. Chem. **208**, 315—318 (1954).
— — BLACK, L.A.: Laboratory synthesis of p-chlorophenyl-L-cysteine and its acetylation by the rat. J. biol. Chem. **193**, 133—135 (1951).
— MILLER, I.H.: The fate of mercapturic acids in the animal body. J. nat. med. Ass. (N.Y.) **54**, 17—21 (1962).
WISHNER, L.A., KEENEY, M.: Comparative study of monocarbonyl compounds formed during deep frying in different fats. J. Amer. Oil. Chem. Soc. **42**, 776—778 (1965).
WIT, J.G., VAN GENDEREN, H.: Metabolism of the herbicide 2,6-dichlorobenzonitrile in rabbits and rats. Biochem. J. **101**, 698—706 (1966).
— LEEUWANGH, P.: Mercapturic acid formation and enzyme-catalyzed conjugations with glutathione in pigeons. Biochim. biophys. Acta (Amst.) **177**, 329—335 (1969).
— SNEL, J.: Enzymatic glutathione conjugations with 2,3-epoxyphenylpropylether and diethylmaleate by wild bird liver supernatant. European J. Pharmacol. **3**, 370—373 (1968).
ZBARSKY, S.H., YOUNG, L.: Mercapturic acids. II. The formation of 1-phenylmercapturic acid from phenyl-1-cysteine *in vivo*. J. biol. Chem. **151**, 217—219 (1943).

Chapter 56

Methyltransferase Enzymes in the Metabolism of Physiologically Active Compounds and Drugs

JULIUS AXELROD

There are a number of methyltransferase enzymes that have been found to be involved in the biosynthesis and inactivation of physiologically active compounds and in the metabolism of drugs. The methyl donor for these reactions is S-adenosylmethionine which is formed from a methionine-activating enzyme as follows (CANTONI and DURELL, 1957):

$$\text{Methionine} + \text{AR-P-P-P} \xrightarrow{Mg^{2+}} \text{S-adenosylmethionine} + \text{pyrophosphate} + \text{Pi}$$

Depending on the enzyme, methyltransferases can transfer the methyl group of S-adenosylmethionine to oxygen or nitrogen to form a methylated product and homocysteine. This report will describe the properties of a number of methyltransferases, their physiological significance and control.

I. Catechol-O-Methyltransferase (COMT)

In 1957 it was found that major metabolic products of noradrenaline are the O-methylated deaminated product 3-methoxy-4-hydroxymandelic acid (ARMSTRONG et al., 1957) and the O-methylated amine normetanephrine (AXELROD, 1957). These observations suggested the presence of an enzyme that can methylate an oxygen group. Enzymes had already been found that could methylate the nitrogen group of nicotinamide (CANTONI, 1951) and guanidoacetic acid (CANTONI and VIGNOS, 1954). S-adenosylmethionine served as the methyl donor for these reactions. These observations prompted a search for an O-methyltransferase in which catecholamines might serve as a substrate. In the initial experiment, a liver homogenate was incubated with S-adenosylmethionine and adrenaline (AXELROD, 1957). Under these conditions adrenaline was metabolized with the formation of a new metabolite, metanephrine (3-methoxy-4-hydroxyphenyl-2-methylamino ethanol).

The properties of this methyltransferase were studied with a partially purified enzyme obtained from rat liver (AXELROD and TOMCHICK, 1958). With ammonium sulfate fractionation and calcium phosphate adsorption and elution the enzyme was purified about 30-fold. Catechol-O-methyltransferase activity from liver has an optimal pH of 7.9 in phosphate buffer. It requires divalent cations such as Mg, Mn, Zn, Co, Fe or Ni. The enzyme O-methylated all catechols examined regardless of the substituent on the aromatic nucleus. The enzyme could O-methylate such normally occurring compounds as noradrenaline, dopamine, adrenaline, dopa, 3,4-dihydroxymandelic acid, 3,4-dihydroxyphenylacetic acid and 2-hydroxyestradiol, and drugs such as 3,4-dihydroxyephedrine, 3,4-dihydroxyamphetamine.

Monophenols could not be O-methylated by COMT. The enzyme showed no stereospecificity to d or l isomers of catecholamines.

Enzymatic O-methylation occurs predominantly on the meta position. However O-methylation by COMT occurs to a small extent on the phenolic group para to the electron deficient as well as nondeficient side chain (SENOH et al., 1959, 1962). Incubation of 3,4-dihydroxyacetophenone with COMT yields 50% each of para and meta O-methylated products while dopamine forms 90% meta and 10% para O-methylated metabolites. 3,4-Dihydroxyacetophenone has a relatively strong nucleophilic para hydroxy group which may explain the increase in para O-methylation. Phenolic compounds having three adjacent hydroxy groups (gallic acid, pyrogallol) are methylated on the middle hydroxy group whether it is in the para or in the meta position. Incubation of 5,6-dihydroxyindoles results in O-methylation mainly on the 6 position (AXELROD and LERNER, 1963). A novel interconversion of the methyl groups of 3-methoxy-4-hydroxyacetophenone to 3-hydroxy-4-methoxy-acetophenone and of the latter compound to 3-methoxy-4-hydroxy-acetophenone occurs *in vivo* (DALY et al., 1960). This interconversion of the *m* and *p* O-methylated catechols ethers is the result of demethylation of the catechol by a NADPH microsomal (AXELROD, 1956) enzyme followed by remethylation by COMT.

COMT can be inhibited reversibly and competitively by polyphenols and catechols such as pyrogallol (AXELROD and LA ROCHE, 1959; BACQ et al., 1959), gallic acid esters, dopacetamide (CARLSSON et al., 1962), dimethylpapaverine, catechol flavonoids, and adnamine and noradnamine, acid degradation products of adrenaline and noradrenaline respectively (ABBS et al., 1967). Tropolones are also potent inhibitors of COMT (BELLEAU and BURBA, 1963). These compounds show an isosterism with catechols, form chelates with divalent cations and may inhibit COMT by displacing the catechol substrate from its complex with enzymes.

The requirement for divalent cations and catechols suggests that the divalent metal may serve as a chelating agent to bring the substrate, S-adenosylmethionine, and catechols together in a bridge complex. The electrophilic methyl group of S-adenosylmethionine is then transferred to one of the hydroxy groups of the catechol by a nucleophilic displacement reaction. In the case of most catechols the 3-hydroxy group is the more strongly nucleophilic so that the transmethylation occurs on this position. The active site on the enzyme surface appears to contain a sulfhydryl group since the enzyme is inhibited by *p*-chloromercuribenzoate and iodoacetic acid (AXELROD and TOMCHICK, 1958). COMT has been purified about 180-fold from rat liver and its molecular weight calculated to be about 29,000 (ANDERSON and D'IORIO, 1968). On starch block electrophoreses COMT appears to be heterogenous (AXELROD and VESSEL, 1970). At least two isozymes have been found in liver and other tissues of rat. The heat stability and K_m values of the two forms of COMT from rat liver were found to be different. There was also a separation of two forms of COMT in human, dog and cat livers. These isozymes appeared to have a different electrophoretic mobility, heat stability and K_m values from those of the rat.

Subcellular studies have shown that COMT is present mainly in the soluble fraction of the cell (AXELROD and TOMCHICK, 1958). A small amount of COMT has been found in the microsomal fraction of the liver (INSCOE et al., 1965). The microsomal COMT appears to be different from that of the soluble fraction with respect to pH optima and species distribution. Cold stress and benzpyrene increase the microsomal COMT but not the soluble enzyme.

COMT is widely distributed in mammalian tissues. It has been found in liver, kidney, spleen, intestines, salivary gland, pituitary, thyroid, pineal, aorta, vena cava and skin (Axelrod and Tomchick, 1958; Bamshad et al., 1964). It is also present in all regions of the central nervous system, peripheral nerves (Axelrod et al., 1961) and in neuroblastoma (La Brosse and Karon, 1962). There is an unequal distribution of the COMT in the brain, highest activity being present in the area postrema and lowest in the cerebellar cortex (Axelrod et al., 1961). In the rat brain COMT is highly localized in synaptic components (Alberici et al., 1965). COMT has also been found in fish (Brandenburger-Brown and Trams, 1968), amphibian and avian tissues (Axelrod and Lauber, 1968).

In newborn rats and chick embryoes COMT activity is very low and rises rapidly after birth (Ignarro and Shideman, 1968). During pregnancy there is a twofold increase in COMT in the rat uterus (Wurtman et al., 1964b). There is an increased COMT activity after cardiac hypertrophy due to congestive heart failure but no change in concentration of the enzyme (Krakoff et al., 1968). Hypophysectomy and large doses of thyroxine reduce COMT activity in rat liver (Landsberg et al., 1969).

COMT serves an important role in the inactivation of circulating catecholamines. Once the neurotransmitter noradrenaline or the hormone adrenaline is released into the bloodstream, they are metabolized mainly by O-methylation in the liver or kidney (Hertting and La Brosse, 1962). The O-methylated products formed and excreted into the urine as a result of the actions of COMT are normetanephrine, metanephrine, N-methylmetanephrine, 3-methoxytyramine, 3-methoxydopa, 3-methoxy-4-hydroxymandelic acid, 3-methoxy-4-hydroxyglycol, homovanillic acid, vanillic acid and 2-methoxyestradiol.

When the neurotransmitter noradrenaline is released from the nerves the principal mechanism for its inactivation is reuptake into sympathetic nerves (Hertting and Axelrod, 1961) but a small fraction of the catecholamine is O-methylated at the effector cell. Another fraction of noradrenaline overflows into the bloodstream and this is ultimately metabolized by COMT in the liver. In studies on the extraneural uptake of noradrenaline it was concluded that COMT was in close juxtaposition to the adrenergic receptor (Eisenfeld et al., 1967). The noradrenaline that is rapidly released from nerves by sympathomimetic amines is also metabolized mainly by O-methylation (Kopin and Gordon, 1962).

Two other catechol-O-methyltransferase enzymes have been found in plants. In fruit plants an O-methylating enzyme is present that methylates catechols mainly on the meta position (Finkle and Nelson, 1963). An enzyme has also been described in flowering bulbs of Nerine bowdenii which methylates the catechol norbelladine mainly on the para position (Mann et al., 1963). An enzyme that O-methylates 2,6-diiodophenols has been found in the liver of mammals. This enzyme differs from COMT since it has a different substrate specificity and has no requirement for Mg^{2+} ions (Tomita et al., 1964).

II. Phenol-O-Methyltransferase

Recently an O-methyltransferase that O-methylates monophenols has been described (Axelrod and Daly, 1968). Phenol, as well as a wide variety of simple alkyl-, methoxy- and halophenols, can be O-methylated by phenol-O-methyltransferase. Hydroxyacetanilide is a good substrate and the enzyme could form the analgesic acetophenetidin with S-adenosylethionine as the alkyl donor. Phenolic amines such as tyramine and 3-methoxy-4-hydroxyphenylethylamine could not serve as substrates for this enzyme. Unlike COMT, phenol-O-methyltransferase is highly localized in the microsomes and is found in liver, lung and other tissues of mammals. Activity of this enzyme is inhibited by SKF 525, a compound that can inhibit enzymes present in the microsomes (COOPER et al., 1954). *p*-Chloromercuribenzoate and N-ethylmaleimide also inhibit phenol-O-methyltransferase indicating the presence of an active SH group. In rats, hypophysectomy increases the activity of phenol-O-methyltransferase in the liver but not in lung or brain.

III. O-Methylation of Hydroxamic Acid

A methylating enzyme has been found that transfers the methyl group of S-adenosylmethionine to the N-O- group of N-hydroxy-2-acetylamino fluorene to form an N-methoxy derivative (LOTIKAR, 1968). This enzyme has an absolute requirement for cysteine and is localized in the soluble fraction of the cell. It is present mainly in the liver of rats and other mammals but small amounts of the N-O-methylating enzyme have been found in the kidney. Other hydroxamic acids such as benzohydroxamic acid, N-hydroxy-4-acetylaminostilbene and propionohydroxamic acid can also serve as substrates. The N-O-methylated metabolite of N-hydroxy-2-acetylaminofluorene is more carcinogenic than the parent compound.

IV. Hydroxyindole-O-Methyl Transferase (HIOMT)

The discovery of HIOMT stemmed from the observation of LERNER et al. (1959) that melatonin (5-methoxy-N-acetyl-tryptamine) is highly localized in the cow pineal gland. The presence of melatonin (a skin lightening agent in amphibians) in the bovine pineal suggested the presence of an enzyme in this organ that can carry out an O-methylation reaction. The two possible substrates for this enzyme were serotonin or N-acetylserotonin. When N-acetylserotonin was incubated with an extract of bovine pineal gland and S-adenosylmethionine, a new compound was formed which was identified as melatonin (AXELROD and WEISSBACH, 1960). These observations suggested the presence of an enzyme in the pineal that can transfer the methyl group from S-adenosylmethionine to the hydroxy group of N-acetylserotonin.

HIOMT was purified about 20-fold from cow pineal glands (AXELROD and WEISSBACH, 1961). The purified enzyme showed an absolute requirement for S-adenosylmethionine but, unlike COMT, did not require metal ions. The enzyme contains an essential sulfhydryl group since its activity was inhibited by *p*-chlormercuribenzoate.

By far the best substrate for mammalian HIOMT is N-acetylserotonin. However, the mammalian enzyme can O-methylate a variety of 5-hydroxyindoles. The rate at which serotonin is O-methylated is less than one twentieth that of N-acetylserotonin suggesting that N-acetylation precedes O-methylation in the formation of melatonin. Other 5-hydroxy indoles such as N-methylserotonin, bufotenine and 5-hydroxyindole are O-methylated, but to a smaller extent. 5,6-Dihydroxy indoles which are both catechols and indoles are O-methylated mainly in the 5 position by HIOMT and in the 6 position by COMT (AXELROD and LERNER, 1963). HIOMT obtained from quail pineal has a somewhat different substrate specificity from that of mammalian HIOMT (AXELROD and LAUBER, 1968). The avian enzyme methylates serotonin as well as N-acetylserotonin. Quail HIOMT also differs from cow HIOMT with respect to electrophoretic mobility, K_m for N-acetylserotonin, and heat stability (AXELROD and VESSEL, 1970). Several N-acetyltryptamine derivatives were found to inhibit HIOMT (BO et al., 1968). The most active compound is phenylacetyltryptamine, which has an affinity for bovine HIOMT six times greater than N-acetylserotonin.

HIOMT is localized mainly in the soluble fraction of the cell. In mammals HIOMT is uniquely located in the pineal gland (AXELROD et al., 1961). The enzyme has been found in all vertebrate species including birds, reptiles, amphibians and fish (AXELROD et al., 1965; BAKER et al., 1965; QUAY, 1965). HIOMT has also been found in the brain of amphibians and the eyes of fish, amphibians, reptiles and some birds (QUAY, 1965). Hamster pineals infected with oncogenic viruses (SV-40, LLE-46 and polyoma) and implanted in homologous hosts formed tumors that contained HIOMT activity (WELLS et al., 1966). HIOMT has been found in pineal tumors of man and has been used as a marker for identifying tumors of pineal origin (WURTMAN et al., 1964c).

HIOMT activity is influenced by environmental lighting and changes in physiological conditions. When animals are kept in continuous darkness, HIOMT activity increases in rat pineal (WURTMAN et al., 1963) and decreases in the hen pineal. The effect of light on pineal HIOMT is not direct in rats but is mediated by the eye, brain and sympathetic nerves (WURTMAN et al., 1964a). Light affects HIOMT in blind as well as ganglionectomized birds (LAUBER et al., 1968). A twofold variation in HIOMT activity was observed during the rat estrus cycle, rising during diestrus and falling during proestrus and estrus (WURTMAN et al., 1965). Pineal glands can be maintained in organ culture (SHEIN et al., 1967). These pineals synthesize melatonin from tryptophan and the neurotransmitter noradrenaline stimulates the formation of melatonin several fold (AXELROD et al., 1969). Noradrenaline also slightly increases the activity of HIOMT in pineal organ culture (KLEIN, 1969).

V. Phenylethanolamine N-Methyl Transferase (PNMT)

PNMT is the enzyme involved in the last step in the metabolism of catecholamines; it N-methylates noradrenaline to adrenaline. The methylation of noradrenaline to adrenaline was first demonstrated in minced adrenal gland in the presence of ATP (BULBRING et al., 1949). *In vivo* studies then showed that the methyl group of methionine is incorporated in the adrenaline isolated from the adrenal gland (KELLER et al., 1950). Later S-adenosylmethionine was shown to be the methyl donor (KIRSHNER and GOODALL, 1957). In 1962 the PNMT enzyme was purified and its properties and distribution studied (AXELROD, 1962b). The enzyme was partially purified about 25-fold by ammonium sulfate precipitation and calcium phosphate gel adsorption and elution. In 0.05 M phosphate buffers optimal activity occurs from pH 7.5—8.0. Increasing the concentration of phosphate ions above 0.05 M caused an inhibition of enzyme activity. There is no stimulation of enzyme activity with Mg^{++} or glutathione. *p*-Chloromercuribenzoate inhibits PNMT indicating the presence of an essential sulfhydryl group. PNMT can methylate phenylethanolamine derivatives but not phenylethylamines. The normally occurring phenylethanolamine derivatives methylated by the enzyme are noradrenaline, normetanephrine, epinephrine, metanephrine and octopamine. Drugs and other foreign compounds are also N-methylated by PNMT. These include phenylethanolamine, neosynephrine, norephedrine, para and dihydroxynorephedrine. The levo isomers are somewhat better substrates than the dextro isomers. PNMT also methylates secondary amines but to a lesser extent than primary amines. Phenylethylamine, phenylethanolamine, noradrenaline and adrenaline inhibit PNMT (FULLER and HUNT, 1965). It has been suggested that adrenaline might control its own synthesis by a negative feedback mechanism. Tranylcypromine and related compounds inhibit PNMT *in vitro* but not *in vivo* (KRAKOFF and AXELROD, 1967).

PNMT is highly localized in the soluble fraction of the adrenal medulla of all mammalian species examined. Small amounts of PNMT activity are present in the heart and brain. In the brain there is an unequal distribution of PNMT (POHO-

RECKY et al., 1969). Highest concentrations are found in the olfactory bulb and the hypothalamus. PNMT has also been found in the parotid gland of *Bufo marinus* along with COMT, histamine-N-methyltransferase and a non-specific N-methyltransferase (MARKI et al., 1962).

PNMT activity in the adrenal medulla is controlled by glucocorticoids arising from the adrenal medulla (WURTMAN and AXELROD, 1966). This relationship was suggested by the juxtaposition of the adrenal medulla and cortex and its influence on the adrenaline content. In the dogfish the chromaffin tissue is outside the adrenal gland and contains no adrenaline (COUPLAND, 1953). Part of the chromaffin tissue is contiguous with the adrenal cortex in the rabbit and this part mainly contains adrenaline. The portion of the adrenal medulla which is not in contact with the cortex contains only noradrenaline. To establish the relationship between the adrenal cortex and PNMT activity, rats were hypophysectomized and the PNMT activity in the adrenal medulla was examined a week later (WURTMAN and AXELROD, 1966). There was an 80% fall in enzyme activity. This could be restored by the administration of ACTH or dexamethasone to the hypophysectomized rats. When protein synthesis was inhibited with puromycin or actinomycin D, dexamethasone was unable to restore PNMT activity. These observations indicated that glucocorticoids present in the adrenal cortex regulate the synthesis of PNMT in the adrenal medulla at the level of RNA transcription from DNA. When fetal rats are hypophysectomized by decapitation neither PNMT nor adrenaline is present in the newborn rat (MARGOLIES et al., 1966). The administration of corticoids or ACTH to the mother of decapitated rat fetuses prevents the fall of PNMT. The administration of corticoids to a normal animal does not increase the activity of PNMT above normal range. However prolonged nerve stimulation causes a small but significant elevation of adrenal PNMT in the rat (THOENEN, MUELLER and AXELROD, 1970).

There are marked species differences in the properties and inducability of PNMT. In mammals there are at least five separate forms of PNMT with respect to electrophoretic mobility and heat stability (AXELROD and VESSEL, 1970). PNMT in the frog adrenal differs from the mammalian enzyme with respect to its pH and temperature optima, ionic strength, heat stability and rate of migration in starch block electrophoresis (WURTMAN et al., 1968). Frog PNMT is present in heart, kidney and brain as well as the adrenal gland. Unlike the mammal, PNMT in the frog adrenal does not decline after hypophysectomy.

VI. Histamine N-Methyltransferase

A major pathway for the metabolism of histamine in mammals involves a methylation reaction to form 1-methyl (β-amino ethyl) imidazole (methylhistamine) (SCHAYER, 1956). These observations prompted the discovery of an enzyme that methylates histamine (BROWN et al., 1959). Histamine N-methyltransferase was partially purified from guinea pig brain and its properties studied. In phosphate buffers optimal pH ranges from 7.2—7.4 while in tris buffer, maximal activity occurs at about pH 9.0. There is an absolute requirement for S-adenosylmethionine. Mg^{++}, reduced glutathione or EDTA does not affect enzyme activity. Histamine N-methyltransferase activity is markedly inhibited by chlorpromazine, bromolysergic acid diethylamide, serotonin, and *p*-chloromercuribenzoate. Antihistaminic agents, LSD, or 48/80 have no inhibiting effect on the enzyme. Chlorpromazine administered *in vivo* inhibits the formation of histamine N-methylated metabolites in cat brains (WHITE, 1960). Chlorpromazine, serotonin or bufotenine slows the disappearance of circulating histamine and the appearance of N-methylhistamine in intact mice (SNYDER and AXELROD, 1964). The product methylhistamine inhibits the enzyme and this can be partially reversed by histamine.

The histamine methylating enzyme is highly specific for histamine (BROWN et al., 1959). The following compounds could not serve as substrates for the enzyme: histidine, methylhistidine, imidazole acetic acid, methylimidazole acetic acid, imidazole, thiolhistidine ergothioneine, N-acetylhistidine and imidazole 4,5-dicarboxylic acid.

Histamine N-methyltransferase is widely distributed in all tissues of mammalian species except the rat. The highest concentration is present in the central nervous system. There is about a 10-fold range of enzyme activity within the brain. The highest activity is present in the neurohypophysis and the lowest in the pons and cerebellum (AXELROD et al., 1961). Histamine N-methyltransferase has also been found in the parotid gland of the South American toad *Bufo marinus* (MARKI et al., 1962). Male rat kidneys have about twice as much histamine N-methyltransferase activity as the female (SNYDER and AXELROD, 1965). The reverse is the case for mouse kidney enzyme. Castration can reduce histamine N-methyltransferase activity in male rats, which can be overcome by the administration of testosterone. Testosterone can elevate histamine N-methyltransferase activity in hyphosectomized female rats. Corticosterone appears to induce the formation of methylhistamine in guinea pig stomachs (KOVACS and HEISLER, 1969).

VII. Non-Specific N-Methyltransferase

It was observed that incubation of the soluble supernatant fractions of rabbit lung with C^{14} S-adenosylmethionine results in the formation of a C^{14}-methylated endogenously occurring compound. To establish the nature of this methyl acceptor a number of possible substrates were added to the lung extract (AXELROD, 1962a). When serotonin was used as a substrate there was a marked increase in the formation of a radioactive substrate that was extractable in isoamyl alcohol. This metabolite was identified as C^{14}-methyl serotonin. These observations suggested the presence of an enzyme in the rabbit lung that methylates serotonin and possibly other amines.

The serotonin methylating enzyme was partially purified, about 10-fold from rabbit lung, and its properties studied. The optimal pH for the enzyme is 8.0 in phosphate buffer and 8.5 in tris buffer. It has an absolute requirement for S-adenosylmethionine and neither Mg^{++} nor glutathione stimulate enzyme activity. Chlorpromazine and imipramine inhibit the serotonin methylating enzyme in concentrations that are in the therapeutic range. LSD and reserpine have no effect on the enzyme but it is inhibited by *p*-chloromercuribenzoate.

The methylating enzyme from rabbit lung was found to methylate a variety of amines although serotonin was the best substrate. Among the normally occurring substrates are tryptamine, tyramine, normetanephrine, metanephrine, 3-methoxytyramine, dopamine, octopamine, noradrenaline and adrenaline. A number of foreign amines are also methylated: amphetamine, norephedrine, ephedrine, neosynephrine, aniline. The rabbit lung enzyme can also convert normorphine and nornicotine to morphine and nicotine respectively. N-methylated compounds also accept a second methyl group in the presence of the enzyme. Thus the nonspecific methylating enzyme can convert normally occurring tryptamine to the psychotomimetic, dimethyl tryptamine (DMT) in two steps (AXELROD, 1961). Recently a similar indolamine N-methyltransferase has been found in chicken and rat brain (MORGAN and MANDELL, 1969).

The rabbit lung also contains an enzyme that can convert adenine to 3-methyl adenine (AXELROD and DALY, 1962). Purines such as 2,6-diamino purine, 7-methyl adenine and 6-methylamino purine are also methylated, but 9-methyl adenine, AMP, ADP and ATP are not.

The nonspecific N-methylating enzyme is highly localized in the soluble supernatant fraction of the rabbit lung. Adrenal gland and kidney have about one fifth the activity of the lung, and the liver and spleen have small but definite amounts of the enzyme. Dialized supernatant fractions of lung from rat, mouse, guinea pig and cat can methylate serotonin. A non-specific N-methyltransferase has been identified in roots of germinating barley (MANN and MUDD, 1963). The normal substrate for this enzyme is tyramine and N-methyltyramine and it forms hordinine.

VIII. Enzymatic Formation of Methanol from S-Adenosylmethionine

In an examination of the distribution of methyltransferases, it was noted that the incubation of C^{14}-S-adenosylmethionine and an extract of the bovine pituitary gland resulted in the formation of a radioactive product that was extracted into organic solvents (AXELROD and DALY, 1965). This compound was identified as C^{14} methanol. When S-adenosylmethionine-2-C^{14} was incubated with the pituitary extract, S-adenosylhomocysteine-2-C^{14} was formed. These results uncovered an enzyme in the pituitary that converts S-adenosylmethionine to methanol and S-adenosylhomocysteine. This reaction proceeds either by methylation of water or by the hydrolytic cleavage of S-adenosylmethionine.

The highest activity of the methanol-forming enzyme was found in the posterior pituitary gland and a smaller amount was present in the anterior pituitary, but all the mammalian pituitaries examined contained the enzyme. Recent work has shown that relatively large amounts of the methanol-forming enzyme are present in red blood cells of all mammalian species (unpublished). Only negligible amounts of this enzyme are present in other tissues.

References

ABBS, E.T., BROADLEY, K.J., ROBERTS, D.J.: Inhibition of catechol-O-methyl transferase by some acid degradation products of adrenaline and noradrenaline. Biochem. Pharmacol. **16**, 279—282 (1967).
ALBERICI, M., RODRIGUEZ, G., DE LORES ARNAIZ, G., DE ROBERTIS, E.: Catechol-O-methyl transferase in nerve endings of the rat brain. Life Sci. **4**, 1951—1960 (1965).
ANDERSON, P.J., D'IORIO, A.: Purification and properties of catechol-O-methyl transferase. Biochem. Pharmacol. **17**, 1943 (1968).
ARMSTRONG, M.D., MCMILLAN, A., SHAW, K.N.F.: 3-methoxy-4-hydroxy d-mandelic acid, a urinary metabolite of norepinephrine. Biochim. biophys. Acta (Amst.) **25**, 422—425 (1957).
AXELROD, J.: The enzymatic cleavage of aromatic ethers. Biochem. J. **63**, 634—639 (1956).
— O-methylation of epinephrine and other catechols *in vitro* and *in vivo*. Science **126**, 400—401 (1957).
— Enzymatic formation of psychotomimetic metabolites from normally occurring compounds. Science **134**, 343 (1961).
— The enzymatic N-methylation of serotonin and other amines. J. Pharmacol. exp. Ther. **138**, 28—33 (1962a).
— Purification and properties of phenylethanol-amine N-methyl transferase. J. biol. Chem. **237**, 1657—1660 (1962b).
— DALY, J.W.: The enzymic conversion of adenine to 3-methyl adenine. Biochim. biophys. Acta (Amst.) **61**, 855—856 (1962).
— — Pituitary gland: Enzymic formation of methanol from S-adenosylmethionine. Science **150**, 892—893 (1965).
— — Phenol-O-methyl transferase. Biochim. biophys. Acta (Amst.) **159**, 472—478 (1968).

AXELROD, J., LA ROCHE, M.J.: Inhibition of O-methylation of epinephrine and norepinephrine *in vitro* and *in vivo*. Science **130**, 800 (1959).
— LAUBER, J.K.: Hydroxyindole-O-methyltransferase in several avian species. Biochem. Pharmacol. **17**, 828—830 (1968).
— LERNER, A.B.: O-methylation in the conversion of tyrosine to melanin. Biochim. biophys. Acta (Amst.) **71**, 650—655 (1963).
— MACLEAN, P.D., ALBERS, R.W., WEISSBACH, H.: Regional distribution of methyl transferase enzymes in the nervous system and glandular tissues. In: Regional Neurochemistry, pp. 307—311. S.S. KETY and J. ELKES (Eds.). Oxford, England: Pergamon Press 1961.
— QUAY, W.B., BAKER, P.C.: Enzymatic synthesis of the skin-lightening agent melatonin in amphibians. Nature (Lond.) **208**, 386 (1965).
— SHEIN, H.M., WURTMAN, R.J.: Stimulation of C^{14}-melatonin synthesis from C^{14}-tryptophan by noradrenaline in rat pineal in organ culture. Proc. nat. Acad. Sci. (Wash.) **62**, 544—549 (1969).
— TOMCHICK, R.: Enzymatic O-methylation of epinephrine and other catechols. J. biol. Chem. **233**, 702—705 (1958).
— VESSEL, E.S.: Heterogeneity of N- and O-Methyltransferases. Molec. Pharmacol. **6**, 78—84 (1970).
— WEISSBACH, H.: Enzymatic O-methylation of N-acetylserotonin to melatonin. Science **131**, 312 (1960).
— — Purification and properties of hydroxyindole-O-methyl transferase. J. biol. Chem. **236**, 211—213 (1961).
— WURTMAN, R.J., WINGET, C.M.: Melatonin synthesis in the hen pineal gland and its control by light. Nature (Lond.) **201**, 1134 (1964).
BACQ, Z.M., GOSSELIN, L., DRESSE, A., RENSON, J.: Inhibition of O-methyltransferase by catechols and sensitization to epinephrine. Science **130**, 453 (1959).
BAKER, P.C., QUAY, W.B., AXELROD, J.: Development of hydroxyindole-O-methyltransferase activity in the eye and brain of the amphibian *Xenopus laevis*. Life Sci. **4**, 1981—1987 (1965).
BAMSHAD, J., LERNER, A.B., MCGUIRE, J.S.: Catechol-O-methyltransferase in skin. J. invest. Derm. **43**, 111—113 (1964).
BELLEAU, B., BURBA, J.: Occupancy of adrenergic receptors and inhibition of catechol-O-methyl transferase by tropolones. J. Med. Chem. **6**, 755—759 (1963).
BO, P.T., MCISAAC, W.M., TANSEY, L.W., KRALIK, P.M.: Hydroxyindole-O-methyltransferase. II. Inhibitory activities of some N-acetyltryptamines. J. pharm. Sci. **57**, 1998—2000 (1968).
BRANDENBURGER-BROWN, A., TRAMS, E.G.: Catecholamine metabolism in elasmobranch interrenal body. Comp. Biochem. Physiol. **25**, 1099—1105 (1968).
BROWN, D.D., TOMCHICK, R., AXELROD, J.: Distribution and properties of a histamine-methylating enzyme. J. biol. Chem. **234**, 2948—2950 (1959).
BULBRING, E.: Methylation of noradrenaline by minced suprarenal tissue. Brit. J. Pharmacol. **4**, 234—244 (1949).
CANTONI, G.L.: Methylation of nicotinamide soluble enzyme system from rat liver. J. biol. Chem. **189**, 203—216 (1951).
— DURELL, J.: Activation of methionine for transmethylation. II. The methionine activating enzyme: Studies on the mechanism of the reaction. J. biol. Chem. **225**, 1033—1048 (1957).
— VIGNOS, P.J.: Enzymatic mechanism of creatine synthesis. J. biol. Chem. **209**, 647—659 (1954).
CARLSSON, A., LINDQVIST, M., FILA-HRODMADKO, S., CORRODI, H.: Synthese von Catechol-O-methyltransferase hemmenden Verbindungen. Helv. chem. Acta **45**, 270 (1962).
COOPER, J.R., AXELROD, J., BRODIE, B.B.: Inhibitory effects of B-diethylaminoethyl diphenylpropylacetate on a variety of drug metabolic pathways *in vitro*. J. Pharmacol. exp. Ther. **112**, 55—63 (1954).
COUPLAND, R.E.: On the morphology and adrenaline-noradrenaline content of chromaffin tissue. J. Endocr. **9**, 194—203 (1953).
DALY, J.W., AXELROD, J., WITKOP, B.: Dynamic aspects of enzymatic O-methylation and demethylation of catechols *in vitro* and *in vivo*. J. biol. Chem. **235**, 1155—1159 (1960).
EISENFELD, A.J., LANDSBERG, L., AXELROD, J.: Effect of drugs on the accumulation and metabolism of extraneuronal norepinephrine in the rat heart. J. Pharmacol. exp. Ther. **158**, 378—385 (1967).
FINKLE, B.J., NELSON, R.F.: Enzyme reaction with phenolic compounds by a meta O-methyl transferase in plants. Biochim. biophys. Acta (Amst.) **78**, 747—749 (1963).
FULLER, R.A., HUNT, J.M.: Substrate specificity of phenethanolamine N-methyl transferase. Biochem. Pharmacol. **4**, 1896 (1965).

Hertting, G., Axelrod, J.: Fate of tritiated noradrenaline at the sympathetic nerve endings. Nature (Lond.) **192**, 172—173 (1961).

— Labrosse, H.: Biliary and urinary excretion of metabolites of 7-H^3-epinephrine in the rat. J. biol. Chem. **237**, 2291—2295 (1962).

Ignarro, L.J., Shideman, F.E.: Catechol-O-methyl transferase and monoamine oxidase activities in the heart and liver of the embryonic and developing chick. J. Pharmacol. exp. Ther. **159**, 29—37 (1968).

Inscoe, J.K., Daly, J., Axelrod, J.: Factors affecting the enzymatic formation of O-methylated dihydroxy derivatives. Biochem. Pharmacol. **14**, 1257—1263 (1965).

Keller, E.B., Boissonas, R.A., Du Vigneaud, V.: The origin of the methyl group of epinephrine. J. biol. Chem. **183**, 627—632 (1950).

Kirshner, N., Goodall, McC.: The formation of adrenaline from noradrenaline. Biochim. biophys. Acta (Amst.) **24**, 658—659 (1957).

Klein, D.C.: Pineal gland: Stimulation of melatonin production by harmine. Fed. Proc. **28**, 734 (1969).

Kopin, I.J., Gordon, E.K.: Metabolism of H_6-norepinephrine released by tyramine and reserpine. J. Pharmacol. exp. Ther. **138**, 351—359 (1962).

Kovacs, E.M., Heisler, S.: The role of N-N-dimethylhistamine in the cortisone induced hypersecretion of guinea pigs. Fed. Proc. **28**, 353 (1969).

Krakoff, L.R., Axelrod, J.: Inhibition of phenylethanolamine N-methyltransferase. Biochem. Pharmacol. **16**, 1384—1386 (1967).

— Buccino, R.A., Spann, J.F., Jr., De Champlain, J.: Cardiac catechol-O-methyltransferase and monoamine oxidase activity in congestive heart failure. Amer. J. Physiol. **215**, 549—552 (1968).

La Brosse, E.H., Karon, M.: Catechol-O-methyltransferase activity in neuroblastoma tumor. Nature (Lond) **196**, 1222—1223 (1962).

Landsberg, L., De Champlain, J., Axelrod, J.: Increased biosynthesis of cardiac norepinephrine after hypophysectomy. J. Pharmacol. exp. Ther. **165**, 102—107 (1969).

Lauber, J.K., Boyd, J.E., Axelrod, J.: Enzymatic synthesis of melatonin in avian pineal body: Extraretinal response to light. Science **161**, 489—490 (1968).

Lerner, A.B., Case, J.D., Heinzelman, R.V.: Structure of melatonin. J. Amer. chem. Soc. **81**, 6084—6086 (1959).

Lotikar, P.D.: Enzymatic N-O-methylation of hydroxyamic acids. Biochim. biophys. Acta (Amst.) **170**, 468—471 (1968).

Mann, J.D., Fales, H.M., Mudd, H.S.: Alkaloids and plant metabolism: O-methylation *in vitro* or norbelladine, a precursor of amaryllіaceae alkaloids. J. biol. Chem. **238**, 3820—3823 (1963).

— Mudd, H.S.: Alkaloids and plant metabolism. IV. The tyramine methylpherase of barley roots. J. biol. Chem. **238**, 381—385 (1963).

Margolies, F.D., Roffi, J., Jost, J.: Norepinephrine methylation in fetal rat adrenals. Science **154**, 275—276 (1966).

Marki, F., Axelrod, J., Witkop, B.: Catecholamines and methyltransferases in the South American toad (*Bufo marinus*). Biochim. biophys. Acta (Amst.) **58**, 367—369 (1962).

Morgan, M., Mandell, A.J.: Indole (ethyl) amine N-methyltransferase in the brain. Science **165**, 492—493 (1969).

Pohorecky, L.A., Zigmond, M.J., Karten, H.J., Wurtman, R.J.: Enzymatic conversion of norepinephrine to epinephrine by the brain. J. Pharmacol. exp. Ther. **165**, 190—195 (1969).

Quay, W.B.: Retinal and pineal hydroxyindole-O-methyltransferase activity in vertebrates. Life Sci. **4**, 983 (1965).

Schayer, R.W.: The metabolism of histamine in various species. Brit. J. Pharmacol. **11**, 472—473 (1956).

Senoh, S., Daly, J., Axelrod, J., Witkop, B.: Enzymatic p-O-methylation by catechol-O-methyltransferase. J. Amer. chem. Soc. **81**, 6240—6245 (1959).

— Tokuyama, Y., Witkop, B.: The role of cations in the non-enzymatic and enzymatic O-methylations of catechol derivatives. J. Amer. chem. Soc. **84**, 1719—1724 (1962).

Shein, H., Wurtman, R.J., Axelrod, J.: Synthesis of serotonin by pineal glands of the rat in organ culture. Nature (Lond.) **213**, 730—731 (1967).

Snyder, S.H., Axelrod, J.: Inhibition of histamine methylation *in vivo* by drugs. Biochem. Pharmacol. **13**, 536—537 (1964).

— — Sex differences and hormonal control of histamine methyltransferase activity. Biochim. biophys. Acta (Amst.) **2**, 416—421 (1965).

Thoenen, H., Mueller, R.A., Axelrod, J.: Neuronally dependent induction of adrenal phenylethanolamine-N-methyltransferase by 6-hydroxydopamine. Biochem. Pharmacol. **19**, 669—673 (1970).

Tomita, E., Macha, E., Lardy, C.A.: Enzymatic O-methylation of iodinated phenols and thyroid hormones. J. biol. Chem. **239**, 1202—1207 (1964).

Wells, S.H., Wurtman, R.J., Rabson, H.S.: Viral neoplastic transformation of hamster pineal cells *in vitro*. Retention of enzymatic function. Science **154**, 278—279 (1966).

White, T.: Formation and catabolism of histamine in cat brain *in vivo*. J. Physiol. (Lond.) **152**, 299—308 (1960).

Wurtman, R.J., Axelrod, J.: Control of enzymatic synthesis of adrenaline in the adrenal medulla by adrenal cortical steroids. J. biol. Chem. **241**, 2301—2305 (1966).

— — Fischer, J.E.: Melatonin synthesis in the pineal gland: Effects of light mediated by the sympathetic nervous system. Science **143**, 1328—1330 (1964a).

— — Phillips, L.S.: Melatonin synthesis in the pineal gland: Control by light. Science **142**, 1071—1073 (1963).

— — Potter, L.T.: The disposition of catecholamines in the rat uterus and the effect of drugs and hormones. J. Pharmacol. exp. Ther. **144**, 150—155 (1964b).

— — Snyder, S.H., Chu, E.W.: Changes in the enzymatic synthesis of melatonin in the pineal during the estrous cycle. Endocrinology **76**, 798—800 (1965).

— — Toch, R.: Demonstration of hydroxyindole-O-methyltransferase, melatonin and serotonin in a metastatic parenchymatous pinealoma. Nature (Lond.) **204**, 1323—1324 (1964c).

— — Vesell, E.S., Ross, G.T.: Species differences in inducibility of phenylethanolamine N-methyltransferase. Endocrinology **82**, 584—590 (1968).

Chapter 57

Enzymes that Inactivate Vasoactive Peptides[1]

E. G. Erdös

With 2 Figures

A. Introduction

This chapter deals with the enzymatic inactivation of two types of vasoactive peptides, plasma kinins and angiotensin II. The metabolic fate of other hormonal or exogenous peptides is not discussed here.

Enzymes that destroy the activity of peptides were found practically simultaneously with the discovery of the agents. The names angiotensinase (hypertensinase, angiotonase) and kininase (bradykininase, kallidinase) were given when the structure of the active peptide was not known yet. Obviously enzymes should not be named after a single substrate. Terms such as kininase or angiotensinase will be used in this chapter for the sake of convenience and as a sort of acceptable scientific jargon. They simply indicate the inactivation of a bradykinin or angiotensin-type peptide by an enzyme or enzymes. According to a recent report of a Committee on Nomenclature for Hypotensive Peptides (Webster, 1966). "The term kininase may be used as a general term to describe enzymes that inactivate kinins. As the various kininases are isolated and the bonds they split are identified, a descriptive trivial name should be assigned by the investigator in an attempt to describe the particular bond split by the enzyme . . ." Much of the same can be said about angiotensinases.

Although commercially available proteolytic enzymes such as chymotrypsin, trypsin, carboxypeptidases A or B have been used by the chemists to help establish the amino acid sequence of the peptides, the enzymes responsible for terminating their actions are different from these. Various kininases and angiotensinases are being gradually characterized by means of investigations *in vitro*, but only since the peptides were synthetized. After the establishment of the mode of action of the enzymes, the next important step is the application of low molecular weight substrates in quantitative chemical assays. Some kininases and angiotensinases have been purified and assays developed for them, but the investigations of other enzymes have not advanced to this state as yet.

It is still difficult to study the metabolism of unlabeled peptides *in vivo*, since the breakdown products, without obvious functions, are very similar to the commonly occurring metabolites in the body. The fairly recent developments in making radioactive peptides available will be of great help in this type of study.

B. Inactivation of Kinins

Kininases are enzymes that inactivate kinins. The rapid disappearance of kinins was observed at the same time when the liberation of kallidin and bradykinin

1 Supported in part by USPHS, NIH Grant HE 08764 and Project THEMIS, Office of Naval Research N00014-68-A-0496.

by enzymes was detected. Subsequently, it was established that the release and inactivation of kinins are independent processes occurring in the same crude system *in vitro*. Kallidin was inactivated by an agent in serum (WERLE et al., 1937). Bradykinin activity was destroyed by chymotrypsin (E.C. 3.4.4.5) contamination in trypsin (E.C. 3.4.4.4) (WERLE and BEREK, 1950; WERLE et al., 1950; WERLE, 1953), by snake venom (ROCHA E SILVA et al., 1949) or by serum (ROCHA E SILVA, 1951).

Kinins occur in blood plasma in the inactive precursor globulin kininogen. Various proteolytic enzymes can release a kinin from this protein (Fig. 1). The most important naturally occurring enzymes are the kallikreins which are found

Fig. 1. *Simplified scheme for the release and inactivation of kinin in plasma*

Activator
+
Prekallikrein ⟶ Kallikrein + Kininogen
↓
Kinin + Kininase
↓
Split Products

mostly in blood plasma, glandular tissues and urine. Plasma kallikrein liberates bradykinin whereas the other kallikreins release kallidin. Bradykinin is a nonapeptide and kallidin is a decapeptide having an additional lysine at the N-terminal end, i.e., Lys-bradykinin. The biological actions of these hypotensive peptides are quite similar (ERDÖS, 1966). A third analogue is the undecapeptide Met-Lys-bradykinin. Kallikrein in the blood plasma and in some tissues frequently exists as an inactive zymogen named prekallikrein (kallikreinogen) and many of the components of the blood coagulation system can participate in the activation of prekallikrein.

Kininases are widely distributed in nature; their sources range from human blood to microorganisms (ERDÖS and YANG, 1970). Some of these enzymes have been purified and the peptide bond cleaved by them identified, but other kininases have been used only as crude extracts in biological experiments.

I. Kininases in Blood

In the circulating blood, red blood cells, leukocytes, thrombocytes and plasma contain active kininases. Bradykinin and kallidin are rapidly inactivated in normal plasma, in contrast to the relative stability of other peptides, such as vasopressin.

II. Carboxypeptidase N

The first kininase characterized was a carboxypeptidase found in fraction IV-1 of human plasma and it was named carboxypeptidase N (ERDÖS, 1961, 1962). The enzyme cleaves the C-terminal arginine of the peptides (Table 1). The inactivation of bradykinin was inhibited by various chelating agents, thus the enzyme is a metallopeptidase. Of the metal ions tested, Co^{2+} enhanced and Cd^{2+} inhibited the *in vitro* hydrolysis of bradykinin (ERDÖS and SLOANE, 1962; ERDÖS et al., 1963b).

From bradykinin substrate 1 ml human blood serum released 0.13 μmole arginine/min, and rabbit serum 0.15 μmole (PASKHINA and TRAPEZNIKOVA, 1967).

Table 1. *Peptide bonds hydrolyzed in bradykinin*

JV — 1 2 3 4 5 6 7 8 9: H-Arg-Pro-Pro-Gly-Phe-Ser-Pro-Phe-Arg-OH

Enzyme	Arg¹-Pro²	Pro²-Pro³	Pro³-Gly⁴	Gly⁴-Phe⁵	Phe⁵-Ser⁶	Ser⁶-Pro⁷	Pro⁷-Phe⁸	Phe⁸-Arg⁹
Chymotrypsin					↑			↑
Carboxypeptidases (B, N, kidney, catheptic)								↑
Kininase II (kidney, plasma)							↑	
Prolidase (imidopeptidase; kidney, erythrocytes)	↑							
Snake venoms				↑	↑			
Bromelain				↑	↑			

The first-order reaction rate constant of the hydrolysis of bradykinin by human fraction IV-1 was $k = 0.024\ min^{-1}$ (ERDÖS and SLOANE, 1962).

In addition to kinins, carboxypeptidase N cleaves shorter peptides (Table 2) including substrates of pancreatic carboxypeptidase B. The rate of hydrolysis of hippuric acid derivatives in human plasma decreased in the order: hippuryl-lysine

Table 2. *Substrates of kininases in chemical assays*

Substrate	Source of Enzyme	Method	Remarks	Ref.
Hip-Lys	Plasma, carboxypeptidase N	UV spectrophotometric	$K_m = 1 \times 10^{-3}$M	1
Hip-argininic acid	Plasma, carboxypeptidase N	UV spectrophotometric, titration	Measures esterase activity $K_m = 1 \times 10^{-4}$	2
Ac-Phe-Arg	Plasma, carboxypeptidase N	Ninhydrin	—	3
Pro-Phe-Arg	Carboxypeptidase N, man, rabbit	Ninhydrin	$K_m = 1 \times 10^{-3}$M	4
Ac-Ser-Pro-Phe-Arg	Plasma, tissues, carboxypeptidase N and kininase II	Ninhydrin	Substrate represents C-terminal tetrapeptide of bradykinin	5
Depsipeptide analogues of bradykinin (e.g., Phenlac⁸-glycyl⁶-bk)	Carboxypeptidase N	Ninhydrin	—	6
Bradykinin	Carboxypeptidase N	Ninhydrin	Measures Arg release	7
Hip-His-Leu	Lung, plasma, kininase II	Ninhydrin, UV spectrophotometric	Substrate of Ang I converting enzyme; Hydrolyzed by kininase II	8, 9
Hip-Gly-Gly t-Boc-Phe(NO_2)-Phe-Gly Cbo-Pro-Leu-Gly	Plasma kininase II, lung and kidney extract	Ninhydrin, UV spectrophotometric	Substrates of Ang I converting enzyme. Hydrolyzed by purified plasma kininase II preparations	9

References: 1. ERDÖS et al. (1964). — 2. ERDÖS et al. (1967). — 3. ERDÖS and YANG (1966). — 4. TRAPEZNIKOVA and PASKHINA (1968). — 5. YANG and ERDÖS (1967), ERDÖS and YANG (1966). — 6. PASKHINA and TRAPEZNIKOVA (1967). — 7. PASKHINA and TRAPEZNIKOVA (1967). — 8. CUSHMAN and CHEUNG (1969), YANG et al. (1970 b, c). — 9. YANG et al. (1970 b, d, e).

(HLL), hippuryl-arginine (HLA), and hippuryl-ornithine. In a routine assay the enzyme activity was determined by measuring the hydrolysis of HLL after the enzyme was pre-equilibrated with $CoCl_2$. This metal ion increases the hydrolysis of HLL about 6-fold in man (ERDÖS et al., 1964) and 1.5-fold in rabbit (SHIMONAEVA, 1967). Differences in the rate of cleavage of lysine from HLL by sera of various animals are smaller than the differences encountered when the inactivation of bradykinin is measured in bioassay (ERDÖS et al., 1964). One ml human plasma cleaves 0.79 μmole of HLL and guinea pig serum cleaves 0.70 μmole per min, though guinea pig serum inactivates bradykinin much faster than human plasma. In a series of experiments, the relative kininase activities of the various untreated serum samples decreased in the order: guinea pig, dog, alligator, and rabbit (ERDÖS et al., 1963b). Rat serum also breaks down bradykinin rapidly (FASCIOLO, 1964), whereas the kininase level in bovine serum is low (WERLE et al., 1937; FREY et al., 1968). It was suspected by the author that some of the discrepancies between the rate of hydrolysis of HLL and the rapidity of inactivation of bradykinin may have been caused by the presence of a second kininase in plasma. (YANG et al., 1970e).

In addition, some peptides representing C-terminal fragments of bradykinin served as substrates not only of carboxypeptidase N but also of other kininases originating from blood or kidney. The N-terminal end of the peptides was acetylated to avoid an unspecific attack by aminopeptidases. Arginine was cleaved from Ac-Phe-Arg and from Ac-Ser-Pro-Phe-Arg (ERDÖS et al., 1964; ERDÖS and YANG, 1966) by plasma and kidney carboxypeptidases (Table 2).

Similar to other peptidases, carboxypeptidase N has an esterase action; it cleaves the ester substrate hippuryl-argininic acid (HLAa; *o*-benzoyl-glycyl-α-L-hydroxyl-δ-guanidino-*n*-valeric acid). For the determination of carboxypeptidase N activity, assaying the esterase instead of the peptidase action offers several advantages, because the assay is faster and the activity can be determined in 5 μl plasma (ERDÖS et al., 1967a). Human serum cleaved HLAa at a rate of 3 μmoles/min per ml serum; swine serum enzyme was more active, splitting 5.2 μmoles. TRAPEZNIKOVA and PASKHINA (1968) used benzyloxycarbonyl (Cbo)-Phe-argininic acid as substrate, and this ester was also hydrolyzed faster than the corresponding peptide substrates.

Carboxypeptidase N was prepared (ERDÖS et al., 1964, 1967a) by precipitating it from plasma with ammonium sulfate, followed by dialysis against cobalt chloride solution. The enzyme was further purified by repeated DEAE-Sephadex column chromatographies. The peptidase activity increased 252-fold over the native plasma, while the esterase activity was enhanced 212-fold. When the ammonium sulfate precipitate was taken as a starting material there was a proportional increase in the kininase activity. The kininase, peptidase, and esterase activities could not be separated because they migrated as a single peak in Pevikon zone electrophoresis at two different pH values. The starting material for electrophoresis was a human globulin fraction precipitated with ammonium sulfate. PASKHINA and TRAPEZNIKOVA (1967) and TRAPEZNIKOVA and PASKHINA (1968) purified carboxypeptidase N from human and from rabbit sera with similar results.

The K_m for carboxypeptidase N of human serum with HLL was 1.4 to 1.6 $\times$ 10^{-3}M (ERDÖS et al., 1964; TRAPEZNIKOVA and PASKHINA, 1968) and with HLAa it was 1×10^{-4} (ERDÖS et al., 1967a). The pH optimum of the carboxypeptidase N with HLL substrate is about 7.5 (ERDÖS et al., 1964; TRAPEZNIKOVA and PASKHINA, 1968) and its activity decreases above pH 8. The optimal pH is slightly higher with the ester substrate and gives a broader peak in the alkaline range. The activity below pH 7 depends on the selection of the buffer (ERDÖS et al., 1964). Metal ions have a different influence upon the peptidase and esterase activities of carboxypeptidase N (ERDÖS et al., 1967a). Like other plasma kininases, carboxypeptidase N is irreversibly inactivated by acid or heat treatment; it loses its activity when incubated at pH 2—3 or at a temperature above 56° (HORTON, 1959; FREY et al., 1968).

Carboxypeptidase N of human or animal plasma can be definitely distinguished from the pancreatic enzyme, although carboxypeptidase N hydrolyzes the peptide bond of basic carboxyl terminal amino acids just as carboxypeptidase B (E.C. 3.4.4.2) does. For example, Zn^{2+} is the cofactor for peptidase activity of the swine pancreatic carboxypeptidase B and Cd^{2+} enhances the esterase activity. Both metal ions, however, inhibit plasma carboxypeptidase N from various sources including swine serum (Erdös et al., 1963b, 1964, 1967a; Erdös, 1966; Yang and Erdös, 1967). In addition EDTA inhibits carboxypeptidase N but not carboxypeptidase B. HLA is hydrolyzed faster than HLL by the pancreatic enzyme, while the opposite is true for the plasma enzyme. Cobalt ions have quantitatively different effects on the two carboxypeptidases. Purified human carboxypeptidase N has an estimated molecular weight of 310.000 (Bokisch and Müller-Eberhard, 1970) a much higher value than carboxypeptidase B has. Rat plasma carboxypeptidase N, because of its higher molecular weight, can be separated from carboxypeptidase B by means of gel-filtration on a Sephadex column (Urbanitz et al., 1969).

Carboxypeptidase N also differs from carboxypeptidase A; indeed, no carboxypeptidase A (E.C. 3.4.2.1) was found in human plasma (Erdös et al., 1964).

In addition to kinins, other peptides may serve as naturally occurring substrates of carboxypeptidase N. For example, blood of animals that do not have plasma kallikrein or kininogen (e.g. frog or carp) still contains kininase activity (Erdös et al., 1964, 1967b, 1968, and unpublished).

III. Kininase II

Carboxypeptidase N was first found in Cohn fraction IV-1 of human plasma (Erdös and Sloane, 1962). The kininase activity of the purified preparation and of the Cohn fraction was caused by the presence of carboxypeptidase N. Later the starting material for the purification of plasma kininase was obtained by means of gel filtration of fresh human plasma through a Sephadex G-200 column. The active fraction hydrolyzed HLL and HLAa, the ester and peptide substrates of carboxypeptidase N; however, the kininase peak was broader than could be expected for the carboxypeptidase N activity alone. When the kininase was further purified on a DEAE-Sephadex column, two enzymes were separated (Yang and Erdös, 1967). One was identical with carboxypeptidase N but the other was different. For the sake of brevity carboxypeptidase N was called kininase I in the report, the second enzyme kininase II. Chromatographic experiments with bradykinin and shorter peptide substrates such as Ac-Ser-Pro-Phe-Arg proved that kininase II inactivates bradykinin by cleaving the link between Pro^7 and Phe^8, thereby removing the dipeptide, phenylalanylarginine, from the C-terminal end of bradykinin. The enzyme was later identified to be a dipeptide hydrolase. It was inhibited by chelating agents although some other inhibitors of kininase I were inactive against kininase II (Section B XIII). The bond specificity and inhibition pattern of kininase II are very similar to those of a swine kidney microsomal enzyme named peptidase P (Erdös and Yang, 1967). Man and most laboratory animals tested seem to have both plasma kininase I and II (Erdös et al., 1968). Highest kininase II (and converting enzyme) activity was found in the guinea pig plasma (Yang et al., 1970e).

IV. Converting Enzyme

Another enzyme that cleaves off a dipeptide at the C-terminal end of a longer peptide is the converting enzyme. This enzyme removes histidylleucine from angiotensin I (Ang I) and thereby converts it into the II form. Plasma kininase II preparations that were purified two hundred-fold contain converting enzyme activity indicating that the two enzymes in blood are identical (YANG et al., 1970b, c, d, e). The dipeptide hydrolase (peptide dipeptidehydrolase) activity can be determined with a variety of substrates since the purified enzyme preparation from swine plasma showed very little specificity. It cleaves a C-terminal dipeptide from the following substrates: hippuryl-histidyl-leucine (CUSHMAN and CHEUNG, 1969), hippuryl-glycyl-glycine (HGG), Cbo-prolyl-leucyl-glycine and *t*-butyloxy-carbonyl (*t*-Boc)-*p*-nitrophenylalanyl-phenylalanyl-glycine (BPG) and bradykinin (Table 2). HGG and BPG were used as substrates in the UV spectrophotometer (YANG et al., 1970b, c, d, e). A partially purified lung enzyme also hydrolyzes most of the above — mentioned substrates suggesting the identity of Ang I converting enzyme with kininase II (YANG et al., 1970e). Thus possibly the same enzyme that liberates the most potent endogenous hypertensive material (Ang II) would also inactivate the endogenous hypotensive peptide (bradykinin). In addition, if the kidney microsomal kininase II (ERDÖS and YANG, 1967) or peptidase P is identical with the converting enzyme, then all the enzymes involved in the metabolism of angiotensins would be present in the various subcellular fractions of the kidney, as suggested by some experiments (YANG et al., 1970e).

V. Kininases in Blood Cells

In addition to plasma, the cellular elements of blood contain kininases. Hemolyzed red blood cells inactivate kinins rapidly at a neutral pH. The enzyme in erythrocytes was inhibited by agents (e.g. $CoCl_2$, *p*-chloromercuriphenyl sulfonic acid; PCMS) which do not block plasma carboxypeptidase (ERDÖS et al., 1963b; AMUNDSEN and NUSTAD, 1964; section B XIII), and conversely, some inhibitors of plasma kininases (e.g. EDTA, ε-amino-*n*-caproic acid, EACA) were inactive against the erythrocyte kininase. 1,10-Phenanthroline, however, is a good inhibitor. Although it was indicated that the kininase in erythrocytes was imidopeptidase (prolidase) (ERDÖS et al., 1963b), it can be safely assumed that erythrocytes contain other kininases besides the imidopeptidase.

Many investigators have studied kininases originating from granulocytes. The enzyme from human or rabbit polymorphonuclear leukocytes is not identical with the plasma enzyme because the leukocyte kininase is inhibited by different agents (SCHWAB, 1962; ZACHARIAE et al., 1966; GREENBAUM and KIM, 1967). Its activity per cell is of the same order of magnitude as that of red blood cell kininase (ZACHARIAE et al., 1966). The optimal pH for rabbit or human leukocyte kininases is around or above the neutral pH (ZACHARIAE et al., 1966; GREENBAUM and KIM, 1967; MELMON and CLINE, 1967). In addition to the "neutral" kininase activity that stayed in the supernatant after fractionating the cells, a granular fraction has a kininase active at pH 5.5 (MELMON and CLINE, 1968). The kininase of granulocytes (YAMAFUJI and CARRARA, 1968) is assumed to cleave bradykinin somewhere in the middle of the peptide chain. Because the kininase activity per white blood cell does not exceed that per erythrocyte (ZACHARIAE et al., 1966), the contribution of leukocyte kininase to the total activity of these enzymes in the blood must be negligible. It may be of greater importance after the extravasation of the cells.

In contrast to granulocytes, human lymphocytes had no kininases (MELMON and CLINE, 1967).

VI. Kininases in Other Biological Fluids

The presence of kininases was also observed in urine (FREY et al., 1950) and lymph (SCHACHTER, 1960). Very little was found in the cerebrospinal fluid (SICUTERI et al., 1965).

Only a few of the kininases of the various fluids were characterized. An ammonium sulfate precipitate of human urine, rat lymph (ERDÖS et al., 1964), and ascites (ERDÖS and MELMON, 1966, unpublished observation) contained a carboxypeptidase, possibly carboxypeptidase N. In addition to carboxypeptidase N (kininase I), human urine has some kininase II activity (YANG and ERDÖS, unpublished observations).

VII. Kininases in Tissues

Homogenized tissues from various sources inactivate kinins (WERLE et al., 1937; ERDÖS, 1966). Some homogenized organ extracts are rich in kininases with higher activity per milligram protein than in plasma. Pancreas, kidney and lung are especially active.

In the homogenized pancreas the kininase action was attributed to three enzymes: chymotrypsin, an aminopeptidase, and a carboxypeptidase (WERLE et al., 1950). Subsequent studies showed pancreatic carboxypeptidase B to be the most potent kininase (ERDÖS, 1962; section B, VIII).

Kidney tissue also contains very active kininases (WERLE et al., 1937; FREY et al., 1950; HAMBERG and ROCHA E SILVA, 1954). Most of the activity of the homogenized rat kidney was concentrated in the microsomal fraction (ERDÖS and YANG, 1966); hardly any kininase was found in the soluble fraction. This is in contrast to the high rate of destruction of bradykinin activity by the soluble, fraction of the homogenized liver (AMUNDSEN and NUSTAD, 1965; ERDÖS and YANG, 1966).

The enzymatic activity in the kidney was much higher than in the liver. Three kininases originating from swine kidney were characterized. One of them is a prolidase (imidopeptidase) that cleaves the Arg^1-Pro^2 bond of the peptide (ERDÖS and YANG, 1966; ZUBER, 1966) (Table 1). The enzyme preparations used (ERDÖS and YANG, 1966) were less active than the two other kininases, which were partially purified from homogenized swine kidney cortex. The first of these is a carboxypeptidase that behaved differently from other carboxypeptidases. Substrate specificity and inhibition pattern of this kidney carboxypeptidase indicated that the enzyme was identical with neither pancreatic carboxypeptidase B (FOLK et al., 1960) nor plasma carboxypeptidase N.

The second enzyme was extracted from a kidney microsomal fraction and was solubilized by repeated gel filtration on a Sephadex G-150 column in the presence of deoxycholate (ERDÖS and YANG, 1967). This kininase was named peptidase P. Similar to plasma kininase II, it inactivated bradykinin by cleaving the Pro^7-Phe^8 bond, thus removing a phenylalanylarginine dipeptide from the C-terminal end. The enzyme may be identical with kininase II (section B, III and IV). The kininases found in the kidney were active at a neutral pH. They were inhibited by chelating agents such as EDTA, 1,10-phenanthroline, and BAL, but were not affected by Trasylol or DFP. 2-Mercaptoethylamine, an activator of cathepsins, inhibited peptidase P (ERDÖS and YANG, 1966).

The hydrolysis of bradykinin by the lung *in vitro* was also recently scrutinized. Homogenized lung inactivates bradykinin somewhat slower than kidney (TRAUTSCHOLD, 1965; FREY et al., 1968). Lung homogenates cleave substrates of kininase II and act as converting enzyme (YANG et al., 1970d, e).

In comparison to other tissues, nervous tissues had less kininase action (FASCIOLO, 1964). Relatively large amounts of kininases were found in the dorsal spinal roots and ganglia (HOOPER, 1963). Kininase activity in an extract from acetone-dried brain was attributed to a carboxypeptidase N-type enzyme (KRIVOY and KROGER, 1964).

Catheptic enzymes also can inactivate kinins at an acid pH. For example, beef spleen contains catheptic carboxypeptidases that are activated by sulfhydryl compounds. The enzyme preparation used cleaved arginine from bradykinin; however, phenylalanine was found in the incubation mixture as well. The release of Phe^8 was attributed to the subsequent action of a second catheptic carboxypeptidase present in the source of enzyme (GREENBAUM and YAMAFUJI, 1966). Another catheptic kininase was discovered in crude extracts of liver (FREY et al., 1968).

VIII. Inactivation of Kinins by Purified Proteases

(peptidyl peptide and peptidyl-amino-acid hydrolases)

Kinins are inactivated by some proteolytic enzymes. The most important among them are two pancreatic enzymes, carboxypeptidase B and chymotrypsin. Other enzymes (some commercially available) that may act as kininases were reviewed by PRADO (1970). These include subtilisin BPN (Nargarse) (E.C. 3.4.4.16), ficin (E.C. 3.4.4.12), papain (E.C. 3.4.4.10), and *St. griseus* protease (Pronase); their site of action in the kinin molecule, however, has not been determined.

In the initial studies when bradykinin was released by trypsin, the enzyme also inactivated the peptide owing to a contamination by chymotrypsin (WERLE et al., 1950; ROCHA E SILVA, 1951; WERLE, 1953). Another kininogenase, commercial kallikrein (Padutin; WERLE et al., 1950; WERLE and BEREK, 1950) destroyed kinin activity because it contained carboxypeptidase B as an impurity (ERDÖS et al., 1962).

Commercially available chymotrypsin was used by many investigators during the 1950's to inactivate the kinin content of crude extracts and thereby to differentiate the peptides from other biologically active substances. Proteolytic enzymes were also applied to degradation studies with purified or synthetic peptides to establish their amino acid sequence. Chymotrypsin (ELLIOTT et al., 1960; BOISSONNAS et al., 1960a, b) hydrolyzes the Phe^8-Arg^9 bond of bradykinin quickly and the Phe^5-Ser^6 bond slowly (Table 1). A carboxypeptidase preparation released Arg^9 first and then Phe^8 from bradykinin (ZUBER and JAQUES, 1960). The first activity was due to carboxypeptidase B and the second to carboxypeptidase A, which must have also been present. Stem bromelain (E.C. 3.4.4.24) destroyed the activity as assayed on the guinea pig ileum and hydrolyzed the peptide at the Phe^5-Ser^6 and Gly^4-Phe^5 bonds (ENOMOTO et al., 1967). Table 1 shows the bonds broken in bradykinin by some of the enzymes mentioned.

In biological studies ERDÖS (1962) and ERDÖS et al. (1963b) noted the very rapid inactivation of bradykinin and kallidin by purified swine pancreatic carboxypeptidase B *in vitro*. If carboxypeptidase B and chymotrypsin were compared on the basis of the same degree of purity, carboxypeptidase B would be several hundred times more active than chymotrypsin. Because of the very fast hydrolysis of the C-terminal arginine of bradykinin by carboxypeptidase B and the relatively higher specificity of the enzyme than that of chymotrypsin, carboxypeptidase B has been frequently employed to identify kinin type peptides in extracts.

Since purified carboxypeptidase B is labile and must be kept frozen, attempts have been made to stabilize the preparations. One approach consists of binding carboxypeptidase B to water-insoluble polymers according to the method of LEVIN et al. (1964). The use of the insoluble derivatives of the enzymes offers numerous advantages (SEKI et al., 1970b); for example, it can be kept without loss of activity in the refrigerator under buffer (CHIANG et al., 1968). Carboxypeptidase B polymer when suspended in solution rapidly inactivated bradykinin (CHIANG et al., 1968; MIWA et al., 1969; ERDÖS et al., 1969). Other methods of stabilizing carboxypeptidase B included binding the enzyme to Sepharose or to the copolymer of *p*-amino-Phe-Leu or adsorbing it on colloidal silica and subsequently cross-linking it with glutaraldehyde (YANG, LEVIN and ERDÖS, unpublished; SEKI et al., 1970a).

IX. Administration of Carboxypeptidase B

Because purified hog pancreatic carboxypeptidase B hydrolyzed bradykinin very rapidly *in vitro* (ERDÖS, 1962), it was tested against the peptide *in vivo* (ERDÖS et al., 1963a, b). Intravenous injection of carboxypeptidase B blocked the hypotensive effects of bradykinin or kallidin in various laboratory animals (ERDÖS et al., 1963a, b; ERDÖS and YANG, 1966). Larger doses were needed, however, to abolish the activity of Met-Lys-bradykinin (ERDÖS and YANG, 1966) or Lys^9-bradykinin (ERDÖS et al., 1967c).

In the cat, after a single i.v. injection of carboxypeptidase B, the level of the enzyme decreases in the blood exponentially. The half-life of the enzyme is about 30 min; it is about 20 min in the rabbit. The decrease in the level of the circulating enzyme and the return of the hypotensive effect of injected bradykinin are closely related. By giving repeated i.v. injections of carboxypeptidase B, the effects of bradykinin can be blocked for several hours (ERDÖS and YANG, 1966). Carboxypeptidase B was also effective against kininogenases such as kallikrein (ERDÖS et al., 1963b) and trypsin.

The very rapid inactivation of kinins by carboxypeptidase B *in vitro* and *in vivo* suggested additional use for the enzyme. Carboxypeptidase B was administered to men and animals under a variety of conditions where the importance of the release of bradykinin or kallidin in a physiological or pathological process was to be established, for example, in vasodilation during muscle contraction in dogs (WEBSTER et al., 1967).

Injection of carboxypeptidase B to rabbits blocked the hypotensive effect of bradykinin but not that of i.v. injection of endotoxin (ERDÖS and MIWA, 1968). From these experiments it was concluded that the endotoxin effect in the rabbit is not connected with kinin release during the initial phase of shock.

MELMON et al. (1967) used carboxypeptidase B to relieve the increase in the temperature of the knee joint that follows intra-articular injection of bradykinin in dogs (PHELPS et al., 1966). Pretreatment of the rat paw with carboxypeptidase B reduced the swelling caused by carrageen in this model of inflammation experiment (VAN ARMAN et al., 1968).

When exogenous carboxypeptidase B disappears from the circulation of various animals, it is taken up by the tissues such as kidneys (ERDÖS and YANG, 1966; ERDÖS et al., 1967c). Large amounts of the enzyme were found in the urine as well. In nephrectomized rats carboxypeptidase B blocked the bradykinin effect for 1—2 hours (CROXATTO and CRUZATT, 1969).

X. Venoms

Snake venoms contain both kininases and kininogenases, but the two activities do not follow parallel courses in the various venoms (DEUTSCH and DINIZ, 1955). The factor that inactivates bradykinin and the one that liberates it can be distinguished by heating snake venom (HAMBERG and ROCHA E SILVA, 1957). *A. halys blomhoffii* venom contains three proteinases. Of these, proteinase B is a kininase because it breaks a glycyl-phenylalanine bond in the peptide (SUZUKI et al., 1966).

In addition some snake venoms cleave the phenylalanyl-serine linkage in bradykinin. *C. atrox*, *C. adamanteus*, and *Trimerusurus flavoridis* split two peptide bonds of the bradykinin molecule whereas the venoms of *A. contortrix*, *Bothrops jararaca*, and *Vipera russellii* hydrolyze only one peptide bond (Table 1) (Suzuki and Iwanaga, 1970).

XI. Microbial Kininases

A commercial, partially purified collagenase preparation from *Clostridium histolyticum* inactivated bradykinin by splitting, among other bonds, the same Pro^7-Phe^8 bond as kininase II of plasma or peptidase P of kidney (Erdös and Sloane cf. Erdös, 1966; Erdös and Yang, 1966). Clostridiopeptidase B (E.C. 3.4.4.20) from *Cl. histolyticum* hydrolyzes the lysyl-arginine and the arginyl-proline bonds in Met-Lys-bradykinin (Mitchell, 1968).

The supernatant fluid of *Pseudomonas aeruginosa (Ps. aer.)* cultures contains strong kininase activity after ultrasonic treatment (Amundsen and Rugstad, 1965). The kininase from *Ps. aer.* was studied in detail by Rugstad (1966, 1967a, b, c), who purified it about 170-fold by gel filtration (Rugstad, 1967a). The molecular weight of this kininase is about 50,000 (Rugstad, 1967a). It is inhibited by *o*-phenanthroline, BAL, $ZnCl_2$, and PCMS (Table 3). The enzyme has a pH optimum of about 7.5. The kininase inactivated bradykinin, kallidin, and phyllokinin (bradykinyl-isoleucyl-tyrosine) as well. Thin-layer chromatography and electrophoresis indicated that either the Phe^5-Ser^6 or the Phe^8-Arg^9 bond of bradykinin may be cleaved first (Rugstad, 1967c).

Intravenous injection of this kininase significantly reduced the effect of bradykinin on the systemic blood pressure of the rat. The enzyme had a half-life of about 20 min in the circulation of the rat (Rugstad, 1967b).

XII. Fate of Kinins *in Vivo*

Bradykinin has a very short half-life in blood. McCarthy et al. (1965) found a $t_1/_2$ of 0.27 min during the passage of dog blood through an extracorporeal system, and the value for kallidin was only slightly higher, 0.32 min. Thus significant amounts of kinins can be inactivated by plasma during one transit of blood through the systemic circulation. The half-life of bradykinin in cat blood was about the same as in dog blood (Ferreira and Vane, 1967a). Based on the circulatory effects of the peptide, Saameli and Eskes (1962) calculated half-life in women to be shorter than 0.5 min.

Bumpus et al. (1964) indicated that infused labeled bradykinin which escaped inactivation in the circulation of the rat was concentrated mainly in the kidney, where it was rapidly inactivated. After half an hour most of the radioactive peptide and its fragments were excreted in the urine. In infused, nephrectomized rats, tritiated bradykinin was taken up mostly by the liver, then by the lung, salivary gland, spleen, heart and uterus respectively (Khairallah, personal communication).

Many organs inactivate kinins if the peptides are injected into the vessel supplying the organ. For example, bradykinin or kallidin had to be given in doses 2—4 times higher into the mesenteric vein than into the femoral vein for an equal hypotension of the systemic arterial blood pressure (Erdös and Yang, 1966). This discrepancy in required doses could probably be explained by the increased inactivation of the peptide during passage through the splanchnic circulation or the liver. Infusion of bradykinin into the artery of human forearm did not increase the peptide level in venous blood for a considerable period. This also suggests a very rapid disappearance of the peptide from the circulation. The capillaries may be important both in the removal and in the inactivation of bradykinin (SICUTERI et al., 1963; ALLWOOD and LEWIS, 1964).

Recent studies showed that, in addition to hydrolysis in blood, the area of the pulmonary circulation plays a prominent role in inactivating kinins after i.v. injection or infusion (KRONEBERG and STOEPEL, 1963). VANE and his associates (1969), with the help of their blood-bathed organ technique, estimated the half-lives of kinins by using a strip of cat jejunum (FERREIRA and VANE, 1967a, b). When bradykinin was infused into various vascular beds of the cat, several areas destroyed the activity of the infused peptide including the head, the liver, and the kidney. They found the lung most impressive, as it rendered 80% of the peptide inactive during a single passage. This was confirmed by BIRON (1968).

The fate of labeled bradykinin in the pulmonary circulation of the rat was studied also by RYAN et al. (1968a). They perfused the lung with Locke's solution instead of blood. Lung rapidly inactivated bradykinin and released metabolites that were collected. The first bond broken in bradykinin in the pulmonary circulation has not been definitely established as yet (STEWART and ROBLERO, 1967; RYAN et al., 1968a). Polistes kinin, the longer analog of bradykinin, was more stable in the pulmonary circulation than the parent compound (STEWART, 1968). Very likely one of the lung kininases is identical with the Ang I converting enzyme and with kininase II (peptidase P; dipeptide hydrolase). (Section B, III and IV).

The rapid inactivation of the peptides in plasma and the effect of passage through the pulmonary circulation may explain in part why after i.v. administration of kinins only a fraction reaches the peripheral vascular bed and why injection of the peptides into the artery of the autoperfused hind limb of the dog requires much smaller amounts to cause vasodilatation than do i.v. injections (ERDÖS, 1966).

XIII. Inhibitors of Kininases

The use of inhibitors *in vitro* played an essential part in characterizing various kininases (ERDÖS, 1961, 1962). The inhibitors found can be grouped as chelating agents, metal ions, compounds structurally related to the products of hydrolysis of the substrates, and miscellaneous compounds. Evidently this classification is somewhat arbitrary because some agents would qualify under various headings (ERDÖS and YANG, 1970; Table 3).

Among the sequestering compounds EDTA is used frequently as an inhibitor (ERDÖS et al., 1963b) but there are differences in the inhibition pattern of the plasma enzymes. Human plasma kininases are inhibited by EDTA (ERDÖS, 1962; YANG and ERDÖS, 1967), while those from some animal serum or plasma are more resistant (ERDÖS et al., 1963b).

1,10-Phenanthroline is a potent inhibitor of various kininases that are metal dependent. These include the exopeptidase-type enzymes (mostly peptidyl amino acid hydrolases) and kininase II (dipeptide hydrolase). This compound has been used frequently to preserve the activity of a kinin after its release *in vitro*, otherwise the kininases present in most crude systems would prevent a quantitative assay of the peptide (ERDÖS et al., 1967b; GARBE, 1967; ERDÖS and MIWA, 1968).

Other sequestering agents, such as 8-hydroxyquinoline or 2,2-dipyridyl, were also employed as inhibitors. The application of cysteine and related SH compounds as kininase blockers can interfere with bioassay *in vitro*, since they potentiate bradykinin effects on isolated smooth muscle preparations (ERDÖS, 1966; ERDÖS and YANG, 1970).

Table 3. *Inhibitors of kininases* (According to ERDÖS and YANG, 1970)

Inhibitor	Source of Enzyme	Substrates
Ethylenediamine tetraacetate (EDTA)	Plasma, carboxypeptidase N; kininase II; kidney	HLL, HLAa, bradykinin
1,10-Phenanthroline and other chelators	Carboxypeptidase N; kininase II; plasma; erythrocytes; tissues; microbial kininase	Bradykinin
Thio compounds	Plasma; tissues; erythrocytes; carboxypeptidase N	Bradykinin
Heavy metal ions	Plasma, erythrocytes; leukocytes; carboxypeptidase N; kininase II; brain	Bradykinin, HLL, HLAa
Products of hydrolysis of substrates and related compounds (e.g., arginine, ε-amino-*n*-caproic acid [EACA])	Carboxypeptidase N; plasma	HLL, HLAa, bradykinin
Miscellaneous compounds, e.g., *p*-chloromercuriphenyl sulfonic acid (PCMS)	Erythrocytes	Bradykinin
Iodosobenzoic acid	Erythrocytes	Bradykinin
Iodoacetic acid	Catheptic carboxypeptidase; spleen	Bradykinin
Bradykinin-potentiating factor (BPF)	Plasma, lung	Bradykinin

The sensitivity of kininases to heavy metal ions varies. For example, kininase I (carboxypeptidase N) is strongly inhibited by $CdSO_4$, whereas kininase II is resistant (YANG and ERDÖS, 1967). $CoCl_2$ accelerates the hydrolysis of bradykinin in plasma but blocks it in the hemolyzed red blood cells (ERDÖS et al., 1963b). $HgCl_2$ seems to be a generally good inhibitor; for example, the I_{50} for carboxypeptidase N is 4×10^{-5}M. $CdSO_4$ has the lowest I_{50}; it inhibited 50% of the hydrolysis of HLAa by carboxypeptidase N, at a 2×10^{-7}M concentration (ERDÖS et al., 1967a). The metal was, however, less effective when used with a purified kininase preparation (TRAPEZNIKOVA and PASKHINA, 1968). Other metal ions such as Zn^{2+} or Cu^{2+} also inhibited some kininases (ERDÖS et al., 1963b), for example, in leucocytes (ZACHARIAE et al., 1966; GREENBAUM and KIM, 1967).

Among compounds that are structurally similar to or identical with the products of hydrolysis of substrates of kininases, arginine (ERDÖS, 1962) and benzoylarginine ($I_{50} = 10^{-4}$M) inhibit carboxypeptidase N (ERDÖS et al., 1964), but arginine is inactive against kininase II of human plasma (YANG and ERDÖS, 1967). The latter enzyme is inhibited by phenylalanylarginine, the dipeptide cleaved from bradykinin. In addition histidylleucine, the split product of the conversion of Ang I, insulin and the B chain of insulin inhibited both the conversion of Ang I and the inactivation of bradykinin by a purified enzyme preparation (YANG et al., 1970e). Argininic acid, the product of the hydrolysis of the ester substrate (HLAa) by carboxypeptidase N, has an I_{50} of 4×10^{-5}M (ERDÖS et al., 1967a). Because of the application of ε-amino-*n*-caproic acid (EACA) to clinical subjects, the inhibition of carboxypeptidase N by this agent is of interest (ERDÖS, 1962; MARGOLIS and BISHOP, 1962; ERDÖS and SLOANE, 1962).

Agents that react with SH group of enzymes, such as *p*-chloromercuriphenyl sulfonate (PCMS), inhibit erythrocyte kininase or some catheptic tissue kininases but not plasma enzymes (ERDÖS et al., 1963b; FREY et al., 1968; GREENBAUM and YAMAFUJI, 1966).

Inhibitors of proteinases (peptidyl peptide hydrolases) are generally inactive against most kininases tested. An exception is the effect of diisopropyl fluorophosphate (DFP) on rabbit granulocyte (GREENBAUM and KIM, 1967) and rabbit brain

(CAMARGO and GRAEFF, 1969) kininases. Venom of *Bothrops jararaca* contains a small molecular weight material, bradykinin-potentiating factor (BPF), that potentiates bradykinin *in vivo*, presumably by inhibition of kininases. This was also shown in various plasmas *in vitro* (FERREIRA, 1966; FERREIRA and VANE, 1967b; see also section B, XIV) and in the lung tissue (BAKHLE, 1968).

XIV. Inhibition of Kininases *in Vivo*

The very rapid inactivation of kinins in the circulation made the search for *in vivo* inhibitors of the kininase obvious. Already in 1939 WERLE and GRUNZ had injected cysteine to enhance the circulatory effects of substance DK (kallidin) in laboratory animals. Inhibition studies *in vitro* led to the application of some of these inhibiting agents to guinea pigs (ERDÖS and WOHLER, 1963a, b) and to other animals (ROCHA E SILVA, 1963). They are mostly metal-binding agents; thiols were especially effective. 2-Mercaptoethanol and mercaptopropionic acid were very well tolerated after i.v. administration to guinea pigs. Because guinea pigs have the highest plasma kininase level among laboratory animals, and these compounds can effectively prevent the *in vitro* enzymatic hydrolysis of kinins, it was assumed that their *in vivo* action is also based on enzyme inhibition. (It should be mentioned, however, that thiol compounds also potentiate the *in vitro* effect of kinins on the smooth muscles. This potentiation cannot be solely attributed to the inhibition of kininases; ERDÖS, 1966.) After the administration of the inhibitors, the drop in systemic arterial blood pressure caused by bradykinin, kallidin or by their homologues (ERDÖS and WOHLER, 1963b; ERDÖS et al., 1967c) was more pronounced and longer lasting. The increased sensitivity to kinins in the guinea pig pretreated with an inhibitor was abolished by an i.v. injection of purified carboxypeptidase B (ERDÖS and WOHLER, 1963b). Because the cardiovascular effects of bradykinin in the guinea pig increase for some time after the injection of an inhibitor such as 2-mercaptoethanol (ERDÖS and WOHLER, unpublished), it can be assumed that in addition to inhibition of the inactivation of kinins in blood, some kininases in tissues are also blocked.

The action of inhibitors is different in the various experimental animals. 2-Mercaptoethanol, for example, is very efficient in the rat, although within a narrower dose range than in the guinea pig (ERDÖS and YANG, 1966). STEWART and his colleagues (STEWART and ROBLERO, 1967; RYAN et al., 1968a) partially blocked the pulmonary inactivation of bradykinin in the rat with 2-mercaptoethanol. Using the blood-bathed organ technique, FERREIRA and VANE (1967b) showed that after i.v. injection more bradykinin reached the arterial side of the circulation in dogs treated with BPF than in control animals.

Recently several peptides were separated from *Bothrops jararaca* venom (GREENE et al., 1970). One of them, the pentapeptide pyrrolidone-5-carboxylic acid (PCA)-Lys-Trp-Ala-Pro, was synthesized. The peptide potentiated the effect of bradykinin *in vitro* but its action *in vivo* was short lasting.

XV. Changes in Kininase Activity

The destruction of bradykinin and kallidin by human blood was studied in a variety of states. Owing to the differences in the methods of determination used, and to the existence of several kininases, some of the data published on the subject are controversial to say the least. Many attempts have been made to link changes in kininases levels to specific pathological conditions, but there is no definite correlation between kininase level in blood and the symptoms observed (ERDÖS and YANG, 1970).

Experiments in which kininase activity was measured in plasma of pregnant women yielded varying results. EFFKEMANN and WERLE (1941) and ARMSTRONG and STEWART (1960) did not observe any increase in blood enzyme level with pregnancy, while CENTARO et al. (1963) and WERLE in a later paper (1960) reported that blood serum or plasma from pregnant women destroys kinins faster than does normal blood. The level of the enzyme in the newborn was lower than in the mother. In the experiments of MELMON et al. (1968), however, the difference between neonatal and adult plasma was not statistically significant.

ERDÖS et al. (1964, 1965) studied the hydrolysis of HLL by carboxypeptidase N in the blood serum of thirty pregnant women. Carboxypeptidase N level was significantly higher (1.07 μmole per min/ml) in pregnant than in nonpregnant subjects (0.77) and lower than normal in the newborn (0.45). When the esterase activity of the enzyme was measured with HLAa, it increased gradually during pregnancy (ERDÖS et al., 1967a) from 3.71 μmole per min/ml in the first trimester to 4.74 in the third trimester.

The hydrolysis of HLL in the blood sera of several hundred clinical subjects was also assayed. Patients with cirrhosis of the liver had lower values, while neoplastic clinical subjects had higher values than healthy individuals. The enzyme level in men suffering from gastrointestinal diseases, allergic conditions, or renal diseases fell within the normal range (ERDÖS et al., 1965).

EDERY and LEWIS (1962) pointed out the importance of the lower activity of carboxypeptidase N below pH 7. In inflammation, the lowered pH of the tissues may lead to the accumulation of the peptides and an aggravation of existing symptoms. Although this hypothesis is an attractive one, it has to be confirmed in a more comprehensive system before it can be generally accepted (ERDÖS and YANG, 1970).

Kininase activity in venous blood of various patients was studied using bioassay to determine the decrease in the bradykinin effect (ABE et al., 1965; WATANABE et al., 1966). Patients with hyperthyroidism and liver diseases had higher than normal values of kininase activity. In pancreatitis, normal enzyme level was found by ERDÖS et al. (1965) and by WATANABE (1967), although NUGENT et al. (1966) reported higher values in blood of dogs.

XVI. Enzymatic Conversion of Kinins

The metabolism of the longer analogs of bradykinin such as kallidin or Met-Lys-bradykinin is somewhat different from that of the nonapeptide, since cleaving off the N-terminal lysine or methionyl-lysine may lead to the release of bradykinin. However, the situation is not analogous to the angiotensin system, where the decapeptide Ang I has to be converted to the octapeptide angiotensin II (Ang II) before becoming active. Kallidin is active in its own right both *in vitro* and *in vivo*, and in some animals it leads to greater hypotension than bradykinin (ERDÖS, 1966). Nevertheless, blood plasma contains an aminopeptidase that can convert kallidin to bradykinin. This was shown simultaneously by WEBSTER and PIERCE (1963) and by ERDÖS et al. (1963b). Probably only a fraction of the available kallidin is converted to bradykinin prior to its inactivation by kininases. Since both kallidin and bradykinin are inactivated equally fast by plasma, kallidin may serve simultaneously as a substrate of the converting aminopeptidase and the inactivating kininases (ERDÖS, 1966).

HOPSU et al. (1966a, b) found in the liver of various laboratory animals an enzyme, called aminopeptidase B, that splits naphthylamides of lysine and arginine. It also occurs in various other tissues and is activated by chloride ions. The enzyme liberated lysine from kallidin but did not hydrolyze bradykinin (HOPSU et al., 1966b).

Some purified proteolytic enzymes can liberate bradykinin not only from the protein substrate kininogen but also from some longer kinin analog peptides. Trypsin can convert kallidin to bradykinin (WEBSTER and PIERCE, 1963; NICOLAIDES et al., 1963; ERDÖS et al., 1963b). Kallidin, however, is a rather poor substrate for trypsin, and not more than 5—14% of a given amount was converted to bradykinin (WEBSTER and PIERCE, 1963; HABERMANN and BLENNEMANN, 1964). Met-Lys-bradykinin can be easily converted to bradykinin by trypsin, serum kallikrein, or snake venom (HABERMANN and BLENNEMANN, 1964; SCHRÖDER, 1964; ELLIOTT and LEWIS, 1965), but the release of bradykinin from kininogen is much faster than that from the undecapeptide (HABERMANN and BLENNEMANN, 1964). Met-Lys-bradykinin is also hydrolyzed by leucine aminopeptidase (E.C. 3.4.1.1); the first two N-terminal bonds of the peptide are broken by the purified enzyme (SCHRÖDER, 1964).

C. Inactivation of Angiotensins

Angiotensin was found simultaneously by two groups of investigators. It was named hypertensin by BRAUN-MENÉNDEZ et al. (1939, 1940) and angiotonin by PAGE and HELMER (1940). Much later the two names were fused into angiotensin. Both pioneering teams noted that renin acts on a plasma globulin to produce a hypertensive substance. This material lost its activity on standing owing to an action of an enzyme or rather enzymes collectively called angiotensinases (angiotonases, hypertensinases). The activity of the enzymes could not be characterized before the structure of the peptide was established. Thus, early experiments were restricted to observing the disappearance of the activity of angiotensin preparations of various degrees of purity during incubation with enzymes. The inactivating enzymes came from various sources, some of them were commercially available as purified enzyme preparations, others were extracted from tissues or from blood. (The pertinent information was summarized in 1946 by BRAUN-MENÉNDEZ et al. and in 1962 by ERDÖS.)

Crude renin was contaminated by angiotensinases that were lost during further purification of renin. On the other hand, renal angiotensinase free of renin could not be prepared at the beginning (BRAUN-MENÉNDEZ et al., 1946).

Angiotensinase activity was expressed in biological units. FASCIOLO et al. (1940) defined the unit of hypertensinase as that amount of enzyme which destroys the activity of 0.5 unit of angiotensin (hypertensin) in 4 hours. The angiotensinase contents of the different organs varied from 1600 units per gram of fresh tissue to 1 unit per ml of plasma. The highest activities were found in intestinal mucosa and the lowest in plasma or serum (BRAUN-MENÉNDEZ et al., 1946). In addition to blood and tissues, angiotensin was inactivated by extracts from plants, mushrooms and yeast or by snake venoms (ERDÖS, 1962). Initial studies with various extracts and with trypsin, chymotrypsin and peptidases suggested that the inactivation was a "proteolytic" process, and that angiotensin is a peptide (BRAUN-MENÉNDEZ et al., 1946).

Finally, the amino acid sequence in angiotensin was established and the mode of angiotensin liberation determined. Subsequently, Ang I and II were synthetized (PAGE and MCCUBBIN, 1968).

Renin splits Leu-Leu bond in the plasma protein precursor angiotensinogen, and thereby releases the decapeptide Ang I. Ang I is converted to the active derivative Ang II by an enzyme, which is not surprisingly called converting enzyme.

Fig. 2. *Simplified scheme for the release and inactivation of angiotensin in plasma*

Renin + Angiotensinogen
↓
Angiotensin I + Converting Enzyme
↓
Angiotensin II + Angiotensinase
↓
Split Product

It cleaves off the C-terminal histidyl-leucine. Figure 2 summarizes the process. Renin occurs in the kidney, but can be found in many other places of the body such as the uterus (PAGE and McCUBBIN, 1968) or the submaxillary gland (WERLE et al., 1957; CHIANG et al., 1968). Numerous other tissues have a renin-like enzyme (SKEGGS et al., 1969). Angiotensins occur in two forms having either valine or isoleucine in the fifth position. Val^5-Asp^1-angiotensin is present in cattle while Ile^5-Asp^1-angiotensin was purified from human, hog and horse plasma (PAGE and McCUBBIN, 1968). In a commercially available synthetic derivative the N-terminal aspartic acid was replaced by asparagine. Val^5-angiotensinII-Asp^1-β-amide (Hypertensin-Ciba; Asn^1-Val^5-angiotensin II; Ang II amide) has been frequently employed in the laboratory as a source of Ang II.

I. Angiotensinases in Blood Plasma

The aminopeptidase character of a plasma angiotensinase was first suggested by CROXATTO and CROXATTO (1946). This was further elaborated by BRUNNER and REGOLI (1962; REGOLI et al., 1963; BRUNNER, 1963). These authors compared first the rate of inactivation of angiotensin homologues in rat serum and in human plasma. The activity of Ang II amide was destroyed faster than that of Ang II. The hydrolysis of α-D-Asp^1, β-L-Asp^1, β-D-Asp^1 and desamino-Ang II was much slower than that of Ang II. Because of the modified N-terminal end, the breakdown of these derivatives could not be attributed to an aminopeptidase but to an endopeptidase. The aminopeptidase would be responsible for about 90% of the total angiotensinase activity of nephrectomized rat serum, but only for 60% in normal human serum.

Removal of Asp^1 or Asn^1 from Ang II does not completely inactivate the peptide. The resulting heptapeptide is about half as active as the unhydrolyzed octapeptide (SCHRÖDER and LÜBKE, 1966).

KHAIRALLAH et al. (1963) incubated various homologues of Ang II with human plasma and measured the residual activity of the peptide in a bioassay. Only Ang II with aspartic acid in the N-terminal position was inactivated. β-Asp^1, Arg^1 or desamino-angiotensin were not hydrolyzed in normal plasma or at a neutral pH. The plasma enzyme was inhibited by EDTA and reactivated by calcium ions. The authors suggested that the plasma enzyme be called angiotensinase A (Table 4).

Table 4. *Peptide bonds hydrolyzed in ang II amide*

	1 H-Asn-	2 Arg-	3 Val-	4 Tyr-	5 Val-	6 His-	7 Pro-	8 Phe-OH
Chymotrypsin					↑			
Trypsin			↑					
Pepsin				↑				
Leucine aminopeptidase		↑	↑	↑	↑	↑		
Carboxypeptidase A, Angiotensinase C								↑
Subtilisin			↑		↑			
Cathepsin C			↑		↑			
Angiotensinase A		↑						

Table 5. *Substrates of angiotensinases in chemical assays*

Substrate	Source of Enzyme	Method	Remarks	Ref.
Ang II amide	Serum, man	Quantitative paper chromatography	Measures Val $K_m = 6 \times 10^{-5}$M	1
Ang II amide	Serum, man	Spectrophotometric	Converts Asn to maleic acid, DPNH dependent reaction $K_m = 2 \times 10^{-4}$M	2
[^{35}S] PTC Ang II amide	Plasma, man	Measurement of radioactivity	Separates products in chromatography	3
Ang II amide	Kidney lysosomes, rat	Amino acid analysis	After short incubation more Phe^8 is released than other amino acids	4
Ang II amide	Liver, rabbit	Spectrophotometric	Measures Phe^8 release; Dialyzed extract against EDTA	5
R_1-Pro-R_2OH (R_1 = blocking group; R_2 amino acid)	Angiotensinase C, kidney lysosomes, hog; urine, leucocytes, man	Ninhydrin assay, Amino acid analysis	Determines the liberated C-terminal amino acid	6
Cbo-Pro-Phe		Ninhydrin assay	Measures Phe	7
Dansyl-Pro-Phe		Fluorometric	Measures dansyl-Pro	8
α-Asp-β-naphthylamide	Serum, man	Colorimetric	Measures naphthylamine release. $K_m = 1 \times 10^{-2}$M	9
Ang II; Ang II amide		Ninhydrin assay	Determines Asp and Asn	9
Leu-β-naphthylamide, Leu-*p*-nitroanilide	Serum, man, rat, hog; kidney, hog	Colorimetric	Presumably shows angiotensinase A_1 activity $K_m = 1$—2×10^{-4}M	10
α-Glu-β-naphthylamide	Serum, man, rat; erythrocytes, kidney, rat	Colorimetric	Enzyme may be identical with angiotensinase A_2, $K_m = 1$—5×10^{-4}M to 7×10^{-3}M	11
α-Glu-*p*-nitroanilide	Serum man, rat; kidney, rat	Colorimetric	Presumably shows A_2 activity $K_m = 1 \times 10^{-4}$M to 3×10^{-2}M	12

References: 1. Klaus et al. (1963). — 2. Oelkers and Goldacker (1967). — 3. Doyle et al. (1967). — 4. Saito et al. (1969). — 5. Johnson and Ryan (1968). — 6. Yang et al. (1968, 1970a), Yang and Erdös (1969a, b). — 7. Yang et al. (1968, 1970a). — 8. Yang et al. (1968, 1970a), Yang and Erdös (1969a, b). — 9. Nagatsu et al. (1965a, b). — 10. Hess (1965), Nagatsu et al. (1965a), Kurtz and Wachsmuth (1969). — 11. Nagatsu et al. (1965a), Hess (1965), Yman and Kulling (1969). — 12. Hess (1965), Yman et al. (1969).

Klaus indicated with the help of a quantitative paper chromatography method (1962; Klaus et al., 1963) that several aminopeptidases may be involved in the breakdown of angiotensin. Unfortunately, his routine method is not suitable for assaying the initial rate of the enzymatic hydrolysis or to observe the cleavage of the first bond in the peptide chain (Table 5).

Nagatsu et al. (1965a, b) distinguished two enzymes in dialyzed human serum. One of them attacks the naturally occurring form of Ang II by cleaving off the N-terminal asparatic acid and is similar to aminopeptidase A of the kidney (Glenner et al., 1962). The mode of action of the enzyme was established in paper chromatography. It also hydrolyzes naphthylamides of glutamic and aspartic acid and requires the presence of calcium ions for its activity. The hydrolysis of

α-aspartyl-β-naphthylamide (α-ANA) substrate by the plasma enzyme can be measured with a colorimetric method. One ml of human serum hydrolyzed 0.88 nmole α-ANA per min. These authors also noticed similarities in the enzymatic cleavage of asparagine from Ang II amide and leucine from leucyl-β-naphthylamide (29.2 nmole/min per ml). Thus the second angiotensinase in plasma would be similar to one of the leucine aminopeptidases (NAGATSU et al., 1970).

Later the two aminopeptidases involved in the metabolism of Ang II amide and Ang II were named angiotensinase A_1 and A_2 (KHAIRALLAH and PAGE 1967). Some initial separation of the two enzymes was carried out by SAMBHI and BARRETT (1966). The angiotensinases were reported to move either with the albumin zone in starch block electrophoresis (KOKUBU et al., 1967a) or with α_1 and α_2 globulins (ASCHEIM et al., 1967). During fractionation of normal human plasma in a DEAE-Sephadex A 50 column, three active peaks were found that destroyed Ang II amide activity. One peak coincided with the appearance of leucyl-β-naphthylamidase activities and D,L-glutamyl-β-naphthylamidase (HIWADA et al., 1966). YMAN and KULLING (1969) and YMAN et al. (1969) purified α-glutamyl-β-naphthylamidase (aminopeptidase A) from human serum. Neither the specific activity nor the purification factor were calculated, but a seemingly significant purification was achieved by the sequential application of ethanol fractionation, hydroxyapatite chromatography and preparative electrophoresis. It was assumed that the purified enzyme was identical with angiotensinase A_2.

Much less is known about the other angiotensinases present in plasma. An angiotensinase active at about pH 5 was detected in human plasma by PICKENS et al. (1965). In contradistinction to angiotensinase A_1 and A_2 that are active at a neutral pH and require calcium as cofactor, the acid angiotensinase is not inhibited by chelating agents but by DFP. Ammonium sulfate fractionation separates the enzyme from the "neutral" angiotensinases (KHAIRALLAH and PAGE 1967); it was named angiotensinase B. The hypothesis was advanced that angiotensinase B acts similarly to chymotrypsin in cleaving angiotensin II into two tetrapeptides. Angiotensinase B may be identical with a rat kidney or serum endopeptidase (REGOLI et al., 1963). Because renin is frequently assayed by incubating it with plasma angiotensinogen at an acid pH (PICKENS et al., 1965; PAGE and MCCUBBIN, 1968) angiotensinase B may interfere with the assay by hydrolyzing the released angiotensin. This would be especially true when small quantities of renin had to be measured after long incubation periods.

A third plasma enzyme, named angiotensinase G, has not yet been completely characterized. It is missing from normal plasma but appears in diseases of the liver. Angiotensinase G was demonstrated in blood after experimental liver damage to rabbits and in blood of patients afflicted with hepatic diseases (KOKUBU, 1966; KOKUBU et al., 1967a, b). Angiotensinase G can be found only when a factor released from the liver acts on a serum protein fraction. This serum protein migrates electrophoretically with the gamma globulin. No angiotensinase G activity was found after separation of plasma and tissue fractions in electrophoresis by ASCHEIM et al. (1967).

The reported values of the K_m of angiotensinases vary according to the method of determination and the substrate used. They range from 10^{-8}M with Ang II substrate (MYERS et al., 1965) to 10^{-2}M with α-ANA (NAGATSU et al., 1965a) (Table 5).

II. Angiotensinases in Blood Cells

Of the cellular elements in blood, erythrocytes destroy Ang II activity, provided they are hemolyzed (SAPIRSTEIN et al., 1946). Intact red cells can only adsorb 6—10% of the available Ang II (BOUCHER et al., 1964), but hemolyzed cells have a hundred times more angiotensinase than plasma has (BRAUN-MENÉNDEZ et al., 1946). A swine erythrocyte preparation was concentrated about 7-fold by gel filtration (DAHLHEIM et al., 1969). The enzyme hydrolyzed Ang II amide 7 times faster than Ang II. It had been assumed that both the plasma and erythrocyte angiotensinases were aminopeptidases (KHAIRALLAH et al., 1963) but some recent experiments do not support this hypothesis. KOKUBU et al. (1969) purified red cell angiotensinase 8,000-fold. After a short incubation period only the C-terminal tetrapeptide of Ang II was found to be intact. This was taken as an indication that the enzyme acts by breaking the Tyr^{4}-Ile^{5} bond in the peptide chain, and that subsequently the other bonds would be cleaved in the N-terminal tetrapeptide fragment. The second possibility is that the Arg^{2}-Val^{3} bond would be cleaved first. In the former case the enzyme would be similar to chymotrypsin, in the latter to trypsin. The authors believe that the chymotrypsin-like action may be the more important one. Strangely the enzyme was inhibited by both EDTA and DFP, and did not hydrolyze some other substrates of trypsin or chymotrypsin.

Leukocytes also contain angiotensinases that inactivate the peptide 200—250 times faster than plasma. This was shown with bovine cells by EBENSPERGER and CROXATTO (1945). YANG et al. (1970a) detected a prolylcarboxypeptidase, called angiotensinase C, in human granulocytes. As in the kidney (section C, IV), angiotensinase C was found in the lysosomal fraction of leukocytes.

III. Angiotensinases in Other Biological Fluids

In addition to blood, angiotensinases appear in other body fluids such as lymph (BRAUN-MENÉNDEZ et al., 1946) or urine (YANG et al., 1968, 1970a). Human urine contains angiotensinase C. In addition, urine hydrolyzes α-glutamyl-β-naphthylamide, presumably through angiotensinase A_2 action (ONO et al., 1968).

IV. Angiotensinases in Tissues

Of the tissue homogenates studied by BRAUN-MENÉNDEZ et al. (1946), only intestinal mucosa destroyed Ang II activity faster than kidney. Crude kidney extract showed two different types of enzymic activities, one with an optimum activity at pH 4 and another at pH 7.5 (PAGE et al., 1943). Because kidney is the origin of renin and is involved in hypertensive diseases, the metabolism of the peptide by this organ was of obvious interest. The activity in kidney was first attributed to an aminopeptidase (CROXATTO, 1943). REGOLI et al. (1963) incubated various Ang II homologues with rat kidney homogenates. When Ang II or Ang II amide were the substrates no large peptide fragments of angiotensin could be identified owing to the very rapid enzymatic breakdown. Thus the first bond broken in the peptide could not be established. When the β derivative was used [(β-*L*-Asp^{1})-angiotensin II] a small amount of N-terminal tetrapeptide was found (RINIKER, 1964). The C-terminal tetrapeptide fragment was not detected; instead the four individual amino acids were seen. This was taken as an indication that an enzyme in the kidney homogenate inactivated Ang II by cleaving the Tyr^{4}-Val^{5} bond. The rate of inactivation by the kidney depended on the structure of the substrate; Ang II amide was hydrolyzed fastest. Other homologues such as β-*L*, α-*D* and desamino-angiotensin II were also degraded, but at a slower rate (RINIKER, 1964). This was explained by the contribution of aminopeptidases in the homogenate to the inactivation of Ang II and Ang II amide. Based on these experiments it was estimated that in the rat kidney homogenate, as in human plasma, the ratio of aminopeptidase to endopeptidase activity was 3:2.

The subcellular distribution of the enzymes in the kidney has also been studied. Particulate fractions of homogenized rat and swine kidney contained 10 times more activity than the final supernatant. About half of the angiotensinase was in a "mitochondrial" fraction (DENGLER and REICHEL, 1960) that presumably contained lysosomes.

The enzymes in the subcellular fractions of the rat kidney were further differentiated by measuring their actions at two pH values. About equal quantities of Ang II amide were inactivated at pH 5 by the lysosomal fraction and at pH 7.6 by the microsomes. The microsomal enzyme was inhibited by EDTA and the lysosomal one by DFP. The activity in the microsomes was attributed to angiotensinase A (MATSUNAGA et al., 1968); the lysosomal enzyme was characterized somewhat later by YANG et al. (1968, 1970a). It acts by cleaving the C-terminal Phe^8 of Ang II at an acid pH and yields a completely inactive derivative, Des-Phe^8-Ang II (SCHRÖDER and LÜBKE, 1966) (Table 4). The enzyme, named angiotensinase C, does not hydrolyze Ang I. The suggested structure for the substrate of angiotensinase C is R_1-Pro-R_2OH. R_1 can be a blocking group such as Cbo or dansyl or another protected amino acid or a peptide. R_2 is an amino acid with a free carboxyl group. Proline has to be in the penultimate position while phenylalanine or another amino acid can form the C-terminal end. Therefore, the enzyme acts as a prolyl-carboxypeptidase (Table 5). It is inhibited by DFP, but not by chelating agents. Activators and inhibitors of catheptic enzymes had no effect on the purified angiotensinase C. The enzyme was purified about 35-fold. A convenient way to determine its action was by using Cbo-Pro-Phe substrate (Table 5). The most specific and sensitive assay was based on employing dansyl-Pro-Phe substrate and determining the liberated dansylproline fluorometrically (YANG and ERDÖS, 1969a, b). Less than 1 nmole can be accurately assayed in this way. Angiotensinase C occurs in hog kidney lysosomes, human urine and in a lysosomal fraction of human granulocytes. The enzyme studied by MATSUNAGA et al. (1968, 1969) may be identical with angiotensinase C, although their preparation still had cathepsin A activity. One of the enzymes in the experiments of SAITO et al. (1969) also might have been identical with angiotensinase C. These authors assayed the amino acids released from Ang II by kidney homogenate. After a short incubation phenylalanine appeared in largest amount followed by proline. Obviously, Ang II is not the only naturally occurring substrate of angiotensinase C. The enzyme could cleave a Pro^7-Phe^8 in bradykinin after the removal of the C-terminal Arg^9 (ERDÖS and YANG, 1966).

Other tissue homogenates also inactivate angiotensin. In contrast to the kidney, in the homogenized liver the supernatant fraction had the highest angiotensinase activity (KOKUBU et al., 1967a; MATSUNAGA et al., 1969). (A similar difference in the intracellular distribution of kininases in liver and in kidney was also observed [section B, VII].)

Angiotensinase activity was also studied in the crude rabbit liver homogenate (JOHNSON and RYAN, 1968). Dialysis against EDTA reduced the activity by 60%, and the EDTA inhibited enzyme was not characterized further. The EDTA resistant activity was tested with [Asn^1, Val^5] and [Asn^1, Ile^5] Ang II. The extract released Phe^8 from the peptide at a neutral pH. Although the conventional carboxypeptidase A substrates were not cleaved by the preparation, the hydrolysis was attributed to a carboxypeptidase. Since angiotensinase C still has a considerable amount of activity above the neutral pH, this enzyme preparation might have contained angiotensinase C.

An angiotensinase that is active at an acid pH but inhibited by DFP (presumably angiotensinase C) is present in many tissues other than the kidney, especially in the liver, spleen, adrenal glands and lung (MATSUNAGA et al., 1969).

Cathepsin C E.C.3.4.4.9 can also inactivate Ang II, as well as many other peptide substrates. The rat liver enzyme tested needed monovalent anions for activity, and it functioned as a dipeptidyl aminopeptidase I. It cleaved off Asn¹-Arg² and subsequently Val³-Tyr⁴ dipeptides from Ang II amide substrate (Table 4) at an acid pH. The C-terminal tetrapeptide was not hydrolyzed by the enzyme (MCDONALD et al., 1969 and 1970). Dipeptidyl aminopeptidase III of bovine pituitary gland cleaves the same bonds at a neutral pH.

V. Use of Purified Proteases in the Determination of Angiotensin Structure

As customary in peptide studies, purified proteolytic enzymes have been used as an aid to elucidate the structure of angiotensins. Table 4 shows the bonds broken by the various purified enzymes.

Leucine aminopeptidase cleaves five bonds sequentially and then stops at His^6-Pro^7. Carboxypeptidase A removes the C-terminal phenylalanine only. Pepsin (E.C. 3.3.4.1) breaks Val^3-Tyr^4 bond slowly and others at an even lower rate; subtilisin cleaves Tyr^4-Val^5 rapidly and Arg^2-Val^3 incompletely. Chymotrypsin hydrolyzed Tyr^4-Val^5 bond at equal speed in 4 analogues tested. In contrast, trypsin splits the naturally occurring Asp^1-Ang II peptide slowest, and the Ang II amide, β and D homologues much faster (RINIKER and SCHWYZER, 1961, 1964; RINIKER, 1964). Trypsin and chymotrypsin have been employed in the past to identify Ang II activity in crude extract because both enzymes destroy it. A convenient way to employ trypsin has been to use an insoluble derivative of the enzyme. Trypsin was bound to the water insoluble copolymer of maleic anhydride and ethylene. The insoluble trypsin preparation inactivated the liberated angiotensin in the incubation mixture and did not interfere with the bioassay (CHIANG et al., 1968).

An enzyme purified from citrus fruit also cleaved the Pro^7-Phe^8 bond in Ang II amide *in vitro*. This enzyme, acting at an acid pH, was named carboxypeptidase C (ZUBER, 1964).

VI. Fate of Angiotensins *in Vivo*

Angiotensins, as many other peptides, disappear from the circulation very rapidly (ERDÖS, 1962). Claims that ^{131}I labeled Ang II has a half-life of 10—15 hours in man (WOLF et al., 1962) were not supported by others. This rapid disappearance was not changed when the N-terminal amino acid had a protective group (DOYLE et al., 1967, 1968) or the β-Asp^1 analogue of the peptide was used (BIRON et al., 1968; LEARY and LEDINGHAM, 1969; KLAUS, 1966). The disappearance was slowed down, however, when a 15,000 molecular weight derivative of the peptide was injected i.a. to unanesthetized dogs (HAAS et al., 1968).

Initial studies pointed out the importance of the liver in the removal of Ang II from the circulation. The peptide is much less effective when administered via the portal or splenic vein is than when infused or injected into the systemic circulation (METHOT et al., 1964; KELLY and NYHUS, 1966; CHAMBERLAIN et al., 1964; COHEN et al., 1967; ABRAMS, 1966; KOKUBU et al., 1967a; BEUZEVILLE and LAUSON, 1965; WERNZE and FUJII, 1966). The extraction of infused Ang II by the liver decreased or disappeared in rats that were pretreated with CCl_4 (BIRON and

MEYER, 1968). Later it was noticed that other vascular beds are also effective and possibly more important in removing the injected peptide from the blood.

The fate of labeled Ang II was studied systematically first by KHAIRALLAH et al. (1962). They infused tritiated Val^5-Ang II amide to rats and determined the radioactivity in the various organs at the end of the infusion and a half an hour later. The breakdown of the angiotensin molecule was indicated by the change in the electrophoretic mobility of the extracted labeled material. The highest concentrations of Ang II were found in the kidney, adrenals and uterus at the end of infusion. Thirty minutes afterwards most of the breakdown products were in the kidney and the urine. After nephrectomy the liver contained most of the Ang II metabolites (BUMPUS et al., 1964).

VANE and his associates (VANE, 1969; HODGE et al., 1967) systematically investigated the metabolism of Ang II *in vivo*. They utilized a bioassay method in which blood is constantly superfused over a sensitive organ such as the rat colon, that contracts in the presence of Ang II. (Others used different techniques with results similar to those of VANE.)

It was noticed that the half-life of angiotensin II homologues in blood is about 2—5 min *in vitro*, but the *in vivo* half-life is about one circulation time (BIRON et al., 1968; HODGE et al., 1967). This excluded the blood as an important site of the inactivation of angiotensin. Perfused dog, cat and rat kidney removed 70—95% of angiotensin II. About $^1/_2$ to $^3/_4$ of the peptide disappeared in perfused head, liver or hind quarters of experimental animal (MORRIS, 1964; GOFFINET and MULROW, 1963; BIRON et al., 1968; HODGE et al., 1967; BAKHLE et al., 1969; VANE, 1969). Others confirmed these results using phenylthiocarbamyl Ang II ^{35}S (DOYLE et al., 1968; OSBORN et al., 1969). The pulmonary circulation was inactive in this respect (GOFFINET and MULROW, 1963; HODGE et al., 1967; LEARY and LEDINGHAM, 1969; BAKHLE et al., 1969; OSBORN et al., 1969). This observation is in contrast to the important role of the lung in converting Ang I into Ang II (VANE, 1969; BIRON et al., 1969).

The nature of Ang II inactivation in the peripheral circulation is not clear. In the rat mesenteric circulation the place of inactivation was suggested to be in the terminal arterioli (MYERS et al., 1965). We do not know how important enzymes are in the initial process of removal, especially since the various low molecular weight derivatives of Ang II disappear with equal rapidity. After i.a. injections, a factor, possibly an adenine derivative, protects angiotensin against disappearance in the hind limb, if it is added to the peptide before injection in the vessels (HAAS et al., 1968, 1969). Studies with enzyme inhibitors in the perfused liver and kidney indicated that the removal of Ang II from perfusion fluid in these organs is related to an enzymatic process (LEARY and LEDINGHAM, 1969). OSBORNE et al. (1970) drew similar conclusions after perfusing the heart and the kidney.

Pregnant women are less sensitive to Ang II infusion than non-pregnant subjects (ABDUL-KARIM and ASSALI, 1961; CHESLEY et al., 1965), although it is unlikely that this can be attributed to the increased blood enzyme level. No difference was observed, however, in pregnant rats, sheep or dogs (DODSON, 1957; ABDUL-KARIM and ASSALI, 1961). Clinical subjects with cirrhosis of the liver are less responsive to Ang II amide infusion than normal persons (KLAUS, 1966).

VII. Inhibitors of Angiotensinases

Because the determination of renin is frequently based on assaying the liberated angiotensin, the inhibition of the enzymatic destruction of the peptide is of prime

Table 6. *Inhibitors of angiotensinases*

Inhibitor	Source of Enzyme	Substrate	Ref.
Diisopropyl fluorophosphate	Serum, plasma man	Ang II amide	1
	Angiotensinase B, G plasma		
	Erythrocytes, rabbit	Ang II	2
	Kidney, hog		
	Angiotensinase C, kidney	Ang II amide	2
	leucocytes, urine	Cbo-Pro-Phe	
		Dansyl-Pro-Phe	
Ethylenediamine tetraacetate	Angiotensinase A_1,A_2,	Ang II amide; Ang II	3
	Plasma, serum		
	Plasma angiotensinase G	Ang II amide	4
	Serum, rat	α-Glu-β-naphthylamide	5
	Erythrocytes, man, hog	Ang II amide	6
	Erythrocytes, rabbit	Ang II	7
	Kidney, microsomes, rat	Ang II amide	8
8-hydroxyquinoline	Plasma	Ang I	9
BAL	Plasma, rabbit	Ang I	10
Cysteine	Serum, man	Ang II amide	11
	Liver, rat	Ang II amide	12
Chlorhexidine gluconate	Plasma, rabbit	Ang I	13
ε-Amino-n-caproic acid	Plasma, man, dog	Ang II,	14
	Tissues, rat	Ang II amide	
Heavy metals	Carboxypeptidase C	Ang II amide	15
	Citrus fruit		
	Serum, rat	α-Glu-β-naphthylamide	16
	Erythrocytes, man, hog	Ang II amide	17
	Tissues, rat, hog		
	Kidney, rat	Ang II amide	18
	Serum, man	Ang II; Asp-β-naphthylamide	19
p-Chloromercaptobenzoate	Erythrocytes, man	Ang II amide	18
Bromosulphophthalein	Serum, rat	α-Glu-β-naphthylamide	5
Ang II and related peptides	Serum, rat	α-Glu-β-naphthylamide	5
	Microsomes, rat kidney	α-Glu-p-nitroanilide	5
Ang II amide	Microsomes, rat kidney	Leu-p-nitroanilide	5
	Serum, rat	Leu-β-naphthylamide	5

References: 1. Klaus et al. (1963), Hiwada (1968), Pickens et al. (1965). — 2. Kokubu et al. (1969), Matsunaga et al. (1968), Nishimura and Sokabe (1968), Yang et al. (1968, 1970a). — 3. Pickens et al. (1965), Khairallah et al. (1963), Khairallah and Page (1967), Zwanzig and Oelkers (1969). — 4. Hiwada (1968). — 5. Hess (1965). — 6. Khairallah et al. (1963), Dahlheim et al. (1969). — 7. Kokubu et al. (1969). — 8. Matsunaga et al. (1968). — 9. Haber et al. (1969). — 10. Ryan et al. (1968b). — 11. Klaus et al. (1963). — 12. Leary and Ledingham (1969). — 13. Ryan et al. (1968b), Boyd et al. (1967). — 14. Itskovitz et al. (1969), Itskovitz and Miller (1967). — 15. Zuber (1964). — 16. Kemp and Rubin (1962), Hess (1965). — 17. Itskovitz and Miller (1967), Dahlheim et al. (1969). — 18. Itskovitz and Miller (1966). — 19. Nagatsu et al. (1965a, b).

importance (Page and McCubbin, 1968). Angiotensinases occur both in the crude substrate, angiotensinogen and in the renin preparations. The angiotensinase activities in plasma can be reduced by lowering the pH below 4 (Braun-Menéndez et al., 1946) and by adding various inhibitors (Pickens et al., 1965). For example, DFP was used to inhibit angiotensinase B active at an acid pH, and EDTA was added to block angiotensinase A active above pH 7, presumably by binding a calcium cofactor. Because renin is usually assayed at an acid pH, both plasma angiotensinase B and kidney angiotensinase C, that may accompany renin during the initial stages of extraction, can interfere with the assay. DFP is an effective inhibitor of both enzymes.

The inhibition of angiotensinases is also prime importance in the immuno-assay of angiotensins. Because Ang II is not degraded at the C-terminal end by plasma enzymes, hydrolysis at the N-terminal end or in the middle of the peptide chain by angiotensinase A and B type enzymes can be similar for both Ang I and II. In addition, sequestering compounds such as EDTA inhibit the plasma converting enzyme (dipeptide hydrolase, section B IV); therefore, they block the cleavage of histidyl-leucine from Ang I and prevent the conversion of the decapeptide into the octapeptide. Added BAL, EDTA and chlorhexidine gluconate block the degradation of Ang I if given in combination (RYAN et al., 1968b; BOYD resin (BOUCHER et al., 1964) or EDTA, BAL and 8-hydroxyquinoline to protect Ang I (HABER et al., 1969).

Presence of BAL or EDTA in the perfusion fluid prevented the loss of Ang II amide in perfused rat liver and kidney (LEARY and LEDINGHAM, 1969). Table 6 lists inhibitors that inhibit the hydrolysis of substrates by angiotensinases.

VIII. Changes in Angiotensinase Activity

Since the discovery of angiotensinases, attempts have been made to correlate their activities with various clinical conditions. It was of obvious interest to link the altered metabolism of Ang II in blood and in tissues with hypertensive diseases. The data obtained by various investigators can be interpreted only very cautiously. For example, it was shown fairly recently (section C, VI) that blood must play a minor role in inactivating angiotensins, although BRAUN-MENÉNDEZ et al. had already stated in 1946 that of all the tissues studied plasma has the lowest angiotensinase levels. It is difficult to compare the results obtained in various laboratories because the methods used differed greatly. For example, some studies did not distinguish between the inactivation of the synthetic (and easily available) Ang II amide and the naturally occurring Asp^1-Ang II, although the former is cleaved much faster by an aminopeptidase. Many of the assays were based on determining the activity of the enzyme in the incubation mixture from a single sample that was withdrawn after incubation of only 10 min by some investigators, or as much as 24 hours by others. Thus the initial steady rate of the reactions was not determined in many cases. In addition, chemical assays have replaced bioassays only recently and only in some of the studies. It has been also questioned whether some of the chemical tests used for the enzyme actually reflect the inactivation of naturally occurring Ang II.

Most authors agree that there is no relationship between the angiotensinase activity in plasma or kidney and experimental renal hypertension, clinical hypertension and toxemic pregnancy (ERDÖS, 1962). Many investigators found the negative data obtained by means of various techniques fascinating enough to be continuously disclosed in publications (GOLDACKER and OELKERS, 1969; HARAKAL and COLLINS, 1956; ITSKOVITZ et al., 1967; LOYKE, 1964; BIRON et al., 1964a; BIRON, 1967; DEXTER, 1942; BLAQUIER et al., 1961; LUBASH et al., 1967; NAGATSU et al., 1965b; OSBORN et al., 1968a, b; SAPIRSTEIN et al., 1946; WERNZE et al., 1968; KLAUS, 1962).

In contrast to these reports a significant elevation of plasma angiotensinase activity was found by HICKLER et al. (1963) and by LAGRUE and MEYER (1963) in hypertension. Similarly to other aminopeptidases or carboxypeptidase N (section B XV), angiotensinase activity increases significantly towards the end of pregnancy (BERGER and LONGHANS, 1967; HICKLER et al., 1963; LUBASH et al., 1969; MANCA et al., 1967; TALLEDO, 1967). In the third trimester of pregnancy, the rate of hydrolysis of α-ANA approximately doubled and that of leucyl-β-naphthylamide was increased about two and a half times (Nagatsu et al., 1965b). Others, however, disagreed with some of these findings (Goldacker and Oelkers, 1969; Klaus, 1962; Klaus et al., 1963; Landesman et al., 1963; Vorherr et al., 1965).

The level of plasma angiotensinase was reported by numerous investigators to be increased in patients afflicted with cirrhosis of the liver and other hepatic diseases (Kokubu, 1966; Biron, 1967; Biron, 1964b; Goldacker and Oelkers, 1969; Hiwada, 1968; Klaus, 1962; Klaus et al., 1963; Lubash et al., 1968). As mentioned elsewhere, some of the activity of plasma after liver damage was attributed to the presence of an angiotensinase G (Hiwada, 1968). Although Ang II amide hydrolysis was increased in the experiments of Lubash et al. (1968) that of α-ANA was not.

Increased inactivation of Ang II amide was observed in plasma of dog during endotoxin shock (Itskovitz et al., 1969). Less α-ANA was split in blood of patients with hyperaldosteronism (Nagatsu et al., 1965b). It was also claimed that rate of inactivation of angiotensin by blood would be genetically controlled in man (Wood, 1962). This statement has not been supported by other authors.

IX. Inactivation of Angiotensin *in Vivo* by Exogenous Enzymes

Because hemolyzed red blood cells have several hundred times more angiotensinase activity than plasma, red cells were hemolyzed and reinjected i.v. to dogs (Sapirstein et al., 1946). The effect of the subsequent administrations of a crude angiotensin preparation was decreased.

A wheat bran extract was a rich source of angiotensinases (Gollan et al., 1948). Injection of this enzyme preparation to dogs i.v. blocked the vasoactivity of renin or angiotensin. Similar to the experiments where carboxypeptidase B was used against kinins in various animals (section B IX), Klaus et al. (1965) administered aminopeptidases and carboxypeptidase A to cats. After i.v. injection of carboxypeptidase A the angiotensinase activity rose 30-fold in plasma over the untreated control, and the effect of a 5 min infusion of angiotensin was significantly decreased. Similar results were obtained when a kidney microsomal aminopeptidase was given to the animals. The half-life of the injected enzyme preparations in blood stream was short, it ranged from 4—80 min. Injection of an aminopeptidase preparation, however, had no influence on the experimental renal hypertension in rats (Klaus and Daum, 1966).

D. Epilogue: The Importance of the Enzymes

Although the enzymes reviewed here hydrolyze angiotensins or plasma kinins, they can cleave susceptible bonds in other naturally occurring peptides. Wherever kallikreins or renin are found in blood and tissues, angiotensinases and kininases are also present; this may contribute to a homeostatic balance in the body. Of the commonly known active peptides, bradykinin and kallidin are inactivated fastest by plasma. This action is partially responsible for the short half-life *in vivo*, but the removal of the peptides from the circulation by various organs and the rapid inactivation during pulmonary passage are of great importance.

The kininases that have been characterized so far may have additional functions. For example, carboxypeptidase N may be involved in the metabolism of fibrino-peptides (Teger-Nilsson, 1968) or protamine (Kleine and Tille, 1969). The human anaphylatoxin inactivator is probably identical with the enzyme, thus anaphylatoxin is a readily hydrolyzed substrate of carboxypeptidase N (Bokisch and MÜLLER-EBERHARD, 1970). Kininase II may have another important activity in converting Ang I into Ang II. If a converting enzyme and kininase II (peptidase P) of plasma, lung and kidney were identical, then the same enzyme could participate in the metabolism of both hypotensive and hypertensive peptides.

Aminopeptidase A cleaves off aspartic acid from Ang II, but it hydrolyzes bonds of N-terminal dicarboxylic acids of other peptides as well (NAGATSU et al., 1970). As mentioned elsewhere in this article, angiotensinases in plasma have a minor role in the metabolism of Ang II under normal conditions; they are of greater significance in tissues. If Ang II were hydrolyzed in plasma very rapidly at the N-terminal end, obviously Ang I would not have a chance to be converted to Ang II in the lung and elsewhere before being inactivated. It has been indicated that plasma angiotensinase A can reverse the tachyphylactic effect of Ang II (KHAIRALLAH et al., 1966), but others disagree (SAMBHI and BARRETT, 1968; OSBORN et al., 1969).

Angiotensinase C (prolylcarboxypeptidase) occurs in lysosomes of kidney and leucocytes, and breaks peptide bonds of proline in the penultimate position. Because of this it may contribute to processes where the metabolism of proline containing peptides is of significance.

References

ABDUL-KARIM, R., ASSALI, N.S.: Pressor response to angiotonin in pregnant and nonpregnant women. Amer. J. Obstet. Gynec. **82**, 246—251 (1961).

ABE, K., WATANABE, N., KUMAGAI, N., MIWA, I., MOURI, K., SEKI, T., OIKAWA, A., YOSHINAGA, K.: Assay of kininase activity in human blood. Tohoku J. exp. Med. **86**, 77—83 (1965).

ABRAMS, J.S.: Blood pressure response to the portal infusion of angiotensin II. Surg. Forum **17**, 133—134 (1966).

ALLWOOD, M.J., LEWIS, G.P.: Bradykinin and forearm blood flow. J. Physiol. (Lond.) **170**, 571—581 (1964).

AMUNDSEN, E., NUSTAD, K.: Kinin-forming and destroying activities of saliva. Brit. J. Pharmacol. **23**, 440—444 (1964).

— — Kinin-forming and destroying activities of cell homogenates. J. Physiol. (Lond.) **179**, 479—488 (1965).

— RUGSTAD, H.E.: Influence of some pathogenic bacteria on kinin formation and destruction. Brit. J. Pharmacol. **25**, 67—73 (1965).

ARMAN, C.G. VAN, NUSS, G.W., WINTER, C.A., FLATAKER, L.: Proteolytic enzymes as mediators of pain. In: Pharmacology of pain, p. 25. Ed. by R.K.S. LIM, D. ARMSTRONG and E.G. PARDO. Oxford: Pergamon Press 1968.

ARMSTRONG, D., STEWART, J.W.: Spontaneous plasma kinin formation in human plasma collected during labour. Nature (Lond.) **188**, 1193 (1960).

ASCHEIM, R.S., HAMMEL, E.C., MEARLES, R.J., LUBASH, G.D.: Human serum, liver and kidney angiotensinases. Biochem. Med. **1**, 288—294 (1967).

BAKHLE, Y.S.: Conversion of angiotensin I to angiotensin II by cell-free extracts of dog lung. Nature (Lond.) **220**, 919—920 (1968).

— REYNARD, A.M., VANE, J.R.: Metabolism of the angiotensins in isolated perfused tissues. Nature (Lond.) **222**, 956—959 (1969).

BERGER, M., LANGHANS, J.: Angiotensinase activity in pregnant and nonpregnant women. Amer. J. Obstet. Gynec. **98**, 215—228 (1967).

BEUZEVILLE, C.A., LAUSON, H.D.: Hepatic clearance of angiotensin from plasma of rats and dogs. Fed. Proc. **24**, 524 (1965).

BIRON, P.: Les angiotensinase du plasma humain. Rev. Canad. Biol. **26**, 43—53 (1967).

— Pulmonary extraction of bradykinin and eledoisin. Rev. Canad. Biol. **27**, 75—76 (1968).

— BALDUS, W.P., SUMMERSKILL, W.H.J.: Plasma angiotensinase activity in cirrhosis. Proc. Soc. exp. Biol. (N.Y.) **116**, 1074—1077 (1964b).

— CAMPEAU, L., DAVID, P.: Fate of angiotensin I and II in the human pulmonary circulation. Amer. J. Cardiol. **24**, 544—547 (1969).

— LANDESMAN, R., HUNT, J.C.: Plasma angiotensinase activity in human hypertension. Nature (Lond.) **204**, 1096 (1964a).

— MEYER, P.: Hepatic extraction of angiotensin after carbon tetrachloride intoxication. Rev. Canad. Biol. **27**, 277—279 (1968).

Biron, P., Baldus, W.P., Panisset, J.-C.: Removal of angiotensins from the systemic circulation. Canad. J. Physiol. Pharmacol. **46**, 175—178 (1968).
Blaquier, P., Bohr, D.F., Taquini, A.C., Jr., Hoobler, S.W.: Renin and angiotensinase content of the kidney of normal and renal hypertensive rats. Proc. Soc. exp. Biol. (N.Y.) **108**, 711—715 (1961).
Boissonnas, R.A., Guttmann, St., Jaquenoud, P.-A.: Synthèse de la L-arginyl-L-prolyl-L-prolyl-glycyl-L-phenylalanyl-L-séryl-L-prolyl-L-phénylalanyl-L-arginine, un nonapetide présentant les proprietés de la bradykinine. Helv. chim. Acta **43**, 1349—1358 (1960a).
— — — Synthèse de la L-arginyl-L-prolyl-L-prolyl-glycyl-L-phenylalanyl-L-seryl-L-phenyl-alanyl-L-arginine. Distinction entre cet octapeptide et la bradykinine. Helv. chim. Acta **43**, 1481—1487 (1960b).
Bokisch, V.A., Müller-Eberhard, H.J.: Anaphylatoxin inactivator of human plasma: its isolation and characterization as a carboxypeptidase. J. exp. Med. (in press) (1970).
Boucher, R., Veyrat, R., Champlain, J. de, Genest, J.: New procedures for measurement of human plasma angiotensin and renin activity levels. Canad. med. Ass. J. **90**, 194—201 (1964).
Boyd, G.W., Landon, J., Peart, W.S.: Radioimmunoassay for determining plasma-levels of angiotensin II in man. Lancet **1967 II**, 1002—1005.
Braun-Menéndez, E., Fasciolo, J.C., Leloir, L.F., Muñoz, J.M.: La substancia hipertensora de la sangre del reñón isquemiado. Rev. Soc. argent. Biol. **15**, 420—425 (1939).
— — — — The substance causing renal hypertension. J. Physiol. (Lond.) **98**, 283—298 (1940).
— — — — Taquini, A.C.: Renal Hypertension. Springfield/Ill.: Charles C. Thomas 1946.
Brunner, H.: Resistenz von verschiedenen Angiotensin-II-Isomeren gegen Inaktivierung durch Plasma oder Nierenhomogenat. Arch. exp. Path. **245**, 283—284 (1963).
— Regoli, D.: Unterschiedliche Empfindlichkeit verschiedener Angiotensinderivate gegen Abbau durch Plasma oder Nierenhomogenat. Experientia (Basel) **18**, 504—505 (1962).
Bumpus, F.M., Smeby, R.R., Page, I.H., Khairallah, P.A.: Distribution and metabolic fate of angiotensin II and various derivatives. Canad. med. Ass. J. **90**, 190—193 (1964).
Camargo, A.C.M., Graeff, F.G.: Subcellular distribution and properties of the bradykinin inactivation system in rabbit brain homogenates. Biochem. Pharmacol. **18**, 548—549 (1969).
Centaro, A., Periti, P., Sicuteri, F.: Bradykininogen and bradykininase in blood of women during labour. Settim. med. **51**, Suppl. I, 70—76 (1963).
Chamberlain, M.J., Browse, N.L., Gibson, D.G., Gleeson, J.A.: Angiotensin and reno-portal anastomosis. Brit. med. J. **2**, 1507—1508 (1964).
Chesley, L.C., Talledo, E., Bohler, C.S., Zuspan, F.P.: Vascular reactivity to antiotensin II and norepinephrine in pregnant and nonpregnant women. Amer. J. Obstet. Gynec. **91**, 837—842 (1965).
Chiang, T.S., Erdös, E.G., Miwa, I., Tague, L.T., Coalson, J.J.: Isolation from a salivary gland of granules containing renin and kallikrein. Circulat. Res. **23**, 507—517 (1968).
Cohen, L.A., Gage, J.O., Kokame, G.M., Creech, O., Jr.: Hepatic inactivation of angiotensin. Bull. Tulane med. Fac. **26**, 295—298 (1967).
Croxatto, H.: La accion hipertensinasica; inactivacion de la hipertensina y de los principios presor y ocitocico de la posthipofisis en el organismo. Rev. Med. Aliment. (Santiago) **5**, 259—271 (1943).
— Cruzatt, H.: Ineffectiveness of carboxypeptidase B in inhibiting the pressor effect of incubated human plasma. Experientia (Basel) **25**, 59—60 (1969).
Croxatto, R., Croxatto, H.: Comparative study of hypertensinase and proteinase activity of blood plasma. Proc. Soc. exp. Biol. (N.Y.) **61**, 330—333 (1946).
Cushman, D.W., Cheung, H.S.: A simple substrate for assay of dog lung angiotensin converting enzyme. Fed. Proc. **28**, 799 (1969).
Dahlheim, H., Petschauer, K., Thurau, K.: Anreicherung und Charakterisierung der Erythrocytenangiotensinase. Pflügers Arch. **305**, 105—117 (1969).
Dengler, H., Reichel, G.: Untersuchungen zur intrazellulären Lokalisation der Renin- und Hypertensinase-Aktivität. Experientia (Basel) **16**, 36—40 (1960).
Deutsch, H.F., Diniz, C.R.: Some proteolytic activities of snake venoms. J. biol. Chem. **216**, 17—26 (1955).
Dexter, L.: The hypertensinase content of plasma of normal, hypertensive and nephrectomized dogs. Ann. intern. Med. **17**, 447—450 (1942).
Dodson, L.F.: The pressor response to hypertensin in pregnant rats. Brit. J. exp. Path. **38**, 635—639 (1957).
Doyle, A.E., Louis, W.J., Osborn, E.C.: Plasma angiotensinase activity on angiotensin II and analogues. Aust. J. exp. Biol. med. Sci. **45**, 41—50 (1967).
— — Jerums, G., Osborn, E.C.: Metabolism and blood levels following infusion of a radioactive analog of angiotensin. Amer. J. Physiol. **215**, 164—168 (1968).

EBENSPERGER, A., CROXATTO, H.: Inactivacion de la hipertensina, de la vasopresina y de la ocitocina por los globulos blancos. Rev. Med. Aliment. (Santiago) **6**, 243—246 (1945).
EDERY, H., LEWIS, G.P.: Inhibition of plasma kininase activity at slightly acid pH. Brit. J. Pharmacol. **19**, 299—305 (1962).
EFFKEMANN, G., WERLE, E.: Die körpereigenen uteruswirksamen und kreislaufaktiven Wirkstoffe im Schwangerenorganismus. Arch. Gynäk. **171**, 1—27 (1941).
ELLIOTT, D.F., LEWIS, G.P.: Methionyl-lysyl-bradykinin, a new kinin from ox blood. Biochem. J. **95**, 437—447 (1965).
— — HORTON, E.W.: The structure of bradykinin — a plasma kinin from ox blood. Biochem. biophys. Res. Commun. **3**, 87—91 (1960).
ENOMOTO, T., MINESHITA, S., OH-ISHI, S., SHIGEI, T.: Kininase activity of stem bromelain. Jap. J. Pharmacol. **17**, 331—332 (1967).
ERDÖS, E.G.: Enzymes that inactive active polypeptides. Biochem. Pharmacol. **8**, 112 (1961).
— Enzymes that inactivate polypeptides. In: Metabolic factors controlling duration of drug actions, pp. 159—178. Ed. by B.B. BRODIE and E.G. ERDÖS. Oxford: Pergamon Press 1962.
— Hypontensive peptides, bradykinin, kallidin and eledoisin. Advanc. Pharmacol. **4**, 1—90 (1966).
— CANO, G., YANG, H.Y.T.: Hypotensive effect of Lys[9]-bradykinin in the guinea pig. Biochem. Pharmacol. **16**, 1035—1041 (1967c).
— McMENNAMIN, M.A., WOHLER, J.R.: Presence of carboxypeptidase B in crude kallikrein (Padutin) preparations. Life Sci. **1**, 765—769 (1962).
— MIWA, I.: Effect of endotoxin shock on the plasma kallikrein-kinin system of the rabbit. Fed. Proc. **27**, 92—95 (1968).
— — GRAHAM, W.J.: Studies on the evolution of plasma kinins. Kinins of reptilian and avian blood. Life Sci. **6**, 2433—2439 (1967b).
— RENFREW, A.G., SLOANE, E.M., WOHLER, J.R.: Enzymatic studies on bradykinin and similar peptides. Ann. N.Y. Acad. Sci. **104**, 222—234 (1963b).
— SEKI, T., YANG, H.Y.T., TAGUE, L.L.: Use of insoluble polymers of enzymes in kinin metabolism. Pharmacol. Res. Commun. **1**, 152 (1969).
— SLOANE, E.M.: An enzyme in human blood plasma that inactivates bradykinin and kallidins. Biochem. Pharmacol. **11**, 585—592 (1962).
— — WOHLER, I.M.: Carboxypeptidase in blood and other fluids. I. Properties, distribution and partial purification of the enzyme. Biochem. Pharmacol. **13**, 893—905 (1964).
— WOHLER, I.M., LEVINE, M.I., WESTERMAN, M.P.: Carboxypeptidase in blood and other fluids. Values in human blood in normal and pathological conditions. Clin. chim. Acta **11**, 39—43 (1965).
— WOHLER, J.R.: Inhibitors of the *in vivo* enzymatic inactivation of bradykinin and kallidin. Life Sci. **2**, 270—274 (1963a).
— — Inhibition *in vivo* of the enzymatic inactivation of bradykinin and kallidin. Biochem. Pharmacol. **12**, 1193—1199 (1963b).
— — LEVINE, M.I.: Blocking of the *in vivo* effects of bradykinin and kallidin with carboxypeptidase B. J. Pharmacol. exp. Ther. **142**, 327—334 (1963a).
— YANG, H.Y.T.: Inactivation and potentiation of the effects of bradykinin. In: Hypotensive peptides, pp. 235—250. Ed. by E.G. ERDÖS, N. BACK and F. SICUTERI. Berlin-Heidelberg-New York: Springer 1966.
— — An enzyme in microsomal fraction of kidney that inactivates bradykinin. Life Sci. **6**, 569—574 (1967).
— — Kininases. In: Bradykinin, kallidin and kallikrein, Handbook of Experimental Pharmacology, p. 289. Ed. by E.G. ERDÖS. Berlin-Heidelberg-New York: Springer 1970.
— — MIWA, I.: Kininases. Hoppe-Seylers Z. physiol. Chem. **349**, 928 (1968).
— — TAGUE, L.L., MANNING, N.: Carboxypeptidase in blood and other fluids. III. The esterase activity of the enzyme. Biochem. Pharmacol. **16**, 1287—1297 (1967a).
FASCIOLO, J.C.: Formation and destruction of plasma kinins. Acta physiol. lat.-amer. **14**, 170—179 (1964).
— LELOIR, L.F., MUÑOZ, J.M., BRAUN-MENÉNDEZ, E.: La hipertensinasa: Su dosaje y distribución. Rev. Soc. argent. Biol. **16**, 643—649 (1940).
FERREIRA, S.H.: Bradykinin-potentiating factor. In: Hypotensive peptides, pp. 356—367. Ed. by E.G. ERDÖS, N. BACK and F. SICUTERI. Berlin-Heidelberg-New York: Springer 1966.
— VANE, J.R.: The disappearance of bradykinin and eledoisin in the circulation and vascular beds of the cat. Brit. J. Pharmacol. **30**, 417—424 (1967a).
— — The detection and estimation of bradykinin in the circulating blood. Brit. J. Pharmacol. **29**, 367—377 (1967b).
FOLK, J.E., PIEZ, K.A., CARROLL, W.R., GLADNER, J.A.: Carboxypeptidase B. IV. Purification and characterization of the porcine enzyme. J. biol. Chem. **235**, 2272—2277 (1960).

Frey, E.K., Kraut, H., Werle, E.: Kallikrein Padutin. Stuttgart: Ferdinand Enke 1950.

— — — Vogel, R., Zickgraf-Rüdel, G., Trautschold, I.: Das Kallikrein-Kinin-System und seine Inhibitoren. Stuttgart: Ferdinand Enke 1968.

Garbe, G.: Quantitative Kininogenbestimmung in menschlichem Plasma. Naunyn-Schmiedeberg's Arch. exp. Path. Pharmak. **256**, 112—118 (1967).

Glenner, G.G., McMillan, P.J., Folk, J.E.: A mammalian peptidase specific for the hydrolysis of N-terminal and α-L-glutamyl and aspartyl residues. Nature (Lond.) **194**, 867 (1962).

Goffinet, J.A., Mulrow, P.J.: Estimation of angiotensin clearance by an *in vivo* assay. Clin. Res. **11**, 408 (1963).

Goldacker, I.U. v., Oelkers, W.: Aminopeptidaseaktivität gegen Angiotensin II-Amid im Serum von Gesunden, Schwangeren, Hypertonikern und Leberkranken. Z. klin. Chem. u. klin. Biochem. **7**, 250—252 (1969).

Gollan, F., Richardson, E., Goldblatt, H.: Studies on plant hypertensinase. J. exp. Med. **87**, 29—39 (1948).

Greenbaum, L.M., Kim, K.S.: The kinin-forming and kininase activities of rabbit polymorphonuclear leucocytes. Brit. J. Pharmacol. **29**, 238—247 (1967).

— Yamafuji, K.: The *in vitro* inactivation and formation of plasma kinins by spleen cathepsins. Brit. J. Pharmacol. **27**, 230—238 (1966).

Greene, L.J., Stewart, J.M., Ferreira, S.H.: Bradykinin-potentiating peptides from the venom of *Bothrops jararaca*. Advanc. exp. Med. Biol. **8**, 81—87 (1970).

Haas, E., Goldblatt, H., Lewis, L., Gipson, E.C.: Inhibition of angiotensin and its protection by a cofactor in blood. Amer. J. Physiol. **215**, 1420—1428 (1968).

— — — — Angiotensin-protective cofactor. Amer. J. Physiol. **217**, 981—987 (1969).

Haber, E., Koerner, T., Page, L.B., Kliman, B., Purnode, A.: Application of a radioimmunoassay for angiotensin I to the physiologic measurements of plasma renin activity in normal human subjects. J. clin. Endocr. **29**, 1349—1355 (1969).

Habermann, E., Blennemann, G.: Über Substrate und Reaktionsprodukte der kininbildenden Enzyme Trypsin, Serum- und Pankreaskallikrein sowie von Crotalusgift. Arch. exp. Pathol. Pharmakol. **249**, 357—373 (1964).

Hamberg, U., Rocha e Silva, M.: Studies on the enzymatic inactivation of bradykinin. Acta physiol. scand. **30**, 215—225 (1954).

— — On the release of bradykinin by trypsin and snake venoms. Arch. int. Pharmacodyn. **110**, 222—238 (1957).

Harakal, C.D., Collins, D.A.: Plasma hypertensinase in experimental renal hypertension. Circulat. Res. **4**, 612—617 (1956).

Hess, R.: Arylamidase activity related to angiotensinase. Biochim. biophys. Acta (Amst.) **99**, 316—324 (1965).

Hickler, R.B., Lauler, D.P., Thorn, G.W.: Plasma angiotensinase activity in patients with hypertension and edema. J. clin. Invest. **42**, 635—648 (1963).

Hiwada, K.: Studies on plasma angiotensinases in liver disease. Jap. Circulat. J. **32**, 1073—1083 (1968).

— Akutsu, H., Fujimoto, S., Kokubu, T., Yamamura, Y.: Separation of plasma angiotensinases by DEAE Sephadex A-50 column chromatography. Clin. chim. Acta **14**, 410—441 (1966).

Hodge, R.L., Ng, K.K.F., Vane, J.R.: Disappearance of angiotensin from the circulation of the dog. Nature (Lond.) **215**, 138—141 (1967).

Hooper, K.C.: The enzymic inactivation of some physiologically active polypeptides by different parts of the nervous system. Biochem. J. **88**, 398—404 (1963).

Hopsu, V.K., Makinen, K.K., Glenner, G.G.: A peptidase (aminopeptidase B) from cat and guinea pig liver selective for N-terminal arginine and lysine residues. I. Purification and substrate specificity. Acta chem. scand. **20**, 1225—1230 (1966a).

— — — Formation of bradykinin from kallidin-10 by aminopeptidase B. Nature (Lond.) **212**, 1271—1272 (1966b).

Horton, E.W.: The estimation of urinary kallikrein. J. Physiol. (Lond.) **148**, 267—282 (1959).

Itskovitz, H.D., Dudrick, S.J., Dyrda, I., Murphy, J.J.: Plasma angiotensinase activity in hypertensive patients. Arch. intern. Med. **119**, 241—246 (1967).

— Miller, L.D.: Renal angiotensinase activity. Circulat. Res. **19**, 507—513 (1966).

— — Differential studies of angiotensinase activities from several tissue sources. Amer. J. med. Sci. **254**, 659—666 (1967).

— — Ural, W., Zapp, J., White, R.: Inactivation of angiotensin in shock. Amer. J. Physiol. **216**, 5—10 (1969).

Johnson, D.C., Ryan, J.W.: Degradation of angiotensin II by a carboxypeptidase of rabbit liver. Biochim. biophys. Acta (Amst.) **160**, 196—203 (1968).

Kelly, K.A., Nyhus, L.M.: Angiotensin and the liver. Amer. J. Physiol. **210**, 305—311 (1966).

KEMP, E., RUBIN, I.: Removal of angiotensinase from a preparation of renin. Arch. Biochem. Biophys. **96**, 56—59 (1962).
KHAIRALLAH, P.A., BUMPUS, F.M., PAGE, I.H., SMEBY, R.R.: Angiotensinase with a high degree of specificity in plasma and red cells. Science **140**, 672—674 (1963).
— PAGE, I.H. Plasma angiotensinases. Biochem. Med. **1**, 1—8 (1967).
— — BUMPUS, F.M., SMEBY, R.R.: Angiotensin II: Its metabolic fate. Science **138**, 523—525 (1962).
— — — TÜRKER, R.K.: Angiotensin tachyphylaxis and its reversal. Circulat. Res. **19**, 247—254 (1966).
KLAUS, D.: Untersuchungen über die Angiotensinase im Serum Gesunder und Kranker. Klin. Wschr. **40**, 701—702 (1962).
— Vergleichende Untersuchungen über die Blutdruckwirkung von α- und β-Angiotensin II bei intravenöser Infusion. Klin. Wschr. **44**, 1044—1046 (1966).
— DAUM, A.: Die Wirkung von Aminopeptidase auf den experimentellen renalen Hochdruck der Ratte. Klin. Wschr. **44**, 903—904 (1966).
— HEIZMANN, A., UEHLEKE, H.: Beeinflussung der Blutdruckwirkung von Angiotensin durch Aminopeptidasen und Carboxypeptidase. Naunyn-Schmiedeberg's Arch. exp. Path. Pharmak. **251**, 28—38 (1965).
— KAFFARNIK, H., PFEIL, H.: Untersuchungen über die Serum-Angiotensinase I, II. Klin. Wschr. **41**, 376—385 (1963).
KLEINE, R., TILLE, D.: Charakterisierung der Protamin hydrolysierenden Enzymwirkung des Rattenserums. Acta biol. med. germ. **22**, 525—535 (1969).
KOKUBU, T.: Renal hypertension and angiotensinase. Jap. J. Med. **5**, 102—104 (1966).
— AKUTSU, H., FUJIMOTO, S., UEDA, E., HIWADA, K., YAMAMURA, Y.: Purification and properties of endopeptidase from rabbit red cells and its process of degradation of angiotensin. Biochim. biophys. Acta (Amst.) **191**, 668—676 (1969).
— FUJIMOTO, S., HIWADA, K., AKUTSU, H., KATO, A., YAMAMURA, Y.: Inactivation of angiotensin II in liver. Jap. Circulat. J. **31**, 879—883 (1967a).
— HIWADA, K., UEDA, E., FUJIMOTO, S., AKUTSU, H., KATO, A., YAMAMURA, Y.: Plasma angiotensinase activity in liver disease. Biochem. Med. **1**, 54—61 (1967b).
KRIVOY, W., KROGER, D.: The preservation of bradykinin by phenothiazines *in vitro*. Brit. J. Pharmacol. **22**, 329—341 (1964).
KRONEBERG, G., STOEPEL, K.: Vergleichende Untersuchungen über die Kreislaufwirkung von Kallikrein (Padutin), Kallidin und Bradykinin. Naunyn-Schmiedeberg's Arch. exp. Path. Pharmak. **245**, 284—285 (1963).
KURTZ, A.B., WACHSMUTH, E.D.: Identification of plasma angiotensinase as aminopeptidase. Nature (Lond.) **221**, 92—93 (1969).
LAGRUE, G., MEYER, P.: Dosage biologique de l'angiotensinase plasmatique. Technique et premiers résultats. Path. et Biol. **11**, 895—897 (1963).
LANDESMAN, R., BIRON, P., CASTELLANOS, R., RUSSA, R.L., WILSON, K.H.: Plasma angiotensinase activity in normal and toxemic pregnancy. Obstet. and Gynec. **22**, 316—323 (1963).
LEARY, W.P., LEDINGHAM, J.G.: Removal of angiotensin by isolated perfused organs of the rat. Nature (Lond.) **222**, 959—960 (1969).
LEVIN, Y., PECHT, M., GOLDSTEIN, L., KATCHALSKI, E.: A water-insoluble polyanionic derivative of trypsin. I. Preparation and properties. Biochemistry **3**, 1905—1913 (1964).
LOYKE, H.F.: Experimental hypertensions treated with CCl_4: Measurements of Adrenal Function, Vascular Responsiveness, Angiotensinase and Converting Enzyme. Proc. Soc. exp. Biol. (N.Y.) **115**, 1035—1040 (1964).
LUBASH, G.D., BARD, R.H., KLINE, J.A.: Serum "angiotensinase activity" and female steroidal hormones. Amer. J. med. Sci. **257**, 155—163 (1969).
— HAMMEL, E.C., MEARLES, R.J.: Serum angiotensinase activity in hypertension. Clin. chim. Acta **18**, 439—445 (1967).
— — — Serum angiotensinase activity in cirrhosis. Amer. J. med. Sci. **255**, 105—112 (1968).
MANCA, P., MORANDINI, G., MANGIONI, C., DIMICH, D.: L'attività angiotensinasica plasmatica nel corso della gravidanza normale e del puerperio. Minerva ginec. **19**, 319—324 (1967).
MARGOLIS, J., BISHOP, E.A.: Interrelations between different mechanisms of release of biologically active peptides from blood plasma. Nature (Lond.) **194**, 749—751 (1962).
MATSUNAGA, M., KIRA, J., SAITO, N., OGINO, K., TAKAYASU, M.: Acid angiotensinase, renin, and acid adenosine triphosphatase in rat kidney lysosomes. Jap. Circulat. J. **32**, 137—143 (1968).
— SAITO, N., KIRA, J., OGINO, K., TAKAYASU, M.: Acid angiotensinase as a lysosomal enzyme. Jap. Circulat. J. **33**, 541—551 (1969).
MCCARTHY, D.A., POTTER, D.E., NICOLAIDES, E.D.: An *in vivo* estimation of the potencies and half-lives of synthetic bradykinin and kallidin. J. Pharmacol. exp. Ther. **148**, 117—122 (1965).

McDonald, J.K., Zeitman, B.B., Reilly, T.J., Ellis, S.: New observations on the substrate specificity of cathepsin C (dipeptidyl aminopeptidase I). J. biol. Chem. **244**, 2693—2709 (1969).

— Callahan, P.X., Ellis, S.: Polypeptide degradation by dipeptidyl aminopeptidase I (cathepsin C) and related peptidases. In: Tissue Proteinases: Enzymology and Biology. Ed. by A.J. Barrett, J.T. Dingle, Amsterdam: North-Holland Publishing Co. (in press).

Melmon, K.L., Cline, M.J.: Interaction of plasma kinins and granulocytes. Nature (Lond.) **217**, 90—92 (1967).

— — The interaction of leukocytes and the kinin system. Biochem. Pharmacol. **17**, Suppl., p. 271—281 (1968).

— — Hughes, T., Nies, A.S.: Kinins: possible mediators of neonatal circulatory changes in man. J. clin. Invest. **47**, 1295—1302 (1968).

Methot, A.L., Meyer, P., Biron, P., Lorain, M.F., Lagrue, G., Milliez, P.: Hepatic inactivation of angiotensin. Nature (Lond.) **203**, 531—532 (1964).

Mitchell, W.M.: Hydrolysis at arginylproline in polypeptides by clostridiopeptidase B. Science **162**, 374—375 (1968).

Miwa, I., Erdös, E.G., Seki, T.: Separation of peptide components of urinary kinin (Substance Z). Proc. Soc. exp. Biol. (N.Y.) **131**, 768—772 (1969).

Morris, R.E.: In discussion. Canad. med. Ass. J. **90**, 194 (1964).

Myers, M.G., Robinson, P.R., Morris, R.E.: Relationships of angiotensinase and angiotensin II. Clin. Res. **13**, 215 (1965).

Nagatsu, I., Gillespie, L., Folk, J.E., Glenner, G.G.: Serum aminopeptidases, "angiotensinase", and hypertension. I. Degradation of angiotensin II by human serum. Biochem. Pharmacol. **14**, 721—728 (1965a).

— — George, J.M., Folk, J.E., Glenner, G.G.: Serum aminopeptidases, "angiotensinase", and hypertension. II. Amino acid β-naphthylamide hydrolysis by normal and hypertensive serum. Biochem. Pharmacol. **14**, 853—861 (1965b).

— Nagatsu, T., Yamamoto, T., Glenner, G.G., Mehl, J.W.: Purification of aminopeptidase A in human serum and degradation of angiotensin II by the purified enzyme. Biochim. biophys. Acta (Amst.) **198**, 255—270 (1970).

Nicolaides, E.D., Dewald, H.A., Craft, M.K.: The synthesis of kinin analogues. Ann. N.Y. Acad. Sci. **104**, 15—22 (1963).

Nishimura, H., Sokabe, H.: Inhibition of angiotensinases in the rat plasma and kidney. Jap. Heart J. **9**, 494—503 (1968).

Nugent, F.W., Atendido, W.A., Bulan, M.B., MacDonald, A.J.: Kininase activity in experimental pancreatitis. Nature (Lond.) **211**, 207—208 (1966).

Oelkers, W., Goldacker, I.U. v.: Bestimmung der Angiotensinase(Aminopeptidase-)-Aktivität im Serum mit einem DPN-abhängigen optischen Test. Klin. Wschr. **45**, 649—653 (1967).

Ono, T., Eto, K., Arakawa, K.: Origin of urinary enzymes hydrolysing β-naphthylamides of L-leucine and L-glutamic acid. Clin. chim. Acta **19**, 257—265 (1968).

Osborn, E.C., Hughes, S.G., Pirie, A.T., Willicombe, P.R., Mahler, R.F.: Clearance studies of angiotensin II and (^{35}S) phenylthiocarbamyl-angiotensin II in the sheep and dog. Cardiovasc. Res. **3**, 134—146 (1969).

— Jerums, G., Jupp, B.A.: Plasma angiotensinase activity in relation to the breakdown of phenylthiocarbamyl-angiotensin II amide in hypertensive and normotensive patients. Cardiovasc. Res. **2**, 31—32 (1968a).

— — — Blood angiotensinase activity in relation to the breakdown of angiotensin II amide and nonisotopic phenylthiocarbamyl-angiotensin II amide in hypertensive and normotensive patients. Cardiovasc. Res. **2**, 33—38 (1968b).

Osborne, M.J., d'Auriac, G.A., Meyer, P., Worcel, M.: Mechanism of Extraction of Angiotensin II in coronary and renal circulations. Life Sci. **9**, 859—867 (1970).

Page, I.H., Helmer, O.M.: A crystalline pressor substance (angiotonin) resulting from the reaction between renin and renin-activator. J. exp. Med. **71**, 29—42 (1940).

— — Kohlstaedt, K.G., Kempf, G.F., Corcoran, A.C., Taylor, R.D.: A progress report on investigations concerned with the experimental treatment of hypertension with kidney extracts. Ann. intern. Med. **18**, 29—42 (1943).

— McCubbin, J.W., editors: Renal Hypertension. Chicago: Year Book Medical Publishers, Inc. 1968.

Paskhina, T.S., Trapeznikova, S.S.: Cleavage of depsipeptide analogs of bradykinin by kininase (carboxypeptidase N) from human and rabbit serum. Biokhimiya **32**, 527 (1967).

Phelps, P., Prockhop, D.J., McCarty, D.J.: Crystal induced inflammation in canine joints. III. Evidence against bradykinin as a mediator of inflammation. J. Lab. clin. Med. **68**, 433—444 (1966).

PICKENS, P.T., BUMPUS, F.M., LLOYD, A.M., SMEBY, R.R., PAGE, I.H.: Measurement of renin activity in human plasma. Circulat. Res. **17**, 438—448 (1965).

PRADO, J.L.: Proteolytic enzymes as kininogenases. In: "Bradykinin, kallidin and kallikrein", Handbook of Experimental Pharmacology, p. 156. Ed. by E.G. ERDÖS. Berlin-Heidelberg-New York: Springer 1970.

REGOLI, D., RINIKER, B., BRUNNER, H.: The enzymatic degradation of various angiotensin II derivatives by serum, plasma or kidney homogenate. Biochem. Pharmacol. **12**, 637—646 (1963).

RINIKER, B.: Recent work on the chemistry and biochemistry of angiotensin II. Metabolism **13**, 283—291 (1964).

— SCHWYZER, R.: Die sterische Einheitlichkeit des synthetischen Val^5-Hypertensin II-Asp^1-β-amids. Helv. chim. Acta **44**, 658—667 (1961).

— — Synthetische Analoge des Hypertensins. V. α-L-, β-L-, α-D- und β-D-Asp^1-Val^5-Hypertensin II; Desamino-Val^5-Hypertensin II. Helv. chim. Acta **47**, 2357—2374 (1964).

ROCHA E SILVA, M.: Bradykinin — mechanism of its release by trypsin and kallikrein. Arch. int. Pharmacodyn. **88**, 271—282 (1951).

— The physiological significance of bradykinin. Ann. N.Y. Acad. Sci. **104**, 190—210 (1963).

— BERALDO, W.T., ROSENFELD, G.: Bradykinin, a hypotensive and smooth muscle stimulating factor released from plasma globulin by snake venoms and by trypsin. Amer. J. Physiol. **156**, 261—273 (1949).

RUGSTAD, H.E.: Kininase production by some microbes. Brit. J. Pharmacol. **28**, 315—323 (1966).

— Purification of a kinin-inactivating enzyme from cultures of *Pseudomonas aeruginosa*. Brit. J. Pharmacol. **30**, 134—142 (1967a).

— Characterization of a plasma kinin-inactivating enzyme produced by *Pseudomonas aeruginosa*. Brit. J. Pharmacol. **30**, 425—435 (1967b).

— Degradation of plasma kinins by an enzyme from *Pseudomonas aeruginosa*. Brit. J. Pharmacol. **31**, 401—406 (1967c).

RYAN, J.W., ROBLERO, J., STEWART, J.M.: Inactivation of bradykinin in the pulmonary circulation. Biochem. J. **110**, 795—797 (1968a).

— MCKENZIE, J.K., LEE, M.R.: A rapid simple method for the assay of renin in rabbit plasma. Biochem. J. **108**, 679—685 (1968b).

SAAMELI, K., ESKES, T.K.A.B.: Bradykinin and cardiovascular system: estimation of half-life. Amer. J. Physiol. **203**, 261—265 (1962).

SAITO, N., SANADA, K., MATSUNAGA, M., KIRA, J., MUKAINO, S., OGINO, K., TAKAYASU, M.: Amino acid analysis after degradation of angiotensin II by rat kidney lysosomes. Jap. Circulat. J. **33**, 87—93 (1969).

SAMBHI, M.P., BARRETT, J.D.: Angiotensinase activity in fractionated human plasma and effect of enzyme inhibitors. Clin. Res. **14**, 149 (1966).

— — Plasma "angiotensinase" activity as a determinant of angiotensin pressor action and tachyphylaxis in the rat. Biochem. Pharmacol. **17**, 787—795 (1968).

SAPIRSTEIN, L.A., REED, R.K., PAGE, E.W.: The site of angiotonin destruction. J. exp. Med. **83**, 425—439 (1946).

SCHACHTER, M.: Some properties of kallidin, bradykinin and wasp venom kinin. In: Polypeptides which affect smooth muscles and blood vessels, pp. 232—246. Ed. by M. SCHACHTER. Oxford 1960.

SCHRÖDER, E.: Über Peptidsynthesen. Synthese von Methionyl-Lysyl-Bradykinin, einem Kinin aus Rinderblut. Experientia (Basel) **20**, 39 (1964).

— LÜBKE, K.: The Peptides. Vol. II. New York: Academic Press 1966.

SCHWAB, J.: Kininases in leucocytes and other tissues. Nature (Lond.) **195**, 345—347 (1962).

SEKI, I., JENSSEN, T.A., LEVIN, Y., ERDÖS, E.G.: Active water-insoluble derivative of renin. Nature (Lond.) **225**, 864—865 (1970b).

— YANG, H.Y.T., LEVIN, Y., JENSSEN, T.A., ERDÖS, E.G.: Application of water-insoluble complexes of kininogenases, inhibitors and kininases to kinin research. Advanc. exp. Med. Biol. (in press) (1970a).

SHIMONAEVA, E.E.: Some properties of carboxypeptidase N from rabbit blood serum. Vop. med. Khim **13**, 105—107 (1967).

SICUTERI, F., FANCIULLACCI, M., DEL BIANCO, P.L., ANSELMI, B.: Bradichininasi nel liquido cefalo-rachidiano dell-uomo. Boll. Soc. ital. Biol. sper. **41**, 464—466 (1965).

— PERITI, P., ANSELMI, B., FANCIULLACCI, M.: Livelli plasmachininici dell'uomo dopo somministrazione endovenosa ed endoarteria di bradichinina sintetica e naturale. Boll. Soc. ital. Biol. sper. **39**, 314—318 (1963).

SKEGGS, L.T., LENTZ, K.E., KAHN, J.R., DORER, F.E., LEVINE, M.: Pseudorenin; a new angiotensin-forming enzyme. Circulat. Res. **25**, 451—462 (1969).

Stewart, J. M.: Synthesis and pharmacology of polistes kinin, a bradykinin homolog. Fed. Proc. **27**, 534 (1968).
— Roblero, J.: Studies on the pulmonary inactivation of bradykinin. In: Symposium on Vasoactive Polypeptides and Inhibitors of Proteolytic Enzymes, pp. 52—55. Tokyo 1967.
Suzuki, T., Iwanaga, S.: Snake venoms. In: Bradykinin, kallidin and kallikrein, Handbook of Experimental Pharmacology, p. 193. Ed. by E. G. Erdös. Berlin-Heidelberg-New York: Springer 1970.
— — Nagasawa, S., Sato, T.: Purification and properties of bradykininogen and of the bradykinin-releasing and -destroying enzymes in snake venom. In: Hypotensive peptides, pp. 149—160. Ed. by E. G. Erdös, N. Back and F. Sicuteri. Berlin-Heidelberg-New York: Springer 1966.
Talledo, O.: Renin-angiotensin system in normal and toxemic pregnancies. II. Inactivation of angiotensin in normal pregnancy. Amer. J. Obstet. Gynec. **97**, 571—572 (1967).
Teger-Nilsson, A.-C.: Degradation of human fibrinopeptides A and B in blood serum *in vitro*. Acta chem. scand. **22**, 3171—3182 (1968).
Trapeznikova, S. S., Paskhina, T. S.: The isolation, purification and properties of carboxypeptidases (kininases) from human and rabbit blood serum. Biokhimiya **33**, 1012—1022 (1968).
Trautschold, I.: Enzyme und Inhibitoren der Bildung und des Abbaues gefäßaktiver Polypeptide (Kinine). Habil.-Schrift Munich 1965.
Urbanitz, D., Wiegand, H., Habermann, E.: Zur Frage der Bedeutung des Kininsystems beim thermischen Odem der Rattenpfote. Naunyn-Schmiedeberg's Arch. **264**, 476—493 (1969).
Vane, J. R.: The release and rate of vasoactive hormones in the circulation. Brit. J. Pharmacol. **35**, 209—242 (1969).
Vorherr, H., Dimitrow, A., Hüter, J.: Biologische Untersuchungen über den Abbau von Hypertensin durch Blutplasma von nichtschwangeren und schwangeren Frauen. Klin. Wschr. **43**, 614—617 (1965).
Watanabe, N.: Kininase activity in human blood in normal and pathological conditions. Tohoku J. exp. Med. **92**, 63—72 (1967).
— Abe, K., Kumagai, N., Mouri, T., Seki, T., Yoshinaga, K.: Kininase activity in human blood. Tohoku J. exp. Med. **89**, 383—386 (1966).
Webster, M. E.: Report of the committee on nomenclature for hypotensive peptides. In: Hypotensive Peptides, pp. 648—653. Ed. by E. G. Erdös, N. Back and F. Sicuteri. Berlin-Heidelberg-New York: Springer 1966.
— Pierce, J. V.: The nature of the kallidins released from human plasma by kallikreins and other enzymes. Ann. N.Y. Acad. Sci. **104**, 91—105 (1963).
— Skinner, N. S., Jr., Powell, W. J., Jr.: Role of the kinins in vasodilatation of skeletal muscle of the dog. Amer. J. Physiol. **212**, 553—558 (1967).
Werle, E.: Über Kallidin und Bradykinin. Arch. int. Pharmacodyn. **92**, 427—431 (1953).
— Kallikrein, kallidin and related substances. In: Polypeptides which affect smooth muscles and blood vessels, pp. 199—209. Ed. by M. Schachter. Oxford 1960.
— Berek, U.: Über Kallidin. Biochem. Z. **320**, 136—145 (1950).
— Götze, W., Keppler, A.: Über die Wirkung des Kallikreins auf den isolierten Darm und über eine neue darmkontrahierende Substanz. Biochem. Z. **289**, 217—233 (1937).
— Grunz, M.: Zur Kenntnis der darmkontrahierenden, uteruserregenden und blutdrucksenkenden Substanz Dk. Biochem. Z. **301**, 429—436 (1939).
— Kehl, R., Koebke, K.: Über Trypsin, Chymotrypsin, Kallidin und Bradykinin. Biochem. Z. **321**, 213—220 (1950).
— Vogel, R., Göldel, L. F.: Über ein blutdrucksteigerndes Prinzip in Extrakten aus der Glandula submaxillaries der weißen Maus. Arch. exp. Path. Pharmakol. **230**, 236—244 (1957).
Wernze, H., Fujii, J.: Hepatische Inaktivierung und pressorische Wirkung von Angiotensin. Z. ges. exp. Med. **140**, 128—135 (1966).
— Hosoda, S., Schölkens, B.: Zur vasopressorischen Wirkung und Inaktivierung von Angiotensin bei essentieller und renaler sowie experimenteller Hypertonie. Arch. Klin. Med. **214**, 286—305 (1968).
Wolf, R. L., Mendlowitz, M., Gitlow, S. E., Naftchi, N.: The metabolism of angiotensin II. Circulat. Res. **11**, 195—208 (1962).
Wood, J. E.: Genetic control of neutralization of angiotensin and its relationship to essential hypertension. Circulation **25**, 225—230 (1962).
Yamafuji, K., Carrara, M. C.: Studies on the kininase activity of rabbit polymorphonuclear leucocytes. Fed. Proc. **27**, 533 (1968).
Yang, H. Y. T., Erdös, E. G.: Second kininase in human blood plasma. Nature (Lond.) **215**, 1402—1403 (1967).

YANG, H.Y.T., ERDÖS, E.G.: Angiotensinase C, characterization and chemical assay. Fourth International Congress on Pharmacology Abstracts, p. 217. Basel 1969a.
— — Fluorometric assay of angiotensinase C activity. Pharmacologist **11**, 217 (1969b).
— — LEVIN, Y.: A dipeptidyl carboxypeptidase that converts angiotensin I and inactivates bradykinin. Biochim. biophys. Acta (Amst.) **214**, 374—376 (1970d).
— — — Characterization of a dipeptide hydrolase. (Kininase II; Angiotensin I converting enzyme). J. Pharmacol. exp. Ther. (in press) (1970e).
— — CHIANG, T.S.: New enzymatic route for the inactivation of angiotensin. Nature (Lond.) **218**, 1224—1226 (1968).
— — JENSSEN, T.A., RODGERS, J.G.: Characteristics of an enzyme that inactivates angiotensin II (angiotensinase C). Biochem. Pharmacol. **19**, 1201 (1970a).
— — — LEVIN, Y.: Characterization of an angiotensin I converting enzyme. Fed. Proc. (in press) (1970c).
— JENSSEN, T.A., ERDÖS, E.G.: Conversion of angiotensin I by a kininase preparation. Clin. Res. **18**, 88 (1970b).
YMAN, L., KULLING, B.: An aminopeptidase from human serum specific for hydrolysis of α-L-dicarboxylic amino acid residues. I. Purification from retroplacental serum by preparative polyacrylamide-gel electrophoresis. Acta Pharm. Suecica **6**, 561—568 (1969).
— — BARTH, T.: An aminopeptidase from human serum specific for hydrolysis of α-L-dicarboxylic amino acid residues. II. Some properties and its relationship to the serum angiotensinase activity. Acta Pharm. Suecica **6**, 569—578 (1969).
ZACHARIAE, H., MALMQUIST, J., OATES, J.A.: Kininase in human polymorphonuclear leukocytes. Life Sci. **5**, 2347—2355 (1966).
ZUBER, H.: Purification and properties of a new carboxypeptidase from citrus fruit. Nature (Lond.) **201**, 613 (1964).
— Observations on the use of enzymes in the analysis of peptides. In: Peptides, p. 189. Ed. by L. ZERVAS. Oxford: Pergamon Press 1966.
— JAQUES, R.: Isolierung von Bradykinin aus Rinderplasma nach Einwirkung von Schlangengift (*Bothrops jararaca*). Helv. chim. Acta **43**, 1128—1130 (1960).
ZWANZIG, M., OELKERS, W.: Untersuchungen über die pH-Abhängigkeit, die Hemmbarkeit und Reaktivierbarkeit von Angiotensin II und Angiotensin II-Amid spaltenden Enzymen des menschlichen Plasmas. Z. klin. Chem. u. klin Biochem. **7**, 253—258 (1969).

Chapter 58

The Metabolism of Analogs of Endogenous Substrates: Wider Application of a Limited Concept[1]

H. GEORGE MANDEL

With 15 Figures

A. Introduction

Substrate analogs may be defined as compounds which bear a close chemical and/or physical resemblance to a constituent of normal tissue and which may replace the latter in one or more of its normal reactions, usually leading to a metabolic block. The substrate analogs, or antimetabolites, usually compete with the natural substrate at the same site on an enzyme. Actually, only a portion of the antimetabolite molecule must be analogous for competition.

Probably the simplest type of substrate analog is represented by an isotopic form of the substrate. This approach has become most useful in our current research in biochemistry and pharmacology since it is generally assumed that the labeled molecule serves as a marker for the normal compound. Because of the physical similarity (and, in this case, chemical identity) of the two compounds, their biological reactivities are usually identical; certain differences in reaction rates have been observed, however, especially as the relative deviation in isotopic weight becomes more pronounced (ELISON et al., 1961).

In general, antimetabolites differ from normal metabolites by small structural substitutions which are isosteric, as, for example, —F for —H; —Cl, —Br or —I for $—CH_3$; —S—, —O— or —NH— for $—CH_2—$; —Se— for —S—; $—CH_3$ for —H; =N— for =CH— in a ring, etc. Numerous other replacements are possible if the functional groups are of similar size and bear corresponding electronic configurations. Whether such a structural analog acts as an antimetabolite requires investigation in individual biological systems.

It is an oversimplification to assume that the metabolism of substrate analogs is unrelated to that of "conventional" drugs, such as aminopyrine, zoxazolamine, hexobarbital, acetophenetidin, codeine, etc. Very frequently, however, investigators interested in following the physiological disposition of metabolite analogs

Abbreviations used in this chapter:

DOPA = Dihydroxyphenylalanine; FU = Fluorouracil; FUdR = Deoxyfluorouridine; FUdRP = Deoxyfluorouridine phosphate (deoxyfluorouridylic acid); FUR = Fluorouridine; FURP = Fluorouridine phosphate (fluorouridylic acid); MMP = S-methylmercaptopurine; MMPR = S-methylmercaptopurine riboside; MP = Mercaptopurine; PRPP = Phosphoribosylpyrophosphate; TG = Thioguanine; U = Uracil.

1 The preparation of this review was supported by USPHS research grants CA 02978 from the National Cancer Institute, and GM-13749 from the National Institute of General Medical Sciences, NIH, Bethesda, Md.

will examine such drugs mainly for their biochemical actions and therapeutic applications, whereas others involved in studying drug metabolism will concentrate on chemical compounds which are known to be the best substrates for enzymes located in select tissues or subcellular components, such as liver microsomes. As a result, there is little information on the similarities and differences in the physiological disposition of substrate analogs and other drugs.

It is now apparent that substrate analogs may follow the metabolic pathway of the corresponding normal substrates, both along biosynthetic and degradative pathways. Although many antineoplastic agents may be substrate analogs, other anticancer drugs are handled by more general schemes of biotransformation. For instance, the alkylating agent, cyclophosphamide, is converted to the active carcinostatic product by enzymes located in the liver microsomes. Although the exact chemical alterations are unclear, they are believed to involve dealkylation, a mixed function oxidase, NADPH and oxygen. SKF 525A, an inhibitor of drug metabolism, decreases the conversion of cyclophosphamide to the active metabolite, whereas phenobarbital or chlordane pretreatment, because of enzyme induction, increases the activation reaction and enhances toxicity (reviewed by Brock and Hohorst, 1967). Another antineoplastic agent, the 3,3-dimethyl-1-triazino derivative of 4-amino-5-imidazolecarboxamide, is metabolized by rat liver microsomes to yield the N-demethylated catabolite plus formaldehyde. Pretreatment with phenobarbital apparently induces this N-demethylation and increases drug degradation (Skibba et al., 1970). In other words, biotransformation along pathways of normal substrates does not apply to the general category of carcinostatic drugs.

It is the purpose of this chapter to describe the metabolism of a few typical substrate analogs and to indicate some of the pharmacological and therapeutic significance resulting from these biochemical conversions. We shall then discuss the metabolism of other drugs not normally classified as antimetabolites which apparently behave as substrate analogs and which use pathways for normal substrates. Lastly, we will examine routes of metabolism reported for substrate analogs which make use of the more conventional routes of drug biotransformation, many of which are mediated by liver microsomes.

In this review special emphasis will not be given to absorption, distribution or excretion of drugs, although a great deal of data is now available on this subject (Mandel, 1959; Oliverio and Zubrod, 1965; Stock, 1966). Some aspects of the role of physiological disposition in the use of agents in therapy have been described previously (Henderson and Mandel, 1963). No attempt is being made to provide a complete account of metabolic alterations, but rather it is hoped to present a characteristic perspective of the metabolism of these drugs.

B. Metabolism of Purine and Pyrimidine Analogs by Pathways of Normal Substrates

I. General Background

Although the actions of numerous structural analogs of vitamins had been recognized by the late 1940's (reviewed by Woolley, 1952), relatively little information on the metabolism of antimetabolites was available at that time. Hitchings et al. had suggested in 1945 that certain analogs might be alternatives to normal substrates in anabolic reactions. One of the first examples is the phosphorylation of deoxypyridoxine (Umbreit and Waddell, 1949) which then combines irreversibly with the corresponding apoenzyme for pyridoxal phosphate to form an inactive compound. The now classical demonstration of PETERS (1952) regarding the "lethal synthesis" of fluoroacetate to fluorocitrate via the tricarboxylic acid cycle, represents another early example in which an antimetabolite uses normal pathways of intermediary metabolism. In this case, the product, fluorocitrate, is the active inhibitor of aconitase.

When the metabolism of tumor-inhibitory purine and pyrimidine analogs was examined, it was observed that 8-azaguanine was deaminated to azaxanthine by the same enzyme which normally degraded guanine (Fig. 1) (ROUSH and NORRIS,

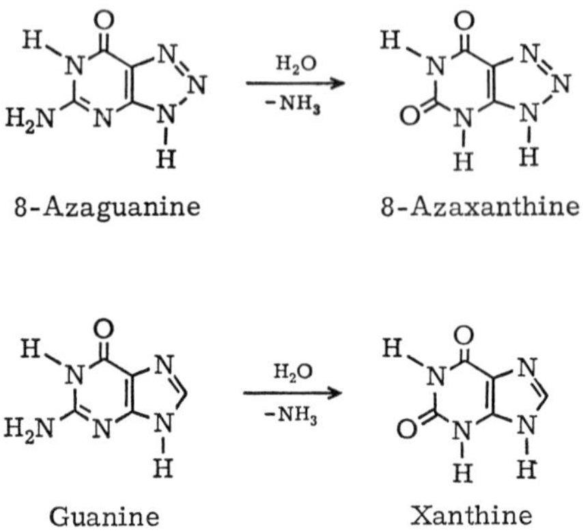

Fig. 1. Parallelism in deamination of 8-azaguanine and guanine to corresponding xanthine derivative, mediated by guanine deaminase

1950). The same conversion *in vivo*, in various animals, including the monkey (MANDEL et al., 1951), revealed the lack of specificity of certain normal biochemical reactions. As might be anticipated, tumor growth inhibition varied inversely with guanine deaminase activity of the tumor since the metabolite, azaxanthine, possessed no carcinostatic activity (HIRSCHBERG et al., 1952). 8-Azaguanine was later shown to make use of the sequence of enzymatic reactions normally used by

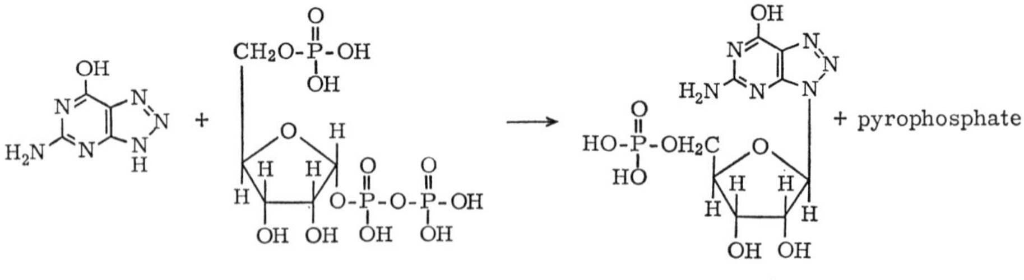

Fig. 2. Conversion of 8-azaguanine to its ribonucleotide. Guanine undergoes the same anabolic reaction

guanine in its anabolism and incorporation into polynucleotides. Some of these reactions of the analog could be demonstrated *in vitro* (WAY and PARKS, 1958) (Fig. 2). The formation of RNA containing 8-azaguanine in several species was conclusively demonstrated by LASNITZKI et al. (1954) who isolated analog-containing nucleotides from this RNA. The utilization of another base analog, 5-bromouracil, for nucleic acid synthesis had already been suggested by WEYGAND et al. (1952).

The metabolism of substrate analogs into more inhibitory products has been the subject of several reviews. MARKHAM (1958) has briefly discussed the actions of antimetabolites in lethal synthesis, and MATTHEWS (1958) has described the utilization of base and amino acid analogs for incorporation into nucleic acids and proteins, respectively; MANDEL (1959) has summarized the degradative and biosynthetic reactions of antimetabolites of interest in cancer chemotherapy. Several other reviews dealing with the biochemical actions and metabolism of these drugs have appeared in the last few years (BROCKMAN and ANDERSON, 1963; ELION and HITCHINGS, 1965; BALIS, 1968; LANGEN, 1968; MANDEL, 1969).

II. Metabolism of a Pyrimidine Analog: 5-Fluorouracil

1. The Pathways of Metabolism

5-Fluorouracil (FU) has been selected for discussion because its metabolism has been studied in great detail. The drug, an analog of uracil (U), is of considerable interest due to its carcinostatic action, and has aided the elucidation of numerous biochemical reaction mechanisms. It was synthesized by HEIDELBERGER and colleagues (1957) since the preferential utilization of U by tumor cells had been reported. Although extensive clinical evaluation has revealed that the antitumor action is not extremely selective, the drug is used clinically in the treatment of a variety of solid tumors (reviewed by HEIDELBERGER, 1965).

The metabolism of 5-fluorouracil is characteristic of a substrate analog using the enzymatic pathways available for uracil (ELION and HITCHINGS, 1965). There is also a resemblance in the mechanism of cell penetration for the two compounds. FU and U have been stated to be absorbed from the intestine of the rat by the same active mediated process, and competition for transport has been demonstrated (SCHANKER and JEFFREY, 1961). In the normal human leukocyte (KESSEL and HALL, 1967) and in Ehrlich ascites cells (JACQUEZ, 1962), however, no active transport mechanism for FU was observed. Like U, FU is subject to the catabolic actions of dihydropyrimidine dehydrogenase to form dihydroFU. This metabolite is further degraded into α-fluoro-β-ureidopropionate, which in turn is excreted as α-fluoro-β-alanine, urea, CO_2 and ammonia (MUKHERJEE and HEIDELBERGER, 1960; CHAUDHURI et al., 1959) (Fig. 3).

FU is also metabolized to compounds of greater complexity after its administration to animals and man. Early attempts to fractionate these products revealed a large number of labeled compounds derived from ^{14}C-FU (Fig. 4) which upon analysis were found to be identical with products obtained *in vitro* (CHAUDHURI et al., 1958). For example, in the presence of uridine phosphorylase, FU reacts with ribose-1-phosphate to yield fluorouridine (FUR). This compound serves as a substrate for uridine kinase, and in the presence of ATP forms fluorouridine phosphate (FURP) (SKÖLD, 1958). This product can also be synthesized *in vitro* from FU in the presence of uridylate pyrophosphorylase (uracil phosphoribosyltransferase) (REYES, 1969). Appropriate kinases then convert the monophosphate derivative to the di- and triphosphates (reviewed by HEIDELBERGER, 1965). The latter compound is a substrate for RNA polymerase, and thus FU is incorporated into RNA (FU-RNA) where it replaces uracil (KAHAN and HURWITZ, 1962). The analog has been reported to be present in ribosomal, transfer and messenger RNA's (reviewed by MANDEL, 1969).

Similarly, with uridine phosphorylase and a source of deoxyribose, such as thymidine, FU is converted to deoxyfluorouridine, FUdR, which is phosphorylated by thymidine kinase and ATP (COHEN et al., 1958). The product, FUdRP,

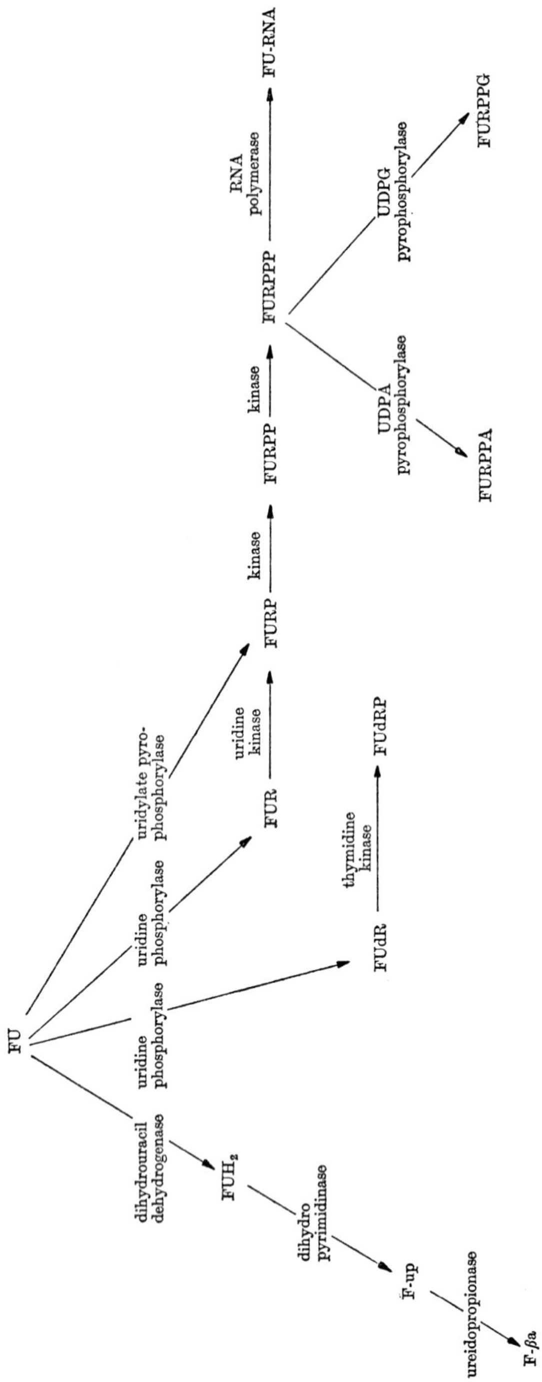

Fig. 3. Pathways of metabolism of 5-fluorouracil (FU); catabolism toward left, anabolism toward right. Symbols: up, ureidopropionate; βa, β-alanine; R, ribose; dR, deoxyribose; P, phosphate; G, glucose; A, acetylglucosamine

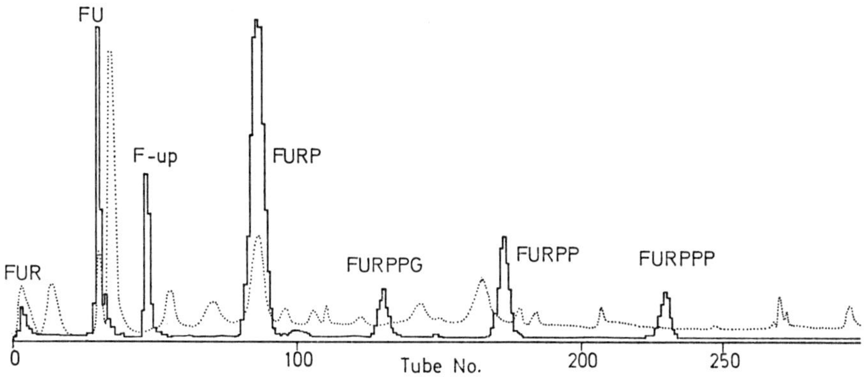

Fig. 4. Characteristic resolution of acid-soluble pools from Ehrlich ascites cells following administration of labeled 5-fluorouracil. The solid line denotes radioactivity, the dashed line represents ultraviolet absorption at 260 mμ. Symbols as in Fig. 3. From CHAUDHURI et al. (1958)

cannot be converted to a thymidylic acid analog because the F atom occupies the position normally methylated. The deoxyribose derivatives are also synthesized by reduction of FUR conjugates, probably at the diphosphate stage (HEIDELBERGER, 1965).

Various other metabolites of FU also are formed *in vivo*, as, for example, fluorouridine diphosphoglucose (FURPPG), fluorouridine diphospho-N-acetylglucosamine (FURPPA), fluorouridine diphospho-muramyl-pentapeptide, and related cofactor analogs (ROGERS and PERKINS, 1960; BROCKMAN et al., 1960). Some of these reaction sequences are shown in Fig. 3.

It is apparent from this scheme of metabolism that FU mimics U in its routes of anabolism. Even though quantitative differences in various reaction rates exist, some qualitative dissimilarities are also noted. In addition to the inability to form the thymidine analog, and thus to be incorporated into DNA, FU is not significantly converted to fluorocytosine and derivatives, whereas uracil readily undergoes such reactions (HEIDELBERGER, 1965).

2. General Interrelationship of Action and Metabolism of FU

Malignant tissue has been reported to possess more limited capacity for FU catabolism, compared to many normal tissues, and therefore relatively more drug is available for anabolic reactions which lead to the active forms of the base analog. In comparing the response to FU by a series of tumors, a correlation exists between formation of FU anabolites and sensitivity to FU, as shown in Fig. 5, although there are some exceptions. Normal tissues with a relatively rapid rate of mitosis, such as the bone marrow and intestine, also anabolize FU, and thus exhibit drug toxicity (MUKHERJEE and HEIDELBERGER, 1960).

Usually when sensitive cell populations are compared with mutants which are drug-resistant, the resistant cell lines have been shown to have lost specific enzyme(s) which mediate the conversion of FU to the pharmacologically active anabolites. Deletion of uridine phosphorylase, for example, prevents the formation of FUR, FUdR and further anabolites, and undoubtedly accounts for the resistance of certain tissues to FU (REICHARD and SKÖLD, 1959). In certain of these cases of acquired insensitivity to FU it has been possible to demonstrate sensitivity to FUR (HEIDELBERGER et al., 1958; HALL et al., 1968). Other enzymes which have been

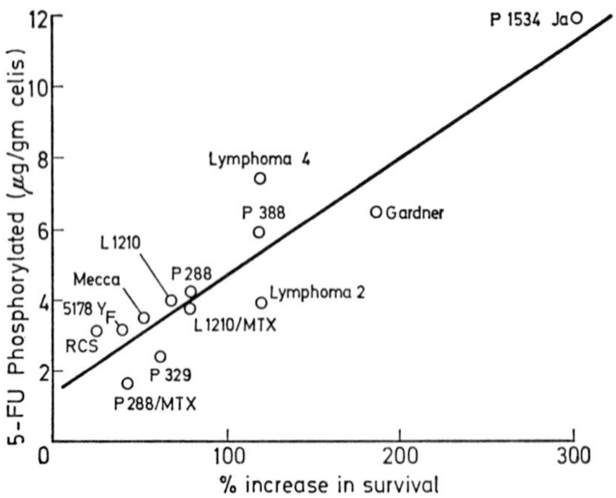

Fig. 5. Correlation between 5-fluorouracil metabolism *in vitro* and drug-promoted survival of tumor-bearing animals. Metabolism was determined by measurement of drug conversion to ribotides plus incorporation into RNA. Each circle represents cells from the tumor strain indicated. From KESSEL et al. (1966)

found to have reduced activity in resistant cells are uridine kinase and uridylate pyrophosphorylase. Treatment with FURP has been unsuccessful, however, because of the failure of nucleotides to enter cells. An alteration in affinity of thymidylate synthetase to FUdRP has also been reported (see HEIDELBERGER, 1965).

3. Actions of Specific Metabolites of FU

FUdRP. The formation of the deoxyribose derivatives of FU, especially in mammalian cells, has important pharmacological consequences. *In vivo,* FUdR is far more potent than FU or FUR in inhibiting the methylation of deoxyuridylate (Fig. 6) (BOSCH et al., 1958), but when thymidylate synthetase is assayed the greatest relative potency is associated with the phosphorylated anabolite, FUdRP. Apparently only the latter metabolite inhibits thymidylate synthetase directly, is a competitive inhibitor of deoxyuridine phosphate and has 1700 times the affinity of the normal substrate (HARTMANN and HEIDELBERGER, 1961). This increased affinity may be related to the greater tendency of enolization of FU compared to U.

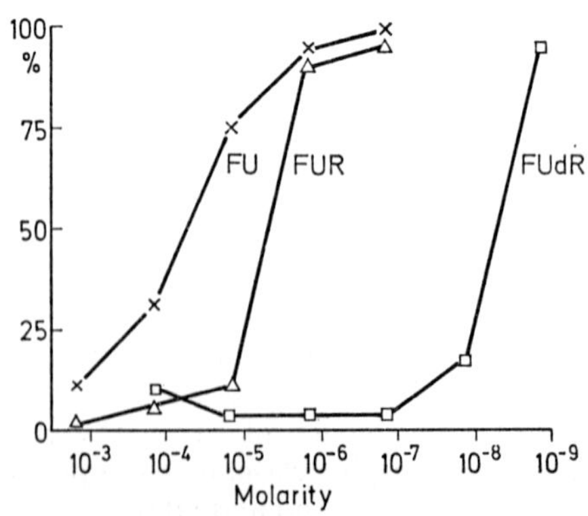

Fig. 6. The effects of fluorinated pyrimidines on the conversion of formate-C^{14} into DNA thymine in suspensions of Ehrlich ascites cells. Per cent of control specific activities is plotted against molarity of inhibitors. FU, 5-fluorouracil; FUR, 5-fluorouridine; FUdR, deoxy-5-fluorouridine. From BOSCH et al. (1958)

Anabolism of FU therefore results in inhibition of DNA synthesis, and selective inhibition of DNA synthesis is known to lead to cell death (COHEN and BARNER, 1954). CHADWICK and ROGERS (1970) have recently reported that twenty-four hours after the administration of FU to tumor-bearing mice the highest levels of FUdRP were found in tumor, small intestine and bone marrow. Thus, a correlation exists between the concentration of this drug anabolite and tissue response to the parent drug.

FU Nucleotides. The biosynthesis of phosphorylated derivatives of FU, such as fluorouridylic acid (FURP), would be expected to alter the cellular control mechanisms which regulate *de novo* pyrimidine biosynthesis. Uridylic acid and related derivatives, for example, react with aspartate carbamyl transferase at an allosteric site to produce feedback inhibition; the corresponding fluorinated compounds exert a pseudo feedback effect and also can reduce normal pyrimidine biosynthesis (BRESNICK, 1962).

FU-RNA. The formation of analog-containing polynucleotides first reported by HEIDELBERGER et al. (1957) and recently reviewed (MANDEL, 1969) has been studied in greatest detail in microorganisms. Investigations have centered on the relative distribution of the antimetabolite within the various subcellular RNA components, in an effort to understand the resulting biochemical alterations. FU has been shown to be incorporated as an integral part of ribosomal and transfer RNA. Ribosomes containing FU differ from normal units in size and physicochemical properties. Selective differences in sensitivity to RNase of the component

Table 1. *Relative composition of RNA fractions from E. coli following treatment with FU for 30 min*

Conditions	RNA preparation	Nucleotide constituents, % of total radioactivity						
		A	G	C	U	FU	U+FU	$\frac{FU \times 100}{U + FU}$
Normal	sRNA	22.1	33.2	29.2	15.5	...	...	...
	16S-RNA	26.7	30.3	22.0	21.0	...	...	...
	23S-RNA	26.3	30.7	21.7	21.2	...	...	...
FU, 30 min . .	sRNA	19.6	30.0	29.8	6.0	14.7	20.7	71.0
	16S-RNA	26.3	28.3	22.7	7.8	14.8	22.6	65.4
	23S-RNA	25.6	30.2	22.3	7.0	14.9	21.9	68.0

After ANDOH and CHARGAFF (1965).

rRNA molecules have also been observed (HAHN and MANDEL, 1971). The synthesis of ribosomes in the presence of the analog is sharply curtailed. Up to 70% replacement of U by FU has been reported for *E. coli* rRNA, the system for which most information is available (Table 1) (ANDOH and CHARGAFF, 1965). Although total amino acid incorporation into polypeptides is not affected by the alteration in ribosomes, binding of such protein to the FU-containing rRNA appears to be impeded. In rat liver also, FU produces a selective depression of ribosome synthesis, probably blocking the transformation of precursors of ribosomal RNA into mature rRNA in nucleoli (STENRAM and WILLÉN, 1967).

Replacement of U by FU in transfer RNA of microorganisms is almost complete, and a disproportionately high proportion of the analog may be incorporated into this subcellular species. Thus, the substitution by FU for U is not uniform. Alterations in composition of some of the minor base constituents of tRNA have been observed, and specific transfer functions of tRNA are altered by FU incorporation (LOWRIE and BERGQUIST, 1968; KAISER, 1969).

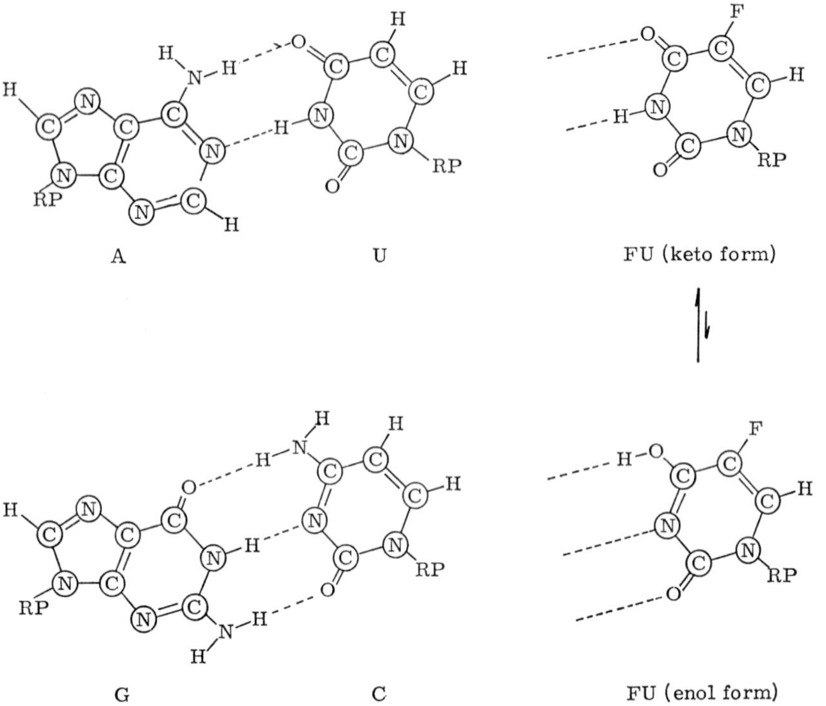

Fig. 7. Potential base pairing of FU in keto form with adenine like uracil, or in enol form with guanine like cytosine. Uracil, with higher pK_a than FU, is entirely in keto form. From Mandel (1969)

Substitution of the analog into messenger RNA of bacteria and plants has been demonstrated, and incorporation of FU into RNA viruses (whose RNA serves as messenger) is extensive. Usually growth and infectivity of the FU-containing virus are reduced, but heavily FU-substituted viruses still retain remarkable infectivity. The somewhat lower pK_a of FU, in comparison with U, has led to the suggestion that the analog, as the enol tautomer at physiological pH, may replace cytosine as well as uracil in base pairing (Fig. 7). The anticipated miscoding (Table 2) undoubtedly explains the formation of virus and phage mutants with altered amino acid composition (Wittmann-Liebold and Wittmann, 1965; Tooze and Weber, 1967). However, reported alterations in protein composition have been highly selective and rather unusual, and could be observed only after careful examination of physical and immunological properties of isolated proteins (reviewed by Mandel, 1969). Enzyme induction in many instances is inhibited by FU, but whether the mechanism involves the altered function of FU-mRNA or catabolite repression is unclear (Horowitz and Kohlmeier, 1967).

FU-Cofactors. The formation of FU-containing nucleotide precursors of cell wall synthesis is responsible for osmotic instability of certain microorganisms, since UDP derivatives function in normal cell wall formation. The replacement of U by FU interferes with this process and causes spheroblast formation and cellular disintegration in *E. coli* (Tomasz and Borek, 1962). FU-containing analogs of normal cell wall precursors, such as FUDP-N-acetylmuramyl-alanyl-glutamyl-lysine exist (Rogers and Perkins, 1960).

Table 2. *Schemes for miscoding due to FU-mRNA*

Condition	Base pairs DNA	Transcribed into mRNA as		Recognized by sRNA as	Alteration from normal in code recognition
I. 1 normal	T—A	U		U	
2 normal	A—T	A		A	
3 normal	G—C	G		G	
4 normal	C—G	C		C	
5 transcription error	C—G [b]	FU	[a]	U	C → U
6 transcription + translation error	C—G [b]	FU	[b]	C	(error corrected)
II. 1 normal	T—A	U		U	
2 translation error	T—A [a]	FU	[b]	C	U → C
3 replacement. . . .	T—A [a]	FU	[9]	U	(none)
		Virus RNA	Replicating form		
III. 1 normal		A	U	U	
2 normal		G	C	C	
3 normal		C	G	G	
4 normal		U	A	A	
5 most likely replication . . .		FU [a]	A	A	(none)
6 replication error		FU [b]	G	G	A → G
7 replication error		G [b]	FU [a]	U	C → U
8 replication error		A [a]	FU [b]	C	U → C

[a] FU pairs like U, [b] FU pairs like C.

From MANDEL (1969).

4. Evaluation of Pharmacological Significance of Various Metabolic Routes

It is difficult to determine which of the many metabolic routes of FU is most closely associated with inhibition of growth of tumors or other cells. The administration of FUdR is more proximally linked to the inhibition of thymidylate synthetase than that of FU or FUR. In addition, the administration of FUR to tumor-bearing mice produces more analog incorporation into nucleic acids and toxicity for comparable carcinostatic activity than does that of FUdR. It is likely, therefore, that the analog's effect on DNA synthesis is of greater therapeutic consequence than that of incorporation into RNA (HEIDELBERGER, 1965). In man, the therapeutic efficacy of FUdR administration may be somewhat greater than that of FU (ANSFIELD and CURRERI, 1963) but this opinion is still controversial (ZUBROD, 1966). The inability in many systems of specifically reversing the effects of FU, as, for instance, by administering thymidine to bypass the blocked thymidylate synthetase reaction and thus to restore DNA synthesis, indicates that even in tumor cells FU acts at more than a single site. These experiments are complicated by the difficulty of dissecting the various drug effects, as well as the reversibility of most of the metabolic pathways; for example, the cleavage of FUdR to FU then permits the re-anabolism to the ribose derivatives of the analog. In microorganisms, the inhibitory properties of FU involve the blockage of DNA synthesis, the inhibition of ribosomal RNA synthesis, the blockage of cell division and the formation of FU-containing RNA. Under appropriate conditions most of these drug effects can be dissociated from each other (DOOLITTLE, HAHN and MANDEL, unpublished).

III. Comparative Metabolism of 5-Halouracil Derivatives

An interesting example of the role of the size of the substituted functional group in a molecule on its metabolism exists amongst the 5-substituted halouracils (Fig. 8). Substitution of the 5-hydrogen by the fluoro atom provides FU, a specific analog of uracil, and results in the described incorporation of this compound into

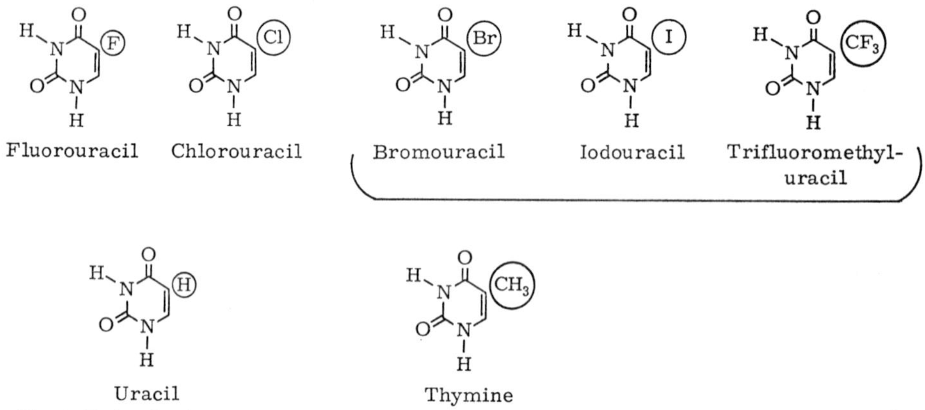

Fig. 8. Role of substituent on C-5 in substrate analog reactions. Van der Waals' radii in Å: F = 1.35; Cl = 1.81; Br = 1.95; I = 2.16; CF_3 = 2.44; H = 1.20; CH_3 = 2.00. Fluorouracil, like uracil, is incorporated into RNA exclusively; bromo, iodo and trifluoromethyluracil, like thymine, are incorporated into DNA exclusively; chlorouracil is incorporated into RNA and DNA

RNA but not DNA. Replacement by a bromo or iodo group, on the other hand, produces compounds that bear greater resemblance to thymine than to uracil, and these drugs act as thymine antagonists. For example, bromo- and iodouracil, or preferably their deoxyribose derivatives, form deoxyribose phosphates and are incorporated into DNA, like anabolites of thymine. Substitution by a chlorine atom which is intermediate in size between fluorine and bromine atoms, produces an antimetabolite which is incorporated into both RNA and DNA (Dunn and Smith, 1957). As might be expected, trifluoromethyldeoxyuridine is incorporated exclusively into DNA (Heidelberger et al., 1965).

IV. Metabolism of a Purine Analog: 6-Thioguanine

The information on thioguanine (TG) is presented in less detail because of a great similarity in the overall concepts of catabolism, anabolism and drug action just described for FU. A parallel exists between the biochemical conversions of thioguanine and guanine (Fig. 9), which differ only in the substituent group on C-6 (Fig. 10).

The analog has been shown to be degraded to thioxanthine and thiouric acid, together with the formation of sulfate (Sartorelli et al., 1958). The cleavage of the sulfur atom from the purine skeleton, at least in microorganisms, leads to the production of guanine or an anabolite of it which is able to antagonize the effects of the original drug. As a result of this reaction, the purine moiety of thioguanine is converted to the purines of nucleic acids, while the sulfur portion is used for sulfur-amino acid formation and subsequent synthesis of protein (Mandel et al., 1965). In man, methylation to S-methylthioguanine is an important route of metabolism (Elion et al., 1962).

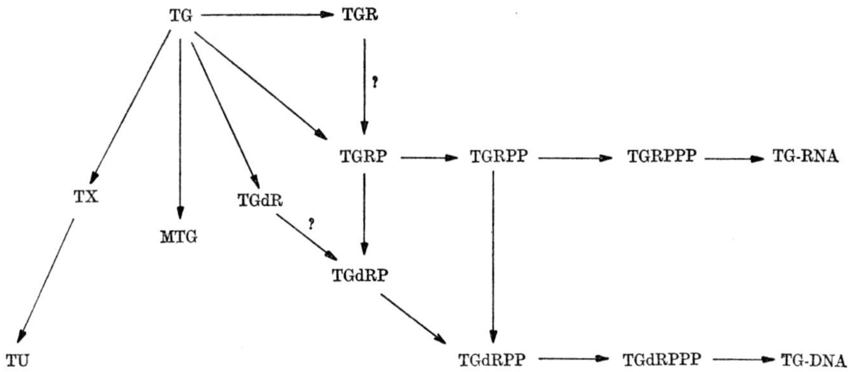

Fig. 9. Routes of metabolism of 6-thioguanine (TG). X, xanthine; U, uric acid; M, S-methyl; R, ribose; dR, deoxyribose; P, phosphate

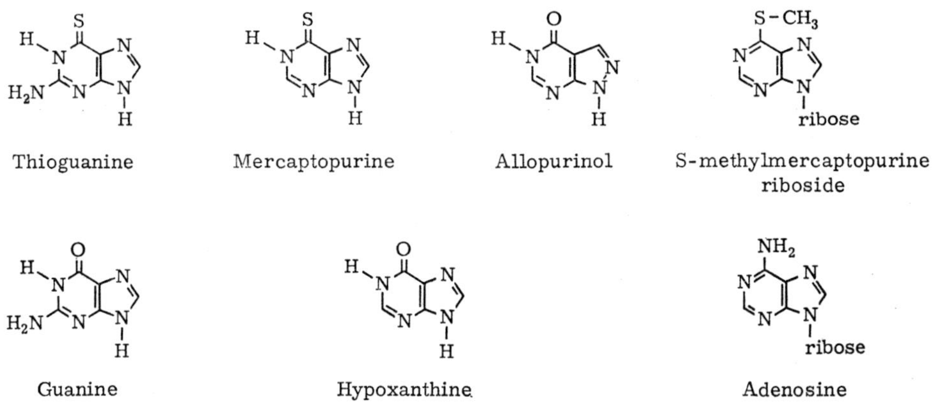

Fig. 10. Substrates and their analogs: guanine and 6-thioguanine; hypoxanthine and mercaptopurine or allopurinol; adenosine and S-methylmercaptopurine riboside

Like the natural purine, thioguanine also forms the nucleotide derivative by reacting with phosphoribosylpyrophosphate (PRPP) and guanine phosphoribosyltransferase; the di- and triphosphate derivatives have been synthesized as well (Moore and Le Page, 1958). These derivatives have also been isolated from tissues following the administration of TG. Evidence has been presented to indicate clearly that the analog also is incorporated into RNA and DNA, particularly of tumor tissue and bone marrow. Thioguanine appears to be distributed in messenger, ribosomal, as well as transfer RNA of Sarcoma 180 ascites cells (Kwan and Mandel, unpublished). The administration of the related anticancer agent, 6-mercaptopurine, also leads to the incorporation of thioguanine into polynucleotides (Scannell and Hitchings, 1966).

A remarkable correlation has been observed between the sensitivity of tissues to thioguanine and the *in vivo* incorporation of the analog into polynucleotides, particularly into DNA (Le Page and Jones, 1961). For example, susceptible tumors contained more drug in the polynucleotides than drug-insensitive neoplasms (Table 3), and spacing of dosages which were more tumor-inhibitory also led to greater incorporation into nucleic acids. Normal tissue, such as bone marrow, had greater levels of the analog, and demonstrated toxic effects; on the other hand,

Table 3. *In vivo incorporation of 6-thioguanine into nucleic acids and tissue response*

Tissue	Survival[a]	DNA[b]	RNA[b]
S-180	160	3.0	3.0
Ehrlich	205	1.9	2.3
Ca-755	195	2.1	1.7
L1210	200	1.3	1.4
TA3	185	1.7	2.7
6C3HED	97	0.06	0.30
Mecca lymphosarcoma	95	0.03	0.27
Ehrlich TGR I	90	0.21	0.55
Ehrlich TGR II	93	0.03	0.33
S-180 TGR	97	0.23	0.47
Ca-755 TGR	88	0.17	0.41
L1210 TGR	89	0.12	0.23
Bone marrow	Toxic	1.3	1.4
Intestinal mucosa	Nontoxic	0	0

[a] Per cent of control. [b] Micrograms of 6-TG per milliliter of cells.

From LE PAGE (1963).

this drug produces little damage to intestinal mucosa, into which there was little or no incorporation of the analog. The co-administration of azaserine, which enhances carcinostatic action, increased thioguanine content in polynucleotides (LE PAGE, 1963). However, whether this incorporation into nucleic acids is directly responsible for tumor growth inhibition is still controversial; in other biological systems such correlation is clearly absent, and drug-resistant tumors contained more TG in nucleic acids than drug-sensitive lines (BIEBER et al., 1961; BALIS, 1968). Again, it has not been possible to dissect all the drug's biochemical effects, or perhaps even to recognize them. Thioguanosine phosphate (TGRP) may also be responsible for some of the growth inhibitory effects of the drug. Among enzymes sensitive to this analog derivative are inosinic acid dehydrogenase, and phosphoribosylpyrosphosphate amido transferase where the nucleotide acts as a pseudo feedback inhibitor of purine biosynthesis.

As with fluorouracil, the loss of enzymes converting the analog to the nucleotide has been associated with resistance of tumor cell lines to the effects of thioguanine, although other mechanisms to explain acquired resistance to thioguanine also have been demonstrated (ELLIS and LE PAGE, 1963). SARTORELLI et al. (1958) have studied a tumor line in which drug-resistant cells exhibited greater catabolism of thioguanine to thiouric acid than in the sensitive cells.

V. Metabolism of Other Purine and Pyrimidine Analogs

The general patterns described for FU and TG exist also for numerous other structural derivatives of the nucleic acid bases (MANDEL, 1959; LANGEN, 1968). However, it should not be assumed that for every substrate analog all of the biochemical pathways are equally available. For example, 6-mercaptopurine and 6-azauracil (or 6-azauridine) which are converted by many mammalian tissues to the ribonucleotide form, do not form sufficient di- and triphosphate derivatives to be incorporated into DNA or RNA (PATERSON, 1959; PASTERNAK and HANDSCHUMACHER, 1959). However, in the cat brain and in certain microorganisms incorporation of 6-azauracil into polynucleotides has been reported (WELLS et al., 1963; HANDSCHUMACHER, 1957). It appears that differences in constituent enzyme patterns in various species, dose and other experimental conditions determine the specific metabolic route of substrate analogs.

It is usually difficult, based on available data, to predict which one of several possible metabolic routes will be used by an untested analog. Some of these structural relationships have recently been clarified by ELION (1969), who reported on the relative affinities of certain purine analogs for specific enzymes in relation to catalytic reaction rates. For example, for adenine phosphoribosyltransferase from monkey liver, the K_M for adenine is 6.9×10^{-7} M. The adenine analog, 2,6-diaminopurine, has a K_I somewhat greater than 10^{-3} M, but its V_{max} is 60% that of the corresponding reaction with adenine. This relatively high V_{max} explains why 2,6-diaminopurine, with a therapeutically effective *in vivo* concentration of only 2.5×10^{-5} M, is anabolized to the nucleotide form in spite of its relatively poor binding to the enzyme. On the other hand, another adenine analog, 4-aminopyrazolopyrimidine, with a K_I of 2.7×10^{-5} M, has a relative V_{max} value only 2% of that for adenine. Thus, at the same *in vivo* level of 2.5×10^{-5} M, 4-aminopyrazolopyrimidine forms about the same amount of nucleotide as does diaminopurine. The availability of data of this type permits reasonable predictions as to the preferred metabolic routes of analogs *in vivo*, and also is helpful in suggesting designs for superior chemotherapeutic agents.

This type of information explains why the hypoxanthine analog, 6-mercaptopurine, forms a nucleotide derivative *in vivo*, whereas the closely related hypoxanthine analog, allopurinol, does not (Fig. 10). Table 4 lists the inhibition constants for these derivatives for human enzymes. 6-MP has low K_I values for the anabolic transferase (KRENITSKY et al., 1969) and the catabolic xanthine oxidase, but unlike hypoxanthine it shows greater affinity for the transferase. These concentrations are in a range normally reached therapeutically. Allopurinol, however, binds preferentially to xanthine oxidase, and its K_I for the transferase enzyme greatly exceeds the drug concentration reached *in vivo*. Thus, allopurinol does not form a nucleotide *in vivo*, but reacts instead with xanthine oxidase to form the xanthine analog, oxipurinol. If present together with 6-MP, it competes with the latter for oxidation by xanthine oxidase. By preventing the catabolic conversion of 6-MP to thiouric acid, relatively more of the 6-MP is available for anabolism to thioinosinic acid (ELION et al., 1963; ELION, 1969).

Table 4. *Binding constants of hypoxanthine analogs*

	Hypoxanthine	6-Mercaptopurine	Allopurinol
	$K_I \times M$	$K_I \times M$	$K_I \times M$
Hypoxanthine phosphoribosyltransferase[a]	2.4×10^{-6}	3.9×10^{-6}	10^{-3}
Xanthine oxidase	3×10^{-6}	1.8×10^{-5}	1.9×10^{-7}

[a] Measured as inhibition of conversion of ^{14}C-hypoxanthine to ^{14}C-inosinate by nonradioactive compounds. For a competitive inhibitor, its K_I value should be equivalent to its K_M value when it is a substrate for the same reaction. After ELION (1969).

Although frequently the antimetabolite drugs have less affinity for specific enzymes compared to normal substrates, numerous examples exist where the reverse is true. For example, for inosinate dehydrogenase, the K_M for inosinate is 1.4×10^{-5} M, whereas the K_I for thioinosinate is 3.6×10^{-6} M. For adenylosuccinate synthetase, however, inosinate has greater affinity than does the thio analog (K_M, 3×10^{-5} M; K_I, 3×10^{-4}, respectively) (ELION, 1969).

VI. Clinical Applications of Knowledge on Metabolism of Purine and Pyrimidine Antimetabolites

An understanding of the action and fate of drugs should increase the usefulness of the agents in their clinical application. Although considerable information is available as to the most active metabolic products of many of the antimetabolites, the lack of sufficient antitumor selectivity has complicated the prediction of optimal dosage schedules. Furthermore, the multiple nature of the biochemical sites of action, together with great variations in the rates of individual metabolic reactions in specific tumors and normal tissues, has resulted in determining optimal drug dosage by clinical response. In the therapy of malignancies, this is a particularly slow and inaccurate measurement. The role of route, dose and schedule of drug administration on the drug's metabolism in various tissues, the biochemical properties of the tumor cell, including the location and number of such cells, as well as the nature of the host, all influence selective toxicity, and should be recognized for optimal therapy (J.F. HENDERSON, 1969). By contrast, chemotherapy of herpes infections of the eye with iododeoxyuridine owes its success to the poor systemic absorption after instillation into the eye, thus limiting systemic toxicity, a major problem of cancer chemotherapy.

Information is being accumulated at the present time on the optimal administration of individual drugs or simple combinations in experimental therapy of animal models, in relation to the maximal concentration of a carcinostatic drug anabolite (e.g., ROGERS et al., 1969; CHADWICK and ROGERS, 1970). In the clinic, however, where multiple drug combinations have been found to be most effective (E.S. HENDERSON and SAMAHA, 1969), there is normally little experimental basis for the chosen drug schedule. Even for a single drug such as FU, which has been extensively studied, it has been difficult to devise a test for predicting the drug's effectiveness against a particular patient's tumor (WOLBERG, 1967).

1. Enhancement of Metabolism

Numerous approaches have permitted increases in the concentration of antimetabolite derivatives in tissues. Unless these changes are selective for the tumor, however, the resulting toxicity usually limits their usefulness. For example, 4-amino-5-imidazolecarboxamide, an inhibitor of guanine deaminase, prevents the rapid catabolism of 8-azaguanine, and permits more of the analog to be anabolized and incorporated into polynucleotides. Unfortunately, this potentiation of tumor growth inhibition is accompanied by enhanced toxicity (CARLÓ and MANDEL, 1954). The combination of 6-mercaptopurine with azaserine, a compound which by blocking *de novo* purine synthesis enhances the anabolism of the thio analog (SARTORELLI and LE PAGE, 1958), has not been of therapeutic benefit in man. By preventing the catabolism of 6-mercaptopurine to thiourate, allopurinol enhances the concentration of 6-MP which can be activated, and in animal tumors potentiates preferentially the carcinostatic actions of 6-MP (ELION et al., 1963). Although in man the benefit of this combination does not appear to be of particular advantage over that of an increased dose of 6-mercaptopurine, this research has led to the development of allopurinol for the treatment of gout. Numerous other examples of limiting degradation by administering agents which compete for the catabolic enzymes have been reported; usually, however, such drug combinations have not been sufficiently selective in therapy.

2. Attempts to Increase Cell Penetrability of Active Metabolites

Since the nucleotide derivatives of purine and pyrimidine analogs appear to be more closely associated with pharmacological activity than the corresponding bases or nucleosides, attempts have been made to exploit their greater inhibitory effect. The use of nucleotide derivatives should be of particular benefit in cases of tumors which have acquired resistance to base analogs by deletion of enzymes catalyzing the formation of these active metabolites. Although preparations from cells resistant to base analogs may be sensitive to the phosphorylated metabolites, these compounds are unable to enter whole cells, and thus are ineffective clinically. Various approaches of overcoming this impenetrability have met with limited success. Mono- and diesters, amides, dinucleoside monophosphates, small nucleotide polymers, and sulfate esters of fluorodeoxyuridine, which were believed to be able to penetrate cells, were not particularly effective as chemotherapeutic agents (MUKHERJEE and HEIDELBERGER, 1962). The dinucleoside monophosphate derivative of 6-MP has been reported to be inhibitory to tumor cells resistant to thioinosinate (MONTGOMERY et al., 1963), but corresponding derivatives of pyrimidine analogs showed no exploitable chemotherapeutic properties. Recently, IUdR incorporation into tumors was reported to be preferentially enhanced when the closely related cytosine derivative, ICdRP, was complexed with polycations, whice apparently enhanced transport into the malignant cells (WOODMAN, 1968).

3. Selectively Increasing the Availability of Active Analog Metabolites

Occasionally the administration of a compound which liberates the active drug *in vivo* may produce a more selective action than the administration of the active drug itself. The greater effectiveness of the immunosuppressive agent, azathioprine, 6-(1-methyl-4 nitro-5 imidazolyl) thiopurine, compared to the closely related drug, 6-mercaptopurine, is believed to be due to the slow release of 6-MP from the former compound (ELION et al., 1961). Sulfhydryl compounds, such as glutathione, have been shown to split azathioprine into 6-MP, which is normally readily catabolized. The administration of azathioprine, therefore, provides 6-MP in such a manner that it is slowly formed by reaction with endogenous sulfhydryl compounds, and therefore it is less subject to oxidation and methylation. Azathioprine is more potent as an immunosuppressant than 6-MP, but pretreatment with glutathione, which increases the *in vivo* conversion of azathioprine to 6-MP, results in the loss of any preferential response to azathioprine (ELION, 1967). Similarly, certain alkoxybromo derivatives of FUdR slowly regenerate FUdR *in vivo* so as to increase potency (DUSCHINSKY et al., 1967).

The triacetyl derivative of 6-azauridine has been found to be more effective after oral administration than azauridine, which is poorly absorbed and is broken down by intestinal bacteria to the neurotoxic base analog, azauracil. Although the triacetyl derivative produces metabolic effects and clinical changes comparable to intravenously administered azauridine, it can be used orally and provides a sustained blood level of azauridine (CREASEY et al., 1963). In a somewhat different approach, BAKER (1967) has been designing substrate analogs which have additional functional groups to interact irreversibly with the same enzyme but at a site other than the active site for the substrate. In this manner, organ and species selectivity may be altered by suitable modification of the additional functional group (BAKER and WOOD, 1969).

4. Spacing of Doses

It has been known for several years that therapeutic effectiveness of drugs can be greatly enhanced by alteration in the route, dose and frequency of administration (GOLDIN et al., 1956). For example, the folate analog, amethopterin (methotrexate) is of greater therapeutic benefit in man when given parenterally twice weekly in large doses than when given daily in smaller oral doses, while toxicity of both schedules was comparable (SELAWRY et al., 1965). It is becoming of increasing importance to understand the factors which control the availability of the active form of antimetabolite drugs so as to provide a selective antitumor effect. For example, the enhanced formation of thioinosinate from 6-MP after prior hourly doses of the base analog appears to rely on the greater availability of PRPP because of reduced *de novo* purine biosynthesis. The PRPP then is used for more thioinosinate synthesis (MELONI and ROGERS, 1969).

The greater percentage of tumor cells in the S phase of the mitotic cycle (DNA synthesis phase), in comparison with cells of the most sensitive tissues of the host, has suggested a more specific dosage regimen for increasing the selectivity of tumor therapy. The DNA polymerase inhibitor, cytosine arabinoside, has been administered in repeated shortly-spaced doses, with appropriate spacing for host recovery, so as to exploit this differential characteristic of tumor cells (SKIPPER et al., 1967). In this manner the blood level of the drug is maintained long enough for as many tumor cells as possible to reach the S phase of their cycle. Synchronization of leukemic cells with a colchicine derivative in order to have all cells sensitive to cytosine arabinoside administered 15 hours later, also has been reported to result in therapeutic potentiation (VADLAMUDI et al., 1968). Synchronization also increases sensitivity to FU. It appears that knowledge of intermitotic times for specific tissues would be most useful in devising optimal drug treatment schedules.

5. Combination Therapy

Only certain additional aspects of combination therapy will be described here which pertain specifically to metabolism of substrate analogs. The importance of proper selection of time intervals in combination therapy to reduce toxicity has been described by LE PAGE and KANEKO (1969). Since normal cells are subject to the influence of corticoids, whereas neoplasms may not respond, these authors have exploited this differential response to depress DNA synthesis in bone marrow and thereby to spare this tissue during the period of peak concentration of thioguanine and its active anabolites. Cortisone-treated mice receiving thioguanine 8 h later were protected from toxicity, whereas toxic effects were evident when the analog had been administered only 4 h after the steroid. The natural diurnal rhythm of corticosteroids in blood undoubtedly accounts for the differential drug effects observed when drugs are administered at different times of the day. Similarly, the incorporation of thioguanine into DNA was greatly altered depending on the relative timing at which the inhibitor of DNA synthesis, cytosine arabinoside, was coadministered.

6-Methylmercaptopurine riboside (6MMPR) which differs from 6-mercaptopurine in being conjugated with ribose while also bearing a methyl group on the sulfur atom (Fig. 10) is an analog of adenosine. Indeed, adenosine kinase converts the drug to the phosphorylated derivative (BENNETT et al., 1965; CALDWELL et al., 1966) which is associated with the drug's growth-inhibitory properties. 6-MP, on the other hand, forms its nucleotide derivatives via the phosphoribosyl transferase reaction described under thioguanine. The differential routes of activation of 6-MP and 6 MMPR, linked to an increase in nucleotide levels of the analogs when in combination (PATERSON and MORIWAKI, 1969), account for the enhancement of carcinostatic activity that has been reported when these drugs have been used in combination (SCHABEL et al., 1967; WANG et al., 1967). The remarkable lack of cross-resistance between these two drugs also relies on this difference in metabolism (BENNETT et al., 1965).

6. Supplying Rescue Agents

The combination of an antimetabolite with the corresponding normal metabolite has occasionally been found effective in selectively "rescuing" normal tissue from toxicity while only minimally affecting the drug's antitumor response. Proper timing and dosage schedules are particularly important for such an approach. Examples of some clinically useful examples of the technique involve the combination of iododeoxyuridine and thymidine, and the use of amethopterin and leucovorin (GOLDIN et al., 1966; MITCHELL et al., 1968). For example, stomatitis and hair loss could be minimized, and bone marrow could be partially protected by the instillation of thymidine into the external carotid artery during treatment of tumors by intravenous doses of iododeoxyuridine (CALABRESI, 1962).

C. Metabolism of Other Analogs by Pathways for Normal Substrates

In addition to purine and pyrimidine analogs, numerous other examples of analogs following the routes of metabolism of the normal substrates exist. Structural alterations of *carbohydrates* have resulted in antimetabolites whose metabolism resembled that of the normal sugars. 2-Deoxy-D-glucose is phosphorylated, forms disaccharides, deoxygluconic acid and nucleotide derivatives like the corresponding reactions of glucose (FARKAŠ et al., 1969). Xylosyl-adenine, like the corresponding ribose derivative, adenosine, has been shown to be converted to the triphosphate derivative (an analog of ATP) and a small amount is incorporated into polynucleotides. The nucleoside analog also is deaminated by adenosine deaminase to the corresponding hypoxanthine compound (ELLIS and LE PAGE, 1966). Cytosine arabinoside is phosphorylated to the nucleotide form and is incorporated into tumor cell RNA and DNA like the corresponding natural ribose and deoxyribose isomers, respectively (Fig. 11) (CHU and FISCHER, 1968). In addition, there is also extensive deamination to the corresponding uracil derivative.

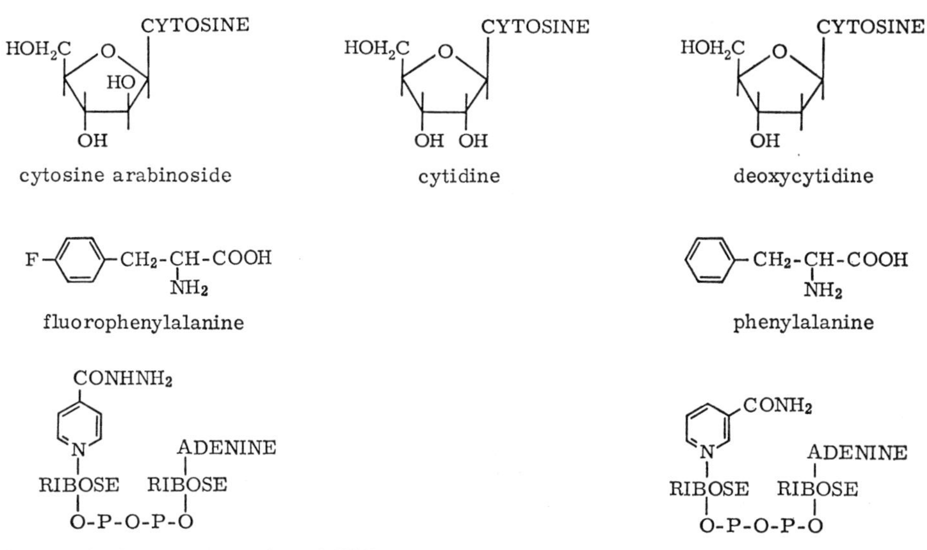

Fig. 11. Analogs and the normal substrates

Numerous examples have been documented where *amino acid* analogs may replace normal amino acids in the activation reactions and in protein synthesis. For example, in *E. coli*, DL-fluorotyrosine may substitute for tyrosine in the ATP-PP exchange reaction, and in reacting with tyrosyl tTNA, with relative K_M values of about 6 and 20 times those for L-tyrosine, respectively (CALENDAR and BERG, 1966). The reduced affinity of the analog for the enzyme, in comparison with that of the normal amino acid, appears to be quite characteristic (NOVELLI, 1967). *p*-Fluorophenylalanine (Fig. 11) is assimilated into bacterial cells by the same route as phenylalanine. Only when the concentration of analog exceeds that of the normal amino acid by a factor of 4 does the fluoro derivative pass into the amino acid pool of *E. coli*. Once in the cell, the amino acid analogs are active in inhibiting the endogenous supply of the natural competitor by interfering with its biosynthesis. Growth is usually decreased from a logarithmic towards a more linear rate, indicating a decrease in biological function of some synthesized enzymes (reviewed by RICHMOND, 1962).

These reactions explain the mechanisms by which amino acid analogs can be incorporated into proteins. Ethionine, probably the first such instance, was shown to be present in protein of tetrahymena following its administration (GROSS and TARVER, 1955), and numerous other analogs have now been demonstrated in microbial or mammalian protein where they replace the normal amino acid, specifically e.g. norleucine, tryptazan, 7-azatryptophan, β-2-thienylalanine, selenomethionine, etc. (RICHMOND, 1962).

In *B. cereus*, *p*-fluorophenylalanine can replace 75% of the phenylalanine of total cell protein, of exocellular protein and of exopenicillinase synthesized. The activity of the latter enzyme is impaired in relation to the replacement of the normal phenylalanine by the analog (Fig. 12), and the immunological properties of the

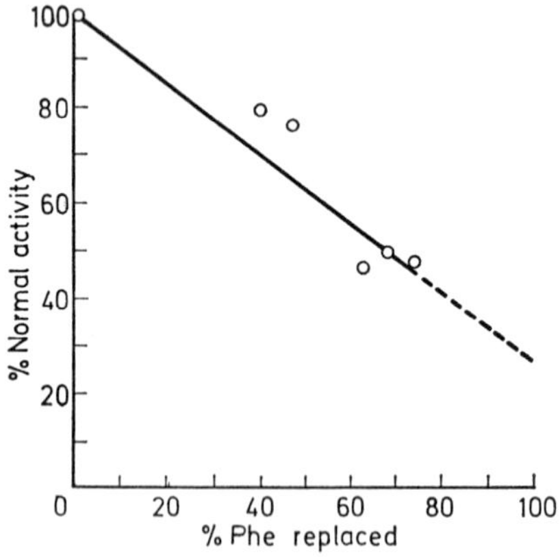

Fig. 12. Effect of replacement of phenylalanine (PHE) by the p-fluoro derivative on the specific enzyme activity of exopenicillinase. From RICHMOND (1962)

enzyme are altered. For other enzymes, however, incorporation of the amino acid antimetabolite does not result in a decrease in specific activity if the amino acid being replaced is not associated with the active center of the enzyme molecule. Indeed, selenomethionine supports the growth of a methionine requiring auxotroph of *E. coli* in the absence of methionine, and is utilized better than methionine in transmethylation reactions in rabbit liver involving Se-adenosyl selenomethionine (MUDD and CANTONI, 1957) (Fig. 13).

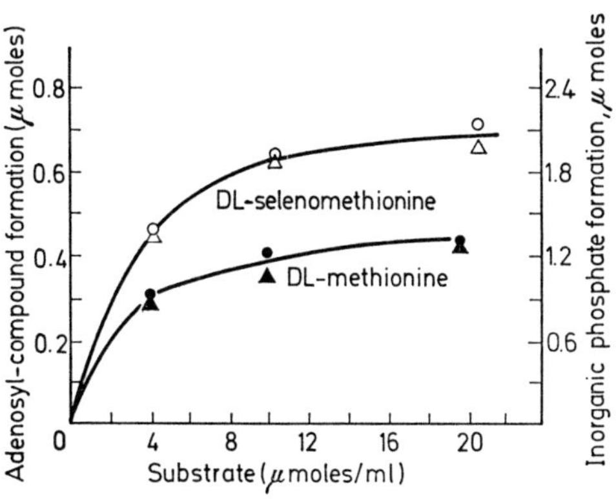

Fig. 13. Activity of methionine and selenomethionine as substrates for yeast methionine-activating enzyme, in presence of ATP. Product measured as adenosyl complex (○, ●) or as inorganic phosphate (△, ▲). From MUDD and CANTONI (1957)

In a similar manner, one may view the disposition of the antibiotic, puromycin, which bears structural resemblance to the amino acyl terminus of a tRNA molecule (Fig. 14). Unlike the latter, however, which is attached to the ribosome at the 30S and 50S sites, puromycin binds to the 50S site only, and becomes attached to the nascent polypeptide chain which then leaves the ribosome prematurely. The resulting product is an abnormally short polypeptide in which puromycin terminates the chain (NATHANS, 1964).

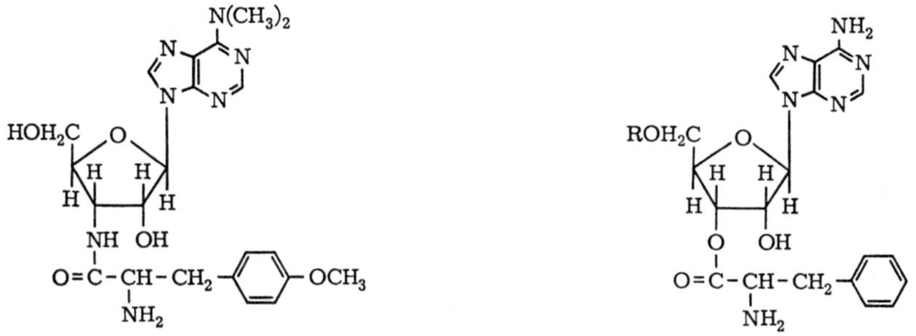

Fig. 14. R represents the remainder of the RNA molecule

There are numerous examples of the biosynthesis of *cofactor* analogs from structurally altered *precursors*. The 3-acetylpyridine analog of NAD has been prepared from 3-acetylpyridine in the presence of NAD and NADase, or following administration of the nicotinamide analog to mice (KAPLAN and CIOTTI, 1956). A corresponding product has been prepared enzymatically when isoniazid was used (ZATMAN et al., 1954) (Fig. 11). These and other NAD analogs participate in the reactions normally mediated by NAD, and the activities of the analog compared to NAD were either diminished or enhanced depending on the enzyme being tested.

Substitution of various groups into fatty acids can lead to toxic products (see GOLDMAN, 1969). The anabolism of fluoroacetate to fluorocitrate has already been mentioned. The breakdown of long chain ω-fluorocarboxylic acids proceeds via β-

Table 5. *The toxicities of ω-fluorocarboxylic acids in mice*

Even members	LD_{50} mg/kg	Odd members	LD_{50} mg/kg
FCH_2COOH	6.6	$F(CH_2)_2COOH$	60
$F(CH_2)_3COOH$	0.65	$F(CH_2)_4COOH$	>100
$F(CH_2)_5COOH$	1.35	$F(CH_2)_6COOH$	40
$F(CH_2)_7COOH$	0.64	$F(CH_2)_8COOH$	>100
$F(CH_2)_9COOH$	1.5	$F(CH_2)_{10}COOH$	57.5
$F(CH_2)_{11}COOH$	1.25		
$F(CH_2)_{15}COOC_2H_5$ [a]	7.0		
$F(CH_2)_{17}COOH$	5.7		

[a] The ester is hydrolyzed to the acid *in vivo*.
From WILLIAMS, Detoxication Mechanisms (1959), after PATTISON et al. (1956).

oxidation, the pathway available for natural long chain fatty acids, and thus leads to the formation of fluoroacetate from analogs having an even number of carbon atoms. These compounds would be expected to be more toxic than ω-fluorocarboxylic acids with an odd number of carbon atoms since the latter cannot be converted to fluoroacetate. Indeed, Table 5 reveals the categorical difference between the toxicities of these compounds in mice.

Evidence has been provided by WACKER et al. (1958) that in microorganisms *p*-aminosalicylic and salicylic acids utilize the enzyme system for *p*-aminobenzoic acid in the synthesis of folic acid derivatives, thus forming ortho-hydroxy analogs.

The similarity between methyl and ethyl *alcohols* extends also to their routes of degradation. Both alcohols serve as substrates of alcohol dehydrogenase, and sufficient competition exists so that ethanol administration is recommended to limit the oxidation of methanol to its toxic metabolites in individuals who have consumed methanol (COOPER and KINI, 1962). The *choline ester*, succinylcholine, is readily hydrolyzed by pseudocholinesterase, for which acetylcholine also is a substrate. The trimethyl*xanthine*, caffeine, is excreted as methylated uric acid derivatives, analogous to the degradation of normal tissue purines (CORNISH and CHRISTMAN, 1957). Various *steroid* interconversions are mediated by enzymes with specificities not restricted to normal substrates exclusively (TOMKINS, 1956).

Over the past few years a situation very reminiscent of the metabolism of antimetabolites has been revealed in the field of adrenergic amines (CREVELING et al., 1962). LOVENBERG et al. (1962) first reported that the decarboxylase which converts dihydroxyphenylalanine (DOPA) to DOPAmine also catalyzes the corresponding decarboxylation for α-methylnorepinephrine, analogous to the formation of norepinephrine. In addition, the brain of animals treated with α-methylDOPA was found to contain α-methylnorepinephrine (CARLSSON and LINDQVIST, 1962) (Fig. 15). In many biological systems investigated, the α-methyl analog is equipotent with norepinephrine (KOPIN, 1968). This "false adrenergic transmitter" is released by sympathetic nerve stimulation of animals administered α-methyl-DOPA (MUSCHOLL and MAITRE, 1963).

There are other closely related examples of adrenergic drugs which are metabolized along the pathways used by adrenergic hormones. α-Methyltyrosine, for example, is converted to α-methylnorepinephrine, presumably via α-methylDOPA (MAITRE, 1965). N-Methylation of α-methylnorepinephrine, to produce the α-methyl derivative of epinephrine, has been observed to take place in the adrenal medulla, and the physiological disposition of this analog corresponds to that of epinephrine (MUSCHOLL, 1965; MUSCHOLL and SPRENGER, 1966). α-Methyl-*m*-tyrosine is converted to metaraminol by a series of reactions analogous to those

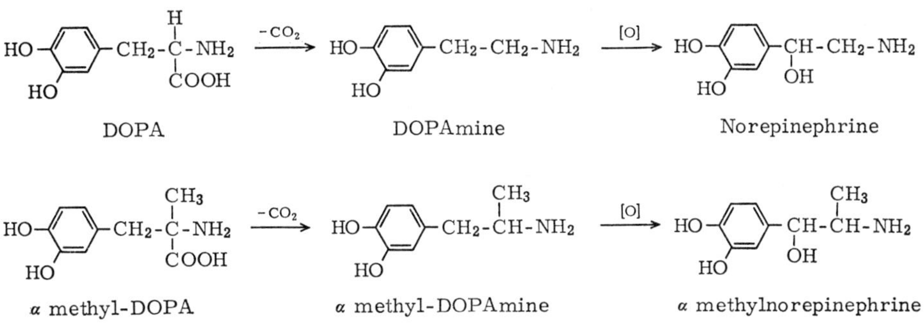

Fig. 15. Route of metabolism of DOPA and its methyl analog

described. This end product is less potent than norepinephrine, and its replacement of norepinephrine upon release of sympathetic nerve stimulation may explain the resulting decrease in adrenergic response (CARLSSON and LINDQVIST, 1962; CROUT et al., 1964; KOPIN, 1968). The exact mechanism of action of all of the above drugs is complicated by the various inhibitory effects associated with the parent compounds and their metabolites, and the decreased formation of normal hormones and their precursors.

D. The Metabolism of Substrate Analogs Along Routes Used by "Conventional" Drugs

In addition to the specific routes of metabolism used by substrate analogs and their corresponding normal substrates, more customary routes of biodegradation are also available to the analogs (WILLIAMS, 1967). This non-selectivity is not really surprising since there is also a great deal of overlap between the pathways of metabolism of "conventional" drugs and normal substrates. For example, naturally occurring compounds such as steroids, thyroxine and bilirubin form glucuronide derivatives, a major conjugation pathway normally associated with microsomes and used for the metabolism of salicylic acid and many other phenolic and carboxylic drugs. Sulfokinases are involved in the formation of endogenous products such as heparin, chondroitin sulfate, various sulfolipids, tyrosine sulfate, the sulfates of epinephrine, norepinephrine, progesterone, estrone, androsterone and bile acids; sulfate conjugation is another important route of metabolism of foreign compounds like aniline and phenol, although some specificity among sulfokinases exists (BORSTRUM, 1965). The mechanism of activation of exogenous benzoic acid to form amides is the same as that used by endogenous fatty acids. Studies on the acetylation of the drug, sulfanilamide, led to the discovery of coenzyme A in intermediary metabolism (LIPMANN, 1945); the hormone, histamine, can also be acetylated by the same mechanism. Methylation occurs with administered pyridine and normorphine as well as various endogenous phenols and amines, such as epinephrine and histamine. Hydroxylation of steroids and numerous drugs is mediated by microsomal hydroxylases. In summary, categorial distinctions between metabolic reactions of drugs and normal substrates are unwarranted, as are those between drugs and substrate analogs (MANDEL, 1971).

There are numerous cases of substrate analogs which are metabolized by the usual pathways of biodegradation, frequently involving microsomes. Relatively little attention has been paid to this field, however. For example, sulfadimethoxine, a long-acting sulfanilamide derivative, forms the N-1 glucuronide in man (BRIDGES et al., 1965). Small amounts of the N-4 glucuronide of this drug also are produced by man, the rabbit, dog and rat (BRIDGES et al., 1964). Trace amounts of sulfasomizole are conjugated to form the N-4 glucuronide in man, dog, rabbit and rat (BRIDGES and WILLIAMS, 1963). Other sulfa drugs which form glucuronide derivatives are sulfadiazine, sulfisoxazole, sulfapyridine, sulfamethazine, sulfamerazine and sulfathiazole (MARSH, 1966; GILLIGAN, 1945). Although the localization of the glucuronyl transferases for these particular drugs has not been reported, it can be assumed by analogy that they are located in the microsomes. In these particular examples it may be said that only a portion of the drug molecule is responsible for the antimetabolic action of the drugs, since it is principally the sulfanilamide moiety of the structure which antagonizes the actions of *p*-aminobenzoic acid. However, it should be noted that the conjugation reactions also take place on that portion of the drug's structure.

Dichloromethotrexate, a folic acid antagonist, is rapidly converted, in part, to the 4-deamino-4, 7-dihydroxy derivative in man and the rodent, but not the dog (OLIVERIO and DAVIDSON, 1962). The hydroxylation reaction is mediated by soluble rather than microsomal enzymes but is inhibited by the microsomal enzyme inhibitor, SKF 525A (LOO and ADAMSON, 1962).

9-Ethyl- and 9-butyl-6-mercaptopurine are excreted into the urine largely as the S-glucuronides in man, even though these products have not actually been identified as such. The ethyl derivative is also converted to the S-glucuronide by Sarcoma-180 ascites cells in mice (HANSEN et al., 1963).

The enhancement of the antitumor effect of 6-MP by phenobarbital and other drugs which may induce enzyme synthesis in liver remains unexplained (MARCHAND and FUJIMOTO, 1962). The binding of 6-methylmercaptopurine riboside (6MMPR) to cytochrome P-450 of rat liver, suggests that this adenosine analog also behaves like many conventional drugs, such as aminopyrine, in its metabolism (JOHNSON et al., 1970). An S-demethylation enzyme in rat liver microsomes removes methyl groups from various thioethers, including 6MMP and methitural, a barbiturate derivative, to form the thiols and formaldehyde (MAZEL et al., 1964). This reaction is inhibited in the presence of carbon monoxide. Pretreatment of rats with 3,4-benzpyrene has led to a threefold increase in S-demethylation of methylthiopurine in the microsomal enzyme system, and SKF 525A produced some inhibition of the system (HENDERSON and MAZEL, 1964b). Demethylation reactions by rodent liver microsomal enzymes also use other purine analogs as substrates, such as 6-methylthioguanine, 6-dimethylaminopurine, 6-methylaminopurine, and, to a lesser extent, the methylated xanthines, caffeine and theophylline. In a similar manner, the antibiotic, puromycin, is also demethylated by rat liver microsomal preparations. Phenobarbital pretreatment of the animals induced the enzyme activity, and SKF 525A inhibited the reaction (HENDERSON and MAZEL, 1964a; MAZEL et al., 1966).

It is sometimes believed that substrate analogs differ from more conventional drugs in being less lipid-soluble, and therefore less likely to be metabolized by microsomal enzymes. However, a comparison of rodent microsomal demethylation and relative lipid solubility of substrates reveals little correlation: very water-soluble compounds, such as puromycin aminonucleoside and 1-methylguanosine, are extensively demethylated, in contrast to much more lipid-soluble drugs, some of which serve poorly as substrates for microsomal demethylation. In this regard, it is remarkable that puromycin and the purine derivative, caffeine, which may be considered substrate analogs, were reported to have partition ratios between chloroform and buffer characteristic of lipid-soluble compounds (MAZEL and HENDERSON, 1965).

It is abundantly clear, therefore, that there are numerous examples of antimetabolite drugs being handled by microsomal enzymes or other pathways normally available for the biodegradation of other drugs. In addition, major classes of drugs, such as the antagonists of histamine, vitamin K, serotonin and steroids, which undoubtedly act as structural analogs of these normal tissue constituents, are metabolized by conventional drug metabolizing enzymes. Many additional drugs may actually be substrate analogs in particular biological systems but have not been recognized as such. For instance, investigations on microorganisms have demonstrated that barbiturates and structurally related CNS depressant and anticonvulsant drugs behave as analogs of orotic acid (MANDEL et al., 1967; MANDEL and RIIS, 1970; MANDEL et al., 1970). With continuing research it may be possible to implicate specific biochemical reactions in which many of our present conventional drugs interfere as antimetabolites. In that case, the distinction between antimetabolites and other drugs would be further diminished, as would that of their metabolic pathways.

E. Summary

Patterns of metabolism of typical substrate analogs have been described. Such compounds may be biotransformed along pathways of metabolism available for the normal substrates, although the relative rates of the corresponding reactions may be different. Many of the substrate analogs owe their pharmacological actions to the formation of anabolic derivatives which may be the truly active form of the drug. Knowledge of the pathways of metabolism available to substrate analogs has permitted the more rational use of these agents in therapy.

Although antimetabolites frequently have carcinostatic properties because they interfere with normal biosynthesis, the described pattern of metabolism is not characteristic for anticancer agents as a group. The similarities in the metabolic pathways of substrate analogs and normal substrates, here described in detail for a pyrimidine and a purine analog, are also valid for sugars, amino acids, aliphatic acids and many other types of compounds, including adrenergic amines. It was suggested that many drugs actually may behave as substrate analogs in still unrecognized reactions. Substrate analogs may also be subject to more conventional metabolic pathways, including those involving liver microsomes. Thus, categorical distinctions between the metabolic reactions of drugs and those of substrate analogs are unwarranted.

References

ANDOH, T., CHARGAFF, E.: Formation and fate of abnormal ribosomes of *E. coli* cells treated with 5-fluorouracil. Proc. nat. Acad. Sci. (Wash.) **54**, 1181—1189 (1965).

ANSFIELD, F.J., CURRERI, A.R.: Further clinical comparison between 5-fluorouracil (5-FU) and 5-fluoro-2′-deoxyuridine (5-FUDR). Cancer Chemother. Reports **32**, 101—105 (1963).

BAKER, B.R.: Design of active-site-directed irreversible enzyme inhibitors. New York: John Wiley & Sons 1967.

— WOOD, W.: Irreversible enzyme inhibitors, CXLVIII. Active-site-directed irreversible inhibitors of guanine deaminase derived from 9-phenyl-guanine bearing a terminal sulfonyl fluoride. J. Med. Chem. **12**, 216—220 (1969).

BALIS, M.E.: Antagonists and nucleic acids. New York: John Wiley & Sons 1968.

BENNETT, L.L., BROCKMAN, R.W., SCHNEBLI, H.P., CHUMLEY, S., DIXON, G.J., SCHABEL, F.M., DULMADGE, E.A., SKIPPER, H.E., MONTGOMERY, J.A., THOMAS, H.J.: Activity and mechanism of action of 6-methylthiopurine ribonucleoside in cancer cells resistant to 6-mercaptopurine. Nature (Lond.) **205**, 1276—1279 (1965).

BIEBER, S., DIETRICH, L.S., ELION, G.B., HITCHINGS, G.H., MARTIN, D.S.: The incorporation of 6-mercaptopurine-S^{35} into the nucleic acids of sensitive and non-sensitive transplantable mouse tumors. Cancer Res. **21**, 228—231 (1961).

BORSTRUM, H.: Sulfate conjugation and conjugated sulfates. (Review). Scand. J. clin. Lab. Invest. **86**, Suppl. 17, 33—52 (1965).
BOSCH, L., HARBERS, E., HEIDELBERGER, C.: Studies on fluorinated pyrimidines. V. Effects on nucleic acid metabolism *in vitro*. Cancer Res. **18**, 335—343 (1958).
BRESNICK, E.: Feedback inhibition of aspartate transcarbamylase in liver and in hepatoma. Cancer Res. **22**, 1246—1251 (1962).
BRIDGES, J.W., KIBBY, M.R., WILLIAMS, R.T.: The nature of the glucuronide of Madribon formed in man. Biochem. J. **91**, 12P (1964).
— — — The structure of the glucuronide of sulfadimethoxine formed in man. Biochem. J. **96**, 829—836 (1965).
— WILLIAMS, R.T.: The metabolism of 5-p-aminobenzenesulphonamido-3-methylisothiazole (sulphasomizole). J. Pharm. Pharmacol. **15**, 565—573 (1963).
BROCK, N., HOHORST, H.-J.: Metabolism of cyclophosphamide. Cancer **20**, 900—904 (1967).
BROCKMAN, R.W., ANDERSON, E.P.: Biochemistry of cancer (metabolic aspects). Ann. Rev. Biochem. **32**, 463—512 (1963).
— DAVIS, J.M., STUTTS, P.: Metabolism of uracil and 5-fluorouracil by drug-sensitive and by drug-resistant bacteria. Biochim. biophys. Acta (Amst.) **40**, 22—32 (1960).
CALABRESI, P.: Regional protection in cancer chemotherapy. I. Infusions of thymidine into external carotid artery of patients receiving systemic 5-iodo-2′-deoxyuridine. J. clin. Invest. **41**, 1484—1491 (1962).
CALDWELL, I.C., HENDERSON, J.F., PATERSON, A.R.P.: The enzymic formation of 6-(methylmercapto)purine ribonucleoside 5′-phosphate. Canad. J. Biochem. **44**, 229—245 (1966).
CALENDAR, R., BERG, P.: The catalytic properties of tyrosyl ribonucleic acid synthetases from *Escherichia coli* and *Bacillus subtilis*. Biochemistry **5**, 1690—1695 (1966).
CARLÓ, P.-E., MANDEL, H.G.: The effect of 4-amino-5-imidazolecarboxamide on the toxicity of 8-azaguanine. Cancer Res. **14**, 459—462 (1954).
CARLSSON, A., LINDQVIST, M.: *In vivo* decarboxylation of α-methylDOPA and α-methyl metatyrosine. Acta physiol. scand. **54**, 87—94 (1962).
CHADWICK, M., ROGERS, W.I.: The distribution of 5-fluoro-2′-deoxyuridine-5′-monophosphate in mice after 5-fluorouracil administration. Proc. Amer. Ass. Cancer Res. **11**, 15 (1970).
CHAUDHURI, N.K., MONTAG, B.J., HEIDELBERGER, C.: Studies on fluorinated pyrimidines. III. The metabolism of 5-fluorouracil-2-C^{14} and 5-fluoroorotic-2-C^{14} acid *in vivo*. Cancer Res. **18**, 318—328 (1958).
— MUKHERJEE, K.L., HEIDELBERGER, C.: Studies on fluorinated pyrimidines. VII. The degradative pathway. Biochem. Pharmacol. **1**, 328—341 (1959).
CHU, M.-Y., FISCHER, G.A.: The incorporation of ^{3}H-cytosine arabinoside and its effects on murine leukemic cells (L5178Y). Biochem. Pharmacol. **17**, 753—767 (1968).
COHEN, S.S., BARNER, H.D.: Studies on unbalanced growth in *Escherichia coli*. Proc. nat. Acad. Sci. (Wash.) **40**, 885—893 (1954).
— FLAKS, J.G., BARNER, H.D., LOEB, M.R., LICHTENSTEIN, J.: The mode of action of 5-fluorouracil and its derivatives. Proc. nat. Acad. Sci. (Wash.) **44**, 1004—1112 (1958).
COOPER, J.R., KINI, M.M.: Biochemical aspects of methanol poisoning — Editorial. Biochem. Pharmacol. **11**, 405—416 (1962).
CORNISH, H.H., CHRISTMAN, A.A.: A study of the metabolism of theobromine, theophylline, and caffeine in man. J. biol. Chem. **228**, 315—323 (1957).
CREASEY, W.A., FINK, M.E., HANDSCHUMACHER, R.E., CALABRESI, P.: Clinical and pharmacological studies with 2′, 3′, 5′-triacetyl-6-azauridine. Cancer Res. **23**, 444—453 (1963).
CREVELING, C.R., DALY, J.W., WITKOP, B., UDENFRIEND, S.: Substrates and inhibitors of dopamine-β-oxidase. Biochim. biophys. Acta (Amst.) **64**, 125—134 (1962).
CROUT, J.R., ALPERS, H.S., TATUM, E.L., SHORE, P.A.: Release of metaraminol (Aramine) from the heart by sympathetic nerve stimulation. Science **145**, 828—829 (1964).
DUNN, D.B., SMITH, J.D.: Effect of 5-halogenated uracils on the growth of *Escherichia coli* and their incorporation into deoxyribonucleic acids. Biochem. J. **67**, 494—506 (1957).
DUSCHINSKY, R., GABRIEL, T., TAUTZ, W., NUSSBAUM, A., HOFFER, M., GRUNBERG, E.: Nucleosides. XXXVII. 5,6-Substituted 5-fluorodihydropyrimidines and their 2′-deoxyribonucleosides. J. Med. Chem. **10**, 47—58 (1967).
ELION, G.B.: Biochemistry and pharmacology of purine analogues. Fed. Proc. **26**, 898—904 (1967).
— Actions of purine analogs: enzyme specificity studies as a basis for interpretation and design. Cancer Res. **29**, 2448—2453 (1969).
— CALLAHAN, S., BIEBER, S., HITCHINGS, G.H., RUNDLES, R.W.: A summary of investigations with [(1-methyl-4-nitro-5-imidazolyl)thio] purine (B.W. 57-322). Cancer Chemother. Reports **14**, 93—98 (1961).
— CALLAHAN, S.W., HITCHINGS, G.H., RUNDLES, R.W., LASZLO, J.: Experimental, clinical, and metabolic studies of thiopurines. Cancer Chemother. Reports **16**, 197—202 (1962).

Elion, G.B., Callahan, S., Nathan, H., Bieber, S., Rundles, R.W., Hitchings, G.H.: Potentiation by inhibition of drug degradation: 6-substituted purines and xanthine oxidase. Biochem. Pharmacol. **12**, 85—93 (1963).

— Hitchings, G.H.: Metabolic basis for the actions of analogs of purines and pyrimidines. Advanc. Chemotherapy **2**, 91—177 (1965).

Elison, C., Rapoport, H., Laursen, R., Elliott, H.W.: Effect of deuteration of N—CH_3 group on potency and enzymatic N-demethylation of morphine. Science **134**, 1078—1079 (1961).

Ellis, D.B., Le Page, G.A.: Biochemical studies of resistance to 6-thioguanine. Cancer Res. **23**, 436—443 (1963).

— — Metabolic fate of 9-β-D-xylofuranosyladenine in mice bearing susceptible tumor cells. Canšer Res. **26**, 893—897 (1966).

Farkas, V., Bauer, S., Zemek, J.: Metabolism of 2-deoxy-D-glucose in Baker's yeast. III. Formation of 2,2′-dideoxy-*a,a*′-trehalose. Biochim. biophys. Acta (Amst.) **84**, 77—82 (1969).

Gilligan, D.R.: Comparative studies of the chemical changes occurring in sulfonamide drugs during therapy in man. J. clin. Invest. **24**, 301—315 (1945).

Goldin, A., Venditti, J.M., Humphreys, S.R., Mantel, N.: Modification of treatment schedules in the management of advanced mouse leukemia with amethopterin. J. nat. Cancer Inst. **17**, 203—212 (1956).

— — Kline, I., Mantel, N.: Eradication of leukaemic cells (L1210) by methotrexate and methotrexate plus citrovorum factor. Nature (Lond.) **212**, 1548—1550 (1966).

Goldman, P.: The carbon-fluorine bond in compounds of biological interest. Science **164**, 1123—1130 (1969).

Gross, D., Tarver, H.: Studies on ethionine. IV. The incorporation of ethionine into the proteins of tetrahymena. J. biol. Chem. **217**, 169—182 (1955).

Hahn, G.A., Mandel, H.G.: The effects of fluorourecil on RNA synthesis in *Bacillus cereus*. Biochem. Pharmacol., in press (1971).

Hall, T.C., Kessel, D., Godsill, A., Roberts, D.: Uridine phosphorylation, an overlooked pathway? 5-Fluorouridine, a neglected drug? Proc. Amer. Ass. Cancer Res. **9**, 27 (1968).

Handschumacher, R.E.: Metabolites of 6-azauracil formed by *Streptococcus faecalis*. Fed. Proc. **16**, 191 (1957).

Hansen, H.J., Giles, W.G., Nadler, S.B.: Metabolism of 9-ethyl-6-MP-S^{35} and 9-butyl-6-MP-S^{35} in humans. Proc. Soc. exp. Biol. (N.Y.) **113**, 163—165 (1963).

Hartmann, K.-U., Heidelberger, C.: Studies on fluorinated pyrimidines. XIII. Inhibition of thymidylate synthetase. J. biol. Chem. **236**, 3006—3013 (1961).

Heidelberger, C.: Fluorinated pyrimidines. Progress in Nucleic Acid Research and Molecular Biology **4**, 1—50 (1965).

— Boohar, J., Kampschroer, B.: Fluorinated pyrimidines. XXIV. *In vivo* metabolism of 5-trifluoromethyluracil-2-C^{14} and 5-trifluoromethyl-2′-deoxyuridine-2-C^{14}. Cancer Res. **25**, 377—381 (1965).

— Chaudhuri, N.K., Danneberg, P., Mooren, D., Griesbach, L., Duschinsky, R., Schnitzer, R.J., Pleven, E., Scheiner, J.: Fluorinated pyrimidines, a new class of tumour-inhibitory compounds. Nature (Lond.) **179**, 663—666 (1957).

— Griesbach, L., Cruz, O., Schnitzer, R.J., Grunberg, E.: Fluorinated pyrimidines. VI. Effects of 5-fluorouridine and 5-fluoro-2′-deoxyuridine on transplanted tumors. Proc. Soc. exp. Biol. (N.Y.) **97**, 470—475 (1958).

Henderson, E.S., Samaha, R.J.: Evidence that drugs in multiple combinations have materially advanced the treatment of human malignancies. Cancer Res. **29**, 2272—2280 (1969).

Henderson, J.F.: Variation in selective toxicity: Causes and consequences. Cancer Res. **29**, 2404—2406 (1969).

— Mandel, H.G.: Purine and pyrimidine antimetabolites in cancer chemotherapy. In: Advances in Pharmacology **2**, 297—343 (1963).

— Mazel, P.: Demethylation of purine analogs by microsomal enzymes from mouse liver. Biochem. Pharmacol. **13**, 207—210 (1964a).

— — Studies on the induction of microsomal S-, N- and O-demethylases. Biochem. Pharmacol. **13**, 1471—1474 (1964b).

Hirschberg, E., Kream, J., Gellhorn, A.: Enzymatic deamination of 8-azaguanine in normal and neoplastic tissues. Cancer Res. **12**, 524—528 (1952).

Hitchings, G.H., Falco, E.A., Sherwood, M.B.: The effects of pyrimidines on the growth of *Lactobacillus casei*. Science **102**, 251—252 (1945).

Horowitz, J., Kohlmeier, V.: Formation of active β-galactosidase by *Escherichia coli* treated with 5-fluorouracil. Biochim. biophys. Acta (Amst.) **142**, 208—218 (1967).

Jacquez, J.A.: Permeability of Ehrlich cells of uracil, thymine and fluorouracil. Proc. Soc. exp. Biol. (N.Y.) **109**, 132—135 (1962).

JOHNSON, R.K., MAZEL, P., DONAHUE, J.D., JONDORF, W.R.: Factors involved in the inhibition of drug metabolism by (—)-emetine. Biochem. Pharmacol. (in press).
KAHAN, F.M., HURWITZ, J.: The role of deoxyribonucleic acid in ribonucleic acid synthesis. IV. The incorporation of pyrimidine and purine analogues into ribonucleic acid. J. biol. Chem. **237**, 3778—3785 (1962).
KAISER, I.I.: Studies on 5-fluorouracil-containing ribonucleic acid. I. Separation and partial characterization of fluorouracil-containing transfer ribonucleic acids from *Escherichia coli*. Biochemistry **8**, 231—238 (1969).
KAPLAN, N.O., CIOTTI, M.M.: Chemistry and properties of the 3-acetylpyridine analogue of diphosphopyridine nucleotide. J. biol. Chem. **221**, 823—832 (1956).
KESSEL, D., HALL, T.C.: Studies on drug transport by normal human leukocytes. Biochem. Pharmacol. **16**, 2395—2403 (1967).
— — WODINSKY, I.: Nucleotide formation as a determinant of 5-fluorouracil response in mouse leukemias. Science **154**, 911—913 (1966).
KOPIN, I.J.: False adrenergic transmitters. Ann. Rev. Pharmacol. **8**, 377—394 (1968).
KRENITSKY, T.A., PAPAIOANNOU, R., ELION, G.B.: Human hypoxanthine phosphoribosyltransferase. I. Purification, properties, and specificity. J. biol. Chem. **244**, 1263—1270 (1969).
LANGEN, P.: Antimetabolite des Nucleinsäure-Stoffwechsels. Berlin: Akademie-Verlag 1968.
LASNITZKI, I., MATTHEWS, R.E.F., SMITH, J.D.: Incorporation of 8-azaguanine into nucleic acids. Nature (Lond.) **173**, 346—349 (1954).
LE PAGE, G.A.: Basic biochemical effects and mechanism of action of 6-thioguanine. Cancer Res. **23**, 1202—1206 (1963).
— JONES, M.: Further studies on the mechanism of action of 6-thioguanine. Cancer Res. **21**, 1590—1594 (1961).
— KANEKO, T.: Effective means of reducing toxicity without concomitant sacrifice of efficacy of carcinostatic therapy. Cancer Res. **29**, 2314—2318 (1969).
LIPMANN, F.: Acetylation of sulfanilamide by liver homogenates and extracts. J. biol. Chem. **160**, 173—190 (1945).
LOO, T.L., ADAMSON, R.H.: The enzymic oxidation of certain folic acid antagonists. Biochem. Pharmacol. **11**, 170—171 (1962).
LOVENBERG, W., WEISSBACH, H., UDENFRIEND, S.: Aromatic L-amino acid decarboxylase. J. biol. Chem. **237**, 89—93 (1962).
LOWRIE, R.J., BERGQUIST, P.L.: Transfer ribonucleic acids from *Escherichia coli* treated with 5-fluorouracil. Biochemistry **7**, 1761—1770 (1968).
MAITRE, L.: Presence of α-methyl-DOPA metabolites in heart and brain of guinea pigs treated with α-methyl-tyrosine. Life Sci. **4**, 2249—2256 (1965).
MANDEL, H.G.: The physiological disposition of some anticancer agents. Pharmacol. Rev. **11**, 743—838 (1959).
— The incorporation of 5-fluorouracil into RNA and its molecular consequences. In: Progress in Molecular and Subcellular Biology, Vol. 1, pp. 82—135 (F.E. HAHN, ed.). Berlin-Heidelberg-New York: Springer 1969.
— Pathways of drug biotransformation: biochemical conjugations. In: Fundamental of drug metabolism and disposition (B.N. LA DU, H.G. MANDEL and E.L. WAY, eds.). Baltimore: Williams & Wilkins 1971.
— ALPEN, E.L., WINTERS, W.D., SMITH, P.K.: The urinary metabolites of 8-azaguanine in the mouse and the monkey. J. biol. Chem. **193**, 63—71 (1951).
— LATIMER, R.G., RIIS, M.: The actions of thioguanine in *Bacillus cereus*. Biochem. Pharmacol. **14**, 661—682 (1965).
— OLIVER, H.M., RIIS, M.: Interference of barbiturates with pyrimidine incorporation. I. Amobarbital inhibition of orotate uptake in *Bacillus cereus*. Molec. Pharmacol. **3**, 537—548 (1967).
— RIIS, M.: Interference of barbiturates with pyrimidine incorporation. II. Structural specificity of the inhibition of orotate uptake in *Bacillus cereus*. Biochem. Pharmacol **19**, 1867—1877 (1970).
— TRIESTER, S.R., SZAPARY, D.: Interference of barbiturates with pyrimidine incorporation. III. Studies on the mechanism of the amobarbital-orotate relationship. Biochem. Pharmacol. **19**, 1879—1892 (1970).
MARCHAND, C., FUJIMOTO, J.M.: The enhancement of the action of 6-mercaptopurine (6MP) on leukemia L1210 by compounds which act on the liver. Fed. Proc. **21**, 165 (1962).
MARKHAM, R.: Lethal synthesis. In: The strategy of chemotherapy. Eighth Symposium of the Society for Gen. Microbiology, pp. 163—177. London: Cambridge University Press 1958.
MARSH, C.A.: Chemistry of D-glucuronic acid and its glycosides. In: Glucuronic acid — free and combined. Chemistry, Biochemistry, Pharmacology and Medicine, pp. 3—136. Ed. by G.J. DUTTON. New York: Academic Press 1966.

MATTHEWS, R.E.F.: Biosynthetic incorporation of metabolite analogs. Pharmacol. Rev. **10**, 359—406 (1958).

MAZEL, P., HENDERSON, J.F.: On the relationship between lipid solubility and microsomal metabolism of drugs. Biochem. Pharmacol. **14**, 92—94 (1965).

— — AXELROD, J.: S-Demethylation by microsomal enzymes. J. Pharmacol. exp. Ther. **143**, 1—6 (1964).

— KERZA-KWIATECKI, A., SIMANIS, J.: Studies on the demethylation of puromycin and related compounds by liver microsomal enzymes. Biochim. biophys. Acta (Amst.) **114**, 72—82 (1966).

MELONI, M.L., ROGERS, W.I.: Enhancement of 6-thioinosine-5′-monophosphate synthesis in solid L-1210 lymphatic leukemia cells by prior exposure to 6-mercaptopurine. Biochem. Pharmacol. **18**, 413—417 (1969).

MITCHELL, M.S., WAWRO, N.W., DE CONTI, R.C., KAPLAN, S.R., PAPAC, R., BERTINO, J.R.: Effectiveness of high-dose infusions of methotrexate followed by leucovorin in carcinoma of the head and neck. Cancer Res. **28**, 1088—1094 (1968).

MONTGOMERY, J.A., DIXON, G.J., DULMAGE, E.A., THOMAS, H.J., BROCKMAN, R.W., SKIPPER, H.E.: Inhibition of 6-mercaptopurine-resistant cancer cells in culture by bis(thioinosine)-5′,5′′′-phosphate. Nature (Lond.) **199**, 769—772 (1963).

MOORE, E.C., LE PAGE, G.A.: The metabolism of 6-thioguanine in normal and neoplastic tissues. Cancer Res. **18**, 1075—1083 (1958).

MUDD, S.H., CANTONI, G.L.: Selenomethionine in enzymatic transmethylations. Nature (Lond.) **180**, 1052 (1957).

MUKHERJEE, K.L., HEIDELBERGER, C.: Studies on fluorinated pyrimidines. IX. The degradation of 5-fluorouracil-6-C^{14}. J. biol. Chem. **235**, 433—437 (1960).

— — Studies on fluorinated pyrimidines. XV. Inhibition of the incorporation of formate-C^{14} into DNA thymine of Ehrlich ascites carcinoma cells by 5-fluoro-2′-deoxyuridine-5′-monophosphate and related compounds. Cancer Res. **22**, 815—822 (1962).

MUSCHOLL, E.: Biosynthese (aus α-Methyldopa), Aufnahme und Freisetzung von α-Methyladrenalin. Arch. exp. Pathol. Pharmakol. **251**, 162—163 (1965).

— MAITRE, L.: Release by sympathetic stimulation of α-methyl-noradrenaline stored in the heart after administration of α-methyldopa. Experientia (Basel) **19**, 658—660 (1963).

— SPRENGER, E.: Vergleichende Untersuchung der Blutdruckwirkung, Aufnahme und Speicherung von Dihydroxyephedrin (α-Methyladrenalin) und Dihydroxypseudoephedrin. Arch. exp. Pathol. Pharmakol. **254**, 109—124 (1966).

NATHANS, D.: Puromycin inhibition of protein synthesis: incorporation of puromycin into peptide chains. Proc. nat. Acad. Sci. (Wash.) **51**, 585—592 (1964).

NOVELLI, G.D.: Amino acid activation for protein synthesis. Annual Review of Biochemistry **36**, 449—484 (1967).

OLIVERIO, V.T., DAVIDSON, J.D.: The physiological disposition of dichloromethotrexate-Cl^{36} in animals. J. Pharmacol. exp. Ther. **137**, 76—83 (1962).

— ZUBROD, C.G.: Clinical pharmacology of the effective anti-tumor drugs. Ann. Rev. Pharmacol. **5**, 335—356 (1965).

PASTERNAK, C.A., HANDSCHUMACHER, R.E.: The biochemical activity of 6-azauridine. Interference with pyrimidine metabolism in transplantable mouse tumors. J. biol. Chem. **234**, 2992—2997 (1959).

PATERSON, A.R.P.: The formation of 6-mercaptopurine riboside phosphate in ascites tumor cells. Canad. J. Biochem. **37**, 1011—1023 (1959).

— MORIWAKI, A.: Combination therapy: Synergistic inhibition of lymphoma L5178Y cells in culture and *in vivo* with 6-mercaptopurine and 6-(methyl-mercapto)purine ribonucleoside. Cancer Res. **29**, 681—686 (1969).

PATTISON, F.L.M., HUNT, S.B.D., STOTHERS, J.B.: Toxic fluorine compounds. IX. ω-Fluorocarboxylic esters and acids. J. Org. Chem. **21**, 883—886 (1956).

PETERS, R.A.: Lethal synthesis. Proc. roy. Soc. B **139**, 143—170 (1952).

REICHARD, P., SKÖLD, O.: Possible enzymic mechanism for the development of resistance against fluorouracil in ascites tumors. Nature (Lond.) **183**, 939—941 (1959).

REYES, P.: Synthesis of 5-fluorouridine 5′-phosphate by pyrimidine phosphoribosyltransferase of mammalian origin. I. Some properties of the enzyme from P 1534J mouse leukemia cells. Biochemistry **8**, 2057—2062 (1969).

RICHMOND, M.H.: The effect of amino acid analogues on growth and protein synthesis in microorganisms. Bact. Rev. **26**, 398—420 (1962).

ROGERS, H.J., PERKINS, H.R.: 5-Fluorouracil and mucopeptide biosynthesis by *Staphylococcus aureus*. Biochem. J. **77**, 448—459 (1960).

ROGERS, W. I., MELONI, M. L., WODINSKY, I., KENSLER, C. J.: Metabolic basis for enhanced chemotherapy of solid L-1210 with 6 MP. Proc. Amer. Ass. Cancer Res. **10**, 74 (1969).

ROUSH, A., NORRIS, E. R.: Deamination of 8-azaguanine by guanase. Arch. Biochem. **29**, 124—129 (1950).

SARTORELLI, A. C., LE PAGE, G. A.: The development and biochemical characterization of resistance to azaserine in a TA-3 ascites carcinoma. Cancer Res. **18**, 457—463 (1958).

— — MOORE, E. C.: Metabolic effects of 6-thioguanine. I. Studies on thioguanine-resistant and -sensitive Ehrlich ascites cells. Cancer Res. **18**, 1232—1239 (1958).

SCANNELL, J. P., HITCHINGS, G. H.: Thioguanine in deoxyribonucleic acid from tumors of 6-mercaptopurine-treated mice. Proc. Soc. exp. Biol. (N.Y.) **122**, 627—629 (1966).

SCHABEL, F. M., JR., LASTER, W. R., JR., SKIPPER, H. E.: Chemotherapy of leukemia L-1210 by 6-mercaptopurine (NSC-755) in combination with 6-methylthiopurine ribonucleoside (NSC 40774). Cancer Chemother. Reports **51**, 111—124 (1967).

SCHANKER, L. S., JEFFREY, J. J.: Active transport of foreign pyrimidines across the intestinal epithelium. Nature (Lond.) **190**, 727—728 (1961).

SELAWRY, O. S., and *Members of Acute Leukemia Group B.*: New treatment schedule with improved survival in childhood leukemia. J. Amer. med. Ass. **194**, 75—80 (1965).

SKIBBA, J. L., BEAL, D. D., RAMIREZ, G., BRYAN, G. T.: N-Demethylation of the antineoplastic agent 4(5)-(3,3-dimethyl-1-triazeno) imidazole-5(4)-carboxamide by rats and man. Cancer Res. **30**, 147—150 (1970).

SKIPPER, H. E., SCHABEL, F. M., JR., WILCOX, W. S.: Experimental evaluation of potential anticancer agents. XXI. Scheduling of arabinosylcytosine to take advantage of its S-phase specificity against leukemia cells. Cancer Chemother. Reports **51**, 125—165 (1967).

SKÖLD, O.: Enzymic ribosidation and ribotidation of 5-fluorouracil by extracts of the Ehrlich-ascites tumor. Biochim. biophys. Acta (Amst.) **29**, 651 (1958).

STENRAM, U., WILLÉN, R.: Radioautographic, ultrastructural and biochemical studies on the effect of fluorouracil on the RNA synthesis in the liver of rats. Z. Zellforsch. **82**, 270—281 (1967).

STOCK, J. A.: Antimetabolites. In: Experimental Chemotherapy, Vol. IV, pp. 79—237, Part 1 (R. J. SCHNITZER and F. HAWKINS, eds.). New York: Academic Press 1966.

TOMASZ, A., BOREK, E.: The mechanism of an osmotic instability induced in *E. coli* K-12 by 5-fluorouracil. Biochemistry **1**, 543—552 (1962).

TOMKINS, G. M.: A mammalian 3 α-hydroxysteroid dehydrogenase. J. biol. Chem. **218**, 437—447 (1956).

TOOZE, J., WEBER, K.: Isolation and characterization of amber mutants of bacteriophage R 17. J. molec. Biol. **28**, 311—330 (1967).

UMBREIT, W. W., WADDELL, J. G.: Mode of action of desoxypyridoxine. Proc. Soc. exp. Biol. (N.Y.) **70**, 293 (1949).

VADLAMUDI, S., FIELDS, L., WARAVDEKAR, V. S., KLINE, I., GOLDIN, A.: Influence of colcemid on therapeutic effectiveness of cytosine arabinoside. Proc. Amer. Ass. Cancer Res. **9**, 73 (1968).

WACKER, A., EBERT, M., KOLM, H.: Metabolism of p-aminosalicylic and salicylic acids by Enterococcus. Z. Naturforsch. **13b**, 147—150 (1958).

WANG, M. C., SIMPSON, A. I., PATERSON, A. R. P.: Combinations of 6-mercaptopurine (NSC-755) and 6-(methylmercapto)purine ribonucleoside (NSC 40774) in the therapy of Ehrlich ascites carcinoma. Cancer Chemother. Reports **51**, 101—109 (1967).

WAY, J. L., PARKS, R. E., JR.: Enzymatic synthesis of 5′-phosphate nucleotides of purine analogues. J. biol. Chem. **231**, 467—480 (1958).

WELLS, W., GAINES, D., KOENIG, H.: Studies of pyrimidine nucleotide metabolism in the central nervous system. I. Metabolic effects and metabolism of 6-azauridine. J. Neurochem. **10**, 709—723 (1963).

WEYGAND, F., WACKER, A., DELLWEG, H.: Stoffwechseluntersuchungen bei Mikroorganismen mit Hilfe radioaktiver Isotope. II. Kompetitive und nicht-kompetitive Enthemmung von 5-^{82}Br-Uracil. Z. Naturforsch. **7b**, 19 (1952).

WILLIAMS, R. T.: Detoxication mechanisms. The metabolism and detoxication of drugs, toxic substances and other organic compounds. New York: John Wiley & Sons 1959.

— The biogenesis of conjugation and detoxication products. In: Biogenesis of natural compounds, 2nd ed., pp. 589—639 (P. BERNFELD, ed.). New York: Pergamon Press 1967.

WITTMANN-LIEBOLD, B., WITTMANN, H. G.: Lokalisierung von Aminosäureaustauschen bei Nitritmutanten des Tabakmosaikvirus. Z. Vererbungsl. **97**, 305—326 (1965).

WOLBERG, W. H.: Determinants of human tumor sensitivity to fluorinated pyrimidine chemotherapy. Ann. Surg. **166**, 609—623 (1967).

WOODMAN, R. J.: Localized incorporation of iododeoxyuridine from polycation-complexed iododeoxycytidylic acid into DNA of several murine and hamster tumors. Cancer Res. **28**, 2007—2016 (1968).

WOOLLEY, D. W.: A study of antimetabolites. New York: John Wiley & Sons, Inc. 1952.

ZATMAN, L. J., KAPLAN, N. O., COLOWICK, S. P., CIOTTI, M. M.: The isolation and properties of the isonicotinic acid hydrazide analogue of diphosphopyridine nucleotide. J. biol. Chem. **209**, 467—484 (1954).

ZUBROD, C. G.: The limited usefulness of 5-fluorouracil (5-FU) and 5-fluorodeoxyuridine (5-FUDR) in the management of patients with adenocarcinoma. In: Controversy in internal medicine, pp. 591—600 (F. J. INGELFINGER, A. S. RELMAN and M. FINLAND, eds.). Philadelphia: W. B. Saunders Co. 1966.

Author Index

Page numbers in *italics* refer to the references.

Subject Index